METAL IONS IN BIOLOGY AND MEDICINE

LES IONS MÉTALLIQUES EN BIOLOGIE ET EN MÉDECINE

Volume 6

The first volume of this series was published in May 1990
Eds. Ph. Collery, L.A. Poirier, M. Manfait, J.C. Étienne

The second volume of this series was published in May 1992
Eds. J. Anastassopoulou, Ph. Collery, J.C. Etienne, T. Theophanides

The third volume of this series was published in May 1994
Eds. Ph. Collery, L.A. Poirier, N.A. Littlefield, J.-C. Etienne

The fourth volume of this series was published in May 1996
Eds. Ph. Collery, J. Corbella, J.L. Domingo, J.-C. Etienne, J.M. Llobet

The fifth volume of this series was publishecd in May 1998
Eds. Ph. Collery, P. Brätter, V. Negretti de Brätter, L. Khassanova, J.-C. Etienne

Editions John Libbey Eurotext
127, avenue de la République, 92120 Montrouge, France
Tél. : (1) 46.73.06.60 – Fax : (1) 40.84.09.99
E-mail : contact@john-libbey-eurotext.fr
http://www.john-libbey-eurotext.fr

John Libbey and Company Ltd
13, Smiths Yard, Summerley Street, London SW 18 4HR, England
Tél. : (01) 947.27.77

John Libbey CIC
Via L. Spallanzani, 11
00161 Rome, Italy
Tel. : (06) 862.289

ISBN 2-7420-0294-4

METAL IONS IN BIOLOGY AND MEDICINE

LES IONS MÉTALLIQUES EN BIOLOGIE ET EN MÉDECINE

Volume 6

Proceedings of the Sixth International Symposium on Metal Ions in Biology and Medicine held in San Juan, Puerto Rico, USA, on May 7-10, 2000

Sixième Symposium International sur les Ions Métalliques en Biologie et en Médecine, San-Juan, Porto-Rico, Etats-Unis, 7-10 mai 2000

Edited by
José A. Centeno
Philippe Collery
Guy Vernet
Robert B. Finkelman
Herman Gibb
Jean-Claude Etienne

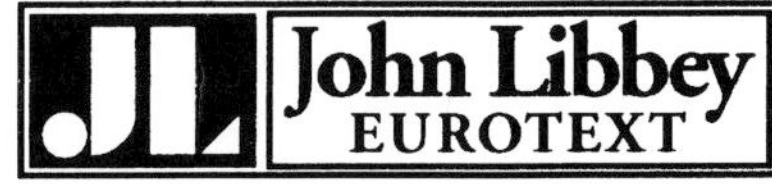

Organizers

American Association for the Advancement of Science – Caribbean Division
American Registry of Pathology (ARP)
Ana G. Méndez University System of Puerto Rico (AGMUS)
Armed Forces Institute of Pathology (AFIP)
Institut International de Recherche sur les Ions Métalliques (IIRIM-Reims, France)
International Institute of Anticancer Research (IIAR)
Jackson State University – School of Science & Technology (JSU)
National Cancer Institute (NCI)
National Institute of Environmental Health Sciences (NIEHS)
Nickel Producers Environmental Research Association (NiPERA)
Ponce School of Medicine, Puerto Rico (PSM-PR)
U.S. Environmental Protection Agency (USEPA)
U.S. Geological Survey (USGS)
University of Puerto Rico at Mayagüez (UPRM)

Contributors

Center for Hemispherical Cooperation on Science and Engineering
Conseil Régional de Champagne Ardenne (CRCA-Reims, France)
Cypress Systems, Inc.
Federation of European Societies on Trace Elements and Minerals (FESTEM)
International Association of Geochemistry and Cosmochemistry
International Copper Association
International Lead and Zinc Research Organization
Journal of Biological Trace Element Research
National Natural Science Foundation of China
Société pour le Développement des Recherches sur le Magnésium
Society of Environmental Toxicology and Chemistry
Society of Toxicologic Pathologist
The International Council on Metals in the Environment
The Nickel Development Institute
Tourism Company of Puerto Rico

The organizing committee wishes to thank the Association Régionale pour l'Enseignement et la Recherche scientifique en Champagne-Ardenne for its support in the realization of this book.

Organizing Committee

José A. Centeno (AFIP)	Chairman
Herman Gibb (USEPA)	Co-Chairman
Michalann Harthill (USGS)	Co-Chairman

Robert B. Finkelman (USGS)
David Reese (USEPA)
Meira Fields (USDA)
Claudia Thompson (NIH-NIEHS)
David Longfellow (NIH-NCI)
Kenneth Cantor (NIH-NCI)

Local Committee

Jaime Matta (PSM)	Co-Chairman

Sylvia Marquéz de Pirazzi (UPRM)
Dulcinia Nuñéz (AGMUS)
Jorge I. Vélez-Arocho (UPRM)
Samuel P. Hernández (UPRM)
Braulio Jímenez (UPR-SM)
Alberto Rivera
Miguel Sastre (UPRH)
José Cintrón (AGMUS)

International Scientific Committee

J.A. Centeno (USA)	Chairman
P. Collery (France)	Co-Chair
L. Khassanova (Russia)	General Secretary
F.G. Mullick (USA)	Honorary Chair
J.C. Etienne (France)	Honorary Chair
G. Vernet (France)	Co-Editor, *Metal Ions* Vol. 6

C. Abernathy (USA)
J. Annastassopoulou (Greece)
V.H. Aposhian (USA)
A. Badawi (Egypt)
G. Beckett (Scotland, UK)
P. Brätter (Germany)
M. Cebrian (Mexico)
B. Conard (Canada)
R. Cornelis (Belgium)
R. Deloncle (France)
F.A. de Wolff (The Netherlands)
J. Durlach (France)
M.F. Flores-Arce (Mexico)
M. Gielen (Belgium)
K. Irgolic (Austria)
K.S. Kasprzak (USA)
J.M. Llobet (Spain)
G. Mendz (Australia)
V. Negretti de Brätter (Germany)
G. Nowak (Poland)
A. Pineau (France)
P. Schramel (Germany)
M. Simonoff (France)
K.T. Suzuki (Japan)
Th. Théophanides (Greece)
M. Vahter (Sweden)
G. Zaray (Hungary)
C. Alpoim (Portugal)
O. Andersen (Denmark)
J.R. Arthur (Scotland, UK)
A. Berthelot (France)
S. Caroli (Italy)
G.F. Combs (USA)
J. Corbella (Spain)
M. Costa (USA)
J.G. Delinassios (Greece)
B. Desoize (France)
J.L. Domingo (Spain)
B. Farzami (Iran)
B. Fowler (USA)
O. Guillard (France)
V. Kalfakakou (Greece)
N.A. Littlefield (USA)
D.N. Guha Mazumder (India)
B. Michalke (Germany)
J. Neve (Belgium)
A.R. Oller (USA)
L.A. Poirier (USA)
S.K. Shukla (Italy)
F.W. Sunderman, Jr. (USA)
T. Tchernitchin (Chile)
D. Templeton (Canada)
M.P. Waalkes (USA)
B.S. Zheng (China)

List and addresses of editors

José A. Centeno, Armed Forces Institute of Pathology, Department of Environmental and Toxicologic Pathology, Division of Environmental Pathology, 16th & Alaska Ave. N.W., Bldg. 54, Room M-093A, Washington, D.C. 20306-6000, USA

Philippe Collery, Institut International de Recherche sur les Ions Métalliques, Université de Reims Champagne-Ardenne, U.F.R. Sciences, B.P. 1039, 51687 Reims Cedex 2, France

Guy Vernet, Institut International de Recherche sur les Ions Métalliques, Université de Reims Champagne-Ardenne, U.F.R. Sciences, B.P. 1039, 51687 Reims Cedex 2, France

Robert B. Finkelman, U.S. Geological Survey, National Center, Mail Stop 956, Reston, VA 20192, USA

Herman Gibb, U.S. Environmental Protection Agency, National Center for Environmental Assessment, Washington, D.C., USA

Jean-Claude Etienne, Institut International de Recherche sur les Ions Métalliques, Université de Reims Champagne-Ardenne, U.F.R. Sciences, B.P. 1039, 51687 Reims Cedex 2, France

Foreword

It has been almost ten years since the first series of this book was published summarizing the proceedings of the ***First International Symposium on Metal Ions in Biology and Medicine*** which was celebrated in Reims, France. Since the beginning of our Symposium series, this biennal conference has provided an international scientific forum by which researchers from all over the world will have the opportunity to share their knowledge, exchange ideas, and discuss scientific, policy and regulatory issues associated with the role of metal ions in biology and medicine. Following this tradition, the ***6th International Symposium on Metal Ions in Biology and Medicine*** (6th ISMIBM) is aimed at promoting interdisciplinary research discussions, to strengthen productive collaborations and to facilitate many new contacts between scientists. In our previous five symposia we have succeeded in bringing together a wide array of researchers from various biomedical disciplines. The sixth symposium in San Juan will mark the first time we brought together the environmental and geoscience communities into this conference series.

The Scientific Program for the 6th ISMIBM is composed of three plenary lectures, 5 short courses and over 300 papers, including invited contributions, oral and poster presentations. The Scientific Program covers a diverse and multidisciplinary research agenda with topics including nutrition, analysis, toxicology, homeostasis, biochemistry, oxidative-reduction processes, mechanisms of metal-induced carcinogenesis, pathology, oncology, gene expression, endocrinology, epidemiology, cardiovascular and neurological effects, reproductive effects and aging, therapy and administration, clinical aspects of selenium, environmental and occupational health aspects, occupational health issues for nickel, and ecotoxicological issues.

For the first time in our Symposium series, the 6th ISMIBM will featured sessions on arsenic health effects, with particular interest on its global impact including presentations on epidemiological studies, toxicology, mechanisms of action, carcinogenesis, and clinico-pathological aspects. Scientists from India, Bangladesh, China, and Chile will present their work on these important issues. We believe that the 6th ISMIBM will be the most dynamic symposium to date and this resulting volume of ***Metal Ions*** represents state-of-the-art advances in metal ion research. We hope that the selection of topics and papers published in volume 6th of ***Metal Ions*** will stimulate further collaborations between scientists working on this field, attract more scientists from all fields in life sciences, and stimulate participation of these groups in the next symposium of this series.

The 6th ISMIBM was organized by the U.S. Armed Forces Institute of Pathology (AFIP), in collaboration with the Institut International de Recherche sur les Ions Métalliques (France), the American Registry of Pathology, the U.S.Geological

Survey, the National Institute of Environmental Health Sciences, the U.S. Environmental Protection Agency, U.S. National Cancer Institute, the Ana G. Méndez University of Puerto Rico, the University of Puerto Rico at Mayagüez, Jackson State University-Mississippi, the Ponce School of Medicine, and the American Association for the Advancement of Science-Caribbean Division. The Institut International de Recherche sur les Ions Métalliques especially wishes to acknowledge the Conseil Régional de Champagne-Ardenne for its constant financial support. Also for their financial support, warm thanks are offered to the Tourism Company of Puerto Rico, Cypress Systems Inc. and the Nickel Producers Environmental Research Association.

Finally, we are grateful not only to the members of the Organizing, International and Local Committees for their valuable advice and suggestions, but also to all the authors for their efforts and willingness to discuss their fine work, and to all the contributors for their support in making the 6th ISMIBM possible. We thank most sincerely and express our gratitude to Dr. Sylvie Biagianti-Risbourg and Dr. Philippe Eullaffroy for their important contribution in editing this book of proceedings. We would also like to express our appreciation to Michalann Harthill (USGS), Dr. Norbert Page (AFIP), Dr. Elena Ladich (AFIP) and Chantal Vezin (John Libbey, Eurotext) for their tireless efforts and dedication to this conference and the successful publication of this book.

Jose A. Centeno
Guy Vernet

May 2000

Préface

Cela fera bientôt dix ans qu'est paru le premier ouvrage de cette collection consacrée aux comptes rendus du premier **Symposium International sur les Ions Métalliques en Biologie et en Médecine** qui s'est tenu à Reims (France) en 1990. Depuis notre tout premier symposium, cette conférence bisannuelle est l'occasion d'un forum scientifique international, permettant aux chercheurs du monde entier de partager leurs connaissances, d'échanger leurs idées et de s'entretenir de toutes les questions scientifiques, politiques ou réglementaires qui ont trait au rôle des ions métalliques en biologie et médecine. Suivant cette tradition, le sixième **Symposium International sur les Ions Métalliques en Biologie et en Médecine** vise à promouvoir des discussions sur les différentes disciplines de la recherche, à renforcer de fructueuses collaborations et à permettre aux scientifiques de nouer de nouveaux contacts. Au cours de nos cinq précédentes rencontres, nous sommes parvenus à réunir un nombre important de chercheurs appartenant aux différentes disciplines biomédicales. Le sixième Symposium de San Juan sera le premier à intégrer dans cette série de rencontres la communauté travaillant sur les sciences de la géologie et de l'environnement.

Le Programme scientifique du 6e Symposium comprend trois conférences plénières, cinq exposés brefs et plus de trois cents communications, incluant celles des orateurs invités ainsi que les présentations orales et les posters. Ce Programme scientifique couvre un large champ de la recherche multidisciplinaire dont les sujets portent sur la nutrition, les techniques d'analyse, la toxicologie, l'homéostasie, la biochimie, les processus d'oxydo-réduction, les mécanismes de la carcinogenèse induite par les métaux, la pathologie, l'oncologie, la génétique, l'endocrinologie, l'épidémiologie, les atteintes cardiovasculaires et neurologiques, les mécanismes de la reproduction et le vieillissement, la thérapie et l'administration, les aspects cliniques du sélénium, les risques sanitaires professionnels et environnementaux, les maladies professionnelles induites par le nickel et les questions d'éco-toxicologie.

Pour la première fois dans ces rencontres, le 6e Symposium consacrera des sessions aux effets de l'arsenic sur la santé, s'intéressant tout particulièrement à son impact global en présentant des études sur son épidémiologie, sa toxicologie ou encore sur ses mécanismes d'action, de carcinogenèse ainsi que sur ses aspects clinico-pathologiques. Des scientifiques venus d'Inde, du Bangladesh, de Chine et du Chili présenteront leurs travaux consacrés à ces points importants. Nous sommes certains que ce 6e Symposium sera particulièrement dynamique et que l'ouvrage qui l'accompagne sera le témoin des avancées récentes de la recherche sur les ions métalliques. Nous espérons que la sélection des sujets et des communications présentés dans le sixième volume de ***Metal Ions*** créera de nouveaux liens entre les chercheurs travaillant dans ce domaine, attirera davantage de scientifiques appartenant à toutes les disciplines et incitera ces derniers à participer au prochain symposium.

Le 6e Symposium est organisé par l'US Armed Forces Institute of Pathology (AFIP) en collaboration avec l'Institut International de Recherche sur les Ions Métalliques (France), l'American Registry of Pathology, l'US Geological Survey, le National Institute of Environnemental Health Sciences, l'US Environmental Protection Agency, l'US National Cancer Institute, l'Ana G. Méndez University of Puerto Rico, l'University of Puerto Rico at Mayagüez, le Jackson State University-Mississippi, la Ponce School of Medicine, et l'American Association for the Advancement of Science-Caribbean Division. L'Institut International de Recherche sur les Ions Métalliques remercie vivement le Conseil Régional de Champagne-Ardenne pour son indéfectible soutien financier. Egalement pour leur soutien financier, nos remerciements chaleureux vont à la Tourism Company of Puerto-Rico, à Cypress Systems Inc., et à la Nickel Producers Environmental Research Association.

Enfin, nous remercions non seulement les membres des comités d'organisation, local et international, pour leurs conseils avisés et leurs suggestions, mais aussi tous les auteurs pour leurs efforts et leur volonté de faire partager leurs connaissances, ainsi qu'à tous ceux dont le soutien a permis ce 6e Symposium. Nous remercions tout particulièrement en leur exprimant notre gratitude le Dr Sylvie Biagianti-Risbourg et le Dr Philippe Eullaffroy pour leur importante contribution à l'édition de ce volume. Nous souhaitons aussi exprimer notre reconnaissance à Michalann Harthill (USGS), au Dr Norbert Page (AFIP), au Dr Elena Ladich (AFIP) et à Chantal Vezin (John Libbey Eurotext) pour leurs efforts inlassables consacrés à la réussite de cette conférence et à la publication de cet ouvrage.

Jose A. Centono
Guy Vernet

Mai 2000

Contents/Sommaire

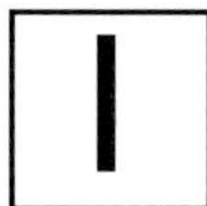

ENVIRONMENTAL PATHOLOGY OF METAL EXPOSURES

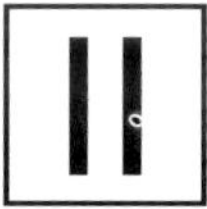

TOXICOLOGY, HEALTH AND REMEDIATION OF SELECTED CONTAMINANTS IN ENVIRONMENTAL TOXICOLOGY

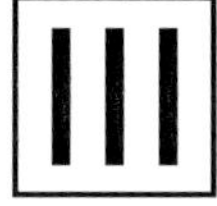

ARSENIC : HUMAN EXPOSURE AND EFFECTS ; MECHANISMS OF ACTION

IV MOLECULAR BIOLOGY OF METAL CARCINOGENESIS

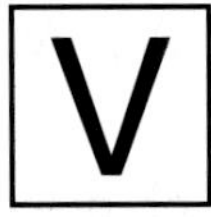

METALS AND HOMEOSTASIS

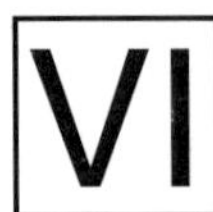

METAL IONS AND ECOLOGICAL STUDIES

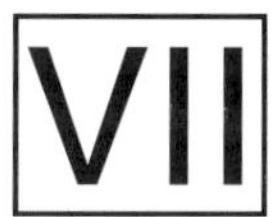

VII METAL IONS AND ONCOLOGY

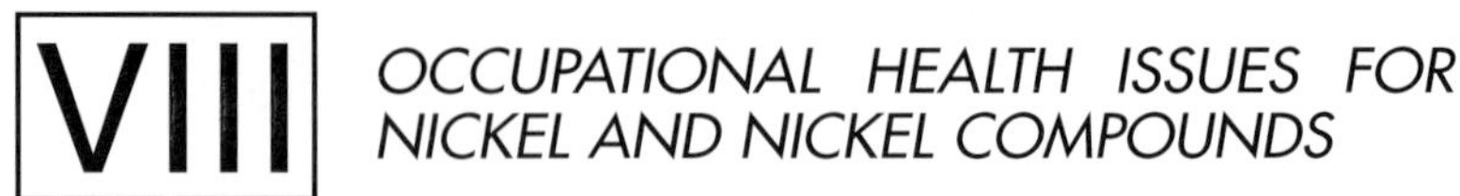

OCCUPATIONAL HEALTH ISSUES FOR NICKEL AND NICKEL COMPOUNDS

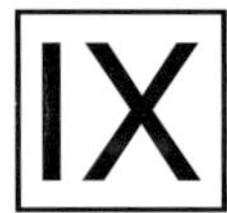

CLINICAL AND MOLECULAR STUDIES OF SELENIUM AND ITS COMPOUNDS

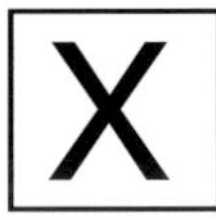

METAL IONS AND TOXICOLOGY

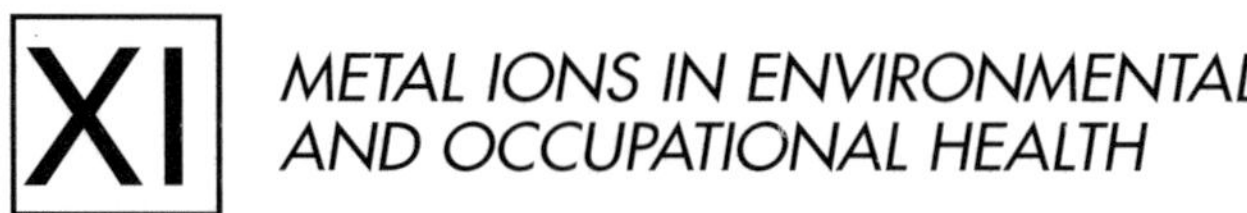

XI METAL IONS IN ENVIRONMENTAL AND OCCUPATIONAL HEALTH

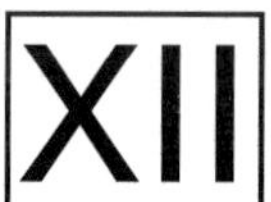

ANALYTICAL ASPECTS

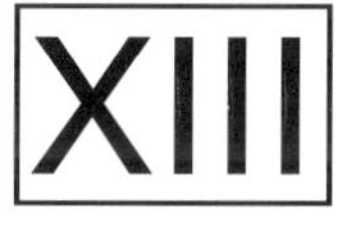

MODERN TRENDS OF METAL ION RESEARCH : SPECIATION, QUALITY ASSURANCE AND REFERENCE MATERIALS

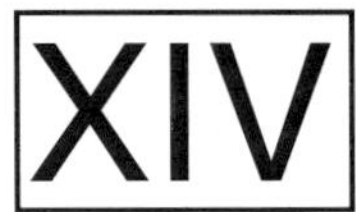

METAL IONS AND NEUROTOXICITY

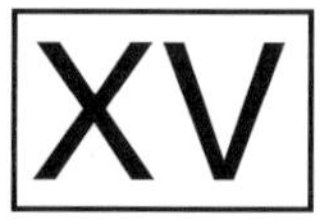

BIOLOGICAL CONDITIONS AFFECTING OXIDATION-REDUCTION OF METAL IONS

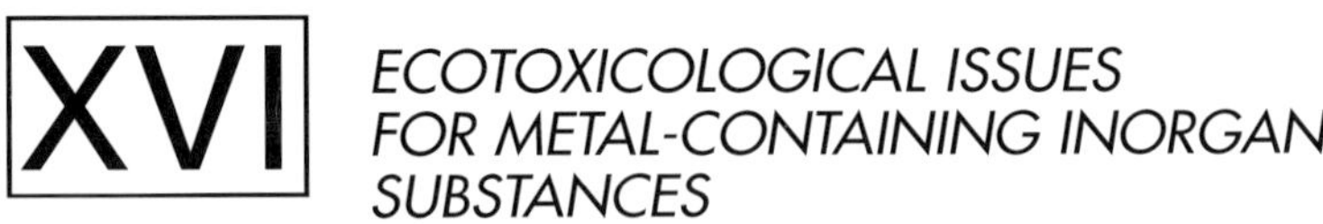

XVI ECOTOXICOLOGICAL ISSUES FOR METAL-CONTAINING INORGANIC SUBSTANCES

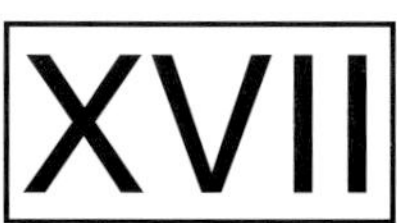

ASSESSMENT OF ELEMENT STATUS : NUTRITIONAL ASPECTS, DEFICIENCIES

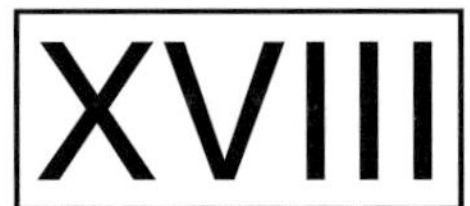

METAL IONS AND HUMAN DISEASE : THERAPY AND ADMINISTRATION

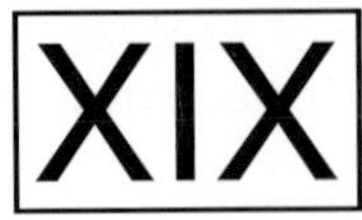

XIX *EFFECTS OF METAL IONS ON THE CARDIOVASCULAR SYSTEM*

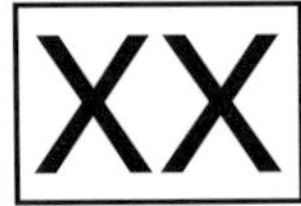

XX *REMEDIATION STRATEGIES FOR METAL ION RESEARCH*

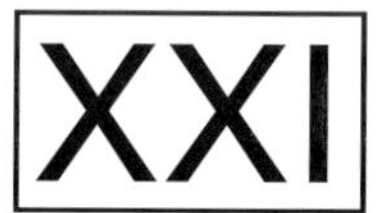

EFFECT OF METAL IONS ON GENE EXPRESSION

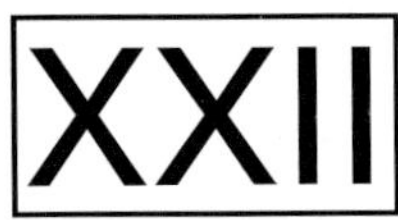

METAL IONS : REPRODUCTIVE EFFECTS AND AGING

Metal Ions in Biology and Medicine; vol 6. Eds. J.A. Centeno, Ph. Collery, G. Vernet, R.B. Finkelman, H. Gibb, J.C. Etienne. John Libbey Eurotext, Paris © 2000, pp. 3-5.

Environmental pathology of metal exposures–skin

Ladich E.R., Mullick F.G., Centeno J.A.

Department of Environmental and Toxicologic Pathology, Armed Forces Institute of Pathology, Washington, DC 20306

Introduction Metals are important in environmental pathology because of their toxic potential to one or more organ systems. The list of metals exhibiting dermal toxicity has been well catalogued. These include metal compounds used in medicinal products, industrial processes, pesticides, cosmetics, dyes, and jewelry. [1] A wide range of injury patterns have been described in association with acute and chronic exposures to metals, which include: pigmentation disorders, spongiotic dermatitis (allergic contact dermatitis and primary irritant dermatitis), granulomatous inflammation, and carcinogenesis.

Carcinogenesis The most widely recognized metal affecting the skin is arsenic. It has been known for many years that arsenic exposure can cause a wide variety of toxic effects ranging from death following acute high-dose exposure to latent effects and cancer from chronic exposure with lower doses. Up until the 1940s, potassium arsenate (1%) Fowler's solution was a popular remedy for treating syphilis and psoriasis, but was discontinued with the introduction of antibiotics and other more effective less toxic therapies. Currently, the use of arsenicals is limited to the treatment of certain tropical diseases, and most recently as an effective therapy for refractory acute promyelocytic leukemia.[2] While the concern for arsenic exposure from its use in medicines has decreased, the concern for arsenic contamination of the environment has increased. Worldwide, some geographical areas have now become heavily contaminated with exceptionally high levels of arsenic in the drinking water and other environmental media.

Epidemiological studies have confirmed the role of arsenic in the induction of cancers of the skin. Of the metals known to exhibit dermal toxicity, only arsenic has been shown conclusively to be carcinogenic to the skin. [3] Arsenic exists in both organic and inorganic forms. The inorganic compounds exhibit the greatest toxicity and carcinogenicity in the skin. Squamous cell carcinomas of the skin and basal cell carcinomas have both been associated with chronic inorganic arsenic ingestion. Arsenical keratosis is a well-established clinical entity characterized by several specific pathologic features. These features include hyperkeratosis, parakeratosis, arsenical pigmentation and squamous cell carcinoma in situ (Bowen's disease). The lesions are normally most pronounced on the palms and soles, although they can occur on the trunk and other areas of the extremities. [4] Furthermore, arsenical skin changes tend to occur in non-sun exposed areas with an absence of dermal solar elastosis noted histologically. The presence of arsenic in tissues was reported in the past using the Osborne stain. [5] Currently, the reliability of this special stain is under investigation. The biological mechanisms by which arsenic induces chronic effects including cancer are not well understood and are the subject of considerable research efforts.

Spongiotic Dermatitis

Allergic contact dermatitis Metals are the most frequent cause of allergic contact dermatitis. Nickel, chromium, and mercury are the most common causes of metal dermatitis in the U.S. and Europe. The organomercurial preservative, thimerosol, is another common sensitizer in dermatologic practice. It is widely used in vaccines and sensitivities are reported in the pediatric population. [6] Histologically, early lesions show a superficial perivascular lymphocytic infiltrate often associated with eosinophils as well as areas of intercellular edema within the epidermal layer (spongiosis). Chronic features include epidermal hyperplasia and excess scale production. [7]

Primary irritant dermatitis A rather large number of metals exhibit primary irritancy in the skin. The pathogenesis of this nonimmunologic inflammatory reaction is not well understood. Histologically, primary irritant dermatitis may be indistinguishable from allergic contact dermatitis. The presence of irregular epidermal hyperplasisa, necrosis, and a neutrophilic infiltrate suggests a diagnosis of primary irritancy. With chronicity, thickened dermal collagen fibers are oriented perpendicular to the overlying epidermis. [8]

Granulomatous dermatitis Foreign body granulomas represent another type of reaction associated with the accumulation of metal ions in dermal or subcutaneous tissues. Histologically, focal aggregations of epithelioid cells, fibroblasts, and multinucleated giant cells are identified associated with a foreign body. Beryllium induces a distinct necrotizing and granulomatous reaction.[9] Other metals known to cause granulomas include talc, aluminum, zirconium, and mercury.

Disorders of pigmentation Deposition of heavy metals or metalloids in the dermis can produce pigmentation. Argyria is a condition caused by prolonged ingestion of silver salts or their application to the mucous membranes of the upper respiratory tract. It is characterized by a permanent slate gray discoloration of the skin. Silver sulfide granules are found in the dermis, as well as increased melanin in the dermis and epidermis. Chrysiasis is a distinctive and permanent pigmentation of light-exposed skin resulting from the administration of parenteral gold salts. Severity of pigmentation correlates with the amount of gold deposited in the dermis.[10] Hyperpigmentation is one of the most common skin changes in people chronically exposed to arsenic. Hypopigmentation occurs as well and may show a characteristic "rain drop" pattern. Application of mercury-containing cosmetic creams may result in hyperpigmentation.[11]

References

1. Lansdown A. Physiological and toxicological changes in the skin resulting from the action and interaction of metal ions. *Crit Rev Tox* 1995; 25: 397-462.
2. Bergstrom S, Gillan E, Quinn J, Altman A. Arsenic trioxide in the treatment of a patient with multiply recurrent, atra-resistant promyelocytic leukemia: a case report. *J Ped.Hem Onc* 1998; 20: 545-7.
3. Mazumder G, De B, Santra A, Dasgupta J, Ghosh N, Roy B, Ghoshal U, Saha J, Chatterjee A, Dutta S, Haque R, Smith A, Chakraborty D, Angle C, Centeno J. Chronic arsenic toxicity:epidemiology, natural history and treatment. In: Chappell W, Abernathy C, Calderon R, eds. *Arsenic exposure and health effects*. Oxford: Elsevier Science, 1999: 335-347.
4. Maloney M. Arsenic in dermatology. *Derm Surg* 1996; 22: 301-4.
5. Osborne E. Microchemical studies of arsenic in arsenical pigmentation and keratoses. *Arch Derm Syph* 1925; 12: 773-788.
6. Patrizi A, Rizzoli L, Vincenzi C, Trevisi P, Tosti A. Sensitization to thimerosal in atopic children. *Contact Derm* 1999; 40: 94-7.
7. Murphy G. Skin. In: Craighead J. ed. *Pathology of environmental and occupational disease*. St. Louis: Mosby, 1995: 437-453.
8. Cohen L, Skopicki D, Harrist T, Clark W. Noninfectious vesiculobullous and vesiculopustular diseases. In: Elder D, Elenitsas R, Jaworsky C, Johnson B, eds. *Lever's histopathology of the skin.* Philadelphia: Lippincott-Raven, 1997: 209-252.
9. Helwig E. Chemical (beryllium) granulomas of the skin. *Milit Surg* 1951; 109: 540-558.
10. Smith R, Leppard B, Barnett N, Millward-Sadler G, McCrae F, Crawley M. Chrysiasis revisited: a clinical and pathological study. *Br J Dermatol* 1995; 133: 671-8.
11. Medina M. The skin. In: Riddell R, ed. *Pathology of drug-induced and toxic diseases.* New York: Churchill Livingstone Inc., 1982: 119-146.

Metal Ions in Biology and Medicine; vol 6. Eds. J.A. Centeno, Ph. Collery, G. Vernet, R.B. Finkelman, H. Gibb, J.C. Etienne. John Libbey Eurotext, Paris © 2000, pp. 6-8.

Pathology of metal exposure in the lung

Teri J. Franks, M.D. and Michael N. Koss, M.D.

Armed Forces Institute of Pathology, Department of Pulmonary and Mediastinal Pathology, Washington, DC, USA

Introduction

Zenker first proposed the term "pneumonokoniosis" in 1867 as a name for lung disease resulting from the inhalation of dust.(1) While many forms of pneumoconioses are known today, each with its own etiologic agent, the definition of pneumoconiosis varies. Some authors restrict the term to non-neoplastic reactions of the lung to inhaled minerals or organic dusts, excluding asthma, bronchitis, and emphysema, while others use the term more broadly to define the accumulation of abnormal amounts of dust and the resulting pathologic reactions.(2) These reactions range from minimal responses to inert dust particles, such as interstitial dust macules, to lethal scarring associated with fibrogenic dusts.

Damage caused by inhaled particles depends on a variety of factors, including the number, size, and physiochemical properties of the particles; the deposition, clearance and retention of particles in the respiratory tract; the host's inflammatory response to the inhaled particles; the duration of exposure and interval since initial exposure, as well as interactions with other inhaled particles, particularly cigarette smoke.(3)

Pathologic Responses to Metals and Metallic Compounds

Metals and metallic compounds, in the form of dusts and fumes, can produce a variety of injury patterns in the lung, which include: diffuse alveolar damage (fume exposure), dust macules with or without small airway fibrosis, diffuse interstitial fibrosis, alveolar proteinosis, granulomatous interstitial pneumonitis, giant-cell and desquamative interstitial pneumonitis, and lung cancer. Generally, these injury patterns lack specific features that implicate a causative agent.

Diffuse alveolar damage (DAD), the histologic correlate to adult respiratory distress syndrome, is the most common serious reaction to inhaled gases and fumes.(4) Microscopically, DAD is characterized by hyaline membranes lining edematous alveolar septa. Virtually any noxious gas or fume, e.g. beryllium and cobalt metal, inhaled in sufficient concentration, can potentially cause DAD.(4) However, numerous other agents, including infectious organisms, drugs, ingestants, shock, and sepsis cause DAD that is microscopically indistinguishable from that produced by gases and fumes.

Dust macules are non-palpable, peribronchiolar interstitial aggregates of pigmented dust and dust-laden macrophages. Initially, macules may have little associated fibrosis, however, with sufficient exposure, peribronchiolar fibrosis may occur. This pattern of injury generally has little functional deficit, but due to the radiodensity of the dust, it is usually associated with an abnormal chest radiograph.(5;6) Agents that produce dust macules include: antimony, barium, chromium ore, iron, rare earths, tin, titanium and tungsten.

Diffuse interstitial fibrosis pattern of injury, an uncommon complication of metal exposure, can be seen with iron (mild fibrosis), aluminum, hard metal (containing cobalt), copper, rare earths, and silicon carbide exposure. Asbestos and mixed dusts containing silicates can also produce interstitial fibrosis.

Alveolar proteinosis pattern is characterized by a relatively uniform filling of alveoli with granular, eosinophilic exudate containing dense bodies and acicular clefts, accompanied by a variable amount of chronic interstitial inflammation and fibrosis.(6) This pattern of injury is usually associated with acute exposure to high levels of silica dust and rarely to aluminum dusts.

Giant cell (GIP) and desquamative interstitial pneumonitis (DIP) patterns of injury can result from exposure to “hard metals.” Patchy interstitial fibrosis with mild chronic inflammatory cell infiltrates, accompanied by striking intraalveolar accumulations of macrophages, characterize these two injury patterns. The presence of enlarged, multinucleated alveolar macrophages, which may contain engulfed inflammatory cells, distinguishes GIP from DIP. Granulomatous interstitial pneumonitis is characterized microscopically by interstitial fibrosis accompanied by non-caseating granulomas. This pattern can be seen in chronic beryllium disease.

Asbestos (particularly when associated with asbestosis), arsenic, beryllium, cadmium, chloromethyl ether, hexavalent chromium compounds, nickel, and radon have been linked to lung cancer. Lung cancer occurring in occupationally exposed individuals is histologically indistinguishable from cancer in non-exposed individuals.

Reference List

1. Zenker F. Iron lung: sclerosis pulmonum. Dtsch Arch Klin Med 1867.

2. Gibbs A. Occupational Lung Disease. In: Hasleton P, ed. Spencer's Pathology of the Lung. New York: McGraw-Hill, 1996;461-506.

3. Roggli V, Shelburne J. Pneumoconioses, Mineral and Vegetable. In: Dail D, Hammar S, eds. Pulmonary Pathology. New York: Springer-Verlag, 1994;867-900.

4. Wright J, Churg A. Diseases caused by gases and fumes. In: Churg A, Green F, eds. Pathology of Occupational Lung Disease. Baltimore: Williams & Wilkins, 1998;57-75.

5. Katzenstein A. Pneumoconiosis. In: Katzenstein A, ed. Non-Neoplastic Lung Disease. Philadelphia: W.B Saunders, 1997;112-137.

6. Churg A, Colby T. Diseases caused by metals and related compounds. In: Churg A, Green F, eds. Pathology of Occupational Lung Disease. Baltimore: Williams & Wilkins, 1998;77-128.

Metal Ions in Biology and Medicine; vol 6. Eds. J.A. Centeno, Ph. Collery, G. Vernet, R.B. Finkelman, H. Gibb, J.C. Etienne. John Libbey Eurotext, Paris © 2000, pp. 9-14.

Pathology of metal exposure in the kidney

Sharda G. Sabnis, M.D.

Introduction:

The kidney an anatomically and physiologically complex organ is primarily involved in excretion of waste matter. It provides homeostasis with regulation of extracellular fluid and electrolytes. It also takes part in formation of hormones, erythropoietin, renin, aldosterone, and several prostaglandins and kinins. Various parts of the nephron have specific functions that may be affected by the nephrotoxins. The vascular elements deliver waste and other materials to the tubules for excretion, return reabsorbed and synthesized materials to the circulation and deliver oxygen and metabolic substrates to the nephron. The renal blood flow is high and the kidneys receive 25% of cardiac output. Therefore higher amounts of any drug or toxin in the circulation is delivered to the kidney. The glomerulus serves as a selective filter. The tubules selectively reabsorb bulk of the filtrate with 98-99% reabsorption of salts and water, and complete reabsorption of sugars and amino acids with selective elimination of waste materials. With reabsorption of salts and water concentrated levels of drugs and nephrotoxins accumulate in the tubules and non-toxic serum levels can become toxic to the tubules. The tubule particularly proximal tubules actively secrete materials into urine. This latter function is responsible for excretion of certain organic compounds and elimination of hydrogen and potassium ions. The tubules actively take part in the synthesis of ammonia and glucose and activation of vitamin D. Although toxic insult can affect any of the functions the toxic effect is commonly reported as alteration in blood urea nitrogen (BUN), creatinine (Cr) and creatinine clearance (CrCl). The response at cellular level to toxic agents can cause minor undetectable physiologic and functional changes. This can result in minor biochemical changes or cell death with necrosis. Functionally toxic effect may reflect as transport abnormalities (glycosuria or aminoaciduria), as decreased concentrating capacity (polyuria), frank anuria or renal failure. 1 can bring about the toxic effect. Vasoconstriction with resultant decreased in renal blood flow and glomerular filtration rate (GFR). 2. Direct effect on the glomerulus altering the permeability affecting GFR, or 3) direct effect on the tubular epithelium affecting reabsorption, secretary function and permeability. Kidney is also sensitive to extra-renal factor such as shock or hemorrhage that decrease blood volume or blood pressure.

Exposure to heavy metals occurs as 1) environmental exposure, 2) used as medicines or 3) occupational exposure. Most metals affect multiple organ systems. The targets for toxicity are specific biochemical processes (enzymes) and and/or membranes of cells and organelles. This occurs with reaction of free metal ions with the target. Most heavy metals are nephrotoxic agents. Low levels of metals produce minor symptoms such as glycosuria, aminoaciduria and polyuria, whereas high levels can produce oliguria, anuria, renal failure and death. Several mechanisms tend to protect the kidney from the effects of metals. Significant levels of metals are seen in the renal tissue prior to development of physiological signs of toxicity. The protective mechanism is by lysosomal binding of metals that can occur via lysosomal endocytosis of metal-protein complex, autophagy of intoxicated organelles such as mitochondria, or by binding of metal to acidic lipoproteins within the lysosomes. In addition apical extrusion of endocytoplasmic reticulum packets eliminate certain metals such as mercury. These protective mechanisms can be overwhelmed by very high concentrations of the metals causing detectable injury. Metals cause toxic effect by: 1) direct effect on nephron components, 2) immunologically induced injury, and by 3) functional changes. The toxic effects are often dose- and duration-related and can cause transient or permanent damage. The renal histologic changes are often nonspecific thus clinical correlation is necessary (1, 2, 3).

Gold:

Gold and its salts have been used in a variety of conditions, however its major use today is limited to rheumatoid arthritis and discoid lupus. Gold is poorly absorbed in the gastro-intestinal (GI) tract. After injection most soluble salts are excreted via the kidney and the GI tract accounts for the excretion of insoluble salts. Gold has a long biological half-life and detectable blood levels can be demonstrated years after the cessation of treatment. Dermatitis and stomatitis are common side effects. Renal toxicity can present as oliguric renal failure or as proteinuria. The proteinuria is associated either with minimal change disease or more commonly as membranous glomerulopathy, an immune complex (IC) deposition disease. The exact mechanism behind the IC disease is not known however, damage to tubules with release of tubular antigen perpetuating an antibody response is suggested. The membranous glomerulopathy consists of thickening of capillary walls by light microscopy (LM), subepithelial and often mesangial deposits by electron microscopy (EM), and IgG and C3 by immunofluorescence microscopy (IM). The renal failure is associated with tubular damage seen as acute tubular necrosis secondary to direct injury. The gold salts have an affinity for mitochondria particularly of proximal tubular epithelium, but can be also seen in glomerular epithelial and mesangial cells. Gold particles can be identified by EM, and appear as electron dense strands associated with granules. They can also be demonstrated by x-ray microanalysis and by histochemical methods (4, 5).

Lithium:

Lithium carbonate is used in the treatment of depression. It is readily absorbed from the GI tract and is distributed equally in all organs. Excretion is mainly through the kidneys and some via the GI tract. The greatest part is present in the cells perhaps competing with sodium and potassium. The therapeutic doses can produce toxic effects. Acute lithium poisoning include CNS and neuromuscular changes (Apathy, sluggishness, tremors rigidity, ataxia, seizures and coma), cardiovascular changes (arrhythmia, hypertension and circulatory collapse), GI changes (anorexia, nausea, and vomiting), and renal changes (acute renal failure, albuminuria and glycosuria). The renal changes are secondary to interference with vasopressin metabolism with resultant diabetes insipidus-like-change. The clinical findings of renal toxicity do not always correspond to histologic changes, but may show distal tubular dilatation and necrosis with swelling of mitochondria and rough endoplasmic reticulum, and rarely acute interstitial nephritis (AIN). More commonly kidney biopsies are performed for possible chronic toxicity that reveal chronic tubulo-interstitial disease (interstitial fibrosis, tubular atrophy, interstitial infiltrates and glomerulosclerosis). Rarely patients may develop nephrotic syndrome with lesions of minimal change disease or focal segmental glomerulosclerosis (6, 7, 8).

Chromium:

Chromium in ambient air comes from industrial sources used in metal industries for ore refining, chemical and refractory processing, combustion of fossil fuels, in cement plants, and for galvanizing. Chromium is also essential in carbohydrate metabolism and is a cofactor in insulin action. It is absorbed by inhalation and is excreted through kidney. Industrial exposure to chromium is associated with respiratory tract malignancies. It also causes ulceration of skin as well as allergic skin reaction. The major toxic effect from ingested chromium (often as suicidal agent) causes acute renal failure with acute tubular necrosis.

Platinum:

Platinum itself is generally harmless, but can cause allergic dermatitis and respiratory allergic reactions in susceptible individuals. Some compounds of platinum such as *cis*-dichlorodiammine, platinum (II), (*cis*-DDP) and various analogs are potent anti-tumor chemicals and are used in the treatment of cancers of head and neck, certain lymphomas and testicular and ovarian tumors. At effective dosage levels these compounds cause severe and persistent inhibition of DNA synthesis and less severe inhibition of RNA synthesis. Although *cis*-DDP has anti-tumor activity, it can also cause tumors such as lung adenomas and skin papillomas and carcinomas in mice. *Cis*-DDP is also nephrotoxic. Ninety percent of administered dose is bound to plasma proteins and the remaining is excreted by kidney. Within tissue platinum is protein bound with largest concentration in the kidney, liver, and spleen and has a half-life of two to three weeks. The renal tubular injury is mainly seen in the proximal and distal tubules of cortico-medullary region where the concentration of platinum is highest. Nephrotoxicity is dose related and is seen with frequent and repeated administration of the drug. Clinical symptoms include proteinuria and commonly azotemia. Renal biopsy reveals dilatation, epithelial necrosis with giant nuclei and cellular atypia of distal and collecting tubules followed by chronic tubulo-interstitial disease (9).

Cadmium:

Cadmium is used in metallurgical industry for galvanizing and electroplating because of its noncorrosive properties. It is absorbed through the respiratory and GI systems. The absorption is enhanced by deficiencies of calcium and iron enhancing the synthesis of calcium binding protein that increases cadmium absorption. About 50-75% of the body burden of cadmium is in liver and kidney. Although exact tissue half-life is not known it is for many years. With continuous accumulation in the kidney a variety of renal manifestations are seen. It affects the proximal tubules and is reflected as increased cadmium in the urine, proteinuria, aminoaciduria, glucosuria and decreased reabsorption of phosphates by the tubules. The morphologic changes are nonspecific. Initially there is tubular cell degeneration progressing to chronic tubulo-interstitial disease when kidney concentrations reach 200 micrograms/gram widely referred to as critical concentration of cadmium. Proteinuria can be either of low molecular weight proteins such as β2 microglobulin and others present in the urine. Proteinuria of high molecular weight with albumin, transferrin etc. suggests glomerular injury and antiglomerular antibodies have been demonstrated in the serum of patients with cadmium toxicity.

Arsenic:

Exposure to arsenic may occur as inorganic arsenicals in the smelting industry. Is associated with lung and hepatic cancers. It was used in asthma and in psoriasis. Long term occupational exposure is associated with neurologic and dermatologic manifestations. Renal involvement is common in acute poisoning and causes renal insufficiency or failure with renal cortical necrosis.

Mercury:

Mercury causes diverse effects dependent on the different biochemical forms. Toxic effects are associated with elemental, organic and inorganic forms. Mercury was used as therapeutic agent, its organic form as diuretic and inorganic form in laxatives and children's teething powder. Ammoniated mercury was used in skin preparations and in cosmetic industry. Various forms of mercury have affinity for certain organ systems. Renal toxicity is rarely seen expect in cases of accidental acute poisoning or when it was used as a suicidal agent or for abortion in the past. Bichloride of mercury is a potent nephrotoxic agent and causes acute tubular necrosis of proximal tubular epithelium. With chronic toxicity due to long term use membranous glomerulopathy has been reported.

Bismuth:

Bismuth was used as anti-syphilis therapy and can cause acute renal failure. Clinically and pathologically it is similar to mercury but in addition yellow brown refractile bodies in the cytoplasm or in nuclei of proximal tubules is found many years after exposure.

Lead:

Humans are exposed to lead in various forms such as ointments (lead acetate, or carbonate), fabrics (lead sulfate), in paints, batteries, solders, ceramics, unglazed china, and insecticides and in the past in gasoline. All forms of lead are toxic depending on the solubility. Lead carbonate and suboxide are most toxic, whereas acetate, chloride and nitrate are less toxic. Conversion of some forms into more toxic forms also occurs. Exposure to lead occurs by inhalation, ingestion, through skin, and can be accidental occupational or medicinal. Absorption is higher in children than in adults and when absorbed it is available as active pool in RBCs (half-life 35 days) and as storage pool in bones (half-life 20-30 years). Blood level depend on exposure. Lead can be measured using biochemical markers such as δ-aminolevulinic acid excretion, or blood porphyrin –

hematocrit determination or by using chemical and analytical methods such as dithizone or dithicarbomate methods, polarographic method or by electrothermal atomic absorption method. Lead is eliminated in urine (75%), and in nails, hair and sweat (25%). It is a biochemical poison that interferes with cellular enzymes, membrane function and oxidative mechanisms. It also combines with sulphydryl groups of proteins including enzymes and causes cell death. The most important toxic effects include neurological, hematological and renal manifestation. Toxic effects of lead on kidney are divided in acute and chronic types. With acute exposure in addition to the neurological symptoms acute renal failure with reversible tubular dysfunction is present. In acute lead toxicity clinical symptoms include functional abnormalities of proximal tubules expressed as aminoaciduria, glycosuria, phosphaturia and renal tubular acidosis. Histologic documentation of renal changes in acute exposure is rare. More commonly renal changes are encountered and documented with chronic lead exposure. The renal morphologic changes include chronic tubulo-interstitial disease and vascular sclerosis and are associated with progressive decrease in the renal function and hypertension. A pathognomonic feature is the presence of intranuclear and rarely intracytoplasmic inclusion bodies. These are commonly seen in the proximal tubular epithelium. By LM these bodies appear eosinophilic dense nuclear inclusions that are acid fast when stained with carbolfuchsin. By EM the bodies have a dense central core and outer fibrillary region. The bodies are made up of lead protein complex (Moore). The protein is acidic and contains large amount of aspartic and glutamic acids and cystine. It is believed that lead attaches loosely to the carboxyl groups of acidic amino acids. Most of the lead in tubular epithelium is bound to the inclusion body and probably protects more susceptible organelles such as mitochondria and endoplasmic reticulum. (Goyer). The pathogenesis of inclusion bodies may be related to tubular transport and excretion of lead. In addition, mitochondria may show degenerative changes with functional changes such as impaired oxidation and phosphorylation abilities. The inclusion bodies are the earliest evidence of exposure to lead before functional changes are apparent as shown in experimental studies. The inclusion bodies are either fewer of absent with chronic histologic changes of advanced nephrosclerosis. Thus clinical correlation is absolutely necessary to make the diagnosis of "Lead nephropathy". The earlier tubular changes are reversible thus early recognition is important to reduce exposure either by removing the source or by chelation therapy. The relationship between lead exposure and hypertension is uncertain however; it may follow the vascular and/or chronic tubulo-interstitial disease (10 -13).

References:

1. Cafruny EJ, Feinfeld DA, Schwartz GJ, Spitzer A. Effects of Drugs toxins, and heavy metals on the kidney. In pediatric Kidney Disease, Edlemann CM (Ed), Little Brown and Company, 1992:1707-1726.
2. Goyer RA. Toxic effects of metals. In Toxicology: The Basic Science of Poisons. Klaassen CD, Amdur MO, Doull J (Eds). New York, NY. Macmillan Publishing Company. 1986.582-635.
3. Hook JB, Hewitt WR. Toxic responses of the kidney. In The Basic Science of Poisons.. Klaassen CD, Amdur MO, Doull J (eds). New York, NY. Macmillan

Publishing Company 1986.310-329.

4. Hall CL. The natural course of gold and penicillamine nephropathy: a longterm study of 54 patients. Adv Exp Med Biol 1989; 252:247-256.
5. Watanabe I, Whittier FC, Moore J, Cuppage FE Gold nephropathy. Ultrastructural, fluorescence, and microanalytic studies of twopatients. Arch Pathol lab Med 1976;100(12):63-635
6. Alexander F, Martin J. Nephrotic syndrome associated with lithium therapy. 1981;15:267-271.
7. Gitlin M. Lithium and the kidney: an updated review. Drug Saf 1999;20(3): 231-243.
8. Tam VK, Green J. Schwieger J, Cohen AH. Nephrotic syndrome and renal insufficiency associated with lithium therapy. Am J Kidney Dis. 1996;27(5):715-720.
9. Choie DD, Longenecker DS, Del Campo AA. Acute and chronic cisplatin nephropathy in rats. Lab Invest 1981; 44:397-402.
10. Choie DD, Richter GW. Lead poisoning: Rapid formation of intranuclear inclusions. Science 1972;177: 1194
11. Goyer RA, Rhyne B. Pathological effect of lead. Int Rev Exp Pathol. 1973;12:1-77.
12. Goyer RA. Lead and the kidney. Curr Topic Pathol., 1971a; 55: 147-76.
13. Goyer RA and Wilson MH. Lead-induced inclusion bodies: results of EDTA treatment. Lab Invest. 1975; 32:149-156.

Metal Ions in Biology and Medicine; vol 6. Eds. J.A. Centeno, Ph. Collery, G. Vernet, R.B. Finkelman, H. Gibb, J.C. Etienne. John Libbey Eurotext, Paris © 2000, pp. 15-17.

Hepatotoxicity of metals

Kamal G. Ishak, M.D., Ph.D.

Armed Forces Institute of Pathology, Department of Hepatic and Gastrointestinal Pathology, Washington, DC, USA

Several metals can injure the liver, by far the most important being iron and copper. The diseases caused by metals may be genetic or acquired, and the effects can be acute or chronic. **Acute Metal Toxicity**: 1. *Hepatocellular Injury.* Ferrous sulfate poisoning in children can lead to coagulative degeneration in zone 1 of the hepatic acinus, and phosphorus poisoning induces lytic necrosis in that zone, as well as steatosis. Copper toxicity causes zone 3 necrosis. 2. *Cholestatic Injury.* Intrahepatic cholestasis has been reported with acute arsenical toxicity, and as an idiosyncratic reaction to the use of gold salts for treatment of rheumatoid arthritis. **Chronic Metal Toxicity**: 1. *Vascular Injury.* Hepatoportal sclerosis is a recognized complication of chronic arsenical toxicity, for example, from ingestion of high levels of As in drinking water (India, Bangladesh). 2. *Chronic Hepatitis.* A stage in the evolution of Wilson's disease. 3. *Fibrosis and Cirrhosis.* These occur in genetic hemochromatosis, Wilson's disease, Indian childhood cirrhosis, acquired Cu toxicosis, neonatal hemochromatosis and Subsaharan hemosiderosis. 4. *Granulomas.* Chronic beryllium toxicity ("berylliosis") in the past was associated with a sarcoidosis-like disease. Exposure of vineyard sprayers to copper sulfate has been reported to lead to granulomas in the lungs and liver. 5. *Malignant Tumors.* Hepatocellular carcinoma is a dreaded complication of genetic hemochromatosis and rarely, of Wilson's disease. Angiosarcoma has been reported after chronic exposure to As and rarely, to Fe or Cu.

Miscellaneous Effects: 1. Hepatic hemosiderosis has been reported after multiple transfusions, chronic hemodialysis, excess ingestion of iron preparations, and prolonged parenteral nutrition in children. 2. Hemosiderin accumulation in the liver in chronic hepatitis C may lead to a poor response to interferon therapy. 3. The presence of Fe in nonalcoholic steatohepatitis may contribute to the hepatic injury.

References

1. Pestaner JP, Ishak KG, Mullick FG, Centeno J. Ferrous sulfate toxicity. A review of autopsy findings. *Biol Trace Elem Res* 1999; 70: 1-8.

2. Chuttani HK, Gupta PS, Gulati S, Gupta DN. Acute copper sulfate poisoning. *Am J Med* 1965; 39:849-854.

3. Diaz-Rivera RS, Collazo PJ, Pons E, Torregrosa MV. Acute phosphorus poisoning in man: A study of 56 cases. *Medicine* 1950; 29:269-298.

4. Zimmerman HJ. Hepatotoxicity. The *adverse effects of drugs and other chemicals on the liver.* 2d Edition. Philadelphia: Lippincott-Williams and Wilkins, 1999.

5. Powell LW, Yapp TR. Hemochromatosis. *Cl Liver Dis* 2000; 4:211-228.

6. Mandishona E, MacPhail AP, Gordeuk VR, Kedda M-A, Paterson AC, Rouault TA, Kew MC. Dietary iron overload as a risk factor for hepatocellular carcinoma in Black Africans. *Hepatology* 1998; 27:1563-1566.

7. Sternlieb I. Wilson's disease. *Cl Liver Dis* 2000, 4:229-239.

8. Tanner S. Disorders of copper metabolism. In: Kelly DA, ed. *Diseases of the liver and biliary system in children.* Oxford: Blackwell Science, 1999: 167-185.

9. Müller T. Feichtinger H, Berger H, Müller W. Endemic Tyrolean infantile cirrhosis: an ecogenetic disorder. *Lancet* 1996; 347: 877-880.

10. Müller-Höcker J, Summer KH, Schramel P, Rodeck B. Different pathomorphologic patterns in exogenous infantile copper intoxication of the liver. *Pathol Res Pract* 1998; 194:377-384.

11. Datta DV, Mitra SK, Chhuttani PN, Chakravarti RN. Chronic oral arsenic intoxication as a possible aetiological factor in idiopathic portal hypertension (non-cirrhotic portal fibrosis) in India. *Gut* 1979; 20:378-384.

12. Roth F. The sequelae of chronic arsenic poisoning in Moselle vintners. *German Med Monthl* 1957; 2:172-175.

Table I
HEPATOTOXICITY OF METALS

Metal	Circumstances	Histopathology	Comments	References
		Acute Toxicity		
Iron	Accidental ingestion by children (usually FeS04)	Zone 1 necrosis	Also severe gastrointestinal injury	1
Copper	Suicidal or accidental	Zone 3 necrosis	Also cholestasis	2
Phosphorus	Suicidal or accidental ingestion of fire crackers, or roach poison	Zone 1 necrosis	Also steatosis	2
Gold	Gold salts used for therapy of rheumatoid arthritis	Intrahepatic cholestasis	Idiosyncratic drug reaction	4
		Chronic Toxicity		
Iron	Genetic hemochromatosis	Hepatic hemosiderosis, fibrosis, cirrhosis, HCC*	C282Y and H63D gene mutations	5
	Bantu or Subsaharan siderosis	Hepatic hemosiderosis + fibrosis or cirrhosis, HCC	Dietary iron overload and genetic factor	6
Copper	Wilson's disease	Cu overload, chronic hepatitis, cirrhosis, fulminant liver failure with necrosis, HCC* (rare)	ATP7B gene mutations	7
	Indian childhood cirrhosis	Cu overload, Mallory body fibrosis, cirrhosis	Excess ingestion of Cu in milk leached from Cu or brass containers	8
	Tyrolean infantile cirrhosis	Cu overload, cirrhosis	Excess ingestion of Cu in milk leached from Cu containers	9
	Hepatic copper toxicosis	Cu overload, Mallory bodies, cirrhosis	Increased ingestion of Cu in drinking water, or idiopathic	10
Arcenic	Excess ingestion of As in drinking water, drugs or exposure to insecticides	Hepatoportal sclerosis, angiosarcoma		11,12

*HCC=Hepatocellular carcinoma

Metal Ions in Biology and Medicine; vol 6. Eds. J.A. Centeno, Ph. Collery, G. Vernet, R.B. Finkelman, H. Gibb, J.C. Etienne. John Libbey Eurotext, Paris © 2000, pp. 18-20.

Toxicity evaluation of arsenic trioxide, and atrazine to three developmental stages of Japanese medaka *(Oryzias latipes)*

P.B. Tchounwou, B. Wilson, A. Ishaque, and D. Sutton

Environmental Toxicology Research Laboratory, NIH-Center for Environmental Health, School of Science and Technology, Jackson State University, Jackson, MS 39217, USA

Abstract: The Japanese medaka fish (*Oryzias latipes*) has been recommended as a model test organism (system) for screening toxicity and carcinogenicity of chemicals, since toxic morphologic and neoplastic changes in this species develop rapidly following administration of relatively small quantities of test materials. In this research, we investigated the acute toxicity of arsenic and atrazine, singly and in combination, to Japanese medaka embryos, fry and adult fish. Ninety-six hours static renewal bioassays were carried out during which 2-3 days old embryos, 2-days old fry, and 2-months old adults were exposed to serial concentrations of arsenic and atrazine. Dimethylsulfoxide-DMSO (2%) was used as a co-solvent for solubilizing atrazine. In the test with chemical mixture a single concentration of atrazine (100 mg/L) was used as solvent to prepare serial concentrations of arsenic. Study results indicated a concentration-response relationship with respect to chemical toxicity. Upon 96 hours of exposure of eggs, arsenic concentrations of 0.08 (0.05 - 0.09) mg/L, 0.15 (0.10-0.18) mg/L, and 0.23 (0.21 - 0.26) mg/L were recorded for NOAEL, LOAEL, and LC_{50}, respectively. No significant difference was found in LC_{50} values between 24 and 96 hours of exposure, indicating that arsenic is a fast acting chemical, with most acute poisoning occurring within 24 hours of exposure. Tests with the fry and adults pointed out a higher tolerance of these stages to arsenic toxicity. On the other hand, atrazine was found to be non toxic to eggs within the range of concentrations tested even at its maximum solubility of 200 mg/L in 2%DMSO. However, results of tests with fry and adults indicated that these developmental stages were more sensitive to atrazine toxicity than the eggs. The mixture of arsenic with 100 mg/L atrazine resulted in 96 hrs-LC_{50} of 0.28 (0.26-0.31) mg/L for the eggs. This LC_{50} was slightly higher than that obtained for arsenic alone (0.23 mg/L), but not statistically significant; indicating a combined toxic effect that is simply additive or slightly antagonistic.

Introduction: Arsenic is the 20th most abundant element in the earth's crust. It is released to the environment from natural sources as a result of natural phenomena such as erosion of mineral deposits and volcanoes, but releases from human activities such as metal melting, coal combustion, chemical production and use, and waste disposal can lead to substantial contamination of the environment. Natural levels of arsenic in soil usually range from 1 to 40 mg/kg, but pesticide application or waste disposal can produce much higher values. In recent years, arsenic contamination of natural resources has emerged as one of the major public health concerns in several countries of the world. A very large number of people are exposed to arsenic chronically throughout the world. This exposure has lead to a significant number of health concerns including hyperkeratosis, jaundice, vascular diseases, and cancer of various organs/tissues including the skin, the liver, the lung and the bladder [1-2]. Arsenic is a known human carcinogen. Its maximum contaminant level (MCL) in drinking water is 50 ppb [3]. Transport and partitioning of arsenic in water depends upon the chemical form of arsenic and on interactions with other materials present. In a contaminated river, sediments can contain substantial amounts of arsenic that are predominantly mobile during water-sediments interactions. Factors influencing the fate of arsenicals in water include the oxido-reduction potential, pH, metal sulfide and sulfide ion concentration, iron concentrations, temperature, salinity, distribution and composition of the biota . Bioconcentration of arsenic occurs in aquatic organisms, primarily algae and lower invertebrates [4].

Atrazine,on the other hand, is one of the most heavily used herbicides in Mississippi, and the United States. It has been widely used on corn and sorghum, especially in the Delta area where most of the agricultural activities are performed. Atrazine is slightly to moderately toxic to humans and other animals. It can be absorbed into the blood stream through oral, dermal, and inhalation exposure. Symptoms of poisoning include: abdominal pain, diarrhea, eye irritation, , irritation of mucuous membranes [5]. At high doses, excitation followed by depression, bradycardia, incoordination, muscle spasms, and hypothermia, as well as muscular weakness, hypoactivity, prostration, convulsion, and death have been observed in studies with laboratory animals [6]. Atrazine is considered as a possible human carcinogen based on the evidence of induction of mammary gland tumors in laboratory animals. The recommended MCL for this compound in drinking water is 3 ppb [6].

Although the effects of arsenic and atrazine on target organisms are well documented, little is known about their effects on non target organisms. Inadvertent contamination of water resources by these chemicals could result in massive destruction of fish populations and other aquatic organisms found in Mississippi wetlands. Using the Japanese medaka fish as a model test organism, this study was designed to investigate the acute toxicity of arsenic and atrazine, singly and in combination.

Experimental Design and Methods: The Japanese medaka (*Oryzias latipes*) fish used in this research were obtained from the Gulf Coast Research Laboratory in Ocean Springs, Mississippi. Ninety-six hours static renewal bioassays were carried out during which 2-3 days old embryos, 2-days old fry, and 2-months old adults were exposed to serial concentrations of arsenic and atrazine. Dimethylsulfoxide-DMSO (2%) was used as a co-solvent for solubilizing atrazine. All bioassays were carried out following standard test protocols [7,8]. In the experiments with chemical mixture using the eggs as test organisms, a single concentration of atrazine (100 mg/L) was used as solvent to prepare serial concentrations of arsenic. For the adult fish, the mixture of arsenic and atrazine was made based on individual LC_{50}s, and the test protocol described by Marking [9] was followed.

Results and Discussion: Study results indicated a concentration-response relationship with respect to chemical toxicity. Upon 96 hours of exposure of eggs, arsenic concentrations of 0.08 (0.05 - 0.09) mg/L, 0.15 (0.10-0.18) mg/L, and 0.23 (0.21 - 0.26) mg/L were recorded for NOAEL, LOAEL, and LC_{50}, respectively. No significant difference ($p > 0.05$) was found in LC_{50} values between 24 and 96 hours of exposure, indicating that arsenic is a fast acting chemical, with most acute poisoning occurring within 24 hours of exposure. Tests with the fry and adults pointed out a higher tolerance of these stages to arsenic toxicity, with 96 hrs-LC_{50}s recorded as 0.37 mg/L (fry), and 0.57 mg/L (adult). In a study of the effects of various metals on *Daphnia magna*, Biesinger and Christensen [10] reported that arsenic in the form of arsenate (As^{+5}) adversely affects the survival, growth, reproduction, and metabolism of this organism. It has also been reported that the mechanism by which arsenic exerts its toxic effect is through impairment of cellular respiration by the inhibition of various mitochondrial enzymes, and the uncoupling of oxidative phosphorylation. Arsenic *in vitro* reacts with protein SH groups to inactivate enzymes such as dihydrolipoyl dehydrogenase and thiolase producing inhibited oxidation of pyruvate and betaoxidation of fatty acids [11].

In the present study, atrazine was found to be non toxic to the Japanese medaka eggs within the range of concentrations tested even at its maximum solubility of 200 mg/L in 2%DMSO. However, results of tests with fry and adults yielded a 96 hrs-LC_{50} of about 25-30 mg/L, indicating that these developmental stages were more sensitive to atrazine toxicity than the eggs. Previous studies on the adverse effects of atrazine indicated that this herbicide is acutely toxic to a significant number of freshwater organisms including phytoplancton, macrophytes, benthic organisms, zooplankton, and fish [121. The degree of toxicity depends on several factors including the toxic endpoint, the duration of exposure, and the biological species involved. In general phytoplancton have been reported to be most sensitive to atrazine toxicity, followed, in decreasing order of sensitivity, by macrophytes, benthic invertebrates, zooplancton, and fish [12].

The mixture of arsenic with 100 mg/L atrazine resulted in 96 hrs-LC_{50} of 0.28 (0.26-0.31) mg/L for the eggs. This LC_{50} was slightly higher than that obtained for arsenic alone (0.23 mg/L), but not statistically significant; indicating a combined toxic effect that is simply additive or slightly antagonistic. Also, the data obtained from bioassays assessing the combined effect of arsenic and atrazine on the adult fish lead to a similar conclusion. Based on the Marking's method of assessment [9], a negative value of additive index was correlated with the sum of toxic action, indicating a reduction in toxicity resulting from the mixture of arsenic and atrazine. These results are in agreement with findings from some studies suggesting that the toxicity of many pesticide mixtures to freshwater organisms is rarely greater than additive [13-15].

Acknowledgments: This research was financially supported by a grant from the National Institutes of Health (No. 1G12RR13459). Additional support during manuscript preparation was provided by a grant from the U.S. Department of Education (Title III Program-Grant No. PO31B440000-98) to Jackson State University.

References:

[1] Tseng WP, Chu HM, How SW, Fong JM, Lin CS, Yeh S. Prevalence of skin cancer in an endemic area of chronic arsenicism in Taiwan. *J Natl Cancer Inst* 1968; 40 : 453 - 463.

[2] Chen CJ, Chen CW, Wu MM, Kuo T-L. Cancer potential in liver lung, bladder and kidney due to ingested inorganic arsenic in drinking water. *Br J Cancer* 1992; 66:888-892.

[3] Tchounwou PB, Wilson B, Ishaque A. Important considerations in the development of public health advisories for arsenic and arsenic-containing compounds in drinking water. *Rev Environ Hlth* 1999; 24 (4) : 1 - 19.

[4] Callahan MA, Slimak MW, Gabel NW. Water-related environmental fate of 129 priority pollutions. Vol. I. Introduction and Technical Background, Metals and Inorganics, Pesticides and PCBs. Report to the U.S. EPA. EPA-440/4-79-029a. EPA Office of Water Planning and Standard. Washington DC, 1979.

[5] Hallenbeck WH, Cummingham B. Pesticides and Human Health. New York, NY. Springer Verlag. 1985.

[6] U.S. EPA. Atrazine Health Advisory. Office of Drinking Water. United States Environmental Protection Agency. Washington DC. 1988.

[7] Johnson WW, Finley MT. Handbook of Acute Toxicity of Chemicals to Fish and Aquatic Invertebrates. Resource Publication No. 137. Wildlife and Fisheries Services. U.S. Department of the Interior. 1980.

[8] Helmstetter MF, Maccubbin AE, Alden RW. The medaka embryo-larval assay: an in vivo assay for toxicity, teratogenicity, and carcinogenicity. In: Ostrander GK ed. Techniques in Aquatic Toxicology. Boca Raton, FL. Lewis Publishers. 1996; 93 - 124.

[9] Marking LL. Method for assessing additive toxicity of chemical mixtures. In: Mayer FL, Hamelink JL, eds. *Aquatic Toxicology and Hazard Evaluation*. Philadephia, PA. American Society for Testing and Materials. 1980; 99 - 108.

[10] Biesinger KE, Christensen GM. Effects of various metals on survival, growth, reproduction, and metabolism of Daphnia magna. *J Fish Res Board Can* 1972; 29 : 1691 - 1700.

[11] Belton JC, Benson NC, Hanna ML, Taylor RT. Growth inhibition and cytotoxic effects of three arsenic compounds on cultured Chinese hamster ovary cells. *J Environ Sci Hlth* 1985; 20A:37-72.

[12] Solomon KR, Baker DB, Richards RP, Dixon KR, Klaine SJ, LaPoint TW, Kendall RJ, Weisskopf CP, Giddings JM, Giesy JP, Hall LW, Williams WM. Ecological risk assessment of atrazine in north american surface waters. *Environ Toxicol Chem* 1996; 15 (1) : 31 -76.

[13] Marking LL, Maulk WL. Toxicity of paired mixtures of candidate forest insecticides to rainbow trout. *Bull Environ Contam Toxicol* 1975; 13 : 518 - 523.

[14] Marking LL. Toxicity of chemical mixtures. In: Rand G, Petrocelli S., eds. *Fundamentals of Aquatic Toxicology*. Washington DC. Hemisphere Publishing Corporation. 1985; 164 - 176.

[15] Abdelghani AA, Tchounwou PB, Anderson AC, Sujono H, Heyer LR, Monkiedje A. Toxicity evaluation of single and chemical mixtures of roundup, garlon-3A, 2,4-D, and Syndets surfactant to channel catfish (*Ictalurus punctatus*), bluegill sunfish (*Lepomis microchirus*), and crawfish (*Procambarus spp.*). *Environ Toxicol Water Qual* 1997; 12 : 237 - 243.

Metal Ions in Biology and Medicine; vol 6. Eds. J.A. Centeno, Ph. Collery, G. Vernet, R.B. Finkelman, H. Gibb, J.C. Etienne. John Libbey Eurotext, Paris © 2000, pp. 21-23.

Health risk assessment and management of arsenic, and other toxic and hazardous metals in drinking water

Paul B. Tchounwou

Environmental Toxicology Research Laboratory, NIH-Center for Environmental Health, School of Science and Technology, Jackson State University, Jackson, MS 39217, USA

Abstract: The National Academy of Sciences (NAS) defines *risk assessment* as the "determination of the probability that an adverse effect will result from a defined exposure". The four major components of the risk assessment framework as recommended by the U.S. Environmental Protection Agency include: *hazard identification*-a process of characterizing the innate toxic effects of a given agent; *dose-response assessment*-a process of characterizing the relationship between the dose and the incidence of adverse effects; *exposure assessment*-a process of estimating the intensity, frequency, and duration of human exposure to the agent; and *risk characterization*-a process of estimating the incidence of health effects under the various conditions of human exposure. *Risk management,* on the other hand, is defined by the NAS as the "process of weighing policy alternatives and selecting the most appropriate regulatory action based on the results of risk assessment and social, economic, and political concerns". In this paper, the author applied these risk assessment and management principles to address important health issues associated with drinking water pollution by toxic and hazardous metals. A special emphasis is put on the arsenic contamination; a major public health problem in several countries around the world. Arsenic is in effect, a systemic toxicant exerting a high degree of toxicity to humans. Recent epidemiologic studies have demonstrated a strong correlation between arsenic exposure and an increase in the incidence of human cancers including skin, and lung neoplasms. A significant number of mutagenic, teratogenic, and reproductive health effects have also been reported with arsenic poisoning.

Introduction: Metals are released to the environment from natural sources as a result of natural phenomena such as erosion of mineral deposits and volcanoes, but releases from human activities such as metal smelting, coal combustion, chemical production and use, and waste disposal can lead to substantial contamination of the environment. The pervasive occurrence of metals as contaminants in drinking water and the great potential for adverse health effects associated with human consumption of contaminated water, have become a major issue facing society, and involving enormous financial and societal implications. In recent years, arsenic contamination of natural resources (ground water) has emerged as one of the major public health concerns in several countries of the world. Outbreaks of arsenosis and other health effects associated with ground water contamination in Argentina, Bangaldesh, Chili, China, Mexico, India, Thailand, and Taiwan are examples of such concerns [1]. As with many other water contaminants, the development of a comprehensive risk assessment (RA) and risk management (RM) protocol for arsenic in drinking water requires a thorough understanding of the four components of the RA paradigm, and an evaluation of RM options related to arsenic contamination [2].

Hazard Identification: There are many case reports of death in humans due to ingestion of high doses of arsenic. The clinical manifestations of arsenic poisoning depend on the type of arsenical involved and on the duration of exposure. Symptoms of acute intoxication usually occur within 30 minutes of ingestion but may be delayed if arsenic is taken with food. In nearly all cases, the most immediate effects are severe nausea and vomiting, colicky abdominal pain, profuse diarrhea with rice stools, gastrointestinal hemorrhage and death may ensue from fluid loss and circulatory collapse. Drowsiness and confusion are often seen along the development of psychosis associated with paranoid delusions, hallucinations and delirium. Finally, seizures, coma and death, usually due to shock, may ensue [3]. Cardiac manifestations include acute cardiomyopathy, subendocardial hemorrhages, and electro cardiographic changes. The pathological lesions described in patients with rapidly fatal arsenic intoxication are fatty degeneration of the liver, hyperemia and hemorrhages of the gastrointestinal tract, renal tubular necrosis, and demyelination of peripheral nerves

[3].Chronic exposure to arsenic affects the gastrointestinal tract, circulatory system, skin, liver kidneys, nervous system and heart. There is clear evidence from epidemiological studies that exposure to inorganic arsenic increases the risk of cancer [4]. When exposure occurs by the oral route, the main carcinogenic effect is increased risk of skin cancer. In addition to skin cancer, increased risk of other internal tumors (mainly of liver, kidney, lung, and bladder) have been reported with arsenic exposure [5,6]. Although, the clinical manifestations of arsenic poisoning appear similar, the toxicity of arsenic compounds depends largely on the chemical species and the form of arsenic involved. Most cases of human toxicity from arsenic have been associated with exposure to inorganic arsenic. Experimentally, arsenicals are fetotoxic and teratogenic in laboratory animals. There are also several epidemiological studies reporting an association between exposure to inorganic arsenic and increased risk of adverse developmental effects such as congenital malformations, low birth weight, and spontaneous abortion. *In vitro* experiments with many arsenicals show that they are powerful clastogens in many cell types. Tests for genotoxicity have indicated that arsenic compounds inhibit DNA repair, and induce chromosomal aberrations, and sister chromatid exchanges [7].

Dose-Response Assessment: It has been demonstrated that the risk of arsenic intoxication increases as a function of exposure level and duration [8]. The National Research Council of Canada reported that 9, 16 and 44% incidence of symptoms of arsenic poisoning are observed at drinking water arsenic concentrations of 50, 50-100, and >100 ug/L, respectively [9]. The frequencies of skin cancer associated with arsenic-contaminated water have been reported by the U.S. EPA as 0.26% and 2.14% at 290 and 600 ug/L, respectively. Also, cancer risks of 10^{-5}, 10^{-6}, and 10^{-7} have been estimated for drinking water containing 0.022, 0.0022, and 0.00022 ug As/L, or for eating aquatic organisms living in contaminated water containing 0.175, 0.0175, and 0.00175 ug As/L [10].

Exposure Assessment: A very large number of people are exposed to arsenic chronically throughout the world. This exposure has lead to a significant number of health concerns including hyperkeratosis, jaundice, vascular diseases, and cancer of various organs/tissues including the skin, the liver, the lung and the bladder [4,5,6]. For most people, the diet is the largest source of arsenic exposure, with an average intake of about 50 ug per day. Intake from air, water and soil are usually much smaller, but exposure from these media may become significant in areas of arsenic contamination. People who produce or use arsenic compounds in occupations such as non-ferrous metal smelting, pesticide manufacturing and application, wood preservation, semiconductor manufacturing, or glass production can be exposed by substantially higher levels of arsenic [7].

Risk Characterization: A review of biological properties and toxic effects of arsenic indicates that this chemical is a systemic toxicant capable of causing a significant number of health effects including: cardiovascular disease, peripheral vascular disease, developmental effects, neurologic and neurobehavioral effects, diabetes, hearing loss, portal fibrosis of the liver, lung fibrosis, hematologic effects (anemia, leukopenia, and eosinophilia), and carcinogenic effects [1]. The oral reference dose (RfD) is $3x10^{-4}$ mg/kg/day, and the cancer potency factor is 1.75 $(mg/kg/day)^{-1}$ [11].The International Agency for Research on Cancer, and the U.S. EPA classify arsenic in Group 1/A-known human carcinogens[11,12]. Studies in Taiwan have also pointed out that in areas where blackfoot disease is endemic, the standardized and cumulative mortality rates were significantly higher for cancer of the bladder, kidney, skin, liver, lung and colon [13].

Risk Management: Because of its high potential to cause adverse effects in exposed persons, a number of regulations and guidelines have been established for various inorganic and organic forms of arsenic by international, federal, and state agencies. The permissible limit for arsenic in drinking water (maximum contaminant level - MCL) has been fixed at 50 ug/L [14,15]. The World Health Organization's tolerable daily intake for inorganic arsenic is 2 ug/kg BW. The action level for arsenic in the air is 5 ug/m^3. The permissible exposure limit-total weighted average (PEL - TWA) is 10 ug/m^3 for inorganic arsenicals, and

500 ug/m^3 for organic arsenicals [16]. British Anti-Lewisite (BAL or 2,3-Dimercaptopropanol) has been used to treat acute dermatitis, and the pulmonary symptoms associated with arsenic exposure. However, because of the side effects associated with BAL, other agents such as DMPS and DMSA are being tested for the chelation therapy of arsenic poisoning [17]. Removal of arsenic by appropriate technologies is one of the most important control and management strategies. Several treatment methods including chemical precipitation (coagulation processes), ion exchange, reverse osmosis/electrodialysis, use of activated alumina or carbon, and oxidation, have therefore been recommended for arsenic removal in water [18,19].

Acknowledgments: This research was financially supported by a grant from the National Institutes of Health (No. 1G12RR13459). The author thanks Dr. A. Mohamed for his technical advise on this project.

References:

[1] Tchounwou PB, Wilson B, Ishaque A. Important considerations in the development of public health advisories for arsenic and arsenic-containing compounds in drinking water. *Rev Environ Hlth* 1999; 14 : 1-19.

[2] NAS. Risk assessment in the federal government: Managing the process. National Academy of Science. Washington DC. 1983.

[3] Gorby MS. Arsenic in human medicine. In: Nriagu JO, ed. *Arsenic in the Environment; Part II: Human Health and Ecosystem Effects*. New York, NY: John Wiley & Sons, Inc., 1994; 1-16.

[4] Tseng WP, Chu HM, How SW, Fong JM., Lin CS, Yeh S. Prevalence of skin Cancer in an endemic area of chronic arsenicism in Taiwan. *J Natl Cancer Inst* 1968; 40 : 453-463.

[5] Hopenhayn- Rich C, Biggs ML, Fuchs A, Bergoglio R, Tello EE, Nicolli H, Smith AH. Bladder cancer mortality associated with arsenic in drinking water in Argentina. *Epidemiol* 1996; 7:117-124.

[6] Chen CJ, Chen CW, Wu MM, Kuo T-L. Cancer potential in liver lung, bladder and kidney due to ingested inorganic arsenic in drinking water. *Br J Cancer* 1992; 66 : 888-892.

[7] ASTDR. Toxicological Profile for Arsenic TP-92/09. Agency for Toxic Substances and Disease Registry. Center for Disease Control, Atlanta, GA, 1993.

[8] Wu MM, Kuo TL, Hwang YH. Dose-response relation between arsenic concentration in well water and mortality from cancers and vascular diseases. *Am J Epidemol* 1989; 130 : 1123-1132.

[9] NRCC. Effects of arsenic in the environment. National Research Council of Canada. *Natl Res Counc Can Publ* 1978; 1-349.

[10] U.S. EPA 1980. Ambient Water Quality Criteria for Arsenic. EPA 400/5-80-021. Environmental Protection Agency. Washington DC. 1980.

[11] IRIS. Integrated Risk Information System. U.S. EPA. Washington, DC, 1992.

[12] IARC. Monographs on the Evaluation of Carcinogenic Risks of Chemicals to Humans. Supplement F. Overall Evaluation of Carcinogenicity. International Agency for Research on Cancer. World Health Organization. Lyon, France, 1987; 29-57.

[13] Chen CJ, Chuang YC, Lin TM, Wu HY. Malignant neoplasms among residents of a blackfoot disease endemic area in Taiwan: High-arsenic artesian well water and cancers. *Cancer Res* 1985; 45 : 5895-5899.

[14] U.S. EPA. National primary drinking water regulations. *Fed Regist* 1985; 50 : 46931-47022.

[15] WHO. Guidelines for Drinking Water Quality. World Health Organization, Geneva, SZD, 1984.

[16] OSHA. Occupational Safety and Health Administration. *Fed Reg* 1989; 54 : 2332-2335.

[17] Goyer RA. Toxic effects of metals. In: Klaassen CD ed., *Cassarett & Doull's Toxicology-The Basic Science of Poisons*. New York, NY: McGraw Hill, 1996; 691-736.

[18] U.S. EPA. Research Plan for Arsenic in Drinking Water. EPA/600/98/042. Office of Research and Development. National Center for Environmental Assessment. Cincinnati, OH.1998.

[19] Jekel MR. Removal of arsenic in drinking water treatment. In Nriagu JO ed. *Arsenic in the Environment, Part I: Cycling and Characterization.* New York, NY: John Wiley & Sons, Inc. 1994; 119-132.

Metal Ions in Biology and Medicine; vol 6. Eds. J.A. Centeno, Ph. Collery, G. Vernet, R.B. Finkelman, H. Gibb, J.C. Etienne. John Libbey Eurotext, Paris © 2000, pp. 25-27.

Cancer incidence and arsenic exposure among residents of Lanyang Basin in Taiwan

Hung-Yi Chiou[a], Yi-Li Chou[a], Hee-Wen Teh[a], Chin-Hsiao Tseng[b], Chien-Jen Chen[c]

[a] *School of Public Health, Taipei Medical College, Taipei, Taiwan;* [b] *Department of Internal Medicine, National Taiwan University Hospital, Taipei, Taiwan;* [c] *Graduate Institute of Epidemiology, College of Public Health, National Taiwan University, Taipei, Taiwan*

Significant dose-response relations between ingested inorganic arsenic and risk of various internal cancers have been reported in our previous studies on residents in southwestern arseniasis-endemic area in Taiwan (1-3), where many households shared few wells in their villages. The arsenic exposure in previous studies was based on the median arsenic concentration in well water of study villages rather than the arsenic concentration in well water of each household. In a newly-identified northeastern arseniasis-endemic area in Taiwan where each household has its own well to supply drinking water (4), we studied cancer risk related to ingested inorganic arsenic measured in a more precise way among a cohort of 8102 residents. Individual exposure to inorganic arsenic of study subjects was based on arsenic concentration in water of their own wells which was determined by hydride generation combined with atomic absorption spectrometry. A standardized interview was used to obtain information on various cancer risk factors including history of cigarette smoking and alcohol drinking. The development of cancers was ascertained by follow-up interview and data linkage with national death certification and cancer registry profiles. Cox's proportional hazards regression analysis was used to estimate the multivariate-adjusted relative risk and its 95% confidence interval (5).

There were 276 residents affected with newly-diagnosed cancer during the five-year follow-up period. Table 1 shows the risk of developing cancers of the all sites combined, nasopharynx, stomach, small intestine, colon and rectum, liver, gallbladder, nasal cavities, lung, female breast, ovary and cervix uteri, and urinary organs among residents were significantly higher than those in the general population in Taiwan. As shown in table 2-4 there was a statistically significant higher risk for development cancers of the all sites combined, lung and urinary organs among residents who drinking well water contained arsenic concentration greater than 100 ug/L after adjustment for age, sex, and cigarette smoking. Compared with residents whose cumulative arsenic exposure was less than 0.1 mg/L * year as the referent group (RR=1.0), a statistically significant higher risk on development of these three cancers was also observed for resident who had long-term arsenic exposure more than 5 mg/L * year after adjustment for age, sex, and cigarette smoking. The biological gradient was even more prominent between cumulative arsenic exposure and cancer risks of lung and urinary organs.

References

1.Chen CJ, Chuang YC, Lin TM, et al. Malignant neoplasms among residents of a blackfoot disease endemic area in Taiwan: high arsenic artesian well water and cancers. Cancer Res 1985;45: 5895-5899.
2.Chen CJ, Wu MM, Kuo, TL. Arsenic and cancers. Lancet, 20: 414-415, 1988.
3.Chiou HY, Hsueh YM, Liaw KF, et al. Incidence of internal cancers and ingested inorganic arsenic: a seven-year follow-up study in Taiwan. Cancer Res 1995;55: 1296-1300.
4. Chiou HY, Huang WI, Su CL, et al. Dose-response relationship between prevalence of cerebrovascular disease and ingested inorganic arsenic. Stroke 1997;28: 1717-1723.
5. Cox DR. Regression models and life tables. J R Stat Soc 1972;34: 187-220.

Table1.Standardized incidence ratio (SIR) with their 95% confidence interval (CI) for various cancers among residents of the arseniasis-endemic area in northeastern Taiwan

Cancer site (ICD-9)	Obs.	SIR	(95% CI)
All sites combined (140~208)	276	200.6	(177.9-226.2)*
Nasopharynx (147)	11	335.7	(167.5-636.7)*
Stomach (151)	44	321.7	(273.1-378.8)*
Small intestine (152)	3	497.7	(102.5-1453.2)*
Colon and rectum (153,154)	37	189.9	(133.9-261.0)*
Liver (155)	29	151.3	(101.4-217.9)*
Gallbladder (156)	6	318.8	(117.0-695.0)*
Nasal cavities (160)	3	492.8	(101.52-1439.1)*
Lung (162)	52	241.3	(179.0-318.5)*
Female breast, overy and cervix uteri (174,180,183)	47	251.7	(183.5-337.3)*
Urinary organs (188,189)	19	216.6	(130.4-337.9)*

*p<0.05

Table 2. Multivariate-adjusted relative risk (RR) and 95% confidence interval (CI) of developing all cancer sites combined among 8102 residents of the arseniasis-endemic area in northeastern Taiwan

		Model I	Model II
Variable	Group	RR (95% C.I.)	RR (95% C.I.)
Age	every one year increment	1.1 (1.0-1.1)***	1.1(1.0-1.1)***
Sex	Female	1.0	1.0
	Male	1.0 (0.7-1.6)	1.1 (0.7-1.6)
Cigarette smoking	No	1.0	1.0
	Yes	1.6 (1.0-2.4)*	1.5 (1.0-2.2)*
Content of arsenic in well water (μ g/L)	0-10.0	1.0	
	10.1-50.0	1.1 (0.8-1.5)	
	50.1-100.0	0.9 (0.6-1.5)	
	>100.0	1.4 (1.0-1.9)[§]	

Cumulative arsenic exposure (mg/L*year)	<0.1		1.0
	0.1-0.9		1.4 (1.0-1.9)[§]
	1.0-4.9		1.2 (0.8-1.6)
	≧5.0		1.7 (1.2-2.5)**

[§] 0.05<p<0.1, * 0.01<p<0.05, ** 0.001<p<0.01, *** p<0.001

Table 3. Multivariate-adjusted relative risk (RR) and 95% confidence interval (CI) of developing lung cancer among 8102 residents of the arseniasis-endemic area in northeastern Taiwan

		Model I	Model II
Variable	Group	RR (95% C.I.)	RR (95% C.I.)
Age	every one year increment	1.1 (1.0-1.1)***	1.1 (1.0-1.1)***
Sex	Female	1.0	1.0
	Male	1.5 (0.5-4.7)	1.4 (0.5-4.0)
Cigarette smoking	No	1.0	1.0
	Yes	3.9 (1.3-12.0)*	3.7 (1.3-10.3)*
Content of arsenic in well water (μg/L)	0-10.0	1.0	
	10.1-50.0	1.1 (0.5-2.5)	
	50.1-100.0	0.6 (0.2-2.2)	
	>100.0	2.5 (1.2-5.1)*	
Cumulative arsenic exposure (mg/L*year)	<0.1		1.0
	0.1-0.9		1.1 (0.5-2.5)
	1.0-4.9		1.1 (0.5-2.3)
	≧5.0		2.6 (1.2-5.5)*

[§] 0.05<p<0.1, * 0.01<p<0.05, ** 0.001<p<0.01, *** p<0.001

Table 4. Multivariate-adjusted relative risk (RR) and 95% confidence interval (CI) of developing urinary cancers among 8102 residents of the arseniasis-endemic area in northeastern Taiwan

		Model I	Model II
Variable	Group	RR (95% C.I.)	RR (95% C.I.)
Age	every one year increment	1.1 (1.0-1.1)*	1.1 (1.0-1.1)*
Sex	Female	1.0	1.0
	Male	0.4 (0.1-2.4)	0.4 (0.1-2.0)
Cigarette smoking	No	1.0	1.0
	Yes	11.3 (1.7-74.9)*	7.4 (1.4-38.1)*
Content of arsenic in well water (μg/L)	0-10.0	1.0[+]	
	10.1-50.0	1.5 (0.3-8.0)	
	50.1-100.0	2.2 (0.4-13.7)	
	>100.0	4.8 (1.2-19.4)*	
Cumulative arsenic exposure (mg/L*year)	<0.1		1.0
	0.1-0.9		2.8 (0.5-15.6)
	1.0-4.9		2.7 (0.5-14.4)
	≧5.0		8.0 (1.6-39.9)*

[§] 0.05<p<0.1, * 0.01<p<0.05, ** 0.001<p<0.01, *** p<0.001

Metal Ions in Biology and Medicine; vol 6. Eds. J.A. Centeno, Ph. Collery, G. Vernet, R.B. Finkelman, H. Gibb, J.C. Etienne. John Libbey Eurotext, Paris © 2000, pp. 28-30.

Designing an arsenic bladder cancer case-control study: what sample size is needed to detect the beginning of a dose response?

Tor D. Tosteson, Margaret R. Karagas

Dartmouth Medical School, 7927 Rubin, One Medical Center Drive, Lebanon NH/USA 03756; tor.tosteson@dartmouth.edu

1) Background: The rationale for studying the cancer dose-response for arsenic differs somewhat from the typical epidemiologic project in that the human carcinogenic potential of arsenic has already been well established in the scientific literature. The case-control studies conducted by the Dartmouth Superfund Program (Karagas et al., 1998) are unique in that they examine the lower range of exposures of currently of greatest regulatory and scientific interest. Arsenic exposure is measured with individual toenail and tap water concentrations. The generally low to moderate water concentrations (0.01-100 ug/L) allow dose response to be studied without resorting to low-dose extrapolations based on unverifiable assumptions about the shape of the dose-response curve.

2) Aims: A statistical method for determining the proper sample size to detect the beginning of the human bladder cancer dose response was devised and applied to the design of a continuing study of bladder cancer in the state of New Hampshire, USA.

3) Methods: Two-segmented logistic regression models provide a convenient way to formalize the statistical problem. They are comprised of two log-linear dose response curves for the odds of bladder cancer incidence joined at a "changepoint". Previously published data from the study of other cancers suggest that the dose-response may be relatively flat until roughly the 75th percentile of the New Hampshire exposure distribution. After that point, these data suggest the possibility of a moderate dose response for the skin cancer.

In preparation for planning the new study, sample size/power calculations were derived based on estimates both for the dose at which a changepoint occurs and for the slope of the linear dose response after the changepoint, expressed as an odds ratio for a logistic regression with a log-transformed exposure variable. Seber and Wild (1989, page 451) give the asymptotic variance of the least squared estimate for the cutpoint α in a two-segmented linear regression model,

$$E(y \mid x) = \beta_1 \text{ if } x < \alpha \text{ and } E(y \mid x) = \beta_1 + \beta_2 (x - \alpha) \text{ if } x > \alpha.$$

After modifying the Seber and Wild variance formula to approximate the variance function for a logistic regression, expressions for the variance of the regression parameters and the cutpoint are obtained as

$$\mathrm{var}(\hat{\beta}_2) = [\pi(1-\pi)n_{x>\alpha}\sigma^2_{x>\alpha}]^{-1}$$

and

$$\begin{aligned}\mathrm{var}(\hat{\beta}_2) = [\pi(1-\pi)\beta_2{}^2]^{-1}\{&E(x^2 \mid x<\alpha)/(n_{x<\alpha}\sigma^2_{x<\alpha}) + E(x^2 \mid x>\alpha)/(n_{x>\alpha}\sigma^2_{x>\alpha}) \\ &+ 2\alpha(E(x \mid x<\alpha)/(n_{x<\alpha}\sigma^2_{x<\alpha}) + E(x \mid x>\alpha)/(n_{x>\alpha}\sigma^2_{x>\alpha})) \\ &+\alpha^2(1/(n_{x<\alpha}\sigma^2_{x<\alpha}) + 1/(n_{x>\alpha}\sigma^2_{x>\alpha}))\}\end{aligned}$$

where $n_{x>\alpha}$ is the number of cases and controls with exposures greater than α; $E(x \mid x<\alpha), E(x^2 \mid x>\alpha)$, and $\sigma^2_{x>\alpha}$ are the mean, mean square, and variance of exposures among cases and controls with exposures greater than α; and π is the proportion of cases in the sample.

The variance expressions above can be used to calculate minimum detectable relative risks for a given change point from a flat to a positively increasing dose response. Also, the *maximum* detectable changepoint for given relative risks parameters can be calculated based on the power of a statistical test for a given null hypothesis changepoint. The figure below illustrates the latter calculation assuming that the relative risk parameter for a 50% increase in toenail concentration is 1.5 after the changepoint.

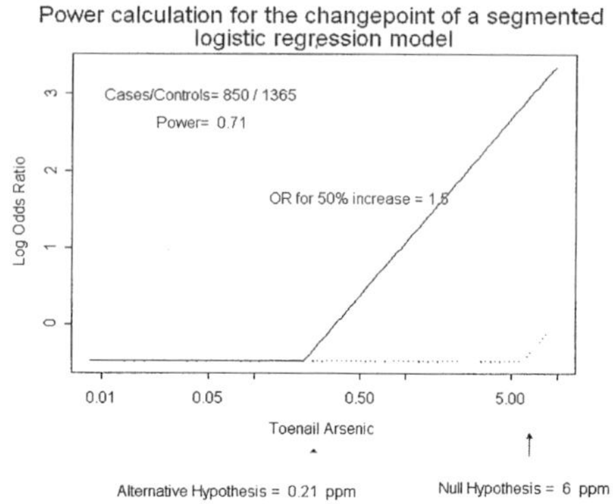

A Web-based program is available for computing this figure at http://biostat.hitchcock.org .

4) Results: The planned study will include 850 bladder cancer cases and approximately 1,365 population controls. Based on this sample size and the current estimates of the distribution of toenail concentrations in the study population, the *maximum* detectable changepoint was calculated for given relative risks parameters for the dose response after the changepoint. The "null hypothesis" changepoint is taken to be 6 ppm in toenails, about what might be expected in the lowest dose group of a Taiwan study of a highly exposed population.

Table 1. Maximum detectable change points for a two-segmented logistic with a null hypothesis of 50 ppm and a slope coefficient corresponding to selected odds ratios for a 100% increase in toenail arsenic. The numbers of subjects (cases and controls combined) assumed to be below and above the changepoints are given as n1 and n2. The assumed significance level is .05.

	Power=.8			Power=.9		
Odds Ratio	Changepoint (ppm in toenail)	n1	n2	Change Point	n1	n2
2.0	0.14	1397	488	0.10	1101	784
2.5	0.20	1639	246	0.17	1540	345

4) Conclusions: The calculations presented give an indication of how small a changepoint can be detected based on the proposed case-control study of bladder cancer and arsenic. It is concluded that the study will provide a useful tool for studying the onset of cancer risk due to arsenic exposure.

References

Karagas MR, Tosteson TD, Blum J, Morris SJ, Baron JA, Klaue B. Design of an epidemiologic study of drinking water arsenic exposure and skin and bladder cancer risk in a US population. Environ Health Persp 1998;106: 1047-1050.

Seber G.A, Wild C.J. (1989). Nonlinear Regression, John Wiley & Sons, New York.

Metal Ions in Biology and Medicine; vol 6. Eds. J.A. Centeno, Ph. Collery, G. Vernet, R.B. Finkelman, H. Gibb, J.C. Etienne. John Libbey Eurotext, Paris © 2000, pp. 31.

Arsenic in ground water of the United States

Alan H. Welch

U.S. Geological Survey, Carson City, NV 89706; 775-887-7609; e-mail: ahwelch@usgs.gov

Although only about 10% of ground water samples in the conterminous United States exceed 10 µg/L, ground water with these high concentrations are found in most parts of the Nation. Widespread high concentrations generally result from natural processes, although human activities can increase arsenic concentrations. The most prevalent causes of widespread high concentrations are release from iron oxide and sulfide mineral oxidation. Upflow of geothermal water and evaporative concentration also can produce high arsenic concentrations in ground water.

Arsenic can be released to ground water by desorption from, and dissolution of, iron oxide. Aquifers with oxic ground water commonly contain iron oxide with arsenic as an impurity. Desorption of arsenic can be promoted by either an increase in pH or the concentration of a competing ion, such as phosphorous. Arsenic also can be released from iron oxide because of chemical reduction of the oxide. Deposition of Fe-coated sediment along with organic matter can lead to the dissolution of the oxide coating with consequent release of arsenic to ground water. Introduction of synthetic organic compounds into aquifers also can lead to reductive dissolution of iron oxide and arsenic release.

Pyrite commonly contains arsenic in trace amounts, although arsenic concentration can exceed five percent. The rate of sulfide-mineral oxidation is limited by the supply of an oxidizing agent, most commonly molecular oxygen. High nitrate concentrations from agricultural activities also can oxidize sulfide minerals. Human activities that increase the supply of oxygen, or another oxidizing agent such as nitrate, to ground water can lead to increased mineral oxidation and, consequently, high arsenic concentrations. Irrigation in arid and semi-arid regions can increase evaporative concentration, which can lead to high arsenic concentrations.

Metal Ions in Biology and Medicine; vol 6. Eds. J.A. Centeno, Ph. Collery, G. Vernet, R.B. Finkelman, H. Gibb, J.C. Etienne. John Libbey Eurotext, Paris © 2000, pp. 32-34.

Researches on the health effects of arsenic in China$

Cheng Zhai[1, 2], Baoshan Zheng[1]

[1] *State Key Lab of Environ Geochemistry, Inst of Geochemistry, Guiyang, Guizhou, P.R. China, 550002;*
[2] *School of Public Health, China Medical University, Shenyang, Liaoning, P.R. China, 110001*

Arsenic is an important part of the traditional Chinese medicine and has been applied to treat diseases for more than 3,000 years. However, arsenic may also cause various adverse health effects in human. In China, more than 2 million people live in the endemic arsenism areas with the potential of being exposed to high levels of arsenic, and more than 6,000 cases of arsenosis have been identified[1]. Altogether, about 5.63 million people in China drink water with arsenic levels above 0.05mg/L[2]. Nonetheless, it took many years to assess the health impacts of arsenic and recognize it as an important public health issue. In the recent years, 130 to160 papers are published annually by researchers in China. Because most of them are published in Chinese, many important findings are unknown to scientists of other countries. We therefore summarized those findings as the following:

I. Endemic arsenosis caused by geochemical sources

1.Blackfoot disease (BFD) caused by drinking water in Taiwan: BFD is a peripheral vascular disease that was prevalent in the southwest coast area of Taiwan where people drank deep pressure water from Quarternary marine sediment. The water contains high concentrations of arsenic and humic acids[3,4].The endemic area of BFD has a popu- lation of around 200,000, and more than 1,990 cases of BFD have been identified. Overall, about 924,000 residents in Taiwan drank water with high arsenic contents[5].

2.Arsenosis caused by drinking water in Xinjiang: People in this area also drink deep pressure water from Quarternary continental sediment containing high levels of arsenic. But, the concentration of humic acids in the water is low. About 100,000 residents are in danger of being exposed to high levels of arsenic, and 523 cases of arsenosis have been identified [6].

3.Arsenosis caused by phreatic water: The endemic areas are in Inner Mongolia, Shanxi, and Ningxia provinces. People drank shallow underground water with high arsenic and humic acid levels from new Quarternary continental sediment. The endemic areas have a total population of more than 400,000 and 3,752 cases of arsenosis have been reported[1,7].

4.Arsenosis caused by indoor combustion of high-arsenic coal in southwestern Guizhou: The coal used by residents in this area is from Longtan coal formation of late Permian, and its arsenic enrichment is related to gold mineralization. The highest arsenic level measured in the coal that caused arsenosis was 9,600mg/kg. About 100,000 residents are still using the coal with high arsenic content. The first case report was in the 1960s, and the total number of patients has reached 1,852[8].

The studies conducted in the endemic arsenosis areas observed significant dose-response relationships between arsenic exposure and the incidence of arsenosis and skin cancer[6,9]. The health effects of arsenic differ among different types of arsenic compounds, dose rates, and routes of entry. Some evidences suggest arsenic may cause internal cancers and liver damages[10], but further epidemiological studies are necessary to confirm the findings.

II.Arsenosis caused by mining and applications of arsenic in industry, agriculture and pasturing

1.Arsenosis caused by mining of realgar and other arsenic-containing minerals: Tin and realgar mining in

Yunnan and Hunan Provinces is the typical example of this category. The standardized mortality rate (SMR) of lung cancer among the tin miners of Gejiu Tin Co. in Yunnan was up to $150*10^{-5}$per person-year. In Hunan, the exposure is from simple arsenic ore dusts during realgar mining. A total of 1,500 cases of arsenosis and 22 cases of lung cancer have been diagnosed, and the SMR ($225*10^{-5}$) of lung cancer was more than that among miners of the Gejiu Tin Co.[11]. Arsenosis and skin cancers caused by illegal mining and processing of arsenic-containing ore have also been reported[12]. Arsenic pollution around mining factories is a serious problem. In 1995, a single arsenosis event in China is caused by high-arsenic drinking water contaminated by mining waste residue, and about 3,000 patients were identified[13].

2.Arsenosis caused by manufacturing and application of preservatives, pesticides, insecticides and chemical fertilizers [14]

III. Arsenosis caused by intentional and unintentional intake of arsenicals

In 1992, 750g of As_2O_3 was mixed into wheat flour intentionally in a college in Zhengzhou city, so that 788 of the staff were diagnosed as arsenic poisoning. [15]

IV. Arsenosis caused by medicine containing arsenic

Medicines containing arsenic have been used in the treatment of skin disorders, dental diseases, leukemia, and other diseases. The etiology included allergy, accumulation of too much arsenic in the body, divulge of the locally sealed arsenic medicines, etc.[16]

V. The value and prospect of arsenic as medicine

Realgar, orpiment, and other arsenic-containing minerals are often used as traditional Chinese medicines in China. In addition, arsenic is the main ingredient of many patent medicines, which are applied in the treatment of psoriasis, asthma, tuberculosis, leukemia, and many other diseases. It took nearly 30 years to identify As_2O_3 as a primary medicine in curing leukemia among patent Chinese herb medicines, Chinese herbs, and pure arsenete salts[17].

In the recent years, regulations of arsenic contents have become a major barrier for traditional Chinese medicines to enter the international markets. Some studies showed that the concentrations of arsenic in some patent Chinese medicines can be reduced without the compromise of their therapeutic effects. But, in most cases, removal of arsenic results in a great loss in curing abilities, which becomes a problem.[18]

In summary, it has become clear that arsenic has a double-blade effect on the health of human beings. Arsenic can promote proliferation of normal cells and tissues as in the development of hyperkeratosis and neoplasm. On the other hand, it can cause the apotosis of over-proligerous cells, such as in the treatment of leukemia. Further studies should be carried out to explore the points of transmission and control of cellular signals, which may help to solve the mystery of the paradoxical effects of arsenic on human's health.

$ The project supported by National Natural Science Foundation of China (49273189 49873007)

1.Hao Y, et al. The Control State of Endemic Arsenism in China. Chin J Contr Ende Dis.1994; 9(3): 169-70

2.Zhang L, et al. Geographic Distribution and Exposure Population of Drinking Water with High Concentration of Arsenic in China. J Hyg Res 1997; 26(5):310-3

3.Chen KP, et al. Epidemiologic Studies on Black-foot disease: 2, A study of source of drinking water in relation to the disease. J Formos Med Assoc 1962; 61:611-8

4.Lu FJ, et al. Black-foot Disease: Arsenic or Humic Acid? The Lancet 1990;336:115-6

5.Gou HR, et al. The Association between Arsenic in Drinking Water and Incidence of Skin Cancer. Environ Res Sec A 1998;79:82-93
6.Wang LF. Research and Control on Damage of Inorganic Arsenic in Xinjiang. Chin J Pub Health (Taipei) 1996; 15(3s):53-7
7.Hu XZ, et al. Epidemiological Investigation of Endemic Arsenic Poisoning in the North of Ningxia. Chin J Endemiol 1999;18(1):23-5
8.Ji RD. Research and Control on Damage of Inorganic Arsenic Poisoning in Guizhou. Chin J Pub Health (Taipei) 1996; 15(3s):40-6
9.Chen CJ, et al. Arsenic and Cancers. *The Lancet.* 1988;2:414-5
10. An D, et al. 30 Years Follow-up of Arsenism in Bazi Village. Chin J Pub Health. 1996;12(7):307-8
11.Yang M, et al. Epidemiological Investigation of Lung Cancer in Relgar Mine, Hunan. J Indus Hyg Occup Dis 1983;9(2):84-6
12.Luo JE, et al. Arsenic Poisoning caused by Illegal Refining of As_2O_3. Chin J Indus Hyg Occup Dis 1987; 5(2):107-9
13.Lin HB, et al. Acute Arsenic Poisoning Caused by Contaminated Water. Guangxi J Prev Med. 1996;2(5):312
14.Shen TH, et al. A Survey on Environmental Pollution Caused by Wood Preservative CCA Using in the Treatment of Crumbs of Wood. Envir Health. 1996;13(3):111-2
15.Dong HQ, et al. A clinical Analysis on 117 Cases of Acute Arsenic Poisoning. Chin J Inter Med. 1993;32(12):813-5
16.Zhang HQ, et al. Keratosis and Melanosis Arsenica caused by Chinese Medicine Relgar: 4 Cases Report. Chin J Dermato. 1983;16(2):132-3
17.Zhang TD, et al. Application of Arsenic Containing Traditional Chinese Medicine in Curing Leukaemia. Chin J Interg Trad West Med. 1998;18(10):581-4
18.Zhang JK, et al. Suggestions on Usage and Dosage of Relgar in *China Pharmacopoeia.* Chin J Chin Materia Med. 1997;22(1):21-3

Metal Ions in Biology and Medicine; vol 6. Eds. J.A. Centeno, Ph. Collery, G. Vernet, R.B. Finkelman, H. Gibb, J.C. Etienne. John Libbey Eurotext, Paris © 2000, pp. 35-37.

The geographical epidemiology of water born As exposure in Inner Mongolia

Xiao-Juan Guo

Institute for Control and Treatment of Endemic Disease in Inner Mongolia

Abstract The waterborne arsenic contamination in the Inner Mongolia area has been caused by many specific geographic environment factors such as geohistory, landform and geology, hydrogeology, and human activities. Arsenic poisoned patients in the Inner Mongolia were found in 1990, who were living in two areas, one is KeSiKeTeng Qi in the east of Inner Mongolia, another is situated on the HeTao Plain in the west. The acreage of arsenic concentration area is nearly 3000 square kilometers. The geological formations are mainly characterized by lake alluvial deposit and alluvial deposit. And the groundwater drainage belt of DaQingShan Mountain in the north and Yellow River in the south is just at the arsenic exposure distribution belt. And 300,000 population lived there. Due to the opening up wasteland and increasing population, the need of drinking water became urgent, so the villages dug wells in their own garden from 1980. The depth of it is about 10-20 meters just at the arsenic rich aquifers. As the result of chronic arsenic exposure, endemic chronic arsenicism (ECA) emerged, which affected human health and became a serious geographic environment problem.

Kei Words: arsenic arsenic/exposure

1. Introduction

Endemic chronic arsenicism (ECA) due to drinking water has widely been existent whether it is through anthropogenic source or natural source of arsenic. As poisoned patients were found in 1990 in two regions in Inner Mongolia. One is KeSiKeTeng Qi in the east. Another region is located on HeTao Plain in the west concluding 11 banners, 64 townships. It is about 1000 kilometers long, 10-40 kilometers wide. The acreage of arsenic concentration expanded into 3000 square kilometers. The author will take HeTao Plain as the main morbid area to analysis the geographical epidemiology of arsenic exposure. Table I

2. The characteristics of landforms

The study area is an arid region, the evaporation capacity is more for 4-20 times than the precipitation and widely contained inland rivers there. This area is plain with an elevation of 1010-1040m,LangShan and DaQingShan Mountains are standing in the north, Yellow River and ErDuoSi Plateau situated in the south. It can be divided into three kinds of landforms, one is in front mountain tilting plain, one is low-lying area showing the belt-like shape from east to west and the other is Yellow River lake alluvial deposit plain. Abandoned fossil river courses and accumulated water depression can be considered to be the microlandforms of HeTao Plain.

3. **The Removal and Distribution of As**

The north mountain area of the He Tao Plain is a well-formed mining area with an arsenic concentration of 10-60 mg/L. It is the origin of the high level arsenic contaminating environment. The arsenic contained in the mineral was dissolved and filtered by weathering and water removing, then it was contained in atmospheric precipitation and groundwater. Consequently, the arsenic moved from the north to the south and reached the low-lying land area. Moreover, the southern riverbed of Yellow River is higher than ground, which makes the groundwater in the south run to the northern low-lying land. In addition, the sluggish flow and dry climate make the groundwater evaporated over a long period time. So, arsenic enriched at this area [1]. 100 wells are used for domestic water supply without any treatment, as a result of water quality analysis, arsenic concentration is low in the area close to the mountain, that is 0.007-0.02mg/l. And in the south of the plain near the Yellow River, arsenic concentration is 0.01mg/l But in the low-lying land of the middle area of the plain, arsenic concentration can reach 0.943mg/l for the highest.

Table I The water-born As exposure in Inner Mongolia

Area	Exposure variety	Exposure concentration (mg/L)	Exposure time	Patients Number	Natural geographical environment
Ke Qi	Hot spring	0.553	1989	97	West Liaohe Plain Arid Endorheism Semi-desert
Tu Qi	Well	1.68	1961	230	Tumote Plain Arid Endorheism Semi-desert
Ba Meng	Well	1.74	1980	1141	Hetao Plain Arid Endorheism Semi-desert
A Meng	Well	1.088	1983	306	Hetao Plain Arid Endorheism Semi-desert

4. **Human environment in the study area**

The study area is an agricultural region, so the occupation, dietary habits, social customs and population distribution are almost the same. Nevertheless, the time of arsenic exposure is in the 1980s, just at the altering period of drinking water through from surface-water (open well) to ground-water (hand-pumping well). The changing was caused by the long-term human activities: such as opening up wasteland, increasing population, so the need of drinking water became urgent. The villagers began to dig wells in their own garden for about 10-20 meters. The depth is just at the arsenic rich aquifers. So arsenic was delivered from geographic environment to human body by dietary chain. Endemic chronic arsenicism arose in this area.

5. The health effect of water-born As exposure

The arsenic exposure area on HeTao Plain involved 11 banners, 64 townships and 300,000 population lived there. According to 10154 checked people, 1800 have been determined to be arsenic poisoned patients. With the study going the number is adding. The author investigated the wells and 1728 population in 15 villages of HeTao Plain area from 1996 to 1999, the result is 96% wells were polluted by arsenic and the highest arsenic concentration is 1.354mg/l, 35.42% people had arsenic poisoned damage. The main clinical symptoms concluded skin and other organ damage. The youngest patient is only ten years old having obvious symptoms on skin and damage in respiratory and neurons system. In the study area, skin cancer and splanchna cancer appeared and the mortality rate of them distinctly higher than the non-exposure area.

6. Discussion

Antecedent to outbreak of endemic chronic arsenicism (ECA), there are recognized a long latent stage of arrangement based on historical, socioeconomical, cultural, geographical and geological background in each endemic area. The major ECA in the world are due chiefly to water-born arsenic and some geographical characteristics common to almost all of the endemic areas are summarized as follows: volcanic zone, dry-inland river basin, delta plain, ancient sea area, deep well, agriculture, mining and smelting [2]. However ancient geography, landforms, geology and human activities caused water-born arsenic contamination in Inner Mongolia. Water-born arsenic contamination had relations with the geological background of abundant arsenic concentration, but it was not the case that such kind of environment can undoubtedly result in arsenic exposure. For it is more important that arsenic transferred, decentralized and accumulated in different geographic environment for the second time. . The geological properties of HeTao Plain are lake illuvial deposit and illuvion. The ground-water drainage belt of DaQingShan Mountains in the north and Yellow River in the south is just at the arsenic exposure distribution belt. Drinking water became urgent because of the opening up wasteland and increasing population. From 1980,villagers began to dig wells at the depth of the arsenic rich aquifers. As a result of long-term drinking such arsenic polluted water, endemic chronic arsenicism appeared, which greatly affected the health of people there. That became a serious geographic environment problem based on the background of population, grain and drinking water.

References

[1] ShuFan.Li, HaoJi.Li. The research of the geological characteristic and forming reasons of arsenic exposure in HeTao area of Inner Mongolia(J). The Research of Endemic Diseases of Inner Mongolia . 1994;19:3

[2] Nobuyuki Hotta. The conditions of drinking water in history and now-a-days in the world(J). Water Report, 1997;17(5):12

Metal Ions in Biology and Medicine; vol 6. Eds. J.A. Centeno, Ph. Collery, G. Vernet, R.B. Finkelman, H. Gibb, J.C. Etienne. John Libbey Eurotext, Paris © 2000, pp. 38-40.

Environmental impact of elevated arsenic in Southern Appalachian Basin coals

Martin B. Goldhaber[1], Elise R. Irwin[2], J. Brian Atkins[3], Rob Lee[1], Humbert Zappia[3], Dee Dee Black[4], and Robert B. Finkelman[5]

[1] U.S. Geological Survey, MS 973, Federal Center, Denver, CO, 80225 USA; [2] U.S. Geological Survey, 331 Funchess Hall, Auburn University, Auburn AL, 36849; [3] U.S. Geological Survey, 2350 Fairlane Drive Suite 120, Montgomery AL, 36116, USA; [4] Auburn University, Auburn AL; 36849, USA; [5] U.S. Geological Survey, MS 956 Reston VA, 20192, USA

The Mobile drainage basin of Alabama, Georgia, and Mississippi is thought to have the highest biodiversity of any such drainage in the lower 48 states (1), and one study reported that this system was as biologically diverse as tropical rain forest areas. Within this drainage, the Warrior Basin of northwestern Alabama is the largest sub-basin within the boundaries of the state. The Warrior Basin contains areas of extensive present and past coal mining within its limits. Our data show that this biologically sensitive environment may be impacted by toxic elements contained in the coal.

The highest arsenic (As) concentrations for all U.S. coals are in the Warrior coalfield. Of all U.S. coals 3 standard deviations above the mean for arsenic concentration, 80 of 99 are from the Warrior basin. The mean arsenic concentration of 72 ppm is three times the mean for all U.S coals (24 ppm) (2,3). Arsenic concentrations in some samples exceed 2500 mg/Kg (ppm) on a whole coal basis. Furthermore, mercury (Hg), selenium (Se), molybdenum (Mo), antimony (Sb) thallium (Tl) and copper (Cu) are present in elevated concentrations compared to other U.S. coals (**3**). Petrologic studies of coal samples collected during this study reveal that As is hosted by the mineral pyrite. Based on ion microprobe and laser ablation ICP Mass Spectrometer studies, the pyrite may contain up to 4.45 weight percent As.

The presence of high concentrations of As in coal beds raises the possibility that natural weathering and/or coal mining will lead to dispersion As into the environment. To evaluate this possibility, a reconnaissance study was conducted. This study utilized archived stream sediment samples from over 2800 sites collected in the late 1970's in northern Alabama during the NURE (National Uranium Resource Investigation) program. These samples were reanalyzed for a suite of elements including As. Stream sediments from the coal mining area are elevated in arsenic (typically 12-50 ppm) compared to adjacent areas (<12 ppm). For comparison, a recent national survey by the USGS of 541 streambed-sediment samples determined that the 75th percentile for As concentration was 9.2 ppm (**4**).

Because As in coal is hosted by the mineral pyrite, we hypothesize that pyrite oxidation, producing acid mine drainage (AMD) is the mechanism of As dispersal to the environment. To test this hypothesis, field studies were conducted of six sites impacted by coal AMD. Grab samples from the coal mine refuse piles that are a major source of the AMD have high concentrations of As with up to 470 ppm. Streams adjacent to these refuse piles have low pH values (3.3-4.2) and are strikingly enriched in arsenic (Table I).

TABLE I

Chemical Analyses of Stream Sediments Impacted by Acid Mine Drainage

Name of Site	Latitude	Longitude	As; ppm	Fe; ppm
Gorgas1	33.6494	-87.2189	180	174000
Gorgas2	33.6494	-87.2189	79	264000
Gorgas3	33.6494	-87.2189	43	104000
Lost Creek 1a	33.6494	-86.9897	14	34900
Lost Creek 1b	33.5067	-86.9897	10	31300
Lost Creek 2a	33.5067	-86.9897	75	105000
Lost Creek 2b	33.5067	-86.9897	45	42100
Lost Creek 3a	33.5067	-86.9897	105	70500
Lost Creek 3b	33.5067	-86.9897	75	58000
Black Branch 1a	33.7356	-87.4297	60	106000
Black Branch 1b	33.7356	-87.4297	55	74200
Black Branch 2a	33.7356	-87.4297	55	437000
Black Branch 2b	33.7356	-87.4297	42	338000
Black Branch 3	33.7356	-87.4297	27	257000
Short Creek 1a	33.5608	-87.0381	10	32100
Short Creek 1b	33.5608	-87.0381	5	14600
Short Creek 2a	33.5608	-87.0381	17	43600
Short Creek 2b	33.5608	-87.0381	16	40900
Short Creek 3	33.5608	-87.0381	150	122000
Goolsby-1	33.5067	-86.9897	52	40000
Goolsby-A	33.5064	-86.9892	20	37700
Goolsby-B	33.5067	-86.9897	14	280000
Blue Creek-2	33.3414	-87.0853	46	25900
Blue Creek-A	33.3414	-87.0853	56	79200
Blue Creek-B	33.3414	-87.0853	38	87100

Selective leaching studies of the stream sediment samples reveals demonstrates that the residence of As is iron oxides. Selective adsorption of As on iron oxides is a well-documented phenomenon. Because of this adsorption, As concentrations in water are low in the AMD impacted streams (generally < 10 μg/liter). However, shallow groundwater in coal tailings may have higher concentrations of As (90 μg/liter).

Formation of toxic mixing zones at the confluence of AMD streams and pH neutral streams is common. Toxic mixing zones are characterized by rapid precipitation of metals, particularly aluminum and iron oxides, caused by abrupt increases in pH. Henry et al. (5) evaluated the toxicity of the mixing zone to fish at one site in Alabama (Cane Creek/Black Branch). They determined that the mixing zone was lethal to fish and sub-lethal effects (i.e., accumulation of Al on gills) were apparent. Studies are under way to determine if toxic metals contribute to detrimental effects on the biota.

The coal environmental impact described above may not be unique to Alabama. High As locally characterizes coal samples from parts of eastern Kentucky, western Pennsylvania and eastern Ohio (2). Given the long (over 100 year) history of coal mining in these areas, the potential exists for environmental impacts in other portions of the Appalachian coal basin.

1. Lydeard, C. and R. L. Mayden. 1995. A diverse and endangered aquatic ecosystem of the southeast United States. Conservation Biology 9:800-805.

2. Bragg, L.J., Oman, J.K., Tewalt S.J, Oman, C.L., Rega, N.H., Washington, P.M., and Finkelman, R.B. 1994. U.S. Geological Survey Coal Quality Database: Version 1.3. U.S. Geological Survey Open File Report 94-205.

3. Goldhaber, M.B., R.C. Bigelow, J.R. Hatch, and J.C. Pashin. 2000; Distribution Of A Suite Of Elements Including Arsenic And Mercury In Alabama Coal; U.S. Geological Survey MF 2333. (Available online at: http://greenwood.cr.usgs.gov/pub/mf-maps/mf-2333/

4. Rice, K.C., 1999; Trace-Element Concentrations in Streambed Sediment Across the Conterminous United States; Environmental Science and Technology; v. 33. Pp 2499-2504.

5. Henry, T. B., E. R. Irwin, J. M. Grizzle, M. L. Wildhaber and W. G. Brumbaugh. *In Press*, Seasonal toxicity of an acid mine drainage mixing zone to juvenile bluegill and largemouth bass. Transactions of the American Fisheries Society.

Metal Ions in Biology and Medicine; vol 6. Eds. J.A. Centeno, Ph. Collery, G. Vernet, R.B. Finkelman, H. Gibb, J.C. Etienne. John Libbey Eurotext, Paris © 2000, pp. 41-43.

Arsenic dissolution and speciation in groundwater of Southeast Michigan

Myoung-Jin Kim[1], Jerome Nriagu[1] and Sheridan Haack[2]

[1] Department of Environmental Health Science, School of Public Health, University of Michigan, Ann Arbor, MI 48109; [2] Water Resources Division, US Geological Survey, Lansing, MI

Abstract

Groundwater samples were collected in nine counties of southeast Michigan in 1997. The highest arsenic concentration detected was 278 μg/L, the average being 29 μg/L. Most of the arsenic was found to be As(III). A new well was drilled in Bad Axe, Huron County, Michigan, and core samples were taken at different depths. Arsenic leaching experiments were conducted with the core samples using several chemicals under various conditions. It was found that arsenic leaching increased with $NaHCO_3$ concentration in water. It is concluded that most arsenic is leached as As(III), As(V) or As-carbonate complex from arsenian pyrite or orpiment into the groundwater of the study area.

The natural occurrence of arsenic in groundwater has been reported all over the world [1-3]. Elevated concentrations of naturally occurring arsenic have also been detected in groundwater of southeast Michigan, with concentrations in some areas exceeding the U.S. Environmental Protection Agency (USEPA) maximum contaminant level (MCL) of 50 μg/L for drinking water. This arsenic occurrence has been associated with arsenic-containing minerals, such as arsenian pyrite and orpiment [4,5]. The main objective of this study is to identify the source of arsenic in groundwater, and to investigate the factors controlling its dissolution, speciation and distribution.

Groundwater samples were collected in nine counties of southeast Michigan in 1997. The highest arsenic concentration detected was 278 μg/L, the average being 29 μg/L. About 12% of the groundwater in the study area exceeded the USEPA arsenic standard. Most (53-98%) of the arsenic was found to be As(III). The total arsenic concentrations are plotted against the percentage of As(III) in Figure 1. As can be seen in the graph, the percentage of As(III) was relatively constant regardless of total arsenic concentrations, but low percentage of As(III) was found when total arsenic was below 50 μg/L. It has been known that the distribution of arsenic species is affected by redox conditions in groundwater; therefore, the low values of dissolved oxygen (0.03 to 2.73 mg/L, average = 0.38 mg/L) and redox potential (-190 to 361 mV, average = 70 mV) as well as the predominance of As(III) in the samples represent consistent results. Since As(III) is much more toxic than As(V), the current guideline of 50 μg/L for total arsenic may not be providing sufficient protection to many Michigan residents who drink the groundwater.

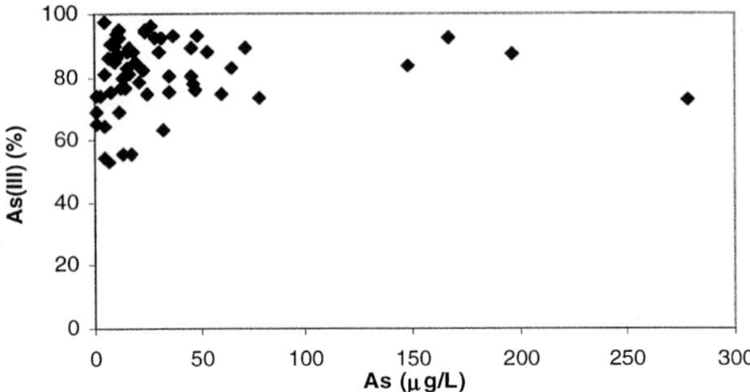

Figure 1. Relation between total arsenic concentration and the percentage of As(III)

A new well was drilled in Bad Axe, Huron County, Michigan in 1997, and core samples were taken at different depths. Total arsenic concentrations in core samples varied from 0.8 mg/kg to 72.1 mg/kg. The arsenic dissolution process from rock into groundwater was investigated. The hypothesis is that the major ions in groundwater affect the dissolution of arsenic from arsenic-containing minerals. Arsenic leaching experiments were conducted with the core samples using several chemicals under various conditions. It was found that arsenic leaching increased with $NaHCO_3$ concentration in water (Figure 2). In addition, noticeable arsenic leaching was found at extremely acidic and basic pHs. The arsenic leaching was also dependent on oxic/anoxic conditions.

It is concluded that most arsenic is leached as As(III), As(V) or As-carbonate complex from arsenian pyrite or orpiment into the groundwater of the study area. Bicarbonate enhances the rate of arsenian pyrite oxidation or orpiment dissolution by producing As-carbonate complex. In shallow groundwater, the solubility of arsenic is controlled by the availability of bicarbonate and oxidants. In deep groundwater, arsenic is dissolved from orpiment and bicarbonate initiates the dissolution reaction. This latter mechanism may explain the high occurrence of arsenic that has been found in groundwater under reduced conditions in many places around the world.

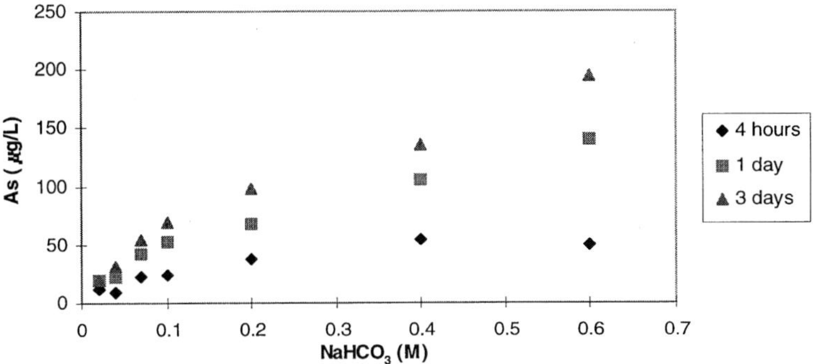

Figure 2. Arsenic leaching rate in different $NaHCO_3$ concentration

References

[1] Acharyya, S.K., Chakraborty, P., Lahiri, S., Raymahashay, B.C., Guha, S., Bhowmik, A. Arsenic poisoning in the Ganges delta. *Nature* 1999: 401:545.

[2] Nickson, R., McArthur, J., Burgess, W., Ahmed, K.M., Ravenscroft, P., and Rahman, M. Arsenic poisoning of Bangladesh groundwater. *Nature* 1998: 395: 338.

[3] Peters, S.C., Blum, J.D., and Karagas, M.R. Arsenic occurrence in New Hampshire drinking water. *Environ Sci & Tech* 1999: 33: 1328-1333.

[4] Kim, M.J. Arsenic dissolution and speciation in groundwater of southeast Michigan. Ph.D. Dissertation thesis. University of Michigan, Ann Arbor, MI. 1999.

[5] Kolker, A., Cannon, W.F., Westjohn, D.B., and Woodruff, L.G. Arsenic-rich pyrite in the Mississippian Marshall Sandstone: source of anomalous arsenic in southeastern Michigan ground water. *Abstract from 1998 National Meeting of the Geological Society of America* Oct. 25-29, Toronto, Ontario, Canada. 1998.

Metal Ions in Biology and Medicine; vol 6. Eds. J.A. Centeno, Ph. Collery, G. Vernet, R.B. Finkelman, H. Gibb, J.C. Etienne. John Libbey Eurotext, Paris © 2000, pp. 44-46.

Molecular mechanism of carcinogenic and anti-cancer effects by arsenic

Zigang Dong

The Hormel Institute, University of Minnesota, 801 16th Avenue NE, Austin, MN 55912

ABSTRACT

Arsenic is a human carcinogen which is associated with cancers of skin, lung, liver and bladder. Interestingly, arsenic has also been used as an effective chemotherapy agent for certain human cancers for hundreds of years in both traditional Chinese medicine and Western medicine. However, the mechanisms by which arsenic causes cancer induction and cancer cell death are not well understood. Recently, we found that exposure of JB6 P^+ cells to low concentrations of arsenic (<25 μM) induces cell transformation, while higher concentrations of arsenite induce cell apoptosis. Arsenite induces Erk phosphorylation and increased Erk activity at doses ranging from 0.8 to 200 μM, while higher doses (more than 50 μM) are required for activation of c-Jun NH_2-terminal kinases (JNKs). Arsenite-induced Erk activation was markedly inhibited by introduction of dominant negative Erk2 into cells, while expression of dominant negative Erk2 did not show inhibition of JNK and $MEK_{1/2}$. Furthermore, arsenite-induced cell transformation was blocked in cells expressing the dominant negative Erk2. In contrast, overexpression of dominant negative JNK1 was shown to increase cell transformation even though it inhibits arsenite-induced JNK activation. Arsenic induces activation of JNKs at a similar dose range for induction of apoptosis in JB6 cells. In addition, we found that arsenic did not induce p53-dependent transactivation. Similarly, there was no difference in apoptosis induction between cells with p53+/+ or p53-/-. In contrast, arsenic-induced apoptosis was almost totally blocked by expression of a dominant-negative mutant of JNK. Taken together with previous findings that p53 mutations are involved in ~50% of all human cancers and nearly all chemotherapeutic agents kill cancer cells mainly by apoptotic induction, we suggest that arsenic may be a useful agent for the treatment of cancer with p53 mutation. These results suggest that the activation of Erk is required for arsenic-induced cell transformation, while the activation of JNKs is involved in arsenic-induced apoptosis of JB6 cells.

Arsenic is a well-documented human carcinogen and is associated with increased risk of human cancers of the skin, lung, kidney, bladder, liver and hematopoietic system. Interestingly, arsenic-containing compounds have been used for treatment of cancer for hundreds of years in both traditional Chinese medicine and Western medicine. Several recent studies confirm that arsenic trioxide ($As_2 O_3$) appears to be a valuable therapeutic tool for patients with acute promyelocytic leukemia.

Although arsenic and its modes of actions have been the subject of reviews and symposia, little data exist regarding specific mechanism(s) of its action as carcinogen to cause cancer and chemotherapeutic agent for treatment of cancer. Recently, our laboratory findings provided the mechanisms of arsenic-induced neoplastic cell transformation and arsenic-induced apoptosis in tumor cells [1-4].

Induction of Cell Transformation by Low Concentration of Arsenic—To study whether arsenite induces cell transformation, we exposed JB6 Cl 41 cells to arsenite in soft agar. Anchorage-independent colonies were observed in the eighth week after arsenite exposure. Cell transformation can only be observed in cells exposed to low concentrations (25 µM) of arsenite, while no cell transformation colonies were observed at high concentrations of arsenite (50-100 µM).

Induction of Apoptosis by Higher Concentration of Arsenic—Treatment of cells with a relatively higher concentration (200 µM) of arsenite or arsenate resulted in apoptosis by 44.5 and 61.5%, respectively.

Differential Activation of Erk and JNK by Arsenite—We found that arsenite could induce activation of both JNK and Erk. However, the activation of each by arsenite is different. During the time course and dose-response studies, marked Erk activation could be observed at 15 min after exposure and at all dosages studied. There was no significant induction of Erk by arsenite after a 30-min exposure. In contrast, activation of JNK was only observed at high dosage (>50 µM) and after 60 min of exposure [1].

Inhibition of Erk Activation Blocks Arsenic-induced Cell Transformation—The results described above revealed that Erk activation by arsenite may be involved in its cell transformation. To test this possibility, we used dominant negative Erk2-K52R stable transfectant [1,2]. Our results demonstrate that Erk activation, but not JNK activation, is required for arsenite-induced cell transformation.

Inhibition of JNK Blocks Arsenic-induced Apoptosis—To investigate the role of the activation of JNKs in arsenic-induced apoptosis, we used JB6 cells and dominant-negative mutant of JNK_1, to test its effects on arsenic-induced apoptosis [2]. Expression of dominant-negative mutant JNK_1 blocked the apoptosis induction by arsenite (4%) or arsenate (7%) as compared with vector-transfected control cells (31.5 and 40.5% for arsenite and arsenate, respectively) [2].

p53 Is Not Involved in Apoptosis Induction by Arsenic—Arsenic had no effect on p53-dependent transcription activity in Cl 41 p53 cells treated with a wide range of arsenic doses [2]. This suggested that p53 may not be involved in arsenic-induced apoptosis. This hypothesis was further tested by studying the effects of arsenic on two fibroblast cell lines, *p53+/+* and *p53-/-*, derived from mouse embryos either containing wild-type *p53* (*p53+/+*) or deficient in *p53* (*p53-/-*). Results showed that treatment with arsenite or arsenate results in apoptosis in both cell lines [2]. Therefore arsenic may be effective in counteracting drug resistance because arsenic appears to be able to induce apoptosis in tumor cells independently of p53 activation and thus could be specifically directed against p53-defective cancer cells.

Involvement of PKC in Arsenic-induced Signal Transduction—Our recent data show that protein kinase C (PKC), upstream from the MAP kinases, may be involved in mediating arsenite-induced signal transduction. Translocation of KC from cytosol to the membrane is a critical step for activation of this enzyme and treatment of JB6 cells with arsenite resulted in an increased translocation of PKC within 15 min. Inhibition of activation of PKC blocked both arsenite-induced AP-1 activity and arsenite-induced phosphorylation of Erks, JNKs, and p38 suggesting that PKC is required for arsenite-induced activation of MAP kinases [3].

REFERENCES

1. Huang C, Ma WY, Li J, Goranson A, Dong Z. Requirement of Erk, but not JNK, for arsenite-induced cell transformation. *J Biol Chem* 1999; 274: 14595-14601.

2. Huang C, Ma WY, Li J, Dong Z. Arsenic induces apoptosis through a c-Jun NH2-terminal kinase-dependent, p53-independent pathway. *Cancer Res* 1999; 59: 3053-3058.

3. Chen NY, Ma WY, Huang C, Ding M, Dong Z. Activation of PKC is required for arsenate-induced signal transduction. *J Environ Pathol Toxicol Oncol* 2000, in press.

4. Bode A, Dong Z. Apoptosis induction by arsenic: mechanisms of action and possible clinical applications for treating therapy-resistant cancer. *Drug Resistance Updates* 2000, in press.

Metal Ions in Biology and Medicine; vol 6. Eds. J.A. Centeno, Ph. Collery, G. Vernet, R.B. Finkelman, H. Gibb, J.C. Etienne. John Libbey Eurotext, Paris © 2000, pp. 47-49.

Oxidant signaling mechanisms initiated by low levels of arsenic in vascular cells

Aaron Barchowsky[1], Linda R. Klei[1], Karol R. Smith[1], and Christopher R. Ross[2]

[1] *Department of Pharmacology and Toxicology, Dartmouth Medical School, 7650 Remsen, Hanover, NH 03755;* and [2] *Department of Anatomy and Physiology, College of Veterinary Medicine, Kansas State University, Manhattan, KS 66506*

Chronic exposure to arsenite in drinking water has been associated with increased risk of cardiovascular and peripheral vascular diseases[1;2]. However, the mechanisms underlying this increased risk are unresolved. Previous work from this laboratory demonstrated that arsenite induced phenotypic change and proliferation in aortic endothelial cells by activating oxidant-sensitive cell signaling. To investigate the hypothesis that the plasma membrane NADPH oxidase complex is the primary source of the reactive oxygen stimulated by arsenite, this enzyme activity was measured in membranes isolated from control cells or cells exposed to 5 μM arsenite. A 1 h exposure to arsenite stimulated a two-fold increase in enzyme activity, relative to control. Immunodepletion of the NADPH oxidase p67^{phox} subunit abolished the arsenite-stimulated activity demonstrating the specificity of the response. The central role of NADPH activity and oxidant formation in arsenite-stimulated signaling cascades was demonstrated by disrupting the activity of the enzyme complex in intact cells with PR-39, a peptide that binds the NADPH oxidase p47^{phox} subunit, or by scavenging the H_2O_2 with catalase. Prior incubation of the cells with either PR-39 or catalase blocked arsenite-induced increases in tyrosine phosphorylation and translocation of the transcription factor NF-κB. These results indicate that activation of NADPH oxidase is a critical initial step in endothelial cell signaling following exposure to environmentally relevant levels of arsenite.

Introduction

Previous studies in this laboratory have demonstrated that exposure of vascular endothelial cells to levels of arsenite that can be found in artesian wells in the United States[3] increased reactive oxygen formation, oxidant-sensitive cell signaling, and gene induction[4-6]. This low level of oxidant formation was insufficient to active stress signaling pathways, but was sufficient to act as a buffer that prevented increased agonist-stimulated nitric oxide formation[5;6]. These data suggest mechanisms through which low level arsenite exposures can affect phenotypic change in vascular cells and disrupt the important role of the endothelium in maintaining normal vascular homeostasis. However, a key question that remained is how arsenite initiates formation of reactive oxygen. Use of pharmacologic inhibitors and examining the kinetics of oxidant release indicated that plasma membrane-bound NADPH oxidase was the primary source of arsenite-stimulated reactive oxygen formation[5;6]. The present studies confirm that endothelial cell NADPH oxidase activity is increased by arsenite and that the resultant oxidants formed are necessary and sufficient for arsenite-induced cell signaling and activation of transcription factors.

Methods

Cell culture: Primary porcine endothelial cells were isolated and cultured in gelatin-coated dishes according to methods established in this laboratory[6]. All cell exposures were conducted with post-confluent cells in the presence of 10% serum. Exposure of the cells and harvest of proteins for Western or electrophoretic mobility shift assays (EMSA) were as previously described[4;5].

NADPH oxidase activity assays: The NADPH oxidase activity in membranes isolated from control or arsenite-exposed cells was measured as superoxide-dependent lucigenin chemiluminescence, as previously described[7]. Briefly 35 μg of membrane protein and 400 μM lucigenin were added to wells of a 96 well luminometer plate. Oxidase assay buffer was added to a final volume of 250 μl and reactions were started by addition of 100 μM NADPH. Luminescence, measured in relative light units (RLU), was monitored during the initial minute of the assay. Antibody inhibition was determined by adding a 1:1000 dilution of either specific antibody to $p67^{phox}$ or non-specific rabbit IgG to the wells prior to adding NADPH.

Results and Discussion

Arsenite increases reactive oxygen generation by NADPH oxidase. To demonstrate that arsenite activates the endothelial cells NADPH oxidase, NADPH-dependent superoxide generation was measured in membranes isolated from control cells or cells exposed to 5 μM arsenite for 1 h. This level of arsenite caused a 2.1 ± 0.5 fold increase in enzyme activity relative to the non-treated controls. There was no activation of the enzyme if arsenite was added directly to the membrane preparation after isolation from the cells, suggesting that arsenite must signal for activation through effectors that are lost when the context of the cell is disrupted. Disruption of the NADPH complex *in vitro* by immunodepleting the p67phox subunit slightly decreased control activity and completely blocked arsenite-stimulated enzyme activity. This confirms NADPH oxidase as the source of the reactive oxygen stimulated by exposure of primary endothelial cells to arsenite.

NADPH oxidase-generated oxidants mediate arsenite-induced cell signaling. PR-39 is a natural peptide synthesized by neutrophils that inhibits assembly and activity of NAD(P)H oxidase of intact cells by binding the SH3 domain of $p47^{phox}$ subunit[8]. To examine the effect of disrupting the NADPH enzyme complex in the intact cells on downstream signaling events, post-confluent cells were incubated with 10 μM PR-39 for 45 minutes prior to adding arsenite (5 μM). After an additional 45 min incubation, total cell protein lysates were prepared. Western analysis with antibodies specific for phosphotyrosine demonstrated that PR-39 blocked arsenite-induced tyrosine phosphorylations (Fig 1A). Pre-treated with 200 U of catalase also inhibited arsenite-stimulated phosphorylation. Finally, EMSA of nuclear proteins isolated from control or arsenite-exposed cells and subsequent densitometric analysis of the resulting gels demonstrated that pre-treatment of the endothelial cells with PR-39 prevented arsenite-induced translocation of NF-κB to the nucleus and its binding to DNA (Fig. 1B). Together these data demonstrated that activation of NADPH oxidase is an essential initial step in the response of vascular cells to non-cytotoxic and environmentally relevant levels of arsenite.

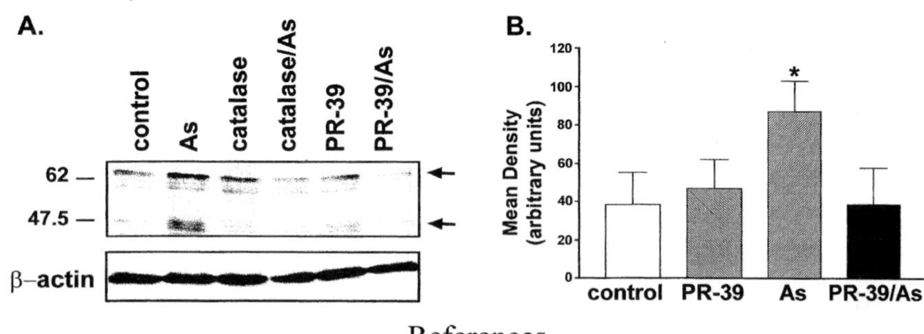

References

1. Engel RR, Smith AH. Arsenic in drinking water and mortality from vascular disease: an ecologic analysis in 30 counties in the United States. *Arch.Environ.Health.* 1994;49418-27.

2. Hertz-Picciotto I, Arrighi HM, Hu SW. Does arsenic exposure increase the risk for circulatory disease? *Am J Epidemiol* 2000;151(2):174-81.

3. Peters SC, Blum JD, Klaue B, Karagas MR. Arsenic occurence in New Hampshire groundwater. *Environ.Sci.Technol.* 1999;33:1328-1333.

4. Barchowsky A, Dudek EJ, Treadwell MD, Wetterhahn KE. Arsenic Induces Oxidant Stress And NF-KappaB Activation In Cultured Aortic Endothelial Cells. *Free Radic.Biol.Med.* 1996;21(6):783-90.

5. Barchowsky A, Roussel RR, Klei LR et al. Low Levels of Arsenic Trioxide Stimulate Proliferative Signals in Primary Vascular Cells without Activating Stress Effector Pathways. *Toxicol Appl Pharmacol* 1999;159(1):65-75.

6. Barchowsky A, Klei LR, Dudek EJ, Swartz HM, James PE. Stimulation of reactive oxygen, but not reactive nitrogen species, in vascular endothelial cells exposed to low levels of arsenite. *Free Radic Biol Med* 1999;271405-12.

7. Pagano PJ, Clark JK, Cifuentes-Pagano ME, Clark SM, Callis GM, Quinn M. Localization of a constitutively active, phagocyte-like NADPH oxidase in rabbit aortic adventitia: enhancement by angiotensin II. *Proc.Natl.Acad.Sci.U.S.A.* 1997;94(26):14483-88.

8. Shi J, Ross CR, Leto T, Blecha F. PR-39, a proline-rich antibacterial peptide that inhibits phagocyte NADPH oxidase activity by binding to Src homology 3 domains of $p47^{phox}$. *Proc.Natl.Acad.Sci.U.S.A.* 1996;936014-18.

Metal Ions in Biology and Medicine; vol 6. Eds. J.A. Centeno, Ph. Collery, G. Vernet, R.B. Finkelman, H. Gibb, J.C. Etienne. John Libbey Eurotext, Paris © 2000, pp. 50-52.

Upregulation of the glutathione-S-transferase, multidrug resistance, and multidrug resistance transporter genes in cells made tolerant to arsenic by chronic low-level exposure

Jie Liu[1], Hua Chen[1], Elizabeth Romach[1], David Miller[2], and Michael Waalkes[1]

[1] *Laboratory of Comparative Carcinogenesis, NCI at NIEHS; and* [2] *Laboratory of Pharmacology and Chemistry, NIEHS, Research Triangle Park, NC, USA*

Abstract. Chronic exposure of rat liver epithelial cells to arsenite produces self-tolerance to arsenicals, with a significant reduction in cellular arsenic (As) accumulation. In chronic As-exposed (CAsE) cells, the expression of glutathione *S*-transferase pi gene (GST) is markedly upregulated. The expression of multidrug resistance protein (Mrp2) and multidrug resistance gene (MDR) that encodes for the transporter P-glycoprotein (P-gp) are also increased, but to a lesser extent than the GST-pi gene. These CAsE cells showed cross-resistance to common anticancer drugs, such as cisplatin, vinblastine, adriamycin, and actinomycin D. These results demonstrate that chronic As exposure not only induces self-tolerance, but also induces cross-tolerance to important anticancer drugs. One of the mechanisms of the tolerance appears to be due to overexpression of GST, which may facilitate the formation of As-glutathione conjugates for efflux by increased Mrp2 and P-gp transporters.

Introduction. We have recently shown that chronic exposure of rat liver epithelial cells to low concentrations of arsenite (125-500 nM), concentrations relevant to environmental As contamination, resulted in malignant transformation of exposed cells which produced tumors capable of metastasis upon inoculation into Nude mice [1]. Global DNA hypomethylation and aberrant gene expression were associated with this As-induced malignant transformation. One of the important features in these chronic As-exposed (CAsE) cells is the development of self-tolerance to arsenicals (arsenite, arsenate, and dimethylarsinic acid), and cross-resistance to other metals, such as antimony, nickel, and cadmium [2].

There are several potential mechanisms for As-induced self-tolerance in these CAsE cells [2]. For instance, there is an increased As metabolism by methylation, and methylation is thought to be a detoxication pathway for inorganic As [2]. Also there is an enhanced inducibility of metallothionein, a protein known to be important in tolerance to other metals like cadmium [2]. However, the most dramatic change in these As-tolerant cells is the reduction of cellular As accumulation (to ~ 12% to that of control), with markedly increased As efflux [2]. Therefore, the current study was designed to further explore the mechanism(s) for the reduced cellular As accumulation in these CAsE cells, focusing on cellular glutathione *S*-transferase (GST) and transporter proteins.

Materials and Methods. The rat liver epithelial cell line TRL 1215 was exposed to arsenite-containing media (0, 125, 250 and 500 nM) for 24 weeks as previously described [1]. Cell monolayers at 70-80% confluence were used throughout. The Atlas cDNA expression microarray and RT-PCR analysis was performed using Clontech Atlas systems according to manufacture's instructions. Western-blot analysis was performed using monoclonal antibodies against Pgp (C219), GST (G172-1138) and rabbit polyclonal antibody against Mrp2. For defining anticancer drug resistance, 70% confluent cells were treated with various concentrations of As and anticancer drugs in triplicates. Cells were then incubated for additional 36 hrs and toxicity was determined using the MTT assay. Data were expressed as metabolic integrity using control as 100%.

Results. The Atlas cDNA expression array indicates the upregulation of the GST-pi (3-fold; Fig. 1), the MDR1 and the multidrug resistance protein gene (~2 fold). The increases in these genes were further confirmed with RT-PCR and Western-blot analysis (not shown).

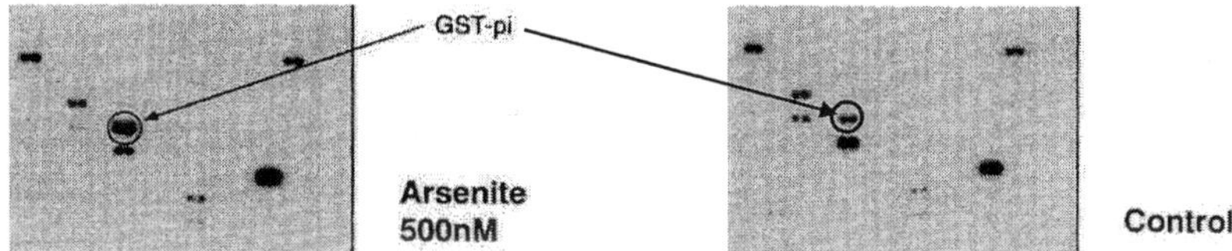

Figure 1. Microarray Analysis Showing Marked Upregulation of GST in CAsE cells.

As a result of increased transporter proteins, cellular As accumulation in CAsE cells was dramatically reduced over 24 hours (3.2 ng total As/10^6 in CAsE cells vs. 25 ng total As/10^6 in control cells). This resulted in increased LC_{50} values in CAsE cells for As as well as common cancer chemotherapeutics (Table 1).

Table 1. Cytotoxicity (LC_{50} in ng/ml) of arsenite and common chemotherapeutic agents in control and CAsE cells and ratios of CAsE/control values.

Agents	Control cells	CAsE	Ratios
Arsenite	2250	6370	2.83
Cisplatin	9000	48000	5.33
Adriamycin	3000	8500	2.83
Vinblastin	25000	95000	3.80
Actinomycin D	500	1350	2.70

Discussion. The results of the present study show that chronic As exposure induces a remarkable self-tolerance, probably associated with GST and transporter overexpression. The overexpression of GST likely plays an important role in acquired As tolerance and in the cross-tolerance to antineoplastic drugs. In As-resistant cells, an increase in GST expression has been reported [3, 4]. Increased GST may facilitate the formation of an As-GSH conjugate which appears to be the favored form for cellular efflux [3, 4]. In this regard, the majority of GS-X conjugates are effluxed by ATP-dependent transporters. This includes multidrug resistance proteins (Mrp), which play a major role in cellular efflux of GSH conjugates. In the present study, a clear upregulation of Mrp 2 protein was detected in microarray analysis, and confirmed by Northern and Western blot analysis, supporting the concept of a role in acquired As tolerance. Arsenite is also known to induce MDR1 gene in various cultured cells, consistent with the present study. Thus, the upregulation of the MDR1 may likewise play an important adaptive role in acquired As tolerance by helping pump As out of the cells.

Beyond issues in development of As resistance, there are important pharmacological implications from this study. The overexpression of GST and the transporter proteins detected in this study not only appear to function in As-induced self-tolerance, but also play important roles in the observed development of anticancer drugs resistance. The CAsE cells showed marked cross-resistant to cisplatin, adriamycin, vinblastin and actinomycin D. These transporter proteins and GST have previously been implicated in acquired resistance to cancer chemotheraputics. The increased expression of transport proteins and GST in CAsE cells has important clinical implications for the current revival of arsenicals as cancer chemotherapeutics.

In summary, the current study demonstrated that in CAsE cells GST-pi, multidrug resistance protein, and multidrug resistance gene encoded for p-glycoprotein, were markedly upregulated. The increases in GST, Mrp, and p-glycoprotein likely are important in acquired As self-tolerance, but also have important implications in cross-resistance to certain anticancer drugs.

REFERENCES:

1 Zhao CQ, Young MR, Diwan BA, Coogan TP, Waalkes MP. Association of arsenic-induced malignant transformation with DNA hypomethylation and aberrant gene expression. *Proc. Natl. Acad. Sci. USA*. 1997; 94 : 10907-10912.

2 Romach, EH, Zhao CQ, Del Razo LM, Cebrian ME, Waalkes MP. Studies on the mechanism of arsenic-induced self tolerance in liver epithelial cells through continuous low-level arsenite exposure. *Toxicol. Sci.* 2000; 54: in press.

3 Wang HF, Lee T-C. Glutathione S-transferase pi facilitates the excretion of arsenic from arsenic-resistant Chinese hamster ovary cells. *Biochem. Biophys. Res. Commun*. 1993; 192 : 1093-1099.

4 Wang Z, Dey S, Rosen BP, Rossman TG. Efflux-mediated resistance to arsenicals in arsenic-resistant and -hypersensitive Chinese hamster cells. *Toxicol. Appl. Pharmacol.* 1996; 137 : 112-119.

Metal Ions in Biology and Medicine; vol 6. Eds. J.A. Centeno, Ph. Collery, G. Vernet, R.B. Finkelman, H. Gibb, J.C. Etienne. John Libbey Eurotext, Paris © 2000, pp. 53-55.

The progress of study on endemic arsenism due to burning arsenic containing coal in Guizhou province

Zhang Aihua[1], Huang Xiaoxin[2], Jiang Xianyao[1], Luo Peng[1], Guo Yucheng[2] and Xue Shouzheng[3]

[1] Department of Toxicology, Guiyang Medical College, Guizhou 550004, China; [2] 44th Hospital of Chinese People's Liberation Army, Guizhou 550009, China; [3] Department of Toxicology, Shangai Medical University, SHanghai 200032, China

Introduction

Endemic arsenism in Guizhou province was caused by coal burning,over 2600 patients have been found since 1976 and population at risk was about 70000 now.The endemic was mainly focused in Jiao-le township,Xin-ren county.1548 cases were reported in 1991 and its percent of all patients in our province is 57.69[1].The existence of coal containing high arsenic was natural reason for arsenism occurring,while burning the coal resulted in food and air pollution made it prevalent as man-made reason.On the basis of epidemiologic research on endemic arsenism in our province, further research was took on the clinical signs、mechanism on causing poisoning、preventive and curative measures of arsenism in March 1998 and 1999.

Methods and subjects

Using cluster sampling and typical investigation,a spot research was took,while experimental indexes were determined by biochemical、genetic、molecular pathologic and toxicologic methods.Consulting the patients who were diagnosised in 1991 by Guizhou Provincial Office of Endemic Disease,we had the numbers of patients、non-patients in endemic area and controls were 200、20 and 60 cases respectively.

Results

1. Environmental arsenic exposure level

Tab Ⅰ Arsenic Content in Food and Environmental Mediator

Items	1999y		1998y		1997y		1991y		Control		Standard
	n	X±SD	n	X±SD	n	X±SD	n	X±SD	n	X±SD	
Hotpepper	13	50.12±37.90	8	45.07±101.6	8	134.9±205.0	35	512.0±300.4	19	0.45±0.19	Food<0.7
Corn	14	2.34± 0.98	8	2.64± 3.41	10	4.24±2.72	32	4.13± 2.76	19	0.37±0.22	
Rice	13	1.19±0.85							13	0.41±0.18	
Bacon	7	53.57±13.21	5	43.97±61.23					7	0.30±0.23	
Water	9	0.010±0.004	6	0.008±0.003			24	0.062±0.015	9	0.003±0.002	Water <0.05
Indoor air	12	0.086±0.028	10	0.088±0.061	8	0.101±0.165	18	0.46±0.30	22	0.0015±0.001	Indoor air <0.03
Out door air	25	0.021±0.007	13	0.022±0.011			4	0.020±0.027	25	0.0005±0.0004	Air <0.003
Soil	13	16.47±6.13	6	15.70±2.10			48	70.4±41.1	13	3.42±1.56	soil <40
Coal	13	368.8±125.6	7	397.2±230.3	35	606.9±1505.1	90	968.5±1024.1	20	3.64±3.03	Coal <45
Tobacco	7	0.42±0.31	4	0.39±0.22					7	0.25±0.15	

* unit of items: water(mg/L), air(mg/m^3), others(mg/kg)

Coal、indoor air、out door air and fried food As content in 1999 and 1998 were still higher than the standard.These suggested arsenic pollution still existed in environment[2].

2. Health effects of arsenic exposure

2.1 Clinical examination

Besides of the typical features of chronic arsenism(dermal hyperpigmentation、 depigmentation and hyperkeratosis),liver、kidney and nerve damages,irritation of respiratory tract were also noticed.The prevalence of hepatomegaly detected with ultrasonic examining was 21.32%.Abnormal features were 46.19%.Rate of thick shadow of lung markings on chest X-ray examination was 21.4%.Alteration of pulmonary function reached 82.2%.Micro circulation of eyes were also abnormal.Dermal histo-pathological examination were took in 70 intermediate、severe poisoning patients.2 cases squamous-cell carcinoma、1 basal-cell carcinoma and 15 cases bowen's disease were found.Malignant patients were all over 40 years old.Major pathological alteration,such as epidermis proliferation、thick cutin、more pigment、derma inflammation change and abnormal cell etc.

2.2 Experimental analysis

2.2.1 Arsenism condition and arsenic body burden

Tab. II Comparison of arsenism condition and As body burden in patients

Subject	n	Urinary arsenic(μg/L) Tot-As	In-As	In-As/Tot-As (%)	n	Hair arsenic (μg/g)
Control	53	45.62±15.71	7.19±4.21	16.27±7.68	45	1.55±1.16
Non-patients in local area	16	76.29±40.75**△	16.79±10.88**	25.18±16.78*	16	5.38±4.90**
Mild arsenism	45	121.14±110.28**△	23.25±20.26**	22.93±16.58**	46	6.72±6.11**
Intermediate arsenism	51	140.15±135.52**△	27.39±32.41**△	25.42±19.06**	48	7.48±6.97**
Severs arsenism	55	145.18±128.53**△	42.55±40.69**△△	31.74±19.06**	62	7.92±7.79**

* Compared with control: * P (0.05, ** P (0.01; Comparison of patients and non-patients: △P (0.05, △△ P (0.01

The concentration of arsenic in urine and hair of patients were higher than the control. The difference were prominently significant With the increase of urinary Tot-As、hair As、In-As/Tot-As in urine also gradually increased, which were coincide with arsenism poisoning[2].

2.2.2 Special experimental examinations

Meanwhile,the research of liver and kidney function、amino acid metabolism、oxidation damage were took.Most of them were abnormal.Such as serum HOP、GST、r-GT、Gly, urine β-sphere protein、creatinine and blood carbamide nitrogen were all much higher than that of the control,which meant liver and kidney function were hurt.But the damages of kidney function were lighter than that of liver.Activity of SOD、GST-Px and content of –SH decreased,while MDA content increased.They suggested that arsenic can destroy the balance of oxidation and anti-oxidation system, and it can induce the ability of anti-oxidation decreased[3].In cytogenetics and molecular genetics detection,we found arsenic pollution from coal-burning could increase SCE(sister chromosome exchange)、CA(chromosome aberration) and MN(micro nucleus) ratio, could induce blood DNA single strand breaks, WBC DNA-protein crosslinks(DPC),and it might make unscheduled DNA synthesis(UDS) increased and DNA spontaneous synthesis obviously decreased in patients.The results showed arsenic can hurt chromosome and DNA, and can restrain DNA synthesis and repair ability[4-6].In this study,we also found that dermal hyperkeratosis might be an indication of malignant change; cell proliferation、anti-apoptosis strengthen and abnormal alteration of $p53^{wt}$、P16、Cyclin D1,together affect dermal malignant changes;abnormal expression of oncogene and tumor suppressor might be an signal of malignant alternation.So its dynamic monitor will help early finding、curing and judging prognosis of dermal cancer[7].

It should be also taken notice:Non-patients in local area had no change in clinical routine examination,but in laboratory analysis,abnormal changes had been found.The results suggested that it has important practical significance to pay attention to non-patients and use corresponding monitor、prevention and curing measures to prevent or control disease happening and developing.

Conclusion

According to all kinds of evidence,including geography、epidemiologic research、clinical and experimental examination,we can make conclusions:

1. Coal containing high-arsenic was the direct reason of endemic arsenism in Guizhou province,totally prohibition digging and burning the coal is the key for eradicating new patients;Building stove with perfect chimney can decrease air pollution indoor, but it may caused second pollution out door,which can not be neglected; 2. The less developed economy、culture and scientific technology indirectly promoted arsenism occurring and developing; 3. Poly-organic and system damages were its clinical features,dermal cancer and liver cirrhosis were major sequels causing death;Dermal cancer occurred on the basis of hyperkeratosis.Ceasing arsenic coal-burning could avoid the new case,but could not stop the progress of already changed dermal and liver lesions; 4. Amino acid metabolism disorder、genetics and oxidation damage、abnormal expression of oncogene、tumor suppressor and protein all play important role during arsenism occurring and developing.

Several proposal

Considering the cumulated experiences for 20 years and our research results, we propose the successful set of preventive means should include:

1. Expedite developing of local economy、improve living condition of residents and popularize health education; 2. Government behavior combine individual action measure, totally prohibiting using high-As coal and get rid of environmental arsenic residues; 3. Examine arsenic content in coal sample before mining and burning it, local recommended limit is 45mg/kg; 4. Change the habit of drying food from heating through direct smoking, building drying room convey heat; 5. Build stove with perfect chimney, improving indoor ventilation especially in cold season; 6. Using sensitive monitor indexes to find patients early, closely dynamic monitor development of patients' condition so that it can be dealt with in time and reasonably; 7. Surgical removal of pre-malignant and malignant dermal lesions and reasonable therapy in vivo and vitro.

Acknowledgement and reference (omit)

Metal Ions in Biology and Medicine; vol 6. Eds. J.A. Centeno, Ph. Collery, G. Vernet, R.B. Finkelman, H. Gibb, J.C. Etienne. John Libbey Eurotext, Paris © 2000, pp. 56-58.

The mode of occurrence of arsenic in high arsenic coals from endemic arsenosis areas in Southwest Guizhou Province, China*

Zhenhua Ding[a], R.B. Finkelman[b], H.E. Belkin[b], Baoshan Zheng[a], Tiandou Hu[c], Yaning Xie[c]

[a] *State key laboratory on environmental geochemistry, institute of geochemistry, Chinese Academy of Sciences, Guiyang 550002, P.R. China;* [b] *956 MS, National center U.S. Geological Survey, Reston VA, 20192, USA;* [c] *BEPC NL, Beijing 100039, P.R. China*

Abstract

Some small coal-mines restricted in small areas have high arsenic content with the highest arsenic content up to 3.5 % in Southwest Guizhou Province, P. R. China, the use of high As-bearing coals has caused near 3,000 cases of arsenic poisoning limited to several villages[1]. Two coal samples were selected from this area, and were determined with sequential leaching experiment, and X-ray absorb fine structure (XASF). Analytical results of leaching experiment showed that more than 50 % of arsenic stayed in residual solid. XAFS showed that arsenic mainly exists in the form of As^{5+}. Combining with the previous work[2], we infer that As in high As coals mainly occurs in the form of As^{5+} combined with organic.

Key word: high As coals, modes of occurrence, Guizhou Province.

1. Introduction

The most serious case of endemic arsenosis caused by domestic coal combustion occurs in the southwest Guizhou Province, China where the local people use high As-coals. The modes of occurrence of arsenic in coals is very important for human being to understand its environmental and health effects, and its real geological significance.[3] It is generally believed that arsenic exists in the form of sulfide in coals,[4-6] but the case of southwest Guizhou is different.

*This work was supported by Natural Science Foundation of China (49873007), key project of the Chinese Academy of Sciences, the venture capitol Foundation (USGS) and partially supported by BEPC NL.

We have conducted laboratory examination of the coals using sequential leaching experiment and XAFS. Combined with the previous work, this paper describes the mode of occurrence of arsenic in the arsenic-rich coals.

2. Samples and methods

Ding et al (1999)[3] and Zheng et al (1999)[7] described geological properties of this area. All these high arsenic coals are anthracitic. Two samples were analyzed for this study. Sample HZ-9 is from Anlong County, J25 from Xingren County.

The sequential leaching procedure used in this study is similar to that described by Palmer et al. (1993)[8]. XAFS for raw and the final residual solid of sequential leaching is used to determine the mode of occurrence of arsenic in coals.

3. Results

The result of sequential leaching is illustrated in figure1. It shows that much arsenic is related to silicates, and that at least 50% arsenic cannot be leached. It also demonstrates that much iron exists in the form of sulfides and oxides.

XAFS indicates most arsenic occurs in the form of As^{5+}. It is the same as what we got before[2].

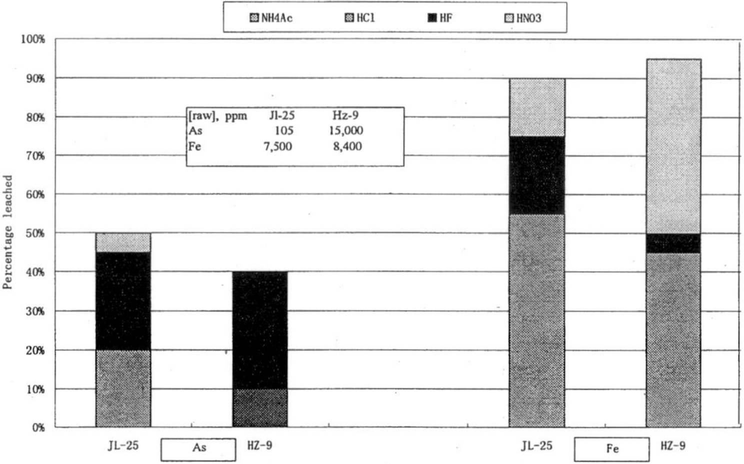

Figure 1 percentage leached for arsenic and iron.

4.Conclusion

Although some As-bearing minerals such as pyrite, arsenopyrite, realgar (?), As-bearing sulfate, and As-bearing clays are found in the high arsenic coals, their contents do not account for the abundance of arsenic in coals. The observation of SEM-EDX (scanning electron microscopy with energy dispersive X-ray analyzer) and TEM (transmission electron microscopy) rules out the possibility of finely dispersed arseno-pyrite or As-bearing pyrite as the origin of the As[2]. Combining the results of sequential leaching and XAFS, we inferred that arsenic in high arsenic coals from Southwest Guizhou Province mainly exists in the form of As^{+5}combined with organisms.

Due to complication of study procedure, many difficulties in identifying and interpreting the results, very few researchers studied the organic mode of the occurrence of trace elements in coals. However it is important to recognize the geochemical behavior of trace elements, the impact of As and organic in the formation of impregnated gold deposits. Much work is yet to be done on the origin and enrichment of arsenic in coals.

Acknowledgement

We wish to thank Drs. Curtis Palmer, Stan Mroczkowski, and Allan Kolker of USGS for their help.

References

1 Belkin H E, Zheng B-S, Finkelman R B. Geochemistry of Coals Causing Arsenism in Southwest China. U.S. Geological Survey Open File Report (97-496) 1997; 4th International Symposium on Environmental Geochemistry, p10.

2 Ding Z- H, Zheng B-S, Zhang J, Belkin H, Finkelman R B, Zhao F H, Zhou D X, Zhou Y S, Chen C G. Preliminary study on the mode of occurrence of arsenic in high arsenic coals from southwest Guizhou Province. Since in China (series D) 1999, 42: 655--61.

3 Finkelman R B. Modes of Occurrences of Trace Elements in Coals. USGS. Open File Report (OFR—81—99) 1981.

4 Bouska V. Geochemistry of Coal. Prague: Academia. 1981.

5 Coleman S L, Bragg L J. Distribution and mode of occurrence of arsenic in coal. In: Chyi L L, and Chou C.-L. ed. Recent Advances in Coal Geochemistry, special paper of the Geological Society of American. 1990, 248: 13-34.

6 Swaine D J. Trace elements in coal. London: Butterworths. 1990.

7 Zheng B-S, Ding, Z- H, Huang R-G, Zhu J-M, Yu X-Y, Wang A-M, Zhou D-X, Mao D-J, Su H-C. Issues of health and disease relating to Coal use in Southwestern China. International Journal of Coal Geology 1999; 40: 119—132.

8 Palmer C A, Krasnow M R, Finkelman R B, D'Angelo W M. An evaluation of leaching to determine modes of occurrence of selected toxic elements in coal. J.Coal Quality 1993; 12: 135—141.

Metal Ions in Biology and Medicine; vol 6. Eds. J.A. Centeno, Ph. Collery, G. Vernet, R.B. Finkelman, H. Gibb, J.C. Etienne. John Libbey Eurotext, Paris © 2000, pp. 59-61.

Exposure to arsenic from soils and dusts in old mining and smelting areas in SW England

Margaret E. Farago[1], Peter J. Kavanagh[1], Iain Thornton[1], Mahmoud Hassanien[2]

[1] Environmental Geochemistry Research Group, The T H Huxley School of Environment, Earth Science and Engineering, Imperial College of Science Technology and Medicine, Royal School of Mines, London SW7 2BP, UK; [2] "Béla Johan" National Institute of Public Health, Gyálí út 2-6, 1097, Budapest, Hungary

The south-western peninsula of England (the South West) consists of the counties of Cornwall to the west, and Devon. The River Tamar forms the boundary between the two counties. This area is extensively contaminated with heavy metals from centuries of mining activity in the region. From about 1860 to 1900, it was the world's major producer of arsenic. These activities have left a legacy of contaminated land, with As- and Cu-rich mine tailings and other wastes, with some 700 km^2 of land affected [1]. Most of the contaminated area is agricultural with villages and small towns; urban development has sometimes taken place on contaminated land. Sources of arsenic in the region and some aspects of the exposure of local populations have been discussed [2]- [4].

On the east (Devon) side of the R. Tamar lies the abandoned Devon Great Consols Mine (DGC), where mining and smelting was carried out. A small number of houses exist on the DGC Mine, close to the abandoned waste tips. On the other (Cornwall) side of the river is the village of Gunnislake, also in close proximity to abandoned waste sites. Dwellings were investigated, from Gunnislake, DGC and Cargreen villages. The last was taken as a control area, being further down the river and away from past mining activities.

A survey of top soils in the area (Table I) demonstrated that the As contamination is very high. The garden soils house dusts and As in urine was investigated for a number of residences in Gunnislake, DCG and Cargreen. The results are shown in Tables II and III. Two methods were used to assess the intake and possible risk to the populations. Firstly, the intakes of inorganic As using published dietary intake, measurement of As in drinking water and an estimation of mean intake from dusts and soils from the houses (Table II). For a child living in the contaminated area, this gave an estimated intake: from soil and dust, 29 μg/day; from food, 11 μg/day; from water, 0.4 μg/day; giving a total intake of about 40 μg/day. Table III shows that the mean urine concentration is 16 μg/g creatinine, assuming an excretion of 1g of cratinine/day, then the daily output is 16 μg. If this represents 40-60% of intake, then the mean intake by a child is ~30-40 μg/day., in reasonable agreement with the estimation. Such as intake would be above the WHO recommended limit of 2 μg/day/kgBW.

Table I. Ranges and geometric means (GM) of concentrations (μg/g) of As in top soils from the Tamar Valley area (ref [5]).

	Range	GM	Mean	N
Cargreen	16-198	37	47	18
Devon Great Consols (DGC)	173-52600	2557	9894	21
Gunnislake Village and surrounding area (excluding GDC)	50-26485	282	819	118

Table II. As (μg/g) in garden soils and housedusts in the Tamar Valley

			Soils			Dusts
Site	N	GM	Range	N	Mean	Range
Gunnislake	71	365	120-1695	9	217	33-1160[a]
DGC	15[b]	4499	345-52600	13	1167	24-3740
Cargreen	18	37	16-198	4	49	20-114

[a]Outlying value of 16700 μg/g ignored; [b]Some samples contain mine wastes.

Table III. Total As (As_i + DMAA + MMAA) concentrations in urine in children and in adults

Total As μg/g creatinine	Cargreen Children N= 4	Gunnislake + DGC Children N= 8	Cargreen Adults N= 3	Gunnislake + DGC Adults N= 16
Mean	5.32	16.36	3.28	12.4
SD	0.07	17.71	1.01	12.50
Median	5.32	11.41	2.95	8.28
Min	5.27	2.65	2.48	5.5
Max	5.37	58.95	4.41	47.3

The second approach used the programme Risk Assistant and the values of As in soils shown in Table I, to calculate the Lifetime Daily Average Dose and the adjusted inhaled concentration. The resulting Hazard Quotient (HQ) in the different areas is shown in Table IV. Table V and VI show the risk estimates and the total risks respectively in the areas investigated.

Table IV. Hazard Quotients (HQ) in the different investigated areas

Area	H.Q.*			
	Child		Adult	
	Mean[1]	Max[2]	Mean[1]	Max[2]
Cargreen, control site	0.91	4.87	0.07	0.36
Great Devon Consols Mine site	79.0	924	5.87	68.6
Gunnislake Village and surrounding areas	6.4	29.7	0.50	2.2

* H.Q> 1→ adverse health effect would be expected and requires actions
[1] Mean soil concentration; [2] Max soil concentration

Table V. Risk estimates in different investigated areas

Area	Risk*(oral)			
	Child		Adult	
	Mean[1]	Max[2]	Mean[1]	Max[2]
Cargreen, control site	4E-5	2E-4	1E-5	7E-5
Great Devon Consols Mine site	3E-3	4E-2	1E-3	1E-2
Gunnislake Village and surrounding areas	2E-4	1E-3	9E-5	4E-4
Area	Risk*(inhalation)			
	Child		Adult	
	Mean[1]	Max[2]	Mean[1]	Max[2]
Cargreen, control site	3E-6	1E-5	3E-6	2E-5
Great Devon Consols Mine site	2E-4	3E-3	3E-4	3E-3
Gunnislake Village and surrounding areas	2E-5	9E-5	2E-5	1E-4

* Risk: Individual probability of getting cancer from this exposure
[1] Mean soil concentration; [2] Max soil concentration

Table VI. Total risks* in the investigated areas

Area	Child		Adult	
	Mean[1]	Max[2]	Mean[1]	Max[2]
Cargreen, control site	4E-5	2E-4	2E-5	9E-5
Great Devon Consols Mine site	3E-3	4E-2	1E-3	2E-2
Gunnislake Village and surrounding areas	3E-4	1E-3	1E-4	5E-4

* Total risks from oral and inhalation [1] Mean soil concentration; [2] Max soil concentration

References

[1]Abrahams, P., Thornton, I., 1987, Distribution and extent of land contaminated by arsenic and associated metals in mining regions of south west England. *Transactionsof the Institute of Mining and Metallurgy (Sheet B: Applied Earth Science)*, 6, B1-B8.

[2] Farago, M.E., Thornton, I., Kavanagh, P., Elliott, P., Leonardi, G., 1997, Health aspects of human exposure to high arsenic concentrations in soil in south-west England, In: *Arsenic; exposure and health effects,* C.O. Abernathy, W.R. R.L. Calderon, W.R Chappell, (eds), 1997,Chapman and Hall, London, pp. 191-209.

[3] Kavanagh, P., Farago, M.E., Thornton, I., Goessler, W., Kuehnelt, D., Schlagenhaufen, C., Irgolic, K.J.,1998, Urinary Arsenic Species in Devon and Cornwall Residents, UK. *The Analyst*, 123(1); 27-30.

[4] Farago, M.E., Kavanagh. P. 1999. High arsenic-containing soils in SW England and human exposure. In: Geochemistry of the Earth's Surface (Ed. H.Armannsson), Balkema, Rotterdam, 181-184.

Metal Ions in Biology and Medicine; vol 6. Eds. J.A. Centeno, Ph. Collery, G. Vernet, R.B. Finkelman, H. Gibb, J.C. Etienne. John Libbey Eurotext, Paris © 2000, pp. 62-64.

Direct and *in situ* speciation of arsenic in microbian mats using X-ray absorption spectroscopy

A.L. Foster, R.A. Ashley, and J.J. Rytuba

U.S. Geological Survey Mineral Resource Program, 345 Middlefield Rd., Menlo Park, CA, 94025-3591 USA

Introduction. The ability of microorganisms and plants to sequester toxic metals and degrade organic compounds is well known. Most studies to date have employed model microorganisms in laboratory studies, but this study examines the uptake of arsenic by natural microbial mats from field settings. Here we report data from 2 sites near the Lava Cap mine complex (Nevada City, CA): one (site 1) where water quality was altered by a mine tailings dam failure in December 1997, and the other (site 2) where seepage from As-bearing tailings has controlled water quality for many years. We used x-ray absorption fine structure spectroscopy (XAFS), an element-specific method, to identify and quantify the arsenic species present in microbial mats. These analyses, coupled with data from mat and water samples, indicate that the mats are very efficient scavengers of arsenic, and that arsenic is primarily associated with precipitated Fe(III) hydroxides that bind the mat together.

Site Characterization, Sampling, and Analysis. Site 1 is a small pond (4-6 feet deep) formed in a tailings delta just below the confluence of Clipper and Little Clipper creeks (Fig. 1). Site 1 water is As(V)-rich, Fe(II)-poor, slightly basic, and contains particulate As (Table 1). A dark-brown mat at the sediment-water interface was collected in a sterile syringe, and placed on ice for transport back to the laboratory. Site 2 is a creek fed by water seeping underneath a second, still-intact tailings dam (Fig. 1). Site 2 water is As(V)-poor, Fe(II)-rich, near-neutral, and contains little particulate As (Table 1). Each summer, an extensive (> 250 ft long, 2-5 ft wide) and thick (up to 6 inches) mat of Fe oxidizing bacteria covers the creek, forming pillowy masses suspended in the water column. We collected the rust-brown mat sample in an acid-washed non-sterile glass jar, and placed it on ice for transport. In the laboratory, samples were stored as collected at 4° C until further analysis.

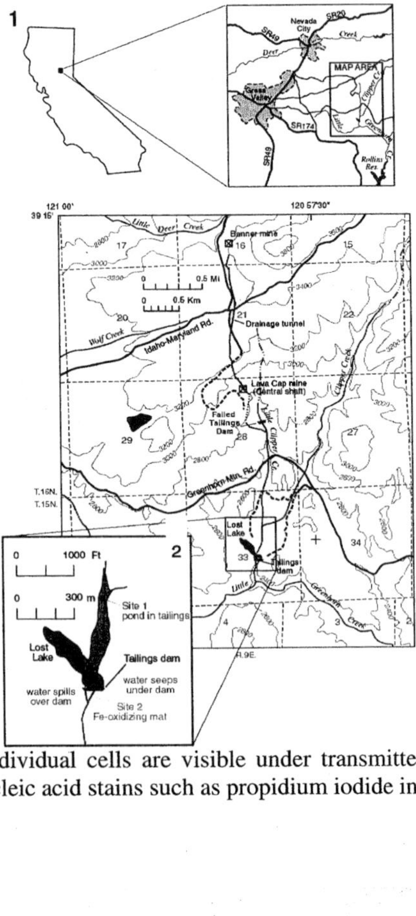

All water samples were collected by sterile syringe, filtered through 0.45 μm, and acidified with ultrapure HNO_3 (for As determinations) or HCL (for Fe determinations).

Characterization of Site 2 Microbial Mat. The total As concentration of oven-dried Site 2 mat material was 5140 mg/kg as determined by ICP-AES after mixed acid digestion, an amount far in excess of the dissolved arsenic concentrations previously measured at this site (Table 1). Unadulterated mat material and formaldehyde-treated, dehydrated mat material were examined with transmitted and epifluoresence light microscopy, respectively. Unadulterated mat material appears under the light microscope as tube-like structures mixed with Fe hydroxide precipitate. Few individual cells are visible under transmitted light. The dehydrated mat was hybridized with several nucleic acid stains such as propidium iodide in

approximately 500 nm in diameter (6b) and chains of cocci or balls < 100 nm wide. It is not known whether the smallest structures represent encrusted bacteria or a growth habit of Fe-oxyhydroxide.

Arsenic Speciation in Microbial Mats. Extended x-ray absorption fine structure spectra of microbial mat material from site 2 is compared with the spectrum of a synthetic sample of arsenic sorbed on Fe-oxyhydroxide in Fig. 4a. Phase-uncorrected Fourier transforms (solid lines) and the non-linear least squares fits (dotted lines) are plotted in Fig. 4b. The mat spectra from Site 1 are not shown because the results are identical to those shown here. The *L. ochracea* mat (site 2) EXAFS spectrum and Fourier transform are qualitatively and quantitatively very similar to those of the model As(V) sorption sample. The fits verify that As in the mat at site 2 and the other mats collected at site 1 is adsorbed to Fe-oxyhydroxide. The predominant sorption complex is a bidentate species composed of 1.5-2.0 Fe atoms at an average distance of 3.30 ±0.02 Å (see model in Fig. 4 b), but we could also fit a minor component of < 0.5 Fe at 2.81-2.89 ±0.02 Å that may represent a monodentate, edge-sharing sorption complex, as has previously been suggested [3].

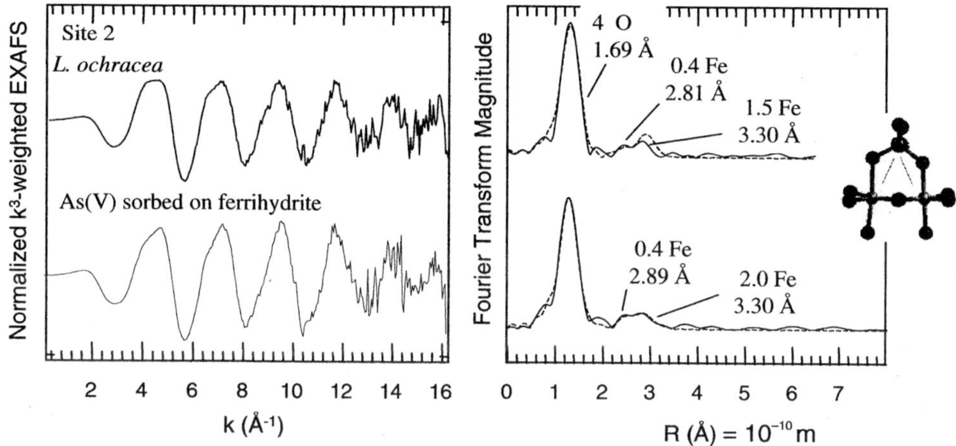

Discussion and Conclusions. The fate of arsenic associated with these mats is not well understood. In particular, the site 2 mat has the potential to release arsenic accumulated during the dry season during winter storm events, when it is almost completely washed away. Dissolution of Fe-oxyhydroxides could lead to the release of mat-associated As. EXAFS spectroscopy indicated that As(V) appears to be the sole accumulated species in the mats, to the limits of detection, but chemical analsyses show that As(III) is the predominant dissolved species at Site 2. We hypothesize that pH is the governing factor in the lack of As(III) accumulation, because laboratory studies suggest low sorption of this ion on mineral surfaces below pH 7 [4]. The EXAFS spectral signature of As(V) sorbed to biogenic Fe-oxyhydroxide is indistinguishable from As(V) sorbed to synthetic Fe-oxyhydroxide, and indicates contributions from bidentate corner-sharing and possibly from mondentate edge-sharing sorbed As(V).

References.

1. van Vleen W L, Mulder E G, Deinema M H. The *Sphaerotilus-Leptothrix* group of bacteria. *Microbio Rev* 1978 ; 42 : 329-56.
2. Emerson D, Revsbech N P. Investigation of an iron-oxidizing microbial mat community located near Aarhus, Denmark: Field studies. *Appl Env Microbiol* 1994 ; 60 : 4022-31.
3. Manceau A. The mechanism of anion adsorption on iron oxides: Evidence for the binding of arsenate tetrahedral on free $Fe(O,OH)_6$ edges. *Geochim Cosmochim Acta* 1995 ; 59 ; 3647-53.
4. Manning B A, Goldberg S. Adsorption and stability of arsenic(III) at the clay mineral-water interface. *Environ Sci Tech* 1997 ; 31 : 2005-11.

Table 1. Representative Analyses of Water from Site 1 and Site 2.

Site	Date	pH	C	As(III)	As(V)	Filtered As	Particulate As	Fe(III)	Fe(II)
			µS	µg/l			µg/l	mg/l	
1	3/24/99	7.84	372	3.1	437	471	239	7.6	< 2.4
	8/24/99	8.12	362	6.1	1334	987	98	4.1	4.4
2	3/24/99*	6.19	62	0.8	0.3			< 2.4	52.5
	8/24/99	6.51	88	97.2	< 0.006			5500	30
Analysis Method				HG-CT-AAS		ICP-MS		Ferrozine	

* the concentration of As and Fe are lower than previous analyses, which we believe reflects dilution by water flowing over the intact tailings dam (see Fig. 1).

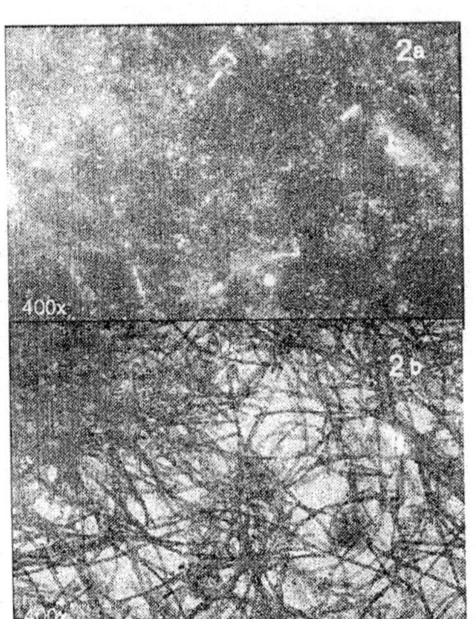

order to render the individual bacteria visible, as seen in Fig. 2a. When the light microscope image is superimposed on the epifluorescent image (Fig. 3b), the spatial relationships between individuals, sheaths, and Fe-oxyhydroxide can be observed. Most of the bacterial sheaths are empty, although some of the sheaths are partially occupied by rod-shaped organisms that appear to grow in pairs. Most of the visible bacteria are much smaller and inhabit the Fe-oxyhydroxide material that is either unassociated with the sheaths or that coats the sheaths (Fig. 2b). In some images filaments of sheathed inhabitants could be observed, and other images showed that empty sheaths were occasionally colonized by alien bacteria (not shown).

According to van Veen et al. [1] the *Sphaerotilus-Lepthothrix* genus of Eubacteria are the most common sheath-forming bacteria found in nutrient-poor (oligotrophic) environments, such as the creek at Site 2. This group is composed of gram-negative, obligately aerobic heterotrophs. *L. ochracea* is the probably the most common Fe-storing sheathed bacterium in the group [1], but has proven difficult to isolate in the laboratory [2]. Several characteristics allow us to tentatively identify the sheath-forming bacterium at site 2 as *L. ochracea* : (1) over 90 % of sheaths are empty, (2) the sheaths are smooth, giving rise to a characteristic "empty drinking straw" morphology, and (3) many of the sheaths are broken, suggesting that they are brittle. These physiological attributes have also been used by other authors to distinguish *L. ochracea* from other members of the *Sphaerotilus-Leptothrix* group, but phylogenetic analysis is needed for unambiguous identification.

Scanning Electron Microscopy (SEM) images show variable sheath encrustation (presumably a reflection of sheath age) (Fig. 3a). Smaller, less common sheaths are also visible in this image and may belong to one of the other members of the *Spaerotilus-Leptothrix* group. Detailed examination of the iron oxyhydroxide mat encrusting one of the sheaths reveals the presence of bacterial-like structures

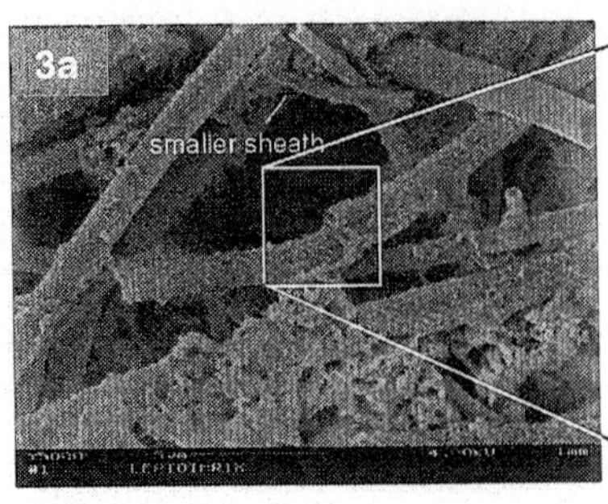

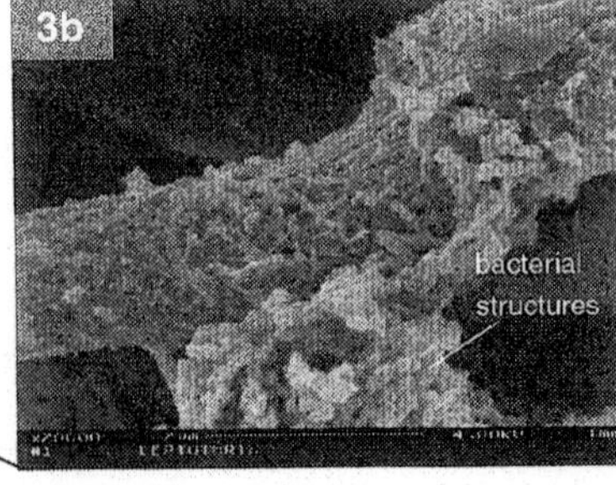

Metal Ions in Biology and Medicine; vol 6. Eds. J.A. Centeno, Ph. Collery, G. Vernet, R.B. Finkelman, H. Gibb, J.C. Etienne. John Libbey Eurotext, Paris © 2000, pp. 65.

Biliary and urinary excretion of inorganic arsenic. Identification of methylarsonous acid (MAsIII) as a major biliary metabolite in rats

Z. Gregus, A. Gyurasics, and I. Csanaky

Department of Pharmacology and Pharmacotherapy, University Medical School of Pécs, H-7643 Pécs, Hungary

In rats exposed to arsenite (AsIII) or arsenate (AsV), the biliary excretion of arsenic depends absolutely on hepatic glutathione availability and is accompanied by a large increase in the biliary output of glutathione (Gyurasics et al., Biochem. Pharmacol. 41: 937, 1991; 42: 465, 1991), suggesting that both AsIII and AsV are transported into bile in thiol-reactive trivalent forms, purportedly as unstable glutathione complexes. To test this hypothesis, the bile and urine of bile duct-cannulated rats injected with AsIII or AsV (50 µmol/kg, i.v.) were collected periodically for two hours and analyzed for arsenic metabolites by HPLC-hydride generation-atomic fluorescence spectrometry. Arsenic was excreted predominantly into bile in AsIII-injected rats, but into urine in the AsV-exposed rats. Injected AsIII was excreted in urine practically unchanged, whereas both AsV and AsIII appeared in urine after administration of AsV. Irrespective of the arsenical administered, the bile contained two main arsenic species, namely AsIII and a hitherto unidentified As metabolite. Formation of this metabolite could be antagonized by pretreatment of rats with the methylation inhibitor periodate-oxidized adenosine, indicating that it is a methylated arsenic compound. This metabolite could be converted in vitro into methylarsonic acid (MAsV) by oxidation, whereas synthetic MAsV could be converted into the unknown metabolite by reduction. Consequently, this biliary metabolite of both AsIII and AsV is MAsIII, a long hypothesized, but never identified, intermedier in the biotransformation of AsIII and AsV. Although MAsIII is thought to be formed from an oxidized precursor, rats injected with MAsV did not excrete MAsIII. In summary, the inorganic arsenicals investigated are transported into bile exclusively in trivalent forms, namely as AsIII and MAsIII, but are excreted in urine in both tri- and pentavalent forms. Identification of MAsIII is signified by the fact that this metabolite is more toxic than AsIII and AsV and thus formation of MAsIII represents toxification of inorganic arsenic.

Metal Ions in Biology and Medicine; vol 6. Eds. J.A. Centeno, Ph. Collery, G. Vernet, R.B. Finkelman, H. Gibb, J.C. Etienne. John Libbey Eurotext, Paris © 2000, pp. 66-68.

Arsenic (III) and chromium (VI) alter glucocorticoid receptor (GR) function and GR-dependent gene regulation

Joshua W. Hamilton, Ronald C. Kaltreider, Alisa M. Davis and Rahshaana A. Green

Department of Pharmacology and Toxicology, Dartmouth Medical School, Hanover NH 03755-3835

Abstract. The effects of arsenic(III) and chromium(VI) on glucocorticoid receptor (GR) function and GR-dependent gene expression were examined in H4IIE rat hepatoma cells. Completely non-cytotoxic treatments with As(III) (3.3 μM) or chromium(VI) (5 μM) decreased both basal and dexamethasone (Dex)-induced expression of transiently transfected luciferase constructs containing an intact hormone-responsive promoter from the mammalian PEPCK gene containing two tandem glucocorticoid response elements (GREs). Arsenic suppressed Dex-inducible expression of a promoter containing two tandem GREs alone, whereas chromium synergistically increased Dex-inducible expression. Western blotting and confocal microscopy of a green fluorescent protein (GFP) tagged-GR fusion protein demonstrated that arsenic or chromium did not significantly alter GR cytoplasmic localization, and pretreatment with either metal did not block the normal Dex-induced nuclear translocation of GR. Therefore, the alteration in GR-dependent gene expression by arsenic and chromium does not appear to be a result of decreased hormone-GR binding or hormone-induced GR activation and nuclear translocation, but rather involves metal-induced changes in the nuclear function of GR as a transcription factor.

Introduction. Chronic human exposures to non-overtly toxic doses of arsenic(III) or chromium(VI) are associated with increased risks of certain cancers. Occupational exposure to either metal is associated with increased risk of lung cancer, and environmental exposure to arsenic is associated with increased risk of lung, skin and bladder cancer [1,2]. The precise mechanisms by which arsenic and chromium may act as human carcinogens are not well understood. Previous studies in our laboratory had demonstrated that single, low dose As(III) or Cr(VI) treatments had profound effects on expression of several inducible genes, including the hormone-regulated phosphoenolpyruvate carboxykinase (PEPCK) gene, in both whole animal and cell culture systems [3]. The effects of each metal on both basal and hormone-inducible PEPCK expression were strongly associated with the glucocorticoid receptor (GR)-mediated regulatory pathway. We therefore specifically examined the effects of low dose As(III) and Cr(VI) treatments on the biochemical function of GR in hormone-responsive rat hepatoma H4IIE cells.

Results and Discussion. Previous experiments had demonstrated that treatment of rat hepatoma H4IIE cells with a single dose of either 3.3 μM As(III) or 10 μM Cr(VI) for 4 hr had little or no effect on cell viability as determined by a colony formation assay [3]. These non-cytotoxic As(III) or Cr(VI) treatments were then used, alone or in combination with 0.05 μM Dex treatments, to examine basal and hormone-inducible expression of several model genetic constructs that were based on the PEPCK hormone-inducible promoter. Arsenic and chromium each significantly altered both basal and Dex-inducible expression of the native rat PEPCK gene in H4IIE cells. Arsenic and chromium also suppressed both basal and Dex-inducible expression of a transiently transfected luciferase constructs under the transcriptional control of the proximal 600 bp of the rat PEPCK promoter which contains two tandem glucocorticoid response elements (GREs) as well as a number of other transcription factor binding sites. This 600 bp promoter construct had previously been shown to demonstrate hormone- and tissue-specific regulation of transgenes in a manner similar to that of the native gene [4]. We then examined a reporter construct under the control of a promoter containing only two tandem GREs. Arsenic also suppressed both basal and Dex-inducible expression of this construct, suggesting that its effects on the intact PEPCK promoter might largely be mediated through the GR pathway. Surprisingly, chromium had no effect on the basal expression of this transgene, while it synergistically increased its Dex-inducible expression, suggesting that, while the GR pathway is also a target for chromium effects, other transcription factors and/or elements within the PEPCK promoter contribute to the overall suppression of native basal and Dex-inducible PEPCK expression by chromium.

Previously, it had been reported that 10 μM or higher arsenic treatment of GR *in vitro* inhibited hormone binding to GR [5] , whereas treatment of cells with 100-200 μM arsenic, which is heat-shock mimetic, caused a translocation of GR to the nucleus independent of hormone[6]. However, when we examined subcellular distribution of GR in H4IIE cells treated with our lower doses of arsenic or chromium which altered PEPCK and PEPCK-luciferase expression, we observed little or no effect on GR localization, which was predominantly cytosolic in control and metal-treated cells and predominantly nuclear in Dex-treated cells with or without metal pre-treatment. To further confirm this, we used confocal microscopy to examine the effects of arsenic and chromium on translocation of a green fluorescent protein (GFP)-tagged GR fusion protein to the nucleus in intact transfected H4IIE cells. The GFP-GR chimeric protein had previously been shown to bind hormone and translocate to the nucleus in a manner identical to native GR [7]. We observed that GFP-GR was predominantly cytosolic in untreated cells, and arsenic and chromium treatments had no effect on GR localization. Dex treatment alone caused an almost total translocation of GFP-GR to the nucleus, and pre-treatment of cells with arsenic or chromium had no apparent effect on this translocation. These results indicate that arsenic and chromium do not significantly alter glucocorticoid binding to GR or its ability to be activated or to translocate to the nucleus. This further indicates that the effects of these metals on GR-mediated gene regulation involve an alteration in its ability to act as a nuclear transciption factor following translocation. Whether this involves alterations in DNA binding, interaction with other proteins or other mechanisms remains to be determined.

Arsenic- and chromium-induced alterations in GR function may play an important role in their mechanism of carcinogenesis. Glucocorticoids have long been known to suppress tumor promotion in the mouse two-stage skin cancer model [8]. This appears to be primarily a result of glucocorticoid-mediated effects on both cell differentiation and suppression of cell proliferation [8]. A progressive loss of hormone responsiveness was observed in later stages of skin cancer in this model, which was associated with both decreased GR expression and altered GR function. Similarly, it has also been shown that mouse lung tumor development can be blocked by glucocorticoids [9,10] . These results suggest that GR mediates suppression of tumor promotion in skin and lung and that down-regulation of GR is permissive to tumor growth. Thus, if chronic exposure to arsenic or chromium is able to alter the normal function of GR as a mediator of gene regulation, as suggested by our results, we hypothesize that this may contribute to its ability to promote tumorigenesis. This unique mechanism would further suggest that arsenic and chromium may be able to act synergistically with other carcinogenic agents such as cigarette smoke to increase cancer risk, which is supported by the epidemiological data (Supported by the Dartmouth Superfund Basic Research Program Project: EPA, NIH-NIEHS ES07373).

References

1. Hamilton JW, Wetterhahn, KE. Chromium. In: Seiler HG, Sigel H, eds. *Handbook on Toxicity of Inorganic Compounds*, New York, NY, Marcel Dekker, Inc., 1987:239-250
2. Bencko V. Arsenic. In: Fishbein L et al., eds. *Genotoxic and Carcinogenic Metals: Environmental and Occupational Occurrence and Exposure*, Princeton NJ: Princeton Sci. Publishing, 1987:1-30
3. Hamilton JW, Kaltreider RC, Bajenova OV, Ihnat MA, McCaffrey J, Turpie BW, Rowell EE, Oh J, Nemeth MJ, Pesce CA, Lariviere JP. Molecular basis for effects of carcinogenic heavy metals on inducible gene expression. *Environ. Hlth. Perspect.* 1998; **106**:1005-1015
4. Imai E, Miner JN, Mitchell JA, Yamamoto KR, Granner DK. Glucocorticoid receptor-cAMP response element-binding protein interaction and the response of the phosphoenolpyruvate carboxykinase gene to glucocorticoids. *J. Biol. Chem.* 1993; **268**:5353-5356
5. Simons SS Jr, Chakraborti PK, Cavanaugh AH. Arsenite and cadmium(II) as probes of glucocorticoid receptor structure and function. *J. Biol. Chem.* 1990; **265**:1938-1945
6. Sanchez ER. Heat shock induces translocation to the nucleus of the unliganded glucocorticoid receptor. *J. Biol. Chem.* 1992; **267**:17-20
7. Carey KL, Richards SA, Lounsbury KM, Macara IG. Evidence using a green fluorescent protein-glucocorticoid receptor chimera that the Ran/TC4 GTPase mediates an essential function independent of nuclear protein import. *J. Cell Biol.* 1996; **133**:985-996
8. Slaga TJ, Fischer SM, Viaje A, Berry DL, Bracken WM, Leclerc S, Miller DR. Inhibition of tumor promotion by antiinflammatory agents: An approach to the biochemical mechanism of promotion. In: Slaga TJ et al., eds. *Mechanisms of Tumor Promotion and Cocarcinogenesis.* New York: Raven Press, 1978:173-195
9. Wattenberg LW, Wiedmann TS, Estensen RD, Zimmerman CL, Steele VE, Kelloff GJ. Chemoprevention of pulmonary carcinogenesis by aerosolized budesonide in female A/J mice. *Cancer Res.* 1997; **57**:5489-92
10. Wattenberg LW, Estensen RD. Studies of chemopreventive effects of budenoside on benzo[a]pyrene-induced neoplasia of the lung of female A/J mice. *Carcinogenesis* 1997; **18**:2015-7

Metal Ions in Biology and Medicine; vol 6. Eds. J.A. Centeno, Ph. Collery, G. Vernet, R.B. Finkelman, H. Gibb, J.C. Etienne. John Libbey Eurotext, Paris © 2000, pp. 69-71.

Induction of p15 gene expression in Molt4 leukemic cells by arsenic trioxide

Harse Jin, Li Yu, FangDing Lou

Hematology Department, PLA General Hospital, 28 Fuxing Road, Beijing, China

P15 gene encodes an inhibitor of cyclin dependent kinase 4 (CDK4),when p15 protein binds to CDK4,progression through the G1 phase of cell cycle is prevented.Deleton or methylaton in this gene result in an abnormal cell growth.[1].Recent studies shown that p15 gene was frequently inactivated by CpG island methylation in leukemia,this is associated with transcriptional loss that was reversed by treatment with the DNA demethylation agent 5-aza-2`-deoxycytidine[2],Arsenic trioxide is a paradoxical drug.72 cases of acute promyelocytic leukemia were treated with intravenous arsenic trioxide.Complete remission rate was 73.3% for the previously untreated group and 52.3% for the refractory or relapsed group[3].But chronic arsenic exposure most frequently produces hyperkeratosis,vascular abnormalities,skin and bladder cancer.Because arsenic is detoxified via methylation using a methyltransferase (Mtase) and s-adenosyl methionine (SAM) as a the methyl donor[4].We hypothesized that a mechanism of treatment of leukemia by arsenic could involve alteration of Mtase/SAM-dependent DNA methylaton of a tumor suppressor gene.In this research we exposed human leukemia cell lines to arsenic trioxide,to determine whether the silencing of growth regulatory genes by de novo methylaton could be reversed,possibly restoring growth control.

Methods

1 Cell culture: Molt4 cell line were grown in RPMI-1640 supplemented with 10% fetal bovine serum in a humidified incubator at 37 ℃in an atmosphere of 5% CO_2 in air.

2 Methylation specific PCR (MSP)[5]:Genomic DNA was obtained from cell lines as routine method.DNA was denatured by NaOH and bisulfite modificated by hydroquinone and sodium bisulfite,then p15 gene was

amplificated.

3 RT-PCR[6]: RNA from molt4 cell line were purified by trizol.Two ug of total RNA was reverse transcribed using random primer.cDNA was amplified.

4 Determinaton of cell cycle profile: Cells were plated and treated with arsenic.cells were fixed with ethanol,treated with Rnasin and stained with propidium iodide.DNA content at each cell cycle stage was determined via flow cytometry.

Results

1 Cultured cells were treated with arsenic. The percentage of viable cells wasdetermined by trypan blue dye exclusion.then cells were analyzed for their DNA conle distribution.

Table 1 Effect of arsenic on molt4 cell lines cell cycle

Drug	concentration	G0-G1phase cell	G2-Mphase cell	S phase cell
As2O3	10^{-6}mol/l	52.14	6.35	41.52
As2O3	20^{-6}mol/l	57.91	3.12	34.28
control		20.75	14.55	64.70

2 Methlation specific PCR of P15,primer sets used for amplification are designated as methylated and unmethylated ,molt4 cell lines p15 gene was methylated(lane 1 methylated and lane 2 unmethylated),U937 (lane 3 methylated and lane 4 unmethylated)cell served as negative control,p15 gene was unmethylated.See figure 1

Figure 1 MSP 0f P15

Marker 1 2 3 4

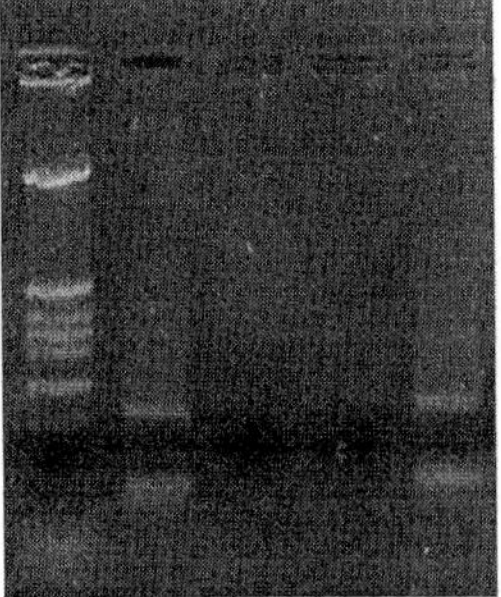

Figure 2 Expression of p15

marker 1 2 3 4

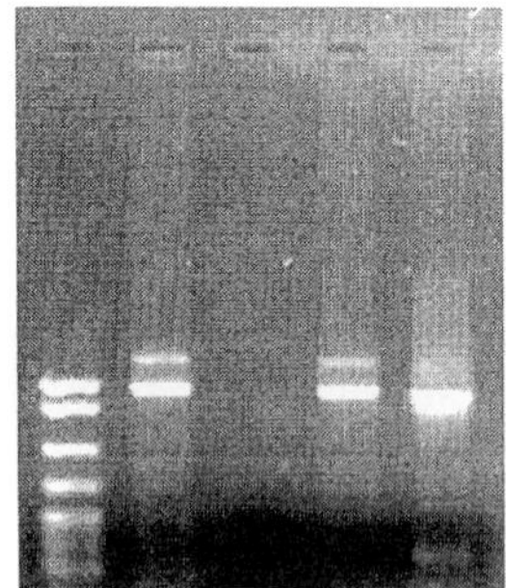

3 RT-PCR was used to examine the expression of p15 gene in molt4 cell lines and normal lymphocytes (served as positive control,lane1),molt4 cell line RNA samples were incubated without(lane 4) or with arsenic(lane 3).after 2 days treatment with arsenic,the p15 mRNA was detectable.Without cDNA sample served as a negative control. β actin was seen readily in all samples,revealing the integrity of cDNA(lane 2).see figure 2

Conclusion

Molt4 cell lines p15 gene was methylated and lose its transcription. After 48 hour arsenic trioxide treatment, the silencing of p15 gene by de novo methylation could be reversed and restored its growth control.

References

1 Ayse Batova, Mitchell B.Diccianni,John C.Yu, Tsutomu Nobori,Michael P.Link,Jeanette Pullen,Alice L.Yu. Frequent and selective methylation of p15 and deletion of both p15 and p16 in T cell acute lymphoblastic leukemia.Cancer Research 1997;57:832—836

2 J-PJ Issa, SB Baylin, IG Herman. DNA methylation changes in hematologic malignancies:biologic and clinical implications. Leukemia 1997;11:s7-s11

3 Peng Zhang, Shuye Wang, Hu Longhu, Fudong Shi, Fengqin Qiu,Luojia Hong,Xueying Han. Treatment of acute promyelocytic leukemia with intravenous arsenic trioxide.Chinese Journal of Hematology 1996;17:58—63

4 Marc J.Mass, Liangjun Wang. Arsenic alters cytosine methylation patterns of the promoter of the tumor suppressor gene p53 in human lung cells: a model for a mechanism of carcinogenesis.Mutation Research 1997;386:263--277

5 James G. herman, Jermy R.Graff, Sanna Myohanen, barry D.Nelkin,Stephen B.Baylin. Methylation specific PCR: A novel PCR assay for methylation status of CpG islands.Proc.natl.acad.sci.USA1996;93:9821-9826

6 James G.Herman,Jin Jen, Adrian Merlo,Stephen B.Baylin. Hypermethylation-associated inactivation indicates a tumor suppressor role for p15.Cancer Research 1996;56:722-727

Metal Ions in Biology and Medicine; vol 6. Eds. J.A. Centeno, Ph. Collery, G. Vernet, R.B. Finkelman, H. Gibb, J.C. Etienne. John Libbey Eurotext, Paris © 2000, pp. 72-73.

Study on injury of the combination of arsenic and fluoride in liver and kidney

Kai-tai Liu, Guo-Quan Wang, Li-Ying Ma, Ping jang, Bi-Yu Xiao, Chen Zhang

Department of Environmental Hygiene, Xinjiang Medical University, Urumqi, Xinjiang, China 830054

SUMMARY: In a subacute animal study, the effects of arsenic and fluoride on liver and kidney of rats were investigated. The results indicated that arsenic, fluoride and their combination affected the activities of superoxide dismutase (SOD) and glutathione peroxidase (GSH-Px) and the contents of malondialdehyde (MDA) and sulphhydryl groups (-SH). Antagonistic effects were found between arsenic and fluoride as well as on Zn, Fe, Ca and Mg in liver and Ca, Mg, Sr and Al in kidney. Arsenic significantly increased the liver and kidney content of Fe. For Mn there seemed to be synergism between arsenic and fluoride. The topic effects of arsenic and fluoride on liver and kidney have two aspects: one is direct action; the other is indirect -- disturbances of free radical balance and abnormal of metabolism of some inorganic elements.

Keywords: Arsenic and fluoride, Lipid peroxidation, metallic element, Liver, Kidney

INTRODUCTION

Arsenic-fluoride poisoning is an exceptional disease in the world. Both domestic and foreign scientific investigators have studied arsenism and fluorosis, and the results indicate that both arsenic and fluoride are able to cause injury to liver and kidney[1-3]. But studies of their combination on liver and kidney, especially in low dose and long-term contact conditions have not been reported. In recent years areas of arsenic-fluoride poisoning have been successively discovered in the provinces of Neimeng and Gueizhou besides Xinjiang. It is therefore highly important to investigate the pattern and mechanism of combined arsenic and fluoride injury on liver and kidney.

MATERIALS AND METHODS

Fifty six healthy Wistar rats (NO.0000569) weighing 140-160 g at the beginning of experiment were obtained from the Laboratory Animal Center of Shanghai Medical University. The rats were randomly divided into four equal groups of 14 animals each: F group, As group, F+As group and control group. All rats were housed in the same room with free access to food and water. The control group was given distilled water in which the fluoride and arsenic concentration was 0 mg/L. The experimental groups were given drinking water containing 150 mg/L sodium fluoride (NaF), 75 mg/L arsenic trioxide (As_2O_3), and 150 mg/L NaF + 75 mg/L As_2O_3, respectively.

After six months the rats were killed. The hepatic and renal tissue (approximately 0.3 g each) were quickly removed, weighed, homogenized, and centrifuged. The supernatant was then assayed for the activities of superoxide dismutase (SOD) and glutathione peroxidase (GSH-Px) and the contents of malondialdehyde (MDA) and sulphhydryl groups (-SH). Other hepatic and renal tissue were baked at 80 □, and then assayed by Inductively Coupled Plasma Atomic Emission Spectrometer (ICP-AES) for metallic elements (Cu, Zn, Fe, Cr, Pb, Sr, Al, Mg and Ca).

RESULTS

Hepatic tissue: Antioxdases levels (SOD, GSH-Px and -SH)decreased significantly by the sixth month in the groups of rats given water containing 150 mg/L NaF and 75 mg/L As_2O_3, respectively. They also decreased in the 150 mg/L NaF plus 75 mg/L As_2O_3 group, but were not significantly different from the controls. The contents of Zn, Fe, Ca and Mg in the liver in the NaF group and the As_2O_3 group were significantly different from the controls. The content of Mg in the NaF + As_2O_3 group was lower than the control. In this study, other elements were not significantly different among the four groups.

Renal tissue: Lipid peroxidation level increased in the As_2O_3 group□but antioxdase levels were lower than in the control group. The content of Fe in the NaF + As_2O_3 group was highest among all 4 groups, and Cr was lowest in the NaF group. The contents of Mg, Ca, Sr and Al in the NaF and As_2O_3 groups were significantly lower than in the control and the NaF + As_2O_3 groups.

DISCUSSION

Activities of many enzymes and the levels of inorganic elements are important factors for keeping in good health. When they become abnormal, the structure and function of internal organs of the body can be disturbed. It has been reported that fluoride and arsenic cause injury to liver and kidney [4-7]. By using the method of subacute animal experimentation, we have examined effects of arsenic, fluoride and arsenic plus fluoride on liver and kidney of rats. Our findings can be summarized as follows:

Effects on liver: Arsenic, fluoride and their combination affected the activities of superoxide dismutase (SOD)and glutathione peroxidase (GSH-Px) and the contents of malondialdehyde(MDA) and sulphhydryl groups(-SH), and of Zn, Fe, Ca and Mg. There were antagonistic effects between arsenic and fluoride. Due to this antagonism between the effects of arsenic plus fluoride on antioxidation, Ca and Mg in rat liver were lower than from the effects of either one when used alone.

Effects on kidney: Arsenic increased the contents of malondialdehyde(MDA) and caused accumulation of Fe. In its effect no Cr, arsenic reduced the action of fluoride. Effects of the combination of arsenic and fluoride on SOD, GSH-Px and -SH in rat kidney were greater than those of arsenic or fluoride alone. The combined action of arsenic and fluoride increased the content of Mn. In this respect, there was synergism between arsenic and fluoride.

As indicated above, the toxicity of arsenic and fluoride in liver and kidney has two aspects. One is the direct action. The other is indirect action – the disturbance of free radical balance and abnormal of metabolism of some inorganic elements. In view of the antagonism found in many indices in liver and kidney, cell metabolism processes were affected. As a result, normal metabolism of cells must have been disturbed with injury to liver and kidney.

REFERENCES

1. Dai Q, Liu WJ, Xei YY et al. Observation of ultrastructural pathology in nephrons of experimental chronic arsenic poisoning mice. Journal of Xinjing University. 1991;Supplement:41-42
2. Kessabi M, Hamliri A, Braun JP. Experimental acute sodium fluoride poisoning in sheep renal, hepatic and metabolic effect. Fluoride. 1987;20(1):41
3. Cittanova ML, Lelongt B, verpont MC et al. Fluoride on toxicity in human kidney collecting duct cells. Anesthesiology. 1996;84(2):428-435
4. Ademuyiwa O, Elsenhars B, Nguyen PT et al. Arsenic-copper ineraction in the kidney of rat. Pharmacol Toxicity. 1996;78(3);154-160
5. Zhao ZL, Wu NP,Gao WH. The influence of fluoride on the content of testosterone and cholesterol in rat. Fluoride. 1995;28(3):128-130
6. Ramos O, Carrizales L, Mejia J et al. Arsenic increased lipid peroxidation in rat tissues by a mechanism independent of glutathione levels. Environmental Health Prespect. 1995;Supplement 1: 85-88
7. Bian XY, Wu ZD, Li H et al. Effect of fluorine and superoxidase on the rat hepatocyte ultrastructure. Chinese Journal of Endemiology. 1993;12(3): 136-137

Metal Ions in Biology and Medicine; vol 6. Eds. J.A. Centeno, Ph. Collery, G. Vernet, R.B. Finkelman, H. Gibb, J.C. Etienne. John Libbey Eurotext, Paris © 2000, pp. 74-76.

40 years follow-up study on mental sequelae to an accidental mass arsenic poisoning in Japan

Akira Kanazawa, Teruhiko Tohyama, Yukari Baba, Ken'ichi Miwa, Masao Nakazawa, Toshio Munesue, Hoichi Matsuda, Takeo Fukuda, Eisaku Ishimura, Nobuyuki Hotta and Naomi Kawasaki

The research group for mental disorders, The Hikari Society. Address of Kanazawa: Faculty of Health Sciences, Ehime University School of Medicine, Shitsukawa, Shigenobu-cho, Ehime, 791-0295, Japan

In the western part of Japan during the spring and summer of 1955, there was an accidental mass poisoning of infant with arsenic in the food supply. An infant formula preparation of dry milk, produced at the Morinaga Milk Company, was contaminated with sodium arsenate, which came from the disodium hydrogen phosphate used in the manufacturing process. According to an announcement of the Ministry of Health and Welfare at the time, 12,131 babies suffered from acute or chronic poisoning, of whom 130 died. Almost all of the arsenic-poisoned babies had displayed initial symptoms of high fever, diarrhea, vomiting and insomnia. They then showed typical symptoms of arsenic, such as exanthema, pigmentation, hepatomegaly and anemia. Many of them suffered cachexia or dehydration as a result of the intoxication and some of them displayed ascites, icterus and convulsions. The frequency and the severity of these symptoms abated upon withdrawal of contaminated powdered milk supplies from market.

In 1956, the Ministry of Health and Welfare instituted a survey of the arsenic poisoned babies' conditions. At the time, nearly all of the babies were judged to have completely recovered from poisoning. The Ministry's ad hoc committee judged at the time that no sequelae would occur in the arsenic poisoned babies. However, in 1969, a group of public health nurses and school nurses noted adverse health consequences in the survivors of the arsenic poisoning. Following the report, a nationwide health screening of the survivors by physicians confirmed some sequelae.

In 1974, a non-governmental relief foundation, the Hikari Society, was established with funding by the milk producer and the Japanese governmental as a result of a court-ordered consent decree issued in response to a lawsuit filed by parents of the victims. The Society provides relief to all victims in the form of regular medical examination, health consultation, social services, underwriting special education needs and guaranteed employment.

As of January 2000, the number of victims totaled 13,419, of whom 839 have died.

The purpose of this report is to survey the social adjustment and neuropsychiatric characteristics of persons with mental disorders, epilepsy and mental retardation who are registered at the Hikari Society.

SUBJECTS AND METHODS

The subjects of this report are victims registered at the head office of the Hikari Society as having had mental disorders, epilepsy or mental retardation.

Of those registered with these disorders, 499 are alive and 79 have died since initial registration. We prepared a questionnaire including items covering physical state during the early stage of the poisoning, the history of education, occupation and marital status, family structure, and family history of illness. The questionnaire also covered history of any present psychiatric illness, history of its therapy, present state of the illness, interpersonal relationship problems, level of daily living skills, current level of social accommodation and adaptation, economic or monetary circumstance and future life prospects.

The questionnaires were completed by case workers who have accumulated detailed data records at the Society's 20 branch offices. Data used in completing the questionnaires was restricted to those gathered from the autumn of 1993 to the spring of 1996. All of the questionnaires were returned completely.

Original diagnosis was made using a variety of diagnostic criteria by the clinician assigned to each patient. Using the data, we categorized cases to conform to the ICD-10.

RESULTS

A 499 living subjects

1) Demographic features

Table I shows the number of male and female subjects in each of the three diagnostic groups.

Table I Sex of the survivors

Sex	Total		Mental Disorders		Epilepsy		Mental Retardation	
	No.	%	No.	%	No.	%	No.	%
Male	296	59.3	128	59.8	32	55.2	136	59.9
Female	203	40.3	86	40.2	26	44.8	91	40.1
Total	499		214		58		227	

Ninety % of the subjects were born in 1954 or 1955 when poisoned infant-formula powdered milk was marketed.

2) History of occupation

Sixty seven (13.4%) of subjects had graduated school for handicapped and 56(11.2%) were exempted from compulsory education.

Three hundred and forty one subjects had obtained at least one job; 108(31.7%) of them did not change their first employment.

3) Marital status and adaptation levels

Marital status is shown in Table II.

Table II Marital status of the survivors

Marital State	Total		Mental Disorders		Epilepsy		Mental Retardation	
	No.	%	No.	%	No.	%	No.	%
Unmarried	368	73.7	133	62.1	50	86.2	185	81.5
Married	107	21.4	63	29.5	7	12.1	37	16.3
Divorced	21	4.2	17	7.9			4	1.8
Widow or Widower	3	0.6	1	0.5	1	1.7	1	0.4
Total	499		214		58		227	

Table III shows levels of social adaptation in these survivors.

Table Ⅲ Present Level of Social Adaptation of the Survivors

ESAS*	Total		Mental Disorders		Epilepsy		Mental Retardation	
	No.	%	No.	%	No.	%	No.	%
Self-Supportive	118	23.6	68	31.8	8	13.8	42	18.5
Semi-Self-Supportive	88	17.6	27	12.6	12	20.7	49	21.6
Socially Adjusted to Family or Community	95	19.0	48	22.4	4	6.9	43	18.9
Maladjusted	53	10.6	26	12.1	11	19.0	16	7.0
Hospitalized	108	21.6	30	14.0	19	32.8	59	26.0
Unknown	37	7.4	15	7.0	4	6.9	18	7.9
Total	499		214		58		227	

*ESAS: Eguma's Social Adjustment Scale. See Reference 1).

B 214 survivors with mental disorders

The number of the survivors with diagnoses by ICD-10 diagnostic Criteria are as follows; F0 Organic Mental Disorders 51(23.8%), F1 Substance Abuse 3(1.4%), F2 Schizophrenic Disorders 110(51.4%), F3 Mood Disorders 12(5.6%), F4 Neurotic Disorders and others 31(14.5%), F6 Personality Disorders 5(2.3%) and Others 2(0.9%). Among 214 survivors with mental disorders, 137 had history of psychiatric hospitalization.

Types of present treatment are as follow; Outpatients at a psychiatric clinic 125(58.4%), Admission to a hospital or other residential facility 32(15.0%), Clients of counseling service 19(8.9%), User of Rehabilitation service 10(4.7%), None 12(5.6%) and Unknown 16(7.5%9)

C Subjects who died

Of the 79 registrants who died, 56(70.9%) were male and 23(29.1%) were female. More than half of the deceased subjects died at 31 years old or over. Cause of death are as follow; Suicide 21(26.6%), Diseases of the Cardiovascular System 17(21.5%), of the respiratory Organs 13(16.5%), of the Central Nervous System 7(8.9%), of the Digestive Organs 4(5.1%), Other Diseases 7(8.9%), Accident 7(8.9%) and Unknown 3(3.8%).

D The social adaptation levels of survivors

The educational achievement of survivors in this survey is somewhat lower than that of the general population in Japan. The marital status of these 499 survivors is very different from that of the general population in Japan, as well. In the same generation, 83.0% of the general population people are married,13.3% are single, 3.2% are divorced and 0.5% are widows or widowers(Reference 2).

Levels of social adaptation of these 499 survivors are low; as shown in Table Ⅲ, only 23.6 % are able to support themselves.

REFERENCES

1) Ogawa K.,Miya M., Watarai A., Nakazawa M., Yuasa S., and Utena H.: A long-term follow-up study of schizophrenia in Japan---With special reference to the course of social adjustment. British J. Psychiat.1987;151:758-765.

2) Statistics and information department, Japanese Ministry of Health and Welfare: Vital statistics of Japan 1993,Vol.1, Tokyo(in Japanese)

Metal Ions in Biology and Medicine; vol 6. Eds. J.A. Centeno, Ph. Collery, G. Vernet, R.B. Finkelman, H. Gibb, J.C. Etienne. John Libbey Eurotext, Paris © 2000, pp. 77-79.

Arsenic species in plants from Yellowknife, NWT, Canada

Iris Koch[a], Chris A. Ollson[a], William R. Cullen[b], Kenneth J. Reimer[a]

[a] *Environmental Sciences Group (ESG), Royal Military College of Canada, 12 Vérité Ave., P.O. Box 17000 Stn. Forces, Kingston, Ontario, Canada, K7K 1B4;* [b] *Department of Chemistry, University of British Columbia, 2036 Main Mall, Vancouver, British Columbia, Canada, V6T 1Z1*

Introduction.

- Arsenic toxicity is dependent on its chemical form (species)—hence the need for speciation analysis of environmental and biological samples.
- Yellowknife, Northwest Territories, has elevated levels of arsenic in soil, water and sediments due to mining activities and natural geology; the community is concerned about potential human health effects.
- Plants from city and mine properties in Yellowknife were previously analyzed for arsenic species by using HPLC-ICP-MS speciation analysis (summary of results in Table I)[1,2].

Table I. Distribution of arsenic species in plants from Yellowknife[1,2].

Plant/Algae type	Arsenic Species[a]	Extraction efficiency (EE)[b]
Vascular plants (terrestrial and emergent)	Mostly inorganic Max. 7% methyl	%EE range 16-130% (median 58%)
Vascular plants (submergent)	Mostly inorganic Max. 7% methyl Max. 11% arsenosugars	%EE range 13-51%
Mosses	Mostly inorganic	%EE range 2-15%
Algae/microbial mats	Mostly inorganic Very little methyl Arsenosugars in most specimens—59% in 1	%EE range 1-41% (max for microbial mats 8.7%)

[a] Inorganic = As III + AsV; Methyl = MMA+DMA+TMAO+ Me_4As^+.
[b] Extraction with $MeOH/H_2O$ (1:1)

Objective. To determine any relationships between the profile of arsenic species in plants and associated soil, porewater, or water characteristics.

Methods. Data that had been previously acquired[1,2,3,4] were analyzed with Microsoft Excel 97 and SYSTAT®8.0. Principal components analysis (PCA) was carried out following $\log_{10}$ transformation of the data.

Results

Total Arsenic. Concentration factors (CFs) were calculated by using the following equation, where all concentrations are total arsenic:

$$CF = [As_{plant\ OR\ algae}]/[As_{soil\ OR\ water}]$$

- When the calculated CFs (from soil) were plotted against the corresponding soil concentrations, a negative non-linear relationship is observed (CF_{soil} vs. As soil concentration). The highest CFs were observed at low As soil concentrations, and the lowest CFs were observed at high As soil concentrations.
- When the CFs (from porewater or water) were plotted against the corresponding porewater/water concentration, a more linear relationship is evident ($r^2 = 0.88$, CF_{water} vs. water concentrations).

Therefore arsenic concentrations in the porewater or water environment of the plant appear to be predictive of the total amount of arsenic taken up by the plant.

Arsenic species. To analyze for arsenic species in environmental samples, a mixture of methanol and water (1:1) was used to extract the water-soluble fractions while preserving the arsenic species as much as possible.

- % Extraction efficiency relates negatively with total arsenic in plants, suggesting that a lower percentage of arsenic may be soluble in plants with high total arsenic concentrations. As arsenic accumulates in plants, it may, for example, be sequestered in cellulose or other cell components that are not available for extraction.

***Figure 1*. AsIII/AsV in plants vs. AsIII/AsV in water/porewater**

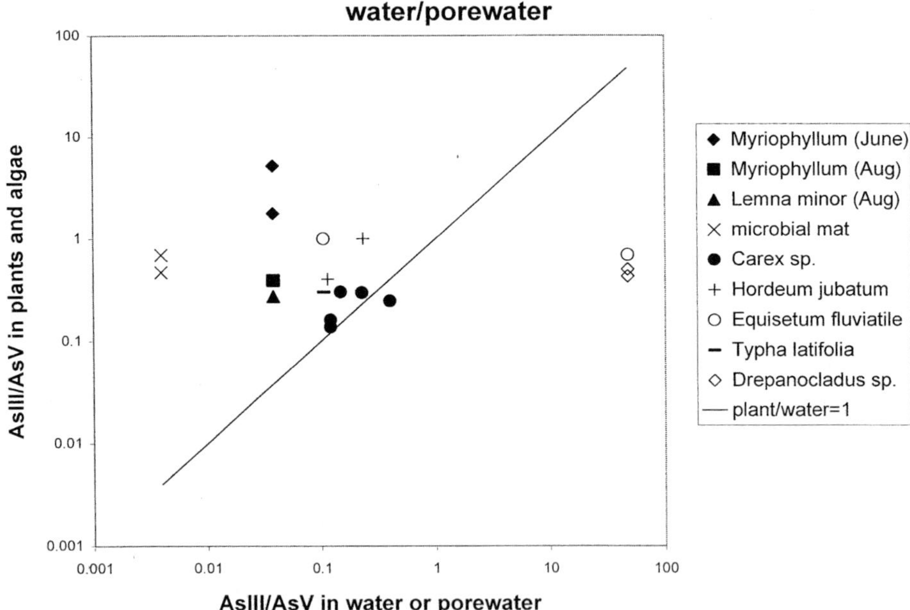

- Having observed the apparent relationship between total arsenic in associated water or porewater and plants or algae, arsenic species (i.e., AsIII/AsV ratios) in these samples were compared (Figure 1). A line representing that which would be seen if the ratios were the same in both media is shown for reference.

(a) The *Carex* sp. samples plot close to the line, suggesting that little or no transformation takes place by this plant or its community.
(b) Two samples of a microbial mat appear to preferentially accumulate AsIII, to transform AsV to AsIII, or to produce reducing conditions that are conducive to the chemical reduction of AsV.
(c) *Hordeum jubatum* and *Typha latifolia* behave similarly to *Carex* sp., possibly with a slight preference for AsIII.
(d) *Myriophyllum* sp. indicates a preference for AsIII when sampled in June, and for AsV in August. The August sample behaves similarly to *Lemna minor*, more closely reflecting the As species profile in water.
(e) *Drepanocladus* sp. contains predominantly AsV in spite of the high AsIII concentrations in its corresponding porewater. AsIII appears to be excluded, perhaps because of possible AsIII toxicity to *Drepanocladus* sp.
(f) *Equisetum fluviatile* seems to retain same ratio of AsIII/AsV regardless of the ratio in water.

- PCA was carried out for plants using the following variables: As species, % extraction efficiency, total arsenic in plants and arsenic in associated soil. The resulting first three factors explained 92% of total variance. The PCA generated values for each plant sample and variable with respect to the first three factors (i.e. new variables). When these values were plotted as a contour plot, the groupings revealed by this PCA were mostly influenced by As levels in plants and associated soil and extraction efficiency, rather than by the As species found.
- Analysis to elucidate relationships between locations and the proportions of arsenic species found in plants or to provide any other information was unsuccessful.

Conclusion. Arsenic speciation and total arsenic in plants appears to be influenced by that in porewater, but relationships between plant arsenic and soil/sediment characteristics appear to be more complicated, probably involving variables not measured in this work.

References

1. Koch, I.; Wang, L.; Ollson, C. A.; Cullen, W. R.; Reimer, K. J. The predominance of inorganic arsenic species in plants from Yellowknife, Northwest Territories, Canada. *Environ. Sci. Technol.* 2000; 34: 22-26.
2. Koch, I. *Arsenic and antimony species in the terrestrial environment*. Ph.D. Thesis, University of British Columbia, Vancouver, 1998.
3. Ollson, C.A. *Arsenic contamination of the terrestrial and freshwater environment impacted by gold mining operations, Yellowknife, NWT*. M.Sc. Thesis, Royal Military College, Kingston, 1999.
4. Environmental Sciences Group, Environmental Chemistry Group, *An Environmental Evaluation of the Miramar Con Mine: Final Report,* June 1999, RMC-CCE-ES-99-18.

Metal Ions in Biology and Medicine; vol 6. Eds. J.A. Centeno, Ph. Collery, G. Vernet, R.B. Finkelman, H. Gibb, J.C. Etienne. John Libbey Eurotext, Paris © 2000, pp. 80-82.

Water arsenic and human life-span

Wang Lianfang, Wang Shenlin, Zhang Lin

Xinjiang Institute for Endemic Disease Control and Research, Urumqi, China 830002

Abstract: In 1980,we found an endemic arsenism area where the drinking water had arsenic level of 0.04-0.75mg/L in Xinjiang, China. For controlling the disease, a project for improving the quality of drinking water was completed in 1984. In order to understand the remote effects of arsenic on human life-span, a follow-up survey among the people of the endemic area was in 1995. In four units surveyed, in which the arsenic level was 0.22-0.75mg/L in original drinking water in A,B,C units and 0.015mg/L in unit D before 1984, a total of 66 inhabitants in A,B and C units was 4.5-5.6 %,and 1.1 % in the unit D. The life-span of the inhabitants died in the four units was inversely proportional to the arsenic content in original drinking water. The malignant tumor is first cause of death. The rate of death from malignant tumor is positively proportional to the arsenic level of original drinking water. The order of constituent ratio of specific causes of death was as follows: malignant tumor>Cardiovascular disease>Cor pulmonale>cerebrovascular disease>digestive tract disease>urinary system disease, and so on. The findings presented in the paper suggest that arsenic is an important factor causing the decrease of human life-span in endemic arsenism area.

Key Words: Water arsenic; Human life-span; Malignant tumor

INTRODUCTION

Endemic arsenism as a result of drinking water with high arsenic level was found in some places of the world in this century. Some papers had reported that arsenic could cause more complications such as malignant tumor, cardiovascular disease, cerebrovascular disease and so on[1-3]. Arsenic could be a factor effecting human life-span in endemic arsenism area. In 1980,an endemic arsenism area where the drinking water had arsenic content of 0.04-0.75mg/L was found in Xinjiang China. For controlling the disease, a project for improving the quality of drinking water was completed in 1984. In order to understand the remote effects of arsenic on human life-span, a follow-up survey among the people of the endemic area was made in 1995. The following is the report of our investigation.

MATERIALS AND METHODS

Four units, in which the arsenic level was 0.22-0.75mg/L in original drinking water in A,B,C units and 0.015mg/L in unit D before 1984, were selected. According to the death data from the health and epidemic prevention station in the area, the family members of the death were visited for verifying the cause of death in further, and the cases of death from injury such as traffic or other accident were excluded. The mortality rate of death of malignant tumor and the average of life-span of death in four units studied in the term of 1989-1995 were calculated, and the relationship between these indexes and the arsenic concentration of original drinking water before 1984 was analyzed, respectively. The constituent of causes of death in two serious arsenism units was calculated from the data in

1980-1995.

RESULTS

1. Mortality and arsenic content of original drinking water

In the period from 1989 to 1995, a total of 66 inhabitants died from all kinds of illness with a range of mortality of 1.1-5.6 % in four units surveyed. The mean of mortality per year of people in A,B,C units was 0.64-0.80 % with 4-5 times that in the unit D(0.16 %). The correlation coefficient between the mean mortality and value of logarithmic transformation of arsenic level in original drinking water was 0.992 showing an obvious positive correlation.

Table 1 Relationship between mortality and arsenic level in original water

Unit	As mg/L(x)	No. of inhabitants	Death	Mortality %	Mean/year % (y)
A	0.75	286	16	5.6	0.80
B	0.56	283	14	4.9	0.70
C	0.22	557	25	4.5	0.64
D	0.015	984	11	1.1	0.16

Lgx vs y: r=0.992, r0.01(2)=0.990, $p<0.01$ y %=0.365 lgx+0.835

2. Average of life-span of inhabitants died

The average of life-span of the death from illness in four units was inversely proportional to the arsenic level in original drinking water, i.e. the higher was the arsenic level in original water, the lower was the length of life-span. Analysis of the water arsenic content in original and the mean of life-span showed a regression equation: y=66.55-14.50x(Table2)

Table 2 Mean of life-span and arsenic level in original water

Unit	As mg/L(x)	No. of death	Age of death(year)	Mean of age year(y)
A	0.75	16	12-17	55.81±16.22
B	0.56	14	5M.-86	57.68±20.91
C	0.22	25	49-87	64.84±11.15
D	0.015	11	23-87	65.45±18.46

R=-0.975,r 0.05(2)=0.950, $p<0.05$, y=66.55-14.50x

3. Rate of death from malignant tumor

During 1989-1995, 19 cases were died from malignant tumor in four units. The rate of death from malignant tumor was positively to proportional to the arsenic concentration of original water with a regression equation:y=496.78x+4.544(x: water arsenic; y: rate of death of malignant tumor).The highest rate of 400 per 10^5 was seen in the unit with a highest arsenic content of 0.75 mg /L.(Table 3)

Table 3 Rate of death of malignant tumor and water arsenic level

Unit	As mg/L(x)	No. of inhabitants	Death	Rate/year per10^5(y)
A	0.75	286	8	400.0
B	0.56	283	5	257.1
C	0.22	557	4	100.0
D	0.015	984	2	28.6

R=0.990, r0.05(2)=0.950, $p<0.05$; y=496.78x+4.554

4. Constituent of causes of death in serious arsenism unit

The constituent of causes of death on two seriously affected units(A&B)was made from the data in 1980-1995. The order of constituent ratio of specific causes of death was as follows: malignant tumor(350 %),cardiovascular disease(22.2 %),Cor pulmonale(11.1 %),cerebrovascular disease(9.3 %),digestive tract disease(7.4 %),urinary system disease(5.6 %),and so on. The malignant tumor is first cause of death in arsenism area.

DISCUSSION

In 1980,an endemic arsenism area where the drinking water had arsenic level of 0.04-0.75mg/L was found in Xinjiang . Some people poisoning and death from arsenic had occurred as a result of drinking water with high arsenic. In order to control the disease, a project for improving the quality of drinking water was completed in 1984.The authors noted that 23 patients had died from cardiovascular disease and malignant neoplasms[4,5]. The second follow-up survey for the endemic area was in 1995. More patients died from malignant tumor, cardiovascular and other disease. In order to understand the remote effects of arsenic on human life-span, four units with arsenic level of 0.015-0.75mg/L in original drinking water before 1984 were investigated for death causes. The mortality of the inhabitants increased with the increase of arsenic content of original drinking water. The life-span of the inhabitants died from all kinds of illness decreased as the arsenic level increased. It showed that the arsenic in the original drinking water was an important factor causing the decrease of human life-span in this area. At the same time, the analysis of the constituent ratio of specific causes of death in serious arsenism unit showed that the malignant tumor was first cause of death. The rate of death from malignant tumor was also positively proportional to the arsenic content in original drinking water in the four units surveyed. It also noted that cardiovascular disease was another main cause of death. As the data presented, we consider that the remote effects of the arsenic still play an important role on promoting malignant tumor and cardiovascular disease after the water with high arsenic had been abandoned, and that arsenic is a main factor causing the decrease of human life-span in endemic arsenism area.

References

1. Chen Cj, Chuang TC, Lin TM, et al. Malignant neoplasms among residents of a blackfoot diseas-endemic area in Taiwan: high-arsenic artesian well water and cancers. Cancer Res 1985;45:5895-5899.
2. Chen CJ, Hsueh YM, Lai MS, et al.Increasel prevalence of hypertension and long-term arsenic exposure. Hypertension 1995;25:53-60
3. Li-Julin, Shan-FA Horng, Kun-Fu Liaw, et al. Arsenic and ischemic heart disease in the blackfoot disease endemic area, Chin J public Health(Taipei):1995;14(6):502-511
4. Wang Lianfang, Liu Hongde,, Lin Fafu, et al. Endemic arsenism in a village of Xinjiang: Epidemiological, Clinical and Preventive studies for 9 years . Endemic Diseases Bulletin,1993; 8(suppl):71-79
5. Wang Lianfang and Huang Jianzhong. Chronic arsenism from drinking water in some areas of Xinjiang, China. In: Arsenic in the Environment, part 11: Human Health and Ecosystem Effects, Edited by J.O.Nriagu, 1994:159-172

Metal Ions in Biology and Medicine; vol 6. Eds. J.A. Centeno, Ph. Collery, G. Vernet, R.B. Finkelman, H. Gibb, J.C. Etienne. John Libbey Eurotext, Paris © 2000, pp. 83-85.

Cholangiocarcinoma presenting as obstruction of sigmoid colon: possible relationship with arsenic exposure during World War II

Ifat A. Shah[1], Osama S. Gani[1], Romeo Esquivel[2], and Joseph R. Salvatore[3]

Department of Pathology and Laboratory Medicine, [1] Internal Medicine, Section of Gastroenterology, [2] and Division of Hematology and Oncology, [3] Veterans Affairs Medical Center, 650 E. Indian School Road Phoenix, AZ 85012, USA

Abstract. We present the history of a World War II Veteran, 72 years, who was a prisoner of war in Germany in an area known for high content of arsenic in the environment. The patient developed a widely metastatic peripheral cholangiocarcinoma (CC) that presented with obstruction of the sigmoid colon. A number of clinical, endoscopic, radiologic, computer-tomographic and laboratory results favored a metatasizing colonic carcinoma; however, normal serum levels for carcinoembryonic antigen(CEA) and CA 19-9; histomorphology of omental tumor, especially its negativity for CEA, and cytokeratin (CK) 20 and its positivity for CK 7; and the absence of malignant changes in the colonic mucosa did not support colon cancer. The autopsy examination revealed in the non-cirrhotic liver a peripheral CC, which had in a unique fashion metastasized to and obstructed the sigmoid colon We discuss the link between the exposure of the patient to arsenic—during WW II imprisonment in Germany—and the causation of CC about 55 years later.

Introduction. The two major types of primary liver cancer (PLC) are HCC and CC, and rarely HCC-CC. In the United States the CC makes up only about one-tenth of HCC.[1-03] Main etiologies of CC include thorotrast exposure, hepatolithiasis, clonorchis sinensis, congenital dilation of the intrahepatic bile duct and chronic inflammatory bowel disease;[4,5] to rare etiologies of CC belong arsenical exposure.[6-9]
To our knowledge, symptoms related mainly to large-bowel obstruction have never been reported in CC. We will discuss, in some detail, arsenic exposure in the development of CC.

History of Patient (Autopsy # 98-37). Mr. RL, 72 years, has been a decorated World War II Veteran who was a prisoner of war for about a year in Germany. For months before the last admission in August 1998, the patient suffered from increased constipation, and occasional melena, nausea, and vomiting. There was no history of ulcerative colitis, sclerosing cholangitis, congenital hepatobilary dilatation, thorotrast exposure, parasitic or viral infection, or of excessive use of tobacco or alcohol.
Barium enema, abdominal ultrasound and computer-tomographic examinations and laparotomy revealed up to 4 cm in diameter tumors in the abdomen, involving sigmoid and descending colons, omentum, peritoneum and a large (about 7 cm across) and multiple small tumor nodules in the liver. An omental biopsy revealed a moderately differentiated carcinoma. Colonoscopy and sigmoid-colon biopsy could not confirm the origin of a tumor from the colonic mucosa. Pertinent laboratory data were as follows: serum CEA, 0.7 (normal, 0-3 ng/ml); CA 19-9, 42 (0-37 U/ml); gamma GT, 1,212 U/L; alkaline phosphtase, 1,319 U/L; total bilirubin, 1.3 mg/dl; AST, 115 U/L; ALT, 151 U/L; and alpha-fetoprotein, 2 ng/ml.The laparotomy was followed by the placement of a loop-diverting ileostomy. Because of the extensive spread of the tumor no curative operation was performed. The patient went a downhill course, developed bronchopneumonia and expired.

Material and Methods. All biopsy and pertinent autopsy specimens were examined with routine hematoxylin-eosin, mucicarmine and periodic-acid Schiff (PAS) reaction. The immunohistochemical procedure by Hsu et al [10] was performed using streptavidine-biotin (SLAB) kit procured from DAKO Corporation, Carpinteria, CA, USA. All antibodies were obtained from DAKO.

Results. The autopsy revealed in the moderately enlarged non-cirrhotic liver a 7-cm across grey-yellow, ill-defined, scirrhous-type infiltrative tumor in the left lobe. There were multiple, up to 3 cm, tumor nodules located subcapsularly and deep in the liver. The larger intra- and extrahepatic bile duct tributaries and the gallbladder were unremarkable. About 20 cm proximal to the anus, a 4-cm in diameter grayish-brown firm tumor involved the wall of and the soft tissue surrounding the sigmoid colon. This segment of the colon was deformed and exhibited an S-form kinking and constriction of the lumen. The tumor in the colon infiltrated all its layers but spared the mucosa. Additional tumor nodules, 0.2 up to 1 cm, were widely distributed in the peritoneum, mesentery, diaphragm, visceral and parietal pleurae, pulmonary parenchyma and peripancreatic area.

Histologic and Immunohistochemical Results. The poorly differentiated tubulopapillary tumor was composed of small, compressed, anastomosing, racemose tubular structures, embedded within fibrous stroma that infiltrated adjacent hepatic cords and sinusoids. The tumor in the colon involved pericolic fat and infiltrated serosa and muscle and submucosal layers but spared the mucosa. Immunocytochemically the tumor cells were strongly and diffusely expressive for CK 7, EMA, and Ber EP 4; weakly and focally for CEA, Leu M 1 and B 72. 3; and non-expressive for CK 20 and PSA.

Elemental Analysis of the Liver. The analysis of the dry-liver tissue provided the following results: copper, 9.81 mcg/g; iron, 272 mcg/g; zinc, 24.4 mcg/g; and arsenic, =< o.1 ng/g. All these concentrations fell within or below the acceptable/ normal reference levels for these elements.

Discussion. Patients with peripheral CC present predominantly with abdominal pain and marked weight loss. Jaundice and ascites are rare. In none of the 112 patients with CC, examined by Altaee et al, [4] was there a colonic obstruction. The main presenting symptoms of our patient were, however, related to lower-colonic obstruction and constipation. This symptomatology was unique for a CC and confirmed only at autopsy. To our knowledge, none of the patients with CC reported in the literature presented with an obstructing tumor in the distal colon. Levels of CEA are increased in 40-60% of patients, while CA 19-9 is elevated in over 80% of patients. [11] Normal serum levels for CEA and CA 19-9 in our patient did not support a primary colonic or pancreatic carcinoma.

CC has, in contrast to HCC, no association with liver cirrhosis, although cirrhosis may be present in a patient with CC. In our patient there was neither cirrhosis, any congenital nor chronic disease of the liver, serving as underlying state to develop a primary liver cancer, especially a CC. Immunocytochemically, normal hepatocytes and HCC express mainly CK 8 and 18 but not CK 7 and 19; on the other hand, CK 7 strongly decorates the normal bile ducts and the CC. [12-14] Almost all CC and none of HCC are reactive for EMA. [12, 15-18] The strong expressivity of the tumors in our patient for CK 7 and EMA, and focally and cytoplasmic for CEA, was a clear evidence for a CC. Moreover, the negative staining of tumor cells for CK 20 was not consistent with primary colon cancer. [19] During the lifetime of the patient the symptoms and clinical picture pointed toward a colonic cancer metastatic to the liver; however, the serologic, immunologic and immunocytochemical results did not support this impression.

Apart from the mode of presentation—obstruction of the sigmoid colon—, another important and unique aspect of our report concerns the etiology of the tumor. A recently proposed pathogenetic mechanism of HCC, CC and combined HCC-CC takes into account that an insult to the hepatocyte, the biliary-epithelial cell, or the intermediate (transitional) cell may effect—in the end—an HCC, a CC or a combined HCC-CC. Further, an HCC may subsequently differentiate into CC, and vice versa.[20] Several etiologic factors have strongly been associated with CC. Among the most cited factors include hepatolithiasis, liver-fluke infestations (clonorchiasis, opisthoorchiasis), congenital biliary cystic diseases, sclerosing cholangitis, and ulcerative colitis. Other lesser known factors include radionuclides, chemical carcinogens and certain drugs.

In our patient none of the above diseases, conditions or factors responsible for the causation of CC were present. Exceedingly rare factors include exposure to substances such as thorotrast (thorium dioxide), polyvinyl chloride (PVC) and arsenic. Arsenic is one of the oldest poisons known.[8] According to Roth,[21] Ayrton was the first to describe in 1820 the occupational malignancy caused by arsenic; this was followed by reports from Hutchinson,[22] Pye-Smith (1913), Leege (1934) and Miyagi (1935). Sommers and McManus[23] reported on the development of cancers of the skin and visceral organs caused by treatment with arsenic. Arsenicals in pesticides cause angiosarcomas and less frequently HCC and cirrhosis in vineyard workers in the Rhineland, Germany.[7-9,]

Occupational, environmental and medicinal exposures to inorganic arsenics were related to cancers of lung, skin and liver.[24-29] High content of arsenic in well water in Taiwan is associated with liver cancer.[6, 30] In 1957, Roth[9] reported on a total of 47 autopsies of vintners in the Moselle region (Germany), thought to have chronic arsenic poisoning; nine had liver tumors, four each were of the predominant hepatocellular variety and hepatic angiosarcomas and one of stenosing papillary and glandular carcinoma of the bile ducts; metastases of the latter carcinoma were found in portal LN, peritoneal carcinosis, mesentery and omentum; there was no cirrhosis and the arsenic content of the liver in this case of central CC was in the normal range.

In patients with arsenical cancer the arsenic-exposure time may be only a few months and the latency period as long as fifty years.[23] Buechner[31] and Liebegott[32] described in 1949 and 1952 arsenic-related 5 tumors (3 carcinomas and 2 sarcomas) of the liver; the latency period ranged between 17-21 years. Interval between arsenic exposure and liver Tumor is estimated to be 20-24 years;[21] 17-21 years;[32] and 13-50 years.[23] The shorter this interval, the higher the arsenic content of different organs harboring malignancy. At autopsy, the arsenic content of the organs of three deceased was in one case each negative, normal, and elevated.[21] The arsenic gets over the years removed from the body. In Moselle vineyard workers, Roth[9] found at autopsy only occasionally abnormal arsenic levels. The liver changes caused by arsenic can continue and progress even after the arsenic has been cleared by the liver.

A person exposed for only a few months to arsenic may develop even after an interval of five decades a CC; the arsenic content of the liver is—after such a long interval—not likely to be higher than reference range. Our patient had no common, uncommon or rare causes or preconditions to develop a CC. We believe our patient, who was a soldier and prisoner of war in Germany for about a year during a period when the people were getting exposed to arsenical agents, may well have been exposed through nutrition or environment to arsenic. The arsenical content of the liver of our patient was in the reference range. As mentioned, the normal arsenical content of the liver does not rule out arsenical exposure more than fifty years earlier.

References. 1) Cancer 1980;45:2663-9; 2) In: Okuda K, Ishak K, eds. Neoplasms of the Liver. Japan: Springer-Verlag 1988;381-96; 3) Cancer 1996; 78:1671-6; 4) Cancer 1991; 68: 2051-5; 5) Seminars in Liver Disease 1995;15:402-13; 6) Cancer Research 1990; 50: 5470-74; 7) Med Welt 1969; 20:557-67; 8) Zeitschr fuer Krebsforschung 1956;61:287-319; 9) Dtsch Med Wschr 1957;82:211-17; 10) J Histochem Cytochem 1981;9:577-58; 11) Neoplasms of the Liver. Tokyo: Springer-Verlag, 1987,381; 12) Cancer 1998; 82: 2145-49; 13) Am J Clin Pathol 1998;110:522; 14) Am J Pathol 1990;136:641-55; 15). Koeppen, H., El Samny, N., Alfsen, C., Nayak, N.C., Shah, I.A.: Value of Epithelial Membrane Antigen (EMA) in the diagnosis of malignant hepatic neoplasms. Scientific Assembly of the American Society of Clinical Pathologists, Chicago, March , 1985; 16) Virchows Arch (Pathol Anat) 1983;401: 307-13; 17) Hum Pathol 1985; 16: 929-40; 18) Histochemical Journal 1983; 15: 645-54; 19) Appl Immunocytochem 1995;3:99-107; 20) Hum Pathol 1995;26:956-64; 21) Zeitschr fuer Krebsforschung 1957;61:468-503; 22) Brit. M. J. 1887; 2:1280-1281; 23) Cancer 1953; 6:347-359; 24) Ger Med Mon 1972; 2:127-128; 25) Environ Health Perspect. 1977; 19:109-119; 26) Prev Med 1976;5:279-294; 27) Toxicol. Environ. Chem 1984;7: 241-50; 28) Arch. Toxicol 1991; 65: 525-3; 29) Pharmac Ther 1992;53:31-65; 30)Cancer Res 1985;45:5895-99; 31) Buechner F. Spezielle Pathologie 1955. Muenchen-Berlin: Urban & Schwarzenberg; 32) Am J Roentgenol 1992;159:503-507.

Metal Ions in Biology and Medicine; vol 6. Eds. J.A. Centeno, Ph. Collery, G. Vernet, R.B. Finkelman, H. Gibb, J.C. Etienne. John Libbey Eurotext, Paris © 2000, pp. 86-88.

The analysis of some cancer markers plasma concentration in people occupationally exposed to arsenic and other metals

Anna Szymańska-Chabowska, Jolanta Antonowicz-Juchniewicz, Ryszard Andrzejak

Dept. of Internal and Occupational Diseases, Wroclaw Medical University, 50-367 Wroclaw, Pasteura 4, Poland

Introduction:

The arsenic is a toxic element of different valences occurring in the organic and inorganic compounds. Arsenic reacts strongly with the sulph-hydryl groups of the enzymes, and causes their inactivation. It attacks the cellular mitochondria, and the succynian dehydrogenase - responsible for oxydative phosphorilation [1]. Besides, the arsenic reveals the mutagenic activity. It causes the clastogenesis, i.e. the chromosomal aberration in peripheral lymphocytes, and it increases the exchange of the sister chromatides. The carcinogenic effect of arsenic follows its inhalation, and concerns mainly lung and skin (squamous cell cancer or basal cell cancer). Arsenic-dependent bladder, liver and kidney cancers are rarely reported [2]. The co-mutagenic (enhancing) effect of arsenic should be also mentioned. Arsenic combined with other metals or UV radiation induces the neoplastic processes in much lower concentration than normally [3].

The development of the neoplasm maintains usually long-lasting process, whereas the first symptoms of the disease are often delayed. The vital question of the contemporary modern oncology is the early diagnosis of the disease, preferably in subclinical phase when there are chances for its successful treatment. The immunological methods, especially the identification of the neoplasm-specific antigens in blood plasma, seem to be promising. Neoplastic markers are the macromolecular substances, mostly proteins or glicolipoproteins, produced by the tumour cells in elevated amounts [4].

The investigation of the potential carcinogenic activity of the arsenic and other heavy metals and the connections between their concentration in constitutional fluids and the level of specific neoplastic markers, which might testify to the occupational malignant disease was the aim of our work.

Material and methods:

Within the Health Program of the Employees of Copper Ironworks “Legnica” 93 people, mean age – 40, mean working time period – 16 years, were examined in June 1998. We have done the following lab tests:

Pb, Cd, Mn, Cu, Zn, Ca, Mg, Fe, As serum, blood and urine concentration – by the spectrophotometric method, and FEP level – by Sergio Piomelli method; the neoplastic markers (AFP, CEA, SCC, PSA) level – by immunoenzymatic method.

Results and discussion:

The mean serum lead level in smelters reached 282,0 ug/l, and was lower than the permissible safe lead concentration. Concomitant low mean FEP (free erythrocyte protoporphyrins) level was revealed. So, the lead overload has not been established in the examined workers.

The levels of the other heavy metals (cadmium and manganese) have not exceeded their permissible safe concentration, as well. Copper, zinc, calcium, and iron reached the middle level of normal concentration. Only magnesium reached lower level of normal concentration.

Generally, the amount of the **excreted arsenic** in urine have not exceeded its permissible safe concentration (80 ug/l). **Only 14 smelters** (15,9%) have excreted **more than 80 ug/l** of arsenic in urine. This group requires careful observation and more frequent follow-ups.

The neoplastic markers (AFP, CEA, SCC, PSA) presented the middle levels of normal concentrations. Individually, the increased level of **CEA** was revealed in **4 smelters** (4,3%) the increased level of **SCC** – in **22 smelters** (23,7%), and **PSA** – in **1 smelter** (1,1%). The increased level of AFP has not been observed.

According to the amount of the excreted arsenic the whole group was divided into several subgroups. The workers who excreted the largest amount of arsenic were the youngest people of the shortest working time period and heavy smokers (it confirms of Lee and Fraumeni observations) [5]. They presented with the largest lead concentration in blood, and magnesium in serum, and the largest amount of FEP in erythrocytes, although still within the permissible safe concentration. This fact means the possibility of complications related to chronic occupational intoxication with lead and arsenic at the work place. Concomitant increased levels of cadmium and magnesium were revealed in the workers, who excreted the increased amount of arsenic in urine.

	Subgroup I As < 80 ug/l	Subgroup II As = 80 ug/l	Level of confidence
age	40,15+/-8,24	36,28+/-9,15	-
work time period	18,27+/-8,57	11,14+/-8,51	$p<0,05$
Pb_b (ug/l)	300+/-131,8	377+/-149,43	-
Cd_b (ug/l	4,01+/-2,5	4,91+/-2,43	-
Mg_s (ug/ml)	19,9+/-1,3	20,11+/-1,57	-
FEP_S (ug/100 ml E	50,5+/-37,3	60,44+/-59,8	-
CEA_S (ng/ml)	1,1+/-1,3	1,15+/-0,81	-
AFP_S (ng/ml	1,92+/-1,1	1,66+/-0,65	-
PSA_S(ng/ml)	0,5+/-0,4	0,72+/-0,92	-
SCC_S(ng/ml)	1,1+/-0,4	1,32+/-0,53	-

The increased level of excreted arsenic has not been accompanied by the increased values of neoplastic markers in serum. Just the opposite - the increased concentration of CEA and PSA in serum accompanied the increased concentration of cadmium in blood and smoking habits.
The increased lead concentration in blood accompanied the increased magnesium concentration in serum and increased level of excreted arsenic. It seems to be the evidence of magnesium protective effect related to arsenic toxicity.

The most important correlations are presented in the table below:

Positive correlations:	
AFP_S - age = +0,40	Mg_S - Pb_B = +0,25
PSA_S - age = +0,35	As_u - Pb_B = +0,36
AFP_S – work time period = +0,38	CEA_S-Cd_B. = +0,34
PSA_S – work time period = +0,36	PSA_S-Cd_B = +0,32
CEA_S – smoking habits = +0,24	

Summary:
Results of our investigations indicate that arsenic is a co-mutagenic factor and neoplastic promoter rather than primary transforming cell factor. The real disposition of young, smoking workers to the accumulating of different metals in the organism might lead to the neoplasm development in future.

References:
1. Arsenic 1998 - draft for public comment. Health effects: 131-132.
2. Magos L.: Epidemiological and experimental aspects of metal carcinogenesis: physiochemical properties, kinetics and the active species. Environ.Health Perspect. 1991, 95: 160-165.
3. Rossman T.G.: Metal mutagenesis. Hand.Exp.Pharm. 1995, 115: 373-409.
4. Lutz W., Krajewska B.: Markery nowotworowe i ich znaczenie w profilaktyce raka zawodowego. Polski Tyg. Lek. 1990, T.XLV, 32-33: 643-646.
5. Thomas D.J., Goyer R.A.: The effects of arsenic, lead and cadmium on the cardiovascular system. Metal.Toxicol. 1997, 10: 265-269.

Metal Ions in Biology and Medicine; vol 6. Eds. J.A. Centeno, Ph. Collery, G. Vernet, R.B. Finkelman, H. Gibb, J.C. Etienne. John Libbey Eurotext, Paris © 2000, pp. 89-91.

Cytogenetic assessment of arsenic trioxide toxicity in the Mutatox, Ames II, and CAT-TOX (L) assays

P.B. Tchounwou[1], B. Wilson[1], J. Schneider[2], and A. Ishaque[1]

[1] *Molecular Toxicology Research Laboratory, NIH-Center for Environmental Health, Jackson State University, Jackson, MS 39217, USA;* [2] *Client Research Laboratory, Xenometrix, Inc., Boulder, CO 80301, USA*

Abstract: The Mutatox, Ames II, and CAT-TOX (L) Assays have recently been developed and validated for use in determining the general genotoxic potential, in identifying a spectrum of point and frameshift mutations, and in detecting and quantifying the specific molecular mechanisms that underlie toxicity of various xenobiotic compounds, respectively. In this research, we performed these assays to determine the mutagenic potential of arsenic trioxide in the Mutatox test with a dark strain of marine bacterium, *Vibrio fischeri*, and in a battery of tests with eight strains of *Salmonella typhimurium* (TA7001-6, TA98, and TA1537), and to assess the transcriptional responses associated with exposure of this chemical to thirteen different recombinant cell lines generated from human liver carcinoma cell lines (HepG2), by creating stable transfectants of mammalian promoter chloramphenicol acetyltransferase (CAT) gene fusions . Study results indicated that arsenic trioxide was genotoxic in the Mutatox Assay, but not mutagenic in the Ames II Assay. Cytotoxicity test with HepG2 cells showed an LC_{50} of 11.94±2.61 ug/mL for cell viability upon 48 hrs of exposure. For most constructs evaluated in the CAT-TOX (L) Assay, a dose-response relationship was recorded with respect to gene induction. For example, induction levels of 2.78±1.41, 12.69±3.53, 57.70±29.00, 78.08±32.32, and 132.41±55.10 were recorded for HMTIIA at 0.3, 0.6, 1.25, 2.5 and 5.0 ug/mL arsenic trioxide, respectively. Overall, eleven out of the 13 tested constructs showed inductions to statistically significant levels ($p < 0.05$). At 5 ug/mL arsenic trioxide, the average levels of induction were 26.27±8.37, 2.92±1.32, 132.41±55.10, 48.23±21.76, 5.56±5.01, 59.51±54.39, 3.03±0.17, 41.17±10.03, 13.26±2.80, 2.72±0.42, and 1.82±0.53 for GST Ya, XRE, HMTIIA, *c-fos*, NF*KB*RE, HSP70, p53RE, GADD153, GADD45, and GRP78, respectively. Induction of CYP 1A1 (1.33±0.05) and RARE (1.00±0.00) were not significant ($p > 0.05$). The implications of these findings in the molecular pharmacology and predictive toxicology of arsenic trioxide are important.

Introduction: Arsenic compounds have been used for at least a century in the treatment of syphilis, yaws, amoebic dysentery, and trypanosomiasis [1]. Arsenical drugs are still used in treating certain tropical diseases such as African sleeping sickness and amoebic dysentery, and in veterinary medicine to treat parasitic diseases, including filariasis in dogs and black head in turkeys and chickens [1]. During the period 1200 to 1650, it was extremely used in homicides [2]. Various phenyl arsonic acids, especially arsanilic acid, sodium arsanilate and 3-nitro-4-hydroxyphenyl arsonic acid, have been used as feed additives for disease control and for improvement of weight gain in swine for almost 40 years. Most importantly, recent data have renewed the interest for arsenic-containing compounds as anticancer agents. In particular, arsenic trioxide has been demonstrated to be an effective drug in the treatment of acute promeylocytic leukemia by inducing programmed cell death (apoptosis) in leukemia cells, both *in vivo*, and *in vitro* [3]. However, the biochemical mechanisms involved in the therapeutic properties of these arsenic compounds are poorly understood. In this research, we performed the Mutatox, and Ames II assays to assess the genotoxicity of arsenic trioxide, and the CAT-TOX assay to determine the transcriptional responses associated with exposure of human liver carcinoma cells to this compound.

Experimental Design and Methods: ***Mutatox Assay:*** This test was carried out using a Microtox/Mutatox Model 500 Toxicity Analyzer System (Azur Environmental, Carlsbad, CA), and conducted according to the protocol described by Azur Environmental [4]. Nonglowing or dark mutant strains of luminescent bacteria were exposed to the test substance, and the amount of light emitted was measured with the Mutatox

Analyzer. The sample-induced reversion from nonglowing to luminescent phenotype was used to indicate the genotoxicity of the sample. The positive response was defined as the light output of at least two times the light intensity of the reagent control blank. A dilution series that contained two or more positive responses at two or more different concentrations was designated "genotoxic"; when the series contained only one positive response, it was designated "suspect or weakly genotoxic"; and when the series contained no positive response, it was designated "negative".

Ames II Assay: This test was performed following a protocol described by Gee and coworkers [5]. The test uses eight different strains of Salmonella tester strains (TA7001-TA7006, TA98, and TA1437) to detect and determine the type of mutations induced by chemical compounds [6].

CAT-Tox Assay: The mammalian Gene Profile Assay was performed for measuring differential gene expression in the human liver hepatoma cell line, HepG2. The test protocol described by Todd and coworkers was followed [7]. This test involves the use of different recombinant human liver cell lines generated by creating stable transfectants of different mammalian promoter-chloramphenicol acetyltransperase (CAT) were used. In summary, thirteen recombinant cell lines and the parental HepG2 Cell line were plated, one row each, over two 96-well microplates. The cell lines were dosed at 6 arsenic trioxide concentrations (0, 19, 38, 75, 150 and 300 ug/mL) and incubated at 37 ^{o}C, 5% CO_2, for 48 hours. After the incubation period, the total protein was measured by the Bradford method at 600nm using a microplate reader. A standard sandwich ELISA was performed and in the final step horse radish peroxidase catalyzed a color change reaction that was measured at 405 nm. The parental Hep G2 cell line was dosed in the same manner as the recombinant cell lines, and was used to perform a MTT-based cellular viability assay at 550 nm. The transcriptional fold inductions for each recombinant cell line at each arsenic trioxide concentration were calculated using the Xenometrix CAT-Tox software based on the optical density readings at 600nm at 405 nm. The software also converted the 550 nm readings to cell viability percentages.

Results and Discussion: The Mutatox assay resulted in a positive genotoxic response, after 20 hours of exposure of *Vibrio fischeri* to arsenic trioxide, indicating that this compound is a potential environmental mutagen. However, experiments using *Salmonella thyphimurium* did not show any significant differences ($p > 0.05$) in reversion rates of any of the eight tester strains (TA7001-TA7006, TA98, and TA1537), indicating that arsenic trioxide is not genotoxic in the Ames II assay. Although the Mutatox is generally non specific in detecting specific types of mutation, this test system appears to be more sensitive in predicting the genotoxicity of arsenic than the Ames II assay. Previous studies on the genotoxicity of arsenic indicate that arsenic compounds inhibit DNA repair, and induce chromosomal aberrations, and sister chromatid exchanges in eucaryotic cells. The mechanism of genotoxicity is not known, but may be due to the ability of arsenite to inhibit DNA replicating or repair enzymes, or the ability of arsenate to act as a phosphate analog [8].

Cytoxicity test with HepG2 cells using the LDH assay for cell viability yielded an LC_{50} of 11.94 ± 2.61 ug/mL, upon 48 hours of exposure. For most constructs evaluated in the CAT-Tox assay, the induction of stress genes was concentration-dependent. Induction levels of 2.78 ± 1.41, 12.69 ± 3.53, 57.70 ± 29.00, 78.08 ± 32.32, and 132.41 ± 55.10 were recorded for HMTIIA at 0.3, 0.6, 1.25, 2.5 and 5.0 ug/mL arsenic trioxide, respectively, indicating a dose-response relationship with respect to metallothionein induction. It has been reported that the synthesis of metallothioneins (MTs) can be induced by a wide variety of metals. This metal-inducible system is of particular importance in metal detoxification since it provides an efficient feedback mechanism for controlling the concentrations of a high-affinity biological ligand which, in turn, controls the speciation of selected metals within the cells [9]. Therefore, MTs may play a central role in protecting cells from potential damage as a result of exposure to arsenic trioxide.

Overall, eleven out of the 13 tested constructs showed inductions to statistically significant levels ($p < 0.05$). At 5 ug/mL arsenic trioxide, the average levels of induction were 26.27 ± 8.37, 2.92 ± 1.32, 132.41 ± 55.10, 48.23 ± 21.76, 5.56 ± 5.01, 59.51 ± 54.39, 3.03 ± 0.17, 41.17 ± 10.03, 13.26 ± 2.80, 2.72 ± 0.42, and 1.82 ± 0.53 for GST Ya, XRE, HMTIIA, *c-fos*, NF*KB*RE, HSP70, p53RE, GADD153, GADD45, and GRP78, respectively. Induction of CYP 1A1 (1.33±0.05) and RARE (1.00±0.00) were not significant ($p > 0.05$).

The relatively weak induction of xenobiotic response element (XRE) compared to glutathion-s-transferase (GSTYa), and the absence of any increase in the activity of cytochrome P450 (CYP1A1), suggests the possibility that the induction of GSTYa may be via the antioxidant response element (ARE), which is also present within the GSTYa promoter sequence. The induction of p53RE appears to be a very important factor in the pharmacology of arsenic trioxide. This tumor suppressor gene with its p53 transcription factor shows a strong activation following exposure to arsenic trioxide. This is indicative of the potential mechanism of action of arsenic trioxide at low doses, and hence, its use as a salvage therapy for relapsed and refractory acute promyelocytic leukemia [10]. From a toxicological standpoint, DNA damage as a consequence of exposure to arsenic trioxide is reflected by strong inductions of *c-fos*, growth arrest DNA damage (GADD153, GADD45), and p53RE. The induction of nuclear factor kappa beta response element (NF*KB*RE) in combination with *c-fos*, is indicative of oxidative damage by arsenic ions. Induction of heat shock protein (HSP70) and glucose regulated protein (GRP78) is indicative of protein perturbation and disturbances. Research has demonstrated that HSP70 prevents incorrect folding of newly synthesized peptides by binding to the growing peptide chain, and maintaining in a loosely folded state until synthesis is complete [9].

Acknowledgment: This research was financially supported by a grant from the National Institutes of Health (Grant No. 1G12RR13459).

References

[1] NAS. Arsenic. National Academy of Science. Washington D C, 1977.

[2] NRCC. Effects of arsenic in the environment. National Research Council of Canada. *Natl Res Counc Can Publ* 1978; 1-349.

[3] Rousselot P, Laboume S, Marolleau JP, Larghero T, Noguera ML, Brouet JC, Fermand JP. Arsenic trioxide and melarsoprol induce apoptosis in plasma cell lines and in plasma cells from myeloma patients. *Cancer Res* 1999; 59 : 1041-1048.

[4] Azur Environmental. Mutatox - Genotoxicity Test. Carlsbad, CA.

[5] Gee P, Maron DM, Ames BN. Detection and classification of mutagens: A set of base-specific *Salmonella* tester strains. *Proc Natl Acad Sci* 1994; 91 : 11606-11610.

[6] Gee P, Sommers CH, Melick AS, Gidrol XM, Todd MD, Burris RB, Nelson ME, Klemm RC, Zeiger E. Comparison of responses of base-specific *Salmonella* tester strains with the traditional strains for identifying mutagens: the results of a validation study. *Mutation Res* 1998; 412 : 115-130.

[7] Todd MD, Lee MJ, Williams JL, Nalenzny JM, Gee P. The CAT-Tox assay: A sensitive and specific measure of stress induced transcription in transformed human liver cells. *Fundamentals Appl Toxicol* 1995; 28 : 118-128.

[8] Li JH, Rossman TC. Inhibition of DNA ligase activity by arsenite: A possible mechanism of its comutagenesis. *Mol Toxicol* 1989; 2 :1-9.

[9] Sanders BM, Goering PL, Jenkins K. The role of general and metal-specific cellular responses in protection and repair of metal-induced damage: stress proteins and metallothioneins. In: Chang LW ed. *Toxicology of Metals*. Boca Raton. Lewis Publishers. 1996; 165-187.

[10] Huang SY, Chan CS, Tang JL, Tien HF, Kuo TL, Huang SF, Yoa YT, Chou WC, Chung CY, Wang CH, Shen MC, Chen YC. Acute and chronic poisoning associated with treatment of acute promyelocytic leukemia. *Br J Haematol* 1998; 103 (4) : 1092-1095.

Metal Ions in Biology and Medicine; vol 6. Eds. J.A. Centeno, Ph. Collery, G. Vernet, R.B. Finkelman, H. Gibb, J.C. Etienne. John Libbey Eurotext, Paris © 2000, pp. 92-93.

Strengthening management and improving the medical value of the use of Realgar

Yali Sun

Bureau of National Traditional Medicine Administration of China, Shanfen Bao and Lin Zhao, Trace Element Research Lab. 301 Hospital, Beijing 100853, P.R. China

1.The history of application of Mineral drug Realgar (Arsenic bisulfide As_2S_2) in China

Minerals drug is one of the important compositions in Chinese Traditional Medicine. China is the first country in the world in discovering and using Realgar. The first record about Realgar was in the earliest extant monograph on meteria medica <*Shen Nong's Herbal Classic*> in China□ which appeared during about the Qin-Han Dynasties. In B.C.475-221 the Realgar was also mentioned more than once in the book <*Shan Hai Jing*>. In the earliest medical classic extant in China - <*The Yellow Emperor's Internal Classic*> which appeared in the Warring States Period (B.C.475-221), the use of Realgar Combined with Orpiment (Arsenic trisulfide As_2S_3) were clearly recorded. Tao Hongjing (452-536), an eminent herbalist and physician, in his book <*Variorum of the Herbal Classic*> introduced the pharmaceutical effects of Realgar as well as its use as dye in drawing. At the beginning of 7th century Lei Xiao in his work <*Treatise on Preparation of Drugs*> described in detail about the special pharmaceutical efficiency, toxicity, preparation and method of processing of Realgar. Tracing back to history, the discovery and application of Realgar in Chinese traditional medicine can be dated up to more than 2000 years ago.

2.The use of Realgar in Medicine

Realgar, or named arsenic yellow, stone yellow, smoke yellow, was formed under the conditions of common effect both low temperature and hot liquid, often coexisting with Orpiment. The main composition of Realgar is As_2S_2 (Arsenic bisulfide). Being ore for refining arsenic, Realgar has been used widely in industry. For example:

(1) Used as insecticide, agent in processing hides and antiseptic of timber

(2) Used in making glass as oxidant , eliminating light green pigment in glass.

(3) Used as raw materials in making semiconductor, alloyed with some metals such as copper, gallium.

(4) The compounds of arsenic can be used as dye, enamel and fireworks.

Apart from the above mentioned uses, the most important application of Realgar in China is in treatment of disease. According to basic theories of Chinese traditional medicine, the diagnosis and treatment are based on the overall analysis of symptoms and signs , nature and location of the illness and patient's physical condition , Chinese traditional prescription is composed of many different kind of herbs, insects and minerals. Realgar is often used as a main component in prescription for treatment of the following diseases:

(1) neuralgia caused by lepra reaction

(2) eczema and zoster

(3) swelling pain induced by rubella virus
(4) epidemic parotitis
(5) snakebite
(6) malaria
(7) pulmonary tuberculosis
(8) anti-dermatomycosis reaction□malignant sore and scabies etc.
(9) In recent years, oral administration of Realgar has been used in treatment of acute promyelocytic leukemia. Now this therapy has been used as the first selected method in radical treatment of acute promyelocytic leukemia in special hematopathy hospital in China , which promote the research and applying of Realgar to a new level.

3 Strenghtening management and ensuring the quality of medicinal Realgar
Realgar is an important mineral drug used universally as both oral or external in Chinese Traditional Medicine. In Chinese pharmacopoeia Realgar is described as pungent in flavor and warm in property, minor toxic. The medicinal main composition of Realgar is As_2S_2, with less toxicity, but the arsenic trioxide (or white arsenic As_2O_3) mixed up with Realgar is hypertoxic with the lethal dose (for man) of 0.1-0.2g. Due to this property, the Ministry of Public Health of China promulgated the "Rule of toxic drug administration in medicine" emphasizing the importance of the strict management for Realgar. Based on this rule, in order to strengthen the management for processing toxic Chinese Traditional medicine and ensure the safety and efficiency of medicine, the Bureau of National Traditional Medicine Administration in 1997 published "The proposal of strengthening management for the appointed place production of toxic sliced medical herbs prepared for decoction " prescribing regulations for 28 kinds of toxic Chinese traditional medicine including Realgar, arsenic (white arsenic and red arsenic), arsenic trioxide and mercury and pointing out clearly that for special kinds of toxic Chinese traditional medicine , the production must be in the appointed special production place controlled by government to meet the market requirement of both domestic and abroad . In 1998 the Bureau of National Traditional Medicine Administration put forward the "Criterion of checking appointed special factories and enterprises processing toxic Chinese traditional medicine" and decided to award with certification to the factories and enterprises which passed the examination and make these factories known to all over the country. In order to strengthen and standardize the management for technological process of sliced medical herbs prepared for decoction of toxic Chinese traditional medicine and to ensure the conformability, strictness and reliability of production process , in 1998, the Bureau of National Traditional Medicine Administration published the"Rule of the record for production in batches of toxic sliced medical herbs prepared for decoction". This rule ensures the strict management for production in batch, standardizing the export channel of Chinese herbs and strengthening the legal administration.

4 **The modernization of Chinese traditional medicine and production of Realgar**
(1) To improve the technological process of preparation
Since ancient time the process of preparation of Realgar has been emphasized because of its pharmacological effect and toxicity. There were a lot of detailed description about the preparation of Realgar in Chinese pharmacopeia of different dynasties. The main purpose of preparation is to remove the arsenic trioxide
(2) To improve the technological process of drying
(3) To improve the technological process of packing

Metal Ions in Biology and Medicine; vol 6. Eds. J.A. Centeno, Ph. Collery, G. Vernet, R.B. Finkelman, H. Gibb, J.C. Etienne. John Libbey Eurotext, Paris © 2000, pp. 95-97.

Transcriptional inactivation of genes by nickel compounds involves inhibition of histone H4 acetylation

Max Costa[1, 2], Konstantin Salnikow[1, 2], Limor Broday[1], Wu Peng[1], Jessica E. Sutherland[1], Maria Zoroddu[3]

[1] *Nelson Institute of Environmental Medicine,* [2] *Kaplan Comprehensive Cancer Center, New York University Medical Center, New York, NY 10016;* [3] *Universita Degli Studi di Sassari, Sassari, Italy*

Carcinogenic nickel compounds including crystalline nickel sulfide and subsulfide are potent carcinogens that induce a wide variety of tumors in experimental animals and have been implicated in the etiology of human respiratory cancer following inhalation exposure [1]. The ability of these water-insoluble nickel compounds to be phagocytized by cancer target cells represents a mechanism that is likely to account for their potent carcinogenic activity. Following the entry of the particles into the cell by phagocytosis, they are dissolved and yield high intracellular levels of nickel, much higher than can be achieved by exposure to water-soluble nickel salts [2]. The major damage produced by carcinogenic nickel particles occurs in heterochromatic regions of chromosomes. Thus, the targeting of nickel to genetically inactive regions may account for the low mutagenic activity exhibited by carcinogenic nickel compounds in classical assays [3].

Exposure of transgenic cells to nickel has selective effects in silencing the transgenes depending upon their chromosomal position [4]. A similar positional effect variegation that caused epigenetic silencing of gene expression in mammalian cells was also demonstrated in the yeast *S. cerevisiae* [5]. This phenomenon, termed telomeric positional effect, was observed with soluble nickel compounds in yeast because yeast cells efficiently took up soluble nickel. DNA is known to be packaged into condensed heterochromatic regions. These regions contain poorly acetylated histones, whereas euchromatic regions contain transcriptionally active genes that are associated with highly acetylated N-terminal lysines of H3 and H4 [6]. This phenomenon is particularly important in the transcriptional regulation of genes because the N-terminal lysines of histone H4 are known to interact with the acidic amino acid tails of H2A and H2B in the absence of lysine acetylation but when the lysines are acetylated, the H4 tails do not bind to the H2A/H2B tails. When this occurs in adjacent nucleosomes, the result is the linking of nucleosomes together by the basic acidic amino acid lysine binding to acidic amino acids [7].

We have studied the effects of nickel compounds on the acetylation status of histone H4 using antibodies specific for H4 lysine acetylation sites. We found that in yeast, nickel is able to inhibit the acetylation of H4 in a dose- and time-dependent manner [8]. In mammalian cells, the nickel subsulfide particles are also able to inhibit histone acetylation but this effect is confined to the lysine at position 12 in histone H4. The lack of effect of nickel on other lysines in mammalian cells may be due to the complexity of the mammalian genome compared to the yeast genome and the difficulty in delivering high concentrations of nickel compounds to the histone N-terminal tails. Interestingly, histone H4 contains a histidine in position 18. We have demonstrated using model peptides with blocked ends that nickel and copper bind tightly to the histidine position 18 of the N-terminal tail of histone H4. Histone H3 does not have a similar histidine in that position and we are examining the effects of nickel and copper on the acetylation of H3. We hypothesize that the binding of nickel to this site represents a mechanism by which inhibition of lysine acetylation occurs. Interestingly, copper also coordinates well to histidine 18 of H4. These studies will be described in greater detail in another manuscript presented at the meeting by Dr. Maria Zoroddu. The ability of nickel to inhibit the acetylation of the N-terminal tail of histone H4 results in the enhanced interactions of the H4 lysines with neighboring H2A and H2B acidic amino acids which condense nucleosomes together, forming a higher order of chromatin structure and thereby decreasing transcription. This is the likely mechanism for the nickel-induced silencing of genes in yeast cells and possibly in mammalian cells as well.

We have previously shown that nickel can induce hypermethylation of DNA in mammalian cells and this is likely the mechanism by which genes are silenced in these cells [9]. The relationship between the inhibition of histone H4 acetylation by nickel in mammalian cells and DNA methylation is currently unknown, but there may be some coordinate mechanism in regulating gene expression. It is known that histone acetylation pattern can be inherited in yeast. Whether histone acetylation patterns determine DNA methylation patterns in mammalian cells or visa versa is an active area of investigation, and whether nickel binds to H4 directly and/or has an effect on histone acetylase or deacetylase enzyme activity to decrease histone acetylation also needs to be further studied.

References

1. International Agency for Research on Cancer. Chromium, Nickel and Welding. IARC Monograph Evaluation of Carcinogenic Risks to Humans, Lyon, France, 1990; Vol. 49.

2. Costa M and Mollenhauer HH. Carcinogenic activity of particulate metal compounds is proportional to their cellular uptake. *Science* 1980; 209 ; 515-7.

3. Fletcher GG, Rossetto FE, Turnbull JD, Nieboer E. Toxicity, uptake, and mutagenicity of particulate and soluble nickel compounds. *Environ Health Perspect* 1994; 102 Suppl. 3: 69-79.

4. Klein CB, Kargacin B, Su L, Cosentino S, Snow ET, Costa M. Metal mutagenesis in transgenic Chinese hamster cell lines. *Environ Health Perspect* 1994; 102 Suppl 3: 63-7.

5. Broday L, Cai J, Costa M. Nickel enhances telomeric silencing in *Saccharomyces cerevisiae*. *Mutat Res* 1999; 440: 121-30.

6. Grunstein M. Histone acetylation in chromatin structure and transcription. *Nature* 1997; 389: 349-52.

7. Luger K, Mäder AW, Richmond RK, Sargent DF, Richmond JJ. Crystal structure of the nucleosome core particle at 2.8 Å resolution. *Nature* 1997; 389: 251-60.

8. Broday L, Peng W, Kuo MH, Salnikow K, Zoroddu M, Costa M. Nickel compounds are novel inhibitors of histone H4 acetylation. *Cancer Res* 2000; 60: 238-41.

9. Lee Y-W, Klein CB, Kargacin B, Salnikow K, Kitahara J, Dowjat K, Zhitkovich A, Christie NT, Costa M. Carcinogenic nickel silences gene expression by chromatin condensation and DNA methylation: a new model for epigenetic carcinogens. *Mol Cell Biol* 1995; 15: 2547-57.

Metal Ions in Biology and Medicine; vol 6. Eds. J.A. Centeno, Ph. Collery, G. Vernet, R.B. Finkelman, H. Gibb, J.C. Etienne. John Libbey Eurotext, Paris © 2000, pp. 98-100.

Identification of signaling pathways affected by nickel compounds

Konstantin Salnikow[1, 2], Max Costa[1, 2], Tomasz Kluz[1], Maria Zoroddu[3]

[1] *Nelson Institute of Environmental Medicine, and* [2] *Kaplan Comprehensive Cancer Center, New York University Medical Center, New York, NY 10016;* [3] *Universita Degli Studi di Sassari, Sassari, Italy*

Nickel (Ni) compounds display *in vitro* immortalizing and transforming capabilities in both human and rodent cell culture systems. IARC has classified all Ni compounds, except for metallic Ni, as carcinogenic to humans [1]. The ability of Ni to transform cells is probably not related to DNA damage since Ni compounds are weakly mutagenic in most of the mutational systems examined thus far. These data suggested that epigenetic rather than genetic changes may be important events in Ni carcinogenesis. To facilitate a better understanding of the mechanisms of Ni carcinogenicity, we identified changes in gene expression patterns in Ni exposed cells to assist us in pinpointing signaling pathways affected by Ni.

Utilizing differential display, we have cloned a new gene that was highly induced by soluble or insoluble Ni compounds in human bronchoepithelial A549 cells [2]. This gene, named *Cap43*, was induced by Ni in all tested human cell lines as well as in tissues of exposed rats. We tested numerous environmental stressors to characterize the regulation of this gene but only hypoxia (1 to 0.5% O_2) appeared to be a potent inducer of gene expression. We found that the transcriptional up-regulation of *Cap43* gene expression by hypoxia or Ni appeared to be actively mediated by the HIF-1 transcription factor because this gene was up-regulated in normal mouse fibroblasts but not in fibroblasts originating from *HIF-1*$\alpha^{-/-}$ mice [3]. Moreover, the induction of HIF-1α protein, an important component of the HIF-1 transcription factor, was observed in cells acutely exposed to Ni [4].

The HIF-1 transcription factor is involved in the coordinated up-regulation of numerous genes including those involved in glucose transport, glycolysis [5], angiogenic vascular-endothelial growth factor, and erythropoietin. Thus, exposure of cells to nickel will produce up-regulation of glycolytic enzymes even in the presence of oxygen. This phenomenon is known as the "Warburg effect" [6] and is characteristic of a cancerous phenotype. If exposure is prolonged, cells with this enhanced glycolytic metabolism will have a selective advantage over other cells because they have higher proliferation rates.

The tumor suppressor p53 is another transcriptional factor which also accumulated in cultured hypoxic cells or tissues [7]. It has been demonstrated that wild type p53 was induced under hypoxic conditions simultaneously with HIF-1α and the binding of these two proteins provided p53 stabilization [8]. Additionally, recent experiments indicated that p53 was involved in the suppression of HIF-1 transcriptional activity [9]. Accumulation of p53 in hypoxic cells resulted in growth arrest due to either p21 up-regulation or activation of an apoptotic signaling pathway via Bax overexpression. In both cases, hypoxia will select against wild-type p53 in tumors since only cells with mutated p53 will continue to proliferate. Nickel exposure, like hypoxia, resulted in the accumulation of wild type p53 protein in A549 and MCF-7 cells. In contrast, Ni exposure did not affect the levels of mutated and non-functional p53 in HOS cells. Acute Ni treatment induced HIF-1α protein regardless of p53 status [4].

Because the HIF-1 transcription factor mediated the up-regulation of genes induced by acute exposure to Ni, we used HIF-1 responsive reporter plasmids to investigate the transcriptional activity of HIF-1 in Ni-transformed human and rodent cells. We found that the transcriptional activity of HIF-1 was significantly elevated in Ni-transformed human and rodent cells. To further elucidate the molecular mechanisms of Ni-induced transformation, we have analyzed p53 transcriptional activity in Ni-transformed cells using p53-responsive reporter plasmids. Transcriptional activity of p53 was found to be decreased in all tested Ni-transformed cells. Finally, the ratio of HIF-1 transcriptional activity to p53 transcriptional activity in the same cell type was found to be significantly increased in Ni-transformed cells. We suggest that this ratio can be conveniently used to identify and characterize the Ni-transformed phenotype.

Many solid tumors *in vivo* experience hypoxia because the rate of growth of the tumor body exceeds the rate of vascularization. Shortage in oxygen supply will turn on angiogenesis following the induction of vascular-endothelial growth factor and some other angiogenic factors. It was shown that tumors in which hypoxia cannot induce HIF-1 transcriptional activity remain small and fail to metastasize [10]. Given the observed shift in the balance between the HIF-1 and p53 transcription factors, we hypothesized that the exposure of cells to Ni will facilitate tumor growth because 1) it will provide selective conditions for cells that lost functional p53; and 2) simultaneously prepare them for survival in hypoxic conditions by turning on angiogenesis and glycolysis. Additionally, Ni will further promote tumor growth by turning off expression of antiangiogenic thrombospondin 1 [11,12].

Further identification of signaling pathways affected by Ni was obtained using gene array screening. We found that the expression of some Ni-inducible genes could be augmented by the elevation of intracellular calcium. This group of genes included *Cap43, Gadd153, VEGF, PDGF-β* and *p21*. Whereas, most of the genes in this group could be induced both by the HIF-1 and the calcium-dependent pathway, the induction of *Gadd153* by Ni was totally HIF-1 independent and was probably mediated entirely by a calcium-dependent pathway. We have previously demonstrated the elevation of intracellular calcium in Ni exposed cells [13], therefore, it is likely that calcium-dependent pathways are also affected by Ni.

In summary, we have identified two signaling pathways that are affected by carcinogenic Ni compounds. One pathway is similar to hypoxic signaling and is mediated by HIF-1 and p53 transcription factors. Another appears to be related to modulation of intracellular calcium homeostasis.

References

1. International Agency for Research on Cancer. Chromium, Nickel and Welding. IARC Monograph Evaluation of Carcinogenic Risks to Humans, Lyon, France, 1990; Vol. 49, 257-445.

2. Zhou D, Salnikow K, Costa M. *Cap43*, a novel gene specifically induced by Ni^{2+} compounds. *Cancer Res* 1998; 58: 2182-89.

3. Salnikow K, Blagosklonny M, Ryan H, Johnson R, Costa M. Carcinogenic nickel induces genes involved with hypoxic stress. *Cancer Res* 2000; 60: 38-41.

4. Salnikow K, An WG, Melillo G, Blagosklonny MV, Costa M. Nickel-induced transformation shifts the balance between HIF-1α and p53 transcription factors. *Carcinogenesis* 1999; 20: 1819-23.

5. Semenza G L. Regulation of mammalian O_2 homeostasis by hypoxia-inducible factor 1. *Annu Rev Cell Dev Biol* 1999; 15: 551-78.

6. Warburg O. On respiratory impairment in cancer cells. *Science* 1956; 123: 309-14.

7. Graeber TG, Osmanian C, Jacks T, Houseman DE, Koch CJ, Lowe SW, Giaccia AJ. Hypoxia-mediated selection of cells with diminished apoptotic potential in solid tumors. *Nature* 1996; 379: 88-91.

8. An WG, Kanekal M, Simon MC, Maltepe E, Blagosklonny MV, Neckers LM. Stabilization of wild-type p53 by hypoxia-inducible factor 1α. *Nature* 1998; 392: 405-8.

9. Blagosklonny MV, An WG, Romanova LY, Trepel J, Fojo T, Neckers LM. p53 inhibits hypoxia-inducible factor-stimulated transcription. *J Biol Chem* 1998; 273: 11995-8.

10. Maxwell PH, Dachs GU, Gleadle JM, Nicholls LG, Harris AL, Stratford IJ, Hankinson O, Pugh CW, Ratcliffe PJ. Hypoxia-inducible factor-1 modulates gene expression in solid tumors and influences both angiogenesis and tumor growth. *Proc Natl Acad Sci USA* 1997; 94: 8104-9.

11. Salnikow K, Cosentino S, Klein C, Costa M. Loss of thrombospondin transcriptional activity in nickel-transformed cells. *Mol Cell Biol* 1994;14: 851-8.

12. Salnikow K, Wang S, Costa M. Induction of activating transcription factor I by nickel and its role as a negative regulator of thrombospondin I gene expression. *Cancer Res* 1997; 57: 5060-6.

13. Salnikow K, Kluz T, Costa M. Role of Ca^{+2} in the regulation of nickel-inducible *Cap43* gene expression. *Toxicol Appl Pharmacol* 1999; 160: 127-32.

Metal Ions in Biology and Medicine; vol 6. Eds. J.A. Centeno, Ph. Collery, G. Vernet, R.B. Finkelman, H. Gibb, J.C. Etienne. John Libbey Eurotext, Paris © 2000, pp. 101-103.

Interaction of Ni(II) and Cu(II) with metal binding sequences of histone H4

Maria Antonietta Zoroddu[1], Teresa Kowalik-Jankowska[2], Henryk Kozlowski[2], Konstantin Salnikow[3], Limor Broday[3], and Max Costa[3]

[1] *Department of Chemistry, University of Sassari, Sassari, Italy;* [2] *Faculty of Chemistry, University of Wroclaw, Wroclaw, Poland;* [3] *Department of Environmental Medicine and Kaplan Comprehensive Cancer Center, New York University School of Medicine, New York, USA*

Ni(II) compounds are well established human carcinogens [1,2]. Ni(II) has been shown to enhance chromatin condensation and increase DNA methylation resulting in down regulation of gene transcription [3]. The molecular mechanism of nickel carcinogenicity, though not fully understood, is believed to involve DNA damage and epigenetic effects in chromatin resulting from nickel binding to cell nucleus [4-6]. It is known that Ni(II) can bind DNA only weakly [7]. Therefore, the nucleus proteins are possible targets for nickel binding. The most abundant proteins of the cell nucleus are histones. Consequently, it is possible that histones may be able to compete for metal ions with even higher affinity metal-binding sites in other, less abundant nuclear proteins or smaller molecules such as glutathione or histidine.

The core histones have multiple domain structures, consisting of globular carboxy terminals and randomly coiled, very basic amino tail regions. Some of the terminal tails are involved in internucleosome contacts in the higher-order structure of the crystals. One of the H4 N-terminal regions (residues 1-23) makes multiple hydrogen bonds between its basic side chain (K_{16}, R_{19}, K_{20}, R_{23}) and acidic side chains of H2A and H2B dimer of a neighboring nucleosome core [8].

Histones are extensively and reversibly post-translationally modified by acetylation, phosphorylation, and methylation. These modifications are confined to the tail regions of the proteins. Of these modification acetylation has generated more interest since gene expression was directly correlated with histone acetylation. The site of acetylation are the lysine residues of the positively charged amino terminal tails where each acetyl group added to a histone reduces its net positive charge weakening and modulating interaction between histones and the surface of the nucleosome. The positive charge of the H4 tail is neutralized by acetylations at lysines 5, 8, 12 and 16, increasing access to transcription factors and making "active chromatin" more available for modifications [9]. Studies involving the amino terminal tail of H4 are of particular interest providing information on the regulation of chromatin structure and function. Characterization of metal ion interactions with an entire histone is a difficult task, therefore we began our investigation with a minimal model of the H4 tail, the sequence AKRHRK (Ala-Lys-Arg-His-Arg-Lys, $A_{15}K_{16}R_{17}H_{18}R_{19}K_{20}$, residues 15-20), and with the sequence SGRGKGGKGLGKGGAKRHRKVL (Ser-Gly-Arg-Gly-Lys-Gly-Gly-Lys-Gly-

Leu-Gly-Lys-Gly-Gly-Ala_{15}-Lys_{16}-Arg_{17}-His_{18}-Arg_{19}-Lys_{20}-Val-Leu, residues 1-22), where an anchoring binding site for metal ions, a histidine (His_{18}), is close to sites for post translational modifications involved in nickel and also in copper toxicity.
The binding study was also extended to Cu (II) in view of the reported [10] toxicity of this metal to yeast cells. In fact, it has been reported that Ni(II) as well as Cu(II) are novel inhibitors of H4 acetylation on the lysines close to histidine 18 of the N-terminal of histone H4.

UV-VIS, CD, EPR and NMR spectroscopic analysis showed that histidine acted as an anchoring metal binding site. A 1N complex was formed between pH=5-7 and 4-6 for Ni(II) and Cu(II), respectively while at a higher pH a series of 4N complexes were formed. Above pH 8, the 2N high-spin octahedral resulted in a 4N low-spin planar Ni(II) complex. The formation of stable five-membered chelate rings by consecutive nitrogens was the driving force of the coordination process.

Although the imidazole nitrogen of the histidine in the H4 model was one order of magnitude more acidic than that for a similar blocked peptide with a histidine in the 4th position Boc-AGGH, the stability constants of the Cu(II) (3N, 4N) and Ni(II) (4N) complexes with the peptide model of the H4 were distinctly higher than those for Boc-AGGH peptide.

This fact suggested that the presence of positively charged side chains of lysines and arginines may have increased the stability of the 3N, 4N complexes [11].

In conclusion, our results show that AKRHRK, a minimal model of the H4 tail could be a competitive binding site for nickel as well as for copper.

References

1. International Agency for Research on Cancer , Monographs on the evaluation of carcinogenic risks to humans. Chromium, Nickel and Welding, IARC Lyon, France 1990; Vol. 49 .
2. Costa M, Molecular mechanisms of nickel carcinogenesis. *Ann. Rev. Pharmacol. Toxicol.* 1991; **31** : 321-37.
3. Lee YW, Klein CB, Kargacin B, Salnikow K, Kitahara J, Dowjat K, Zhitkovich A, and Costa M. Carcinogenic nickel silences gene expression by chromatin condensation and DNA methylation : a new model for epigenetic carcinogens. *Mol. Cell. Biol.* 1995; **15** : 2547-57.
4. Salnikow K, Cosentino S, Klein C and Costa M. Loss of thrombospondin transcriptional activity in nickel-transformed cells. *Mol. Cell. Biol.* 1994; **14** : 851-8.
5. Huang X, Kitahara J, Zhitkovich A, Dowjat K, and Costa M. Heterochromatic proteins specifically enhance nickel-induced 8-oxo-dG formation. *Carcinogenesis* 1995; **16** : 1753-59.

6. Bal W, and Kasprzak KS, In Hadjiliadis, N.D. Ed., Cytotoxic, mutagenic and carcinogenic potential of heavy metals related to human environment, Kluwer Academic Publishers, Dordrecht, 1997, Vol. 26, pp. 107-21, NATO ASI Ser. 2, Environment.
7. Lee JE, Ciccarelli RB, and Wetterhahn JK. Solubilization of the carcinogen nickel subsulfide and its interaction with deoxynucleic acid and protein. *Biochem.* 1982; **21** : 771-78.
8. Luger K, Mader AW, Richmond RK, Sargent DF and Richmond TJ. Crystal structure of the nucleosome core particle at 2.8 A resolution. *Nature* 1997; **389** : 251-60.
9. Grunstein M. Histone acetylation in chromatin structure and transcription *Nature* 1997; **389** : 349-52.
10. Broday L, Peng W, Kuo MH, Salnikow K, Zoroddu MA, Costa M. Nickel compounds are novel inhibitors of histone H4 acetylation. *Cancer Res.* 2000; 60: 238-41
11. Bal W, Lukszo J, Bialkowski K, and Kasprzak KS. Binding of nickel(II) and copper(II) to the N-terminal sequence of human protamine HP2 *Chem. Res. Toxicol.* 1997; **10** : 906-14

Metal Ions in Biology and Medicine; vol 6. Eds. J.A. Centeno, Ph. Collery, G. Vernet, R.B. Finkelman, H. Gibb, J.C. Etienne. John Libbey Eurotext, Paris © 2000, pp. 104-106.

Genetic events associated with arsenite-induced malignant transformation: application of cDNA microarray technology

Hua Chen[1], Jie Liu[1], Alex Merrick[2], and Michael P. Waalkes[1]

[1] *Laboratory of Comparative Carcinogenesis, NCI at NIEHS;* [2] *Laboratory of Molecular Carcinogenesis, NIEHS, Research Triangle Park, NC, USA*

Abstract. Arsenic is a human carcinogen with studies linking exposure to cancers of the skin, lung, liver and other organs. However, inorganic arsenic has not been unequivocally established as an animal carcinogen and its carcinogenic mechanism remains unknown. Our prior work showed that chronic (>18 weeks), low level exposure (125 to 500 nM) to sodium arsenite induces malignant transformation in a rat liver epithelial cell line [1]. DNA methylation is significantly reduced and aberrant expression of the oncogene, c-*myc*, is increased in these transformed cells. To further examine aberrant gene expression linked to arsenic carcinogenesis, the Clontech Atlas cDNA expression microarray was used. Results show that the expression of more than 50 genes were altered in arsenite-transformed cells. For example, several oncogenes (c-*myc*, c-*jun* and c-*met,* etc.) were upregulated, and expression of the cell cycle related genes CyclinD1, cyclin-dependent kinase 4 and PCNA were also increased in arsenite-transformed cells. The Western Blot and RT-PCR analysis of *c-myc*, CyclinD1, and PCNA agreed with gene expression analysis. These results revealed important aberrant gene expression patterns occurring in arsenite-induced malignant transformation. These initial gene array studies could be critical in future studies designed to more fully elucidate the molecular mechanisms of arsenic carcinogenesis.

Introduction. Inorganic arsenic is a common environmental pollutant and a high priority hazardous substance around the world. Human studies show that inorganic arsenic exposure causes skin, bladder, liver and lung tumors, which develop in dose and exposure duration related pattern. However, as inorganic arsenic has not been unequivocally established as an animal carcinogen, its mechanism remains unknown. Our prior work showed that chronic treatment of a normal rat liver epithelial cell line (TRL 1215) with low level arsenite produced malignant transformation [1]. This effect was related to the depletion of the cellular S-adenosyl-methionine (SAM) pool resulting from arsenic metabolism, which undergoes enzymatic methylation with SAM as the methyl donor. This chronic depletion of SAM appears to result in global DNA hypomethylation and aberrant gene expression of at least two genes, namely c-*myc* and *MT*. However, the precise pattern of altered gene expression in arsenic-induced malignant transformation is not fully understood.

The cDNA microarray is a high-throughput method, allowing expression profiling of a wide variety of genes important in cancer. Thus, in this study we used the microarray to define gene expression patterns in control and arsenite-transformed cells to further examine aberrant gene expression associated with arsenic carcinogenesis.

Material and methods. The rat liver epithelial cell line (TRL 1215) and its arsenite transformant, which had been chronically exposed to arsenite (125, 250 and 500 nM) for 24 weeks) as described in [1] were used. The Clontech cDNA microarray, RT-PCR and Western blot analysis were used to analyzed gene expression.

Results. Chronic arsenite exposure (125-500 nM; 24 weeks) markedly increased cell proliferation in a dose-dependent manner (Fig. 1), a sign of transformation. At the highest arsenite concentration cell proliferation increased 4.7-fold over control.

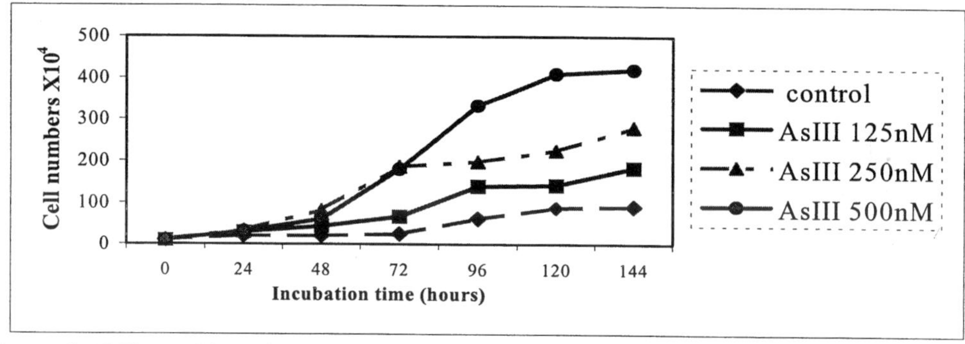

Figure 1. Effects Chronic Arsenite Exposure on Cell Proliferation.

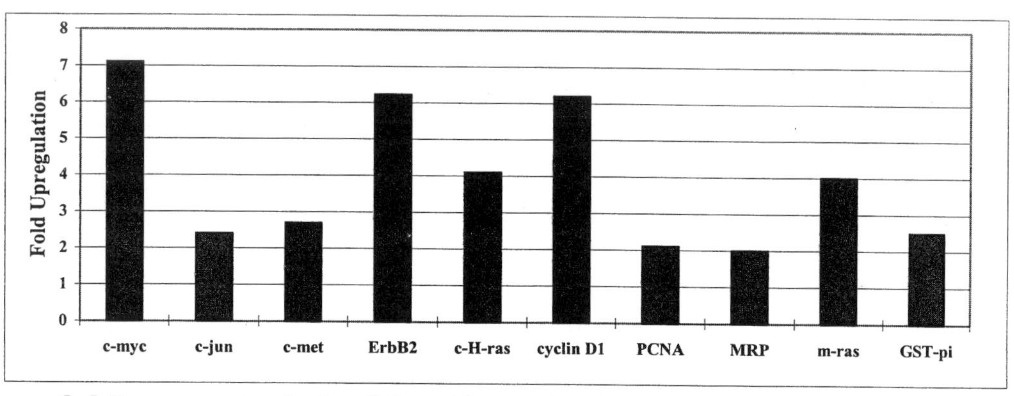

Figure 2. Microarray Analysis of Gene Expression in Arsenite-transformed Cells.

Microarray results showed the expression of more than 50 genes were altered in arsenite-transformed cells, including up regulation of known oncogenes (c-*myc,* c-*jun,* c-*met,* etc.) and the cell cycle related genes cyclin D1, and PCNA (Fig. 2). The microarray results with c-*myc*, cyclin D1, and PCNA in arsenite transformed cells were further confirmed by RT-PCR (Fig. 3) and Western blot analysis (not shown).

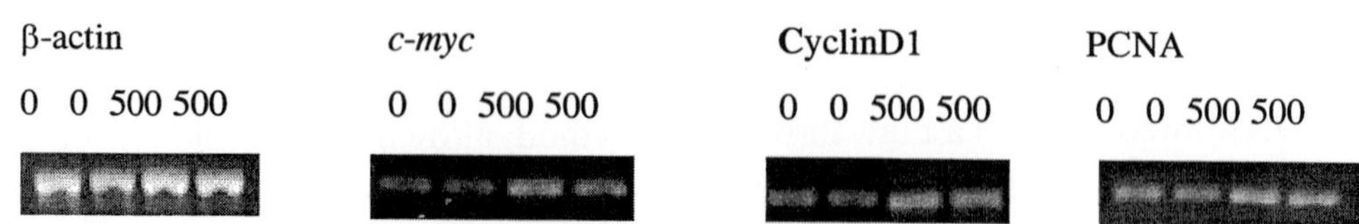

Figure 3. RT-PCR Analysis of Gene Expression in Control and Arsenite-transformed Cells

Discussion. This study used the cDNA microarray to define gene expression changes in arsenite-transformed cells. Arsenite transformation produced a dramatic, dose-dependent increase in cell proliferation consistent with transformation and altered the expression of more than 50 genes. For example, the oncogenes c-*myc*, c-*jun*, c-*met*, c-ErbA, *c-fos*, *m-ras*, and ErbB2 were all upregulated. The cell cycle related genes, cyclin D1, cyclin-dependent kinase 4 and PCNA were also increased in arsenite-transformed cells. The over expression of c-*myc* could be particularly important in arsenite-transformation. Expression of c-*myc* strongly stimulates cellular proliferation, prompting cells to exit G0/G1 and enter the cell cycle, and the Myc protein prevents growth arrest and drives cell cycle progression through the transcriptional regulation of target genes [2]. The ability of c-*myc* expression to cause cell-cycle progression likely contributes to its strong transformational and oncogenic potential. In addition, the cell cycle is regulated by the periodic synthesis and destruction of cyclins that associate with and activate cyclin dependent kinases. The D-types cyclins are also likely important in arsenite transformation as these are the first cyclins to be induced as G0 cells are stimulated to enter the cell cycle. When D-type cyclin synthesis becomes independent of the presence of growth factors, the cell cycle machinery may perceive this as a signal that growth factors are constantly present, and so cells would proliferate rather than differentiate. This cellular change clearly promotes oncogenesis. Aberrant expression of cyclin D1 would be expected to co-operate with other oncogenes in transformation. For instance, cyclin D1 can co-operate with *myc* in transgenic mice [3] and with cellular growth-related genes including *c-myc, c-jun* and *ras* in cultured cells. Therefore, these changes in cell cycle genes and oncogenes may play an integral role in arsenic carcinogenesis.

References:

1. Zhao CQ, Young MR, Diwan BA, Coogan TP, Waalkes MP. Association of arsenic-induced malignant transformation with DNA hypomethylation and aberrant gene expression. *Proc Natl Acad Sci USA* 1997; 94 : 10907-10912.
2. Marhin WW, Chen S, Facchini LM, Fornace AJ, Penn LZ. Myc represses the growth arrest gene gadd45. Oncogene 1997; 14 : 2825-2834.
3. Bodrug S, Warner B, Bath M, Adams J. CyclinD1 transgene impedes lymphocyte maturation and collaborates in lymphomagenesis with the *myc* gene. Embo J 1994; 13 : 2124-2130.

Metal Ions in Biology and Medicine; vol 6. Eds. J.A. Centeno, Ph. Collery, G. Vernet, R.B. Finkelman, H. Gibb, J.C. Etienne. John Libbey Eurotext, Paris © 2000, pp. 107-109.

Genes over-expressed in lead resistant rat glioma cells

Toby G. Rossman and Ping Li

Nelson Institute of Environmental Medicine, New York University School of Medicine, 57 Old Forge Road, Tuxedo, New York, NY 10987 USA

ABSTRACT

Glial cells are thought to protect neurons against lead toxicity [1]. As a model for studying the molecular targets of lead, lead-resistant C6 rat glioma cells have been isolated. Using cell fusion, we have demonstrated that lead-resistance is a dominant genetic trait [2].

To identify and analyze altered gene expression in resistant glioma line PbR11, suppression subtractive hybridization (SSH) between mRNAs of wild type and PbR11 cells was performed. 200 random recombinant clones were analyzed and 7 sequences were found up-regulated in lead-resistant cells. Sequencing and data base searches identified two sequences as novel genes. Five sequences matched known genes: 2 genes involved in the ubiquitin-proteosome system, 2 genes involved in angiogenesis and axon growth, and 1 identified as rat endogenous retrovirus. Which of these genes confer lead resistance is now under investigation. It is possible that some of the proteins encoded by these genes might serve as biomarkers of exposure in lead-exposed individuals, or may be suitable candidates for human susceptibility markers.

INTRODUCTION

The central nervous system undergoes development during the first few years of life. During this time, it is especially sensitive to lead toxicity [3]. Inter-individual variability in sensitivity to chemicals has been known to exist for some time, and is expected to exist also for lead exposure.

Molecular cloning techniques make it possible to identify specific genes that contribute to an increase in resistance or sensitivity to toxic agents. Long-term treatment of a toxicant, particularly if there has been selection for toxicant-resistance, can cause permanent alterations in gene expression. Identification of these genes can give important information about biochemical targets of lead as well as cellular defense mechanisms.

We have isolated lead-resistant rat C6 glioma cell lines and have shown that resistance is a dominant trait [2]. Here we report on the first 7 genes found to be up-regulated in the lead-resistant cell line PbR11.

RESULTS AND DISCUSSION

The details of molecular cloning, based on suppression subtractive hybridization [4] are the subject of a paper in preparation. We have subtracted wild type C6 sequences from those of lead-resistant PbR11 cells. Out of 200 random subtracted recombinant clones examined, 7 sequences were found to be up-regulated in PbR11 cells (Table 1). Data base searching for homologs and translation products was via the Internet (http://www.ncbi.nlm.nih.gov/).

Table 1
Sequences overexpressed in PbR11 cells

Clone number(s)	Homolog	Gene
54	*HSP90*	Heat shock protein 90
102	*UBA3*	Ubiquitin-like-activating enzyme Ube1c
42, 83		*TSP-1* Thrombospondin 1:
1	*NRP-1*	Neuropilin:
191	*pBUS19*	Rat-specific endogenous retrovirus
63, 82, 43	novel 2C9	Similar to sequence 2C9 (unknown gene)
87	novel 87	Homologous to sequences 5′ of heparin sulphate 6-sulphotransferase gene

The types of genes that are overexpressed in PbR11 cells give clues as to possible targets of lead toxicity or protective mechanisms. We suspect that HSP90 and UBA3 may be important in lead resistance, as these proteins are needed for protein processing. TSP-1 plays a role in control of angiogenesis and NRP-1 is responsible for controlling axon growth. Interference of these proteins by lead may be important in developmental neuropathology. Activation of retrovirus may give clues as to possible carcinogenic mechanisms. The characterization of the novel proteins could yield further clues about lead toxicology or defense systems.

Inter-individual variability in sensitivity to chemicals has been known to exist for some time [5]. Unlike inbred strains of animals, human populations are genetically heterogeneous. Differences in individual susceptibility may result from differences in the activation levels of particular genes as well as polymorphisms in these genes. By integrating mechanistically plausible genes into epidemiological studies, insight will be obtained on gene-environment interactions.

1. Lindahl LS, Bird L, Legare ME, Mikeska G, Bratton GR, Tiffany-Castiglioni E. Differential ability of astroglia and neuronal cells to accumulate lead: Dependence on cell type and on degree of differentiation. *Toxicol Sci* 1999; 50 : 236-243.

2. Dolzhanskaya N, Goncharova EI, Rossman TG. Isolation and properties of lead-resistant rat glioma cells. *Biological Trace Element Res* 1998; 65 : 31-43.

3. Holtzman D, DeVries C, Nguyen H, Olson J, Bensch K. Maturation of resistance to lead encephalopathy: Cellular and subcellular mechanisms. *Neurotoxicology* 1984; 5 : 97-124.

4. Diatchenko L, Lau YF, Campbell AP, Chenchik A, Moqadam, F, Huang B, Lukyanov S, Lukyanov K, Gurskaya N, Sverdlov ED, Siebert PD. . Suppression subtractive hybridization: a method for generating differentially regulated or tissue-specific cDNA probes and libraries. *Proc Natl Acad Sci USA* 1996; 93 : 6025-6030.

5. Calabrese EJ. . Biochemical individuality: The next generation. *Regul Toxicol Pharmacol* 1996; 24 : S58-S67.

Supported by EPA Grant R82-0984 and NIEHS Grant ES08453.

Metal Ions in Biology and Medicine; vol 6. Eds. J.A. Centeno, Ph. Collery, G. Vernet, R.B. Finkelman, H. Gibb, J.C. Etienne. John Libbey Eurotext, Paris © 2000, pp. 110-112.

Molecular mechanism of Cr(VI)-induced carcinogenesis

Xianglin Shi, Vince Castranova, and Val Vallyathan

Pathology and Physiology Research Branch, Health Effects Laboratory Division, National Institute for Occupational Safety and Health, Morgantown, WV 26505

Abstract: We hypothesize that reduction of Cr(VI) to its low oxidation states, Cr(V) and Cr(IV), is an important step in the mechanism of Cr(VI)-induced carcinogenesis. These chromium intermediates are able to generate reactive oxygen species (ROS), which initiate Cr(VI)-induced carcinogenesis. Through free radical reactions, Cr(VI) can activate multiple carcinogenic processes. (1) Cr(VI) causes activation of nuclear transcription factor kappa B (NF-κB). Among ROS, hydroxyl radicals (•OH) are responsible for Cr(VI)-induced NF-κB activation. (2) Cr(VI) is able to activate activator protein-1 (AP-1). (3) Cr(VI) causes p53 activation and •OH radicals function as messengers for the activation of this tumor suppressor protein. (4) Cr(VI) is capable of inducing apoptosis via both p53 and ROS-mediated reactions. (5) Cr(VI) causes over-expression of oncogenes (jun-B and raf), up-regulation of antioxidants (glutathione peroxidase), activation of certain enzymes involved in mitogen-activated protein kinase (MAP kinase) signal pathways (MAPKAP kinase), stimulation of enzymes involved in cell cycle control and checkpoint mechanisms (checkpoint suppressor 1), and activation of enzymes responsible for Cr(VI) reduction, such as NAD(P)H dependent dihydrolipoamide dehydrogenase.

Cr(VI)-containing compounds are considered to be well established carcinogens (1). They are potent inducers of tumors in experimental animals and active agents in causing DNA damage such as DNA strand breakage. We have hypothesized that reduction of Cr(VI) to its low oxidation states, Cr(V) and Cr(IV), is an important step (2). These chromium intermediates are able to generate ROS, which initiate Cr(VI)-induced carcinogenesis. This article summarizes our studies on Cr(VI) reduction and related free radical generation and the role of free radical reactions in various potential mechanisms for the initiation of carcinogenesis induced by this metal.

Cr(VI) reduction: Various low-molecular-weight cellular constituents have been shown to be able to reduce Cr(VI) *in vitro* at physiological pH. A variety of enzymatic and nonenzymatic factors function as Cr(VI) reductants (2, 3). These factors include microsomes, mitochondria, cytochromes, and several flavoenzymes, such as glutathione reductase.

Using electron spin resonance (ESR) with a low-frequency microwave bridge and a cylinder-shaped loop gap resonator, we were able to show that a Cr(V) intermediate can be generated by one electron reduction of Cr(VI) in living animals (4). The Cr(V) was found predominantly in the liver with a small amount in the blood. The Cr(V) intermediate was identified to be a Cr(V)-NADPH complex with an oxygen bond to Cr(V). Pretreatment of the animals with ascorbate or GSH decreased the Cr(V) formation, while pretreatment with NADPH enhanced it. These results suggest that NADPH/flavoenzymes and not GSH or ascorbate are the major one-electron Cr(VI) reductants *in vivo*.

Free radical generation: Chromium is able to generate many different kinds of free radicals through its reactive intermediates, Cr(V), Cr(IV), Cr(III), and Cr(II), upon reactions with different agents. For example, reaction of Cr(VI) with glutathione (GSH) generates GSH-derived free radicals, while reaction with ascorbate generates ascorbate-derived free radicals (3, 5). Although all of these radicals can cause cell injury, hydroxyl radical (•OH) is especially important due to its high reactivity. In our earlier studies on the enzymatic reduction of Cr(VI), we have found that ${}^{\bullet}OH$ can be generated upon reaction of Cr(V) with hydrogen peroxide (H_2O_2) through a Fenton-like reaction. It has been suggested that this radical may be the species responsible for Cr(VI)-induced carcinogenesis (2). Further studies have demonstrated that various chromium oxidation states can be reduced by superoxide radical ($O_2^{\bullet-}$) to generate chromium intermediates at lower oxidation states, which react with H_2O_2 to generate ${}^{\bullet}OH$ through Haber-weiss reactions (2). The scheme that summarizes chromium-mediated ${}^{\bullet}OH$ generation is illustrated in Figure 1.

DNA damage by free radical reactions: Using λ Hind III DNA digest, our laboratory assessed DNA damage induced by a mixture of Cr(VI) and ascorbate. A significant amount of DNA strand breaks occurred when the DNA was incubated with Cr(VI) and ascorbate. Ascorbate-derived free radicals play a major role in this type of DNA damage. Addition of H_2O_2 to the reaction mixture generated ${}^{\bullet}OH$ radical and drastically enhanced the DNA damage. In addition to strand breaks, ${}^{\bullet}OH$ radicals can also react with guanine residues at several positions to generate a range of products, of which the most studied one is 8-hydroxyl-deoxyguanosine (8-OHdG). The formation of this adduct is considered a biomarker to implicate ROS in the mechanism of carcinogenesis induced by a variety of agents. Using HPLC with electrochemical detection, we have found that ${}^{\bullet}OH$ radicals generated by Cr(V) and Cr(IV)-mediated reaction caused 2'-deoxyguanosine (dG) hydroxylation to form 8-OHdG.

NF-κB activation: Nuclear transcription factor (NF)-κB is considered a primary oxidative response factor that functions to enhance the transcription of a variety of genes. In several cell types, ROS have been shown to activate this transcription factor. It has been shown that Cr(VI) is able to induce NF-κB activation (6). The reduction of Cr(VI) to low oxidation states is required for the NF-κB activation. Hydroxyl radicals generated by Cr(V)- and Cr(IV)-mediated Fenton-like reactions play a prominent role in the mechanism of Cr(VI)-induced NF-κB activation. It is possible that NF-κB activation and a subsequent expression of proto-oncogenes, such as c-*myc*, may play a role in the induction of neoplastic transformation by Cr(VI).

AP-1 activation: Nuclear transcription factor AP-1 is also an oxidative stress response transcription factor. It is a complex protein composed of homodimers and heterodimers of oncogene proteins of the Jun and Fos families. The results obtained from our recent studies have shown that Cr(VI) is able to induce activation of this transcription factor. This induction requires mitogen activated protein (MAP) kinase p38 and c-jun-N-terminal kinase (JNK), but not extracellular-signal-regulated kinase (ERK). Aspirin, a newly established antioxidant, inhibited the AP-1 activation. Inhibition of p38 and IκB kinase (IKK) attenuated the Cr(VI)-induced AP-1 activation. The results suggest that ROS may serve as a common up-stream signal initiating the AP-1 activation in response to Cr(VI) stimulation, whereas p38 and IKK act as down-stream executive kinases for the activation of this transcription factor.

Activation of p53: The p53 is also an important oxidative response transcription factor. It is involved in various biological processes, such as regulation of genes in the cell cycle, cell growth arrest after DNA damage, and apoptosis. Our recent studies have shown that Cr(VI) is able to induce the activation of p53 protein in the epithelial cell line, A549. Hydroxyl radical plays a key role in this Cr(VI)-induced p53 activation. Hydroxyl radical is generated by a Cr(VI)-mediated Fenton-like reaction. H_2O_2 was generated via $O_2^{\bullet-}$ dismutation. The $O_2^{\bullet-}$ radical was produced from molecular oxygen during the Cr(VI) reduction.

Apoptosis: Apoptosis is a programmed cell death mechanism to control cell number in tissues and to

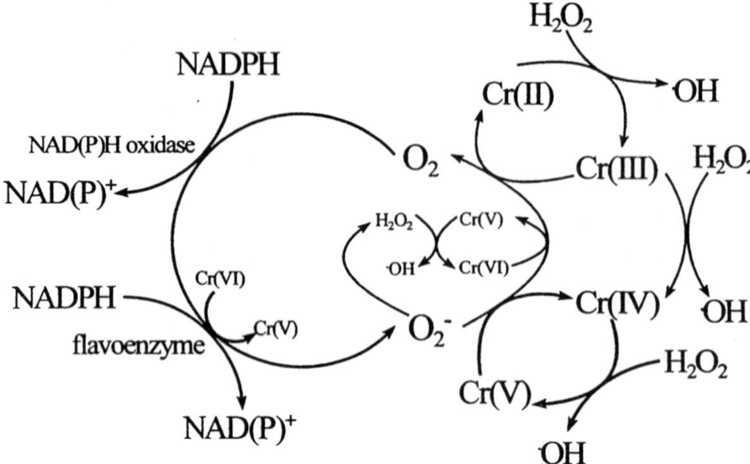

Figure 1. A scheme of chroimium-mediated ·OH generation.

eliminate individual cells that may lead to disease states. Because of the fundamental importance of apoptosis in the regulation of tissue growth, alteration of this pathway is important in carcinogenesis. Our study has shown that Cr(VI) is able to induce apoptosis (8). In the apoptotic signaling pathway, ROS generated from both Cr(VI) reduction and p53 activation play an important role. The Cr(VI)-derived ROS initiate apoptosis before activation of p53 protein. Cr(VI) induces apoptosis through both p53-dependent and p53 independent pathways. ROS generated by Cr(VI) may play a dual role in the mechanism of Cr(VI)-induced carcinogenesis: genetic damage and apoptosis. The cancer development may depend on the delicate balance of these two opposite processes.

References

1. De Flora, S., Bagnasco, M., Serra, D., and Zanacchi, P. (1990) Genotoxicity of chromium compounds: a review. *Mutat. Res.* **238**, 99-172.
2. Shi, X., Chiu, A., Chen, C.T., Halliwell, B., Castranova, V., and Vallyathan, V. Reduction of chromium(VI) and its relationship to carcinogenesis. *J Toxicol Environ Health* **2**, 87-104, 1999.
3. Shi, X., and Dalal, N.S. On the hydroxyl radical formation in the reaction between hydrogen peroxide and biologically generated chromium (V) species. *Arch Biochem Biophys* **277**, 342-350, 1990.
4. Liu, K.J., Shi, X., Jiang, J.J., Goda, F., Dalal, N.S., and Swartz, H.M. Chromate-induced chromium(V) formation in live mice and its control by cellular antioxidants: an L-band EPR study. *Arch Biochem Biophys* **323**, 33-39, 1995.
5. Shi, X., Ding, M., Ye, J., Wang, S., Leonard, S.S., Zang, L., Castranova, V., Valyathan, V., Chiu, A., Dalal, N.S., and Liu, K. Cr(IV) causes activation of nuclear transcription factors-κB, DNA strand breaks and dG hydroxylation via free radical reactions. J Inorg Biochem 75, 37-44, 1999.
6. Ye, J., Zhang, X., Young, H.A., Mao, Y., and Shi, X. Chromium(VI)-induced nuclear factor-κB activation in intact cells via free radical reactions. *Carcinogenesis* **16**, 2401-2405, 1995..
7. Ye, J., Wang, S., Leonard, S.S., Sun, Y., Butterworth, L., Antonini, J., Ding, M., Vallyathan, V., Castranova, V., and Shi, X. Role of reactive oxygen species and p53 in chromium(VI)-induced apoptosis. *J Biol Chem* **274**, 34974-34980, 1999.

Metal Ions in Biology and Medicine; vol 6. Eds. J.A. Centeno, Ph. Collery, G. Vernet, R.B. Finkelman, H. Gibb, J.C. Etienne. John Libbey Eurotext, Paris © 2000, pp. 113-115.

Chromium(III)-DNA adducts are the major form of mutagenic DNA lesions produced during reductive metabolism of chromate by cysteine

Anatoly Zhitkovich, Victoria Voitkun, Yi Song, George Quievryn and Angela DeLucia

Department of Pathology and Laboratory Medicine, Brown University, Providence, RI 02906

Abstract. Hexavalent Cr compounds are established mutagens and human carcinogens. Induction of genetic damage by Cr(VI) results from the reductive conversion of Cr(VI) to Cr(III), a process accomponied by the formation of unstable intermediates. In this work, we analyzed formation of mutagenic DNA damage during Cr(VI) reduction by cysteine. Reduction of Cr(VI) led to a dose-dependent binding of Cr(III) to DNA producing binary Cr-DNA and ternary cysteine-Cr-DNA adducts. Reductive metabolism of Cr(VI) by cysteine has also resulted in the induction of mutations in a shuttle-vector following its replication in human cells. Elimination of Cr-DNA binding abolished mutagenic responses indicating that the formation of mutagenic DNA damage during reduction of Cr(VI) is caused by Cr-DNA adducts.

Genotoxic activity of Cr(VI) compounds is known to be dependent on its reductive metabolism. In the absence of reducing compounds, chromate is unreactive toward DNA and other macromolecules. Predominant reducers of Cr(VI) in cells are believed to be ascorbate and low-molecular weight thiols, such as cysteine (Cys) and glutathione (1,2). Intracellular metabolism of Cr(VI) leads to the formation of stable Cr(III) form and this process is potentially associated with production of oxidative DNA damage. Exposure of cells to Cr(VI) has been shown to result in the formation of several types of Cr-DNA adducts. These include binary Cr-DNA adducts, DNA-protein crosslinks and Cr(III)-mediated DNA crosslinks with His, Cys or glutathione (3). DNA crosslinks with amino acids and glutathione formed in the reaction with Cr(III) has recently been shown to be mutagenic in human cells pointing to a potential importance of Cr(III)-dependent pathway in chromate genotoxicity (4). However, formation of Cr-DNA adducts may be somewhat different if the starting material is Cr(VI) which is subsequently converted into Cr(III) in the reduction reaction. In addition, this reduction process may also lead to the formation of potentially mutagenic forms of oxidative DNA damage. In order to determine a relative importance of Cr-dependent reactions in mutagenicity of chromate, we analyzed spectrum of DNA lesions produced during reduction with Cys and studied induction of mutagenic damage.

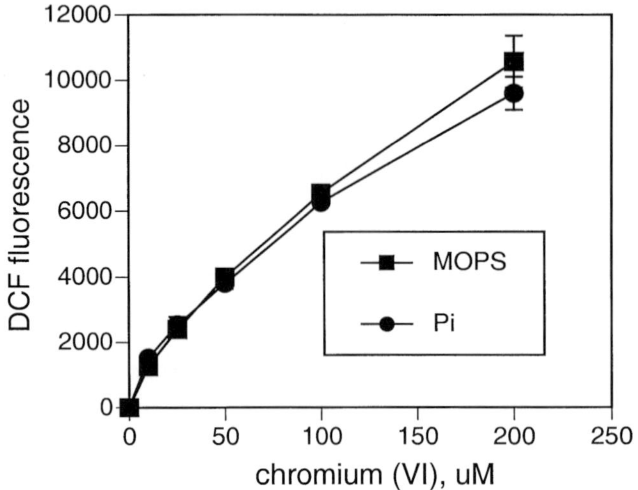

Figure 1. Production of oxidizing species during reduction of Cr(VI) as determined by the DCF fluorescence.

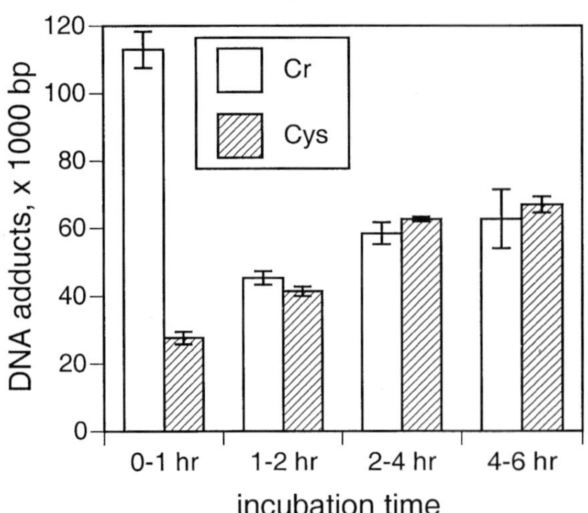

Figure 2. Formation of DNA adducts with Cr and cysteine at different times after the start of Cr(VI) reduction.

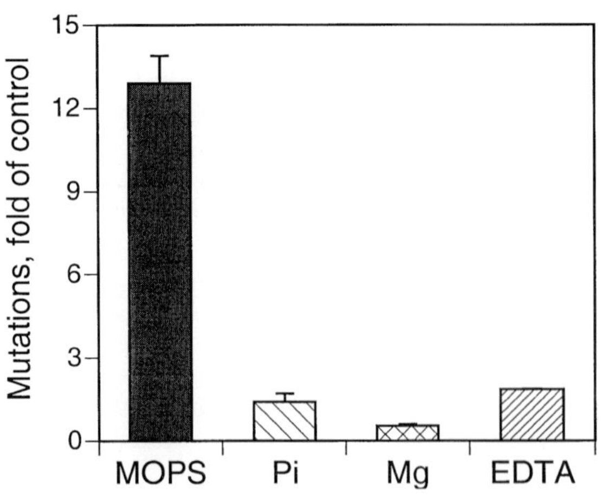

Figure 3. Induction of mutagenic DNA damage during reduction of Cr(VI) by cysteine.

Reduction reactions of Cr(VI) were performed with 2 mM cysteine in 25 mM MOPS or phosphate buffer, pH 7.0. All reagents used in these studies were rigorously purified from trace amounts of redox-active metals by Chelex-100 chromatography. The kinetics of Cr(VI) reduction was followed by absorbance measurements at 372 nm. Formation of oxidizing species was registered by fluorescence of 2',7'-dichlorofluorescein (DCF). A number of DNA adducts was determined using radiolabeled chromate and ^{35}S-cysteine. DNA binding experiments were carried out in the presence of 400 μM Cr(VI) and MOPS buffer. Induction of mutagenic DNA lesions was tested in the pSP189 shuttle-vector system as described earlier (4).

In our initial experiments, we determined that in the presence of 2 mM Cys more than 95% of Cr(VI) was reduced after just 1 hr incubation. The reduction process was accompanied by the production of oxidizing species as evidenced by an extensive formation of fluorescent form of oxidant-sensitive dye DCFH after 30 min after the start of the reaction (Fig. 1). DCF fluorescence was similar among samples containing either phosphate or MOPS buffer. Reduction of Cr(VI) also led to the formation of binary Cr-DNA adducts and DNA crosslinks with cysteine (Fig. 2). The most active formation of binary Cr-DNA adducts was observed during the initial incubation time. At later time points, overall Cr-DNA binding was significantly lower and was associated with almost equimolar crosslinking of Cys. In contrast to binary Cr adducts, DNA crosslinks with Cys were more actively formed after the completion of Cr(VI) reduction. The later finding is consistent with the previous results that crosslinking of Cys occurs through attack of DNA by Cr(III)-Cys complexes (5). Lower yield of Cr-DNA adducts at post-reduction time is likely to result from complexation of Cr(III) with Cys. Complexes of Cr(III) with two cysteines are expected to have a substantially diminished reactivity toward DNA (6). Oxidative DNA damage was not detected under buffer conditions studied.

Mutational activity of plasmids was tested following 1 hr reduction of 50 μM Cr(VI). In the preliminary experiments, we found that a number Cr-DNA adducts was severely decreased in the presence of Mg^{2+}, phosphate or EDTA. Reduction of Cr(VI) in MOPS buffer led to a substantial increase in the mutation frequency of pSP189 plasmids (Fig. 3). Incubation of plasmids in the presence of phosphate, Mg ions or EDTA essentially eliminated mutagenic activity of Cr(VI)/cysteine mixtures. Phosphate and EDTA prevent formation of Cr-DNA adducts by binding Cr(III), whereas Mg^{2+} blocks DNA phosphates needed for Cr(III) attachment. We concluded that Cr-DNA adducts were largely responsible for mutagenic DNA damage produced during reduction of Cr(VI) by Cys.

References

1. DeFlora S. and Wetterhahn K. E.*Life Chemistry Reports*, **7:** 169-244 (1989).
2. Suzuki Y. and Fukuda K. *Arch. Tox.*, **64:** 169-176 (1990).
3. Zhitkovich A., Voitkun V. and Costa M. *Carcinogenesis*, **16**: 907-913 (1995).
4. Voitkun V., Zhitkovich A. and Costa M. *Nucl. Acids Res.*, **26**: 2024-2030 (1998).
5. Zhitkovich A., Voitkun V. and Costa M. *Biochemistry*, **35**: 7275-7282 (1996).
6. Hneihen A.S., Standeven A.M. and Wetterhahn K.E. *Carcinogenesis*, **14**: 1795-803 (1993).

Metal Ions in Biology and Medicine; vol 6. Eds. J.A. Centeno, Ph. Collery, G. Vernet, R.B. Finkelman, H. Gibb, J.C. Etienne. John Libbey Eurotext, Paris © 2000, pp. 117-119.

Evaluation of apoptosis in a cell culture exposed to low doses of lead acetate

Iavicoli I., Carelli G., Masci O., Castellino N.

Institute of Occupational Health (Director: Prof. N. Castellino), Università Cattolica del Sacro Cuore, Largo F. Vito, 1-00168 Roma Italy

Introduction

In the literature lead-related cell toxicity studies refer principally to primary cultured cells isolated from lab animals after intoxication at different doses (1). Following epidemiological investigations into the effects of low doses of lead on the central nervous system in children (2,3), this type of research was aimed mainly at ascertaining the action mechanisms, and particularly, the effects of lead on nerve cells.

The aim of this study is to evaluate the effects of lead on fibroblast cell vitality and to identify the eventual type of cell death that occurs as a result of lead toxicity.

Materials and methods

Cell vitality assessment

Cultured rat fibroblasts (RAT-1) were placed in dishes containing 24 wells (10^4 cells/well) with Eagle's minimum essential medium (EMEM) supplemented with 10% fetal bovine. These were then incubated at 37°C in a 5% CO_2 atmosphere. When cells were subconfluent, the medium in each well was replaced by 1 ml medium supplemented with lead (Lead (II) acetate trihydrate for analysis, Merck, Germany) at the following concentrations: 0.078, 0.156, 0.312, 0.625, 1.25, 2.5, 5.0, 10.0 μM. These cells were then incubated for 48h at 37°C. The experiment was repeated seven times for each concentration and results are presented as a percentage value. The MTT test was used to assess cell vitality (4).

Apoptosis assessment

Apoptosis (5), evaluated by cytosolic DNA fragments, was quantified with a cell death detection ELISA assay (6) (Boehringer Mannheim GmbH, Germany). Briefly, the assay is based on a quantitative sandwich-enzyme-immunoassay-principle using mouse monoclonal antibodies directed against DNA and histones, respectively. This permits the specific determination of mono- and oligonucleosomes in the cytoplasmatic fraction of cell lysates.

Lead assessment in cells, in the medium and in PBS

Lead was calculated in cells in the medium to which no lead had been added and also in cells whose medium had received a 0.156 µM lead dose. In both the control and the 0.156 µM dose, cultured rat fibroblasts (RAT-1) were plated on two polystyrene dishes (diam 15mm, Greiner) in EMEM without or with lead added for 48h after subconfluence occurred. After plating the medium was removed by sterile glass Pasteur pipette. The cells were washed twice in the dishes with Phosphate Buffered Salin (PBS) and then collected with a Falcon's scraper. Subsequently the cells (10^7) were centrifuged for 5 min at 1250 rpm in 15 ml polypropylene vessels (Greiner) at 40°C and the supernatant was discharged. After a further washing with PBS, the cells were centrifuged in 1.5 ml plastic vessels (Eppendorf) under the same centrifugation conditions. The supernatant was completely removed avoiding cell loss, and the pellet was stored at -80°C until analysis.

Lead analyses in cells, medium and PBS were performed after nitric acid digestion by flameless atomic absorption spectrometry with Zeeman background correction. The recovery of added lead ranged between 91.0 and 109.0 (average±SD = 97.4±5.0, n = 9).

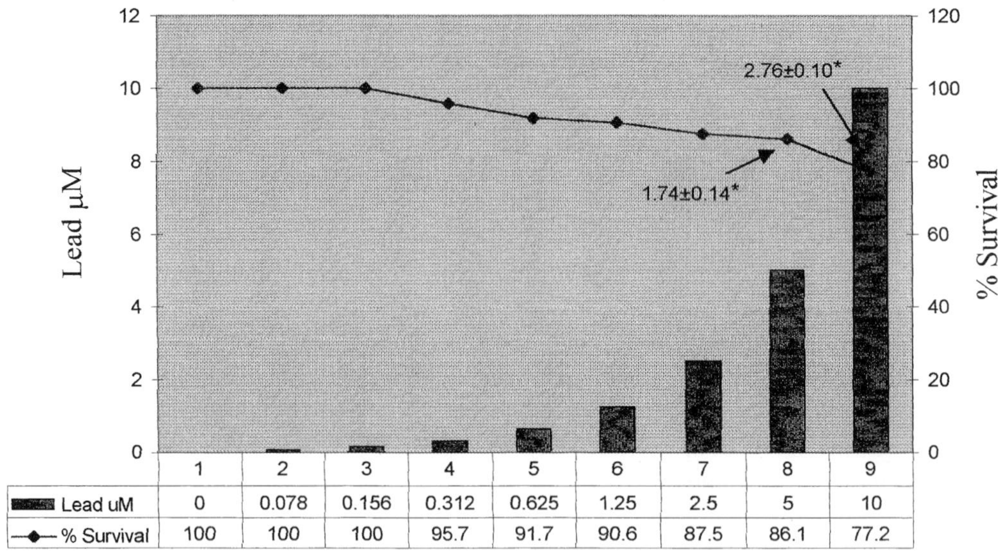

	1	2	3	4	5	6	7	8	9
Lead uM	0	0.078	0.156	0.312	0.625	1.25	2.5	5	10
% Survival	100	100	100	95.7	91.7	90.6	87.5	86.1	77.2

Results

Evaluation of vitality by means of the MTT test on RAT-1 fibroblasts exposed to different concentrations of lead acetate is expressed as a percentage in figure. The t-Test revealed significant differences in survival rate between the control and concentrations ranging from 0.625 to 10 µM.

This figure also illustrates apoptosis as an enrichment factor (DNA fragmentation) at two exposure concentrations (5 μM e 10 μM). The experiment was repeated seven times for each concentration and results are presented as the mean ± SE.
Vitality therefore remains unimpaired in relation to control values at a concentration of 0.156 μM, although mineralization of fibroblast samples (10^7 cells) exposed to this dose demonstrated the presence of a 7.1 ng lead concentration, i.e. above the 3.1 ng control value based on a medium to which no lead had been added. EMEM and PBS lead levels are quite similar (approx. 0.05 μM)

Conclusions

The experiments performed on rat fibroblasts indicated that:

-there is a decline in vitality at medium concentrations of 0,312 μM and over. In medium concentrations of up to 0.156 μM there is No Observed Effect

-lead uptake in culture cells occurs even at concentrations below the action concentration.

-assessment of programmed death or necrotic death is important in understanding the final effects of low dose lead toxicity on biological systems.

References

1. Kern M, Audesirk G. Inorganic lead may inhibit neurite development in cultured rat hippocampal neurons through hyperphosphorylation. Toxicol Appl Pharmacol 1995, 134, 111-23.
2. Banks EC, Ferretti LE, Shucard DW. Effects of low level lead exposure on cognitive function in children: a review of behavioral, neuropsychological and biological evidence. Neurotoxicology 1997, 18(1), 237-81.
3. Dudek B, Merecz D. Impairment of psychological functions in children environmentally exposed to lead. Int J Occup Med Environ Health 1997, 10(1), 37-46.
4. Mosmann T. Rapid colorimetric assay for cellular growth and survival: application to proliferation and cytotoxicity assays. J Immunol Methods 1983, 65(1-2), 55-63.
5. Green DR, Reed JC. Mithocondria and apoptosis. Science 1998, 281(5381), 1309-12.
6. Sandoval M, Zhang XJ, Liu X, Mannick EE, Clark DA, Miller MJ. Peroxynitrite-induced apoptosis in T84 and RAW 264.7 cells: attenuation by L-ascorbic acid. Free Radic Biol Med 1997 22(3) 489-95.

Metal Ions in Biology and Medicine; vol 6. Eds. J.A. Centeno, Ph. Collery, G. Vernet, R.B. Finkelman, H. Gibb, J.C. Etienne. John Libbey Eurotext, Paris © 2000, pp. 120-122.

The biological methylation of bismuth; evidence for the involvement of polydimethylsiloxanes in the biologically-mediated methylation of metals

Eugene B. Wickenheiser[1], Klaus Michalke[2], Alfred V. Hirner[3], Reinhard Hensel[2], and Daniela Flassbeck[3]

[1] Department of Biochemistry, Northern Michigan University, Marquette, MI 49855; [2] Microbiology Department, University of Essen, 45117 Essen, Germany; [3] Institute for Environmental and Analytical Chemistry, University of Essen, 45117 Essen, Germany

Abstract
We present evidence that chemicals in household products aid in the mobilization of metals from waste deposit sites. Two commonly used polydimethylsiloxanes (D4 and D5) stimulate the microbial production of trimethylbismuth.

Introduction
The methylation of elements in the environment is well documented, and the presence of volatile methyl- and hydride derivatives of heavy metals in the gases released from waste deposits and sewage treatment facilities indicates that similar processes also occur there [1]. Although the chemical pathways producing the methylated compounds the gases are unknown, microbial activity can account for the production of several of the species [2,3]. Environmental methylation can be attributed to methyl transfer from biologically-derived sources (methylcobalamine, S-adenosylmethionine); however, we have investigated the possibility that materials of anthropogenic origin, namely polydimethylsiloxanes (PDMS), may be involved in biological methylation processes, and have chosen the metal bismuth, and the organism *Methanosarcina barkeri* (*M. Barkeri*), to pursue this question. Trimethylbismuth (TMBi) is a volatile bismuth species that has been identified in environmental gases [4], and *M. Barkeri* is a cobalamine-producing archaea commonly found in sewage [2]. Bismuth and PDMS are present in domestic waste as a result of their use in household products; the PDMS examined here, octamethylcyclotetrasiloxane(D4; $(CH_3)_8Si_4O_4$) and decamethylcyclopentasiloxane (D5; $(CH_3)_{10}Si_5O_5$), have a combined annual US production exceeding 1 million pounds [5].

Experimental Section
Experiments were conducted with pure cultures of *Methanosarcina barkeri* in 100mL serum bottles at 37°C in the dark, with 50 mL medium (DSMZ-Medium 120, without sludge fluid) in an atmosphere of CO_2/H_2 (80/20%; P=2atm). The samples were spiked with to give concentrations of 4ppm Bi^{3+} and 100ppm of D4 or D5. Sewage sludge

samples were incubated in an atmosphere of CO_2/H_2 (80/20%; P=2atm) at 37°C in the dark without the addition of Bi^{3+} and/or siloxanes. Gases were analyzed using a gas chromatographic separation system coupled to an inductively-coupled plasma mass spectrometer [3], and gas constituents were identified by their characteristic masses (e.g. Bi, 209m/z; Si, 28m/z, 29m/z; SiOH, 47m/z) and retention time comparison with commercially obtained D4 and D5 (Gelest, Germany) and synthesized TMBi [6]. The deuterium labeling studies were conducted using synthesized D4-d_{24} [7] and a Hewlett Packard GC-MS for TMBi analysis (HP 5890II GC, HP 5 column; HP 5989 detector).

Results and Discussion

A series of experiments sheds light on the biological activity of the siloxanes D4 and D5 in sewage. First of all, several of the volatile metal- and metalloid-containing compounds found in waste deposit gases can be readily observed in the gas phase above incubated sewage sludge (Figure 1a). These samples also revealed the presence of D4 and D5 in the gas phase, consistent with their volatility, and their common occurrence in sewage sludge [8]. As mentioned earlier, *M. barkeri* produces the methylating agent cobalamine; however, experiments in which pure cultures were spiked with bismuth produced no detectable quantities of TMBi. When cultures of *M. barkeri* were spiked with both bismuth and D4 or D5, TMBi was produced at levels comparable to those observed in sewage sludge (Figure 1b). TMBi was not detected in control experiments, where bismuth and D4 or D5 were incubated in sterile growth medium, implying that PDMS is involved in the biological methylation of bismuth.

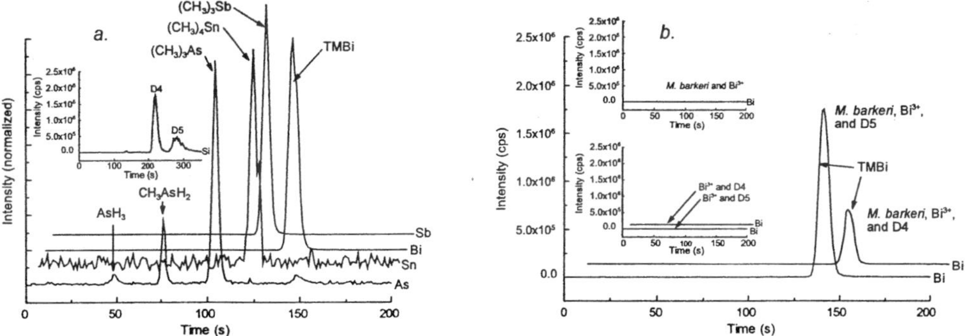

FIGURE 1*a*. Gases detected above incubated sewage sludge; *b*. ^{209}Bi chromatographs indicating TMBi production by *M. barkeri* in the presence of Bi^{3+}(aq) and D4 (below), and D5 (above). Insets show the absence of TMBi in control experiments.

The environmental degradation of PDMS produces low molecular weight oligomers, dimethylsilanediol, and trimethylsilanol [9], and ultimately the inorganic compounds carbon dioxide and silicic acid [10]. In order to test the possibility of biologically-mediated methyl-group transfer from PDMS to bismuth during PDMS degradation, we conducted experiments with deuterium-labeled PDMS. Following the same protocol for non-labeled PDMS, cultures of *M. barkeri* were spiked with bismuth and D4-d_{24}. In this case, the TMBi in the headspace gases were analyzed with electron ionization GC-MS to obtain molecular and fragment masses, which were found to be identical in fragment and parent-ion masses to the unlabelled TMBi, indicating that the methyl groups of the TMBi do not originate from the D4, or its degradation products.

Based on this work, PDMS compounds, which were initially thought to be environmentally inert, are involved in the mobilization of bismuth in pure cultures of an organism known to be a part of the microbiological flora in waste treatment settings. The broader implications of these results are that polymethylated siloxanes may be involved in chemical reactions of metals when biological activity, metals and PDMS are present. The process by which the methylation occurs is unknown, but the PDMS are not the methyl-group donors in the formation of trimethylbismuth as studied here. Given that siloxanes in sludge partition primarily onto the microbial biomass [11], it may be that their activity lies in the modification of bacterial cell membranes.

Acknowledgments
We thank the Deutsche Forschungs Gemeinschaft for the financial support.

Literature Cited

1. Feldmann J, Grümping R, Hirner A. Determination of volatile metal and metalloid compounds in gases from domestic waste deposits with GC/ICP-MS. *Fresenius J Anal Chem* 1994; 350: 228-34.
2. Gadd G, Microbial formation and transformation of organometallic and organometalloid compounds. *FEMS Microbiol Rev* 1993; 11: 297-316.
3. Wickenheiser E, Michalke K, Drescher C, Hirner A, Hensel R.The study of anaerobic arsenic metabolism by the application of liquid and gas chromatographic speciation techniques with element specific detection. *Fresenius J Anal Chem* 1998; 362: 498-501.
4. Feldmann, J., E. M. Krupp, D. Glindemann, A. V. Hirner, and W. R. Cullen. 1999. Methylated bismuth in the environment. *Appl Organometal Chem* 1999; 13: 1-10.
5. High Production Volume Chemical List, Office of Pollution Prevention and Toxics, United States Environmental Protection Agency, 1998.
6. Wieber M, Gmelin Handbuch der Anorganischen Chemie. New York: Springer Verlag. 1977.
7. *a.* Beltzung M, Picot C, Rempp P, Herz J. Investigation of the conformation of elastic chains in poly(dimethylsiloxane) networks by small-angle neutron-scattering, *Macromol* 1982; 15: 1594-1600; *b.* Gilliam W, Liebhasfky H, Winslow A. Dimethyl silicon dichloride and methyl silicon trichloride. *J Am Chem Soc* 1941; 63: 801-3.
8. Fendinger N, McAvoy D, Eckhoff W, Price B. Environmental occurrence of polydimethylsiloxanes. *Environ Sci Technol* 1997; 31: 1555-63.
9. Grümping R, Mikolajczak D, Hirner A. Determination of trimethylsilanol in the environment by LT-GC/ICP-OES and GC-MS. *Fresenius J Anal Chem* 1998; 31: 133-9.
10. Stevens C. Environmental degradation pathways for the breakdown of polydimethylsiloxanes. *J Inorg Biochem* 1998; 69: 203-7.
11. Watts R, Kong S, Haling C, Gearhart L, Frye C, Vigon B. Fate and effects of polydimethylsiloxanes on pilot and bench-top activated sludge reactors and anaerobic/aerobic digesters. *Wat Res* 1995; 29: 2405-11.

Metal Ions in Biology and Medicine; vol 6. Eds. J.A. Centeno, Ph. Collery, G. Vernet, R.B. Finkelman, H. Gibb, J.C. Etienne. John Libbey Eurotext, Paris © 2000, pp. 123-125.

Iron accumulation in hypotransferrinemic mouse brain

Atsushi Takeda, Keiko Takatsuka, James R Connor* and Naoto Oku

*Department of Radiobiochemistry, School of Pharmaceutical Sciences, University of Shizuoka, 52-1 Yada, Shizuoka 422-8526, Japan, * Department of Neuroscience & Anatomy, M.S. Hershey Medical Center, Pennsylvania State University College of Medicine, Hershey, PA 17033, USA*

Iron is an essential trace metal for brain development and also a toxicant in excessive amounts. Transferrin, a serum glycoprotein, has been considered as critical for the transport of iron. Transferrin is synthesized primarily in the liver but significant amounts are also produced in the brain. Iron can generate free radicals because of its strength as a reducing agent. Alteration of iron metabolism in the brain has been associated with neurological disorders such as Alzheimer's disease and Parkinson's disease. Ttansferrin levels in brain decrease with age and the decrease is more dramatic when Alzheimer's or Parkinson's diseases are superimposed on the aging process. The transferrin/iron ratio, an index of iron mobilization capacity, is decreased in the globus pallidus and caudate putamen in both Alzheimer's and Parkinson's diseases. The decrease in Transferrin in neurological diseases has been suggested as the cause of increased brain iron accumulation in these diseases.

The HP mouse, a naturally occurring mouse mutant, has a point mutation or small deletion in the transferrin gene that results in defective splicing of transferrin precursor mRNA. As a consequence of this mutation, the HP mouse produces <1 % of the normal circulating level of plasma transferrin. The affected animals are small, pale and severely anemic at birth and require weekly injections of transferrin for survival. The cellular and regional distribution of iron, transferrin, transferrin receptor and ferritin in the brain of HP adult mice injected with transferrin is similar to normal brain and transferrin in the brain of the former is of exogeneous origin. Iron is found predominantly in oligodendrocytes in the brain and required for myelin production. There is evidence of hypomyelination in the brain of HP mice.

The purpose of the present study is to examine the participation of non-transferrin-mediated uptake system in iron acquisition by the brain of 7-day-old Hp mutant mice without injection of transferrin. Iron uptake is the highest during postnatal development at a time period that coincides with peaks in brain growth and myelinogenesis.

HP mutant and non-mutant mice were subcutaneously injected with $^{59}FeCl_3$ and subjected to brain autoradiography 24 h after injection. In the brain of HP mice, ^{59}Fe was largely concentrated in the lateral, the third and the fourth ventricles, including the choroid plexus, with only small amounts in the cerebral aqueduct. On the other hand, in the brain of non-mutant mice, ^{59}Fe was extensively distributed in the brain. When radioactivity distribution in the brain autoradiograms was measured quantitatively with a Bio-imaging Analyzer, the radioactivity in the choroid plexus in the lateral ventricles of HP mutant brain was approximately 7 times higher than that of non-mutant brain. The radioactivity in other brain regions of the former was a little lower than that of the latter and the radioactivity in the hippocampus, substantia nigra and inferior colliculi of the former was significantly lower. The radioactivity in the cerebellum was relatively high in non-mutant brain. When binding of ^{59}Fe to serum proteins of HP mutant and non-mutant mice was examined in vitro, HPLC analysis indicated that most ^{59}Fe was bound to proteins of molecular weights of <80 kDa in HP mutant serum. Transferrin was not detected in HP mutant serum by the HPLC analysis. These results indicate that non-transferrin-mediated iron uptake system is present in the brain of HP mice.

Non-transferrin-bound iron might be interact with DMT1, a divalent metal transporter, which is localized in the choroidal epithelial cells. If the non-transferrin-bound iron is reduced to ferrous iron via a ferrireductase on the choroidal epithelial cells, the iron could be taken up by the cells. There may be also another mechanism that non-transferrin-bound iron is transported into the brain via p97 (melanotransferrin), an iron binding protein, which is localized in human brain capillary endothelium. In the brain, DMT1 is also found in most neurons, but not glial or ependymal cells. On the other hand, non-transferrin mediated iron uptake is demonstrated in glial cell cultures from neonatal HP mutant mice (1).

Because blood radioactivity of HP mice was approximately one-fifth of that of non-mutant mice 24 h after injection of $^{59}FeCl_3$, brain uptake ratio expressed relative to blood radioactivity was calculated to correct the brain uptake for change in the blood radioactivity. ^{59}Fe uptake ratio of HP mutant mice was remarkably higher in any brain region than in that of non-mutant mice. These results suggest that iron is readily taken up in the brain of HP mice via non-transferrin mediated uptake system. Moreover, iron concentration in the brain of HP mice was measured with a flameless atomic absorption spectrophotometer. It was approximately three times higher than that of non-mutant mice. It is likely that iron is not properly utilized in the brain of HP mice without injection of transferrin. Therefore, transferrin produced by oligodendrocytes may be important for iron utilization in myelinogenesis. These results suggest that non-transferrin mediated iron uptake is involved in iron deposit in the brain.

In glial cell cultures from normal neonatal mice, ^{59}Fe uptake was facilitated in the media without transferrin suggesting that non-transferrin-mediated iron uptake system is also present in the normal brain.

In conclusion, non-transferrin-mediated iron uptake may be involved in iron deposit in the brain, which is associated with pathogenesis of neurodegenration.

Reference

1. Takeda A, Devenyi A, Connor JR, Evidence for non-transferrin-mediated uptake and release of iron and manganese in glial cell cultures from hypotransferinemic mice. J. Neurosci. Res. 51, 454-462 (1998)

Metal Ions in Biology and Medicine; vol 6. Eds. J.A. Centeno, Ph. Collery, G. Vernet, R.B. Finkelman, H. Gibb, J.C. Etienne. John Libbey Eurotext, Paris © 2000, pp. 126-128.

Bicarbonate effects on Zn, Cu, Cd, Ca, Mg transport in the rat's isolated urinary bladder

Dimitris Giannakis[2], Angelos Evangelou[1], Xenophon Giannakopoulos[2], Angeliki Galani[1] and Vicky Kalfakakou[1]

[1] Laboratory of Experimental Physiology, [2] Urology Clinic, Faculty of Medicine, University of Ioannina, Ioannina 45110, Greece

Background: Zinc as an essential metal participates several enzymatic systems, possesses a protective role against Cd toxicity and presents antagonism with Cu, Ca and Mg in many tissues. Bicarbonates regulate Zn transport in the red blood cells rich in carbonic anhydrase, a Zn enzyme and may interfere the metal's transport in tissues with similar bicarbonate management.

Aim: The elucidation of bicarbonate related mechanisms regulating Zn,Cu,Cd,Ca,Mg transport in the urinary bladder wall.

Methods: The urinary bladders and urine samples of male wistar rats were determined for their Zn,Cu,Cd,Ca,Mg content. Isolated urinary bladders were then incubated in Chenoweth based medium, pH:7.8, resembling the urine content in the above metals, for 20 and 60 min in different bicarbonate and furosemide – a carbonic anhydrase inhibitor-concentrations.

Results: Bicarbonate presence reduces significantly (68.3%) urinary bladder's zinc content and increases Cu and Cd (95% and 213% correspondingly)concentrations. Furosemide (0.1mg/ml) induced Cd eflux.

Conclusions: Bicarbonates may enhance the incorporation of carcinogenic metals such as Cd and the efflux of essential and protective ones such as Zn in the rat's urinary bladder.

Key words: zinc,cadmium,transport, bicarbonates,furosemide

Introduction

Bladder undergoes active transport of ions such as, Na^+ absorption, H^+ and HCO_3^- excretion from cells rich in carbonic anhydrase (CA) and Cl^- reabsorption.[1].Zinc- bicarbonate- chloride anionic complexes influx easily across red blood cell membrane.[2] Furthermore an exchange reaction between Zn^{2+} and Ca^{2+} helps zinc upgradient transport in human red cells.[3] There are though contradictory reports on Zn and Cu effects related to Cd transport across membranes .[4,5]

Since bladder and red cells exhibit similar bicarbonate management we investigated bicarbonate relations to cationic metals in rat's urinary bladder.

Materials and Methods

A model-incubation medium, based on Chenoweth solution and resembling the rat urine conditions, according to analysis of Na+, K+, Cl-, HCO3-, pH, PO2, Zn, Cu, Mg, Ca and Cd, in 24h urine collections of a control group of male rats, was prepared (control group: N=12, age: 9-10 weeks, b.w: 190-200g).

Determination of serum and bladder Zn, Cu, Cd , Ca and Mg concentrations of control rats were also performed by means of atomic absorption spectrophotometry (AAS).(Perkin-Elmer 560 with

HGA and background corrector).The urinary bladders of the experimental group of rats were subsequently isolated and incubated at pH=7.8 , in various conditions as follows:

a. in absence of HCO_3^-
b. in normal HCO_3^- concs($2.5x10^{-2}$ M) and
c. (2xnormal) HCO_3^- concs.

Subsequently incubations a, b, c were repeated after furosemide (0.1 mg/ml=pharmacological levels) addition. Each set of incubations included six (6) urinary bladders, three (3) for 20 min and three (3) for 60 min of incubation.All bladders after acid digestion were determined for their Zn, Cu, Cd, Ca and Mg content.

Results

Urinary bladders incubated without bicarbonates manifested a time depended increase in Cd and Cu incorporation whereas bladder's Zn, Mg, and Ca content was decreased.

Time	**Cu**	**Zn**	**Ca**	**Cd**	**Mg**
0-20 '	153% ↑	34.9%↓	47.3%↓	205.9%↑	95.7%↓
0-60 '	208% ↑	45.5%↓	37.6%↓	222.0%↑	93.9%↓

Table1.Changes (%) of metal concs in rat's bladder wall after incubation without bicarbonates at pH=7.8

Bladders incubated in bicarbonates ($2.5x10^{-2}$ M and $5x10^{-2}$) revealed increased Cd incorporation and zinc efflux.The effects were not dose dependent.

Time	**Cu**	**Zn**	**Ca**	**Cd**	**Mg**
0-20'	118.7%↑	59.6%↓	36.9%↓	278%↑	92.8%↓
0-60'	95.0%↑	68.3%↓	31.2%↓	213%↑	93.9%↓

Table 2.Changes (%) of metal concs in rat's bladder wall after incubation with bicarbonates($2.5.10^{-2}$ M) at pH=7.8

Furosemide decreased bicarbonate induced incorporation of Cu and Cd while Zn excretion was not affected.

Time	**Cu**	**Zn**	**Ca**	**Cd**	**Mg**
0-20'	38.2%↑	63.8%↓	69.2%↓	140%↑	87%↓
0-60'	42.4%↑	65.7%↓	54.6%↓	49.5%↑	89%↓

Table 3.Changes (%) of metal concs in rat's bladder wall after incubation with bicarbonates($2.5.10^{-2}$ M) and furosemide (0.1mg/m) at pH=7.8

Discussion

Carbonic anhydrase (CA), an enzymatic system producing bicarbonates, is abudantly met in RBCs and urinary system.Zinc in presence of bicarbonates and chlorides forms an anionic complex passively and rapidly transported into the RBCs.[2]It is reported that in turtle's bladder exist 2 cell species: a-cells excreting H+ and b-cells excreting HCO_3^- and reabsorbing Cl^-.[1] In our results zinc release from bladder wall in presence of bicarbonates is significantly increased ($p=0.04$ at 20 min and $p=0.002$ at 60 min) while Cd incorporation is, in contrast ,significantly increased(Table 1,2).

No significant differences between the two bicarbonate concentrations ,$2.5.10^{-2}$M and 5.10^{-2}M used in our study, on the transport of both metals were observed, indicating that the maximum effect on both metals transport was achieved with the lower conc. Furosemide-induced inhibition of carbonic anhydrase, is consequently producing no effect on both metals' transport. In addition there are reports suggesting that elevated extracellullar concs of bicarbonates inhibit carbonic anhydrase and H+ ATPase.[1] Bicarbonates is also reported to increase Cd influx and accumulation in renal epethelial cells via an inorganic anion exchanger, whereas Cd efflux is mainly served via a H+-antiport system.[6,7] Furosemide a Na^+ K^+Cl^- cotransporter inhibitor also, decreased Cd incorporation, in presence of bicarbonates. (Table 3)

Furosemide's effects thus may not be attributed to carbonic anhydrase inhibition but rather to the enhancement of Cd efflux, through a direct or indirect effect on the H+ antiport system..It is obvious that further investigation is needed in order to elucidate bicarbonate effects on metal transport and /or accumulation in the bladder wall.

References

1.Stetson DL.Turtle urinary bladder: regulation of ion transport by dynamic changes in plasma membrane area.*Am.J.Physiology* 1989;257:R973-81.

2.Kalfakakou V, Simons TJ.Anionic mechanisms of zinc uptake across the human red cell membrane.*J Physiol(Lond)* 1990;421:485-97.

3.Simons TJ.Calcium-dependent zinc efflux in human red blood cells.*J Membr.Biol* 1991;123:73-82

4.Garty M,Bracken WM, Klaassen Cd.Cadmium uptake by rat red blood cells.Toxicology 1986;15,42:111-9.

5.Nguyen QH,Chien PK.Cadmium uptake kinetics in human erythrocytes.*Biol Trace Elem Res* 1989;22:119-29.

6.EndoT,Kimura O,Sakakta M.Bidirectional transport of cadmium across apical membrane of renal epithelial cell lines via H^+-antiporter and inorganic anion exchanger. *Toxicology* 1998;131:183-92.

7.Endo T,Kimura O,Sakata M.Further analysis of cadmium uptake from apical membrane of LLC-PK1 cells via inorganic anion exchanger.*Pharmacol Toxicol* 1999; 84:187-92.

Metal Ions in Biology and Medicine; vol 6. Eds. J.A. Centeno, Ph. Collery, G. Vernet, R.B. Finkelman, H. Gibb, J.C. Etienne. John Libbey Eurotext, Paris © 2000, pp. 129-132.

Activation of *Helicobacter pylori* aconitase by interactions with the cell wall

George L. Mendz

School of Biochemistry and Molecular Genetics, The University of New South Wales, Sydney, NSW 2052, Australia

ABSTRACT

The catalytic properties of the aconitase of the pathogenic bacterium *Helicobacter pylori* were studied *in vivo, in situ* and in cell extracts. The bacterial enzyme was activated by thiols and Fe^{2+} like other aconitases, and was less oxygen labile than porcine aconitase. The activity of the enzyme was not abolished completely at millimolar concentrations of metal chelators such as EDTA, NTA, or 1,10-phenantroline. The *H. pylori* enzyme was cytosolic and was stimulated by interactions with the bacterial cell-wall without addition of exogenous iron. In contrast, the activity of pig heart aconitase was not modulated by interactions with the bacterial cell wall. The aconitase activity of *H. pylori* cytosolic extracts did not change in the presence of cell envelopes of *Campylobacter coli* or *Escherichia coli.* The *in situ* and *in silico* results for *H. pylori* aconitase suggested that together with the formation of catalytically active Fe-S centres, stimulation of the enzyme required conformational changes in the protein molecule which took place on interacting with components of the cell wall.

INTRODUCTION

Aconitase (Acn; EC 4.2.1.3) is a TCA cycle enzyme which employs an Fe-S cluster to catalyse reversibly the conversion of citrate to isocitrate via *cis*-aconitate in a dehydration/rehydration reaction. In *Escherichia coli* two aconitases have been identified: AcnA is an aerobic-stationary-phase enzyme more stable than AcnB, the catabolic enzyme which modulates energy metabolism. Bacterial aconitases are closely related to the mammalian enzymes: AcnA resembles cytosolic aconitase, and AcnB is similar to mitochondrial aconitase [1]. Like the mammalian proteins, bacterial aconitases are bifunctional enzymes mediating a post-transcriptional iron-sulphur-cluster-dependent autoregulatory switch, in which the apoenzymes lacking the cluster are able to bind mRNA iron-response elements and modulate the expression of genes involved in iron metabolism [2,3].

The catalytic activity of aconitases is activated by addition of reductants and Fe^{2+}. The inactive form of the holoenzyme has a {3Fe-4S} cluster in which a solvent-exposed iron atom has been released. It can be activated anaerobically to the active {4Fe-4S} form by reducing agents without addition of iron, in a process in which active clusters are rebuilt at the expense of a fraction of the 3Fe clusters present. Thiols facilitate cluster interconversions, and the iron ion acquired to form the fully active 4Fe clusters is readily lost on oxidation of the cluster to form inactive 3Fe clusters which decay further more slowly [4]. Thus, Acn has an essential requirement for a {4Fe-4S} to catalyse a reaction which does not require oxidation-reduction chemistry.

The aconitase of the human pathogen bacterium *Helicobacter pylori* is a single polypeptide which shows very low similarity to most other aconitases of eukaryote or prokaryote, with the exception of *E. coli* AcnB with which it shows 64% amino acid sequence identity. Investigations of the TCA cycle of *H. pylori* showed no differences in aconitase activity between aerobic or anaerobic assay conditions, indicating that it is much more stable that *E. coli* AcnB [5]. An unusual property of the *H. pylori* enzyme is that after lysate fractionation only about a third of its activity is present in the cytosolic fraction and no activity is observed in the cell envelope fraction [5]. Employing ^{1}H-NMR spectroscopy the properties of *H. pylori* AcnB were investigated, as well as its interactions with cell components, and with cell envelopes extracted from other bacteria.

MATERIALS AND METHODS

cis-Aconitate, porcine heart aconitase, EDTA, DTT, NTA and 10-phenantroline were obtained from Sigma (St. Louis, MO). All other reagents were of analytical grade.

Campylobacter coli strain ATCC 33559, *E. coli* K-12 and several strains of *H. pylori* cells were grown on Blood Agar Base No. 2 plates (Oxoid, Basingstoke, UK) supplemented with 5% (v/v) horse blood and antibiotics, and incubated in an atmosphere of 10% CO_2 in air, 95% humidity at 37 °C. Cell suspensions were prepared by harvesting cells in sterile NaCl (150 mM) and centrifuging them at 17,000 x *g* (6 °C, 8 min), the supernatant was discarded and the pellet was collected and resuspended in NaCl. The procedure was repeated three times. Following the final wash, packed cells were resuspended to a concentration of approximately 10^8-10^9 cells/ml in sterile KCl. Lysates were prepared by twice freezing cell suspensions in liquid nitrogen and thawing them. Cell-free supernatants were obtained by centrifuging the lysates.

For NMR measurements samples were placed into 5 mm tubes (Wilmad, Buena, NJ) and the substrate was added. Free induction decays were collected using a Bruker DMX-500 NMR spectrometer, operating in the pulsed Fourier transform mode with quadrature detection. Measurements were carried out at 37 °C. One-dimensional ^{1}H-NMR spectra were acquired at 500.13 MHz with presaturation of the water resonance. The instrumental parameters were: spectral width 5000 Hz, memory size 16 K, acquisition time 1.64 s, number of transients 64, and relaxation delay with solvent presaturation 1.4 s. A Gaussian multiplication window function with line-broadening of -0.6 Hz and Gaussian parameter of 0.19 was applied prior to Fourier transformation.

Aconitase activity was measured employing ^{1}H-NMR spectroscopy in suspensions of packed cells, lysates or supernatants suspended in phosphate (65 mM, pH 7), NaCl (65 mM) buffer. Suspensions were placed in 5 mm tubes, and *cis*-aconitate was added to start the reaction. The time-evolution of metabolites was followed by acquiring sequential spectra in which the resonances arising from aconitate decreased in intensity and those corresponding to isocitrate and citrate increased in intensity. Progress curves were obtained by measuring the integrals of the *cis*-aconitate methine resonance at *ca.* 5.75 ppm, which does not overlap with any other resonances arising from either substrates or products of the reaction.

RESULTS AND DISCUSSION

Rates of aconitase activity were measured *in vivo, in situ* and in cell-free extracts from progress curves which were linear for about 20 min (Fig. 1). *In situ,* in whole cell lysates, the K_m of the enzyme was 6.8 ± 0.8 mM; and the V_{max} 301 ± 12 nmol/min/mg protein.

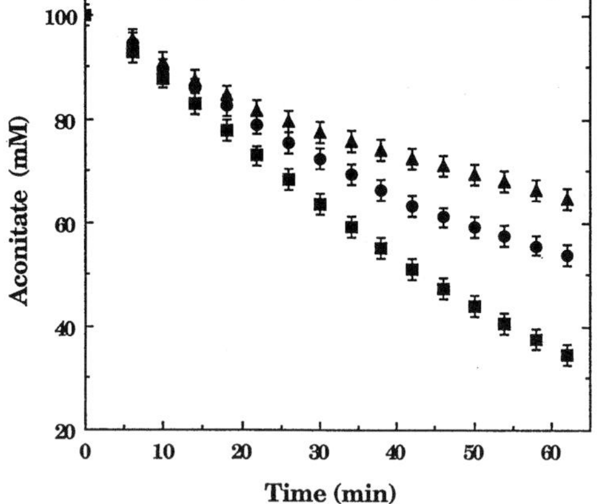

Figure 1. Time-evolution of cis-*aconitate in the reaction catalyzed by* H. pylori *aconitase in the presence of EDTA at concentrations of 0* (■), *2* (●), *and 5* (▲) *mM.*

Fractionation of whole lysates by centrifugation resulted into a pellet containing the cell envelope, and supernatants containing the cytosol. Most of the enzyme activity was found in the cytosol. In whole cell lysates and cytosolic fractions, maximal activity was observed at pH 8.85 ± 0.15. *H. pylori* aconitase was activated by thiol-bearing compounds and Fe^{2+} like other aconitases, but was less oxygen labile than the porcine enzyme. Similar rates were observed in suspensions of cells or whole lysates prepared in buffers which were either fully aerated or saturated with argon.

The metal chelators EDTA, NTA or 1,10-phenantroline decreased the rates of enzyme activity (Fig. 1), with IC_{50} of approximately 5, >25, and 2 mM, respectively.

Addition of the cell-envelope fraction increased cytosolic *H. pylori* AcnB activity (Fig. 2). This activation of the enzyme depended on the amount of pellet added, and it reached a maximum of about twice the value of the activity measured for whole lysates. In contrast, the addition of cell envelopes of *Campylobacter coli* or *Escherichia coli* obtained by similar procedures did not affect the activity of *H. pylori* AcnB in cytosolic fractions. At variance with the *H. pylori* enzyme, the activity of purified porcine heart aconitase was not modulated by the presence of cell-wall fractions. These data suggested that the activation of *H. pylori* AcnB arose from specific interactions with its own cell envelope.

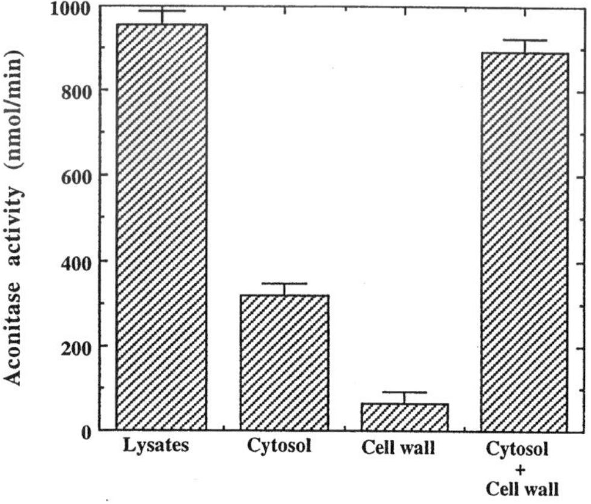

Figure 2. H. pylori *AcnB activities measured in three cell fractions, showing the modulation of the cytosolic enzyme by interactions with the cell wall.*

To investigate the factors involved in *H. pylori* AcnB activation two candidates were examined. Iron is a ubiquitous contaminant, and the increase of activity observed in the presence of the cell envelope could arise from trace iron present the pellet fractions. However, the fact that porcine aconitase was not stimulated by these fractions suggested it was unlikely that trace iron was causing the effect on the enzyme of the bacterium. It has been proposed that *H. pylori* has an iron uptake system involving the reduction of ferric iron to ferrous iron [6]. The iron reductase enzyme present in *H. pylori* may increase the levels of Fe^{2+}, and induce an activation of AcnB. To elucidate this possibility, cell-wall fractions were denatured by heating pellets at 80 °C for 2 h, and their effect on aconitase activity examined. Heat-denatured cell-envelopes also activated *H. pylori* AcnB indicating that the increase in activity did not take place through the action of the iron reductase or of any other enzyme. In a control with heat-treated supernatants and cell-wall fractions, enzyme activity was abolished almost completely. Interactions with other factors, such as cell-wall lipids, peptidoglycans, lipopolysaccharides and proteins (even denatured) could induce conformational changes in AcnB resulting in enhanced catalytic activity. However, the effects of such factors remain to be measured.

Besides establishing the cellular factors involved in the modulation of *H. pylori* AcnB, it is of interest also to examine the protein itself, and attempt to identify elements of its sequence which could account for its special properties. AcnA and mammalian cytoplasmic aconitase contain four domains; the first three (1-2-3) from the *N*-terminus are tightly associated about the Fe-S cluster, and all three cysteine ligands to the cluster are located in domain 3. Association of the larger *C*-terminal domain with the first three creates an extensive interface with a cleft which is the principal access of the solvent to the cluster. A linker peptide connects domains 3 and 4, and the quaternary structure of the molecule suggests the possibility of a hinge motion about this peptide which will vary the separation between domains 1-2-3 and 4, thus modulating the accessibility of the the solvent to the Fe-S cluster. All four domains contribute residues to the active site [7]. *E. coli* AcnB has very low similarity to AcnA, and the identity between both proteins is only 17%, even after the AcnB domain organisation has been rearranged in a 4-1-2-3 order in which sequence homology is maximised, but 16 of the 20 catalytic residues are conserved between the two enzymes, including the three cysteinyls involved in ligand binding the Fe-S centre [8]. The similarity of *H. pylori* AcnB to other aconitases can be maximised also by arranging its domains in a 4-1-2-3 form, indicating that both enzymes represent a distinct class of aconitase. Aconitases homologous to these two are found in *Neisseria meningiditis* and *Synechocystis* spp. It is possible, but presently it is only speculation, that the different location of domain 4 in the protein molecule endows AcnB with a capacity to interact with other cellular components that is missing in AcnA.

In conclusion, *in situ* stimulation of and *H. pylori* aconitase suggested that together with the formation of catalytically active Fe-S centres, the enzyme required conformational changes in the protein molecule which took place on interacting with components of the cell wall.

REFERENCES

1. Jordan, PA, Tang, Y, Bradbury, AJ, Thomson, AJ, GUest, JR. Biochemical and spectroscopic characterization of *Escherichia coli* aconitases (AcnA, AcnB). *Biochem J* 1999; 344 : 739-746.
2. Tang, Y, Guest, JR. Direct evidence for mRNA binding and post-transcriptional regulation by *Escherichia coli* aconitases. *Microbiology* 1999; 145 : 3069-3079.
3. Alen, C, Sonenshein, AL. *Bacillus subtilis* aconitase is an RNA-binding protein. *Proc Natl Acad Sci USA* 1999; 96 : 10412-10417.
4. Kennedy, CC, Emptage, MH, Dreyer, JL, Beinert H. The role of iron in the activation of aconitase. *J Biol Chem* 1983; 258 : 11098-11105.
5. Pitson, SM, Mendz, GL, Srinivasan, S, Hazell, SL. The tricarboxylic acid cycle of *Helicobacter pylori. Eur J Biochem* 1999; 260 : 258-267.
6. Worst, DJ, Gerrits, MM, Vandenbroucke-Grauls, CMJE, Kusters, JG. *Helicobacter pylori ribBA*-mediated riboflavin production is involved in iron acquisition. *J Bacteriol* 1998; 180 : 1473-1479.
7. Robbins, AH, Stout, CD. The Structure of aconitase. *Prot Struc Function Genet* 1989; 5 : 289-312.
8. Bradbury, AJ, Gruer, MJ, Rudd, KE, Guest JR. The second aconitase (AcnB) of *Escherichia coli. Microbiology* 1996; 142 : 389-400.

Metal Ions in Biology and Medicine; vol 6. Eds. J.A. Centeno, Ph. Collery, G. Vernet, R.B. Finkelman, H. Gibb, J.C. Etienne. John Libbey Eurotext, Paris © 2000, pp. 133-136.

Copper homeostasis in *Enterococcus hirae*: pumps, repressor, chaperone

Karl-Dimiter Bissig, Haibo Wunderli-Ye, and Marc Solioz

Department of Clinical Pharmacology, University of Berne, 3010 Berne, Switzerland

Enterococcus hirae **is a convenient model system for the study of copper homeostasis. Its *cop* operon encodes two copper ATPases, CopA and CopB, that serve in the import and the export of copper(I), respectively. The copper chaperone, CopZ, effects the intracellular routing of copper and the copper responsive repressor, CopY, regulates the expression of the four genes. All components of the system have been purified and are under structural and functional investigation.**

Since the first report of ATP-driven copper transport in the Gram-positive *Enterococcus hirae* in 1992 [1], our understanding of cellular copper metabolism has virtually exploded. Today, we have molecular information on key steps and components of cellular copper homeostasis, stemming from the study of bacteria, yeast and mammalian cells. In the unraveling of cellular copper circulation, *E. hirae* has proven to be an excellent model system [2].

In *E. hirae*, the *cop* operon encodes four key components of copper metabolism, namely two copper pumps, a repressor, and a copper chaperone. The two copper ATPases, CopA and CopB, accomplish transmembranous copper transport, with CopA serving in the uptake of copper under limiting conditions, and CopB in copper secretion when it reaches toxic levels [3]. CopA and CopB share 35 to 40% sequence identity with the human copper ATPases which are associated with two inherited disorders of copper metabolism, Menkes and Wilson disease, respectively, but also with cadmium ATPases of bacterial resistance systems.

Based on the protein sequences, CopA, CopB, cadmium ATPases, and the human copper ATPases are P-type ATPases, classically represented by Ca- and Na,K-ATPases. P-type ATPases share the conserved sequence motif DKTGT. The aspartic acid residue of this motif forms a high-energy acylphosphate intermediate in the course of the reaction cycle - hence the name P-type ATPases. As more copper ATPases were discovered, it became apparent that they, together with the cadmium ATPases, had a secondary structure and a predicted membrane topology quite distinct from the non-heavy metal ATPases. Phylogenetic analysis revealed that the ion-motive ATPases branched into heavy metal and non-heavy metal ATPases early in evolution, probably before the division into prokaryotes and eukaryotes. To date, over 30 heavy metal ATPases have been cloned and ion specificities include Cu^{+},

Ag^+, Zn^{2+}, Cd^{2+}, and Pb^{2+}. Due to their different structures, the heavy metal ATPases have been assigned to a subclass of the P-type ATPases, called CPx-type or P1-type ATPases [4,5].

The evidence for copper uptake through the action of the *E. hirae* CopA ATPase is so far indirect: first, knock-out mutants in CopA are unable to grow in copper depleted media and, secondly, such mutants can grow in 5 μM $AgNO_3$, which completely inhibits the growth of wild-type cells [3]. This suggests that CopA serves as a pathway for the entry of copper(I), but also silver(I), into the cell. CopA ATPase endowed with an N-terminal, cleavable histidine-tag was expressed in *E. coli* and purified to homogeneity by affinity chromatography on a nickel resin. Isolated CopA, when reconstituted into proteoliposomes, formed an acylphosphate intermediate and therefor belongs to the supergroup of P-type ATPases. The purified, reconstituted CopA ATPase serves as an ideal model system for the study of ATP-driven copper transport.

The function of CopB of *E. hirae* in copper export is supported by three lines of evidence. First, CopB knock-out mutants are sensitive to micromolar concentrations of copper, while wild-type *E. hirae* tolerates up to 8 mM copper. Secondly, when cells are loaded with $^{110m}Ag^+$, ΔCopB mutants do not extrude the silver while wild-type cells do. Third, native inside-out membrane vesicles of *E. hirae* exhibit ATP-driven accumulation of copper(I) or silver(I) [6]. Thus, CopB appears to serve in the extrusion of copper from cells if copper is excessive. Silver(I), which has an ionic radius similar to that of copper(I), is a substrate for both, the CopA and the CopB ATPase.

CopB was purified from an *E. hirae* mutant with up-regulated expression of the *cop* operon. Since the N-terminus of CopB is very rich in histidine residues, it could be affinity purified on a nickel affinity resin without the need of adding a histidine tag. Purified CopB, reconstituted into proteoliposomes, formed an acylphosphate intermediate, was inhibited by vanadate, and showed a limited copper dependence [7].

The CopB experimental system proved valuable for the analysis of the functional role of amino acid residues. A CPH or CPC motif is found in the sixth transmembranous helix of all CPx-type ATPases (hence the name) and is believed to serve in the translocation of ions across the membrane. The cysteine of the CPH motif of CopB was mutated to serine (C396S). This mutation abolished copper transport function *in vivo*, as assessed by the complementation of a CopB knock-out strain. However, C390S-CopB was still able to form an acylphosphate intermediate from ATP. The partial function of this mutant enzyme indeed suggests a direct role of the CPH motif in transport, but not in ATP hydrolysis.

CopY is a copper responsive repressor that regulates the expression of the *cop* operon. In normal media that contain approximately 10 μM copper, expression of the *cop* genes is minimal. Higher as well as lower copper levels induce the operon. We could show that this regulation was effected by the binding of CopY to two binding sites upstream of the coding region [8]. Mutation of both CopY binding sites to weaken CopY binding, lead to hyperinduction by excess copper, but did not affect induction by a lack of copper. This suggests that two different mechanisms are responsible for the induction of the *cop* operon by high and low copper [9].

Since copper ions can undergo a Fenton type reaction with the generation of radicals, copper ions are probably never free in the cytoplasm. This requires specialized proteins to route copper intracellularly [10]. In *E. hirae* CopZ appears to fulfill this role. With an *in vitro* band-shift assay, we could show that copper(I)-CopZ can donate copper to the CopY repressor, thereby releasing it from the DNA. This copper transfer appeared to be specific, as a similar copper binding protein was unable to donate copper to CopY [11].

The structure of CopZ was elucidated by NMR spectroscopy. It exhibits a βαββαβ-fold, with the four β-strands forming an antiparallel β-sheet and the two α-helices lying on top of it. The copper binding motif CxxC lies between the first β-strand and the beginning of the first α-helix [12]. This structure closely resembles those of the bacterial mercury chaperone MerP [13], the yeast copper chaperone Atx1 [14], and the fourth copper binding motifs of the human Menkes copper ATPase [15]. Upon the binding of copper, the NMR signals from the vicinity of the copper binding region were lost, probably due to dimerization of Cu(I)-CopZ. No major structural changes could be observed in the remainder of the protein.

Study of the *E. hirae cop* operon has so far considerably contributed to our understanding of copper homeostasis. Using purified components of this system promises to provide further insight into nature's dealing with copper.

References

[1] Odermatt A, Suter H, Krapf R, Solioz M. An ATPase operon involved in copper resistance by *Enterococcus hirae*. *Ann N Y Acad Sci* 1992; 671 : 484-486.

[2] Lu ZH, Cobine P, Dameron CT, Solioz M. How cells handle copper: A view from microbes. *J Trace Elem Exp Med* 1999; 12 : 347-360.

[3] Odermatt A, Suter H, Krapf R, Solioz M. Primary structure of two P-type ATPases involved in copper homeostasis in *Enterococcus hirae*. *J Biol Chem* 1993; 268 : 12775-12779.

[4] Solioz M, Vulpe C. CPx-type ATPases: a class of P-type ATPases that pump heavy metals. *Trends Biochem Sci* 1996; 21 : 237-241.

[5] Lutsenko S, Kaplan JH. Organization of P-type ATPases: Significance of structural diversity. *Biochemistry* 1995; 34 : 15607-15613.

[6] Solioz M, Odermatt A. Copper and silver transport by CopB-ATPase in membrane vesicles of *Enterococcus hirae*. *J Biol Chem* 1995; 270 : 9217-9221.

[7] Wyler-Duda P, Solioz M. Phosphoenzyme formation by purified, reconstituted copper ATPase of *Enterococcus hirae* . *FEBS Lett* 1996; 399 : 143-146.

[8] Strausak D, Solioz M. CopY is a copper-inducible repressor of the *Enterococcus hirae* copper ATPases. *J Biol Chem* 1997; 272 : 8932-8936.

[9] Wunderli-Ye H, Solioz M. Effects of promoter mutations on the *in vivo* regulation of the *cop* operon of *Enterococcus hirae* by copper(I) and copper(II). *Biochem Biophys Res Commun* 1999; 259 : 443-449.

[10] Pufahl RA, Singer CP, Peariso KL, Lin S, Schmidt PJ, Fahrni CJ et al. Metal ion chaperone function of the soluble Cu(I) receptor Atx1. *Science* 1997; 278 : 853-856.

[11] Cobine P, Wickramasinghe WA, Harrison MD, Weber T, Solioz M, Dameron CT. The *Enterococcus hirae* copper chaperone CopZ delivers copper(I) to the CopY repressor. *FEBS Lett* 1999; 445 : 27-30.

[12] Wimmer R, Herrmann T, Solioz M, Wüthrich K. NMR structure and metal interactions of the CopZ copper chaperone. *J Biol Chem* 1999; 274 : 22597-22603.

[13] Steele RA, Opella SJ. Structures of the reduced and mercury-bound forms of MerP, the periplasmic protein from the bacterial mercury detoxification system. *Biochemistry* 1997; 36 : 6885-6895.

[14] Rosenzweig AC, Huffman DL, Hou MY, Wernimont AK, Pufahl RA, O'Halloran TV. Crystal structure of the Atx1 metallochaperone protein at 1.02 Å resolution. *Structure* 1999; 7 : 605-617.

[15] Gitschier J, Moffat B, Reilly D, Wood WI, Fairbrother WJ. Solution structure of the fourth metal-binding domain from the Menkes copper-transporting ATPase. *Nat Struct Biol* 1998; 5 : 47-54.

Metal Ions in Biology and Medicine; vol 6. Eds. J.A. Centeno, Ph. Collery, G. Vernet, R.B. Finkelman, H. Gibb, J.C. Etienne. John Libbey Eurotext, Paris © 2000, pp. 137-139.

Interaction of chromium (III) ions and their cysteine coplex with bilayers

Kylyvnyk K.E., Sushenko C.A., Bovykin B.A., Zegzhda G.D.

The Ukrainian State Chemical Technology University, Dnepropetrovsk, Ukraine

The physiological value of chromium for animals and human beings was first ascertained by Schwarz and Mertz. They detected that chromium deficiency in an animal's nutrition results in a deceleration in growth, reduction in life span and damaging of sugar metabolism [1]. These investigations stimulated increasing interest in studying the biological activity of chromium and its compounds [2-6].

It was determined that chromium have positive influence on ferment systems and participates in the stabilisation of nucleic acids[3], have high hemogenic activity in the presence of hemolytic anaemia [4]. Information exists about the role of chromium and its compounds [5] in infringement of thyroid gland function and antitumoural activity.

In the diversity of investigations of the chromium compounds' biological activity only a few are dedicated to their interaction with biological membranes. In these was shown that the Cr^{+3} ions render the same inhibiting effect on interlinking Ca^{+2} with membranes of erythrocytes as do divalent metal ions, and the adsorptive capacity of chromium (III) ions on the BLM is stacked in a series: $In^{+3} > Ga^{+3} > Cr^{+3}$ [7].

Materials and methods. $CrCl_3*6H_2O$ was chemically pure and the $[Cr(H_2L)_6]Cl_3*3H_2O$ complex was obtained by direct interaction of $CrCl_3$ with neutral cysteine molecules [8]. The BLM are formed from the n-octane solutions of ox brain lipids with concentration 20 mg/ml on a aperture (Ø=1,1 mm) in a teflon septum parting two aqueous spaces (the Mueller procedure [9]). The electrolyte was 0,01 M KCl with adding of the acetate buffer (pH was equal 4,0 and 6,0). The experiments took place at the 20°C. The conductivity and capacity of the BLM was measured by a method of cyclic volt-ampere characteristics (VAC)[10] at a scanning rate 4 mV/s in a voltage range ± 100 mV.

The magnitude of transmembrane potential difference ($\Delta\varphi$) was measured with the help of a potentiadynamic method with recording of a current of 2nd harmonic [11]. In this method the slow sawtooth voltage and sinusoidal voltage with 500 Hz frequency was simultaneously applied to the membrane. The change of the $\Delta\varphi$ on addition of the investigated substances was determined on the amplitude minimum shift of a second harmonic current $i(2\omega)$. Each point on the curves is the average value of 4-5 experiments. After adding the next portion of substances the measurement was conducted after 15 min period, indispensable for achievement of equilibrium.

Results and discussion. The VACs have shown that cysteine, Cr^{3+} ions and cysteine complex in concentrations up to $1*10^{-3}$ M do not change the conductivity and capacity of the BLM in electrolytes with pH equal 4,0 and 6,0.

However, the VACs for the complex differed from those for ions Cr^{+3}. This difference consisted in the current fluctuations which arose in the field of positive scanning voltages after adding the complex. Their amplitude and frequency depended on

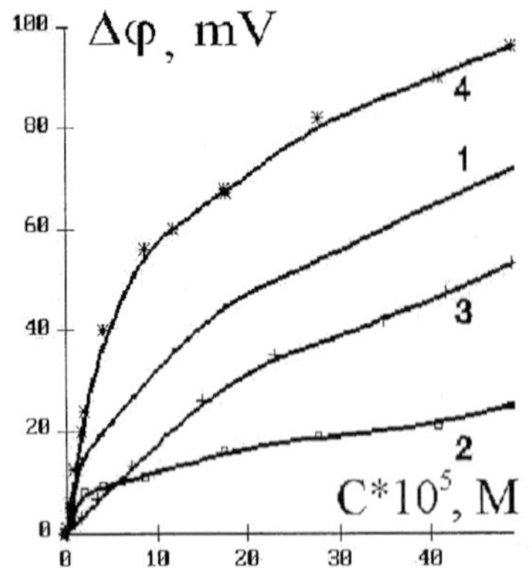

Fig.1. The change of transmembrane potential difference Δφ at the addition of Cr^{3+} ions(1,2) and $[Cr(H_2L)_6]^{3+}$ complex (3,4) Curves 1 and 3 - pH 4; 2 and 4 pH 6

mechanical influences on the BLM caused of mixing the solution with a magnetic stirrer.

A scanning voltage shift into the positive area (the electrode posed in the interior of the membrane is under a zero potential) resulted in increased amplitude of fluctuations and, frequently, to break up of the membrane. During voltage shift into negative area, the current fluctuation stopped and the course of the volt-ampere curve was completely identical to the unmodified membrane and to the membrane with addition of Cr^{3+} salt.

Such BLM behaviour testifies, that the added complex is adsorbed on the membrane surface reversibly. This adsorption is strengthened in the field of positive potentials corresponding to the positive charge of a complex ion $[Cr(H_2L)_6]^{3+}$. Probably surface compartments which has a rigid structures are formed on the membrane alter the elastic properties [12]. For confirmation of this hypothesis the adsorption of Cr^{+3} ions and complex $[Cr(H_2L)_6]Cl_3*3H_2O$ on BLM by the method of 2nd harmonic current was investigated.

The addition of various quantities of Cr^{3+} ions and complex resulted in a shift of the 2nd harmonic current amplitude minimum (i(2ω)) to the negative area, which testified to generation of a positive Δφ and adsorption on the BLM of positively charged particles (fig.1)

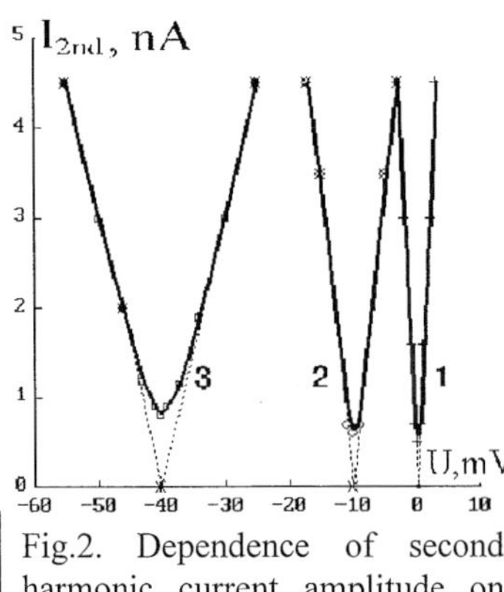

Fig.2. Dependence of second harmonic current amplitude on the voltage at the addition of various concentration of $[Cr(H_2L)_6]^{3+}$ complex pH=4. The complex concentration 1 - 0: 2 - $5*10^{-5}$: 3 - $2.7*10^{-4}$ M.

In figure 1 we can see that, in the solution with pH=4, the addition of Cr^{3+} ions (the curve 1) resulted in a bigger change of the Δφ, i.e. to stronger adsorption than with the addition of $[Cr(H_2L)_6]^{3+}$ complex (curve 3). This is the result of a positive charge density with reduction at transition from the smaller ion Cr^{3+} to the large complex ion $[Cr(H_2L)_6]^{3+}$. The change of pH solution from 4 to 6 resulted in the decrease of Cr^{3+} ions adsorption (curve 2) and the increase of the complex adsorption (curve 4). It is possible to explain the given phenomenon by simultaneous action of two processes: - the Cr^{3+} ions transition to hydroxide and in polynuclear hydroxo-substances with a pH increase; - the increasing dissociation of phosphate and carboxylic phospholipid groups of membrane, resulting in increase of a negative surface charge.

The curve shape of the second harmonic current amplitude on addition chrome chloride $1*10^{-3}$ mol/l varies little. The adding of $[Cr(H_2L)_6]Cl_3*3H_2O$ complex results in a considerable change of curve shape (fig. 2).

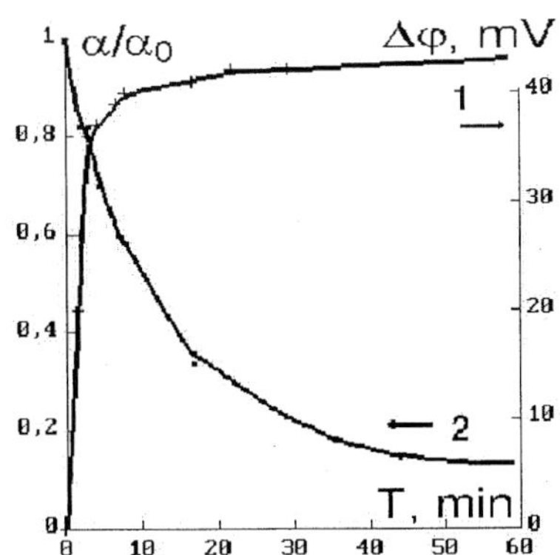

Fig. 3. The dynamics of change of transmembrane potential difference (1) and the relative change of α electrostriction coefficient (2) at addition $2,7*10^{-4}$ M complex. pH=4.

Taking into account that the investigated substances do not change conductivity and capacity of the membranes, and that the amplitude and frequency of a sine wave signal during the experiment remain constant, by the change of the form of these curves it is possible to calculate the change of electrostriction coefficient α describing the elastic property of bilayer lipid membranes:

$$i(2\omega) = 3\,\alpha\,\varphi\,V^2 \sin(2\omega t) \qquad (1)$$

where: φ is the constant voltage component which creates pressure compressing a membrane; V - amplitude and ω - frequency of sinusoidal voltage. The α coefficient shows how the membrane thickness varies when the electric voltage φ is applied and is proportional to the Young elastic modulus in the perpendicular direction of the membrane plane. In the given conditions the coefficient α determines the form of dependence of the i(2ω) amplitude on the voltage.

The dependence of the 2nd harmonic current amplitude on the voltage at various times after addition of $2,7*10^{-4}$ mol/l of the $[Cr(H_2L)_6]^{3+}$ complex shows that the complex is fast adsorbing on the membrane surface, changing its potential (fig. 3. Carve1). Then there is a slower process resulting in reduction of the electrostriction coefficient α (curve 2). It testifies to a weakening of the elastic properties of the membrane.

A similar effect is observed on the BLM on addition of insulin. The addition of insulin 10^{-9} mol/l results in a 150% increase of the Young elastic module [13]. As is evident from fig.3 the addition of $2,7*10^{-4}$ mol/l of $[Cr(H_2L)_6]^{3+}$ complex ions results in a lager change in the elastic properties of the membrane.

On the basis of our research it is possible to conclude that the biological activity of the complex is higher than that of inorganic salts. This explained by the hydrolysis of Cr^{3+} and their transformation into insoluble and poorly assimilable hydroxide. The presence of organic ligands interferes with the hydrolysis, and the change of hydrophilic-hydrophobic balance results in the intensification of influence on model membranes.

1. Mertz W., Roginiski E.E., Schwarz K.//J. Biol. Chem. 1961. V.236, N.2, p.318-322.
2. Акбаров А.Б.//Ж.неорган.химии,1990,Т.35,N 3,с.660-664.
3. Roginski E.E., Mertz W.//J.Nutz.1969,V.97, N.4, p.525-530.
4. Смирнов М.И.//Гигиена окружающей среды. М. : Медицина, 1987,С.78-79.
5. Хухрянский В.Г., Циганенко А.Я. Химия биогенных элементов.-Киев:Вища школа,1990,206.
6. Offenbaher Esther G., Pi-Sunyer F.,//Annu. Rev. Nutr.V.8.-Palo Alto (Calif.), 1988, p. 543-563.
7. Омельченко А.М.//Итоги науки и техники. сер. Биофизика. М.:ВИНИТИ, 1991, т.41, с.47-50
8. Виниченко И.Г., Зегжда Г.Д.// Журн. неорган. химии, 1993, Т.38, N1, С.87-91.
9. Mueller P., Rudin P., Tien M.In: Recent progress in surface science. N.Y.-Lond.,1964,p. 379-393.
10. Tien H.T.//J. Phys. Chim.1984,V.88, N15, p. 3172-3174.
11. Соколов В.С., Кузьмин В.Г.//Биофизика.1980,Т.25, N1, с.170-172.
12. Blank M.//Structure and function in excitable cells,1983,p.435-450.
13. Kavecansky J., Hianik T., Zorad S., Macho Z.//Gen. Physiol. Biophys, 1988, V.7, p. 537-542.

Metal Ions in Biology and Medicine; vol 6. Eds. J.A. Centeno, Ph. Collery, G. Vernet, R.B. Finkelman, H. Gibb, J.C. Etienne. John Libbey Eurotext, Paris © 2000, pp. 140-143.

Perturbations induced by a sublethal concentration of platinum in the anterior intestine of the teleost *Brachydanio rerio:* an ultrastructural study

S. Biagianti-Risbourg[1, 2], F. Arnoult[1, 2], S. Betoulle[1], J.-C. Etienne[2] and G. Vernet[1, 2]

[1] *Laboratoire d'Eco-Toxicologie and* [2] *Institut International de Recherche sur les Ions Métalliques, Université de Reims Champagne-Ardenne, BP 1039, 51687 Reims Cedex 02, France*

More than 10% of the Pt salts emitted from automobile exhaust converters are soluble in water and thus potentially bioavailable to aquatic organisms [1]. Pt therefore should be assessed as a potential environmental toxicant. The fish intestine whose surface is constantly exposed to the qualitative variations of the aquatic environment constitutes both a barrier and a site of uptake of aquatic pollutants particularly heavy metals [2].
We have previously shown histological effects produced by various concentrations of Pt in the anterior part of *Brachydanio rerio* intestine [3]. The intestinal responses were time and concentration dependent. Some of them were analysed as degenerative (necrosis and lysis of some enterocytes at the villi apex, changes in submucosal structures) or adaptative (fusion between adjacent villi). The next logical step was therefore a detailed study at the ultrastructural level.
This study evaluates after 2, 7 and 14 days exposure, the ultrastructural effects of an actual water concentration of 16 $\mu g.l^{-1}$ Pt (H_2PtCl_6, $4.5H_20$) in *Brachydanio rerio* anterior intestine. The protocole of fish exposure to Pt and the methods for electron microscopy have been previously detailed in [3]. The number of microvilli was counted on electron micrographs within 1 µm of the enterocyte apical pole (number of measurements: 25 ± 4).

Results and discussion

A number of abnormalities were found in the liver of the Pt-treated fish that were never observed in control fish. At the ultrastructural level, progressive loss of enterocytic polarity (Fig. 3) and obvious cellular perturbations were induced. The main subcellular effects concerned the plasma membrane (microvilli of the brush border), nuclei, mitochondria, dictyosomes and lipid content.
The most original response was the rapid and clear decrease in the microvilli number of the brush border during all the exposure period (Fig. 1). This could reflect an adaptive response by reduction of the absorptive surface and consequently limitation of the metallic uptake.
From day 2 to day 14 a number of degenerative events occurred. Vesiculation and disruption of the enterocyte plasma membrane were revealed at the brush

border level (Fig. 2). The lysis of the apical enterocyte plasma membrane (Fig. 5) provoked the release of numerous cellular components (mitochondria, endoplasmic reticulum...) in the intestinal lumen (Fig. 2). This membrane response is not specific of the metallic contamination since similar alteration has been shown under various other deleterious environmental conditions (starvation, exposure to organic pollutants). However, the membrane injuries seen in this study could result from lipidic peroxidation, since heavy metals, particularly Pt, are known to induce ROS formation [4; 5].
Vacuolization of numerous mitochondria and mitochondria cristae lysis were also seen in nearly all enterocytes (Figs. 2 and 3). According to [2], mitochondria can be considered as one of the most important target of heavy metals, and Pt has been shown to provoke severe mitochondria dysfunction [6].
The number of enterocytes with nuclei at various stages of pycnosis increased with exposure time (Fig. 4). It is generally accepted that nuclear DNA is the target involved in the cytotoxic action of platinum compounds [7].
Increase in dictyosome number, fragmentation and vacuolisation of dictyosome saccules were rapidly induced and observable during all the exposure period (Figs. 2 and 4). Such changes have been previously revealed in hepatocytes of fish submitted to cadmium [8]. Delayed lipid accumulation in enterocytes (Fig. 3) could be due to functional impairment of organelles (endoplasmic reticulum, mitochondria, Golgi apparatus) involved in intestinal lipid metabolism. Lipid stagnation in enterocytes could be due to a decrease or a cessation of the synthesis of apoproteins and/or enzymes involved in lipid transformation and transfer mechanisms.
These alterations were unspecific but revealed important impairment of intestinal function and thus alteration of the health status of the fish. The characterisation of intestine responses in fish experimentally exposed to Pt can provide a basis for recognition of toxicity syndromes and should *in fine* be useful in the early prognosis of the deleterious effects of aquatic pollution.

Aknowledgement

This work was supported by the Conseil Régional de Champagne-Ardenne.

Legends

Fig. 1: Reduction of the enterocyte microvilli number induced by 16 $\mu g.l^{-1}$ Pt. CO: control; C2: two days exposure; C7: seven days exposure; C 14: fourteen days exposure.

Fig. 2: Ultrastructural perturbations induced in the anterior intestine of danios after 2 days exposure to Pt. *: mitochondria vacuolisation; cd: cellular debris; D: dictyosome; m: mitochondria; mv: microvilli; N: nucleus; ser: smooth endoplasmic reticulum; tw: terminal web. (scale bar = 1 µm)

Fig. 3: Ultrastructural alterations induced in the anterior intestine of danios after 14 days exposure to Pt. Er: endoplasmic reticulum; L: lipid droplets; m: mitochondria; mv: microvilli; N: nucleus. (scale bar = 1 μm)

Fig. 4: Alterations of enterocyte nuclei and dictyosomes after 14 days exposure to Pt. D: dictyosome; N: nucleus. (scale bar = 0.5 μm)

Fig. 5: Enterocyte lysis (rupture of the apical plasma membrane) induced by 7 days exposure to Pt. Er: endoplasmic reticulum; L: lipid droplets; Ly: lysosome; Lys: lysis; m: mitochondria; mv: microvilli. (scale bar = 2 μm)

References

[1] Hodge V.F. and Stallard M.O. Platinum and palladium in roadside dusts. *Env Sci Technol* 1986 ; **20**(10) : 1058-1060.

[2] Viarengo A. Biochemical effects of trace metals. *Mar Poll Bull* 1985 ; **16**(4) : 153-158.

[3] Jouhaud R., Biagianti-Risbourg S., Arsac F. and Vernet G. Effets du platine chez *Brachydanio rerio* (Téléostéen, cyprinidé). I- Toxicité aiguë, bioaccumulation et histopathologie intestinales. *J. Appl Ichthyol* 1999 ; **15** : 41-48.

[4] Sadzuka Y., Shoji T. and Takino Y. Mechanism of increase in lipid peroxide induced by cisplatin in the kidneys of rats. *Toxicolog Letters* 1992 ; **62** : 293-300.

[5] Torii Y., Mutoh M., Saito H. and Matsuki N. Involvement of free radicals in cisplatin-induced emesis in *Suncus murinus. Europ J Pharmacol, Environ Toxicol Pharmacol Section* 1993 ; **248** : 131-135.

[6] Brady H.R., Zeidel M.L., Kone B.C., Geibisch G. and Gullans S.R. Differencial actions of cisplatin on renal proximal tubule and inner medullary collecting duct cells. *J Pharmacol Exp Therapeutics* 1993 ; **265**(3) : 1421-1428.

[7] Yasumasu T., Ueda T., Uozumi J., Mihara Y., Koikawa Y. and Kamazawa J. Ultrastructural alterations and DNA synthesis of renal cell nuclei following cisplatin or carboplatin injection in rats. *J Pharm Pharmacol* 1992 ; **44** : 885-887.

[8] Ferri S. Effects of cadmium on Golgi complex of freshwater teleost *(Pimelodus maculatus)* hepatocytes. *Protoplasma* 1980 ; **103** : 99-103.

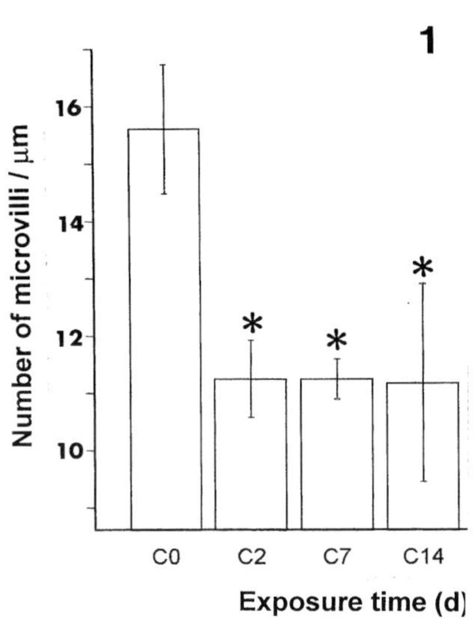

* Significatively different from control (Student test, p<00.5)

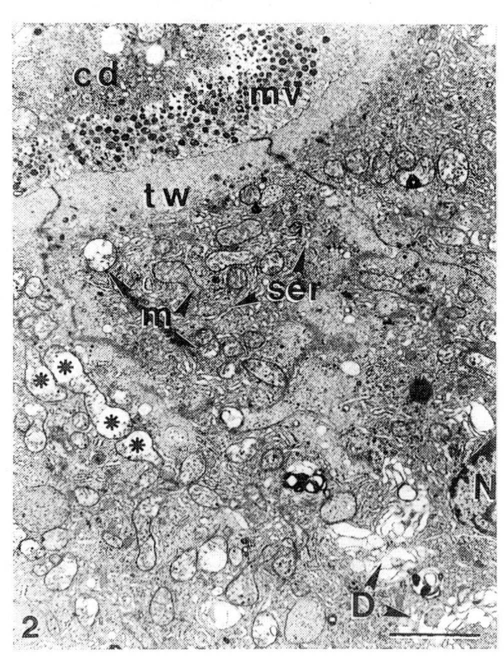

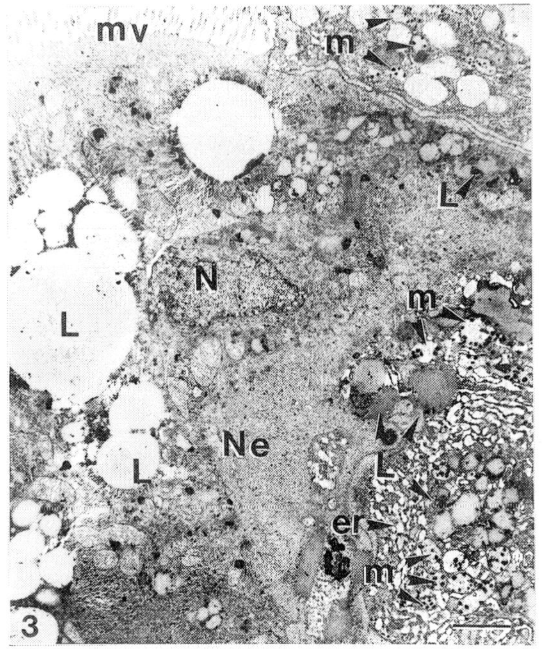

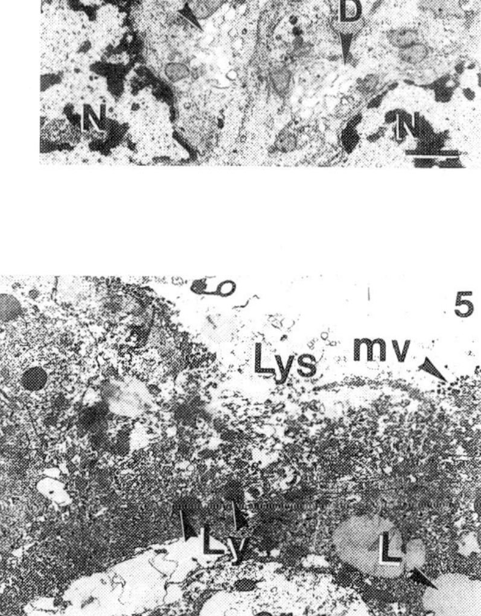

Metal Ions in Biology and Medicine; vol 6. Eds. J.A. Centeno, Ph. Collery, G. Vernet, R.B. Finkelman, H. Gibb, J.C. Etienne. John Libbey Eurotext, Paris © 2000, pp. 144-146.

Effects of atrial natriuretic peptide (ANP) and furosemide on zinc transport through the red cell membrane

Angeliki Galani, Patra Vezyraki, Angelos Evangelou and Vicky Kalfakakou

Dept. of Exp. Physiology, Faculty of Medicine, University of Ioannina, 45110, Ioannina Greece

Abstract

Atrial- natriuretic- peptide (ANP) and furosemide are both Na-K-Cl co-transpoter inhibitors and natriuretic factors. ANP synthesis, release and degradation is Zn related whereas furosemide is a Zn-carbonic anhydrase inhibitor and a zincuretic factor. Zinc is transported across the red blood cell (RBC) membrane as a bicarbonate-chloride anion complex implicated probably to ANP and furosemide mechanisms of action.The present work aims the investigation of the effects of ANP and furosemide on zinc influx into the human RBCs and elucidation of the physiological mechanisms involved in Zn transport across red cell membrane. Human blood bank red cells were incubated with $ZnCl_2$ (1mM) in presence and absence of $KHCO_3$ (5mM) at 37° for 0, 20, 40, 60 and 80 minutes. The same procedure was followed in presence of ANP (20, 60, and 200pM) or Furosemide (0.1, 0.3 and 1mM). Zinc content of RBCs was consequently determinted by means of atomic absorption spectrophotometry. Furosemide at pharmacological concentrations (0.1-0.3mM) induced Zn transport inhibition across RBC membrane. Bicarbonates (5mM) counteracted furosemide action at the above levels but failed to restore the actions of higher furosemide concentrations (1mM). ANP at concentrations 200pM enchanced Zn influx to RBCs and this effect was not bicarbonate depented.It was concluded that Zn influx to RBC is bicarbonate depented and may be inhibited by carbonic anydrase inhibitors such as furosemide but not from Na- K- Cl contransporter inhibitors such as ANP which on the contrary acts as a promoter of Zn influx to RBCs.

Key words: Atrial- Natriuretic-peptide (ANP), Furosemide, Red Cell Membrane, Zinc

Introduction

Atrial natriuretic peptide (ANP) is a resently discovered hormone secreted primarily by atrial myocytes in response to local wall stretch. The combined actions of ANP on vasculature, kidneys and adrenal serve both acutely and chronically to reduce systemic blood pressure as well as intravascular volume in various animal species and humans [1, 2].Zinc is a trace metal related to the synthesis and release of ANP as well as to ANP degradation through zinc mettalopeptidases, such as neutral endopeptidase 24.11.[3,4]. Furosemide is a synthetic natriuretic compound , possessing almost 1000 fold weaker natriuretic effects than ANP. Both substances induce, also, increased zincuresis through kidneys [5].ANP and furosemide are as well Na-K- Cl co-transporter inhibitors, while furosemide is also a bicarbonate inhibitor. Zincuresis hence may be due to bicarbonate or chloride inhibition. In the present study the effects of ANP and furosemide on zinc influx through the red cell membrane, as well as the possible mechanisms of zinc transport are investigated.

Materials and Methods

Blood (Hospital Blood Bank) was centrifuged at 0° for 10 min by means of a refrigerated centrifuge (Heraceus Sepatech Biofuge HRS1) and washed by a buffered solution (KCl 150nM, k/Hepes 5mM, EDTA 1ml at PH=7.45). RBCs were counted in a isotonic solution by means of a Coulter counter (Industrial D).Then the RBCs were spread into tubes containing an incubation solution (K_3 citrate 2mM, K/Hepes 5mM, 150mM KCl), under the following conditions:
A (1ml RBC and 1mM of Zn) in absence and presence of $KHCO_3$.
B: (**A** and 20pM, 60pM and 200pM of ANP) and
C: (**A** and 0.1mM, 0.3mM and 1mM furosemide).
All were incubated at 37° C for 0, 20, 40, 60 and 80 minutes. Samples as above were washed by the washing solution and the RBC sediment was mixed with $HCLO_4$ 15%. After centrifugation the supernatant was removed and the zinc concentration was estimated in a flame Atomic Absorption Spectrophotometer (Perkin Elmer Mod.560). The results expressed in μmol/l of RBC were statistically evaluated by t-student's test.

Results

Zinc influx through the red cell membrane during incubation (1mM $ZnCl_2$) is significantly increased in presence of bicarbonates ($KHCO_3$). Non-significant differences, in intracellular zinc concentrations, between 5mM and 8mM $KHCO_3$ incubations, indicate that zinc influx becomes maximum at 5mM $KHCO_3$ incubation. Zinc influx during incubation with 1mM $ZnCl_2$ and 0.1mM furosemide showed a remarkable inhibition of zinc influx ($p<0.001$) at any time of incubation. Incubation of 1mM $ZnCl_2$ and 0.1mM , 0.3mM furosemide in the presence of bicarbonates (5mM $KHCO_3$), induced Zn transport across RBC membrane. Higher furosemide concentration (1mM) inhibiting effects, on zinc transport were not counteracted by the presence of bicarbonates (5mM $KHCO_3$) at any time of incubation ($p\leq0.000$).Incubation with 1mM $ZnCl_2$ and ANP at concentrations 20pM, 60pM and 200pM in presence of bicarbonates (5mM$KHCO_3$) showed that 200pM ANP resulted in significant increase of zinc influx at any time of incubation ($p<0.005$).

Table I. Intracellular Zinc (%) changes under different conditions.

Incubation (min)	1mM $ZnCl_2$	1mM $ZnCl_2$ 5mM $KHCO_3$	1mM $ZnCl_2$ 5mM $KHCO_3$ 0.1mM Furos	1mM$ZnCl_2$ 5mM $KHCO_3$ 1mM Furos.	1mM $ZnCl_2$ 5mM $KHCO_3$ 200pM ANP
0	100%	100%	100%	100%	100%
20	170%	214%	202%	172%	205%
40	217%	326%	287%	232%	444%
60	290%	382%	379%	282%	498%
80	348%	453%	442%	310%	567%

Discussion

Furosemide is a well known inhibitor of carbonic anhydrase. Inhibition of carbonic anhydrase decreases zinc influx through RBC's membrane, due to decreased production of bicarbonates, and hence zinc-bicarbonate complexes formation that facilitates zinc influx to RBCs [6].

Bicarbonates at cons (5mM), producing otherwise maximum zinc influx, failed to counteract high furosemide cons (1mM) inhibiting effects on zinc influx. Furosemide high cons effect cannot be attributed to RBC membrane changes since furosemide exerts no influence on human erythrocyte shape in vitro [7]. Furosemide is also a well known Na-K-Cl co-transporter inhibitor and if zinc transport across RBC membrane was depended on this mechanism, as well as on bicarbonates, this could explain our results. ANP a Na-K-Cl co-transporter inhibitor induced zinc influx instead of inhibition [8,9]. It was resently reported that increased plasma ANP levels are related to increased zinc content in heart tissue in Wistar rats during cold acclimatization [4]. ANP acts also as an erythrocyte Na^{+}/K^{+} exchange stimulator [10]. Whether this action is reversely related to Na-K-Cl co-transporter inhibition and to zinc transport, remains to be investigated.

References

1.De Bold J, Heart atrial granularity:effects of changes in water-electrolyte balances. *Proc.Soc.Exp.Biol.Med.* 1979; 161:133-138

2.Brenner B, Ballermann B, GunningM, and Zeidel M, Diverse Biological Actions of Atrial Natriuretic peptides. *Physiological Rev.* 1990; 70(3) :665-699

3..Achilihu G., Frishman W.H., Landau A., Neutral endopeptidase and atrial natriuretic peptide. *J.Clin.Pharmacol* 1991;31:758-762

4.Vezyraki P,Kalfakakou V, Papagiannis J, and Evangelou A, Atrial Natriuretic Peptide relation to plasma and heart zinc concentrations of wistar rats exposed to cold and hot ambients. *Biol Trace Elem Res* 1999; 10: 215-223

5.Cohen N, Goli K.A, Dishi V.,.Zaidenstein R, .Weissgarden J., Averbukh Z, Modai D, Effects of furosemide oral solution, versus furosemide tablets on diuresis and electrolytes in patients with moderate congestive heart failure, *Miner Electrolyte Metabol* 1996;22 : 248-252

6.Kalfakakou V, and Simons T, Anionic mechanisms on zinc uptake across the human red cell membrane *J.Physiol*, 1990; 37(8) 1070-1083

7.Hasler R, Reinhart H, No influence of furosemide on human etythrocyte shape and blood viscosity in vitro. *Clin Hemorheol Microcirc* .1998; 18: 43-46

8.O'Grady S, Field M, Nash N, Rao M, Atrial natriuretic factor inhibits Na-K-Cl cotransport in teleost intestine , *Am.J.Physiol.* 1985 ; 249: 531-534

9.O'Donell M, Regulation of Na-K-Cl cotransporter in endithelial cells by atrial natriuretc factor, *Am.J.Physiol* . 1989; 257:36-44

10.Petrov V, Amery A, Lijen P, Role of cyclic GMP in Atrial-natriuretic-peptide stimulation of erythrocyte Na+/ H+ exchange, *Eur.J.Biochem.* 1994 ;1: 195-199

Metal Ions in Biology and Medicine; vol 6. Eds. J.A. Centeno, Ph. Collery, G. Vernet, R.B. Finkelman, H. Gibb, J.C. Etienne. John Libbey Eurotext, Paris © 2000, pp. 147-149.

Effects of heavy metals on dielectrical properties of tissues at microwave frequencies

Olga García Arribas[1], Mar Pérez Calvo[1], José L. Sebastián[2], Sagrario Muñoz[2], Miguel Sancho[2], José M. Miranda[2], José M. Escribano[3], Luis P. Rodríguez[4], Bartolomé Ribas[1]

[1] Department of Toxicology, Instituto de Salud Carlos III, Madrid; [2] Department of Applied Physics III, Faculty of Physics; and [4] Department of Physical Medicine, Complutense University, Madrid; [3] Institut of Cardiology, Autonomous Community of Madrid, Spain

Abstract

The industrial production is increasing the prevalence in our environment of heavy metals as iron, lead, cadmium and mercury. The aim of this work is to establish the variation of the dielectrical properties (conductivity and permittivity) of treated organs with different metals, cadmium, lead and mercury in order to characterize the effect of microwave radiations such as those from mobile telephones. For this work 65 male Wistar rats were used. Several groups of animals were treated intraperitoneally with each toxic metal. Another group of rats was used as control. The animals were sacrified and samples of each tissue of 2mm thick were cut and introduced in the center of a methacrylate block filling a section of WR 430 waveguide to measure the permittivity and conductivity at 2.45 GHz. It is shown that exposure of biological tissues to heavy metal pollutants alter their electric properties. Statistically significant differences are found in tissues overloaded with different toxic metals compared to untreated tissues. For each metal, the variations observed in the permittivity and conductivity on the exposed tissues are explained and correlated with the variations of various biochemical and hematological parameters. The effects of heavy metals could be combined with those from the environmental electromagnetic fields and with human pathological conditions. This technique may be a very practical tool for the future evaluation of metal exposure.

Keywords: dielectrical properties, microwave frequencies, heavy metals.

Introduction

Small quantities of several metallic elements are essential for health. However, the growing industrial activity is leading to a higher environmental toxicity. Heavy metals, lead, cadmium and mercury are attracting a lot of interest because the issues are raised both by occupational environmental exposures and environmental pollution. Early experimental studies (Yannai, 1993) show that heavy concentration of these metals induce proteinemia, nephropathy, homeostatic disregulation and have influence on the metabolism of erythrocytes. A living body is made up of a complex structure of biological tissues with very dissimilar electric properties (dielectric permittivity ε and conductivity σ), (Juutilainen, 1998, Repacholi, 1998, Azanza, 1994, Linet,1997). As tissues and cells are exposed to metal polllutants, toxic chemicals and hazardous waste, they are poisoned to a point where their electric properties may be severely altered and therefore, the biological tissues can no longer fuction properly. (Gabriel, 1996a, Gabriel, 1996b). The objetive of this work is the determination of the variation of the electrical properties of poisoned organs with pollutant metals. And also, it's shown that the variations observed in ε and σ may be associated to the variations of various biochemical and hematological parameters that are found in blood analysis.

Material and Methods

For this work, 65 male Wistar rats, with average weight ranging from 170g to 220 g were maintained in metabolic cages with water and food "ad libitum". There are two groups of rats, the control group, and the group treated daily with intraperitoneal doses from 0.05 to 0.14 mg/gbw of different disolutions of heavy metals. The animals were killed by a total extraction by a cardiac puncture under ether anesthesia. A blood analysis is made of each animal. Liver, lung, kidney, pancreas and muscle were dissected, and samples up to 2mm thick were maintained at 0ºC.

The experimental characterization is performed by measuring the reflection and transmission complex coefficients of the acutal biological sample at the industrial frequency of 2.45 GHz. For this purpose, the rectangular sample of biological tissue is placed in the center of a methacrylate block filling a section of WR430 waveguide suitable for work with the range 1.7 to 2.6 GHz. The reflection S_{11} and transmission S_{21} complex coefficients of the sample at RF are measured by using a network analyzer (VNA). For the calibration of the measuring system the sample cut of biological tissue was replaced by a piece of methacrylate of the same dimensions. The same structure (tissue inside the waveguide) was analyzed using the HP HFSS simulator. The simulator makes it possible to detemine the value of the complex dielectric permittivity of a tissue that produces the same values for S_{11} and S_{21} that have been experimentally determined.

Results

Table 1. The table shows the blood analysis (hematological, biochemical and enzymatic) for the control group and for the treated group for each toxic metal.

TISSUE	CONTROL	Hg	Pb	Cd
Erytrocytes (10^6/mm^3)	7'05±0'49	5'54±0'5	5'5±0'7	5'7±1
Hemoglobin (g/dL)	12'75±0'35	10'4±1'5	10'76±0'97	9'97±1'50
Hemathocryte (%)	37'30±0'8	31'8±3'07	31'46±4'12	31'8±6'10
Platelets (10^3/mm^3)	896±48'9	789'3±213	1.136±108	1.214±41
Glucose (g/100mL)	166±13	123'6±17	110'6±4'7	109±3'5
Total Protein (g/100mL)	6'3±0'2	5'3±1'66	5'62±0'35	5'96±0'61
Albumin (mg/100mL)	3'7±0'12	2'4±0'64	2'8±0'2	2'35±0'2
Urea (mg/100mL)	33±2	37'3±4'49	24'25±1'47	39±15'26
Total Bilirubin (mg/100mL)	0'25±0'05	0'3±0'08	0'375±0'24	0'575±0'54
Calcium serum (mg/100mL)	11'7±0'9	9'4±2'39	0'85±1'30	10'17±1'17
Iron serum (μg/100mL)	116'6±13	93'4±11'3	155'25±33	100'5±28'8
Phosphor (mg/100mL)	7'5±1'3	6'2±1'2	8'05±0'55	7'55±0'25
Magnesium (mg/100mL)	2'2±0'33	1'87±0'38	2'25±0'2	2'65±0'47
GOT (U/L)	93'5±12'5	99'25±13'7	110'5±8'55	275'2±17'3
GPT (U/L)	81±12'9	67'8±31'5	77'5±18	47'75±17
Gamma- GT (U/L)	0	1'6±0'48	0'6±0'4	2±1'22
LDH (U/L)	252'5±30'5	578±50	447'6±60'4	1004±55'7
CPK (U/L)	277'5±59'5	262±70	381'3±60'0	651'5±58'4

Table 2. Dielectric properties of tissues for the control group and the treated groups with different pollutant metals.

Tissue		Control	Hg	Pb	Cd
Liver	ε	42,6±0,96	43,7±1,36	45,40±1,38*	42,50±0,8**
	σ	1,52±0,08	1,17±0,05*	1,20±0,16*	1,35±0,18**
Kidney	ε	49,84±1,09	47,50±1,23*	45,70±1,18*	44,17±0,98*
	σ	1,77±0,21	1,42±0,18*	1,21±0,20*	1,08±0,10*
Lung	ε	47,36±0,69	41,25±1,23	38,99±1,34*	40,75±1,33**
	σ	1,64±0,09	1,27±0,18	1,19±0,10*	1,19±0,09*

* Extremely significant difference with the control group ($p<0.001$).
** Significant difference with the control group ($p<0.05$).

Discussion

For lung, statistically significant differences in the permittivity with respect to the control group were observed for lead and cadmium. Mercury have tendency to concentrate electrical fields.This is a biophysical effect and explains the extremely significant chage produced in the conductivity of the treated tissue.

The kidney is the major target tissue for metal toxicity and this fact could explain the changes observed in its complex permittivity. In particular, the renal cortex is preferred target tissue for cadmium toxicity, provoking proximal tubular disfunction. Lead treated tissues show a decrease in hemoglobin synthesis. This can lead to mocrocytic anemia and may explain the extremely significant differences found in both permittivity and conductivity of treated tissues.

In liver the cadmium produces high acute liver toxicity, the significant differences found in both permittivity and conductivity for the cadmium are in agreement with the increase observed in the oxalacetic glutamic transaminase, GOT and the decrease of the structural integrity of hepatocytes. The blood analysis shows that the rats treated with cadmium have lower than normal values of hematocryte and hemoglobin, since the cadmium treatment affects the erytrocyte metabolism.

It has been shown that the exposure of biological tissues to heavy metal pollutants alter their electric properties. Statistically extremely significant differences are found in tissues treated with different toxic metals compared to untreated tissues.

References

Juutilainen J. and De Seze R. (1998). Biological effects of amplituded-modulated rediofrequency radiation. Scand. J. Work Environ. Health. 24, 245-254.

Repacholi M.H. (1998). Low-level exposure to radiofrequency electromagnetic fields: health effects and research needs. Biolectromag. 19, 1-19.

Linet M.S., Hatch E.E., Kleinerman R.A., Robison L.L., Kaune W.T., Friedman D.R., Severson R.K., Haines C.M. et al. (1997). Residential exposure to magnetic fields and acute lymphoblastic leukemia in children. New Engl. J. Med. 337, 1-7.

Azanza M.J., Del Moral A. (1994). Cell membrane biochemistry and neurobiological approach to biomagnetism. Prog. Neurobiol. 44, 517-601.

Gabriel C., Gabriel S. and Corthout E. (1996)[a]. The dielectric properties of biological tissues: I. Literature Survey. Phys. Med. Biol. 41, 2231-2249.

Gabriel S., Lau R. W. and Gabriel C.(1996)[b]. The dielectric properties of biological tissues: III. Parametric models for the dielectric spectrum of tissues. Phys. Med. Biol. 41, 2271-2293.

Yannai S., and Sachs K. M. (1993). Absorption and accumulation of cadmium, lead and mercury from foods by rats. Fd. Chem. Toxic. 31, 351-355.

Metal Ions in Biology and Medicine; vol 6. Eds. J.A. Centeno, Ph. Collery, G. Vernet, R.B. Finkelman, H. Gibb, J.C. Etienne. John Libbey Eurotext, Paris © 2000, pp. 150-153.

Metallothioneins and extrathymic functions (liver natural killer activity) during the circadian cycle in young and old mice

Eugenio Mocchegiani, Mario Muzzioli, Catia Cipriano, Robertina Giacconi

Immunology Crt., Research Department INRCA, Via Birarelli 8, 60121 Ancona, Italy. Correspondence: e.mocchegiani@inrca.it

Abstract

Metallothioneins (MTs) are proteins especially produced in the liver and involved in zinc homeostasis, which, in turn, is relevant for immune efficiency including Natural Killer (NK) activity of also extrathymic (liver) origin. This is a T-cell pathway prominent in ageing. High MTs levels have been found in the atrophic thymus and liver of old mice suggesting a possible MTs different role between young and old age: from protective to dangerous for immune efficiency, respectively. In order to further suggest this different role, MTmRNA, liver NK activity and IL-6 are tested in young and old mice during the circadian cycle because immune differences between young and old age are present in the dark period as compared to the light period. IL-6 plasma levels are tested because MTmRNA is under the control of this interleukin. High IL-6 levels are associated with high MTmRNA during the circadian cycle more evident in old age. Concomitantly reduced liver NK activity is observed. Because of zinc requirement for NK activity, augmented expression of MTmRNA may induce a continuos sequester of zinc with consequent impaired liver NK activity also during the circadian cycle especially in the light period. Therefore increased MTs in ageing may be deleterious for entire immune efficiency representing, as such, a possible novel diagnostic and genetic marker for the ageing process.

Introduction

Metallothioneins (MTs), a proteins' class containing cystein and mainly produced in the liver, play pivotal roles in metal-related cell homeostasis because of their high affinity for metals. The main MTs functional role is to sequester and /or dispense metal ions participating primarily in zinc homeostasis [1], which is relevant for the efficiency of entire immune functions especially for Natural Killer (NK) activity from thymic and extrathymic (liver) origin [2]. Consistent with this role, MTs protect the cells against cytotoxic effect of reactive oxigen species forming "clusters" due to the presence in their molecules of reduced thiols groups [1]. As such, MTs gene expression in higher eukaryotic species are transcriptionally induced by a variety of stressor agents. In this context a peculiar role is exerted by MTs in inducing the secretion by macrophages for a prompt immune responses by stressor agents of some interleukins, such as IL-6, which is, in turn, involved in new synthesis of MTs in the liver [3]. Such MTs role is peculiar in young-adult age but it may be questioned in ageing for the following points. **i)** High MTs levels are found in atrophic thymus of old mice [2]; **ii)** high MTs levels are present in the liver of old mice associated with impaired NK activity [4]. Following that, the role of MTs may become from protective in young-adult age to dangerous in ageing because of the continuos sequester of zinc inducing, as such, low zinc ions bioavailability with subsequent impaired peripheral immune efficiency [2]. In order to further suggest this possible different role, MTmRNA in the liver, plasma IL-6 levels and NK activity of liver origin are tested in young and old mice during the circadian cycle because of very significant differences in thymic functions and plasma zinc levels between young and old age during the nocturnal period as compared to the light period [5]. The choice to test NK activity of liver origin because of its relevance in liver extrathymic T-cell pathway prominent in ageing (6) and because MTs are especially produced in the liver [1].

Materials and Methods

Mice

Inbred male Balb/c mice of 3 months (young) and 20 months (old) of age were used. Time intervals during the circadian cycle were: 9am, 2pm, 7pm, 2am and 9am. 5 young and 5 old mice were sacrificed under ether anaesthesia for each time interval. Plasma and tissue liver were frozen at -80 °C until used.

IL-6 plasma determination

Plasma IL-6 was tested using mouse interleukin-6 ELISA kit (Endogen, USA). The data were expressed in pg/ml. The sensitivity of kit is ≤7 pg/ml.

MTmRNA determination (semiquantitative RT-PCR)

Total RNA was extracted by the liver using Tri-Reagent according manufacture's protocol (Sigma,USA). 1μg of total RNA was reverse trascripted using oligo-dT primer and MuMLV (Gibco/BRL, USA). Semiquantitative RT-PCR was performed using specific primers for MT-I [7] and β-actin. The data are expressed as a relative unit determined by normalisation of the density of MT-I band to that of β-actin band [8].

Liver NK activity determination

The separation of lymphocytes from the liver was performed using the method of Watanabe et al. [9]. NK activity was measured using lymphoma cell line YAC-1 as target. NK activity was tested in liver lymphocytes using $1x10^5$ cells as target and $2x10^6$ liver lymphocytes. 100μCi of ^{51}Cr was used as marker for NK lysis. The data are expressed in Lytic Unit $20/10^7$ cells.

Statistical analysis

Analysis of IL-6, MTmRNA and liver NK rhythmicity was performed according to the cosinor method [10]. Paired Student's t test and ANOVA (two-way) were used where appropriate. Correlations were determined by linear regression analysis by the least square method. Differences were considered significant when $p< 0.05$.

Results

Table I shows the existence of a circadian cycle of IL-6, liver MTmRNA and liver NK activity in young and old mice with no significant variations during the light period but with significant peaks (increments or decrements) during the night period . In particular significant increments of IL-6 and liver MTmRNA are observed at 9.00 am in old mice as compared to young mice ($p<0.01$).

Table I. IL-6 plasma levels, liver MTmRNA and liver NK activity in young and old mice during the circadian cycle

YOUNG		9.00 am	2.00 pm	7.00 pm	2.00 am	9.00 am
	IL-6 (pg/ml)	7.8±3.9	9.9±6.3	8.4±2.2	20.1±2.8§	8.1±2.8
	liver MTmRNA	0.31±0.02	0.5±0.03	0.27±0.03	0.8±0.04§	0.36±0.03
	liver NK activity (LU)	48.42±4.3	30.49±3.5	29.79±3.0	20.26±2.9§	46.74±6.1

§ p<0.001 as compared to the values of the light period in circadian cycle (ANOVA)

OLD		9.00 am	2.00 pm	7.00 pm	2.00 am	9.00 am
	IL-6 (pg/ml)	25.8±10.9*	30.9±14.6*	41.5±3.1*	9.3±3.2°	22.4±8.4*
	liver MTmRNA	0.96±0.05*	0.95±0.04*	0.96±0.05*	0.32±0.02°	1.00±0.05*
	liver NK activity (LU)	37.06±3.6+	33.78±4.8	32.86±4.9	43.87±4.3+	34.35±5.3+

*p< 0.01 as compared to young mice ; +p< 0.01 as compared to young mice (Paired Student's t test)
°p<0.001 as compared to values of the light period in circadian cycle (ANOVA).

Such increments are associated with significant decrements of liver NK activity at the same time of observation (9.00 am) in old mice as compared to young ($p<0.01$).

Significant decrements of IL-6 production and MTmRNA gene expression are observed during the night period (2.00 am) associated with significant increments of liver NK activity as compared to the light period in old mice ($p< 0.01$). Concomitantly the high increments of IL-6 and MTmRNA at 2.00am are associated with a loss of liver NK activity as compared to the light period in young mice ($p<0.001$) (Table I). Significant variations of liver NK activity are present during the circadian cycle in young mice (from 9.00am to 9.00am of the next day) ($p<0.001$), whereas no significant or modest variations occur during the circadian cycle in old mice. Significant positive correlations exist between IL-6 and MTmRNA in young and old mice ($r=0.75$, $p<0.01$ and $r=0.72$, $p<0.01$ respectively) during the circadian cycle. Significant inverse correlations exist between MTmRNA and liver NK activity in young and old mice ($r= -0.73$ $p<0.01$ and $r= -0.78$, $p<0.01$, respectively) during the circadian cycle.

Discussion

In agreement with other authors for old people [11], IL-6 is also increased in old mice as compared to young with variations during the circadian cycle. Such increments are associated with augmented MTmRNA gene expression and impaired liver NK activity in old mice during the light period. However a loss of IL-6 production is observed in the dark period (2.00 am) in old mice. Such a loss is associated with decrements of MTmRNA and increments on liver NK activity as compared to values of the light period. Conversely increments of IL-6 in the dark period are associated with increments of MTmRNA and decrements of liver NK activity in young mice. These data while one hand confirm that the MTmRNA gene expression is under the control of IL-6 [3], on the other hand suggest the existence of a link between MTs and immune functions as documented by the existence of significant correlations between MTmRNA and immune parameters tested during the circadian cycle in young and old mice. Moreover increments of MTmRNA impair liver NK activity of extrathymic origin, which is prominent in ageing [6]. Such an impairment may be largely due to the fact that MTs bind preferentially zinc, rather than copper, in ageing [2] inducing, as such, low zinc ions bioavailability for immune efficiency, especially for NK activity of thymic and extrathymic origin [2]. In fact high zinc content is present in the liver of old mice as compared to young [2]. Since AAS tests zinc bound and zinc unbound, while one hand it may justify high zinc content in the liver of old mice [2] because zinc is bound to MTs, on the other hand it suggests that circadian variations of liver MTmRNA are crucial for the zinc ions bioavailability and consequent efficiency of the liver extrathymic T-cell pathway. Indeed MTs are involved either as sequesters of zinc or as reservoir of zinc during zinc toxicity or zinc deficiency, respectively [12]. This task of MTs is more evident in young age where circadian variations of MTmRNA is associated with more significant circadian variations of liver NK activity. This phenomenon is less evident in old mice despite the loss of MTmRNA gene expression is associated with increments of liver NK activity in the dark period. In fact the liver NK activity during the dark period in old mice is quite similar to that one found in the light period (9.00am) where high MTmRNA are associated with lower NK activity as compared to young (Table I) and low zinc ions bioavailability is always present during the circadian cycle in old mice [5]. These findings suggest that zinc ions bioavailability by means of MTs production is crucial for liver NK activity also during the circadian cycle in particular in old age. Following that, MTs may not completely transfer zinc in ageing passing, as such, from beneficial role in young-adult age to deleterious one for immune efficiency in ageing. Because both MTs production (3] and NK activity [13] are also under the control of glucocorticoids, which are, in turn, always high during the circadian cycle [5], it is a further support for a different role of MTs for immune efficiency between young and old age: from protective to dangerous, respectively. On the other hand high MTs levels are present in the atrophic thymus and liver of old mice [2] and transgenic MTs mice show thymic involution and melanoma development [14]. Therefore high zinc-bound MTs migh induce to a lack of the plasticity of the liver extrathymic functions in old age, and immune plasticity is fundamental to maintain good immune homeostasis, as it occurs in young-adult age [15]. As such, the old organism may become a low responder to external noxae with subsequent rising of age-related pathologies (cancer and infections) despite the MTmRNA expression is higher in old than in young age. On the other hand high MTs levels are an index of poor prognosis in cancer and infections [2]. Thus MTmRNA may represent a novel diagnostic and genetic marker of ageing and age-related diseases. Further clinical and experimental studies are currently in progress in our laboratory.

Acknowledgements

This paper was supported by INRCA and by Italian Health Ministry. The authors thank Mrs. Nazzarena Gasparini for her excellent technical assistance.

References

1. Kagi RHJ. Evolution, structure and chemical activity of class I metallothioneins: an overview. In: Suzuki KT, Imura N, Kimura M eds. *Metallothioneins III.* Basel, Switzerland: Birkhauser Verlag Publisher, 1993: 29-56.
2. Mocchegiani E, Muzzioli M, Cipriano C, Giacconi R. Zinc, T-cell pathways, ageing : role of metallothioneins. *Mechanism Ageing Develop.* 1998; 106: 183-204.
3. Grider A, Cousins RJ. Role of metallothioneins in copper and zinc metabolism: special reference to inflammatory condition. In: Milanino R, Rainsford KD, Velo GP eds. *Copper and zinc in inflammation.* Lancaster, U.K.: Kluwer Academic Publisher, 1989: 21-32.
4. Mocchegiani E, Verbanac D, Santarelli L, Tibaldi A, Muzzioli M, Radosevic-Stasic B, Milin C. Zinc and metallothioneins on cellular immune effectiveness during liver regeneration in young and old mice. *Life Sciences* 1997; 61: 1125-1145.
5. Mocchegiani E, Santarelli L, Tibaldi A, Muzzioli M, Bulian D, Cipriano C, Olivieri F, Fabris N. Presence of links between zinc and melatonin during the circadian cycle in old mice : effects on thymic endocrine activity and on the survival. *J. Neuroimmunology* 1998; 86: 111-122.
6. Abo T. Extrathymic pathways of T-cell differentiation : a primitive and fundamental immune system. *Microbiol. Immunol.* 1993; 37: 247-258.
7. Andrews GK, Huet-Hudson YM, Paria BC, McMaster MT, De SK, Dey SK. Metallothionein gene expression and metal regulation during preimplantation mouse embryo development (MT mRNA during early development). *Developmental Biology* 1991; 145: 13-27.
8. Okuda Y, Nakatsuji Y, Fujimura H, Esumi H, Ogura T, Yanagihara T, Sakoda S. Expression of the inducible isoform od nitric oxide synthase in the central nervous system of mice correlates with the severity of actively induced experimental allergic encephalomyelitis. *J. Neuroimmunol.* 1995; 62: 103-112.
9. Watanabe H, Ohtsuka K, Kimura M, Ikarashi Y, Ohmori K, Kusumi A, Ohteki T, Seki S, Abo T. Details of an isolation method for hepatic lymphocytes in mice. *J. Immunol. Methods* 1992; 146: 145-154.
10. Nelson W, Tong JL, Lee JK, Halberg F. Methods for cosinor-rhythmometry. *Chronobiologia* 1979; 6: 305-323.
11. Fagiolo U, Cossarizza A, Scala E, Fanales-Belasio E, Ortolani C, Cozzi D, Monti D, Franceschi C, Paganelli R. Increased cytokine production in mononuclear cells of healthy and elderly people. *Eur. J. Immunol.* 1993; 23: 2375-2378.
12. Kelly EJ, Quaife CF, Froelik GJ, Palmiter RD. Metallothionein I and II against zinc deficiency and zinc toxicity. *J. Nutr.* 1996; 126: 1782-1790.
13. McGlone JJ, Lumpkin EA, Norman RL. Adrenocorticotropin stimulates natural killer cell activity. *Endocrinology* 1991; 129: 1653-1658.
14. Iia T, Watanabe H, Iwamoto T, Nakashima I, Abo T. Predominant activation of extrathymic T cells during melanoma development of metallothionein/ret transgenic mice. *Cellular Immunology* 1994; 153: 412-427.
15. Fabris N, Mocchegiani E, Provinciali M. Plasticity of neuroendocrine-immune interactions during ageing. *Exp. Gerontol.* 1997; 32: 415-429.

Metal Ions in Biology and Medicine; vol 6. Eds. J.A. Centeno, Ph. Collery, G. Vernet, R.B. Finkelman, H. Gibb, J.C. Etienne. John Libbey Eurotext, Paris © 2000, pp. 154-156.

Effect of chronic magnesium deficiency on mitochondrial Zn content in different rat brain structures

Elena Planells, Nuria Sánchez-Morito, Mª José Moreno, Pilar Aranda, Juan Llopis

Department of Physiology, School of Pharmacy and Institute of Nutrition and Food Tecnology, University of Granada, 18071 Granada, Spain

INTRODUCTION

Magnesium deficiency is known to be linked with cardiovascular alterations and many renal, gastrointestinal, neurological and muscular disorders (1) . The symptoms and signs of Mg deficiency have been traced, in large part, to complex electrolytic alterations secondary to the mineral deficit.

In addition to these findings there is evidence from epidemiological studies that Mg intake in a large proportion (from 15 to 20%) of the population in industrialized countries is approximately 30% below the Recommended Daily Allowances, and that Mg deficiency, together with inadequate dietary habits, can lead to many disease states (2, 3, 4).

In previous studies we reported that Mg deficit alters the bioavailability and tissue distribution of a number of elements such as calcium and phosphorus (5,6), zinc (7), iron (8), copper (9), manganese (10) and selenium (11). Mg deficiency significantly increased intestinal absorption of Zn, Zn balance, and Zn concentration in femur and kidney, decreased Zn concentration in heart, but no change was found in brain Zn concentration (7).

The present study was designed to investigate the effect of dietary magnesium deficiency on mitochondrial Zn content in different rat cerebral structures: cortex, cerebellum, striatum and hippocampus.

MATERIAL AND METHODS

Animals and diets

Recently-weaned male Wistar rats consumed a standard commercial diet (Panlab, Barcelona) until they reached a body weight of 100 g. Thereafter they were allowed access *ad libitum* to double-distilled water and a semisynthetic diet deficient in Mg. The diet contained (g/kg) casein (Musal & Chemical, Granada, Spain) 140; cystine (Roche SA, Madrid) 1.8; sucrose (Musal & Chemical) 100; wheat starch (Musal & Chemical) 622; fiber (cellulose) (Musal & Chemical) 50; olive oil 40; AIN-93 mineral mix (12) (without magnesium oxide) 35; AIN-93 (21) vitamin mix 10; and choline bitartrate (Merck) 2.5. In all, these components provide 129 mg Mg.

To study the development of Mg-deficiency, 6 groups of 5 deficient rats were killed after feeding with the diet for 5 and 10 weeks. Different structures were dissected from the rat brain. The mitochondria of the cortex, cerebellum, striatum and hippocampus were isolated.

The results were compared with those for a group of control rats (5 y 10 weeks) fed the same diet, except that the amount of Mg was adequate to cover their nutritional requirements (480 mg/kg food). Control animals were pair-fed with the deficient rats.

Throughout the 70-day experimental period the control and Mg-deficient rats were housed in individual metabolic cages in a well-ventilated, temperature-controlled room (21±2ºC) with a light:dark period of 12 h.

Analytical techniques

The mitochondria of the different brain structures were isolated following the Fleischer et al. procedure (13). Protein concentration of all samples were assayed according to Lowry method and Zn were determined by atomic absorption spectrophotometry (AAS) (Perkin Elmer 1100B), in wet-mineralized samples (NO_3H/ClO_4H).

Bovine liver (Certified Reference Material CRM 185, Community Bureau of Reference, Brussels, Belgium) was used for quality control assays.

Statistical analyses

The data for control and Mg-deficient animals were compared with Student's *t* test . All analyses were done with the SPSS software package. Differences were considered significant at the 5% probability level.

RESULTS

TABLE 1.- MITOCHONDRIA ZINC CONTENT (mg/g proteín)

	5 WEEKS		10 WEEKS	
	CONTROL	DEFICIENT	CONTROL	DEFICIENT
STRIATUM	0.60±0.01	0.70±0.01 d	0.90±0.05 *	1.40±0.08 d
HIPOCAMPUS	0.48±0.03	0.74±0.05 c	1.03±0.14 *	1.65±0.19 d
CEREBELLUM	0.81±0.08	0.80±0.07	0.90±0.05	0.98±0.08
CORTEX	0.87±0.10	1.02±0.08	1.03±0.06	1.29±0.09

Mean values for 6 pools (5 rats/pool) ±SEM.
Significant difference between control and deficient rats. c $p<0.01$; d $p<0.001$.
Significant difference between 5 and 10 weeks control rats. * $p<0.001$.

Mitochondrial Zn concentrations in the striatum and hippocampus of control rats was significantly higher in week 10. These results may be related to changes in age. In our experimental conditions, feeding with an Mg-deficient diet significantly increased mitochondrial Zn content in the striatum and hippocampus, measured on weeks 5 ($p<0.001$ and $p<0.01$, respectively) and 10 ($p<0.001$, both). However, we found no changes, related to age and/or magnesium deficiency, in Zn mitochondia in the cortex and cerebellum.

REFERENCES

1. Shils ME: Magnesium. In: Ziegler EE, Filer LJ (eds). Present Knowledge in Nutrition. Washington, DC: ILSI Press, pp 307-319, 1996.
2. Wester PO: Magnesium. Am J Clin Nutr 45: 1305- 1312,1987
3. Schimatschek HF, Classen HG. Age, sex and seasonal effects on plasma and calcium levels of 4859 children. *Mag Res* 1993; 6: 65-66
4.Wong ET, Rude RK, Singer FR. A high prevalence of hypomagnesemia and hypermagnesemia in hospitalized patients. *Am J Clin Pathol* 1983;79: 348-352.
5. Planells E, Aranda P, Peran F, LLopis. Changes in calcium and phosphorus absorption and retention during long-term magnesium deficiency in rats. *Nutr Res* 1993;13: 691- 699.
6. Planells E, LLopis J, Perán F, Aranda P. Changes in tissue calcium and phosphorus content and plasma concentration of parathyroid hormone and calcitonin after long-term magnesium deficiency in rats. *J Am Coll Nutr* 1995; 14:292-298.
7. Planells E, Aranda P, Lerma A, LLopis J. Changes in bioavailability and tissue distribution of zinc caused by magnesium deficiency in rats. *Br J Nutr* 1994; 72:315-323.
8. Sanchez-Morito N, Planells E, Aranda P, Llopis J. Influence of magnesium deficiency on the bioavailability and tissue distribution of iron in the rat. *J Nutr Biochem* 2000, (in press)
9. Jiménez A, Planells E, Aranda P, Sánchez-Viñas M, Llopis J. Changes in bioavailability and tissue distribution of copper caused by magnesium deficiency in rats. *J Agric Food Chem* 1997; 45: 4023-4027.
10. Sanchez-Morito N, Planells E, Aranda P, Llopis J. Magnesium-Manganese interactions caused by magnesium deficiency in rats. *J Am Coll Nutr* 1999; 18: 475-480.
11. Jiménez A, Planells E, Aranda P, Sánchez-Viñas M, Llopis J. Changes in bioavailability and tissue distribution of selenium caused by magnesium deficiency in rats. *J Am Coll Nutr* 1997; 16: 175-180.
12. Reeves PG, Nielsen FH, Fahey GC. AIN-93 purifieds diets for laboratory rodents: Final report of the American Institute of Nutrition ad hoc writing Committe on the reformulation of the AIN-76 rodent diet. *J Nutr* 1993; 123:1939-1951.
13. Fleisher S, McIntyre IO, Vidal JC. Large scale preparation of rat liver mitochondria in high yield. *Methods Enzymol* 1979; 55:32.

Metal Ions in Biology and Medicine; vol 6. Eds. J.A. Centeno, Ph. Collery, G. Vernet, R.B. Finkelman, H. Gibb, J.C. Etienne. John Libbey Eurotext, Paris © 2000, pp. 157-159.

Potential cesium chelators: *in vitro* evaluation in octanol/water systems and rat erythrocytes

A. Torres[1], A. Raya[2], J.M. Llobet[2, 3], J.L. Domingo[3]

[1] *Biochemistry Unit, School of Medicine, Rovira i Virgili University, c/Sant Llorenç 21, 43201, Reus, Spain;* [2] *Toxicology Unit, School of Pharmacy, University of Barcelona, Av. Joan XXIII s/n, 08028, Barcelona, Spain, and* [3] *Laboratory of Toxicology and Environmental Health, c/Sant Llorenç 21, 43201 Reus, Spain*

Due to its physical and biological properties, ^{137}Cs is one of the most dangerous radionuclides released in nuclear accidents [1-3]. Prussian blue derivatives can be given to absorb Cs and to reduce its gastrointestinal absorption [4-7], these compounds are not able to remove internal Cs. To date, there is not effective treatment to remove Cs from contaminated people. The aim of the present study was to provide comparable data on a series of chelating agents in two *in vitro* models. The octanol/water system [6-7] and a rat erythrocyte suspension [8] were used to select chelators and pairs of chelators to be subsequebtly tested in *in vivo* studies.

Materials and Methods

Animals and chemicals: Male Sprague-Dawley rats (Interfauna Ibérica, Barcelona, Spain) weighing 315 ± 15 g were used. CsCl (E. Merck, Darmstadt, Germany); CDTA, Tiron, sodium salicylate (SS) (Sigma Chemical Co, St. Louis, MO, USA); Kryptofix® 222 (K-222), 15-Crown-5, 12-Crown-4, 1,3,5-trithiane (6-S-3) (Aldrich, Steinheim, Germany); desferrioxamine (DFOA) (Ciba-Geigy, Basel, Switzerland); L1 (gift from Professor Mark M. Jones, Vanderbilt University, Nashville, TN, USA).

Octanol/water systems (O/W): Two O/W systems were developed. To simulate the relative composition of K^+ and Na^+ in the extra and intracellular media, two physiological incubation mediums were used as aqueous phases: $CaCl_2$ 0.9 mM, KH_2PO_4 1.5 mM, Na_2HPO_4 8.1 mM, $MgCl_2$ 0.5 mM and NaCl 136.8 mM, KCl 2.7 mM (solution A), and NaCl 2.7 mM, KCl 136.8 mM (solution B). The organic phase consisted of n-octanol saturated with the corresponding aqueous phase. Each chelator was dissolved at a concentration 1mM in the corresponding aqueous phase (to which 5 g/l of Cs were added). Four ml of aqueous solution were mixed with 4 ml of n-octanol, shaked at 37°C for 24 h and centrifuged. The octanol layer was removed and Cs was extracted by incubation with a concentrated KCl solution. Cs concentrations in the samples were determined by atomic emission spectrophotometry (Philips PU 9200X).

Rat erythrocyte suspension: Animals were Cs loaded by two i.p. injections of 0.3 g CsCl/kg/injection 48 and 24 h previous to the blood extraction. Venous blood was obtained and erythrocytes isolated by standard centrifugation procedures. All erythrocytes were mixed, preincubated in an isotonic medium (NaCl 115 mM, KCl 20 mM,

Na_3PO_4 4.75 mM, dextrose 10 mM; pH 7.4), washed and centrifuged. Portions of 1 ml of the erythrocyte precipitated were incubated for 2 h with 4 ml of the media containing 0.5 mM of each chelator and centrifuged. Extracellular medias were finally obtained. Cs concentrations and the absorbances (at 415 nm, to measure hemolytic rates) were determined. After initial screening, some combinations of two chelators were tested at a concentration of 0.5 mM each.

Results and Discussion

The effects of the chelating agents on Cs distribution in the two *in vitro* models of the study are shown in Tables 1 and 2.

Table 1. The effect of the indicated chelating agents on Cs distribution in the O/W and rat erythrocyte system. Results are expressed as mg Cs/l

	Cs in organic phase (aqueous solution A)	Cs in organic phase (aqueous solution B)	extracellular Cs
Control	2.91 ± 1.87	1.47 ± 0.15	0.68 ± 0.06
CDTA	13.28 ± 9.49^c	1.99 ± 0.83	0.68 ± 0.10
Tiron	9.24 ± 8.03^c	1.49 ± 0.23	0.91 ± 0.18^b
SS	4.97 ± 2.54^b	8.57 ± 9.52^c	0.59 ± 0.05^a
K-222	1.52 ± 0.99^a	1.79 ± 0.62	0.66 ± 0.06
15-Crown-5	12.07 ± 10.32^a	2.21 ± 0.93^a	0.89 ± 0.20^a
12-Crown-4	7.11 ± 4.61^a	3.88 ± 3.51^a	0.66 ± 0.04
6-S-3	7.97 ± 5.97^a	2.88 ± 1.20^b	1.07 ± 0.31^b
DFOA	1.52 ± 0.62^a	5.50 ± 4.72^c	0.63 ± 0.06
L1	3.48 ± 0.90^a	4.26 ± 3.32^a	0.59 ± 0.04^a

[a] Significantly different from control, $p < 0.05$, [b] Significantly different from control, $p < 0.01$
[c] Significantly different from control, $p < 0.001$

Table 2. The effect of the indicated pairs of chelating agents on Cs distribution in the rat erythrocyte system. Results are expressed as mg Cs/l

	extracellular Cs
Control	0.78 ± 0.03
DFOA/Tiron	0.79 ± 0.06
DFOA/15-Crown-5	0.80 ± 0.03
DFOA/6-S-3	0.97 ± 0.24^a
K-222/Tiron	0.99 ± 0.27^a
K-222/15-Crown-5	1.04 ± 0.21^b
K-222/6-S-3	1.19 ± 0.49^b
DFOA/SS	0.81 ± 0.13
DFOA/L1	0.94 ± 0.08^b

[a] Significantly different from control, $p < 0.05$
[b] Significantly different from control, $p < 0.01$

When in the O/W system, the aqueous solution A, with higher amounts of Na^+ (simulating the extracellular media) was used, only DFOA and K-222 produced significant decreases of Cs concentration in the octanol phase. Consequently, it would be expected that DFOA and K-222, placed in the extracellular side of a membrane, would be able to extract Cs from the membrane. When the aqueous solution B with higher amounts of K^+(simulating the intracellular media) was used, significant increases on Cs concentration were found in the octanol phase in the presence of SS, 15-Crown-5, 12-Crown-4, 6-S-3, DFOA and L1.

From these results, it could be expected that these compounds, placed in the intracellular side of a membrane, would be able to remove Cs from the intracellular media and to place this element into the membrane structure.
An hypotheses of the current study was that a couple of compounds might act in collaboration to enhance Cs excretion from the body. One of the compounds would be placed inside the cell, whereas the other would be placed in the extracellular side. If the compound placed in the extracellular side had higher affinity for Cs than that placed in the intracellular side, both chelators could stablish an hypothetical "channel" between the intra and the extracellular media. Cs could be then eliminated from the cell according to its own gradient of concentration.
The erythrocyte suspension method is a more realistic procedure because in this system Cs is accumulated in the cells and the compounds to be tested are initially placed outside the cell. Using single chelating agents, an increased extracellular Cs concentration for TIRON, 15-Crown-5 and 6-S-3 was found. The present results show that although some pairs of compounds could be effective in removing Cs from the cell, only the system DFOA/L1 was more effective than the individual use of these chelators. Taking into account the effectiviness of DFOA and L1 as well as thier acceptance in clinical use (treatment in Fe and Al intoxication) [9-10]. The concurrent use of DFOA plus L1 could be tested for the removal of Cs in vivo.

Acknowledgements: The authors thank Ms. Amparo Aguilar and Ms. Anabel Diez for valuable technical assistance.

REFERENCES

1. Catsch A, Harmuth-Hoene AE. Parmacology and therapeutic applications of agents used in heavy metal poisoning. In: Levine WG, ed. *The chelation of Heavy Metals.* Oxford: Pergamon Press, 1979: 190-3.
2. Dahlgaard H. Sources of ^{137}Cs, ^{90}Sr and ^{99}Tc in the east Greenland current. *J Environ Radioact* 1994; 25: 37-55.
3. Higgit DL, Rowan JS, Walling DE. Catchment-scale deposition and redistribution of Chernobyl radiocaesium in upland Britain. *Environ Int* 1993; 19: 155-66.
4. Dresow B, Nielsen P, Fischer R, Pfau AA, Heinrich HC. In vivo binding of radiocesium by two forms of Prussian blue and by ammonium iron hexacyanoferrate (II). *Clin Toxicol* 1993; 31:563-69.
5. Lipsztein JL, Bertelli L, Oliveira CA, Dantas BM. Studies of Cs retention in the human body related to body parameters and Prussian blue administration. *Health Phys* 1991; 60:57-61.
6. Llobet JM, Colomina MT, Domingo JL, Corbella J. Evaluation of potential strontium chelators in an octanol/water system. *Health Phys* 1993; 65: 541-44.
7. Yokel RA, Kostenbauder HB. Assessment of potential aluminum chelators in an octanol/aqueous system and in the aluminum-loaded rabbit. *Toxicol Appl Pharmacol* 1987; 91:281-94.
8. Bramham J, Riddell FG. Cesium uptake studies on human erythrocytes. *J Inorg Biochem* 1994; 53: 169-76.
9. Domingo JL. Adverse effects of aluminum-chelating compounds for clinical use. *Adverse Drug React Toxicol Rev* 1996. 15: 145-65.
10. Olivieri NF, Brittenham GM, McLaren CE, Templeton DM, Cameron RG, McClelland RA, Burt AD, Fleming KA. Long term safety and effectiveness of iron-chelation therapy with deferiprone for thalassemia major. *N Engl J Med* 1998; 339: 417-23.

Metal Ions in Biology and Medicine; vol 6. Eds. J.A. Centeno, Ph. Collery, G. Vernet, R.B. Finkelman, H. Gibb, J.C. Etienne. John Libbey Eurotext, Paris © 2000, pp. 160-162.

Serum aluminium in haemodialysis patients

Pérez Beriain R.M., García de Jalón A., Zapatero González M.D., Escanero Marcén J.F., Calvo Ruata M.L., García de Jalón Martínez A.

Servicio de Bioquímica Clínica, Sección de Nutrición y Metales, Hospital Universitario Miguel Servet, Calle Calamita n° 3, 50009 Zaragoza, Spain

INTRODUCTION

Encephalopathy, osteopathy and anaemie are associated with the accumulation of aluminium in patients with chronic renal failure undergoing dialysis programmes [1].

Contamination through dialysis solutions is controlled and minimized, so it is important to know the influence of other factors in the impregnation with aluminium [2,3].

The aluminium hydroxide (Al (OH3)) has been the most widespread treatment for hyperphosphoremia given its efficacy, but it involves exposing the patient to aluminium [4,5].

In order to eliminate this risk other phosphor chelatings have been tested, among others calcium carbonate ($CaCO_3$) [1,5].

AIMS

The following work attempts to establish the link between the aluminaemia in haemodialysis patients and the type of phosphor chelating used, in relation to their duration in the dialysis programme.

MATERIALS AND METHODS

Aragon has a population of 1.200.000 of which 338 annually under go dialysis programmes owing to chronic renal failure (CRF).

The determination of serum aluminium for the control of these patients from public hospitals in the Autonomous Region of Aragon was carried out in our unit, by the method of atomic absorption spectrometry (AAS) with a graphite camera and Zeeman background corrector (*Perkin Elmer 4110 ZL*).

The serum aluminium concentration was determined in 273 patients in the period from 1 January 1999 to 31 December 1999, from whom the dialysis treatment duration and chelating used was recorded for 193, and the remainder were discarded.

The statistical calculations were carried out using SPSS statistics program. The statistical test used, has been the analysis of variance.

RESULTS

A relation between aluminium concentrations and months in haemodialysis programme (fig.1) was demonstrated.

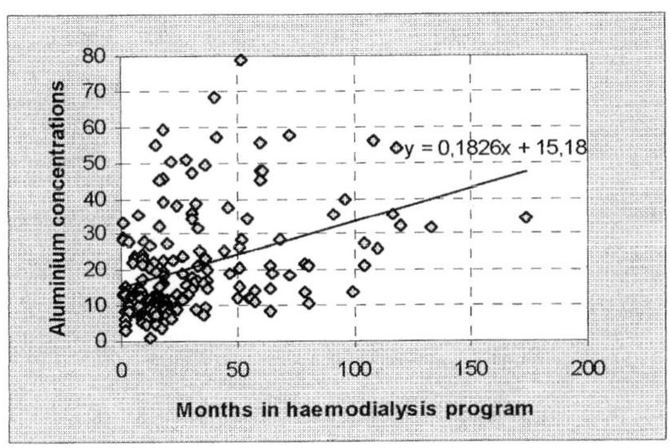

Figure 1.

In order to avoid factors of confusion, the serum aluminium concentrations of the patients have been grouped in the following way:

	<2 years on dialysis	>2 years on dialysis	
$Al(OH)_3$ as Phosphor chelating	N=39 Mean=27.1 µg/l D.S.=15.7	N=47 Mean=33.5 µg/l D.S.=20.2	N=86
Other non aluminium chelatings	N=69 Mean=13.9 µg/l D.S.= 11.7	N=38 Mean=17.6 µg/l D.S.=12.5	N=107
	N=108	N=85	N=193

Table 1.

The result is a contingency table, and the analysis of variance shows a statistically significant difference with a value for $p=0.027$.

Confidence intervals for mean of the groups in study are shown at the following illustration (fig 2):

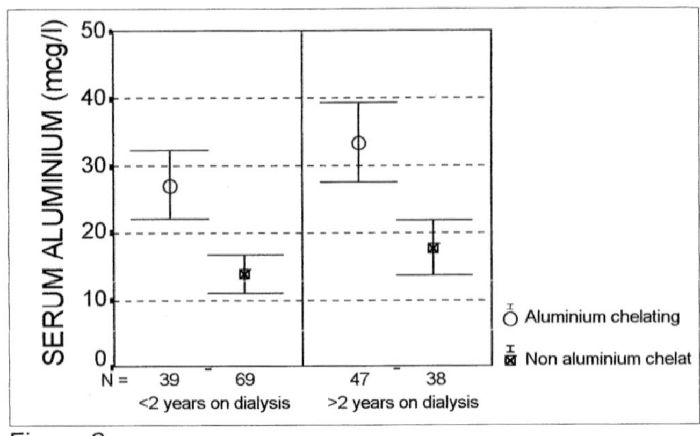

Figure 2.

CONCLUSIONS

Factors exist which influence the level of aluminium in blood such as dialysis duration and chelating type.

It is important that the factors which can be modified (the use of $CaCO_3$ unstead of Al $(OH)_3$ whenever possible) should be taken into account by the specialists monitoring those patients.

REFERENCES

1. Gonzalez Enguita M. Alteraciones metabólicas del aluminio y otros elementos traza (Zn, Cu y Fe) en pacientes hemodializados. Universidad de Zaragoza 1992. Tesis Doctoral.
2. Cannata JB, Serrano M, Fernández I, Fernández JL, Olaizola I. Minimizing the risk of oral aluminium exposure in chronic renal failure. In: Traeger J, Cantarovich F, Olmer M (eds.). *Present-day concepts in the treatment of chronic renal failure*. Contrib. Nephrol. 1989. Vol 71 : 81-89.
3. Reglamentación técnico-sanitaria para el abastecimiento y control de calidad de las aguas potables de consumo público. B.O.E. de 20 de septiembre de 1990; 27489-97.
4. D'Haese PC, Van de Vyver FL, De Wolff FA, De Broe ME. Measurement of aluminium in serum, blood, urine and tissue of chronic hemodialysed patients by use of electrotermal atomic absorption spectrometry. *Clin Chem* 1985; 31 : 24-29.
5. Zapatero Gónzalez MD. Niveles de aaluminio sérico en la población de Zaragoza: Estudio transversal y factores relacionables. . Universidad de Zaragoza 1995. Tesis Doctoral.

ACKNOWLEDGMENTS

This work has been supported by the Asociación para la Promoción de la Fundación Miguel Servet.

Metal Ions in Biology and Medicine; vol 6. Eds. J.A. Centeno, Ph. Collery, G. Vernet, R.B. Finkelman, H. Gibb, J.C. Etienne. John Libbey Eurotext, Paris © 2000, pp. 163-165.

Disturbances of the magnesemia in operated patients

Z. Kopański[1], W. Piekoszewski[2], M. Schlegel-Zawadzka[3], K. Sadlik[2], B. Witkowska[1]

[1] Clinical Military Hospital, [2] Institute of Forensic Research, [3] Jagiellonian University; Kraków, Poland

SUMMARY

The analysis included 98 patients operated for different abdominal diseases. Post-operative changes of the magnesemia in relation to sex, age, duration and extent of the procedure were estimated. The magnesium concentration in the serum was determined using the FAAS method. It was confirmed that mainly men over 60 years old were predisposed to deep disturbances in the magnesium concentration of the serum in the post-operative period. The deficiencies of that bioelement were statistically significantly influenced by procedures lasting over 60 minutes as well as by extensive operations carried out on the large intestine and the stomach.

Key words: magnesium concentration in the blood, sex, patient age, duration and extent of the surgical procedure, FAAS

INTRODUCTION

Post-operative complications depend on many factors, including the basic disease, the existing illness, age, sex, duration of the operation and method of anesthesia. Some authors emphasize that the complicated post-operative course may also be linked in many patients with disturbances of the magnesium metabolism in the preoperative period [1-3]. Yet so far, studying to what extent selected epidemiological-clinical traits such as sex, age, duration of the operation and extent of the procedure influence the changes of the magnesium concentration in the blood has rarely been tried. The existing thematic gap inclined the authors to analyse their own material to determine the degree of the disturbances of the magnesium concentration in the serum and evaluate the significance of those epidemiological-clinical traits in the generation of a dysmagnesemia in patients subjected to surgical treatment for different diseases of the abdominal organs.

MATERIAL AND METHOD

The analysis included 98 patients (58 men and 40 women) aged 45 to 76 years operated for different abdominal diseases. The group included 36 persons operated for cholelithiasis, 29 for cancer of the large intestine, 20 for acute appendicitis, 7 for ovarian tumours and 6 for cancer of the stomach. In all the patients the determination of the magnesium concentration in the serum was conducted with FAAS [4] before the procedure as well as in the following post-operative days up to the discharge from the clinic. Conditions were standardized.

On analysing the age of the patients, two groups were considered: up to 60 years of age and over 60 years. The durations of the operations were divided as follows: up to 30 minutes, from 31 to 60 minutes, over 60 minutes. Then the procedures were divided into three groups considering the magnitude of the „trauma" to which the patients had been subjected: I - laparoscopic procedures, removal of the appendix or the ovary through laparotomy, II - procedures on the bile ducts or segmentary excision of the large bowel through laparotomy, III - total gastrectomy, extensive excision of the large intestine or abdomino-perineal amputation of the rectum [5].

RESULTS

In patients having undergone on abdominal organs the magnesium concentration varied from 4.03 to 23.11 ug/ml (average 16.86±6.26 ug/ml).

The changes of the magnesium concentration during the post-operative course in relation to different factors are presented Table I.

Table I. Post-operative changes of the magnesemia in relation to sex, age and type of the procedure.

Factor	Group of patients	Magnesium concentration in the serum [ug/ml] Average mean±Standard deviation
Sex	Men	15.83±4.21
	Women	17.89±5.12
Age	To 60 years	19.41±3.47*
	Above 60 years	14.31±4.34**
Type of procedure	Group I	19.03±4.82*
	Group II	17.62±5.38*
	Group III	13.93±6.11**

* to ** - difference statistically significant

DISCUSSION

Magnesium in preponderant quantity is an intracellular element. Over half of that element is located in the bones, about 1/4 in the skeletic muscles, the rest is spread throughout the whole organism, mainly in the nervous systems and in the organs of high metabolic activity. 30 % of magnesium in the blood occurs in ionised form (as a free magnesium ion) and the remaining 70% is bound in the form of salt or compounds with proteins and lipids [3,6]. From our studies it follows that after a surgical procedure there comes a decrease in the magnesium concentration in the serum. Mainly men over 60 are predisposed to hypomagnesemia developing after the operation. The deficiencies of that bioelement are statistically significantly influenced by procedures lasting over 60 minutes as well as by extensive procedures carried out on the large intestine and on the stomach. Other authors have also paid attention to the magnesium insufficiencies forming after procedures [3]. It appears, however, that the direction of studies proposed in this work has not been followed through yet, hence for fully estimation the observations we registered further examinations in other clinical centres are necessary.

REFERENCES

1. Appleby J, Lawrence VA. Anesthesia. *J Gen Intern Med.* 1994; 9:635-647.
2. Brown FH. Perioperative Medicine. New York, NY: McGraw-Hill Book Co., 1999.
3. Durlach J. Magnesium in clinical practice. London Paris, John Libbey 1988.
4. Kopański Z, Piekoszewski W, Schlegel-Zawadzka M, Sibiga W, Lewandowski T, Habiniak J, Bruchnalska A. Influence of some epidemiologico-clinical factors on serum magnesium levels in patients with gastrointestinal tract cancer. *Trace Elem Electrol.* 2000; 17:36-39
5. Shoemaker WC. Pathophysiology, monitoring, outcome prediction, and therapy of shock states. *Critical Care Clinics.* 1987; 3:307-357.
6. Mertz W. The essential trace elements. *Science* 1981; 213:1332-1338.

Metal Ions in Biology and Medicine; vol 6. Eds. J.A. Centeno, Ph. Collery, G. Vernet, R.B. Finkelman, H. Gibb, J.C. Etienne. John Libbey Eurotext, Paris © 2000, pp. 166-168.

Effect of detoxification on serum level of selected microelements in addicts

Wojciech Piekoszewski[1, 3], Janusz Pach[2], Krystyna Sadlik[1], Lidia Winnik[2]

[1] Institute of Forensic Research, 9 Westerplatte, 31-033 Krakow, Poland; [2] Department of Clinical Toxicology, Jagiellonian University, 2 Zlota Jesien, 31-826 Krakow, Poland; [3] Laboratory of Clinical Toxicology and Pharmacokinetics, Rydyger's Hospital, 2 Zlota Jesien, 31-826 Krakow, Poland

Abstract

The aim of the study was to investigate the influence of chronic opiates taking on the serum level of selected microelements (zinc, copper and magnesium). Except of amphetamine the opiates are the most popular illicit drugs among polish addicts. Blood samples were taken from 30 acutely poisoned opiates addicts. As a control the blood samples taken from 22 young health, drugs free, male voluntaries were used. The microelements' concentrations were measured by the means of atomic absorption spectrophotometric method.

The present result demonstrate that, in the examined group before therapy, zinc level was reduced (by 27.8%) when compared to the control and only slightly increased after detoxification process. Opposite effect was observed in copper serum concentrations. The increased copper level (1.35 mg/l) during admission to hospital (control group 1.11 mg/l) was lowering during hospitalisation (1.18 mg/l). The concentration of magnesium in plasma of drug addicts was in the same range as in the control and did not change during therapy.

Introduction

Changes of serum trice elements levels in alcoholics are well-documented *(1),* but the information about these changes after taking the illicit drugs is scarce. In heroin addicts the whole blood copper concentration was higher and zinc lower than in the control group *(3)*. However Iyengar et al. *(2)* reported the higher urinary excretion of zinc and copper; the amount of eliminated copper was in the normally observed range. Most of polish opiates users take home-made heroin intravenously - this drug is produced in primitive condition, by acetylation of morphine extracted from poppy straw. Except of heroine, morphine and codeine this product contains an unknown amount and other chemicals used during drug production.

The aim of the study was to check the influence of using home-made heroin and detoxification therapy on the serum copper levels.

Material and methods

33 acutely poisoned male patients aged 17 – 46 years (the mean ages was 22), with a history of drug use ranging from one year to more then ten years, participate in the study. The clinical diagnosis was on the basis of: patents interview, a physical, psychological and psychiatric examination, and determination of opiates, amphetamine cocaine and cannabinols in urine. During admission all patients were amphetamine, cocaine and canabinnols free. The liver was examined on the basis of biochemical probes Patients were not HIV-infected.

Blood samples were taken after admission to the Clinic and next after treatment. The period of detoxification was from 3 to 20 days and during these time patients received: hemiton, bioxetin, cyclobarbital, dormicum and mefacit. As a control the blood samples taken from 22 young (23-27 years), healthy male volunteers were used. The zinc, copper and magnesium concentrations were measured by means of the atomic absorption spectrophotometric method. The accuracy and inter-run precision of the method were obtained against an international standard Seronorm (Nycomed, Oslo, Norway). RSD [%] in single bunch (n-10) was: Zn – 2.2, Cu – 2.9, Mg – 0.8 and between bunches (n=10): Zn – 2.7, Cu - 4.2, Mg –2.5.

For statistical evaluation analyses of variance was used.

Result and discussion

The results obtained in this study are shown in table 1.

Table 1. The concentration of Zn, Cu and Mg in the serum of drug addicts and healthy volunteers

Element	Patients	Mean ± SD	Median	Range
Zinc [mg/l]	On admission	0.815±0.144*	0805	0.550-1.160
	End of hospitalisation	0.859±0.205*	0.820	0.860-1.920
	Healthy volunteers	1.118±0.114	1.180	1.000-1.300
Copper [mg/l]	On admission	1.351±0.273*	1.265	0.860-1.920
	End of hospitalisation	1.179±0.252	1.135	0.760-1.830
	Healthy volunteers	1.106±0.119	1.080	0.900-1.320
Magnesium [mg/l]	On admission	20.33±1.30	20.08	18.27-23.42
	End of hospitalisation	20.24±1.90	19.95	17.20-25.56
	Healthy volunteers	20.56±1.37	20.55	17.40±24.00

*statistically significant difference from the control group, $p>0.05$

During admission to hospital patients were acutely poisoned and analysis revealed the presence of morphine, but any other illicit drugs were not found in their urine. The physical, psychological and psychiatric examinations confirmed drug addiction of patients. A liver examination showed a slight increase in SGPT (65.4 ± 46.7 U/l) and SGOT (55.9 ± 49.6 U/l) activity above normal values. The mean concentration of zinc was lower than concentration in the control blood serum and slightly increased during detoxification, however did not reached normal concentration. Copper serum concentrations 1.35 ± 0.27 mg/l measured during admission to the hospital were higher than in the control group 1.11 ± 0.12 mg/l. During therapy the concentration decreased and reached a level similar to the control group. The changes in copper concentration during hospitalisation ranged from –0.58 to 0.42 mg/l, however only four results increased after detoxification. Magnesium did not differ significantly from concentration in serum of control group. These results indicate a slight tendency of zinc to be lower and strong tendency for the concentration of copper to be higher in serum of people addicted to opiates in relation to healthy volunteers; furthermore, the concentration of magnesium was similar to that in control. In the case of copper the process of detoxification and several days of abstinence leads to lowering in the (elevated) concentrations of copper are able to change the serum level of copper, however a quick return to the normal concentration.
This study concern only opiate addicts, a further study in patients poisoned by other drugs is needed.

References

1. C. C. Cook, r. j. Walden, B. R. Graham, C. Gillham, S. Davies, B. N. Prichard, Trace elements and vitamin deficiency in alcoholic and control subjects, *Alcohol Alcoholism*, 26, 541-548, (1991)
2. V. Iyengar, P. P. Chou, A. G. Constantino, C. B. Cook, Excessive urinary excretion of zinc in drug addicts: a preliminary study during methadone detoxification, *J. Trace Elem. Electrolytes Health Dis*. 8, 213-215, (1994)
3. T. Elnimr, A. Hashem, R Assar, Heroin dependence effects on some major and trace elements. *Biol. Trace Elem. Res*. 54, 153-162 (1996)

Metal Ions in Biology and Medicine; vol 6. Eds. J.A. Centeno, Ph. Collery, G. Vernet, R.B. Finkelman, H. Gibb, J.C. Etienne. John Libbey Eurotext, Paris © 2000, pp. 169-172.

Heavy metals in sediments and water from San Jose and Joyuda Lagoons in Puerto Rico

David Acevedo[1, 2], Carlos J. Rodríguez-Sierra[1, 2], Darwin R. Reyes[1, 3], Braulio D. Jiménez[1, 3]

[1] Center for Environmental and Toxicological Research, [2] Department of Environmental Health, [3] Department of Biochemistry, Medical Sciences Campus, University of Puerto Rico, San Juan, Puerto Rico

Introduction

Heavy metal concentrations in contaminated sediments and water are essential for performing risk assessment for aquatic organisms and humans. Environmental monitoring of metal pollution in bodies of water should be assessed in order to control inputs of hazardous compounds, which can be bioaccumulated and cause direct toxic effects on organisms. Metal concentrations in water tend to have strong fluctuations due to many environmental variables such as: daily and seasonal variations in water flow and freshwater inputs, changes in pH and redox conditions, and temperature among others [1]. Sediments act as a source of contaminants long after the pollution of waterways has been abated, representing one of the largest risks to the aquatic environment [2] since it represents the sink to many pollutants and little regulation exits on their levels in ecosystems. Metals are redistributed naturally in the environment by both geologic and biologic cycles. They can be directly incorporated from the water by organisms or once they precipitate and fall to sediments they could be bioavailable and transfer through the food chain to man via contaminated fishfood. Metals are naturally found in the environment [3] at different concentrations depending on the geology of the area, however, human activities can increase their natural background concentrations and hence their potential for health effects. The objective of this study was to evaluate the levels of seven heavy metals (known as anthropogenic contaminants in water and sediment), in two distinct estuaries in Puerto Rico. The San José Lagoon (SJL) is a lagoon highly influenced by urban and industrial development and contained a long history of environmental pollution, and the Joyuda Lagoon, a natural reserve relatively undisturbed by development. This study provides the bases for heavy metal concentration comparisons in sediment and water from two aquatic habitats in the island.

Methodology

Samples were collected from 11 stations at the SJL located on the North coast and from 4 stations at the Joyuda Lagoon, located on the West coast. Surface sediments samples were obtained using a Ponar dredge and placed on a glass tray. Samples were homogenized with a spatula and any organic matter (leaves, twings or snails) discarded and transferred to plastic bags. Water samples were collected using a Wildco water sampler and transferred to 500 mL plastic bottles. The water pH was lowered to < 2 using concentrated nitric acid. All samples were stored in a cooler at 4°C until transported to the laboratory. In the laboratory, sediments were stored in a freezer at –20°C while water samples were stored in a refrigerator at 4°C until further analysis. Physico-chemical parameters such as pH, temperature, salinity, dissolved oxygen, conductivity and turbidity were measured *in-situ* at the surface and the bottom of the water column for every station using a Horiba Water Quality U-10 instrument.

Water samples were filtered through a Whatman 41 filter for the analysis of As, Cd, Cu, Pb, Se and Zn. For the analysis of Hg in water the EPA method 7470A was used [4]. The preparation of sediments samples for As, Cd, Cu, Pb and Zn was made based on the methodology of the EPA Method 3051, while Hg was performed using the EPA Method 7471A [4]. Metals concentrations were measured with an atomic absorption spectrophotometer. A standard reference material of estuarine sediment, method and field blanks, spikes samples and a rigorous cleaning procedure of the materials were used for quality control.

Unpaired t-tests or Mann-Whitney tests were used to evaluate statistical differences between SJL and Joyuda samples. The probability value of $p < 0.05$ was established as the level for statistical significance.

Results and Discussion

Based on the physico-chemical characteristics of both lagoons one can conclude that SJL showed vertical and horizontal variations in most of the parameters while Joyuda exhibited uniform values throughout the system. This can be explained by the differences in water depth and fresh water inputs (SJL being deeper and receiving more fresh water inputs than Joyuda). In SJL, the pH values ranged from 7.10 to 8.75, with a tendency of lower pH values at the bottom of the water column, while in Joyuda the pH values remained relatively constant through the lagoon (8.05-8.15). The dissolved oxygen also remained relatively constant at Joyuda with an average value of 6.49 mg/L, but in the SJL anoxic values as low as 0.05 mg/L were found. The dissolved oxygen at SJL shows the same tendency of the pH values (lower values at the bottom). Oxygen values ranged from 0.05 to 12.5 mg/L. The turbidity and conductivity in the SJL range from 6-60 NTU and 2.10-8.70 mS/cm, while in Joyuda it remained around 10 NTU and 13 mS/cm, respectively.

Concentrations of arsenic, cadmium and lead in water were significantly higher at the Joyuda system when compared to those obtained at the SJL (Table I). This finding can be attributed to the presence of mineral deposits located at the Northeast section of the lagoon. These mineral deposits of laterite serpentinite are rich in metals, such as nickel, cobalt, iron and chromium [5]. It is possible for many of these metals to remain in solution

Table I: Average Concentrations and Standard Errors for Sediment and Water Samples at San José and Joyuda Lagoon

Sample	As	Cd	Cu	Hg	Pb	Se	Zn
SJL water (n=11)	1.1 ± 0.1*	0.99 ± 0.07*	5.0 ± 0.6	< 0.4	2.7 ± 0.4*	< 0.5	21.9 ± 0.9
Joy water (n=17)	13 ± 1*	5.4 ± 0.3*	7 ± 1	< 0.4	15 ± 1*	< 0.5	< 20
SJL sed (n=4)	13 ± 2	1.8 ± 0.4*	102 ± 14*	1.4 ± 0.4*	219 ± 50*	NA	531 ± 121*
Joy sed (n=4)	18 ± 4	0.10 ± 0.03*	22 ± 5*	0.17 ± 0.04*	8 ± 2*	NA	52 ± 11*

Concentrations are in μg/L for water and μg/g dry weight for sediment.
NA = not analyzed; Joy =Joyuda; sed = sediment
When water samples were not detected, the detection limit was used as the sample concentration value.
* Statistical difference ($p < 0.05$)

due to the high oxygen content in water, limiting their accumulation in sediments (Table 1). Conversely, most of the metals analyzed in sediments were significantly higher at the SJL (Cd, Cu, Hg, Pb and Zn). Levels of Hg, Pb and Zn in sediments from the SJL could represent a possible threat to aquatic organisms because their levels were higher than sediment guideline concentrations above which toxic effect frequently occur in marine organisms. The sediment guideline concentration, in μg/g, are 0.71 for Hg, 218 for Pb and 410 for Zn [6]. There were also spatial differences at the SJL in metal concentrations, while at Joyuda variations were minimal with almost constant concentrations. The highest average metal concentration found in sediments at any given station for the SJL were; 211 for Cu, 4.9 for Hg, 548 for Pb and 1530 for Zn, all in μg/g dry weight (dw). Average metal concentrations (except for As) in sediment at Joyuda were below the world average shale values, while at SJL all concentrations were frequently higher than the world average shale values (except As as well). The world average shale values represent the background concentrations of metals in sedimentary rocks formed by clay or argillaceous material worlwide [7].
In conclusion, the SJL has relatively high metal concentrations in sediments probably due to anthropogenic activities. These levels shoud be a matter of concern because the threat they represent to the aquatic environment, and to humans if they are bioaccumalate through the food chain. The results obtained from this work shows the value of the research and urges an additional study that evaluates the levels of these metals in aquatic organisms from this system . We suggest that species locally consumed by the population be analyzed in order to determine the possible risk of transfer of these pollutants and adverse effects to humans.

References

1. Förstner U. Assessment of Metal Pollution in Rivers and Estuaries. In: Thornton I, ed. Applied Environmental Geochemistry. London: Academic Press, 1983: 395-423.
2. Burton GA. Assessing Contaminated Aquatic Sediments. Environ Sci Technol 1992; 26: 1862.
3. Goyer R. Toxic Effects of Metals. In: Klaassen CD, ed. Casarett & Doulll's Toxicology, The Basic Science of Poisons. New York: McGraw-Hill, 1996: 691-736.
4. U.S. Environmental Protection Agency, " Test Methods for Evaluating Solid Waste, Physical/Chemical Methods", SW-846, 3rd edition, 1992.
5. Carvajal J, Cintrón G, Pérez M. Estudio de la Laguna de Joyuda: Un Ecosistema Marino. Programa de Zona Costanera de Puerto Rico, Departamento de Recursos Naturales 1978-1979.
6. Long E, Mac Donald D, Smith S, Calder F. Incidence of Adverse Biological Effects Within Ranges of Chemical Concentrations in Marine and Estuarine Sediments. Environmental Management 1995; 19: 81-97.
7. Krauskoft K, Bird D. Introduction to Geochemistry third edition. New York: McGraw-Hill, 1995.

Metal Ions in Biology and Medicine; vol 6. Eds. J.A. Centeno, Ph. Collery, G. Vernet, R.B. Finkelman, H. Gibb, J.C. Etienne. John Libbey Eurotext, Paris © 2000, pp. 173-176.

Trace elements concentration in sediments and some commercially important marine fishes & shell fishes of Chittagong Coast, Bangladesh

Mohammed Abul Kashem[1], Yusuf Sharif Ahmed Khan[1], Mohammed Alamgir[2]

[1] *Institute of Marine Sciences, University of Chittagong, Chittagong, Bangladesh;* [2] *Chief Scientific Officer, Institute of Nuclear Science & Technology, Atomic Energy Research Establishment, Savar, Dhaka-1000, Bangladesh*

Abstract

*A study was carried out to determine distribution of trace metals (Cd, Zn, Ni, Pb, Cu, Mn, Fe, Cr) concentration in sediment and in some commercially important marine fishes (Hg, Pb, As, Se, Cd, Zn, Cr, Fe, Ni, Cu) of the Chittagong Coast by employing Neutron Activation Analysis (NAA) and Atomic Absorption Spectrophotometer. In sediments metal concentration ($\mu g.g^{-1}$ dry weight) were found to range from 0.49 to 0.89 for Cd, 62.80 to 162.30 for Zn, 23.29 to 68.11 for Ni, 16.00 to 142.90 for Pb, 18.05 to 48.30 for Cu, 276.88 to 954.43 for Zn, 852.50 to 5250.90 for Fe and 18.30 to 121.30 for Cr. The mean values of Cd, Zn, Pb, Cu and Cr were recorded higher level in the investigated region than those of GESAMP Standards. Five species of fishes (**Setpinna phassa, Harpodon nehereus, Lates Calcarifer, Pangasius pangasius, Johnius argentatus**) were collected from the investigated area. Metal concentration in muscle of the fishes were performed seasonally. In muscle of the fishes, metal levels ($\mu g.g^{-1}$ dry weight) ranged from 0.069 to 0.637 for Hg, 0.677 to 4.019 for Pb, 0.025 to 3.582 for As, 1.926 to 6.725 for Se, 0.075 to 0.743 for Cd, 25.76 to 121.03 for Zn, 0.446 to 10.182 for Cr, 31.029 to 278.550 for Fe, 0.723 to 6.414 for Ni and 0.647 to 7.610 for Cu. The levels obtained for trace metals were found much higher in the ship-breaking area in comparison with the karnaphuli River Estuary. As per analysis and subsequent determinations the ship-breaking area has been indicated as polluted zone.*

Introduction

The marine & coastal environment of Bangladesh are degrading alarmingly from a wide range of marine and land activities. Major threats come from the urban effluents discharged into the sea or estuary from sea-front or river side cities, municipal, agriculture and industrial ventures, other activities like human settlements, urban development and tourism, increase in water consumption, irrational expansion of coastal shrimp farming, port & shipping activities, deforestation, unplanned construction of coastal dikes and dams and salinity intrusion are also insidiously contributing to the coastal pollution.

The coastal zone of Bangladesh, stretching along 720 km long coastline, encompassing vast area at the land and water interface, including an expanse of marine waters, is economically highly productive and endowed with rich bio-diversity. The Bay of Bengal is considered as busy shipping routes and is a lucrative commercial fishing area. Historically, shipping & commercial fishing vessels are responsible to pollute the sea through accidental and deliberate discharge of wastes and dirty oil products. Marine pollution in port areas can originate from wastes products and dirty oil produced by ships, from infrastructure wastes, from normal port operations including loading and discharge, from ballast water and from some ships protective antifouling paints (Ministry of shipping, 1996 & ANZECC, 1995). The main input of trace elements in the coastal water & sediments come from the rivers and atmospheric deposition (Tyler & Buckney, 1984).Most of the industries and factories are situated on the bank of the rivers or very close to river system. Annually about 1200 ships and 50-60 oil tankers are handled in the Chittagong port. and power driven trawlers and boats engaged in fishing is about 3000 in the coastal area of Bangladesh (Majumder, 1992).

Study Area

About 1252 manufacturing industries are situated in the study areas which is about 27.67% of the total industries of the country. None of these industries have waste treatment facilities and they discharge their untreated wastes into the nearest water bodies which finally find their way into the Bay of Bengal (Paul & Rahman, 1992).

At present ship breaking has turned into a vital industry along the sea coast, Chittagong creating job opportunities for thousands of workers & private enterprises. The activities of ship breaking is concentrated along the sea beach from Fauzderhat to Kumira in Chittagong. There are about 50 firms under the banner of association, engaged in ship-breaking. The main pollutants are waste oil, sludge, blast oil, lubricant, asbestos assorted junk and many kinds of metals. These pollutants are contaminating the soil, water and organisms (Kashem & Khan Y.S.A., 1998).

Materials & Method

Sampling and Analysis

Twenty surface (10cm) sediment samples were collected from the investigated area using Ekman Grab Sampler. The sediment samples were prepared for AAS (Pye Unicam 2900) measurement by using nitric-perchloric-hydropluoric acid digestion method.

Five varieties of common marine fishes (Table-2) selected in accordance with public favor were collected from the investigated area and sun-dried after removal of internal organs, head, skin & tails. The samples were dried at 105 - 110°C in an oven until a constant weight was obtained (Dry Weight). 200mg of fish flesh sample were heat-sealed in glass bottle and irradiated along with a known amount of MA-A-2 (TM). The fish flesh was homogenated following standard of IAEA in the CIRUS reactor at Bhabha Atomic Research Center, Trombay, Bombay, India at a flux of about (0.5 to 1). 10^{12} n.Cm^{-2}.5^{-1} for 20 hours.

Result & Discussion

The results of trace metal concentration in sediment are shown in Table-1. The concentrations of different trace metals at all the stations are not uniform. The lowest concentration of Zn is 68.80μg g^{-1} and the highest being 162.30 μg g^{-1} found in sample no-1&18 respectively. The marine sediment contains higher amount of Zn than almost all the marine sediments of the world analyzed so far (Salomons & Froster, 1984 GESAMP, 1982). The presence of high amount of metals may be due to discharge of huge metal-rich waste from Galvanization Plants situated in the port city of Chittagong.

The concentration of Cd was always higher in all the stations compared to the other metals. The mean value of Cd concentration was 0.70μg g^{-1} and the range is 0.49-0.89μg g^{-1} which is 6 times higher than the recommended value (0.11μg g^{-1}) of unpolluted marine sediments (GESAMP

1982; Salomons & Forster, 1984; IAEA). The high percentage of Cd may be attributed to the gypsum wastes of TSP Complex to the estuarine zone.
The average copper content (34.37μg g^{-1}) of marine sediment is quite lower than the values found in other areas of the world, except that found in Arabian Gulf near to Iraq (2.59 μg g^{-1})
The mean concentration of total nickel in the sediment samples examined is 52.03 μg g^{-1}, which is slightly less than that of recommended values (IEAE.?).
The mean concentration of Pb in the sediment samples examined is 57.95 μg g^{-1} but this is mainly due to high concentration found only in six sampling stations. The mean value of the other 14 stations is 41.34μg g^{-1}. This behavior is not understood but, it could be possibly attributed to the uneven distribution of this metals due to heavy traffic and activities due to ship-breaking industries nearby.
Cr concentration in the investigated area was very complex in nature. The concentration of Cr in the study area is higher than the recommended values. The mean value (70.74μg g^{-1}) is almost similar in the coastal & estuarine sediments of the Seto Inland Sea, Japan (Hirata, 1992).
The mean concentration of Fe 2853.53 μg g^{-1} did not exceed the recommended values. Although industrial effluents & wastes were discharged into the Bay of Bengal, fishes do not seem to be contaminated at present as far as Pb and Cd are concerned (Sharif et al., 1993).
From the above discussion, it seems that trace metal concentrations around the Karnafully River mouth and Ship—breaking areas (Fauzderhat to Kumira) are higher than the Sitakundah coastal belt, which may be due to the influence of untreated effluents discharged by various small and large industries located in the bank of the Karnafully.
Almost all the elements in the muscle are being reported for the first time in some marine & estuarine fishes at the mouth of the Karnafully River Estuary and north – west coast of Chittagong, Bangladesh.

Table : 1 Trace metal concentrations in sediments collected from the Karnafully River mouth to North-West Coast of the Bay of Bengal (μg.g^{-1})

Sample collection site no	Cd	Zn	Ni	Pb	Cu	Mn	Fe	Cr
1	**0.89**	**62.80**	51.05	19.70	46.90	523.40	3950.17	77.90
2	0.68	119.70	53.29	40.93	48.10	625.00	3738.00	136.00
3	0.61	122.90	43.32	16.33	39.35	704.10	2769.79	67.41
4	0.66	130.00	58.12	**142.90**	51.60	599.20	4000.60	85.53
5	0.65	146.00	49.88	41.30	**48.30**	**276.88**	3980.15	57.42
6	**0.49**	137.50	60.83	59.43	42.11	370.50	1289.54	83.14
7	0.88	151.10	38.96	126.50	26.08	843.25	3840.20	102.20
8	0.54	108.90	57.18	110.50	32.05	**954.43**	3800.00	116.50
9	0.64	76.58	**68.11**	91.14	44.05	467.18	942.79	94.36
10	0.71	139.51	50.93	103.67	29.60	410.50	1012.00	**121.30**
11	0.83	114.70	54.71	114.73	46.23	560.16	1800.00	73.50
12	0.88	139.00	53.20	26.60	32.90	321.00	**5250.90**	94.70
13	0.64	149.74	35.69	35.50	33.09	310.50	2810.00	21.30
14	0.61	74.86	37.86	36.60	22.06	456.60	2530.80	BDL
15	0.58	101.60	57.23	42.50	**18.05**	285.90	3980.20	41.88
16	0.55	137.50	51.97	28.80	30.94	578.50	3820.00	19.90
17	0.88	120.40	**23.29**	29.60	47.80	455.60	**852.50**	70.29
18	0.67	**162.30**	43.33	16.60	30.70	302.35	3300.00	46.80
19	0.89	88.90	40.89	59.60	39.60	492.20	4108.57	86.00
20	0.78	121.80	49.81	**16.00**	32.04	305.10	3094.42	**18.80**
Average	**0.70**	**120.29**	**52.03**	57.95	**34.37**	**429.57**	**2853.53**	**70.74**
Range	**(0.49-0.89)**	**(62.80-162.30)**	**(23.29-68.11)**	**(16.00-142.90)**	**(18.05-48.30)**	**(276.88-954.43)**	**(852.50-5250.90)**	**(18.30-121.30)**

- BDL = Below Detection Level.

Table –2 : Seasonal variation of trace metal concentrations (μg.g^{-1} dry weight) in muscle of the selected fishes of the investigated area.

Types of Fishes		Season	METAL CONCENTRATION									
Local or Bangladeshi Name	Scientific Name		Hg	Pb	As	Se	Cd	Zn	Cr	Fe	Ni	Cu
Phassa	***Setipinna Phassa***	Pre-monsoon	0.637	4.019	3.259	3.793	0.698	52.715	1.031	278.550	6.414	3.031
		Monsoon	0.501	2.079	1.021	3.002	0.075	50.230	0.872	49.172	2.439	2.900
		Post-monsoon	0.603	3.611	2.932	2.594	0.479	55.012	0991	138.257	3.178	2.972
Latia	***Harpodon nehereus***	Pre-monsoon	0.295	2.215	3.173	6.725	0.743	108.14	2.789	383.40	5.009	6.542
		Monsoon	0.172	0.783	0.025	3.013	0.518	121.03	0.865	245.173	3.123	3.526
		Post-monsoon	0.358	1.648	1.591	4.729	0.523	79.83	5.393	101.751	4.672	4.104
Bhetki/Koral	***Lates calcarifer***	Pre-monsoon	0.531	0.635	0.521	3.005	0.089	35.017	10.782	119.581	0.895	1.760
		Monsoon	0.069	0.677	0.238	2.956	0.091	43.951	5.514	31.029	0.723	0.643
		Post-monsoon	0.085	0.912	0.981	4.092	0.256	10.064	7.362	81.207	0.912	1.879
Fatty Catfish Pangus	***Pangasius pangasius***	Pre-monsoon	0.127	3.075			0.197	58.091	1.728	116.563	6.125	7.610
		Monsoon	0.096	1.519	ND	ND	0.203	43.213	1.005	40.002	5.204	4.219
		Post-monsoon	0.258	2.624			0.132	39.641	0.913	37.141	2.035	3.514
Phoua	***Johnius argentatus***	Pre-monsoon	0.547	1.856	3.582	3.467	0.143	37.010	0.795	276.34	5.439	3.421
		Monsoon	0.475	2.037	2.921	1.926	0.098	25.761	0.446	35.625	2.375	1.980
		Post-monsoon	0.123	0.722	3.005	3.003	0.619	35.574	0.515	173.053	3.249	1.003

ND = Not Detected

REFERENCES

Izquierdo C, Gracia I, Usero J. Speciation of Heavy Metals in Sediments from Salt marshes on the Southern Atlantic Coast of Spain. *Mar. Poll. Bull.* 1997; 34(2) : 123-128.

Khan Y S A, Talukder A. Pollution in Coastal Waters of Bangladesh. *The Journal of NOAMI*. 1993; 10(1) : 1-11

Hirata S. Trace metal in humic substances of coastal sediments of the Seto Inland Sea, Japan. Sci. *Total Environ.* 1992; 117/117:325-333

Laxem DPH. The Chemistry of metal pollution in water. In : Roy MH, ed. Pollution Causes, Effect & Control. London : WIVOBN; 1983 : 103-104

Sharif AKH, Mustafa AI, Hossain MA, Amin MN and Safiullah S. Lead and cadmium contents in ten species of tropical marine fish from the Bay of Bangal, *Sci. Total Environ*; 1993; 133 : 193-199.

Subramanian V, Jha PK and Jergrieken R. Heavy metals in the Ganges estuary. *Mar. Pollut. Bull.* 1988; 19(6) : 290-293.

Uthe JF and Blish EG. Preliminary survey of heavy metal contamination of Canadian fresh water fish. 1971; *J. Fish. Res. Bd. Can.* 28: 786-788.

Brooks RR, Presley BJ & Kaplan IR. Trace elements in interstitial waters of marine sediments. *Geochim. Cosmochim.* 1968; Acta, 32: 399-414.

Chester R and Stoner JH. Trace elements in sediments from lower Seven Estuary and Bristol Channel. *Mar. Pollut. Bull.* 1975; 6: 92-95.

Coleman JM. “Brahmaputra river : Channel processes and sedimentation”. *Sedimentary Geology*. 1969; 1 3/2-3:129-238.

Patel B, Bangera V, Patel S and Balani MC. Heavy metal in the Bombay Harbour Area. *Mar. Pollu. Bull.* 1993; 16: 22-28.

Mahmood N, Khan YSA & Ahmed MK. Studies on the hydrology of the Karnafully estuary. *Asiatic Soc. of Bangladesh.* 1976; 2(1) : 89-99.

Verma DD, Rao AT & Dasari MR. Trace element geochemistry of Clay fraction and bulk sediments from Vamasadhala River basin, east coast of India. *Indian J. of Mar. Sci.* 1993; 22: 247-251.

Rule JH. Assessment of trace elements geochemistry of Hampton Roads and lower Chesapeake Bay area sediments. *Environ. Geol. Waker Sci*, 1986; 8 : 209-219.

Martincic D, Kwokal Z, Stoeppler M & Branica M. Trace metal in sediment from the Adriatic Sea. *Sci. Total Environ*, 1989; 84: 135-147.

Metal Ions in Biology and Medicine; vol 6. Eds. J.A. Centeno, Ph. Collery, G. Vernet, R.B. Finkelman, H. Gibb, J.C. Etienne. John Libbey Eurotext, Paris © 2000, pp. 177-179.

Cadmium accumulation in native vegetation of Alaska and Colorado

James G. Crock[1], James R. Larison[2], and L.P. Gough[3]

[1] U.S. Geological Survey, M.S. 973, D.F.C., Denver, CO 80225; [2] 138 Strand Hall, Oregon State University, Corvallis, OR 97331; [3] U.S. Geological Survey, 4200 University Dr., Anchorage, AK 99508

Cadmium is known to be extremely toxic to most life forms and is usually present in the environment in measurable concentrations. Typically, Cd is found in the 0.1-0.5 µg/g range for most non-contaminated soils and rocks and is usually associated with Zn in the ratio of approximately 500:1 (Zn: Cd). Our current investigations show that this ratio is not necessarily true for plant tissue and where some vegetation may biomagnify Cd up to two orders of magnitude over the parent soil and neighboring vegetation.

Baseline investigations of native vegetation, soils, and rocks in Alaska and Colorado are in progress. The studies in Alaska are biogeochemical investigations of Cd, As, and other trace elements in the gold-rich Fortymile Mining District of east-central Alaska. Using detailed geologic and hydrologic framework studies, the cycling of trace elements is under examination in the sub-arctic boreal forest ecosystem of the Interior Highlands Ecoregion. These studies seek to define the relative contribution to the ecosystem of various geogenic (natural) sources (e.g., Crock and others, 1999, 2000; Gough and others, 2000). These studies also provide a regional framework and interpretive data for land management agencies involved in assessing the relative contribution of geogenic vs. anthropogenic geochemical landscape patterns and processes. Relations between the chemistry of A, B, and C soil horizons, willow (*Salix glauca*) and alder (*Alnus crispa*) leaf and twig tissue, and feather moss (*Hylocomium splendens*) tissue were examined and correlated with the geochemistry of the underlying bedrock units. Additionally, baseline information is presented for feather moss, *Peltigera apthosa* (ground lichen), *Picea glauca* (white spruce), willow, and alder. In general, elemental concentration differences were more easily defined for As than for Cd among both the rock units and the soils developed from these rock units. Arsenic concentrations are much higher in the C soil horizon than in any of the rock units studied and trend to increase with increasing soil depth and soil horizon. The opposite trend is true for Cd in soils--decreasing Cd concentrations with increasing soil depth and soil horizon. The total Cd concentration in plant tissue was not strongly correlated with rock units. The variability of Cd is large (nearly two orders of magnitude) in the vegetation sampled (Table I). This variability is due mainly to the ability of willow to act as a bioaccumulator for Cd. This concentration of Cd by willows has implications to Cd's mobility in terrestrial ecosystems and to the food chain, especially for the ptarmigan and other animals that browse heavily on willow during the winter months when other vegetation is not available. The calculated baselines for the various media for Cd in this watershed are generally below levels found in similar materials statewide.

Cadmium within the Alaska study area soils is derived from the weathering of the primary metasedimentary and metavolcanic bedrock. In these types of residual soils, Cd is commonly adsorbed by various clay minerals and also by Ca- and Mg-carbonates. Cadmium does not form highly stable complexes with most organic matter. In addition, in these cold boreal forest soils where microbial decomposition rates are low, the Cd that is tied up in organic matter probably remains immobile for some time. Cadmium can form many compounds of low solubility by precipitation as carbonates, hydroxides, and phosphates. This process is less important, however, in our low pH, generally low-carbonate soils. Cadmium is readily leached from soils at pH values below about 5.0, especially if the soils have a sandy texture. However, its increased solubility and bioavailability in acidic soils may potentially result in an increase in the amount of Cd absorbed and translocated by plants in this area. Zinc has close geochemical similarities with Cd and competes for exchange sites in soil. The soils of both study areas are not particularly high in Zn however, and therefore it probably has a minimal influence on cadmium bioavailability.

Table I. Summary statistics for Cd in vegetation and soils, Fortymile River watershed, Alaska (dry weight basis, μg/g).

Material	GM[1]	GD[2]	Observed Range	Expected 95% Range (Baseline)[3]
Alder twig	0.029	1.83	0.010 – 0.029	0.009 – 0.097
Alder leaf	0.031	1.70	0.011 – 0.093	0.011 – 0.090
Willow twig	0.78	1.97	0.17 – 3.5	0.20 – 3.0
Willow leaf	1.00	1.78	0.22 – 2.4	0.32 – 3.2
Moss	0.14	1.68	0.046 – 0.42	0.05 – 0.40
A Horizon soil	0.43	1.92	0.14 – 2.7	0.11 – 1.6
B Horizon soil	0.25	1.89	0.08 – 1.5	0.07 – 0.89
C Horizon soil	0.20	2.08	0.08 – 2.5	0.05 – 0.86
	Average	Deviation	Observed Range	
Ground lichen (n=28)	0.217	0.204	0.06 – 0.94	
White spruce (n=13)	0.017	0.007	0.01 – 0.03	

[1] Geometric mean
[2] Geometric deviation
[3] GM/GD^2 to $GM \times GD^2$

Studies in Colorado were initiated to investigate the occurrence of fragile-boned ptarmigan (*Lagopus leucurus*) inhabiting the Animas River watershed, near Silverton, Colorado, a well-known mining district. We hypothesized that this condition might be related to chronic, long-term exposure to toxic metals in the food chain, possibly exacerbated by past or present mining activities. Vegetation samples that represented the food web of the ptarmigan were sampled (Larison and others, 2000). Only Cd and Zn were accumulated in sufficient quantities, especially by one genus of plants, to cause possible health affects in ptarmigan. Willows, all species, whether ground hugging or free standing, and whether growing in the alpine or in the montane marshes of this region tend to accumulate Cd at levels that are up to two orders of magnitude greater than levels in native soils. Preliminary summary statistics for this study are given in Table II.

Table II. Summary statistics for Cd in vegetation (dry weight basis, μg/g) from the Colorado Mineral Belt study area.

Material	Number of Samples	Mean	Standard Deviation	Observed Range
Acomastylis rossi	13	0.23	0.195	0.07 – 0.52
Bistorta b.	9	0.14	0.099	0.04 – 0.35
Carex ebenea	1	0.15		
Dryas octopetela	1	0.20		
Trifolium sp.	11	0.21	0.040	0.15 – 0.30
Salix spp. (leaves and twigs, summer sampling)	47	2.11	1.80	0.08 – 9.67
Salix spp. (buds and twigs, winter sampling)	17	3.09	1.26	1.3 – 5.1

References

Crock, J.G., Gough, L.P., Wanty, R.B., Day, W.C., Wang, B., Gamble, B.M., Henning, M., Brown, Z.A., and Meier, A.L., 1999, Regional geochemical results from the analyses of rock, water, soil, stream sediment, and vegetation samples—Fortymile River watershed, east-central, Alaska: U.S. Geological Survey Open File Report 99-33, 82 pp.

Crock, J.G., Gough, L.P., Wanty, R.B., Day, W.C., Wang, B., Gamble, B.M., Henning, M., Brown, Z.A., and Meier, A.L., 2000, Regional geochemical results from the analyses of rock, water, soil, stream sediment, and vegetation samples—Fortymile River watershed, east-central, Alaska, 1999 sampling: U.S. Geological Survey Open File Report, in press.

Gough, L.P., Crock, J.G., Day, W.C., and Vohden, J., 2000, Biogeochemistry of As and Cd, Fortymile River watershed, East-central Alaska: Geologic Studies in Alaska by the U.S. Geological Survey, 1998: U.S.G.S. Professional Paper, in press.

Larison, J.R., Likens, E.E., Fitzpatrick, J.W., and Crock, J.G., 2000, Cadmium toxicity among wildlife in the Colorado Rocky Mountains: Nature, in press.

Metal Ions in Biology and Medicine; vol 6. Eds. J.A. Centeno, Ph. Collery, G. Vernet, R.B. Finkelman, H. Gibb, J.C. Etienne. John Libbey Eurotext, Paris © 2000, pp. 180-182.

Potential for selenium exposure in livestock grazed on reclaimed strip mine sites in the Western United States

Abdel-Razak M. Kadry, In Suk Kim, Aron M. Yoffe, Michael K. Hoffman

Food Safety and Inspection Service, United States Department of Agriculture, Washington DC

Abstract

Recently, cases of selenium (Se) toxicosis were identified in livestock that had been grazed on, or adjacent to, several reclaimed phosphate strip mine sites in the western United States. As a result, several environmental studies have been initiated at these sites. Our analysis of the available data from these studies indicates the presence of highly elevated levels of Se and some heavy metals in rocks used to backfill open pits, sediment, ground water and vegetation.

The levels of metals in these livestock could be assessed by sampling and analysis. Furthermore, useful scientific information may be generated by an investigation of the nationwide practice of grazing food animals on reclaimed mine sites.

Introduction

In the winter of 1996, toxic levels of selenium were reported in a total of seven horses grazing downstream from phosphate mining activities in a region of the western United States. Because of the severity of the toxicity, it was necessary to euthanize six of these animals.

Five phosphate mining companies collectively implemented a sampling survey at 70 sites, including those at which toxicity occurred in the horses. This survey was carried out by Montgomery Watson, Inc. (Steamboat Springs, CO, 1998), under the oversight of the United States Department of Agriculture-Forest Service, the Bureau of Land Management, and local governmental authorities. In this publication, we highlight some of the findings from the above survey that may be applicable to the safety of animals raised for human food consumption.

Results and Discussion

The concentration of selenium, cadmium, vanadium and zinc in the rock used to backfill the open pits at each mine site are illustrated in Fig. 1. The selenium concentrations are 280 and 800-fold higher than the continental crust average in the carbonate and mudstone rocks, respectively. Cadmium concentrations in these rocks were elevated by 250 and 200-fold, respectively.

Analyses of water samples indicated the presence of higher levels of selenium than the cold water criterion of 0.005 ppm. The highest concentrations, found in the dump seeps, were 280-fold above this criterion (Fig. 2).

Table 1. describes the selenium levels in the tested soils relative to those of control soils obtained from the same region, but not exposed to mining operations. Over 65% of the potentially exposed soils contained elevated levels of selenium, varying between 5 and 100-fold higher than the mean selenium level of the control samples. However, by comparison with the level of selenium in the single highest control sample, only 9% of the potentially exposed soils demonstrated selenium levels between 5 and 20-fold greater than the level of the highest control.

Approximately 67% of the samples of potentially exposed vegetation contained selenium levels that range from 5 to 500-fold greater than the mean control level. Two percent of the tested vegetation samples contained selenium levels more than 500-fold greater that of the mean control vegetation level (Table 2). Even by comparison with the level of selenium in the single highest control sample, 62% of the potentially exposed vegetation demonstrated selenium levels between 5 and 500-fold greater than the level of the highest control.

While selenium is an essential nutrient, excessive selenium has been shown to cause toxicity in humans and animals (Combs,1994; Lemly, 1997). High environmental levels of selenium, and livestock toxicosis, have been identified at and near these reclaimed mine sites.

Continued cooperation among the mining industry, ranchers, and local, state and federal agencies is needed to ensure the continued safety of animals raised for human food consumption.

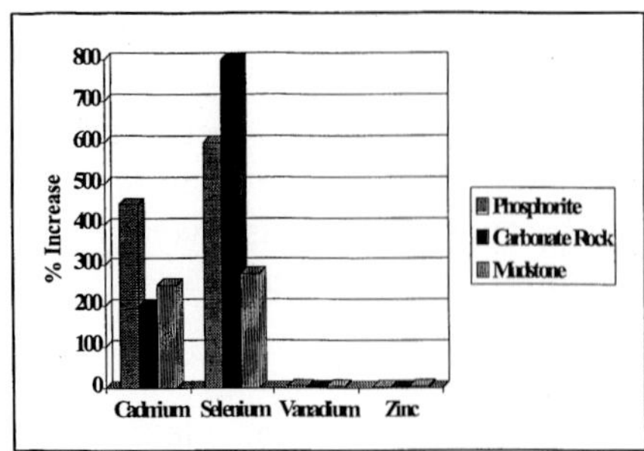

Fig.1 : Elevation of Metal Concentrations in Phosphatic ShaleTest Group Relative to Mean Continental Crust Levels (Montgomery Watson, 1998)

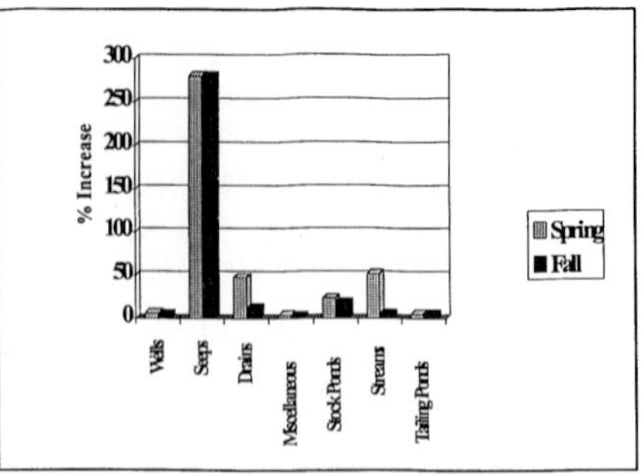

Fig. 2: Elevation of Selenium Concentrations in Surface Water Samples Relative to 0.005 ppm Cold Water Criterion (Montgomery Watson, 1998)

Table 1

Relative Selenium Concentrations in Soil, from 1998 Montgomery Watson Survey

Test Sample Levels as Multiples of Control Group Levels	*% of Samples (Relative to Mean of Control Group)*	*% of Samples (Relative to Highest Control Sample with Highest Concentration)*
≤ 1		
Waste Rock Dumps	4.44	42.22
Waste Rock Dump Seeps	20.00	40
1-5		
Waste Rock Dumps	28.89	48.89
Waste Rock Dump Seeps	20.00	20.00
5-10		
Waste Rock Dumps	31.11	6.67
Waste Rock Dump Seeps	00	00
10 - 20		
Waste Rock Dumps	20.00	2.22
Waste Rock Dump Seeps	00	20
20 - 50		
Waste Rock Dumps	11.11	0
Waste Rock Dump Seeps	20	0
51 – 100		
Waste Rock Dumps	4.44	0
Waste Rock Dump Seeps	20	0
100 - 500		
Waste Rock Dumps	0	0
Waste Rock Dump Seeps	20	20

Table 2

Relative Selenium Concentrations in Vegetation, from 1998 Montgomery Watson Survey

Test Sample Levels as Multiples of Control Group Levels	*% of Samples (Relative to Mean of Control Group)*	*% of Samples (Relative to Highest Control Sample with Highest Concentration)*
≤1		
Waste Rock Dumps	0	13.33
Waste Rock Dump Seeps	0	20
1 - 5		
Waste Rock Dumps	13.33	22.22
Waste Rock Dump Seeps	20.00	0
5-10		
Waste Rock Dumps	11.11	20
Waste Rock Dump Seeps	0	20
10 - 20		
Waste Rock Dumps	4.44	6.67
Waste Rock Dump Seeps	0	0
20 - 50		
Waste Rock Dumps	24.44	26.67
Waste Rock Dump Seeps	20	40
51 - 100		
Waste Rock Dumps	8.89	6.67
Waste Rock Dump Seeps	0	20
100 - 500		
Waste Rock Dumps	17.78	2.22
Waste Rock Dump Seeps	60	0
>500		
Waste Rock Dumps	2.22	0
Waste Rock Dump Seeps	0	0

References

Combs G. Essentiality and toxicity of selenium: a critique of the Recommended Dietary Allowances and the Reference Dose. In Mertz, C., Abernathy, C. & Olin, S.S., eds. Risk Assessment of Essential Elements. Washington, DC: International Life Sciences Institute Press,1994: 167-183.

Lemly A. Environmental implications of excessive selenium: a review. Biomed Environ Sci 1997 ;10:415-35.

Montgomery Watson. Draft – 1998 Regional Investigation Report, Southeast Idaho Phosphate Resource Area Selenium Project. Montogomery Watson, Steamboat Springs, CO.

Metal Ions in Biology and Medicine; vol 6. Eds. J.A. Centeno, Ph. Collery, G. Vernet, R.B. Finkelman, H. Gibb, J.C. Etienne. John Libbey Eurotext, Paris © 2000, pp. 183-185.

Biological effects of copper on the oligochaete *Tubifex tubifex*

F. Arnoult[1, 2], S. Biagianti-Risbourg[1, 2], M. Couderchet[1, 2], J.C. Etienne[2], and G. Vernet[1, 2]

[1] *Laboratoire d'Eco-Toxicologie and* [2] *Institut International de Recherche sur les Ions Métalliques, Université de Reims Champagne-Ardenne, BP 1039, 51687 Reims 02, France*

Introduction

The quality of aquatic ecosystems often has to be monitored to assess ecotoxicological impact of pollutants, and this requires methods that have to be simple and reliable [1]. Bioindicators and or biomarkers can be used for this purpose. The identification and description of biomarkers is a new approach that can be used to assess the effect of chronic exposure to pollutants on populations in their environment. *Tubifex tubifex* is an aquatic oligochaete known to be very resistant to pollution and is often the last to disappear from a contaminated site [2]. As a result, it has been used as a bioindicator of pollution [3]. We have shown that *T. tubifex* is abundant on sites severely contaminated by copper. We have also analyzed some of the phenomena by which the worms adapt to the toxic impact induced by copper (Cu) and examined how they could be used as biomarkers of contamination. Part of the work was done in the field on *T. tubifex* harvested at the contaminated site, and part in the laboratory where the worms were exposed to acute and subacute Cu concentrations.

Materials and methods

Worms were harvested from a retention basin (Reuil, Marne, France) that receives and confines runoff water from a vineyard. Copper (Cu), used on vines as a fungicide for over 100 years, represents a major metallic contaminant in Champagne. The Cu concentration in the retention basin may reach 500 $mg.kg^{-1}$ in the sediment and 100 $\mu g.l^{-1}$ in the water. Some worms were fixed for examination in scanning electron microscopy (SEM), and others were analyzed by atomic absorption spectrometry. A third group was cultured for 15 months before being exposed to Cu.

The worms were maintained in two-liter aquaria containing spring water (Source des Grands Bois, Fismes, France; hardness: 300 ± 10 $mg.l^{-1}$ $CaCO_3$; pH: 7 ± 0.1), which was changed weekly, and fed with TetraMin flakes once a week. Culture conditions were: 20 ± 2°C, 12 h light 12 h darkness and 60% oxygen saturation.

Since Cu is rapidly precipitated in spring water [4], experiments were done in distilled water [5]. Groups of ten worms were placed in distilled water for 10 days and exposed for 96 h to acute concentrations of Cu (0.2; 0.5; 1 $mg.l^{-1}$) and to subacute concentrations Cu (0.005; 0.01; 0.02 $mg.l^{-1}$). Experiments were conducted in triplicate. During the experiments, the worms were not fed. Worms that survived the

96 h exposure to 0.01 and 0.02 $mg.l^{-1}$ Cu were fixed for examinations by SEM. The metal concentrations in worms exposed to 0.005 $mg.l^{-1}$ Cu was determined.
For Cu determination, the whole worms were washed several times and transferred to spring water for 48 h, to empty the gut and remove heavy metals weakly bound to their outer surface [6]. The worms were then cut into three pieces, and the anterior ("heads") and the posterior sections ("tails") were assayed for Cu concentrations (Varian atomic absorption spectrometer). For SEM, worms were examined in a Jeol scanning electron microscope.

Results
Results showed a LC50-96 h of 0.014 $mg.l^{-1}$ in semi static conditions (with daily renewal of the medium) and 0.126 $mg.l^{-1}$ in static conditions (without renewal of the medium). In semi static conditions, mortality was 30% and 100% after 96 h exposure to respectively 0.01 $mg.l^{-1}$ and 0.05 $mg.l^{-1}$.
The control worms have undergone no morphological alterations. The morphology of the anterior part of the worms collected at the study-site was similar to that of the controls. In contrast, many of the worms (about 75%) had abnormal caudal regions. Half of them, completely lacked a posterior part and it was regenerating in the remainder.
Worms kept for 96 h in subacute concentrations of Cu (in static conditions) showed no visible morphological alteration of the chetae. But exposure to Cu caused them to lose their tails. The frequency of this loss was concentration-dependent (79 ± 9% for 0.01 $mg.l^{-1}$ and 100 ± 0% for 0.02 $mg.l^{-1}$ Cu). It was induced by Cu concentrations close to those detected in the water column of the study-basin. It is interesting to note that the worms retained their ability to regenerate even in contaminated water: this was confirmed in the field study.
The Cu concentrations in the Reuil basin were high enough for Cu to accumulate in the oligochaetes. The Cu concentrations in these worms were greater than those of the controls. Furthermore, there was an anterior-posterior concentration gradient, with the posterior region containing twice as much Cu as the anterior region.
Exposure of the worms for 96 h (0.005 $mg.l^{-1}$ Cu) was sufficient to detect differences in Cu concentrations between the contaminated worms and the controls showing that this toxic metal was rapidly accumulated. The majority of the metal was accumulated in the posterior part of the organisms, so that the Cu concentrations in the distal end were twice those of the anterior part.

Discussion
Experimental contamination with subacute concentrations of copper and data from worms collected at a contaminated site, all indicate that *T. tubifex* responds to toxic stress induced by Cu by the autotomy of the caudal region, in which the toxic metals accumulated. This is clearly a mean by which the animal may protect itself against the increase of internal concentrations of toxic metals that would otherwise be fatal. These protection mechanisms appear to be effective, since they led to rapid decontamination of the worms. The capacity of the worms to regenerate was not impaired in contaminated medium.

Crustaceans concentrate metals in their exoskeleton, which is then eliminated during moulting [7]. The fundamental difference between the two processes is that the crustaceans eliminate metals via a normal physiological phenomenon, moulting, whereas *T. tubifex* worms use amputation process to adapt to contaminated media.
It has been suggested that some oligochaetes undergo spontaneous fragmentation, as a mean of detoxication mechanism [8]. Other studies have related the fragmentation of *T. tubifex* exposed to metals including Cu, but did not link the event to an adaptation process to toxic stress [5].
The loss of the tail due to experimental contamination with Cu also occurs in the field. This loss could therefore be a biomarker of contamination by heavy metals. Ecotoxicological research is now focusing on biomarkers that may be used in the field [9]. Most of the studies concern biochemical markers, the induction of metallothioneins or structural markers [1]. Detecting these biomarkers requires fairly complex methods, whereas the loss of a tail by *T. tubifex* is easily and rapidly observed. It is also concentration-dependent. These present great advantages in ecotoxicology.
This loss of the caudal region of *T. tubifex* appears to be a good candidate to be used as a biomarker.

References

1 Lagadic L, Caquet T, Amiard JC, Ramade F. Biomarqueurs en écotoxicologie. Aspects fondamentaux. Paris: Masson, 1997.
2 Milbrink G. Biological characterization of sediments by standardized tubificid bioassays. *Hydrobiologia* 1987; 155 : 267-75.
3 Chapman PM Churchland LM Thomson PA Michnowski E. Heavy metals studies with oligochaetes. In : Brinkhurst RO, Look DG, eds. *Aquatic oligochaetes biology*. New York : Plenum Press, 1980 : 477-502.
4 Lucan-Bouché ML, Arsac F, Biagianti-Risbourg S, Habets F, Vernet G. Etude expérimentale des effets létaux induits par le cuivre et ou le plomb chez l'oligochète *Tubifex tubifex*. *Bull Soc zool Fr* 1997; 122 : 389-92.
5 Brkovic-Popovic I, Popovic M. Effects of heavy metals on survival and respiration rate of tubificid worms. Part I. Effetcs on survival. *Environ Pollut* 1977; 13 : 65-72.
6 Lucan-Bouché ML. Contribution à l'étude de la biodisponibilité et de l'impact biologique chez *Tubifex tubifex* de contaminants du pool sédimentaire de l'environnement champardennais. PhD thesis, Reims, France, 1997.
7 Dhainaut-Courtois N, Demuynck S, Salzet-Raveillon B. Mécanismes de détoxication chez les poissons et invertébrés marins. *Océanis* 1991; 17 : 403-19.
8 Jamieson BG. The ultrastructure of the oligochaeta. London : Academic Press, 1981.
9 Lagadic L, Caquet T, Amiard JC, Ramade F. Utilisation de biomarqueurs pour la surveillance de la qualité de l'environnement. Paris : Tec & Doc Lavoisier, 1998.

Metal Ions in Biology and Medicine; vol 6. Eds. J.A. Centeno, Ph. Collery, G. Vernet, R.B. Finkelman, H. Gibb, J.C. Etienne. John Libbey Eurotext, Paris © 2000, pp. 186-188.

Mercury, lead, cadmium and selenium in blood from pilot whales and sperm whales

J.B. Nielsen[1], F. Nielsen[1], P.-J. Jørgensen[2], P. Grandjean[1]

[1] *Dept. of Environmental Medicine, SDU, Odense University, Winsløwparken 17, DK-5000 Odense C, Denmark;* [2] *Dept. of Clinical Chemistry, Odense University Hospital, DK-5000 Odense C, Denmark*

Abstract
Mercury, lead, cadmium and selenium were measured in blood from pilot whales (*Globicephala melas*) caught on the Faeroe islands and in blood from four sperm whales (*Physeter catodon*) stranded in Denmark. The median whole-blood concentration of Hg in pilot whales was 229 µg/L with a positive correlation to the corresponding Se concentrations with a molar ratio between Se and Hg close to ten. Blood concentrations of Hg and Cd up to 2421 µg/L and 31100 µg/L, respectively, were found in the sperm whales. Cd concentration was on average 500-1000 times higher in stranded sperm whales than in the pilot whales. The Hg and Cd concentrations dramatically exceed levels which are associated with severe toxicity in several other mammal species including man.

Introduction
Concentration of heavy metals in tissues from different species of whales have been used as biological indicators of pollution of the marine environment, but access to blood samples has been limited. However, information on blood concentrations may be useful for comparison with exposures in humans and other mammals. We collected blood from 17 pilot whales caught during landing of one school in 1996 at the Faroe Islands and from four male sperm whales stranded in Denmark in 1997. All blood samples were analysed for mercury (Hg), lead (Pb), cadmium (Cd) and selenium (Se).

Materials and methods
Blood samples: The pilot whales (*Globicephala melas*) were killed immediately after beaching and blood was collected directly from the carotid artery. Blood was sampled from 17 pilot whales. The length of the pilot whales varied between 381 cm and 530 cm, reflecting a mixed school of juvenile and mature individuals. From four sperm whales (*Physeter catodon*) stranded in Denmark whole-blood was sampled directly from an artery. During sampling, the utmost care was taken to avoid contamination of blood samples with salt water. Blood was sampled and and kept at -20°C until analysis.

Chemical analysis: Electrothermal AAS was used for determination of lead in blood (B-Pb), cadmium in blood (B-Cd) and selenium in blood (B-Se). Mercury analyses were performed by flow-injection cold vapour atomic absorption spectrometry. Methods are described and referenced in (1).

Table 1. Whole-blood concentration of Hg, Se, Cd, and Pb in 6 pilot whales.

Sex	male	male	female	female	female	female
B-Hg (µg/L)	253.9	428.6	166.0	291.2	203.7	172.0
B-Se (µg/L)	983.1	1449.2	664.9	994.5	956.6	907.4
B-Cd (µg/L)	33.4	13.3	13.1	25.0	9.2	9.8
B-Pb (µg/L)	12.0	8.0	8.0	12.0	12.0	8.0

Results

Serum Hg concentrations from 17 pilot whales (11 females and 6 males) averaged 18.7 µg/L (SD=6.4 µg/L). Serum concentrations of Hg correlated only weakly with the length of the whales (r=0.29) and no gender-related differences in Hg concentration in serum were observed. Three pregnant whales had serum concentrations of 10.9; 13.5; and 19.9 µg Hg/L, i.e. slightly lower (p=0.1, Mann-Whitney) than the serum levels in non-pregnant females (N=8; median= 20.5 µg Hg/L, range 14.9-34.1 µg Hg/L).

The average whole-blood concentrations (N=6) of metals in pilot whales were 228.8 µg Hg/L, 969.9 µg Se/L, 13.2 µg Cd/L, and 10 µg Pb/L (Table 1). There was a strong and positive correlation between Hg and Se in whole-blood (r=0.93; p<0.001, Spearman). The ratio between Se and Hg concentrations (µg/L) in whole-blood was close to four (range 3.4 - 5.2) corresponding to a molar ratio of 10 (Table 1).

Despite comparable lengths, very different concentrations of especially mercury and cadmium were observed in the sperm whales (Table 2). Thus, the sperm whale with the highest concentration of Hg (2421 µg Hg/L) and Cd (31100 µg Cd/L) had 11 times and 31 times higher concentrations than the sperm whale with the lowest whole-blood concentrations. There was no obvious association between Hg and Se concentrations in the sperm whales; the molar ratios between Se and Hg varying between 0.7 and 2.9. Variations in whole-blood Se levels in the sperm whales were less than the variations in the concentration of the other metals (Table 2).

Table 2. Whole-blood concentration of Hg, Se, Cd, and Pb in 4 male sperm whales.

B-Hg (µg/L)	2421	638	889	221
B-Se (µg/L)	638	729	585	324
B-Cd (µg/L)	31100	6190	5050	930
B-Pb (µg/L)	60	46	39	15

Discussion

Variations in organ levels of Hg are often observed within as well as between pods and probably reflect different ages and feeding behaviours. In 17 pilot whales from the same pod we observed a much smaller coefficient of variation than previously observed on tissue samples, which is probably due to the fact that the blood concentrations reflect recent exposure and that whales from the same pod are likely to have fed on the same prey. The indication that pregnant pilot whales had less Hg in the serum than non-pregnant female pilot whales is intriguing. An increased elimination could be due to transplacental transfer of Hg to the fetus, but a change in exposure, i.e. diet, is also possible. Squid is normally the major food item in pilot whales, but lactating pilot whales are thought to eat a greater proportion of fish (2).

A ratio of 20 between Hg in erythrocytes and Hg in plasma found in the present study (data not shown) supports the notion that Hg exposure is primarily in the form of methylmercury (MeHg). Blood is used as indicator medium for MeHg exposure in humans. Current evidence suggests that concentrations above 200 µg Hg/L are associated with early manifestations of neurotoxicity (3). Direct comparison of dose-response relationships may be inappropriate, but the high concentrations of metals in blood of the whales and the absence of apparent toxicity indicate an ability to detoxify the metals. In pilot whales, the present study demonstrated a strong correlation between Se and Hg and a molar ratio close to 10, i.e., 4-fold higher than in the stranded sperm whales. Marine food is a good source for Se, and inorganic Se is known to form insoluble complexes with Hg and in this way detoxify the Hg (4).

High concentrations of MeHg in whale meat result in worrisome exposures among humans who eat marine mammals (5). The excessively high levels of Hg in sperm whales without a concomitant increase in Se might be an indication of metal neurotoxicity in the whales. Thus, the present study adds emphasis to the notion that marine pollution with both Cd and Hg may result in adverse effects in the whales themselves.

References

1. Grandjean P, Nielsen GD, Jørgensen PJ, Hørder M. Reference intervals for trace elements in blood: significance of risk factors. *Scand J Clin Lab Invest 1992a;* **52**, 321-37.
2. Desportes G, Mouritsen R. Diet of the pilot whale, Globicephala melas around the Faroe Islands. ICES Report No. C.M. 1988/No 12 (mimeo).
3 IPCS (International Programme on Chemical Safety). (1990) Environmental Health Criteria for Methylmercury (EHC 101). pp. 1-144. Geneva: WHO.
4. Nielsen JB, Andersen O. A comparison of the effects of sodium selenite and seleno-L-methionine on disposition of orally administered mercuric chloride. *J Trace Elem Electrol Health 1991;* **5**, 245-50.
5. Grandjean P, Weihe P, Jørgensen PJ, Clarkson T, Cernichiari E, Viderø T. Impact of maternal seafood diet on fetal exposure to mercury, selenium, and lead. *Arch Environ Health 1992b;* **47**, 185-95.

Metal Ions in Biology and Medicine; vol 6. Eds. J.A. Centeno, Ph. Collery, G. Vernet, R.B. Finkelman, H. Gibb, J.C. Etienne. John Libbey Eurotext, Paris © 2000, pp. 189-192.

Assessing the environmental toxicity of copper

M. Couderchet[1, 2], F. Arnoult[1, 2], S. Biagianti-Risbourg[1, 2], P. Eullaffroy[1, 2], J.-C. Etienne[2], and G. Vernet[1, 2]

[1] Laboratoire d'Eco-Toxicologie, [2] Institut International de Recherches sur les Ions Métalliques, Université de Reims Champagne-Ardenne, BP 1039, 51687 Reims 02, France

Introduction

Copper has been used as Bordeaux mixture to control fungal diseases in vineyards for over 100 years. Since that time it has been accumulating and runoff, which is important on the steep slopes of Champagne's vineyards, has brought this metal in contact with the aquatic flora and fauna. Indeed, copper concentrations in some areas may be relatively high, for example in basins collecting vineyard runoff water it may be as high as 500 $mg.kg^{-1}$ in the sediment and 100 $\mu g.L^{-1}$ in the water.

Assessing the toxicity of a pesticide or a metal is often restricted to acute toxicity and determination of lethal doses or concentrations. For plants effective or inhibitory concentration is preferred to lethal concentration since determination of death is not always easy. Another more innovative way to assess toxicity is the use of biomarkers. Biomarkers are defined as any behavioral, physiological, cellular, biochemical, or molecular change that can be observed and/or measured which indicates an organism has been exposed to at least one polluting chemical compound [1].

Therefore, in order to assess the toxicity of copper, our laboratory has developed several biomarkers using various organisms, a unicellular green alga *Scenedesmus acutus*, a floating macrophyte *Lemna minor*, two worms *Lumbriculus variegatus* and *Tubifex tubifex*, and two fish *Brachydanio rerio* and *Rutilus rutilus*.

Acute toxicity of copper

Acute toxicity of copper was determined after exposure to the metal as inhibition of growth (IC) for plants and death (LC) for animals (Table 1).

Table 1: Acute toxicity of Copper for various organisms as determined by its inhibitory (IC) or lethal (LC) concentrations (mg.L^{-1}). Copper was given as CuSO4 and concentration was set at the beginning of experiments.

	Test duration	IC_{10} or LC_{10}	IC_{50} or LC_{50}	IC_{90} or LC_{90}
Scenedesmus acutus	48 h	1.42	3.25	7.50
Lemna minor	7 d	0.03	0.16	0.95
Lumbriculus variegatus	96 h		0.062	
Tubifex tubifex	96 h		0.126	
Brachydanio rerio	96 h		0.43	

Sublethal effects of copper

Plants

Metals and pesticides often lead to the accumulation of reactive oxygen species (ROS) in plants [2], this accumulation may be directly responsible for plant death or only be a side effect. Generation of ROS (O_2^-, •OH, H_2O_2) in response to copper exposure induces several detoxification reactions in the plant such as accumulation of antioxidants and stimulation of antioxidative enzymes [3]. This could be confirmed in *L. minor*. In this plant, copper induced the accumulation of ascorbate. After 48h the level of this antioxidant has increased by 53% with 0.50 mg.L^{-1} copper. The metal also induced an increase in several antioxidative enzymes in the plant. After 24h the activity of pyrogaloll peroxidase, guaiacol peroxidase and catalase was stimulated with the lowest copper concentration tested (16 µg.L^{-1}) and stimulation reached 67%, 276%, and 247% at the highest metal concentration tested (640 µg.L^{-1}). The activity of ascorbate peroxidase and glutathione-*S*-transferase was only slightly stimulated at low copper concentration and inhibited at 320 µg.L^{-1} and above and that of glutathion reductase was slightly inhibited [4]. The stimulation of pyrogaloll peroxidase, guaiacol peroxidase and catalase activity were found to be interesting biomarkers of copper contamination since they are sensitive (16 µg.L^{-1}) and rapid, 24h of incubation is sufficient.

In *S. acutus* and *L. minor*, chlorophyll (Chl) concentration and the ratio Chl a/b were also envisioned as a biomarker. In both organisms, Chl content and the ratio Chl a/b decreased in response to copper. However, the inhibitory concentrations and time of incubation were very much comparable to those of growth inhibition, except for the ratio Chl a/b in the alga that was very sensitive to the metal, it decreased from approximately 2.50 in the control to 1.00 when the algae were incubated 24h with 10 mg.L^{-1} of the metal. This ratio is an indirect quantification of Light Harvesting Complex II of the chloroplast [5], its decrease indicating more destruction of photosystem I than photosystem II in the algae.

The alterations of photosynthesis can also be used as a biomarker of copper contamination. These alterations were measured with a fluorescence-based method giving some indications on the quantum efficiency of photosynthesis, photochemical and non-photochemical quenching. With this biomarker it was possible to demonstrate interactions between copper and organic fungicides [6].

Worms

In nature, sissiparity followed by regeneration of the missing part is the only mean of reproduction of the oligochaete worm *L. variegatus*. In presence of copper this regeneration was found to be strongly delayed. Incubating the worms in spring water containing 0.05 $mg.L^{-1}$ of copper during 7 days had no effect on worm survival, however regeneration was delayed in over 20 % of the worms. Therefore, this property appeared to be an interesting biomarker [7].

The aquatic oligochaete *T. tubifex* is known to be very resistant to pollution, especially by copper. It seems that this worm is able to protect itself against the increase of internal concentration of metal by the autotomy of its caudal region [8]. This loss occurred at relatively low concentration since over 50% of the worms had lost their tails after 96h in the presence of only 10 $\mu g.L^{-1}$ of copper, indicating that this property is a sensitive biomarker [9].

Fish

In the teleost fish *R. rutilus*, the exposure to sublethal concentrations of copper (40 to 140 $\mu g.L^{-1}$) during 14 days induced several degenerative processes [10]. Liver of the fish displayed large lyzed areas after 7 days. However, after 4 or 7 days, protein content increased together with antioxidative defenses. In this species, it seems that the (ultra)structural disorders and also antioxidative activity may be used as biomarker of copper contamination in this organism. It can be noted that such biomarkers have also been used to demonstrate the effects of platinum in another fish, *Brachydanio rerio* [11].

Conclusion

Copper induced sublethal effects in all organisms presented here. Most of these sublethal effects could be used as biomarkers of copper contamination. However, the effects of copper in organisms in their natural environment may be influenced by other environmental factors. Thus, determining copper concentration in the environment does not allow any conclusion on the toxicity of the metal since copper may be sequestered and not bio-available, but also because its effect may be synergized or antagonized by other contaminants in the ecosystem.

Acknowledgment

This work was supported by the Conseil Régional de Champagne-Ardenne.

References

1. Lagadic L, Caquet T, Amiard JC, Ramade F. Biomarqueurs en écotoxicologie. Aspects fondamentaux. Paris: Masson, 1997.

2. McKersie BD, Leshem YY. Stress and stress coping in cultivated plants. Dordrecht, Kluwer Academic Publishers, 1994.
3. Foyer CH, Lelandais M, Kunert KJ. Photooxidative stress in plants. *Physiol Plant* 1994; 92: 696-717.
4. Teisseire H. Toxicologie et écotoxicologie des pesticides et des métaux lourds susceptibles d'être présents dans le vignoble champenois: études de leur impact physiologique et biochimique sur *Lemna minor*. Doctorate Thesis, University of Reims, 1999.
5. Busheva M, Garab G, Liker E, Toth Z, Szèll M, Nagy F. Diurnal fluctuations in the content and functional properties of the light harvesting complex in thylakoid membranes. *Plant Physiol* 1991; 95: 997-1003.
6. Frankart C, Eullaffroy P, Couderchet M, Dautremepuits C, Etienne JC, Vernet G. Influence of copper on the toxicity of fungicides on *Lemna minor*. This Volume, 2000.
7. Veltz-Balatre. Contribution à l'étude, chez un invertébré d'eau douce *Lumbriculus variegatus* (Annélide, Oligochète), de la toxicité de divers contaminants métalliques susceptibles d'être présents dans l'environnement champardennais. Doctorate Thesis, University of Reims, 1998.
8. Lucan-Bouché ML, Biagianti-Risbourg S, Arsac F, Vernet G. An original decontamination process developed by the aquatic oligochaete *Tubifex tubifex* exposed to copper and lead. *Aquat Toxicol* 1999; 45: 9-17.
9. Arnoult F, Biagianti-Risbourg S., Couderchet M, Etienne JC, Vernet G. Biological effects of copper on the oligochaete *Tubifex tubifex*. This volume, 2000
10. Paris-Palacios S, Biagianti-Risbourg S, Eullaffroy P, Etienne JC, Vernet G. Biochemical and (ultra)structural alterations induced by sublethal concentrations of copper in the liver of the teleost *Rutilus rutilus*. This volume, 2000.
11. Biagianti-Risbourg S, Arnoult F, Betoulle S, Etienne JC, Vernet G. Perturbations induced by a sublethal concentration of platinum in the anterior intestine of the teleost *Brachydanio rerio*: an ultra structural study. This volume, 2000.

Metal Ions in Biology and Medicine; vol 6. Eds. J.A. Centeno, Ph. Collery, G. Vernet, R.B. Finkelman, H. Gibb, J.C. Etienne. John Libbey Eurotext, Paris © 2000, pp. 193-197.

Effects of gallium nitrate on the immune system of carp (*Cyprinus carpio* L.)

Stéphane Betoulle[1, 2], Sylvie Biagianti-Risbourg[1, 2], Séverine Paris-Palacios[1, 2], Jean-Claude Etienne[2] and Guy Vernet[1, 2]

[1] *Laboratoire d'Eco-Toxicologie and* [2] *Institut International de Recherche sur les Ions Métalliques, Université de Reims Champagne-Ardenne, BP 1039, 51687 Reims cedex 2, France*

Introduction

Gallium nitrate is an antitumor agent which shows efficacy in the treatment of several medical disorders such as cancers and infectious diseases [1] [2]. Furthermore, gallium has specific immunomodulating activities. Several *in vivo* or *in vitro* studies have shown gallium to suppress certain immune functions without being generally immunosuppressive or cytotoxic [3]. All the immunomodulating effects of gallium are not fully understood yet and many questions about the biological activities of this metal remain unanswered. The immune system of fish is simpler than that of mammals and can be used as a simplified tool to better understand the mechanisms involved in the modulation of the immune responses by drugs and chemicals in higher vertebrates.

We studied the impact of gallium nitrate on macrophages, one of the major immune defenses in fish. As well as being accessory cells with an important role in initiating specific immune responses, macrophages are also potent effector cells of the nonspecific immune response, capable of killing a wide range of pathogens by generating reactive oxygen species (ROS) [4]. We monitored the generation of ROS by macrophages of carps exposed or not to gallium nitrate in water. Simultaneously, the total number of blood leucocytes was determined. In a second part, *in vitro* effects of gallium nitrate on the ROS production of macrophages isolated from healthy carps and cytotoxicity of macrophages exposed to gallium nitrate was examined.

Materials and methods

Acute toxicity of Gallium nitrate in carp

Common carps (*Cyprinus carpio* L.) (20 ± 3 g) were transfered in water containing gallium nitrate (Sigma) (0, 5, 10, 25, 50, 100, 250 and 500 $mg.l^{-1}$ corresponding to 19.5, 39.1, 97.7, 195.5, 391, 977, 1955 µM). Controls were fishes transfered in fresh water (Aurele source, Ardennes, France) without gallium nitrate. The fish mortality was estimated by counting the number of dead fishes every 12 hours. The 96-h LC_{50} was estimated using the method of Litchfield and Wilcoxon [5].

Exposition of carp to sublethal concentrations of gallium nitrate in water

Carps were placed in water containing gallium nitrate at sublethal concentrations (0, 5 or 50 $mg.l^{-1}$ corresponding to 19.5 or 195.5 µM). At different times (0, 24, 48 or 96 hours), fishes were sacrified and were bled to isolate peripheral blood leucocytes from blood [6]. The number of total viable leucocytes was estimated by Trypan blue test and were counted using an hemocytometer. At the same time, macrophages were isolated from head kidneys [7]. The oxidative response of these macrophages was estimated by chemiluminescence using a liquid scintillation biocounter (Packard) [8]. Data were collected in terms of counts per minutes (cpm) taken from readings every 5 minutes for 25 min and the maximal value reached was recorded.

Exposition of carp macrophages to gallium nitrate in vitro

Macrophages (20 x 10^6 cells/ml) isolated from healthy fishes were incubated at +20°C, for 5 or 15 minutes in culture medium (Leibowitz, L15, Gibco-Brl) containing 0, 50, 500 nM, 5, 50, 100 or 200 µM of gallium nitrate (corresponding to 0, 0.013, 0.13, 1.3, 12.8, 25.6 or 51.1 $mg.l^{-1}$). Controls were carried out with culture medium only. Macrophages were then washed in a buffer (PBS, Gibco-Brl) (centrifugation 800g, 10 min, + 4°C) and percentages of cytotoxicity were determinated by counting the number of viable cells by Trypan blue test using an hemocytometer. The macrophagic ROS production was measured by the chemiluminescence assay.

Results and discussion

The 96 h LC50 of gallium nitrate for common carp was 95.25 $mg.l^{-1}$ (372.5 µM). This value was very high comparatively to those estimated for other heavy metals [9]. Carps exposed to 50 $mg.l^{-1}$ gallium nitrate in water for 96 h, had a significantly lower number of peripheral leucocytes in blood than controls (table I). No significant difference was observed for the other time tested (24 or 48 h) and for the other concentration of gallium nitrate used (5 $mg.l^{-1}$) (Table I). ROS production of macrophages isolated from gallium nitrate-contaminated carps for 96 h was significantly low comparatively to ROS production measured in macrophages of controls at 96 h (53943 ± 8747 cpm and 88220 ± 4599 cpm respectively, $p<0.01$) (Fig 1). A similar result was observed for carps maintained in water containing 50 $mg.l^{-1}$ gallium nitrate for 48 h. Thus, carps elevated for 96 h in a water containing 50 $mg.l^{-1}$ gallium nitrate have a significantly lower number of total leucocytes in blood and a lower macrophagic oxidative response than carps elevated in fresh water. When macrophages isolated from healthy fish were incubated *in vitro* with gallium nitrate, their ROS production was significantly increased after a contact with 50 or 500 nM gallium nitrate for 15 minutes and after a contact with 500 nM for 5 minutes (Fig 2). After an incubation with 50, 100 or 200 µM gallium nitrate in culture medium, ROS productions of carp macrophages were significantly decreased whatever the incubation time tested. The oxidative response of fish macrophages treated with gallium nitrate was related to the concentration used. Moreover, Gallium nitrate was cytotoxic for carp macrophages only at 200 µM after 15 min of contact with cells (Table II). However, in mammals, gallium nitrate from 12.5 to 100 µM displays a dose –dependent growth inhibition and apoptosis of leukemic cells after 48 h of incubation [10].

Actually, no data are available concerning effects of gallium nitrate on the immune system of fish. In mammals, gallium reduces some immune functions and appears to induce specific inflammatory and proliferative responses particularly those mediated by T lymphocytes and macrophages [11] [3]. The dominant mechanism underlying most of gallium's diverse activities is its ability to act as a chemically irreducible ferric iron analog in a wide variety of systems. Iron is an essential element in some immune cells activations (lymphocytes...) and there are numerous interactions between iron and immunity in mammals [12]. In organisms, Fe^{3+} is generally linked to transferrin and iron-associated transferrin enters into cells via transferrin receptors [13]. In mammals, macrophages may express large amounts of transferrin receptors and have high iron requirements [14]. Iron as other metallic ions, interferes in ROS production reactions in macrophages. In cells, Fe^{3+} is reduced in Fe^{2+} and in presence of reduced iron, hydroxyle radicals (OH^-) are produced from reaction between hydrogene peroxyde and superoxide anion (O_2^-) (Haber Weiss and Fenton reaction). Thus, in mammals, iron can be used by macrophages to enhance ROS production during inflammatory processes. In our study on fish immune system, we speculate that gallium ion, which can act as a ferric analog but can not be reduced to a divalent form, can be linked to iron-transport molecules (transferrin...) and then, can block the iron uptake in macrophages and decrease in part the ROS production as observed here on carp macrophages *in vivo* and only for the highest concentrations used *in vitro*. This hypothesis is not valable to explain some of our data obtained *in vitro*, where gallium nitrate at 50 or 500 nM increases significantly the macrophagic ROS production. Thus, cellular mechanisms responsible for ROS production by macrophages in fish would be different in part with those observed in mammals.

Gallium nitrate remains undetectable in continental freshwater ecosystems. Our study shows that this marginal metal ion presents a low toxicity against carp . However, this study of comparative immunology would permit a best understanding of fish immune response and immunomodulating activities of gallium nitrate in highest vertebrates.

References

[1] Adamson RH, Canellos GP, Sieber SM. Studies on the antitumor activity of gallium nitrate and other group IIIa metal salts. *Cancer Chemother. Rep.* 1975; 59 : 599-610.

[2] Katsir O, Malik Z. Toxic effect of gallium nitrate on Friend erythroleukemia cells. *Cancer J.* 1997; 10 : 43-48.

[3] Bernstein LR. Mechanisms for therapeutic activity for gallium. *Pharmacol. Rev.* 1998; 50 : 665-681.

[4] Secombes CJ. Enhancement of fish phagocyte activity. *Fish Shellfish Immunol.* 1994; 4 : 421-436.

[5] Litchfield JT, Wilcoxon F. A simplified method of evaluating dose-effect experiments. *J. Pharmacol. Exp. Ther.* 1949; 96 : 99-113.

[6] Sakai DK. Separation of lymphocytes from the peripheral blood of rainbow trout and goldfish. *Bull. Jap. Soc. Sci. Fish.* 1981; 47 : 1281-1288.

[7] Secombes CJ. Isolation of Salmonid macrophages and analysis of their killing activity. In : Stolen JS, Fletcher TC, Anderson DP, Roberson BS, Van Muiswinkel WB, eds. *Techniques in fish immunology* 1990 : 137-153.

[8] Stave, JW, Roberson BS, Hetrick FM. Chemiluminescence of phagocytic cells isolated from the pronephros of Striped Bass. *Dev. Comp. Immunol.* 1983; 7 : 269-276.

[9] Leland HV, Kuwabara JS. Trace metals. In : Rand GM, Petrocelli SR, eds. *Fundamentals in aquatic toxicology*. 1985 : 374-404.

[10] Ul-Haq R, Wereley JP, Chitambar CR. Induction of apoptosis by iron deprivation in human leukemic CCRF-CEM cells. *Exp. Hematol.* 1995; 23 : 428-432.

[11] Matkovic V, Balboa A, Clinchot D, Whitacre C, Zwilling B, Brown D, Weisbrode SE, Apseloff G, Gerber N. Gallium prevents adjuvant arthritis in rats and interferes with macrophage/T cell function in the immune response. *Curr. Ther. Res.* 1991; 50 : 255-267.

[12] Seligman PA, Kovar J, Gelfand EW. Lymphocyte proliferation is controlled by both iron availability and regulation of iron uptake pathways. *Pathobiol.* 1992; 60 : 19-26.

[13] Huebers HA, Finch CA. The physiology of transferrin and transferrin receptors. *Physiol. Rev.* 1987; 67 : 520-582.

[14] Gatter KC, Brown B, Trowbridge IS, Woolston R, Mason DY. Transferin receptors in human tissue: their distribution and possible clinical relevance. *J. Clin. Pathol.* 1983; 36 : 539-545.

Acknowledgements

We thank the Conseil Régional de Champagne-Ardenne (France) for its financial help in making this study possible.

Time (hours)	Number of Peripheral Blood Leucocytes (x 10^6 cells.ml^{-1})		
	0	**[GaNO$_3$]=5 mg.l^{-1}**	**[GaNO$_3$]=50 mg.l^{-1}**
0	11.2±0.9	10.4±0.96	12.7±1.6
24	9.2±1	8.3±1.3	10.2±1.5
48	10.75±1.1	11.4±2.2	9.4±1.5
96	13.6±1.5	10.8±1.04	7.95±1 **(p<0.05)**(**)

Table I : Numbers of peripheral leucocytes in blood of carps exposed or not to gallium nitrate in water.
Each value was mean ± SD obtained from ten fishes exposed to the same treatment and environmental conditions. For each treatment, means obtained at 24, 48 or 96 h were compared to mean of controls (0 hour) by the two-tailed Student's t test (significance : **p<0.05**). For each time of prelevement, means obtained from fish exposed to gallium nitrate (5 or 50 mg.l^{-1}) were compared to means obtained in controls (no gallium nitrate in water (0)) by the two-tailed Student's t test (** : p<0.01).

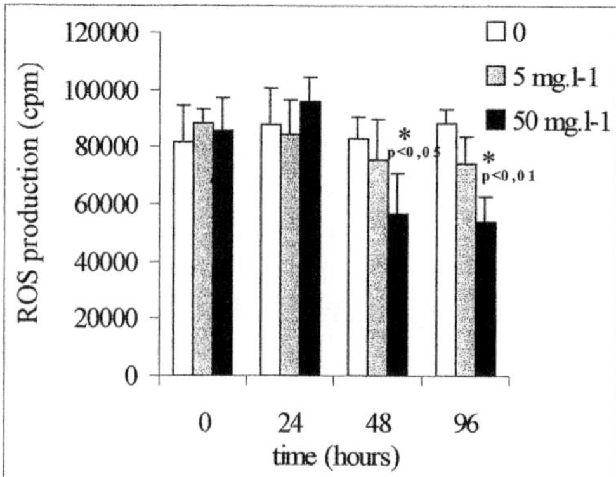

Figure 1 : ROS production of macrophages of carps exposed or not to gallium nitrate in water.
Each bar was mean ± SD of maximal ROS production obtained from ten fishes exposed to the same treatment and environmental conditions. For each treatment, means obtained at 24, 48 or 96 h were compared to mean of controls (0 hour) by the two-tailed Student's t test (significance : **p<0.05**). For each time of prelevement, means obtained from fish exposed to gallium nitrate (5 or 50 mg.l^{-1}) were compared to means obtained in controls (no gallium nitrate in water (0)) by the two-tailed Student's t test (* : p<0.05).

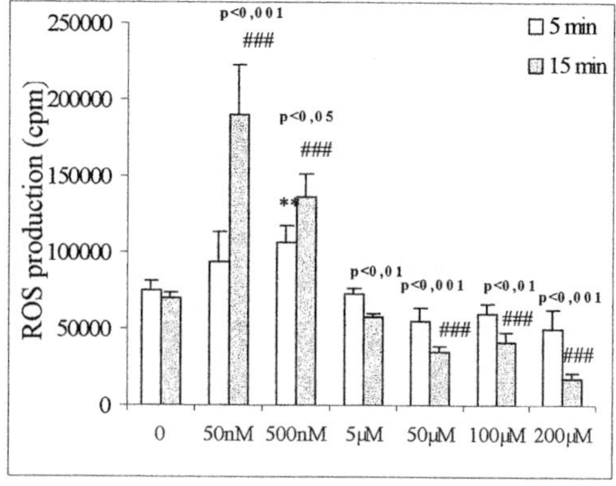

Figure 2 : ROS production of carp macrophages exposed or not to gallium nitrate.
Each bar was mean ± SD of maximal ROS production obtained from eight identical experiments. For each treatment, means obtained at 5 or 15 min were compared each other by the two-tailed Student's t test (significance : **p<0.05**). For each time, means obtained from fish exposed to gallium nitrate (from 50 nM to 200 µM) were compared to means obtained in controls (no gallium nitrate in water (0)) by the two-tailed Student's t test (* : p<0.05, after 5 min; # : p<0.05, after 15 min).

Time (min)	[GaNO$_3$]						
	0	50 nM	500 nM	5 µM	50 µM	100 µM	200 µM
5	-15.6±6	-7.2±2.9	-9.5±7.8	-13.3±1.4	-28.3±4.7	-20.8±4.8	-25.3±8.6
15	-10.2±4.3	-12.0±7.2	-10.5±2.6	-12.3±5.4	-25.3±7.8	-21.7±6.1	-78.5±13.3 (##)(**)

Table II : Cytotoxicity in macrophage cell suspensions exposed or not to gallium nitrate.
Each value was mean ± SD of percentages of cell mortality observed in cell suspension treated or not with gallium nitrate. Means were calculated from eight identical experiments. For each treatment, means obtained after 5 or 15 min were compared each other by the two-tailed Student's t test (##: p<0.01). For each time of prelevement, means obtained from fish exposed to gallium nitrate (from 50 nM to 200 µM) were compared to means obtained in controls (no gallium nitrate in water (0)) by the two-tailed Student's t test (** : p<0.01).

Metal Ions in Biology and Medicine; vol 6. Eds. J.A. Centeno, Ph. Collery, G. Vernet, R.B. Finkelman, H. Gibb, J.C. Etienne. John Libbey Eurotext, Paris © 2000, pp. 198-201.

Influence of copper on the toxicity of fungicides on *Lemna minor*

C. Frankart[1, 2], P. Eullafroy[1, 2], M. Couderchet[1, 2], C. Dautremepuits[1, 2], J.-C. Etienne[2], and G. Vernet[1, 2]

[1] *Laboratoire d'Eco-Toxicologie;* [2] *Institut International de Recherche sur les Ions Métalliques, Université de Reims Champagne-Ardenne, BP 1039, 51687 Reims 02 France*

INTRODUCTION

Copper is an essential micronutrient for plant life, playing an irreplaceable role in a large number of enzymes vital to cell metabolism [1]. However, in excessive quantities copper becomes toxic as it interferes with photosynthetic and respiratory processes, protein synthesis and development of plant organelles [2], [3], [4]. Copper is also known as a pesticide to control mildew and other fungal diseases in grape and then is generously sprayed on vineyards in Champagne (France). It belongs with two other fungicides (procymidone and pyrimethanil) to the most widely used agrochemical in those fields. These three pesticides are anti-botrytic fungicides used against the development of *Botrytis cinerea*, phytopathogen mushroom responsible for a disease named "gray rot" or *Botrytis*. Because the vineyard in Champagne are established on hillsides, runoff and leaching are particularly important phenomena in this area. Then copper and fungicides can be found in the environment and can potentially damaged aquatic ecosystem.

In this study, we investigated, by using a chlorophyll fluorescence based method, the interaction between copper and these two fungicides in *Lemna minor*, an aquatic plant regularly used for ecotoxicological studies [5].

MATERIALS AND METHODS

Plant material: *Lemna minor* commonly named duckweed were collected from ponds in Ardennes (France). They were cultured in mineral medium (pH 6.5). All the aquaria were maintained in growth chamber at 22°C under continuous light (100 μmoles.m^{-2}.s^{-1}). The experiments were carried out in Erlenmeyer's containing 100 ml of mineral solution The plants were exposed to copper as cupric sulfate at concentrations of 0.1, 0.5 and 1 mg.L^{-1} added to 0.2, 2 and 20 mg.L^{-1} of one of the two fungicides as their commercial form (Scala and Sumisclex for procymidone and pyrimethanil respectively). Plants without added copper and pesticide served as control. Three replicate groups of plants were exposed to contaminant for 3 days.

Chlorophyll fluorescence measurements: Room temperature signals were generated by a pulse amplitude modulated fluorometer (PAM-FMS1 Hansatech, England). For each experiment, three fully developed leaves were taken and placed in darkness for 15 minutes at 22°C before onset of measurement. After recording the dark signal level, the probing light beam was turned on (1,6 kHz, 0.02 μmoles.m^{-2}.s^{-1}) and a stable Fo-level recorded. A single saturating flash of 17000 μmoles.m^{-2}.s^{-1}, 1s duration, was then applied to reach Fm, whereupon the white actinic light (1140 μmoles.m^{-2}.s^{-1})

was turned on. The photosynthetic capacity of *Lemna minor* was determined as Fv / Fm = (Fm – Fo) / Fm.

Combination of copper and pyrimethanil or procymidone: When *L. minor* was exposed to mixture of copper and pyrimethanil or procymidone under static conditions, possible interaction between them were estimated using Abott's formula [6]. In this widely used model, the expected inhibition of the mixture, expressed as percent C_{exp}, can be predicted as:

$$C_{exp} = A + B - (AB / 100)$$

Where A and B represent the inhibition levels given by the single chemicals (respectively copper and pyrimethanil or procymidone). The ratio of inhibition (RI) was then calculated as follows for each pesticide combination:

$$RI = C_{exp} / \text{experimentally observed efficacy}$$

A $RI < 1$ indicated synergism between the two contaminants and a $RI > 1$ antagonism between the chemicals.

RESULTS AND DISCUSSION

To characterize the influence of cupric ions, pyrimethanil and procymidone on photosynthesis activity of *Lemna minor,* measurements of *in vivo* chlorophyll fluorescence were conducted. The photochemical activity was only slightly inhibited after addition of 0.1 mg/L Cu^{2+} (-3% at 72 h) when this decrease was important in *Lemna* exposed to 0.5 and 1 mg/L Cu^{2+} (-14 and -42% respectively at 72 h). Although copper is known as an essential constituent of many proteins and enzymes [7] [8], our experiment shows that the photosynthetic apparatus of *Lemna* is particularly sensitive to copper. It is known that copper may interfere with numerous physiological processes in leaves [9], [10] and especially at the oxygen evolving complex site [11].
Pyrimethanil and procymidone seems to have no effect or to induce a slight activation of the photosynthetic capacity of *Lemna* (table I). Pyrimethanil and procymidone are known to inhibit growth of *Botritys cinerea* mycelium by decreasing secretion of enzymes, triglycerides synthesis and by inducing oxidative stress [12]. But since pyrimethanil and procymidone are fungicides, little or none data are available on the effect of these xenobiotics on plants. A stimulation of growth response has been reported in plants [13] [14]. The observed activation can be due to the active ingredient by itself or by the formulation of the commercial product.

Table I: Kinetics of Fv/Fm changes in *Lemna*, in percentage (mean ± SE) after pesticide exposition. The level measured at t = 0 hour was taken as 100 %.

	Copper (mg.L^{-1})			**Pyrimethanil** (mg.L^{-1})			**Procymidone** (mg.L^{-1})		
	0.1	**0.5**	**1**	**0.2**	**2**	**20**	**0.2**	**2**	**20**
0 hour	100	100	100	100	100	1,00	100	100	100
4 hours	99 ± 2	99 ± 2	100 ± 1	102 ± 1	102 ± 1	100 ± 1	101 ± 2	101 ± 1	102 ± 1
24 hours	97 ± 3	93 ± 1	90 ± 6	101 ±1	102 ± 1	102 ± 1	104 ± 1	103 ± 1	104 ± 1
48 hours	96 ± 2	91 ± 4	70 ± 11	100 ± 0	102 ± 1	101 ± 1	103 ± 1	103 ± 3	106 ± 3
72 hours	97 ± 3	86 ± 8	58 ± 14	102 ± 3	107 ± 1	107 ± 1	104 ± 0	103 ± 1	105 ± 2

Lemna minor was also exposed to mixtures of copper and pyrimethanil or procymidone and possible interaction between them were estimated using Abott's formula [7].

Concerning the mixture of copper and pyrimethanil, the comparison between the Fv/Fm expected inhibition (C_{exp}) and experimentally observed inhibition revealed two different responses (table II). For the lowest pyrimethanil concentration (0.2 and 2 $mg.L^{-1}$) the experimentally observed photosynthetic capacity inhibition values were superior to C_{exp} and the RIs were less than 1 (0.57 and 0.7 respectively) indicating a potential synergism between copper and pyrimethanil. In contrast for the highest pyrimethanil concentration tested (20 $mg.L^{-1}$), the ratio was greater than 1, indicating antagonism between the two chemicals.

When *Lemna* was exposed to a combination of copper and procymidone, we observed an antagonism between the two. Even at the lowest studied concentration of procymidone, this antagonism was noticed with a RI upper than 1 (RI=2.26 at 72 h for mixture of 0.5 mg/L Cu^{2+} and 0.2 mg/L procymidone).

Table II: Kinetics of Fv/Fm changes in Lemna (mean ± SE) exposed to mixture of copper (0.5 $mg.L^{-1}$) and pyrimethanil or procymidone at different concentrations. The level measured at t = 0 hour was taken as 100 %.

	Copper + Pyrimethanil ($mg.L^{-1}$)			**Copper + Procymidone** ($mg.L^{-1}$)		
	0.2	**2**	**20**	**0.2**	**2**	**20**
0 hour	100	100	100	100	100	100
4 hours	98 ± 3	96 ± 6	95 ± 5	103 ± 2	105 ± 2	107 ± 3
24 hours	83 ± 1	90 ± 7	99 ± 1	98 ± 1	111 ± 3	108 ± 1
48 hours	70 ± 4	85 ± 2	100 ± 0	90 ± 4	112 ± 7	106 ± 5
72 hours	51 ±11	75 ± 10	97.± 0	90 ± 3	109 ± 5	94 ± 7

To explain the synergism observed at 0.5 mg/L Cu^{2+} and 0.2 mg/L pyrimethanil it is possible that the formulation facilitates the penetration of the cupric ions in the leaves. However at higher concentration of pyrimethanil and in mixtures of copper and procymidone the observed antagonism can be explain by a complexation of copper by pyrimethanil or procymidone which would reduce the bioavailability of copper and lowering or suppressing its toxicity. Such complexation of copper was described with other pesticides such as glyphosate [15].

This study demonstrated that copper is toxic to *Lemna minor* but that pyrimethanil and procymidone can be considered as poorly or none toxic to duckweed. However, synergism of copper and pyrimethanil at low concentration may reinforce the ecotoxicological risk of both pollutants.

Acknowledgment: This work was supported by the Conseil Régional de Champagne-Ardenne.

REFERENCES

[1] Baron M, Sandmann G. Activities of copper-containing proteins in copper-depleted pea leaves. *Physiol Plant* 1988; 72: 801-806.

[2] Wainwright S J, Woolhouse H W. Some physiological aspects of copper and zinc tolerance in *Agrostis teneuis* Sibth: Cell elongation and membrane damage. *J Exp Bot* 1977; 28: 1029-1036.
[3] Argawala S C, Nautiyal B D, Chatterjee C, Nautiyal N. Variations in copper and zinc supply influence growth and activities of some enzyme in maize. *Soil Sci Plant Nutr* 1995; 41: 329-335.
[4] Mousatakas M, Ouzounidiou G, Symeonidis L, Karataglis S. Field study of the effects of excess copper on wheat photosynthesis and productivity. *Soil Sci Plant Nutr* 1997; 43 (3): 531-539.
[5] Lewis M A. Freshwater primary producers, in *Handbook of Ecotoxicology,* P.Calow, Oxford Blackwell Scientific Publications, London, Edinburg, Boston, Melbourne, Paris, Berlin, Vienna, 1993: 28-50.
[6] GISI U. Synergic interaction of fungicides in mixture. *Phythopath* 1996; 86: 1273-1279.
[7] Fernandes J C, Henriques F S. Biochemical, physiological and structural effects of excess copper in plants. *Bot Rev* 1991; 57: 246-273.
[8] Arellano J B, Lazaro J J, Lopez-Gorgé J, Baron M. The donor side of photosystem II as the copper-inhibitory binding site. *Photosynth. Res* 1995; 45: 127-134.
[9] Lidon F C, Henriques F S. Copper-mediated oxygen toxicity in rice chloroplasts. *Photosynthetica* 1993; 29: 385-400.
[10] Navari-Izzo F, Quartacci M F, Pinzino C, Balla Vecchia F, Sgherri C L M. Thylakoid-bound and stromal antioxydative enzymes in wheat treated with excess copper. *Physiol Plant* 1998; 104: 630-638.
[11] Samson G, Popovic R. Use of algal fluorescence for determination of phytotoxicity of heavy metals and pesticides as environmental pollutants. *Ecotox Environ Safe* 1998; 16: 272-278.
[12] Tomlin C. *The Pesticide Manual* C. Tomlin Ed., 10th ed., Crop Protection Publ., Farnham, UK, 1994; 518-519.
[13] Teisseire H, Couderchet M, Vernet G. Toxic response and catalase activity of *Lemna minor* L. exposed to folpet, copper and their combination. *Ecotox Environ Safe* 1998; 40: 194-200.
[14] Buchenauer H. Physiological reactions in the inhibition of plant pathogenic fungi. In *Chemistry of Plant Protection* (W S Bowers, W Ebing, D Martin, R Wegler, Eds) Springer-Verlag, Berlin 1990; Vol 6: 217-292.
[15] Undabeytia T, Ceshire M V, Mc Phail D. Interaction of the herbicide glyphosate with copper in humic complexes. *Chemosphere* 1996; 32: 1245-1250.

Metal Ions in Biology and Medicine; vol 6. Eds. J.A. Centeno, Ph. Collery, G. Vernet, R.B. Finkelman, H. Gibb, J.C. Etienne. John Libbey Eurotext, Paris © 2000, pp. 202-204.

Determining the source(s) of metals in the environment using microanalysis

Allan Kolker, Harvey E. Belkin, and Robert B. Finkelman

U.S. Geological Survey, 956 National Center, Reston, VA 20192 USA

Introduction

Microbeam analytical instruments such as the electron microprobe, scanning electron microscope (SEM), and ion probe play an important role in helping to determine the source(s), concentration(s), and micro-scale distribution of toxic elements in the environment. This knowledge is essential to understanding biogeochemical interactions of organisms with metals from natural and anthropogenic sources, and predicting where toxicity is likely to occur. The electron microprobe has been especially useful in determining arsenic concentrations in sulfide minerals such as pyrite, which upon weathering, becomes a major natural source of arsenic in arsenic-contaminated ground water. Microbeam methods have also been used to determine the nature of metal-enrichment in coal, in order to understand the contribution of metals from coal combustion to the environment. This paper summarizes these recent and ongoing investigations in which microanalysis plays a significant role.

Arsenic in Ground Water

In the Marshall Aquifer of southeastern Michigan, USA, domestic wells exceed the current EPA drinking water standard (50 μg/L) by as much as a factor of eight. Our studies show that individual pyrite grains in the Marshall sandstone have micro-scale compositional domains with as much as 7 weight percent arsenic (Fig.1). Oxidation of this material, or of glacial deposits containing fragments of it, is the most likely source of arsenic contamination in southeastern Michigan ground water [1].

Preliminary electron microprobe/SEM studies of pyrite grains from Ganges-Brahmaputra-Meghna delta sediments show that arsenic-rich pyrite is present in the area of India and Bangladesh where millions suffer from arsenic toxicity (Fig. 2). In this study, it is apparent that arsenic is sequestered from natural waters by pyritization of organic matter under reducing conditions, in addition to possibly being released by pyrite oxidation. Reduction of arsenic-rich iron oxides, derived from arsenic-rich pyrite, and sorption of As onto mineral surfaces are other known mechanisms that add or subtract aqueous As. Additional work, including microanalysis, is needed to determine the role of pyrite oxidation vs. reduction of iron oxides in arsenic-contaminated ground water of the Ganges-Bramaputra-Meghna delta [2].

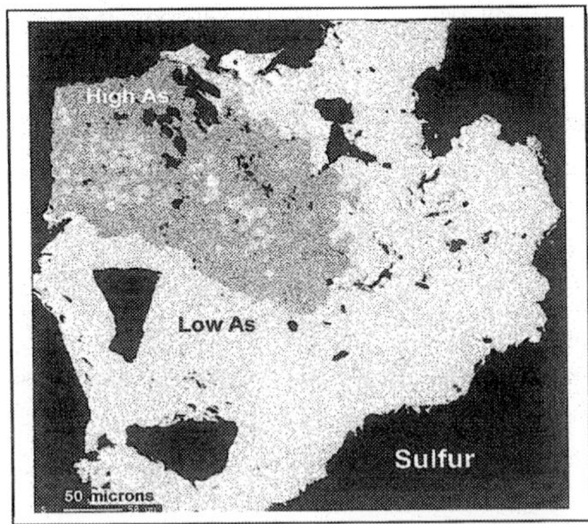

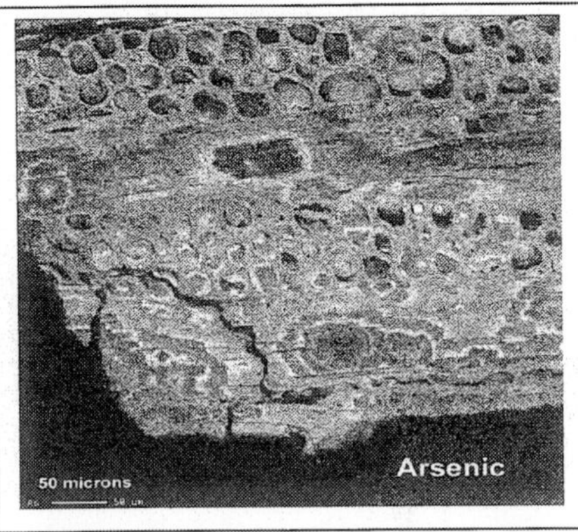

Figure 1. (left) Sulfur map of Michigan pyrite (FeS_2) showing arsenic-rich and arsenic-poor domains (dark and bright, respectively). Figure 2. (right) Arsenic map of a West Bengal pyrite showing arsenic-enrichment (bright bands) in pyritized woody fragment.

Trace Metals in Coal

Microanalytical techniques are used to investigate the concentrations and modes of occurrence of potentially harmful elements in coals used in the U.S. and abroad. In one such study, we investigated extreme arsenic-enriched coals in southwestern Guizhou Province, China, where domestic coal use has resulted in acute arsenic toxicity. The most arsenic-enriched coal samples have bulk As concentrations greater than one weight percent; some samples exceed three percent As [3]. In these samples, As is diffused throughout the organic coal structure, as confirmed by back-scattered electron SEM images and transmission electron microscopy (Fig. 3).

The distribution of metals in U.S. coals used for electric power generation is being investigated to help develop a predictive model for trace-element transformations during coal combustion. Here the emphasis is on a range of potentially toxic elements including Cr, Mn, Co, Ni, As, Se, Cd, Sb, Hg, and Pb. The electron microprobe has been used in combination with the Stanford University/USGS SHRIMP-RG ion microprobe to make direct determinations of the modes of occurrence of these elements in coal. Results for chromium, obtained using the SHRIMP-RG, show that clay minerals, important inorganic constituents of coal, are also significant sources of chromium emitted during coal burning (Fig. 4). Some of the chromium in coal combustion products may be present in the highly toxic hexavalent form [4]. In future studies, the ion probe will be used to investigate Hg distribution in sulfides in coal, and metal distribution in fly ash.

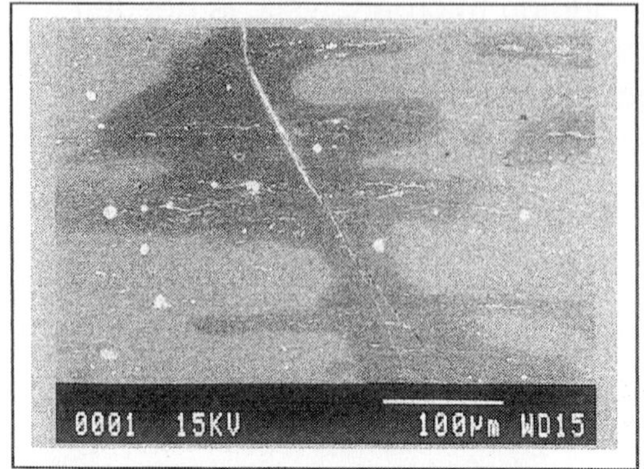

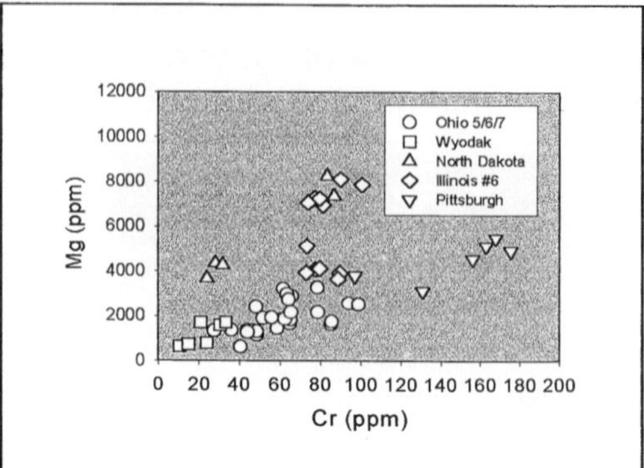

Figure 3. (left) Back-scattered electron image showing arsenic-enrichment (milky areas) in a Guizhou (China) coal sample. Figure 4. (right) Ion probe data plot of Mg vs Cr (in ppm) for illite (clay) in samples of selected coals used for commercial power generation.

Conclusions

Determination of potentially toxic elements in natural materials provides basic information on the distribution of metals that can enter the environment and be taken up by organisms. Microanalysis allows these distributions to be determined on a micrometer scale, thereby identifying the geologic sources of potentially available metal ions.

[1] Kolker, A, Cannon, WF, Westjohn, DB, and Woodruff, LG, Arsenic-rich pyrite in the Mississippian Marshall Sandstone: Source of anomalous arsenic in southeastern Michigan ground water. *Geological Society of America, Abstracts with Programs*, 1998; 30, #7: A-59.

[2] Chowdhury, TR, Basu, GK, Mandal, BK, Samanta, G, Roy, SL, Chakraborti, D., Breit, GN, Kolker, A, Welch, AH, and Nordstrom, DK, Characterization of arsenic-bearing sediments of West Bengal, India: manuscript in preparation.

[3] Belkin, HE, Warwick, PD, Zheng, B, Zhou, D, and Finkelman, RB, High arsenic coals related to sedimentary rock hosted gold deposition in southwestern Guizhou Province, People's Republic of China. *Proceedings of the Fifteenth Pittsburgh Coal Conference*, 1998; 4 p. (CD-ROM).

[4] Sheps, S, Finkelman, RB, Councell, TB, and Cohen, H, Leaching of hexavalent chromium from fly ash. *Proceedings of the 9th International Conference on Coal Science*, Essen, Germany, 1997, p. 1883-1886.

Acquisition of a portion of our results was supported by U.S. Department of Energy Interagency Agreement DE-AI22-95PC95145.

Metal Ions in Biology and Medicine; vol 6. Eds. J.A. Centeno, Ph. Collery, G. Vernet, R.B. Finkelman, H. Gibb, J.C. Etienne. John Libbey Eurotext, Paris © 2000, pp. 205-207.

Hepatic perturbations of the teleost *Rutilus rutilus* induced by sublethal concentrations of Cu^{2+}: a biochemical and (ultra)structural study

Paris-Palacios S.[1], Biagianti-Risbourg S.[1, 2], Eullaffroy P.[1], Etienne J.-C.[2] and Vernet G.[1, 2]

[1] *Laboratoire d'Eco-Toxicologie and* [2] *Institut International de Recherches sur les Ions Métalliques, Université de Reims Champagne-Ardenne, Moulin de la Housse, B.P. 1039, 51687 Reims cedex 2, France*

Copper sulfate is frequently used in viticulture as fungicide and thus can contaminate aquatic ecosystems. Toxicological effects of Cu^{2+} on fish are well documented but the variability of reported results is large [1]. The (ultra)structural reported changes are either adaptive (reticulum and chondriom development; lysosomal proliferation...) or degenerative (losses in integrity of mitochondria, plasma or nuclear membranes; fragmentation of endoplasmic reticulum...) depending on Cu^{2+} concentration and exposure duration [1, 2, 3]. Some metals are known as promoters of oxidative stress and can either increase or decrease hepatic protein content and the activity of anti-oxidative enzymes such as catalase (Cat), superoxide dismutase (SOD) or glutathione reductase (GRd) depending on metal type and concentration, length of exposure, fish species, and water hardness [4, 5]. The simultaneous analysis of both biochemical and ultrastructural responses of fish liver to metallic stress are particularly scarse. Thus, it is difficult to assess if the ultrastructural events interpreted as liver adaptive responses are associated to decide whether the development of anti-oxidative protective systems and enhanced protein synthesis. This study concerns the chronological analysis of the oxidative stress and the structural perturbations induced by sublethal concentrations of Cu^{2+} in liver of roach *Rutilus rutilus.*

Materials and Methods: Roach (90 females) were acclimatized 3 weeks to laboratory conditions in bottled spring water (eau Cristaline, source des Grands Bois, 51170 Fismes France); pH 8 ± 0.5; temperature 8 ± 0.5°C; hardness 300 mg/l; $[Ca^{2+}]$ 124 mg/l. Two series of 3 groups of 15 fish (control, fish exposed to actual concentrations of 40 ± 10 or 140 ± 30 µgCu/l) were kept in aquaria with a density of 1.5 fish/l. $[Cu^{2+}]$ was monitored every 5 hours by atomic absorption spectrometry. Tests were conducted in semi-static conditions (water renewed every 2 days). After a 14-d exposure 9 fish of each groups were replaced in clean water. After 4, 7, 14 d of exposure and 14 d exposure followed by 14 or 20 d depuration, fish were killed by decapitation and their liver used for histo-cytology and biochemical studies. Histo-cytological procedures were conducted according to Paris-Palacios *et al.* [3]. For each sampling 4 livers were examined in histology and 3 in cytology. For biochemical procedures 2 pools of 3 livers were used and each measurement was made 3 times (n=6). Livers were homogenized in phosphate buffer and centrifugated 15 min at 2300 g (4°C) [3]. The supernatant was used to determine total protein content, Cat and GRd activity and total glutathione content according to Paris-Palacios [5].

Results: Toxicity of Cu^{2+} was clearly demonstrated as liver developed large lyzed zones (Fig. 1). Hepatic parenchyma showed clear hepatocytes (Fig. 1) which ultrastructural response was degenerative in nature: severe mitochondrial alterations, decreased number of rough endoplasmic reticulum cisternae (Fig. 2). However, after 4 or 7 days of exposure large parenchymal zones were composed of basophilic hepatocytes displaying typical structural features of increased metabolism (development of rough endoplasmic reticulum and chondriom; increased size of nucleus and nucleolus: Fig. 3, Table I). Increased protein content and anti-oxidative defenses (Cat and GRd activities, total glutathione content: Table II) indicated that the overall response of the liver was adaptive.

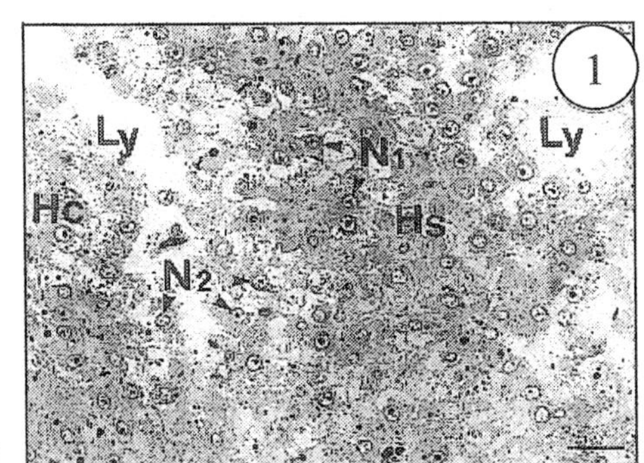

] **140 µgCu^{2+}/l.** Hc: clear hepatocytes; Hs: basophile hepatocyte; Ly: lyzis; N1 : nucleus of Hs; N2: nucleus of Hc. (bar = 30 µm)

For longer exposure duration the number of basophylic hepatocytes decreased (Table I). Large zones of the parenchyma were lyzed or composed of clear degenerative hepatocytes (Fig. 1, Table I). Simultaneously hepatic protein content decreased to control values and anti-oxidative defenses were reduced (decrease of total glutathione content, GRd and Cat activities: Table II) indicating that livers had lost their adaptive capacity. Therefore the overall hepatic response of the roaches exposed to Cu^{2+} became degenerative.

	Roach exposed to 40 µgCu^{2+}/l					**Roach exposed to 140 µgCu^{2+}/l**				
	4 d	7 d	14 d	14 d + dep. of: 14 d	20 d	4 d	7 d	14 d	14 d + dep. of: 14 d	20 d
Hl	15 ± 5	25 ± 5*	40 ± 10*	40 ± 10*	20 ± 10	15 ± 5	35 ± 5*	55 ± 5*	60 ± 10*	20 ± 10
Hc	10 ± 5*	15 ± 5*	30 ± 10*	30 ± 10*	20 ± 10*	15 ± 5*	25 ± 5*	30 ± 10*	30 ± 10*	20 ± 10*
Hs	75 ± 5*	65 ± 5*	30 ± 10*	30 ± 10*	60 ± 10*	70 ± 5*	40 ± 5*	20 ± 10*	20 ± 10*	50 ± 10*

Table I: Percentage of lyzed (Hl), clear (Hc) and basophilic hepatocytes (Hs) in the liver of roach during Cu exposure and depuration (dep.). * significantly different from control (student test, $p<0.01$)

A 14-day depuration was not sufficient to produce any modification of the (ultra)structural and biochemical responses in the liver. However, after 20 d of depuration, the hepatic parenchyma presented clear increase of the basophilic hepatocyte number (Table I); reduction of perturbations (decreased of lyzed zone surface) and development of granular endoplasmic reticulum and chondriom in numerous hepatocytes. The reversibility of perturbations was confirmed by a new increase of anti-oxidative defenses (Table II).

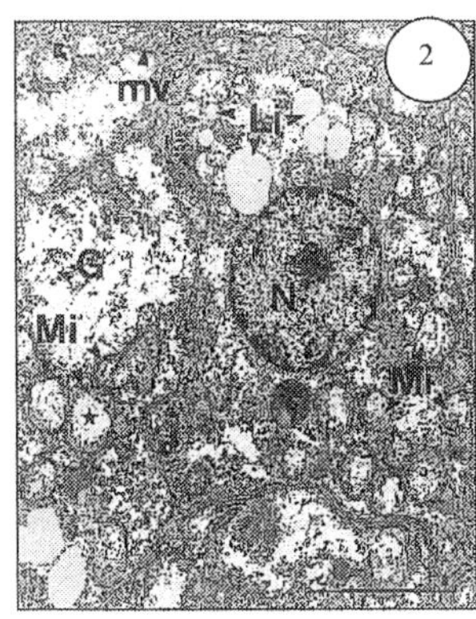

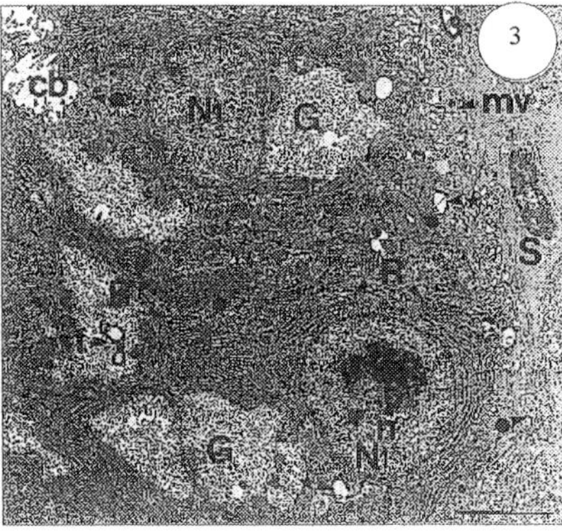

Fig. 2: Degenerative hepatocyte (Hc) in roach exposed 14 d to 140 µgCu^{2+}/l

Fig. 3: Basophile hepatocytes (Hs) in roach exposed 14 d to 140 µgCu^{2+}/l

cb: bile canaliculus G: glygogen; Li: lipid; Mi: mitochondria; mv: microvillies; N: nucleus; n: nucleolus; R: rough endoplasmic reticulum; S: sinusoide; ★: vacuolized Mi.
(bar = 6 µm)

Conclusions: These results showed that (ultra)structural and biochemical studies are complementary to describe fish hepatic perturbations induced by Cu^{2+}. Liver of danio exposed in comparable conditions to copper still showed, even after 14 d exposure, hepatocyte adaptive responses [3, 5]. Thus we can conclude that roach were more sensitive to Cu^{2+} than danio. This observation shows that it is difficult to extrapolate from one fish species to the other as far as liver responses are concerned.

	Roach exposed to 40 µgCu^{2+}/l					**Roach exposed to 140 µgCu^{2+}/l**				
	4 d	7 d	14 d	14 d + dep. of: 14 d	20 d	4 d	7 d	14 d	14 d + dep. of: 14 d	20 d
Protein tot.	+ 258*	+ 46*	+ 29*	0	0	+ 188*	+ 50*	0	-54*	-15*
Cat	+ 400*	+ 480*	+ 200*	+ 413*	+ 1260*	+ 9*	-20*	- 30*	+ 400*	+ 1000*
GRd	+ 129*	+ 182*	+ 128*	+ 328*		+ 178*	+ 15	- 15	+ 10	+ 15
Glutathione	+ 90*	+ 133*	+ 150*	+ 180*	+ 170*	+ 90*	+ 40*	0	+ 40*	+60*

Table. II: Percentage of increase or of reduction of hepatic protein and glutathione contents and of Cat and GRd activities of roach exposed to Cu^{2+} as compared to control liver. * significantly different from control (student test, $p<0.01$)

References

[1] Segner H, Braunbeck T. Qualitative and quantitative assessment of the response of milkfish, *Chanos chanos* fry to low level copper exposure. In: Perkins FO, Cheng TC, ed. *Pathology in marine science*. San Diego: Academic press, 1990; 347-368;

[2] Roncero V, Duràn E, Soler F, Masot J, Gómez L. Morphometric, structural and ultrastructural studies of tench (*Tinca tinca L.*) hepatocytes after copper sulfate administration. *Environ Res* 1992; 57: 45-58

[3] Paris-Palacios S, Biagianti-Risbourg S, Vernet G. Biochemical and (ultra)structural hepatic perturbations of *Brachydanio rerio* exposed to two sublethal concentrations of copper sulfate. *Aquatic Toxicol* 2000, (in press).

[4] Tóth L, Juhasz M, Varga T, Csikkel-Szolnoki A, Nemcsok J. Some effect of $CuSO_4$ in carp. *J. Environ. Sci. Health* 1996; B31, 3: 627-635.

[5] Paris-Palacios S. Ecotoxicologie des pesticides et des métaux lourds susceptibles d'être présents dans le vignoble champenois: Etude de leur impact hépatique chez les Cyprinidés. PhD Thesis, 1999, Reims, France.

Metal Ions in Biology and Medicine; vol 6. Eds. J.A. Centeno, Ph. Collery, G. Vernet, R.B. Finkelman, H. Gibb, J.C. Etienne. John Libbey Eurotext, Paris © 2000, pp. 209-211.

Potential health effects of the heavy metals, depleted uranium and tungsten, used in amor-piercing munitions: comparison of neoplastic transformation, mutagenicity, genomic instability, and oncogenesis

Alexandra C. Miller, Jiaquan Xu, Michael Stewart, Christine Emond, Shelly Hodge, Consuelo Matthews, John Kalanich, David McClain

Armed Forces Radiobiology Research Institute (AFRRI), Bethesda, MD 20889

Abstract: The use of the heavy metals, depleted uranium (DU) and tungsten alloys (HMTA) in military applications worldwide could result in soldiers with imbedded heavy metal shrapnel. The acute and long-term health effects of exposure to these heavy metals are unknown. We have used both an *in vitro* human cell-model and rodent studies to examine the potential late health effects of these heavy metals. Data demonstrate that DU and HMTA are transforming and genotoxic agents *in vitro*. The *in vivo* effects of internalized DU include enhancement of mutagenicity and oncogene activation. Further carcinogenesis studies are warranted.

Introduction Limited data exist to permit an accurate assessment of risks for carcinogenesis and mutagenesis from depleted uranium (DU) embedded fragments or inhaled particulates. Ongoing studies are designed to provide information about the carcinogenic potential of DU using *in vitro* and *in vivo* assessments of morphological transformation, cytogenetic, mutagenic, and oncogenic effects (1-5). As a comparison, other military-projectile metals, i.e., tungsten alloys, and the known carcinogen, i.e., nickel, are being examined.

Materials and Methods: Human osteoblast cells (HOS) were cultured and used as previously described (1-5). DU-uranium oxide (50mg powder/ml) was used in all experiments. To mimic the tungsten alloy used in military applications, a pure mixture of W (92%), Ni (5%), and Co (3%) particles (made in the laboratory without extensive milling) was used This mixture is hereafter called HMTA. All other methods are detailed elsewhere (1-5).

Results and Discussion Quantitative and qualitative *in vitro* transformation studies were done to assess the carcinogenic potential of radiation and chemical hazards. Using a human cell model (HOS), we demonstrated that soluble and insoluble DU compounds can transform cells to the tumorigenic phenotype, characterized by morphological, biochemical, and oncogenic changes consistent with tumor cell behavior (Table I and 2,5). Specific changes include altered saturation density and increased clonability in soft-agar. Similarly, tungsten alloys, and nickel were also shown to be neoplastic transforming agents, although at a reduced frequency than DU (Table I). Furthermore, DU and tungsten alloys were shown to be genotoxic using the sister chromatid exchange (SCE), micronuclei, and alkaline filter elution assays. Exposure to a nontoxic, nontransforming dose of DU did induce a small but statistically significant increase in the number of dicentrics formed in cells.

Table I. HEAVY METAL-INDUCED NEOPLASTIC TRANSFORMATION, MUTAGENICITY, CYTOGENICITY, AND ONCOGENESIS : IN VITRO AND IN VIVO STUDIES

In vitro studies	DU	HMTA	Nickel	Tantalum
Transformation Frequency	↑	↑	↑	No change
Growth Rate	↑	↑	↑	No change
Tumorigenicity	↑	↑	↑	No change
Mutagenicity	↑	↑	↑	No change
Micronuclei	↑	↑	↑	No change
Chromosome Aberration	↑	↑	↑	No change
DNA Breakage	↑	↑	↑	No change
Dicentric Formation	↑	none	none	Nd[1]
***In vivo* studies**				
Uranium levels	↑	Nd	Nd	No change
Mutagenic Urine	↑	Nd	Nd	Nd
Ras Oncogene	↑	Nd	Nd	Nd
P53 Alteration	↑	Nd	Nd	Nd
BCl2 Alteration	↑	Nd	Nd	Nd

[1]Nd, not done

DU was shown to induce genomic instability, possibly linked to its tumorigenic potential or its ability to induce a short-term increased resistance to oxidative stress.

Studies with animals with embedded DU pellets demonstrated that increased tissue uranium content is associated with aberrant activation of several oncogenes and tumor suppressor genes associated with human carcinogenesis (Table I). Northern blot analysis of mRNA obtained from muscle tissue proximal to the implanted DU, showed an elevation in k*ras*, *bcl*-2 , and p53 gene expression. In contrast, tissues from animals with tantalum implants did not show this aberrant oncogene pattern. Using the Ames bacterial reversion assay, the mutagenic activity of DU was evaluated. Mutagenicity tests with animal urine indicate that urine with a high uranium content is mutagenic. This enhanced DU-induced mutagenicity in urine was both DU-dose and time- dependent (1).

The results in this study demonstrate that insoluble DU and HMTA can transform human cells to the tumorigenic phenotype. The mechanism of this transformation involves DNA damage induction and chromosomal damage. DU can induce chromosomal aberrations that are distinctly characteristic of radiation exposure suggesting that the alpha particle component of DU exposure may play a role in the transformation and genotoxic process. Interestingly, the results with DU and HMTA are consistent with those obtained with the known carcinogen, nickel. In contrast, the inert metal, tantalum, did not induce tumorigenic, mutagenic, or cytogenetic effects.

The *in vivo* results demonstrate that 1) DU is a mutagen and 2) that the enhanced urine-mutagenicity may be a useful marker of DU exposure. While the changes in oncogene and tumor suppressor gene status are inconclusive, this altered activity could indeed be a preneoplastic marker. Further studies are warranted to fully understand the potential late health effects caused by exposure to DU or tungsten alloys used in armor-piercing munitions. Taken together, these results suggest that long-term exposure to DU or HMTAs could potentially be critical to the development of neoplastic disease in humans.

References

1 Miller AC, Fuciarelli AF, Jackson WE, Ejnik EJ, Emond C, Strocko S, Hogan J, Page N, Pellmar T, Urinary and Serum Muatagenicity Studies with Rats Implanted with Depleted Uranium or Tantalum Pellets, *Mutagenesis*, 13(6):101-106, 1998.

2 Miller AC, Blakely WF, et al., Transformation of human osteoblast cells to the tumorigenic phenotype by depleted uranium-uranyl chloride, *Environmental Health Perspectives* 106:465-471, 1998.

3 Miller AC, Whittaker T, Hogan J, McBride S, and Benson K, Oncogenes as Biomarkers for Low Dose Radiation-induced Health effects. *Cancer Detection and Prevention*, 20(5), 1996.

4 Pellmar TC, Fuciarelli AF, Ejnik JW, Hamilton M, Hogan J, Strocko S, Emond C, Mottaz HM, Landauer MR (1999) Distribution of uranium in rats implanted with depleted uranium pellets. *Toxicological Sciences* **49**, 29-39.

5 Miller AC. Suppression of depleted uranium-induced neoplastic transformation by the phenyl fatty acid, phenylacetate. *Radiation Research* (in press).

Acknowledgements: The authors would like to thank Dr Terry Pellmar, Dr David Livengood, and Dr. John Ejnik for their invaluable assistance. This research was supported in part by the Armed Forces Radiobiology Research Institute. The views presented are those of the authors and do not reflect the official views of the Department of Defense or the U.S. government.

Metal Ions in Biology and Medicine; vol 6. Eds. J.A. Centeno, Ph. Collery, G. Vernet, R.B. Finkelman, H. Gibb, J.C. Etienne. John Libbey Eurotext, Paris © 2000, pp. 212-214.

Calcium nutriture and cancer risk; determination by bone mineral density in the NHANES-I follow-up

Richard Nelson, Victoria Persky, Mary Turyk, Jane Kim

Epidemiology/Biometry Division, University of Illinois School of Public Health, and Department of Surgery, University of Illinois College of Medicine at Chicago, Room 2204 (M/C) 957 University of Illinois Hospital, 1740 West Taylor, Chicago, Illinois 60612 USA, e. altohorn@uic.edu; p. 312 996 6935; F 312 996 2704

INTRODUCTION

Dietary calcium has long been thought to have an ameliorating effect on colorectal cancer risk. Some of the most powerful, meticulously designed and well conducted analytical studies in human epidemiology have been done in order to establish this relationship, so that, if supported, public health recommendations concerning cancer prevention might be made. However the data and analyses to date have been inconsistent in establishing dietary calcium as a colorectal cancer preventer [1,2]. This may have arisen for several reasons. One reason might be that calcium is not effective as a cancer preventative agent. This leaves the positive studies difficult to explain. Other reasons include inaccuracy in dietary recall in retrospective case/control studies, variations in subsequent intake when data are collected prospectively in cohort studies, separation of the effects of calcium from other components of dairy products, since it is dairy intake that is the primary source of measured calcium intake. In addition the intake or exposure to many other items greatly effect dietary calcium absorption including vitamin D, ethanol, vitamin C, lactose intolerance, fecal pH, physical activity [3], body mass index and estrogen. Variations in any of these not clearly separated from calcium intake would confound measures of calcium exposure. Prospective randomized studies of calcium supplementation, the ultimate test of effectiveness, have for a variety of reasons chosen many different end points as surrogates of colorectal cancer incidence, such as adenoma recurrence or mitotic activity of colonis mucosa. These have their own problems in establishing a direct relationship of calcium to colorectal cancer risk.

Might it not be better to determine if calcium is effective in the prevention of colorectal cancer by assessing the long term effect of dietary calcium exposure, using a technique which also assesses the effect of confounding variables in calcium nutriture: measuring bone mineral density and its relationship to subsequent colorectal cancer risk? Bone density has recently been reported in relation to breast cancer [4,5], with a weak relationship found between those with the highest bone density and subsequent breast cancer risk. These have been interpreted as establishing a relationship of breast cancer risk to estrogen exposure, also a difficult variable to quantify due to estrogens many sources: from ovaries, adipose tissue, dietary plant sources or pharmacologic sources [6]. In the following report a third cohort is examined, the NHANES I follow up, for the relationship of bone mineral density, measured at recruitment in 1971-1974, and subsequent cancer risk both of the breast and colorectum.

METHODS

The National Health and Nutrition Examination Surveys (NHANES) program was comprised of a series of cross sectional surveys by the National Center for Health Statistics. It was designed to provide nationally representative reference data and prevalence estimates for a variety of dietary and health measures and conditions. NHANES I data collection took place in 1971 - 1974. A subset of subjects aged 25-74 at the initial recruitment received a more detailed health examination which continued through 1975. This group was sampled as well in order to be representative of the United States population aged 25-74. This examination included a hand-wrist x-ray in 6413 subjects. Details of the x-ray technique can be obtained from NHANES public use files. The bone density of these x-rays has been read twice, initially by photodensitometry measurements of the phalanx and radius, and more recently the films were re-read by a technique called osteogram radiographic absorptiometry at Compumed, Inc. 153 films could not be read and a additional 213 more subjects were lost to follow-up, so the cohort described herein is comprised of 6046 NHANES follow-up subjects.

Both incidence and mortality of several cancers were obtained from NHANES public use files including cancers of the breast, colorectum, prostate, ovary and uterus. Additional data include gender, date of birth, height, weight and body mass index. The relationship of bone density to subsequent cancer risk was assessed for breast and colorectum, controlling for age. The analysis was then limited to individuals over the age of 60 years at the time of hand-wrist x-ray.

RESULTS

At the date of most recent follow up data, 1992, 93 colorectal cancers had occurred within the 6046 subjects of the bone density cohort, 67 breast cancers and 63 prostate cancers. Looking only at the 854 women who were over 60 years of age at the time of hand-wrist x-ray, only 21 breast cancers and 32 colorectal cancers have been reported. Contrary to previous reports, the number of breast cancers in those in the highest quartile of bone mineral density was lower (3) than the number seen in the lowest quartile (7). The odds ratio is 0.44, 95% confidence interval is 0.11 to 1.8. For colorectal cancer a similar trend was noted with fewer cancers (5) in the highest quartile compared to the lowest (8); OR=0.67, 0.21-2.1. An eight fold increase in the number of colorectal cancers, if these ratios were maintained, and a four fold increase in the number of breast cancers would have resulted in a statistically significant trend towards diminishing cancer risk with increasing bone mineral density.

DISCUSSION

The power of this study is hindered by the small number of cancers reported in follow-up in women past menopause at the time of hand-wrist x-ray. As more recent follow-up data become available, it will be most interesting to see if the relationships found in this preliminary analysis are maintained. If they are, the protective effect of calcium in colorectal cancer is strengthened and the balanced effect of calcium and estrogen in breast cancer risk made more complicated.

REFERENCES

1 Martinez ME, Willett WC. Calcium, vitamin-D, and colorectal cancer: a review of the epidemiologic evidence. Can Epid, Biomark & Prev.1998;7:163-8.

2 Nelson RL, Persky V, Turyk M. Determination of factors responsible for the declining incidence of colorectal cancer. Dis. Colon & Rectum. 1999;42:741-752.

3 Branca F. Physical activity, diet and skeletal health. Public Health Nutr. 1999;2(3A):391-6.

4 Cauley JA, Lucas FL, Kuller LH, Vogt MT, Browner WS, Cummings SR,. Bone mineral density and risk of breast cancer in older women; the study of osteoporotic fractures. JAMA.1996;276:1404-8.

5 Zhang Y, Kiel DP, Kreger BE, Cupples LA, Ellison RC, Dorgan JF, Schatzkin A, Levy D, Felson DT. Bone mass and the risk of breast cancer among postmenopausal women. N Eng J Med.1997;336:611-7.

6 Grodstein F, Newcomb PA, Stampfer MJ. Postmenopausal hormone therapy and the risk of colorectal cancer: a review and meta-analysis. Am J Med.1999;106:574-82.

Metal Ions in Biology and Medicine; vol 6. Eds. J.A. Centeno, Ph. Collery, G. Vernet, R.B. Finkelman, H. Gibb, J.C. Etienne. John Libbey Eurotext, Paris © 2000, pp. 215-217.

Trace metals in differentiated neuroblasts treated with retinoic acid, an anti-cancer drug

B. Gouget, C. Sergeant, Ch. Hamon, Y. Llabador, J. Bénard, M. Simonoff

Laboratoire de Chimie Nucléaire Analytique et Bioenvironnementale, CNRS UMR 5084, Le Haut Vigneau, BP 120, 33175 Gradignan cedex, France

Abstract

Fe and Zn contents have been measured by PIXE analysis in 3 human neuroblastoma cell lines treated with retinoic acid [RA] and expressing various amounts of the N-myc protein. RA-treatment does not modify trace metal contents in non-amplified neuroblasts but highly increases Fe and Zn levels in N-*myc* amplified cells. These results indicate that a relationship exists between intracellular trace metals and N-myc expression, and may suggest a role of trace metals in RA antitumor activity.

Introduction

Neuroblastoma [NB], a common solid tumor of childhood, can be characterized by specific genetic abnormalities, such as the amplification of the N-*myc* oncogene, a transcription factor regulating cell proliferation. The level of the N-myc protein synthesized by NB cells is directly related to the number of N-*myc* copies per haploid genome. *In vitro*, the incubation of NB cells with RA leads to inhibition of cell growth and reduces tumorigenicity. RA is a differentiating agent that transforms neuroblasts to neural cells with neuritis outgrowth. Cell differentiation by RA has been shown to down-regulate the N-myc transcript levels.

Previous studies have shown that a deregulation of intracellular trace metal contents can affect cell proliferation, gene expression and can even lead to oncogenesis. In a foregoing study, we compared Fe and Zn contents in monolayers of 3 human NB cell lines characterized by various degrees of N-*myc* oncogene amplification [1]. A relationship was found to exist between intracellular trace metals and N-*myc* oncogene amplification and our work confirmed the determinant role of trace elements in mechanisms of NB oncogenesis, whereby N-*myc* amplified cell lines represented more aggressive phenotypes of the disease. In order to investigate further the relationship between the N-myc expression and intracellular Fe and Zn concentrations in the same line, we determined trace metal contents in both RA-differentiated and non-differentiated neuroblasts. This procedure led to a better understanding of the mechanism of action of RA in NB regression.

The particle-induced X-ray emission technique [PIXE] that we used in this study is of particular interest in the biological field [2]. Various advantages such as multi-elemental response, high X-ray production efficiency coupled to a low radiation background and a good sensitivity (minimum detection limits of μg/g) make this method very competitive for the analysis of intracellular Fe and Zn trace metal concentrations.

Materials and Methods

IGR-N-91, IMR-32 and SK-N-SH NB cell lines, presenting respectively 60, 25 and 1 copies of the N-*myc* oncogene, were grown as referenced in [3]. All-trans retinoic acid, diluted in dimethyl sulfoxide [DMSO] was added directly to the growth medium to a final concentration of 10 or 20 μM. Control cultures contained the same volume of the solvent alone (DMSO).

For PIXE analysis of NB cell pellets, an original protocol has been set up in the laboratory. It is based on a concentration of the sample to a minimal volume (up to 10^7 cells in 150 μl). Briefly, cells were cultivated in Petri dishes, with or without RA. They were harvested with a scraper at the end of the exponential growth phase (48 hr after seeding) and washed by suspension in Eagle's salt solution. Cells were counted with a haemocytometer and centrifuged. The cell pellet was resuspended in 100 μl of ultra-pure water completed with 50 μl of yttrium solution as internal standard. Drops of the suspension were deposited onto a thin polycarbonate film and desiccated at 45°C. The target was then bombarded with a 2.5 MeV proton beam of 80 nA, from the Bordeaux CENG facility. Elemental concentrations were deduced from the X-ray intensities and normalized to the yttrium signal. Statistical analysis of trace metal contents in the three cell lines was carried out with the non-parametric Mann-Whitney test.

Results

As already described, we observed that RA induced morphologic differentiation of NB cells: SK-N-SH neuroblasts (neural cells) developed long neurites and IGR-N-91 cells (substrate-adherent cells) transformed morphotype to a neural type. Moreover, PIXE analysis allowed a quantitative measure of Fe and Zn contents of SK-N-SH, IMR-32 and IGR-N-91 neuroblasts, incubated with 10 or 20 μM RA for 24 and 48 hr. As presented in Table 1, incubation of IMR-32 (25 copies of N-*myc*) or IGR-N-91 cells (60 copies of N-*myc*) with 20 μM RA highly increased Fe and Zn concentrations as compared to DMSO alone (respectively 7- and 3-fold higher for IMR-32 cells and 7-fold higher for the IGR-N-91 cell line). On the other hand, Fe and Zn contents in the SK-N-SH cell line (1 copy of N-*myc*) were not modified by a 48-hr treatment with 20 μM RA. Moreover, the incubation of the three NB lines with 20 μM RA for 24 hr, or a treatment with 10 μM RA for 24 or 48 hr were not sufficient to modify trace metal contents (data not shown).

Discussion

Retinoic acid has been shown to induce cell morphological differentiation and to reverse the malignant phenotype of various tumors, such as neuroblastoma. *In vitro*, neuroblasts of the SK-N-SH and IGR-N-91 cell lines present a neuritic outgrowth and an inhibited proliferation after incubation with RA. N-myc transcript levels gradually decrease up to 95% in IGR-N-91 N-*myc* amplified cells treated with 10 μM RA, whereas they are unchanged in the non-amplified SK-N-SH cell line [4]. RA highly decreases N-myc expression in N-*myc* amplified cell lines: cells acquire the morphotype of non-aggressive NB cells (neural cells) and intracellular Fe and Zn contents tend to increase as in the non-amplified cell line. The increase in Fe and Zn concentrations of NB cells cultivated with RA is directly correlated with the degree of N-*myc* amplification in the cell line. Conversely, the N-myc protein is only weakly synthesized in cells of the non-amplified cell line and RA cannot highly decrease its expression. Trace metal concentrations are not significantly modified.

The morphological transformation of NB cultured cells by RA (from the S- to the N-type) is correlated with an alteration of the extracellular matrix [ECM]. Indeed, cell differentiation leads to an increase in the activity of zinc-metalloenzymes: the matrix metalloproteinases [MMP]. A major target gene for RA is the collagenase MMP-1, an enzyme which can degrade one of the principal components of ECM, the interstitial collagen. In a previous study, we established an oncogenic concept, which explains the correlations between trace metals and NB genesis in terms of MMP expression and

formation of metastases. In the course of NB carcinogenesis, neuroblasts first synthesize large amounts of Tissue Inhibitors of Metalloproteinases [TIMP] which protect cells against an aggressive phenotype. In a second stage, NB cells overexpress N-myc and the MMP counter-balance the TIMP. RA-treated SK-N-SH cells do not express MMP activators like MT-MMP and cannot activate the Zn-metalloproteinase MMP-2 [5]. Thus, SK-N-SH cells incubated with RA do not present high Zn concentrations compared to controls. Kikkawa showed that RA inhibits tumor invasion by preventing MMP secretion [6]. The MMP are then sequestered into the cells. Thus, N-*myc* amplified cells treated with RA present very high Zn concentrations. RA could be partially responsible for a decrease in N-*myc* carcinogen properties by inhibiting MMP activation.
In conclusion, this study shows for the first time the influence of retinoic acid, an anticancer drug used for the treatment of neuroblastoma, on intracellular trace metal concentrations. It enables the comparison of trace metal contents in cells of the same cell line presenting various degrees of oncogene expression.

Acknowledgments

The authors thank Professor J. MacCordick for critical reading of the manuscript.

References

[1] Gouget B, Sergeant C, Llabador Y, Bénard J, Simonoff M. N-*myc* oncogene amplification is correlated with trace metal concentrations in neuroblastoma cultured cells. *Nucl Instr Meth Phys Res B* Submitted.
[2] Llabador Y, Moretto Ph. Nuclear microprobes in the life sciences. Singapore: World Scientific, 1998.
[3] Ferrandis E, Bénard J. Activation of the human MDR1 gene promoter in differentiated neuroblasts. *Int J Cancer* 1993; 54: 987-991.
[4] Ikegaki N, Temeles G, Kennett RH. Modulation of protein expression associated with chemically induced differentiation of neuroblastoma cells. *Adv Neuroblastoma Res* 1991; 3: 157-163.

[5] Tiberio A, Farina AR, Tacconelli A, Cappabianca L, Gulino A, Mackay AR. Retinoic acid-enhanced invasion through reconstituted basement membrane by human SK-N-SH neuroblastoma cells involves membrane-associated tissue-type plasminogen activator. *Int J Cancer* 1997; 73: 740-748.
[6] Kikkawa F. Regulation of matrix-degrading enzymes in gynecologic cancer tissues and cells. *Nippon Sanka Fujinka Gakkai Zasshi* 1996; 48: 618-622.

Cell line	Content	**No treatment**	**DMSO**	**RA 20 µM**
SK-N-SH	Fe	$24{,}4 \pm 7{,}0^{a}$	$23{,}8 \pm 9{,}7^{b}$	$21{,}8 \pm 7{,}7^{b}$
	Zn	$43{,}8 \pm 11{,}7^{a}$	$49{,}1 \pm 3{,}2^{b}$	$52{,}5 \pm 17{,}0^{b}$
IMR-32	Fe	$26{,}4 \pm 6{,}5^{c}$	$16{,}7 \pm 6{,}9^{b}$	$111{,}5 \pm 4{,}4^{b*}$
	Zn	$71{,}8 \pm 21{,}8^{c}$	$78{,}3 \pm 26{,}0^{b}$	$246{,}3 \pm 9{,}9^{b*}$
IGR-N-91	Fe	$20{,}2 \pm 4{,}6^{a}$	$50{,}2 \pm 14{,}4^{b}$	$407{,}1 \pm 70{,}0^{b*}$
	Zn	$58{,}7 \pm 11{,}7^{a}$	$64{,}3 \pm 20{,}0^{b}$	$435{,}9 \pm 74{,}0^{b*}$

Table 1: Means ± SD ([a]14, [b]3 and [c]10 analyses) of Fe and Zn concentrations, in µg/g of proteins, in neuroblasts incubated without treatment, after 48 hr-incubation with 20 µM RA in DMSO and after a treatment with the correspondent volume of DMSO (controls).
-Significant levels p<1‰ of RA vs. DMSO are represented by asterisks-

Metal Ions in Biology and Medicine; vol 6. Eds. J.A. Centeno, Ph. Collery, G. Vernet, R.B. Finkelman, H. Gibb, J.C. Etienne. John Libbey Eurotext, Paris © 2000, pp. 218-220.

Tumor growth after subcutaneous injection is affected by hepatic zinc-metallothionein level

Haruna Tamano, Shuichi Enomoto, Emi Igasaki[1], Naoto Oku[1], Norio Itoh[2], Keiichi Tanaka[2], and Atsushi Takeda[1]

Riken (The Institute of Physical and Chemical Research), Wako, Saitama, Japan, [1] Department of Radiobiochemistry, School of Pharmaceutical Sciences, University of Shizuoka, Shizuoka, Japan, [2] Department of Toxicology, Graduate School of Pharmaceutical Sciences, Osaka University, Suita, Osaka, Japan

Metallothionein (MT) is an intracellular zinc-binding protein and may be involved in cellular zinc homeostasis. The increases of hepatic zinc and MT, without an appreciable change in copper level, were found in murines after transplantation of tumors such as Ehrlich carcinoma, sarcoma 180 and ascites hepatoma 7974F into the inguinal region (1). This increase occurs only in the liver, and is inhibited by the feeding with zinc-deficient diet (2). The characteristic increase of hepatic MT was also observed in carcinogen-treated murines (3). The mechanism of MT induction in the liver by tumor transplantation is different from those by administration of inflammation-inducing materials and immobilization stress; zinc may play a key role for MT induction in the liver after tumor transplantation (2). Zinc is an important nutrient for malignant tissues and abnormal growth of malignant tissues is effectively inhibited by dietary zinc deprivation (4). Therefore, it is considered that a scramble for zinc occurs between host and malignant tissue. Clarification of zinc metabolism in tumor-bearing animals is important to understand zinc homeostasis in the vertebrate.

Because the prefeeding with zinc-deficient diet for 1 week suppressed the increases of zinc and MT in the liver after tumor transplantation (2), zinc level in hepatic cytosolic MT fraction was determined 9 days after subcutaneous transplantation of Ehrlich carcinoma by means of Sephadex G-75 gel filtration. The increase of zinc in hepatic cytosolic MT fraction of tumor-bearing mice was inhibited by the dietary zinc deprivation (5). These results suggest that dietary zinc absorbed from the gut is necessary for apo-MT induction in the liver after tumor transplantation and is incorporated into the induced apo-MT.

One hour after i.v. injection of $^{65}ZnCl_2$, ^{65}Zn uptake in the liver of tumor-bearing mice was higher than that of control mice and that of the former was increased with the increase of tumor weight (6). On the other hand, ^{65}Zn uptake and zinc concentration in the liver of mice injected with turpentine or carrageenan were increased transiently; the mechanism of zinc uptake in the liver of inflammation-induced mice may be different from that of tumor-bearing mice. Zinc may be preferentially accumulated in the liver of tumor-bearing mice in the form of zinc-MT (7,8).

In the present study, ^{65}Zn distribution in the liver, pancreas and blood was compared between control and tumor-bearing mice after intravenous injection of $^{65}ZnCl_2$ (5). Ten minutes after injection, ^{65}Zn uptake in the liver of tumor-bearing mice was remarkably higher than that of control mice, whereas ^{65}Zn uptake in the pancreas and ^{65}Zn level in the blood of the former were much lower than those of the latter. The high uptake of zinc in the liver may lead to apo-MT induction. ^{65}Zn level in the liver of tumor-bearing mice was higher than that of control mice until 72 h after injection, suggesting that the ^{65}Zn taken up in the liver is incorporated into the induced apo-MT and that ^{65}Zn-MT formed is retained in the liver. On the other hand, ^{65}Zn levels in the pancreas and blood of the tumor-bearing mice were lower than those of the control mice until 24 h and 6 h, respectively, after injection. Judging from the clearance of ^{65}Zn from the blood, ^{65}Zn distribution in normal mice may be completed around 24 h after injection, whereas that in tumor-bearing mice may be completed around 6 h after injection. These results indicate that hepatic zinc response via MT induction influences zinc metabolism in the body after tumor transplantation. It is likely that the formation of zinc-MT in the liver of tumor-bearing mice makes blood zinc less available for other tissues such as pancreas.

^{65}Zn uptake in the liver of tumor-bearing mice treated with cadmium chloride, which induced MT synthesis in the liver of tumor-bearing mice, was significantly higher than that of control tumor-bearing mice. On the other hand, ^{65}Zn uptake in the tumor and ^{65}Zn level in the blood of the former were significantly lower than those of the latter (4). To study the influence of hepatic MT induction on zinc metabolism in tumor-bearing mice, ^{65}Zn distribution was determined using MT-deficient tumor-bearing mice. ^{65}Zn uptake in the liver of MT-deficient tumor-bearing mice was lower than that of control tumor-bearing mice 1 h after injection. The increase of hepatic MT was not observed in MT-deficient mice after tumor transplantation. On the other hand, ^{65}Zn uptake in the tumor and ^{65}Zn level in the blood of MT-deficient tumor-bearing mice were higher than those of control tumor-bearing mice. Dietary zinc taken up in the liver may not be stored in MT-deficient tumor-bearing mice and more zinc may be secreted from the liver to the blood. There might be more exchangeable zinc in the blood of MT-deficient tumor-bearing mice than in that of control tumor-bearing mice. Zinc level in the plasma of MT-deficient mice is higher than that of control mice. The high level of zinc in the plasma of MT-deficient mice would be due to the disruption of zinc homeostasis. Therefore, MT would be useful for zinc homeostasis in the body. Moreover, tumor weight increased significantly ($p<0.05$) in MT-deficient mice than in control mice 12 days after tumor transplantation, indicating that MT deficiency promotes tumor growth.

There is a possibility that factors secreted from tumor cells induce MT synthesis in the liver after tumor transplantation. Media (0.2 ml) cultured with Ehrlich carcinoma and AH7974F cells were subcutaneously injected into mice and rats, respectively, once a day for 4 days and hepatic MT levels were determined 24 h after the last injection. Hepatic MT was increased by neither administration, suggesting that factors secreted from tumor cells do not cause hepatic MT induction. Hepatic MT may be induced as a host defense against the growth of tumor.

In conclusion, hepatic zinc response via MT induction influences zinc metabolism in the body after tumor transplantation. The formation of zinc-MT in the liver of tumor-bearing mice may make blood zinc less available for other tissues including tumor.

References

1. Takeda, A., Sato, T., Tamano. H., Okada, S., Biochem. Biophys. Res. Commun. 189, 645-649 (1992)

2. Takeda, A., Tamano, H., Sato, T., Goto, K., Okada, S., Biochim. Biophys. Acta 1243, 325-328 (1995)

3. Takeda, A., Tamano, H., Hoshino, A., Okada, S., Biol. Trace Elem. Res. 41, 157-164 (1994)

4. Takeda, A., Goto, K., Okada, S., Biol. Trace Elem. Res. 59, 23-29 (1997)

5. Tamano, H., Igasaki, E., Enomoto, S., Oku, N., Itoh, N., Kimura, T., Tanaka, K., Takeda, A., submitted

6. Takeda, A., Sato, T., Okada S., Nucl. Med. Biol. 21, 71-75 (1994)

7. Takeda, A., Tamano H., Okada S., Nucl. Med. Biol. 22, 133-136 (1995)

8. Takeda, A., Goto, K., Sato T., Tamano H., Okada, S., J. Trace Elem. Exp. Med. 10, 243-248 (1997)

Metal Ions in Biology and Medicine; vol 6. Eds. J.A. Centeno, Ph. Collery, G. Vernet, R.B. Finkelman, H. Gibb, J.C. Etienne. John Libbey Eurotext, Paris © 2000, pp. 221-223.

Iron chelators as potential anti-neoplastic agents: their effect on molecules involved in proliferation

Lovejoy D., Gao J. and Richardson D.R.

The Heart Research Institute, 145 Missenden Rd, Camperdown, Sydney, 2050, Australia

Introduction

We have demonstrated that some analogues of the iron (Fe) chelator, pyridoxal isonicotinoyl hydrazone (PIH), show high anti-tumour activity being far more effective than desferrioxamine (DFO) [1-4]. These studies have been initiated due to observations that DFO can markedly inhibit the growth of the childhood cancer neuroblastoma both *in vitro* in cell culture studies and also in clinical trials [for reviews see 3].

In this investigation we have assessed the effect of DFO and one of the most active chelators (2-hydroxy-1-naphthylaldehyde isonicotinoyl hydrazone; 311) on molecular targets involved in proliferation. In particular, we have assessed the effect of the chelators on the RNA-binding activity of the iron-regulatory protein 1 (IRP1) that is a master regulator of intracellular Fe metabolism [3]. Since very little is known concerning the effect of chelators on the cell cycle, we have examined the p53-responsive genes *WAF1* (wild-type p53 activating fragment 1 gene), *GADD-45* (growth arrest and DNA damage gene), and human *mdm-2* (murine double minute gene). WAF-1 is a potent universal inhibitor of cyclin-dependent kinases, and can induce a G_1/S arrest and possibly a G_2/M arrest [5]. GADD-45 is induced upon DNA damage and can arrest the cell cycle and is also involved in DNA nucleotide excision repair [5]. On the other hand, p53-mediated transactivation of *mdm-2* results in a feedback control mechanism of p53 activity [5]. Interestingly, both the expression of *WAF1* and *GADD45* can also be controlled by p53-independent pathways.

Materials and Methods

A variety of techniques have been used in the present study including ligand-binding assays (^{59}Fe-transferrin), gel-retardation analysis, plus Western and Northern analysis.

Results and Discussion

Ligand 311 was far more active than DFO at increasing ^{59}Fe mobilization and preventing ^{59}Fe uptake from ^{59}Fe-transferrin (Tf) by SK-N-MC neuroepithelioma and BE-2 neuroblastoma (NB) cells [1,2,4]. For example, at a chelator concentration of 2.5 μM, 311 increased cellular ^{59}Fe release from prelabelled SK-N-MC cells to 35%, while DFO released 4%.

Like DFO, 311 increased the RNA-binding activity of the iron-regulatory proteins (IRPs). However, despite the far greater Fe chelation efficacy of 311 compared to DFO, a similar increase in IRP RNA-binding activity occurred after a 2-4 h incubation with either chelator [4]. These results suggest that irrespective of the Fe chelation efficacy of a ligand, an increase in IRP-RNA-binding activity occurred via a time-dependent step [4]. Furthermore, the increase in IRP-RNA binding activity occurred in the presence of the protein synthesis inhibitor, cycloheximide. These latter results suggest that the increase in RNA-binding activity observed after exposure to the chelators was not due to an elevation in IRP synthesis [4].

Further studies examined the effect of 311 and DFO on the expression of p53-transactivated genes that are crucial for cell cycle control and DNA repair, namely *WAF1*, *GADD45*, and *mdm-2* [4]. Incubation of 3 different cell lines (SK-N-MC neuroblastoma, BE-2 neuroblastoma, or K562 erythroleukemia) with DFO or 311 caused a pronounced concentration- and time-dependent increase in the expression of *WAF1* and *GADD45* mRNA, but not *mdm-2* mRNA [4]. In accordance with the distinct differences in Fe chelation efficacy and anti-proliferative activity of DFO and 311, much higher levels of DFO (150 μM) than 311 (2.5-5 μM) were required to increase *GADD45* and *WAF1* mRNA levels. The increase in *GADD45* and *WAF1* mRNA expression was seen only after a 20 h exposure to the ligands and was reversible [4]. In contrast to the chelators, the Fe(III) complexes of DFO and 311 had no effect on increasing *GADD45* and *WAF1* mRNA levels. The increase in *GADD45* and *WAF1* mRNAs appeared to occur by a p53-independent pathway in SK-N-MC and K562 cells, as these cell lines lack functional p53 [4].

The increase in *WAF1* mRNA expression after exposure to 311 was observed in a number of other cell lines including IMR-32 neuroblastoma cells, SK-N-SH neuroblastoma cells, and MCF-7 breast cancer cells. These latter cell lines have native p53, much of which is sequestered. In cell lines with and without wild-type p53, the level of *p53* mRNA or protein was not significantly affected by 311. Further studies are essential in order to determine if the chelator-mediated increase in WAF1 and GADD45 expression can occur by both p53-dependent and p53-independent pathways.

Since DFO and the PIH analogues act at G1/S of the cell cycle [2-4], it is important to understand the effect of the chelators on the molecular mechanisms which control progression through this important regulatory region. The proliferating cell nuclear antigen (PCNA), retinoblastoma protein (Rb), and cyclins D1 and E, are essential for progression through the G_1/S phase of the cell cycle [5]. Western blot analysis demonstrated that neither chelator had any effect on the expression of PCNA. However, on a molar basis, 311 was far more effective than DFO at causing hypophosphorylation of Rb and at decreasing cyclin D1 levels. For example, cyclin D1 was undetectable after a 30 h incubation of SK-N-MC cells with 75-150 μM DFO, whereas similar results were observed with 311 at only 2.5 μM. In contrast to these latter results, cyclin E was increased as a function of chelator concentration.

The paradoxical effects of the chelators on cyclins D1 and E was unexpected, but may be related to the different functions of these molecules in G_1/S progression. It can be speculated that the increase in cyclin E levels may be a response in order to overcome the G_1/S arrest induced by the chelators. Together with our results on *GADD45* and *WAF1* expression, these latter data demonstrate that Fe plays a crucial role in controlling the expression of molecules that play important functions in regulating the cell cycle.

The present study has clearly demonstrated that DFO and 311 effect a variety of molecular targets involved in the cell cycle and proliferation. Moreover, 311 is far more potent than DFO and may have potential as an effective anti-neoplastic agent.

References

1. Richardson DR, Tran E, Ponka P. The potential of iron chelators of the pyridoxal isonicotinoyl hydrazone class as effective anti-proliferative agents. *Blood* 1995; 86: 4295-306.

2. Richardson DR, Milnes K. The potential of iron chelators of the pyridoxal isonicotinoyl hydrazone class as effective antiproliferative agents II. The mechanism of action of ligands derived from salicylaldehyde benzoyl hydrazone and 2-hydroxy-1-naphthylaldehyde benzoyl hydrazone. *Blood* 1997; 89 :3025-38.

3. Richardson DR. Potential of iron chelators as effective anti-proliferative agents. *Can J Physiol Pharmacol* 1997; 75: 1164-80.

4. Darnell G, Richardson DR. The potential of iron chelators of the pyridoxal isonicotinoyl hydrazone class as effective antiproliferative agents III. The effect of the ligands on molecular targets involved in proliferation. *Blood* 1999; 94: 781-92.

5. Agarwal ML, Taylor WR, Chernov MV, Chernova OB, Stark GR. The p53 network. J Biol Chem 1998; 273 : 1-4.

Metal Ions in Biology and Medicine; vol 6. Eds. J.A. Centeno, Ph. Collery, G. Vernet, R.B. Finkelman, H. Gibb, J.C. Etienne. John Libbey Eurotext, Paris © 2000, pp. 224-226.

Structure-activity relationships of novel chelators with anti-cancer activity: the "NT" series

Lovejoy D.[a], Bernhardt P.V.[b], and Richardson D.R.[a]

[a] *The Heart Research Institute, 145 Missenden Rd Camperdown 2050, Australia;* [b] *Department of Chemistry, University of Queensland, Brisbane, 4072, Australia*

Introduction

Our previous investigations have demonstrated that cellular iron (Fe) is a major molecular target of the chelator pyridoxal isonicotinoyl hydrazone (PIH) and its analogues [1-3]. Compared to desferrioxamine (DFO) which is the Fe chelator currently used to treat Fe-overload, PIH and many of its analogues are far more efficient at removing intracellular Fe and preventing cellular Fe uptake from transferrin. Anti-tumour properties of DFO, particularly against neuroblastoma and leukemia, have been well described both in cell culture studies and in clinical trials [for review see 4]. Importantly, the PIH analogue 2-hydroxy-1-naphthaldehyde isonicotinoyl hydrazone (311; see Figure 1) and several related chelators possess *in vitro* anti-tumour activity that is much greater than DFO [1-4].

Fig. 1

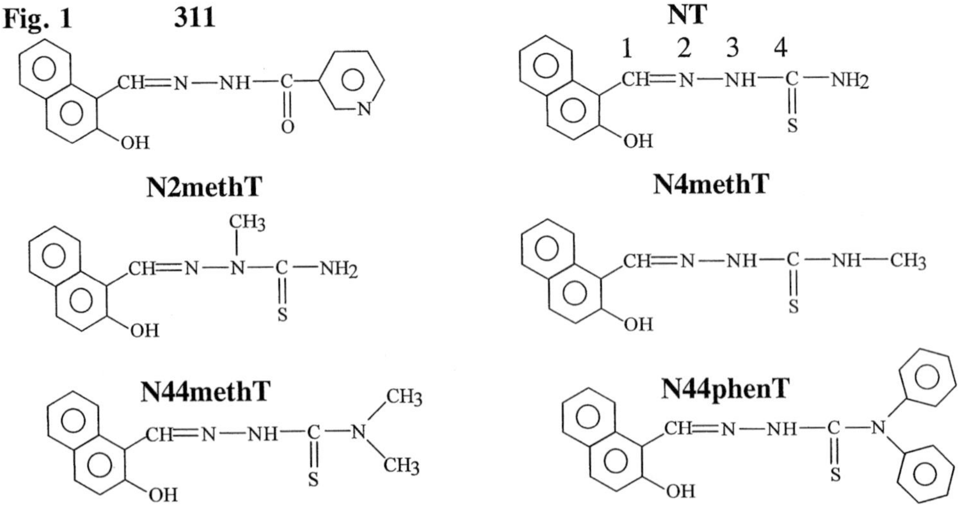

From our studies of the PIH analogues, we have identified the salicylaldehyde and 2-hydroxy-1-naphthylaldehyde moeities as structural components which infer anti-neoplastic activity [1]. Since a related group of chelators known as the thiosemicarbazones also demonstrate anti-tumour activity, we have designed and synthesized a new group of ligands by condensation of the aldehydes described above with a range of thiosemicarbazides. In the present investigation, the effect of these chelators on Fe uptake from Tf and Fe release from SK-N-MC neuroepithelioma cells has been examined together with their effect on cellular proliferation.

Materials and Methods

Several techniques have been used in the present study including ligand-binding experiments (^{59}Fe-transferrin; ^{59}Fe-Tf) and cellular proliferation assays (ie., MTT assay).

Results and Discussion

The parent compound of this new series of chelators, 2-hydroxy-1-naphthlaldehyde thiosemicarbazone (NT; Fig. 1), showed anti-tumour activity (IC_{50} = 0.5 μM) that was very similar to the most effective aroylhydrazone ligand yet identified, namely chelator 311 (IC_{50} = 0.3 μM). The anti-proliferative activity observed for these ligands was far greater than that seen with DFO (IC_{50} = 45 μM).

The anti-proliferative activity of 311 or NT was not correlated with their ability to inhibit ^{59}Fe uptake from ^{59}Fe-Tf or increase ^{59}Fe efflux from cells. Comparing the ability of these two chelators to increase ^{59}Fe mobilization from cells prelabelled with ^{59}Fe-Tf, NT resulted in the release of 13% of cellular ^{59}Fe, whereas NIH released 43%. Additionally, NT inhibited ^{59}Fe uptake from ^{59}Fe-transferrin (Tf) by only 20%, whereas NIH decreased it to over 90%. The NT analogue N44methT, which has lower anti-proliferative activity than NT, effluxed 43% of cellular ^{59}Fe and inhibited ^{59}Fe uptake by 95%.

To further assess the anti-proliferative mechanism of NT, the Fe(III) complex of the ligand was synthesized. In marked contrast to the NIH-Fe(III) complex which shows little anti-proliferative action [3,5], the Fe(III)-complex of NT demonstrated similar activity to NT alone. These data suggest that the anti-proliferative activity of NT may be due to the formation of the Fe(III) complex which could possibly redox cycle or interact directly with crucial biological targets.

Substitution of a methyl group at the 2-position of NT, leading to the chelator N2methT (Fig. 1), resulted in a marked decrease in anti-proliferative activity (IC_{50} > 12.5 μM). This substitution also resulted in a decrease in the ability of the chelator to mobilise ^{59}Fe from prelabelled cells. However, methyl group substitution at the 4-position of NT, producing the ligand N4methT (Fig. 1), led to an analogue with comparable activity to NT (IC_{50} = 0.5 μM) and a considerable increase in Fe chelation activity. These data suggest that substitution of a methyl group at the 2-position hinders delocalisation of the conjugate bond system, and hence, metal ion binding. These results are additional evidence that the anti-proliferative activity of NT may be due to its ability to form a metal ion complex.

In further exploring the structure-activity relationships of this new series, we found that anti-proliferative activity decreased as hydrophobic bulk increased at the 4-position of NT (Fig. 1). For example, 2-hydroxy-1-naphthylaldehyde-4,4-dimethyl thiosemicarbazone (N44methT; Fig. 1) demonstrates pronounced Fe chelation efficacy but slightly lower anti-proliferative activity than NT (IC_{50} = 1.5 μM). A further increase in hydrophobic bulk results in an additional decrease in anti-proliferative activity. For example, 2-hydroxy-1-naphthylaldehyde-4,4-diphenyl thiosemicarbazone (N44phenT; Fig. 1) has an IC_{50} of 5 μM. However, both N44methT and N44phenT are appreciably more effective than NT at mobilizing ^{59}Fe from SK-N-MC neuroepithelioma cells. In fact, the N44methT analogue is one of the most effective ligands yet screened in terms of its Fe chelation efficacy. By understanding the structure-activity relationships of these ligands, effective chelators for clinical use may be designed.

References

1. Richardson DR, Tran E, Ponka P. The potential of iron chelators of the pyridoxal isonicotinoyl hydrazone class as effective anti-proliferative agents. *Blood* 1995; 86: 4295-306.

2. Richardson DR, Milnes K. The potential of iron chelators of the pyridoxal isonicotinoyl hydrazone class as effective antiproliferative agents II. The mechanism of action of ligands derived from salicylaldehyde benzoyl hydrazone and 2-hydroxy-1-naphthylaldehyde benzoyl hydrazone. *Blood* 1997; 89 :3025-38.

3. Darnell G, Richardson DR. The potential of iron chelators of the pyridoxal isonicotinoyl hydrazone class as effective antiproliferative agents III. The effect of the ligands on molecular targets involved in proliferation. *Blood* 1999; 94 :781-92.

4. Richardson DR. Potential of iron chelators as effective anti-proliferative agents. *Can J Physiol Pharmacol* 1997; 75: 1164-80.

5. Richardson, D.R. and Bernhardt, P. Crystal and molecular structure of 2-hydroxy-1-naphthylaldehyde isonicotinoyl hydrazone (NIH) and its iron(III) complex: An iron chelator with anti-proliferative activity. *J. Biol. Inorg. Chem.* 1999; 4: 266-73.

Metal Ions in Biology and Medicine; vol 6. Eds. J.A. Centeno, Ph. Collery, G. Vernet, R.B. Finkelman, H. Gibb, J.C. Etienne. John Libbey Eurotext, Paris © 2000, pp. 227-229.

Modern principles for the characterisation of worker's exposure in nickel refineries

Yngvar Thomassen[1], Siri Hetland[1], Wolfgang Koch[2], Evert Nieboer[3], Hugo M. Ortner[4], James H. Vincent[5] and Valeri Tchatchtchine[6]

[1] National Institute of Occupational Health, P.O. Box 8149 Dep, N-0033 Oslo, Norway; [2] Fraunhofer Institute of Toxicology and Aerosol Research, D-30625 Hannover, Germany; [3] Department of Biochemistry and Occupational Health Program, McMaster University, Health Science Centre, 1200 Main Street West, Hamilton, ON, Canada, L8N 3Z5; [4] Material Science Department, Technical University of Darmstadt, D-64287 Darmstadt, Germany; [5] Department of Environmental and Industrial Health, School of Public Health, 109 S. Observatory Street, Ann Arbor, MI 48109, U.S.A.; [6] Kola Research Laboratory for Occupational Health, Kirovsk, Russia

The cancer risk in the nickel refining industry appears to depend on the nickel species inhaled. Exposure to nickel oxides and sulfides, which are relatively insoluble in water, figures prominently in the epidemiology of nickel-related lung and nasal cancer and the International Committee on Nickel Carcinogenesis in Man (ICNCM) identified four classes of nickel compounds as having different intrinsic activity or biological availability as cancer causing agents [1]. The specific categories were sulfidic, oxidic, metallic and water-soluble nickel. Since these categories are operationally defined, they do not provide detailed information about the specific chemical composition and morphological characteristics of individual aerosol particles. Such knowledge would improve our understanding of the basis for the reported different health risks. A parallel development was the adoption of particle size-selective criteria by the International Standard Organisation (ISO)/American Conference of Governmental and Industrial Hygienists (ACGIH)/Comité Europeén Normalisation (CEN) guidelines for workplace exposure. In the light of the demand from standards setting bodies worldwide, the need for a realistic assessment of occupational aerosol exposures in relation to specific disease outcomes has stimulated the development of sampling instruments to measure these health related aerosol fractions (inhalable, extrathoracic, thoracic, tracheobronchial and respirable).

Until recently, reproductive and developmental effects in humans have not been reported in conjuction with occupational exposure to nickel compounds. Russian studies have, however, expressed concern about an apparent increase in spontaneous abortions among females employed in the nickel refinery at Monchegorsk [2].

Our aim is to illustrate how modern technology used in aerosol measurement and characterisation can provide detailed information about the specific particle-size distribution, time-resolved concentration monitoring of particle-size fractions, chemical composition and morphological characteristics of workroom aerosols collected during production of nickel.

Methods

Particle-size distribution measurements were made with personal inhalable dust spectrometer (PIDS). This instrument is based on an 8-stage cascade impactor with an additional entry stage at the top and a backing filter at the bottom, requiring the gravimetric and/or chemical analysis of 10 individual samples.

A novel instrument for personal, time-resolved concentration monitoring and sampling of the five above defined health-related aerosol fractions has been developed. This instrument combines inertial classification, filter sampling and photometric aerosol detection. It consists of a two-stage virtual impactor, three filters and three light scattering photometers and the optical sensors are calibrated in-situ via mass concentrations obtained by gravimetrical or elemental analysis of the filter samples (Respicon photometric multi-stage virtual impactor, HUND, Wetzlar, Germany).

The inhalable aerosol sampler employed was the IOM personal inhalable sampler (from SKC, Inc., Eighty-Four, PA, USA).

Chemical speciation of the water-soluble, sulfidic, metallic and oxidic fractions by the procedure devised by Zatka et al. was used [3].

The quantitative measurements of 13 elements (O, Na, Mg, Al, Si, S, Cl, K, Ca, Fe, Co, Ni and Cu) *in 1170 individual aerosol particles* has been made by wavelenght-dispersive electron-probe microanalysis [4].

Results and conclusions

The results of the particle-size distribution measurements in two different nickel refineries indicate that there is differences between worksites with respect to the relative coarseness of aerosol [5,6]. Unexpected findings were that the respirable weight fraction was small (about 5% of total) in all departments of the refineries. Nevertheless, particles of d_{ae} below 2 μm were abundant. The extrathoracic aerosol fraction is largely responsible for the actual dust and nickel exposure experienced by the workers, althought the presence of small particles may result in unique toxicologic consequences. The mass particle-distribution described also applies to cobalt and copper.

The Respicon photometric monitoring of workers exposure have identified a temporal pattern of exposure with both high episode peaks and lenghts. This observation of time variability of the exposure raises the issue of how such information should be used in workers exposure monitoring.

Recent comparisons between 'total' and inhalable aerosol sampling indicates that inhalable exposures were, on average, nearly twice as high as corresponding 'total' aerosol measurements for dust, nickel and several other elements in nickel refineries. Thus, for nickel refinery exposure measurements a replacement of the 'total' aerosol sampling approach is recommended [6].

Nickel speciation results showed that the predominant chemical form in electrorefining department (Monchegorsk refinery) workroom air was soluble nickel (55-99%); oxidic and sulfidic nickel constituted, respectively, <0.6-34% and 1-19% for various jobs, with very little in the metallic form. The amount of sulfidic was reduced substantially during matte roasting with a concomitant increase in the oxidic and metallic fractions. It was

also noticeable that in the early stages of the roasting process, the amount of soluble nickel increased and that the workroom air concentration of soluble nickel was higher at the top of the roaster than in the electrolytic department [5].
Although the majority of the individual particles had significant nickel content, both copper, iron, and cobalt were consistently present. The absence of well-defined phases and simple stoichiometries was however, suprising. Clearly, exposures to pure substances such as nickel subsulfide, other nickel sulfides, and specific nickel oxides appeared not to occur [4]. This observation calls into question the relevance of the focus in animal studies and regulatory considerations on exposure to single nickel compounds. The heterogeneous composition of individual particles may well influence the results obtained in chemical speciation procedures that involve consecutive leaching.

References:

[1] Doll R (Author-in Chief). Report on the international committee on nickel carcinogenesis in man. *Scand J Work Environ Health* 1990; 16: 1-82.

[2] Chashschin VP, Artunina GP, Norseth T. Congential-defects, abortion and other health-effects in nickel refinery workers. *Sci total Environ* 1994; 148 (2-3): 287-291.

[3] Zatka VJ, Warner JS, Maskery D. Chemical speciation of nickel in airborne dusts - Analytical method and results of an interlaboratory test program. *Environ Sci Technol* 1992; 26: 138-144.

[4] Höflich BLW, Wentzel M, Ortner HM, Weinbruch S, Skogstad A, Hetland S, Thomassen Y, Tchachtchine VP, Nieboer E. Chemical composition of individual aerosol particles from working areas in a nickel refinery. *J Environ Monit* 2000; 2: in press.

[5] Thomassen Y, Nieboer E, Ellingsen D, Hetland S, Norseth T, Odland JØ, Romanova N, Chernova S, Tchatchtchine VP. Characterisation of workers' exposure in a Russian nickel refinery. *J Environ Monit* 1991; 1: 15-22.

[6] Werner MA, Vincent JH, Thomassen Y, Hetland S, Berge S. Inhalable and "total" metal amd metal compound aerosol exposures for nickel refinery workers. *Occup Hyg* 1999; 5(2): 93-109.

Metal Ions in Biology and Medicine; vol 6. Eds. J.A. Centeno, Ph. Collery, G. Vernet, R.B. Finkelman, H. Gibb, J.C. Etienne. John Libbey Eurotext, Paris © 2000, pp. 230-232.

Evaluation of nickel compounds for listing in the report on carcinogens

Michael P. Waalkes[1], and C. William Jameson[2]

[1] *Laboratory of Comparative Carcinogenesis, NCI at NIEHS and* [2] *ETP, NIEHS, Research Triangle Park, NC 27709 USA*

Abstract. The 8th Edition of the Report on Carcinogens (RoC) lists Nickel (Ni) and Certain Ni Compounds as *reasonably anticipated to be human carcinogens*. The RoC is a Congressionally mandated listing of *known* and *reasonably anticipated* human carcinogens prepared by the NTP. A 1990 IARC Monograph evaluated Ni compounds and classified them as *carcinogenic to humans,* prompting the 1998 evaluation for the listing for Ni compounds in the RoC. This did not include metallic Ni and Ni alloys, which will be considered separately. Ni is found in many EPA National Priority List sites and is on the priority List of Hazardous Substances. Significant numbers of US residents are exposed to Ni. Studies of workers exposed to Ni compounds show elevated risks for death from lung and nasal cancer. Although the precise Ni compound responsible for the carcinogenic effects is not always clear, studies indicate that Ni compounds encountered in the Ni refining industries, including sulfates (soluble), and combinations of sulfides and oxides (insoluble), are human carcinogens. Both soluble and insoluble Ni compounds are multi-species, multi-route animal carcinogens causing tumors at the site of application and at distant sites. Based on the activity of a multitude of Ni compounds at various sites, it was concluded that Ni compounds act by presenting Ni ions to target sites. Ni compounds are genotoxic and mechanisms based around ionic Ni were considered most likely. The review groups for the RoC (NIEHS/NTP Review Committee, NTP Executive Committee Interagency Working Group, NTP Board of Scientific Counselors' Subcommittee for the RoC) all recommended that Ni compounds be listed in the RoC as *known to be human carcinogens*. This recommendation was based on the combined results of epidemiological studies, rodent carcinogenesis studies, and mechanistic data that support the concept that Ni compounds act by presenting Ni ions to critical sites in target cells and allow evaluation of these compounds as a single group.

Discussion. The 8th Edition of the Report on Carcinogens (RoC) lists Nickel and Certain Nickel Compounds as *reasonably anticipated to be human carcinogens* [1].

This Report is a Congressionally mandated listing of known and reasonably anticipated human carcinogens and its preparation is delegated to the National Toxicology Program (NTP) by the Secretary, Department of Health and Human Services (DHHS). Section 301 (b) (4) of the Public Health Service Act, as amended, provides that the Secretary, DHHS, shall publish a biennial report which contains a list of all substances which either are known to be human carcinogens or may reasonably be anticipated to be human carcinogens and to which a significant number of persons residing in the United States (US) are exposed. In 1990 the International Agency for Research on Cancer (IARC) evaluated Nickel and Nickel Compounds and classified Nickel compounds as *carcinogenic to humans* [2]. This classification was based on epidemiological data indicating there was sufficient evidence in humans for the carcinogenicity of nickel sulfate, and the combination of nickel sulfides and oxides encountered in the nickel refining industry together with sufficient evidence of rodent carcinogenesis resulting from exposure to a variety of nickel compounds and several types of other relevant data supported by the underlying concept that nickel compounds act by presenting nickel ions to critical sites in target cells [2].

The 1990 IARC classification [2] prompted a 1998 evaluation for the listing for Nickel Compounds in the RoC. This evaluation did not include metallic Nickel and Nickel Alloys, which are to be considered separately. Nickel and nickel compounds are found in many US Environmental Protection Agency National Priority List sites and are on the Agency for Toxic Substances and Disease Registry Priority List of Hazardous Substances to the population of the US. A significant number of US residents are exposed to nickel compounds in a variety of forms. Thus, there is a significant population in the US exposed to nickel compounds which is a criteria to list in the RoC.

Cohort studies evaluated by the IARC in 1990 of workers that had been exposed to nickel compounds in occupational settings show clearly elevated risks for death from both nasal and lung cancer [2]. Additional cohort studies published after this evaluation confirm that occupational nickel exposure is associated with an elevated risk of nasal and/or lung cancers in exposed workers and confirmed the carcinogenic potential of soluble nickel compounds [3, 4]. The linkage between soluble nickel compounds and nasal and lung tumors in exposed workers was dose-related and was significant even after adjusting for potential confounding factors including smoking, age and exposure to insoluble nickel compounds [4]. Thus, even though the precise nickel compound responsible for the carcinogenic effects is not always entirely clear, studies both before and after the 1990 IARC evaluation [2-4] indicate that nickel compounds encountered in the nickel refining industries, including sulfates (soluble), and combinations of sulfides and oxides (insoluble), are human carcinogens.

Both soluble and insoluble nickel compounds are multi-species, multi-route animal carcinogens, inducing tumors at the site of application and at distant sites as well [2].

Recently, several NTP chronic bioassay inhalation studies confirmed the carcinogenicity of various nickel compounds both in the lungs and in the adrenal medulla of rats [5, 6]. Another recent study showed that brief transplacental exposure to soluble nickel acetate caused malignant pituitary tumors in the offspring [7]. Based on the activity of a multitude of nickel compounds at various sites, including sites at some distance to the original point of entry, it was concluded that nickel compounds act by presenting nickel ions to sensitive target sites. Nickel compounds are clearly genotoxic [1, 2] and mechanisms based around ionic nickel are considered most likely the cause of these genotoxic effects.

The review groups for the Report on Carcinogens, including the NIEHS/NTP Review Committee, the NTP Executive Committee Interagency Working Group, and the NTP Board of Scientific Counselors' Subcommittee for the Report on Carcinogens all recommended that Nickel Compounds be listed in the Report on Carcinogens as *known to be human carcinogens*. This recommendation was based on the combined results of epidemiological studies, rodent carcinogenesis studies, and mechanistic data that support the concept that nickel compounds act by presenting nickel ions to critical sites in target cells and allow evaluation of these compounds as a single group.

References:

1. The 8th Report on Carcinogens. Research Triangle Park: NTP, 1998: 146-149.
2. International Agency for Research on Cancer Monographs on the Evaluation of the Carcinogenic Risks to Humans: Volume 49, Chromium, Nickel and Welding. Lyon: IARC Scientific Publications, 1990: 257-445.
3. Anttila A, Pukkala E, Aitio A, Rantanen T, Karjalainen S. Update of cancer incidence among workers at a copper/nickel smelter and nickel refinery. *Int Arch Occup Environ Health* 1998; 71 : 245-250.
4. Andersen A, Berge S, Engeland A, Norseth T. Exposure to nickel compounds and smoking in relation to incidence of lung and nasal cancer among nickel refinery workers. *Occup Environ Med* 1996; 53 : 708-713.
5. National Toxicology Program: Toxicology and Carcinogenesis Studies of Nickel Oxide (CAS No. 1313-99-1) in F344 Rats and B6C3F1 Mice (Inhalation Studies); Report No. TR-451. Research Triangle Park: NTP, 1996.
6. National Toxicology Program: Toxicology and Carcinogenesis Studies of Nickel Subsulfide (CAS No. 12035-72-2) in F344 Rats and B6C3F1 Mice (Inhalation Studies); Report No. TR-453. Research Triangle Park: NTP, 1996.
7. Diwan B A, Kasprzak K S, and Rice, J M. Transplacental carcinogenic effects of nickel(II) in the renal cortex, renal pelvis and adenohypophysis in F344/NCr. *Carcinogenesis* 1992; 13 : 1351-1357.

Metal Ions in Biology and Medicine; vol 6. Eds. J.A. Centeno, Ph. Collery, G. Vernet, R.B. Finkelman, H. Gibb, J.C. Etienne. John Libbey Eurotext, Paris © 2000, pp. 233-235.

Cancer and noncancer assessments of ingested and inhaled soluble nickel salts

Lynne T. Haber and Michael L. Dourson

Toxicology Excellence for Risk Assessment, 1757 Chase Ave., Cincinnati, OH, USA 45223

This paper summarizes the findings of a *Toxicological Review* of the human health effects of environmental exposure to *soluble nickel compounds* [1]; insoluble forms of nickel were not addressed. The results were also presented more concisely by Haber et al. [2,3].*

A substantial body of occupational epidemiology data has shown that exposure to mixed soluble and insoluble nickel causes the development of lung and nasal cancer. These epidemiology data are reviewed in ICNCM [4]. More recent epidemiology studies of nickel refinery workers and a cohort of British electroplaters (who are exposed primarily to soluble nickel salts, in the absence of insoluble nickel compounds) were also evaluated. Although extensive data are available, the contribution of soluble nickel is difficult to determine, due to coexposure of these populations to soluble and insoluble forms of nickel, and limitations in exposure measurements. Soluble nickel was negative in an NTP inhalation bioassay [5,6], while there was some evidence for tumorigenicity in rats for less soluble nickel oxide [7], and there was clear evidence for tumorigenicity of insoluble nickel subsulfide in rats [8]. Results of parenteral assays follow a similar pattern, but provide evidence of weak carcinogenicity of soluble nickel. Kinetic factors also indicate that exposure to soluble nickel alone has a low carcinogenic potential. Overall, we conclude that the carcinogenic activity of insoluble nickel compounds should not be used to predict the carcinogenic potential of water-soluble nickel salts. The overall data suggest a nonlinear dose-response relationship for carcinogenicity, but the data are insufficient to determine the doses

* This work was performed under contract to the Metal Finishing Association of Southern California, Inc., the U.S. Environmental Protection Agency (EPA), and Health Canada. The conclusions of the *Toxicological Review* and opinions expressed in that document and this paper are those of the authors, and do not necessarily represent the views of the sponsors. After U.S. EPA review, the conclusions of the assessment will also be summarized for EPA's Integrated Risk Information System (http://www.epa.gov/iris), which will also make available the revised *Toxicological Review*.

at which such nonlinearities occur. Under the U.S. EPA's 1996 Proposed Guidelines for Carcinogen Risk Assessment, inhaled soluble nickel compounds would be classified as "*cannot be determined,*" because the existing evidence is composed of conflicting data. There are a number of negative animal bioassays with soluble nickel salts, but all of them have deficiencies that preclude a definitive conclusion. According to EPA's 1996 draft cancer guidelines, the carcinogenic potential of oral exposure to soluble nickel "*cannot be determined* because there are *inadequate data* to perform an assessment".

A Reference Concentration (RfC) of 2E-4 mg Ni/cu.m was calculated, based on lung fibrosis in male rats observed in the chronic inhalation study [6]. This RfC was calculated as follows. The human equivalent concentration (HEC) for the experimental exposures was calculated using the dosimetry in the U.S. EPA methods. The lower bound on the concentration corresponding to 10% extra risk was calculated using benchmark concentration modeling, resulting in a $BMCL_{10}$(HEC) of 0.0017 mg Ni/cu.m. In the absence of sufficient data on sensitive human subpopulations, an uncertainty factor of 10 was applied to account for intrahuman variability. A factor of 1 (instead of the standard factor of 3 when using EPA dosimetry) was used to extrapolate from animals to humans, based on minimal effects seen in humans under occupational exposures [9] that were higher than exposures that resulted in significant respiratory toxicity in the chronic rat bioassay [6]. The Muir et al. [9] study was not used as the basis for the RfC, due to numerous study uncertainties, including very crude exposure measurements.

A reference dose (RfD) of 8E-3 mg Ni/kg/day *in addition to the amount in food* was calculated, based on albuminuria in female rats exposed to nickel sulfate in drinking water for 6 months [10], with a minimal LOAEL of 7.6 mg Ni/kg-day. This RfD is comparable to the current RfD on EPA's IRIS, based on decreased body weight in a chronic feeding study in rats [11]. Both studies have uncertainties and limitations. The proposed RfD was based on the Vyskocil et al. [10] study, because the uncertainties in the study were insufficient to discount the observed effects, and the RfD based on the Vyskocil study would likely be more health-protective than an RfD derived based on the Ambrose study [11]. Two full uncertainty factors of 10 (for intrahuman variability and for interspecies extrapolation) and a combined factor of 10 (for subchronic-to-chronic extrapolation, an insufficient database, and use of a minimal LOAEL) were used. A composite factor of 1000 results.

References

1. TERA. Toxicological review of soluble nickel salts. Toxicology Excellence for Risk Assessment. Cincinnati, OH. 1999. Available online at http://www.tera.org/vera

2. Haber L, Erdreich L, Diamond G, Maier A, Ratney R, Zhao Q, Dourson M. Hazard identification and dose-response of inhaled nickel soluble salts. *Regul Toxicol Pharmacol* 2000; in press.

3. Haber L, Diamond G, Zhao Q, Erdreich L, Dourson M. Hazard identification and dose-response of ingested nickel soluble salts. *Regul Toxicol Pharmacol* 2000; in press.

4. ICNCM. Report of the International Committee on Nickel Carcinogenesis in Man. *Scand J Work Environ Health* 1990; 16(1): 1-82.

5. Dunnick J, Elwell M, Radovsky A, Benson J, Hahn F, Nikula K, Barr E, Hobbs C. Comparative carcinogenic effects of nickel subsulfide, nickel oxide, or nickel sulfate hexahydrate chronic exposures in the lung. *Cancer Res* 1995; 55: 5251-5256.

6. NTP (National Toxicology Program). Toxicology and carcinogenesis studies of nickel sulfate hexahydrate (CAS NO. 10101-97-0) in F344/N rats and B6C3F1 mice (Inhalation Studies). U. S. Department of Health and Human Services. NTP TR 454. NIH Publication No. 96-3370. 1996a.

7. NTP (National Toxicology Program). Toxicology and carcinogenesis studies of nickel oxide (CAS NO. 1313-99-1) in F344/N rats and B6C3F1 mice (Inhalation Studies). U. S. Department of Health and Human Services. NTP TR 451. NIH Publication No. 96-3367. 1996b.

8. NTP (National Toxicology Program). Toxicology and carcinogenesis studies of nickel subsulfide (CAS NO. 12035-72-2) in F344/N rats and B6C3F1 mice (Inhalation Studies). U.S. Department of Health and Human Services. NTP TR 453. NIH Publication No. 96-3369. 1996c.

9. Muir D, Julian J, Jadon N, Roberts R, Roos J, Chan J, Maehle W, Morgan W. Prevalence of small opacities in chest radiographs of nickel sinter plant workers. *Br J Ind Med* 1993; 50: 428-31.

10. Vyskocil A, Viau C, Cizkova M. Chronic nephrotoxicity of soluble nickel in rats. *Hum Exp Toxicol* 1994; 13: 689-693.

11. Ambrose A, Larson P, Borzelleca J, Hennigar G Jr. Long term toxicologic assessment of nickel in rats and dogs. *J Food Sci Technol* 1976; 13: 181-187.

Metal Ions in Biology and Medicine; vol 6. Eds. J.A. Centeno, Ph. Collery, G. Vernet, R.B. Finkelman, H. Gibb, J.C. Etienne. John Libbey Eurotext, Paris © 2000, pp. 237-240.

Nonprotein bound selenium in plasma: relevance in assessing selenium status

G.F. Combs, Jr., T. Hyun and W.P. Gray

Division of Nutritional Sciences, Cornell University, Ithaca, NY, USA 14853

ABSTRACT

A new, sensitive analytical technique, hydride generation-atomic flame fluorescence spectrometry, facilitated the detection of a previously unrecognized form(s) of selenium (Se) in plasma. This form is not covalently bound to proteins, although about half appears to be associated non-covalently with plasma proteins. The fraction comprised 1.4-10.2% of total plasma Se in cows, sheep, pigs, rats and chicks. In humans, it comprised an average or 2.7% of total plasma Se. In both rats and chicks, the fraction responded more to supplementation with selenite than with L-seleno-methionine (SeMet), suggesting that it may contain reduced and, perhaps, methylated Se-metabolites. It is proposed that the non-protein Se fraction may valuable in assessing Se status, particularly for purposes of cancer chemoprevention.

INTRODUCTION

Selenium (Se) status is currently assessed, for the purposes of detecting nutritional deficiencies and toxicity, by measurement of the total Se concentrations in accessible tissues, particularly, whole blood, serum or plasma. In serum/plasma, is has been generally accepted that Se exists exclusively in protein-bound form. In particular, it has been assumed that serum/plasma Se is bound to proteins that depend on the element for their expression and contain it in the form of selenocysteine (SeCys) (glutathione peroxidase [GPX], selenoprotein P [SeP]) and others that contain the element in non-specific forms as selenomethionine (SeMet) (e.g., albumin). Because the Se contents of these major components are not regulated similarly, various dietary forms of Se can affect serum/plasma total in different ways. This fact diminishes the inferential value of serum/plasma Se as a parameter of Se status, particularly at supranutritional levels of Se intake, as might be considered for cancer chemoprevention. Therefore, the following studies were conducted for the purpose of developing a parameter of Se status that might be more useful in surveillance of high-level Se exposure.

MATERIALS AND METHODS

Rats and chicks were raised in separate experiments using low-Se, vitamin E-adequate semi-purified diets based on Torula yeast [1]. These were supplemented with graded levels of Se either as sodium selenite (Na_2SeO_3) or L-selenomethionine. Blood samples were obtained from various other ongoing experiments involving other livestock species or humans through the generous cooperation of several investigators.

Non-protein-bound Se in plasma from various sources was determined in ultrafiltrates of de-proteinated samples. This was accomplished by treating plasma with 5% trichloroacetic acid (TCA) and subjecting the filtrate (Whatman 45) to ultrafiltration using tubes fitted with 10 kD cut-off membranes (Lida Manufacturing Co., WI) under low-speed centrifugation (5,000 x g for 3 hrs at $4^{o}C$). The ultrafiltrate was analyzed then for Se by hydride-generation, atomic flame fluorescence (AFFS) spectrometry (Millenium Excalibur, P. S. Analytical Co. Mississagua, Canada) after nitric-perchloric acid digestion. Rat plasma samples were also fractionated into the major Se-containing protein fractions (GPX, SeP, albumin) using the tandem affinity column chromatography system method of Deagen et al [2]. Total Se concentrations of plasma were measured by electrothermal atomic absorption spectrophotometry (AAS) with Zeeman-effect background correction (Cary 3030, Varian Instruments, Walnut Creek, CA) using a reduced palladium matrix modifier.

RESULTS AND DISCUSSION

The use of AFFS yielded a limit of detection of Se of at least two orders of magnitude greater than has been possible using AAS methods. When coupled to hydride-generation, this method was free of spectral interferences, such that Se could be detected at concentrations that hitherto have not been possible. Thus, using a fairly straight-forward approach to removing the protein-containing components from plasma, ultrafiltration, it was possible to detect low amounts of Se in the non-protein fraction. These amounts increased by a factor of 2 if plasma proteins were denatured in TCA prior to ultrafiltration, indicating that about half of the non-protein Se is normally associated non-covalently with proteins. Non-protein Se was found in casual samples of plasma from each of five mammalian and one avian species tested (Table 1), comprising as little as 1.39% and as much as 10.21% of total plasma Se in chicks and cows, respectively.

Table 1. Non-protein-bound Se present in plasma of all species tested

Species	n	Total Se ng/ml	Non-Protein Bound Se ng/ml	%
Cow	4	72.07±11.19	7.26±0.51	10.21±1.18
Sheep	4	151.39±18.40	9.43±1.97	6.21±0.86
Pig	5	172.28±17.15	2.25±0.42	1.31±0.18
Rat	5	32.83±4.62	1.46±0.24	4.81±0.75
Chick	4	218.55±18.04	2.03±1.81	1.39±1.00
Human	4	142.32±28.36	3.33±0.27	2.34±0.32

Table 2. Effect of dietary Se on plasma Se concentrations

Dietary Se*		Whole	Plasma fraction			
form	Level ppm	Plasma	GPX	SeP	Albumin	Non-protein
None	0	28.9± 2.3a	6.9± 0.4a	7.9± 0.5a	6.6± 0.5a	1.40±0.31a
Selenite	1	476.5±78.9b	127.5±20.7bc	244.0±34.4c	41.7± 5.1b	9.21±3.29b
	2	466.3±74.7b	127.3± 7.8bc	255.3±17.1c	51.2± 1.3b	6.29±0.20b
	5	470.8±97.1b	112.0± 3.7b	273.6± 6.2c	62.1± 6.5b	9.09±6.15b
	10	525.2±15.1b	110.7±58.3bc	291.9±18.6cd	54.6± 3.8b	6.58±1.40b
L-SeMet	1	522.7±31.8bc	87.3± 9.1b	20.7± 3.4b	66.1±10.5b	4.87±2.44ab
	2	598.8±32.49c	121.4±16.4c	352.3± 4.4e	94.3±16.7bcd	6.82±2.54b
	5	630.3±86.91c	181.3±16.7d	371.3±18.1e	106.5±11.1d	7.69±3.18b
	10	596.7±91.56bc	129.0±27.2cd	331.5±44.4cde	86.9± 7.8cd	13.41±6.68b

*Basal diet contained 0.05 ppm Se.

The non-protein Se fraction responded to Se-feeding in both the rat (Table 2) and the chick (Fig. 1). In both cases, the relative response (*vs.* other plasma Se-fractions) to selenite was greater than that to SeMet; yet the non-protein Se fraction was maintained in apparent first-order relationship with other plasma Se-fractions and with total plasma Se. Humans participating in a study involving long-term supplementation with putatively anti-carcinogenic doses of Se (as Se-enriched yeast) also showed this relationship (Fig. 2), with non-protein Se comprised an average of 2.7% of total plasma Se.

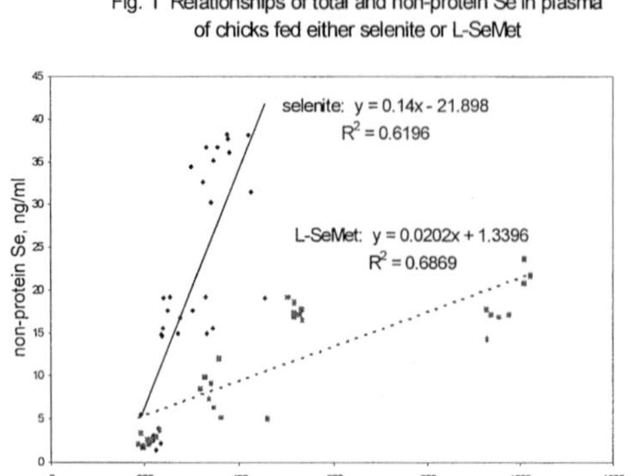

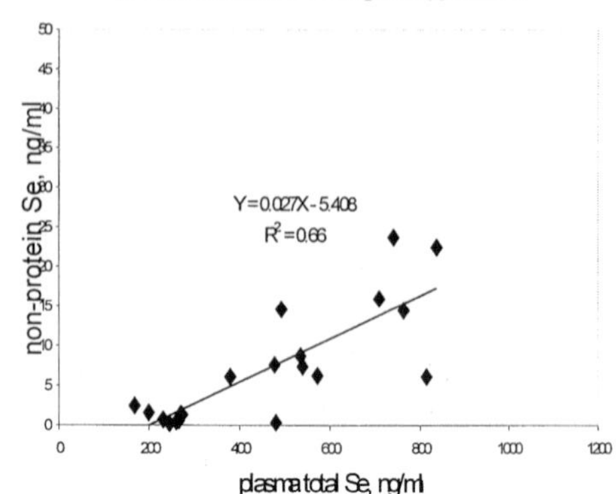

CONCLUSIONS

The non-protein Se fraction of plasma exists at levels just below the limits of detection of most current analytical procedures and has therefore been invisible to investigators concerned with the assessment of Se status. With the added sensitivity of AAFS, this fraction is now clear, and one would expect that it contains the low molecular weight forms of Se involved in transport as well as those involved in Se-anti-carcinogensis and toxicity. It will, thus, be important to speciate this fraction in order to determine the full extent of its utility in the assessment and surveillance and surveillance of Se status.

REFERENCES

[1] Combs, Jr., G.F. and Combs, S.B., The Role of Selenium in Nutrition, Academic Press, 1986, p. 120.

[2] Deagan, J. T., Butler, J. A., Zachara, B. A., and Whanger, P. D. 1993. Determination of the Distribution of Se between Glutathione Peroxidase, Selenoprotein P, and Albumin in Plasma. *Anal. Biochem.* 208: 176-181.

Metal Ions in Biology and Medicine; vol 6. Eds. J.A. Centeno, Ph. Collery, G. Vernet, R.B. Finkelman, H. Gibb, J.C. Etienne. John Libbey Eurotext, Paris © 2000, pp. 241-243.

Selenium levels in placental tissue and in maternal blood in first and third trimester of pregnancy

M. Kantola[1], R. Purkunen[2], P. Kröger[1a], A. Tooming[3], J. Juravskaja[4], M. Pasanen[5], S. Saarikoski[6], T. Vartiainen[2, 7]

[1] Department of Chemistry, University of Kuopio a) présent address: Pharmadata Oy, Helsinki, Finland; [2] Department of Chemistry, National Public Health Institute, Kuopio; [3] Central Hospital of Rakvere, Estonia; [4] Institute for Advanced Training of Physicians, St. Petersburg, Russia; [5] Department of Pharmacology and Toxicology, University of Oulu, and National Agency for Medicines, Finland; [6] Clinic of Gynaecology and Obstetrics, University Hospital of Kuopio; [7] Department of Environmental Sciences, University of Kuopio, Kuopio, Finland

Introduction

During the last years, a lot of new findings of possible selenium containing enzymes and proteins have been published and some of them seem to have importance also in pregnancy. The selenoprotein p has been found to express in the placenta of mice in late pregnancy (1) and it may play role in the transplacental transport of selenium to the fetus, during late pregnancy. It has been suggested that combined deficiencies of iodine and selenium may have adverse effects on neonatal growth, development and survival (2) by decreasing in liver type I outer ring 5' deionase, containing selenium, both in the mother and fetus. Both extracellular and cellular glutathione peroxidases are synthesized in placenta (3).
Sodium selenate has been supplemented to all agricultural fertilizers used in Finland since 1984 and it has increased human milk and serum selenium levels in Finland. In Estonia selenium levels in serum and human milk are as low as they were in Finland before supplementation (4).
In this research we studied selenium levels in placental tissue and maternal blood during the first and third trimesters of pregnancy and transportation of selenium to the fetus by measuring cord blood selenium levels at delivery. We compared selenium status of mothers during pregnancy in Finland, Estonia and St. Petersburg. We also studied the possible interactions and relations between selenium, zinc, cadmium and copper concentrations in placenta and in mothers blood.

Material and methods

Study materials: Placentas, serum, whole blood, and cord blood samples at delivery and placentas, serum and whole blood samples of abortion patients at 8-12 weeks of pregnancy. *Study subjects*: 216 healthy, voluntary women. *Analytical methods:* Microwave digestions and atomic absorption methods. The detailed methods and results of the zinc, copper and cadmium measurements have been published earlier (5). *Statistical methods:* Analyses of variances, with Sheffe's multiple range test were used to study the equality of means. Multiple regression was used for partial association between various elements and concentrations in different study materials.

Results

The mean selenium levels in placental tissue, in blood serum and in whole blood were higher during the first trimester of pregnancy comparing to the time of delivery both in Finland and in Estonia. In St. Petersburg the differences were not significant (Table 1). The mean selenium concentrations in cord blood were significantly higher comparing to whole-blood selenium and serum selenium both in Finland and in Estonia. The number of samples was too small in St.Petersburg for comparison. The mean selenium concentrations in placentas at term were higher in smokers comparing to nonsmokers, the statistically significant difference was found only among the Finnish mothers. Selenium levels were highest in all studied materials in Finnish mothers and lowest in Estonia. In the whole material strong single correlations were found between selenium concentrations in all studied materials. In the multivariate regression analysis for the nonsmoking Finnish mothers, the whole-blood selenium and the placental copper were the most powerful determinants for serum selenium at the time of delivery (β = 0.302, P = 0.044 and β = 0.310, P = 0.039, n=34 respectively). Placental selenium, zinc, copper and cadmium, whole-blood selenium and cadmium, serum zinc and copper, cord-blood selenium and cadmium were included to the model. The model accounted 16% of the variation. For the whole-blood selenium, the strongest determinants were serum zinc and placental cadmium, serum zinc having strong positive association and placental cadmium negative association (β = 0.548, P = 0.000 and β = - 0.274, P = 0.044, n= 34 respectively). The same variables as above and serum selenium instead of whole-blood selenium were included to the model. This model accounted 33% of the variation.

Discussion

Our results demonstrate the significant decrease in mothers' selenium levels in all studied materials during the pregnancy. The decrease was significant both among Estonian mothers with low selenium status and among Finnish mothers with higher selenium levels as a consequence of selenium supplementation. This and the high cord-blood selenium levels comparing to mothers' whole blood selenium levels suggest that an active selenium transportation takes place from the mother to the fetus. The higher placental selenium concentrations of smoking mothers might be a part of the mothers defending system against the oxidative stress caused by smoking. Although our results show that the intake of selenium seems to have the strongest influence on the selenium concentrations in all studied material, the results of multivariate analyses among the Finnish mothers show that blood selenium concentrations have association with zinc and copper concentrations in serum and placenta. Previously, the possible connections between selenium and zinc and selenium and copper have been reported in human milk (6,7). In animal experiments selenium has been found to decrease the toxic effects of cadmium possibly by binding cadmium to the selenides (8). Our results demonstrate that high whole blood selenium concentrations might decrease the transportation of cadmium to the placenta.

References

1.Kasik JW, Rice EJ. Selenoprotein p expression in liver, uterus and placenta during late pregnancy. *Placenta* 1995; 16:67-74.

2.Vanderpas JB, Contempre B, Duale NL, et al. Iodine and selenium deficiency associated with cretinism in northern Zaire. *Am J Clin Nutr* 1990;52:1087-93.

3. Avissar N, Eisenman C, Breen JG, Horowitz S, Miller RK, Harvey JC. Human placenta makes extracellular glutathione peroxidase and secretes it into maternal circulation. *Am J Physiol* 1994;267 (Endocrinol Metab 30): E68-76.
4. Kantola M, Mand E, Viitak A, Juravskaja J, Purkunen R, Saarikoski S, Pasanen M. Selenium content of serum and human milk from Finland and neighbouring countries. *J Trace Elem Expl Med* 1997; 10:225-232.
5. Kantola M, Kröger P, Purkunen R, Tooming A, Juravskaja J, Pasanen M, Vartiainen T. Accumulation of cadmium, zinc and copper in maternal blood and developemental Placental tissue: Differencies between Finland, Estonia and St. Petersburg. *Env Res* 2000 ; in press
6. Brätter P, Negreti de Brätter VE, Recknagel S, Brunetto R. Maternal selenium status influences the concentration and binding pattern of zinc in human milk. *J Trace Elem Med Biol* 1997; 11:203-9.
7. Perrone L, Di Palma L, Di Toro R, Gialanella G, Moro R. Interaction of trace elements in a longitudinal study of human milk from full-term and preterm mothers. *Biol Trace ElemRes* 1994; 41:1-30.
8. Magos L, Webb M. The interactions of selenium with cadmium and mercury. *Crit Rev Toxicol* 1980: 1-42.

Table 1. The mean selenium concentrations and standard deviations in placental tissue serum (S-Se), whole blood (W-Se), and cord blood (C-Se) in different study sites according to the gestational age and smoking habits.

	First trimester		**At delivery**	
Variable	**Non smokers Mean ± SD (n)**	**Smokers Mean ± SD (n)**	**Non smokers Mean ± SD (n)**	**Smokers Mean ± SD (n)**
***Finland*:**				
P-Se (µg/g)	1.34 ± 0.13 (11)	1.33 ± 0.17 (13)	1.01 ± 0.12[a] (66)	1.13 ± 011[a] (16)
S-Se (µg/L)	121.4 ± 18 (18)	115.1 ± 14 (14)	109.7 ± 20[c] (63)	110.9 ± 20.1 (15)
W-Se(µg/L)	119.9 ± 12 (18)	114.6 ± 17 (15)	109.7± 17[b] (61)	108.7 ± 17 (16)
C-Se (µg/L)	n.d.	n.d.	118.3 ±16 (67)	123.6 ± 23 (15)
***Estonia*:**				
P-Se (µg/g)	0.92 ± 0.22 (7)	0.99 ± 0.19 (11)	0.62 ± 0.07[a] (17)	0.71 ± 0.20[c] (6)
S-Se (µg/L)	63 ± 8 (9)	65 ± 10 (11)	53 ± 9[c] (14)	55 ± 11 (5)
W-Se (µg/L)	63 ± 7 (9)	68 ± 10 (12)	54 ±10[c] (17)	57 ± 10[c] (6)
C- Se (µg/L)	n.d.	n.d.	75 ±12 (17)	73 ±15 (6)
***St. Petersburg*:**				
P-Se (µg/g)	0.80 ± 0.11 (4)	1.02 ± 0.01 (2)	0.83 ± 0.10 (22)	0.81 ±0.19 (4)
S-Se (µg/L)	81 ± 27 (3)	108 ± 32 (2)	86 ± 22 (11)	90 (1)
W-Se (µg/L)	98 ± 30 (4)	115 ± 42 (2)	83 ±19 (20)	96 ±28 (3)
C- Se (µg/L)	n.d.	n.d.	126 ± 30 (2)	131± 12 (3)

a Statistical significance comparing to the mean in the first trimester ; ($P<0.001$).
b Statistical significance comparing to the mean in the first trimester ; ($P<0.01$).
c Statistical significance comparing to the mean in the first trimester ; ($P<0.05$).

Metal Ions in Biology and Medicine; vol 6. Eds. J.A. Centeno, Ph. Collery, G. Vernet, R.B. Finkelman, H. Gibb, J.C. Etienne. John Libbey Eurotext, Paris © 2000, pp. 244-247.

Maternal selenium status influences the concentration and binding form of iodine in human milk

P. Brätter, V.E. Negretti de Brätter, I. Navarro Blasco*, A. Raab

*Hahn-Meitner-Institut Berlin, Department of Molecular Trace Element Research for Health and Nutrition, Glienicker Str. 100. D-14109 Berlin, Germany, * Universidad de Navarra, Department of Chemistry and Soil Science, Irunlarrea s/n, E-31080 Pamplona, Spain*

Abstract

Effects of dietary selenium intake (range of 40-870 µg/d) on the content and binding form of iodine in breast milk of European an Venezuelan mothers were studied. Se and I were found to be correlated in breast milk but not in maternal serum. The organic-bound iodine fraction increased with rising selenium intake. At selenium intake levels higher than 400 mg/d the correlation was ended and the organic fraction becomes depressed. We assume that a metabolic relationship between iodine and selenium in the mammary gland exists which change at high dietary selenium intake. **Keywords:** selenium, iodine, human milk, speciation, metabolic changes.

Introduction

Iodine is essential for the synthesis of thyroid hormones. Deficiency of iodine during the fetal period and/or the early infancy is a cause of a variety of disorders including brain damage and irreversible mental retardation. The iodine intake of newborns is completely dependent on the iodine content of breast milk or adapted formulas. Iodine in breast milk is significantly higher concentrated than in the maternal serum. The reverse relationship is known for selenium. The serum/milk-ratio of selenium is nearly constant and independent of the maternal selenium intake level (1). That indicates different transfer mechanisms for both elements. It is suggested that both an iodide transporter and a peroxidase enzyme are involved in the accumulation of iodide in mammary cells during lactation (2) similar to that reported for thyroid tissues. Associated with the discovery that deiodinases are selenoproteins, the link between selenium- and iodine metabolism was established (3).

Aims: The present study was performed to assess the iodine content of breast milk samples from different geographic regions and to investigate the responsiveness of iodine to variations in the regional maternal selenium status. In order to cover a wide range of daily maternal dietary selenium intake (40 - 800 µg) mature breast milk samples were collected in Spain, Germany and Venezuela including its seleniferous area of the Portuguesa province.

Methods:

Total selenium was determined by instrumental neutron activation analysis (INAA). Total iodine was determined by means of ICP-MS after dilution of the sample in suprapure ammonia solution. Quality control was carried out using RNAA as independent analytical method as well as certified reference materials (Tab. 1)

Tab.1: Determination of iodine and selenium in certified reference materials (mean±SD)

Reference Material	I (μg/g)		Se (ng/g)	
	Mean	Certified	Mean	Certified
BCR 150	1,26 ± 0,013	1,29 ± 0,09	---	---
SRM 1549	3,38 ± 0,05	3,38 ± 0,02	129,4± 5,6	110 ±10
IAEA 155	0,372± 0,005	---	65,6 ± 3	64 (51-77)

By online coupling of ICP-MS with a chromatographic column for protein separation (SEC) the binding pattern of iodine and selenium in milk whey were studied. The breast milk samples were collected 20-24 days post partum. Details of the analytical methods and sample collection has been given elsewhere (4,5).

Results and Discussion

The breast milk level of selenium is strongly correlated with the maternal intake (1). There was no correlation between selenium and iodine in serum (Tab.2) whereas selenium in serum and iodine in breast milk were significant positively correlated. With respect to the iodine level in breast milk literature data regarding its correlation with the maternal iodine dietary intake are contradictory (6). In our study the iodine concentration in serum of women from Europe and Venezuela (mean: 63,2± 2,4 and 71±12 μg/L respectively) was found within the same range indicating a comparable iodine status. According to the mean selenium content of breast milk in Tab.3 three groups of lactating mothers were defined: Europe 16 ± 4 μg/L, Venezuela Yaracuy 42 ± 10 μg/L and Venezuela Portuguesa (seleniferous area) 84 ± 40 μg/L. A positive

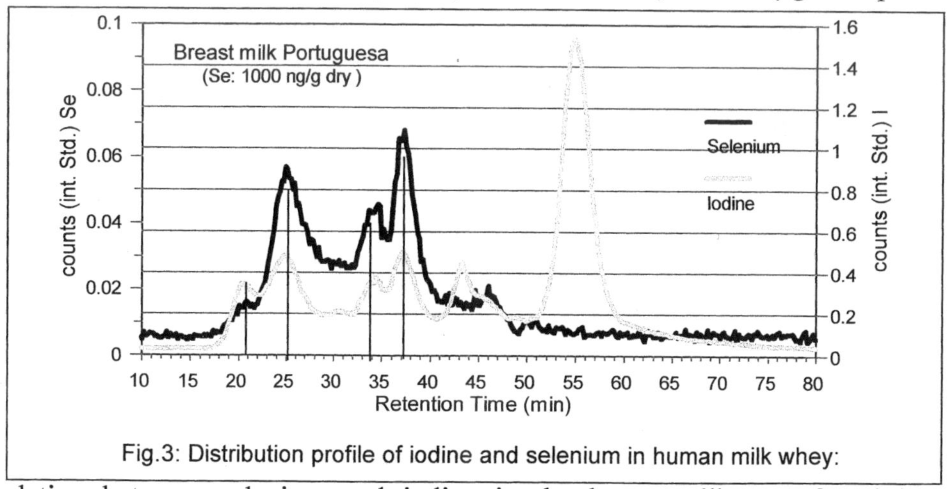

Fig.3: Distribution profile of iodine and selenium in human milk whey:

correlation between selenium and iodine in the breast milk was found in all population groups (Fig.1) within the range 10-70μg/L selenium. Speciation analysis of iodine in human milk whey showed besides the iodide peak up to six iodine-binding ligands present in the molecular mass range 5 - 300 kD (Fig.3). Coelution with three of the four Se-binding proteins was observed. The species remained to be identified.

From the elution profiles of iodine the percentages of inorganic and organic bound iodine were calculated. The total iodine of the European breast milk samples was 95±60 μg/L showing about 80 % of the iodine as inorganic bound (Tab.3). This findings are consistent with those given for France (7). Towards the higher selenium level of the Venezuelan samples a significant increase of the organic bound iodine (up to 60%) was found (Fig.2). But at selenium breast milk levels higher than 80 μg/L - which correspond to about 400 μg/d Se-intake - an inverse correlation between the selenium and the organic-bound iodine and simultaneously no changes in the total iodine content (Fig.4) were observed. This means that an excess of selenium may impair the synthesis of the iodine binding organic components. Our previous results (8) showed that at the same high range of dietary selenium intake (350-400μg/d), the activity of the selenoenzyme type I iodothyronine 5′-diodinase which catalyzes the production of the biologically active hormone T3 from T4 becomes depressed . Both selenium-dependent functional changes can be used to estimate the upper range of the safe dietary selenium intake.

Tab.2: Correlation of iodine and selenium in breast milk (BM) and serum of lactating mothers (Spearman rank test)

Serum-Se vs. Serum-I	not significant	BM-organic I vs. BM-Se (< 70 ng/ml)
Serum-Se vs. BM-Se	p< 0.01	n=42, r=0,8290, p<0,001
Serum-Se vs. BM-I	p< 0,01	BM-total I vs. BM-Se (<70 ng/ml)
Serum -I vs. BM-I	p< 0,01	n=46, r= 0,5113, p<0,001

Tab.3: Concentration (mean ± SD) of Se and I in breast milk from Germany, Spain and Venezuela Calculation of the Se-intake by means of the Se concentration in breast milk according to the correlation BM-Se (μg/L)=1,75 +0,2 Se-intake (μg/d). (1)

Human milk	Total Iodine (mg/L)	Ionic Iodide (mg/L)	(%)	Organic Iodine (mg/L)	(%)	Selenium (μg/L)	Se - intake (μg per day)
Spain	0,093±0,063	0,082±0,074	76,7	0,037±0,093	23,3	16,2±4,6	38-136
Germany	0,109±0,082	0,096±0,068	86,6	0,014±0,017	13.4	15,9±2,6	54-91
Europe	0.095±0,066	0.084±0,073	78,1	0,034±0,087	21,9	16,2±4,4	38-136
Venezuela Yaracuy	0,204±0,103	0,144±0,084	72,4	0,061±0,049	27,6	42,0±10,7	137-311
Portuguesa	0,165±0,072	0,068±0,042	49,7	0,079±0,042	50,3	83,5±40,0	203-878

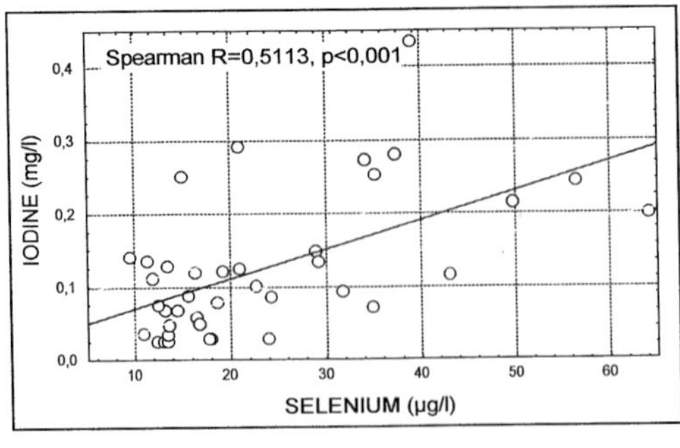

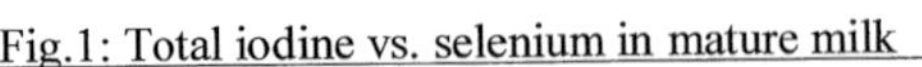

Fig.1: Total iodine vs. selenium in mature milk

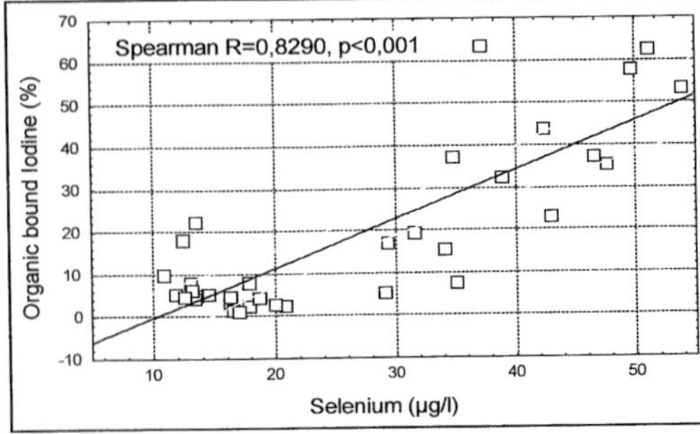

Fig. 2: Percentage of organic bound iodine vs. selenium in breast milk

Conclusions

From our results it is hypothesized that the effect of high dietary selenium intake on the iodine level in breast milk is associated with the depression of the activity of selenoenzymes involved in the iodine metabolism of the mammary secretory cells. This effect can be of interest for estimation of the safe dietary intake level of selenium. Furthermore, the influence of the maternal selenium status on the iodine content of breast milk can be of interest in the discussion of endemic nutritional deficiency manifestations of both elements. With respect to the severity of iodine deficiency diseases dietary selenium is regarded as an additional factor (9) Concerning the mechanisms of trace element transfer to the mammary gland and metabolic interaction many questions remain open for research.

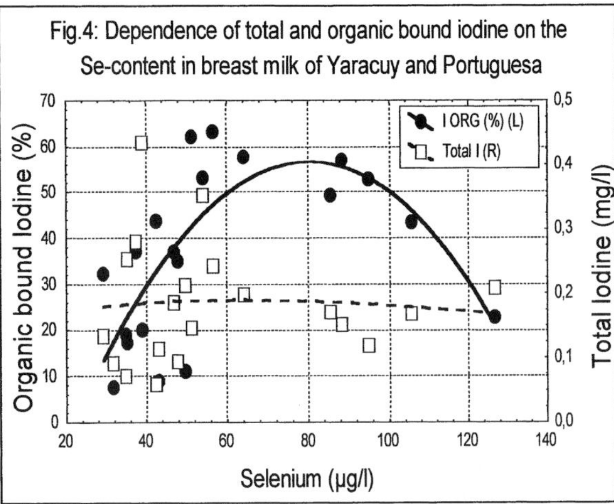

References:

1. Brätter, P., Negretti de Brätter, V.E., Rösick, U., von Stockhausen, H.B.. Selenium in the nutrition of infants: Influence of the maternal selenium status. In:*Trace elements in the nutrition of children II*. Chandra R.J. ed. Nestlé Nutrition Workshop Series Vol.23. Nestec Ltd. Vevey/Raven Press. New York. 1991; 79-90
2. Rilema J.A. and Rowady D.L. Characteristic of the prolactin stimulation of iodide uptake iinto mouse mammary gland explants.*P.S.E.B.M.* 1997; 215:366-9
3. Arthur J.R., Nicol, F., Beckett G.J. Selenium deficiency, thyroid hormone metabolism and thyroid hormone deiodinase. *Am.J.Clin.Nutr.* 1993; 57: 236S-9S
4. Brätter, P., Navarro-Blasco I., Negretti de Brätter, V.E., Raab, A. Speciation as an analytical aid in trace element research, *Analyst* 1998; 123:821-6
5. Brätter, P. Negretti de Brätter, V.E., Recknagel, S., Brunetto, R. Maternal selenium status influences the concentration and binding pattern of zinc in human milk. *J. Trace Elements Med.Biol.* 1997; 11:203-209
6. Chierici, R., Saccomandi, D., Vigi, V. Dietary supplements for the lactating mother: influence on the trace element content of milk. Acta Paediatr Suppl 1999; 88 (430): 7-13
7. Etling, N., Gehin-Fouque, F. Iodinated compounds and thyroxine binding to albumin in human breast milk. *Pediatric Res.* 1984; 18(9): 901-3
8. Brätter, P., Negretti de Brätter, V.E. Influence of high dietary selenium intake on the thyroid hormone level in human serum. *J. Trace Elements Med.Biol.* 1996; 10: 163-6
9. Ma, T., Guo, J., Wang, F. The epidemiology of iodine deficiency in China. *Am.J.Clin.Nutr.* 1993; 57:264S-6S

Metal Ions in Biology and Medicine; vol 6. Eds. J.A. Centeno, Ph. Collery, G. Vernet, R.B. Finkelman, H. Gibb, J.C. Etienne. John Libbey Eurotext, Paris © 2000, pp. 248-250.

Selenium balance in healthy American and Hungarian children living in Budapest, Hungary

Mária Ágnes Cser[1], Ibolya Sziklai-László[2], Nóra Adányi[3], Pamela Snyder[4] and Robert David Snyder[4]

[1] Bethesda Children's Hospital, 1146 Budapest, Bethesda St.3; [2] Atomic Energy Research Institute, 1525 Budapest 114. P.O.B. 49; [3] Central Food Research Institute, 1537 Budapest, P.O.B. 393; [4] Thomas Jefferson University, Philadelphia, PA, 19107 USA

Abstract. Blood selenium (Se) status of healthy Hungarians proved to be lower than that of others in Europe or USA. The aim of this study was to determine Se balance of healthy, 8-17 years old Americans living in Hungary on mixed food compared to those of healthy Hungarians consuming solely local food products. Over 3 days food intake was recorded, and total Se intake was determined by INAA analysis of duplicate diets. Urine and blood Se were measured by AAS. Results showed, that the daily caloric intake was similar in Americans and Hungarians, but Americans consumed more protein and carbohydrates and Hungarians had higher fat intake. Se intake and the Se content of food consumed were higher in Americans compared to the Hungarians. Se concentrations of erythrocytes, whole blood and plasma were significantly higher in Americans (p values <0.001). Urinary Se output was nearly 3 times higher in Americans compared to Hungarian children. In conclusion: locally produced Hungarian food provided a lower Se supply. Americans consumed foreign cereals, took more brown bread, milk and meat, their protein intake was higher resulting higher Se intake. Se balance was positive in both groups and Se output as fraction of intake was much higher in Americans than in Hungarians indicating to significant Se retention in order to maintain Se balance.

Introduction Se status depends mainly on Se intake(1) which is determined by the Se content in the diet provided by the complete food chain. Hungarian soil has been proven to be low in Se(2), and the Se status of healthy Hungarian population is lower than those of other healthy Europeans(3,4). Se requirements for children could vary between 50-200 mcg/day(5). Thus the contribution of various food groups to the overall dietary intake of selenium can differ markedly from one country to another and general dietary patterns could be very different. The principal route of non absorbed Se is the urinary excretion, which takes 50-60% of a wide range of the intake(6), and associated with the plasma Se concentration(1,7) as well as with dietary Se intake(8,9) of patients with different Se status. The aim of the present study was to compare Se balances of healthy group of children with different eating patterns, based on their habitual Se intake and output.

Material and methods 10 American and 15 Hungarian children recorded, individually weighed their diet, food duplicates and urine collected in trace element free plastic containers over two consecutive week days and on weekend, blood was taken on the third day. Body weights were 25-97 percentiles, all children were healthy, none had proteinuria. The total daily food was mixed, weighed, homogenised, lyophilised, aliquotes weighed before freezing in order to determine the conversion ratios from fresh to dry weight. Food Se contents were determined by Instrumental Neutron Activation Analysis (INAA), blood and urine Se measured by atomic absorption. Seven reference materials were applied, coefficients of variation were 4.5% for INAA and 1.5% for blood, 2.8% for urine with AAS method. Urine protein tested by Quantimetrix (Diagnosticum Hungary), creatinine measured by Jaffe, both by automated photometry.

Results Total daily Se intake varied between 36.2 to 97.3 mcg with an 18% coefficient of variance in the Americans and from 26.8 to 52.1 mcg in the Hungarians with only 7% c.v., the mean intake was higher in the Americans, 62 versus 41 mcg/day ($p<0.001$). Se intake calculated for body weight, resulted even greater differences, being 1.54 v. 0.91 mcg/kg/day respectively ($p<0.001$). Food consumed reached 0.14 mcg Se/g dry weight in the Americans and it was only 0.08 in the Hungarians ($p<0.01$). Caloric intake was similar in both groups: 2320±175 and 2280±128 kcal/day respectively. Americans consumed more protein (1.8±0.42 versus 0.72±0.32 g/kg b.w.) and carbohydrates (8.3±0.4 v 5.8±0.9 g/kg b.w.), and Hungarians had higher fat intake (2.9 ±0.3 vs. 1.5±0.6 g/kg b.w.). Caloric intake increased with age, but no such association was found in relation with Se intake. Se concentrations (μmol/L) of erythrocytes (1.69±0.21 vs. 1.14±0.20), of whole blood (1.13±0.17 vs. 0.83±12) and of plasma (0.85±0.16 vs. 0.64±0.1) were significantly higher in Americans (p values<0.001). Urinary Se excretion was remarkably less in Hungarians, 6.9 mcg/day compared to 24 mcg/day in Americans, similar differences were observed when Se output was calculated per g creatinin, 11±5 vs. 27± 9 mcg respectively, or for body weight, 0.36±0.11 vs. 0.15±0.08 μmol/kg. Se balance was considered as the difference between intake and urinary output resulted 39±22 mcg/day or 1.01±0.72 mcg/kg b.w. in Americans and 33±7 mcg/day or 0.75±0.18 mcg/kg b.w. in Hungarians. Se output as percentage of intake was 41% in the Americans and only 17% in the Hungarians.

Discussion Selenium balance studies revealed that they are not suitable to define requirements since humans maintain Se balance over a broad range of intake(10). Factors affecting either Se inflow or outflow, such as disturbed mucosal, intestinal, kidney or hormonal functions were carefully excluded. Therefore the comparison of the balance results of the two healthy groups of children may give some information associated with habitual metabolic patterns. It has been shown, that on average 1 mcg of Se/kg body weight maintains a zero balance and Se pools in American adults(11). The American children living longer than a year in Hungary had a Se intake above this value, but the Hungarians were below that level and in those under ten years of age it did not reach the sum of basal and normative Se requirement suggested by the WHO(12). The Se content in their diet was different and this can be explained by analyzing the composition of diet samples. The American children consumed more protein, first of all meat and more cereals and wholemeal bread, the later known to have higher bioavailability than white bread. Hungarians had a similar caloric intake, but fat consumption revealed a larger fraction of their diet. The fact that all blood compartments showed higher Se concentrations in the Americans suggest that their tissue Se sources could be higher than that of the Hungarian children. The most striking difference between the two groups was observed concerning the daily urinary Se excretion. Americans excreted similar amounts as German(13) or Polish(14) children but Hungarians as little as penylketonurics or people in Keshan area(15). In many studies Se excretion correlated with Se intake(16), in our study the higher intake also associated with higher output. However Se intake of the Americans was 30% igher than that of the Hungarians, a much smaller fraction of intake was excreted with urine in this group showing a lower Se status. This disproportion might indicate a less than optimal tissue Se sources inducing renal retention of selenium. The present observations could promote to encourage the Hungarians to change their eating patterns in order to increase their selenium status.

Literature

1.Thomson, C.D., Robinson M.F., Campbell D.R., Rea H.M. Effect of prolonged supplementation with daily supplements of selenomethionine and sodium selenite on glutathione peroxidase avtivity in blood of New Zealand residents. Am. Nutr. 1982; 36: 24-31.

2. Gondi F., Pantó Gy., Fehér J., Bogye G.,Alfthan G. Seleniumin Hungary. The rock-soil-human system. Biol Trace Elem Res. 1992; 35: 299-306.

3. Cser M.Á., Sziklai-László I., Menzel H., Lombeck I. Selenium and glutathione peroxidases in healthy Hungarian children and adults.J. Ped. Hun. 1996; 47: 384-394.

4. Cser M.Á., Sziklai-László I., Menzel H., Lombeck I. Selenium and glutathione peroxidase activity in Hungarian children. J Trace Elem Med Biol 1996; 10: 167-173.

5. Levander O.A. Clinical consequences of low selenium intake and its relationship to vitamin E. Annals of N.Y Acad. Sci. 1982; 39: 70-80.

6. Levander O.A., Sutherland B., Morris V.C., King J.C. Selenium balance in young men during selenium depletion and repletion. Am. J. Clin. Nutr. 1981; 34: 2662-2669.

7. Robinson M.F., Rea H.M., Friend G.M., Stewart R.D., Snow P.G., Thomson C.D. On supplementing the selenium intake of New Zealanders. 2. prolonged metabolic experiments with daily supplements of selenomethionine, selenite and fish. Br J Nutr 1978; 39: 589-600

8. Thomson C.D., Robinson M.F. Selenium in human health with emphasis on those aspects peculiar to New Zealand. Am. J. Clin. Nutr. 1980; 33: 303- 323.

9. Néve J., Vertongen F., Capel P. Selenium supplementation in healthy Belgium adults: response in platelet glutathione peroxidase activity and other blood indices. Am J Clin. Nutr. 1988; 48: 139-143.

10. Mertz W. Use and misuse of balance studies. J.Nutr. 1987; 117: 1811-1813.

11. Levander O.A., Morris V.C. Dietary slenium levels needed to maintain balance in North American adults consuming self-selected diets. Am.J.Clin. Nutr. 1984; 39: 809-815

12. WHO Geneva Trace elements in human nutrition and health. 1996; pp 105-122.

13. Jochum F., Terwolbeck K., Meinhold H., Behne D., Menzel H., Lombeck I. Effects of low selenium state in patients with phenylketonuria.Acta Paediatr. 1997; 86: 775-777.

14. Wasowicz W., Golebiowska M., Chlebna-Sokol D. Increased urinary excretion of selenium in children-a response to surplus fluorine in drinking water. Trace Elem.Med. 1988; 5: 43-46.

15. Yang G., Wang S., Zhou R., Sun S. Endemic selenium intoxication of humans in China Am.J.Clin.Nutr. 1983; 37: 872- 881

16. Oster O., Prellwitz W. The renal excretion of selenium Biol.Trace Elem.Res. 1990; 24: 119-146.

Metal Ions in Biology and Medicine; vol 6. Eds. J.A. Centeno, Ph. Collery, G. Vernet, R.B. Finkelman, H. Gibb, J.C. Etienne. John Libbey Eurotext, Paris © 2000, pp. 251-253.

Selenium and thyroid hormones status during a year of selenium and iodine supplementation

Jan Kvíčala[1], Václav Zamrazil[1], Miloš Beran[2]

[1] *Institute of endocrinology, Národní 8, 116 94 Praha 1, Czech Republic;* [2] *VUPP, Radiová 7, 10231 Praha 10, Czech Republic*

SUMMARY

Two groups of participants of the supplemental trial were followed during one year of supplementation by 50 μg Se/day and 100 μg I/day in the form of yeast lysate. Se in serum and urine were detected as Se indexes as well as thyroid volume and serum thyroid hormones for the detection of its status. Serum Se of the supplemented persons increased significantly after 2 weeks and reached the values between 80 and 90 μg/l serum. Se in urine increased significantly in the same time. Se stores in organisms were probably filled during one year of the supplementation and so daily Se excretion reached value 44μg Se/day, which seems to be in agreement with the theory of 50-60% excretion of Se intake by urine. Supplemented and placebo group varied in the volume of thyroid significantly after one year of the trial and also trend in difference of serum TSH between the groups was visible, even when not significant. Reached values of Se indexes are not yet in the range of optimal Se status but increase of Se status is significant and the method used seems sufficient for substantial improvement of Se status and so its beneficial effects upon the Se deficient organism.

INTRODUCTION

Selenium is an essential trace element with many regulatory and protective functions, like detoxification of heavy metals and carcinogenic organic compounds, antioxidative protection, control of synthesis of prostaglandins, prostacyclines, leucotrienes and tromboxanes, or immunomodulation. Deiodination of thyroxine to thyromimetically active triiodothyronine by selenoprotein Deiodinase is one of the most important Se functions. Whole Europe is more or less Se-deficient and in the Czech Republic several regions with substantial Se deficiency were found (1-5). The aim of this study was: 1) To assess possibilities to increase Se status of our low Se population by food supplement on the basis of Se enriched yeast's lysate.

2) To follow state of thyroid and thyroid hormones after combined supplementation of Se and I to the group of inhabitants with low Se intake and marginal I intake.

MATERIALS AND METHODS

Chemicals, biological reference materials, and instruments were used as stated elsewhere [1]. Blood serum was analysed by neutron activation analysis (NAA) [2]. Human serum of the second generation and IAEA standard reference material H-4 were coanalysed for quality assurance of Se analyses, with the results of 1.06 μg /g dry serum (declared 1.05 μg/g) and 0.29 μg/g dry muscle (declared 0.28 μg/g). Urine Se was detected by fluorimetry as a complex with 2,3-diaminonaphthalene hydrochloride after one-tube wet ashing [1]. The precision was checked by Lyphocheck Urine analysis with the results 63.4 μg/l (declared 69.3 μg/l with acceptable values 55.4 – 83.2 μg/l). Analytical results were evaluated by the usual statistical methods.

RESULTS AND DISCUSSION

Serious Se deficiency of subpopulations in more regions of the Czech Republic has been found, with average serum Se between 42 – 63 μg/l and average urine Se between 7.6 – 12.6 μg/l for inhabitants 6 to 65 years old.50 persons chosen for this study were high school and university graduated inhabitants of Prague in the age of 18 to 65 years. They were divided into two groups of 27 persons supplemented by 50 μg Se and 100 μg I per day and placebo group of 23 persons. Starting Se indexes of both groups were identical (63.5 μg Se/l serum, 62.2 μg Se/l serum resp., and 20.2 μg Se/l urine, 19.2 μg Se/l urine resp.). Their average Se daily intake was assessed at about 40 μg per day according to the daily urine Se of 19.8 μg. Thyroid and thyroid hormone serum concentrations were in normal ranges. Blood for serum and 24 hours collections of urine were collected a week before and at the start of the supplementation. The next days of the collections were after 1, 2, 4, 9, 13, 29, 43 and 56 weeks of duration of the supplementation.15 persons withdrew from the trial after 13 weeks so the groups were reduced to 17 supplemented and 18 controls in the next duration of the trial. The course of both selenium indexes of both groups is shown on the figure 1.

Serum Se of placebo group varied in the range of 60 – 70 μg/l probably according to the Se intake in the diet whereas serum Se values of the supplemented group continually increased from the 2nd week of supplementation to the 9th one and then average Se concentration maintained the level between 80 and 90 μg Se/l serum. Differences between placebo and supplemented groups were highly significant ($p<0.01$ and better) from the 2nd week of supplementation till the end of the supplementation trial. The increase from 60 to 90 μg Se/l serum is substantial and reached concentration is on the average value of West-European countries. Even when it did not reach optimal values of 100 – 150 μg/l, values between 80 and 90 μg Se/l plasma are much better then values of placebo group. Moreover, placebo group represents higher standard of our population concerning this Se index. This fact emphasize necessity to increase Se status of our population and the result obtained shows one of the possible ways to this aim.

As for urine Se, the curve of Se excretion in the placebo group oscillates around the value of 20 μg Se per day, which represents daily intake of about 40 μg Se. Significant increase ($p<0.05$) has been detected after 2 and 4 weeks of Se supplementation even when low increase on 90% probability level ($p<0.1$) was found

Fig. 1 - Serum And Urine Se Concentration During Supplementation (50 ug/day)

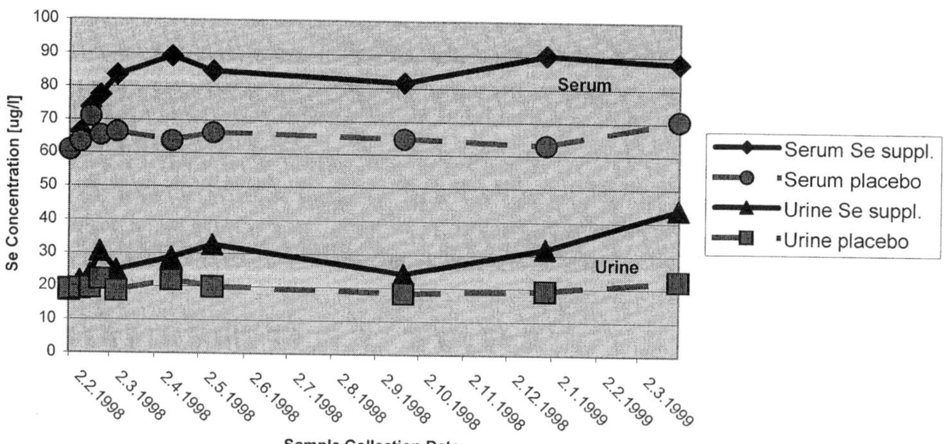

already after one week of supplementation. The decrease of urine Se excretion between 2nd and 4th week was probably due to the lower Se in the diet of both groups, whereas the decrease of the Se excretion in 29th week in supplemented group was due to irregular consumption of supplement (holidays, travelling etc.). Final increase of Se excretion to 44 μg/day in the group of supplemented persons might be explained by the completment of the body Se reserves, after which steady state between daily intake and excretion should be established. According the literature, 50 – 60 % of daily intake is excreted by urine. 22 μg increase of daily urine Se excretion in the supplementation group fits well with supplement of 50 μg Se per day.

Significant correlations between selenium and thyroid metabolism were published for low Se and marginal I intake [1]. Attention was paid in this trial to the thyroid and thyroid hormones. Thyroid volume was detected by sonography before the trial, after 29 weeks, and at the end of the supplementation. Significant differences ($p<0.01$) between thyroid volumes of the two groups were found at the end of trial. Overall changes of thyroid hormones were insignificant. Difference between TSH value of the supplemented participants and placebo group reached 80% probability level after one year of supplementation. These results show some trend of beneficial influence of Se and I increase upon organism.

ACKNOWLEDGMENT: This work was partly supported by grants IGA MZ CR No. 4845-3 and Research intention MZ CR No. MZ:000000023761.

REFERENCES

1. Kvicala J, Zamrazil V, Soutorova M, Tomiska F. Correlations between parameters of body selenium status and peripheral thyroid parameters in the low selenium region. *Analyst* 1995; 120: 959-65.

2. Kvicala J, Havelka J. Frequency of concentrations of some trace elements in serum by INAA. *J Radioanal NuclChem* 1988; 121: 261-70.

Metal Ions in Biology and Medicine; vol 6. Eds. J.A. Centeno, Ph. Collery, G. Vernet, R.B. Finkelman, H. Gibb, J.C. Etienne. John Libbey Eurotext, Paris © 2000, pp. 254-256.

Selenium status affects arsenic deprivation in rats

Eric O Uthus, Junquan Gao*, John W Finley, Cindy D Davis and Forrest H Nielsen

*USDA, ARS Grand Forks Human Nutrition Research Center, 2420 2nd Avenue North, Grand Forks, ND 58202-9034, USA and * Institute of Nutrition and Food Hygiene, Chinese Academy of Preventive Medicine, 29 Nan Wei Road, Beijing 100050, China*

Since 1938 when it was found that arsenic (As) counteracted the toxicity of seleniferous grains, it has been recognized that As and selenium (Se) can affect the metabolism of each other. Furthermore, there is evidence that As and Se can substitute for each other to prevent signs of deficiency. Thus, two experiments were performed to ascertain whether high or low dietary As would affect the signs of Se deficiency and whether high or low dietary Se would affect the signs of As deficiency.

Methods In experiment 1, male weanling Fisher-344 rats were fed a torula yeast-sucrose based diet containing about 3.9 ng of Se and 85 ng of As per g for 56 days. In experiment 2, female Sprague Dawley rats were fed a casein-sucrose based diet containing about 49 ng of Se and 3.1 ng of As per g diet for 63 days. Each experiment was factorially arranged. In experiment 1, the dietary variables were supplements of 0, 0.1 or 2.0 μg Se/g diet as selenite or selenomethionine (SeMeth) and 0 or 5 μg As/g diet as sodium arsenite. In experiment 2, the dietary variables were supplements of 0, 0.25 or 2.5 μg Se/g diet as selenite and 0 or 0.25 μg As/g diet as sodium arsenite. Standard methods were used for all analyses. Data were statistically compared by using analysis of variance contained in the statistical package SAS; differences were considered significant when $p<0.05$.

Results In experiment 1, Se deficiency decreased liver glutathione peroxidase (GPx); As did not affect this change (Table 1). However, in rats fed high dietary As, GPX was increased in animals fed 2.0 μg selenite/g compared to other Se-supplemented groups; in rats fed no supplemental As, no Se-supplemented groups were different. Plasma total homocysteine (tHcy) was decreased by 50% in Se-deficient rats; As did not affect this change. On the other hand, when high SeMeth was fed, high dietary As increased tHcy (Table 1). Incorporation of ^{3}H-methyl into liver DNA was increased by Se deprivation (^{3}H-methyl incorporation as measured by dpm/μg DNA is inversely related to methylation status of the DNA).

Table 2 (experiment 2) shows that marginal Se deficiency decreased liver GPx. An interaction between Se and As affected GPx and kidney molybdenum (K-Mo). Compared to rats fed 0.25 μg Se/g, those fed 2.5 μg Se/g had a decrease in

GPx activity in As-deprived, but not As-supplemented rats. As deprivation did not affect on K-Mo in rats fed no supplemental Se but decreased K-Mo in rats fed 0.25 μgSe/g diet. As deprivation decreased tHcy. Blood As was decreased by As deprivation; in rats fed 0.25 μg As/g, blood As tended to be lowest in rats fed 0.25 μg Se/g compared to rats fed either no supplemental Se or 2.5 μg Se/g.

Table 1. The effect of As and Se on GPx, tHcy, DNA methylation, and whole blood As (Experiment 1).

Se	As	GPx	tHcy	DNA methylation	Blood As
μg/g[a]		U/mg protein	μmol/L	dpm/μg DNA	μg/ml
0	0	21.4±9.0[b]	3.07±0.34	47110±13970	0.66 (0.60, 0.73)[c]
0	5	21.8±11.9	3.17±0.21	53330±10750	119 (102, 139)
0.1, selenite	0	1033±92.0	7.27±0.39	21120±3200	0.64 (0.55, 0.73)
0.1, selenite	5	826±232	6.82±1.35	29310±12310	121 (96, 152)
2.0, selenite	0	1161±226	6.91±0.89	19130±7400	0.63 (0.53, 0.75)
2.0, selenite	5	1579±327	6.30±0.40	20450±5910	121 (100, 142)
0.1, SeMeth	0	1046±358	6.87±1.06	25070±10980	0.80 (0.72, 0.89)
0.1, SeMeth	5	961±191	6.31±0.86	28200±14450	99 (46, 215)
2.0, SeMeth	0	1019±219	6.19±0.63	24130±11510	0.50 (0.32, 0.80)
2.0, SeMeth	5	1159±241	7.77±0.65	31260±15880	129 (104, 161)
Analysis of variance p values		Se=0.0001 As·Se=0.013	Se=0.0001 As·Se=0.01	Se=0.0001, As=0.08	As=0.0001

[a]Amount of Se or As supplemented to basal diet. [b]Mean ± standard deviation (N=6 per group). [c]Data were natural log-transformed prior to statistical analysis. Range given: (-1 SD, +1 SD).

Discussion Whole blood As, an indicator of As status, shows that rats fed no supplemental As averaged about 0.66 μg As/ml blood in experiment 1 (Table 1) and about 0.12 μg As/ml blood in experiment 2 (Table 2). The basal diets in experiment 1 and 2 contained approximately 85 ng As/g diet and 3.1 ng As/g diet, respectively. As indicated by As concentration in whole blood and diet, the diet from experiment 1 was only marginally deficient in As. As deprivation studies are typically done with diets containing <10 ng As/g diet.

The torula yeast-based diet is an excellent diet for Se deficiency studies. However, it contains an amount of As that does not allow for proper studies of As deprivation. Likewise, the diet used in experiment 2 is easily used to study As deprivation. However, it contains amounts of Se that do not allow for a marked Se deficiency. Thus, these experiments were not designed to study the effect of a marked As deprivation on a marked Se deficiency and vice versa.

Table 2. The effect of As and Se on GPx, kidney Mo, tHcy, and whole blood As (Experiment 2).

Se	As	GPx	K-Mo	tHcy	Blood As
µg/g[a]		U/mg protein	µg/g	µmol/L	µg/ml
0	0	956±49.3[b]	1.07±0.13	3.78±1.18	0.13 (0.11, 0.15)[c]
0	0.25	909±101	1.04±0.06	5.59±1.34	10.6 (7.9, 14.3)
0.25	0	1427±98.1	1.00±0.10	5.09±1.73	0.12 (0.10, 0.15)
0.25	0.25	1297±137	1.32±0.10	7.13±4.59	8.73 (7.77, 9.81)
2.5	0	1087±127	1.37±0.18	3.85±0.94	0.11 (0.09, 0.14)
2.5	0.25	1184±109	1.50±0.05	4.80±1.89	11.1 (10.4, 11.9)
Analysis of variance p values		Se=0.0001, As·Se=0.02	As,Se <0.001 As·Se=0.001	As=0.02	As=0.0001 As·Se=0.08

[a]Amount of Se or As supplemented to basal diet. [b]Mean ± standard deviation (N=7 – 8 per group). [c]Data were natural log-transformed prior to statistical analysis. Range given: (-1 SD, +1 SD).

There are several novel findings obtained in these experiments. The first is that Se deprivation decreased tHcy in rats. The reason for this decrease is presently unknown. Liver S-adenosylmethionine and S-adenosylhomocysteine were not affected by Se status (data not shown). Bunk and Combs (1) showed that plasma free homocysteine concentrations were decreased in Se-deprived chicks. They suggested that Se may be involved in the conversion of methionine to cysteine. As also has been shown to influence the metabolism of methionine and molybdenum. Molybdenum, which was affected by an interaction between As and Se, is needed in transsulfuration. Hypomethylated DNA has been associated with increased risk of cancer. Thus, the effect of Se on DNA methylation may, in part, explain some of the reported protective effects of Se on cancer.

The findings from experiment 1 indicate that although high dietary As (5 µg As/g diet) does not exacerbate signs of Se deficiency, both low and high dietary Se alter the response of rats fed a diet marginally deficient in As. Results from experiment 2 show that Se, at adequate or excess intake, can affect the response of rats to As deprivation.

Reference 1. Bunk MJ and Combs GF Jr. Evidence for an impairment in the conversion of methionine to cysteine in the selenium-deficient chick. *Proc Soc Exper Biol Med* 1981; 167: 87-93.

Metal Ions in Biology and Medicine; vol 6. Eds. J.A. Centeno, Ph. Collery, G. Vernet, R.B. Finkelman, H. Gibb, J.C. Etienne. John Libbey Eurotext, Paris © 2000, pp. 257-260.

Inhibitory potential of selenomethionine in dimethylhydrazine-induced rat colon cancer

Santa Ghosh, Mitali Basu, Sunil Srivastawa and Malay Chatterjee*

Division of Biochemistry, Department of Pharmaceutical Technology, Jadavpur University, Calcutta 700 032, India

Abstract

A single DMH injection (20mg/kg body weight, intraperitoneally) was given for DNA single strand break study from rat colon tissue according to Basak 1996[1]. SeM (8ppm) was administered *ad libitum* through drinking water. Transmission electron microscopy (TEM) of colon tissue sections were performed after 32 weeks of SeM treatment and 16 DMH injections (once/week). More than 10-fold increase in DNA strand break was observed in DMH treated rat tissue (P<0.001). SeM significantly (P<0.001) reduced strand break to a mere 2.3-fold in DMH treated samples. SeM effectively reduced the single strand break and also does improve ultrastructural changes associated with carcinogenic development.

Introduction:

Administration of selenium in the diet or drinking water to animals exposed to a wide variety of chemical carcinogens has resulted in reduced tumor incidence and/or tumor numbers [2,3]. Our study was extended to Electronic Microscopic (TEM) observation to ascertain the potential of Selenium as SeM on the ultrastructural changes associated with development of DMH induced colon-carcinogenesis.

Materials and Method

Animals and Diet: Male Sprague-Dawley rats obtained from the Indian Institute of Chemical Biology (Calcutta, India) and weighing 80-100g at the beginning of the experiment were used. After an initial acclimatization animals are divided into two sets of various experimental and control groups. Group A, comprised of DMH-induced carcinogen control animals to which 1,2 DMH was administered intraperitoneally at 20mg/Kg body weight in 0.9% Nacl solution for a total period of 16 weeks. Group B, normal control animals received saline vehicle intraperitoneally. Group C, include animals supplemented with selenium as SeM at the dose of 8ppm *ad libitum* to drinking water following 24 hours after the carcinogen exposure. Group D animals comprised of SeM control and received only SeM at a dose of 8ppm *ad libitum* through drinking water.

Treatment of animals up for DNA-chain break: For the DNA chain break study, rats in group A and C were injected intraperitoneally with a single dose of DMH dissolved in 0.9% Nacl. DNA was isolated and purified from all the groups and number of single strand break per DNA fragment and the extent of the DNA unwinding were estimated according to Basak 1996[1]. Data were analyzed statistically for differences between the means using Student's t-test.

Treatment of Tissues for TEM: TEM of colon tissue sections were performed after 32 weeks of SeM treatment and 16 DMH injection (once/week). Specimens are processed according to Luft 1961[5] and examined in a Philips CM 10 electron microscope at an accelerating voltage of 60 kv. After TEM viewing for 2hours per sample, photographs were taken.

Results and Discussion:

DMH induced carcinogen control animals (Group A) resulted in a significant rise in the colonic single strand break in comparison to their normal control counterparts (Group B). Where as the single strand break of DNA of experimental group (Group C) was 2.3 fold less ($P<0.001$) compare to DMH control (Group A)(Fig.1). This inhibition in the number of single strand breaks of the DNA at the initiation stage of colon carcinogenesis explain antitumor efficacy of SeM through modulation of cytogenetic change.

From the previous study it has revealed that in electron microscopic investigation of neoplastic colonocytes in DMH induced rat colon carcinogenesis the proliferative lesions displayed a mixture of several alteration. In contrast normal colonic feature the DMH induced preneoplastic colonic cell displayed visual indications of cellular proliferation. While in Group C animals displayed feature closely resembling those of the normal control. The loosening of cells was arrested only feeble loosening between the cells were noted. Thus chemopreventive potential of SeM was reaffirmed through electron microscopic studies. Our present investigation supports the molecular basis of the anticarcinogenic action of selenium on rat liver, mamary, intestine fore stomach and finally on colon carcinogenesis.

Reference:

[1] Basak J. Estimation of single-strand breaks induced in the dried film of DNA by high energy alpha particle from a cyclotron. *Ind. J Biochem. Biophys*. 1996; **33**:35-38.

[2] Cekan E, Slanina P, Bergman K, Tribukait B. Effect of dietary supplementation with selenomethionine on the tetratogenic effect of isonising radiation in mice. *Acta Radiol. Oncol*. 1985; **24**:459-63.

[3] Beems RB. Dietary selenium and benzo(a) pyrene induced respiratory tract tumors in hamsters. Carcinogenesis.1986; **7**:485-63.

[4] Popescu NC, Ansbaugh SC and Dipaolo JA. Correlation of morphological transformation to sister chromatid exchanges induced by split doses of chemical or physical carcinogens on cultured syrian Hamster cells. *Cancer Res*.1984; **44**: 1933-1938.

[5] Luft HT, Symrck TC, Watson P, Lanspa SJ, Lynch JF, Lyrnch PM, Cavalieri RJ and Boland CR. Genetics, natural history, tumor spectrum and pathology of hereditary no-polyposis colorectal cancer-An updated review. *Gastroentology*. 1993; **104**: 1535.

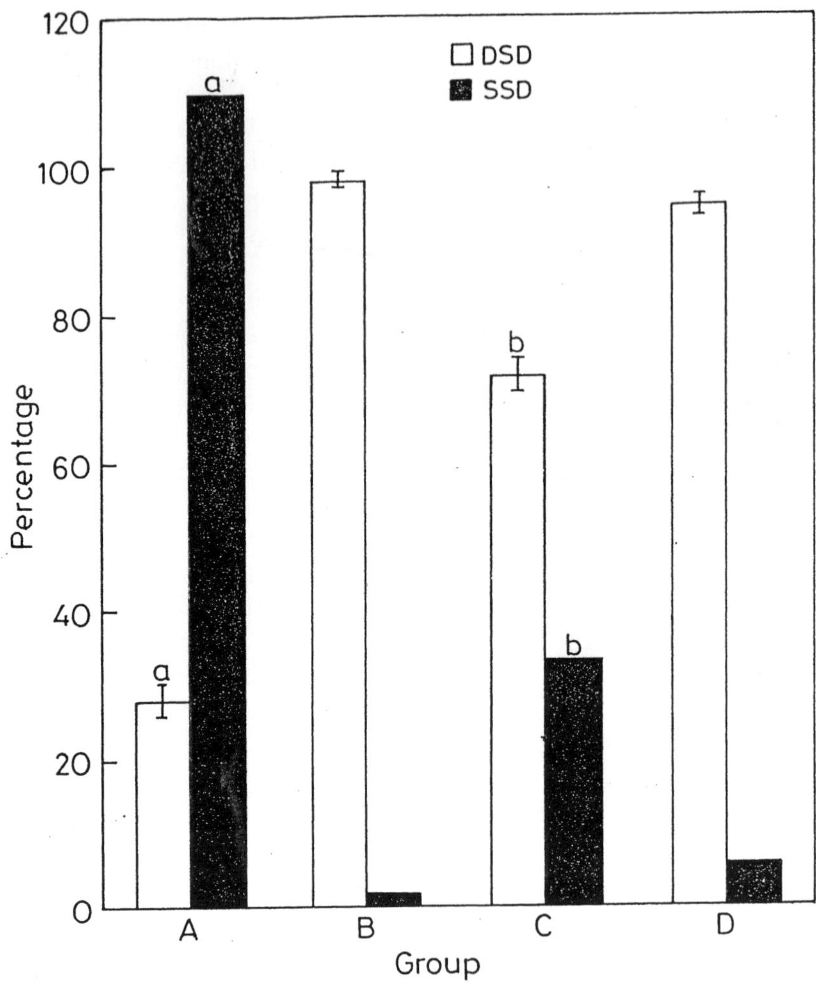

Fig. I. Effect of SeM (a ppm) supplementation on the generation of DNA-chain breaks in the presence/ absence of DMH treatment.

Metal Ions in Biology and Medicine; vol 6. Eds. J.A. Centeno, Ph. Collery, G. Vernet, R.B. Finkelman, H. Gibb, J.C. Etienne. John Libbey Eurotext, Paris © 2000, pp. 261-263.

Peroxidase activity in selenium and copper treated liver

Kralj-Klobučar N. and M. Gorup

Department of Biology, Faculty of Science, Rooseveltov trg 6, 10000 Zagreb, Croatia

Carp (*Cyprinus carpio L.*) were treated with selenium and copper in final concentation of 0,1 mg/L water. Concentration of proteins and peroxidase activity were spectrophotometrically determined in the liver during sixteen days of contamination. Treatment led to decrease of protein concentration. Peroxidase activity were increased by copper and decreased by selenium treatment.

Introduction

Introduced in organism, selenium bounds in the blood to the transport protein albumin which transports it to the liver. In the liver selenium is incorporated into selenoprotein as a part of the enzyme glutathione-peroxidase (GSH-Px). GSH-Px is an antioxidative enzyme which reduces hydrogen peroxid and organic peroxides and diminishes oxidative stress. The aim of the present study was to investigate effect of selenium and copper contamination on peroxidase activity.

Material and methods

Research was conducted on carp (*Cyprinus carpio L.*) treated separately with $Na_2SeO_3x5H_2O$ and $CuSO_4x5H_2O$ in final concetrations of 0,1 mg Se and Cu/L water, during sixteen days. The liver samples were taken for analysis every day during first four days, and after that period, in intervals of two or three days. The peroxidase activity was determined spectrophotometrically by measuring the values of absorbancy at 470 nm [1] and concentration of total proteins at 595 nm [2].

Results

Selenium and copper intoxication led to a slowly decrease of protein concentration in tissue (Fig. I). Mean value of protein concentration in the nontreated tissue was 10,29447 mg/gFW, by copper treatment 9,282474 mg/gFW , and by selenium treatment 8,691202 mg/gFW. Results suggested that elements brought in organism inhibited syntesis of proteins and the effect was more strongly expressed in selenium intoxication. Both elements showed considerable influence on peroxidase activity in tissue (Fig. II). Increase of peroxidase activity during first 48 hours apparently presented a quick response to the intoxication responsible for preventing peroxidative damage. After the initial growth which was concordant for both elements, activity was noticeably distinguished. Copper contamination led to increase and selenium contamination to decrease of peroxidase activity in relation to control specimens. In the copper treated tissue maen value was 1,073867 nm/min·mg which presented increase in relation to activity of nontreated tissue which was 0,883934 nm/min·mg. In selenium treatment mean value of peroxidase activity was 0,850078 nm/min·mg and presented value lower than in nontreated tissue.

Discussion

Increased peroxidase activity during copper intoxication found in our investigation represented defensive reaction of organism to the oxidative stress caused by intensified metal intake. Protection against reactive oxigen generated by copper was attained perhaps by sequestration of copper in the metallothioneins [3]. The metallothionein level and its inducibility following administration of the heavy metals have been demonstrated in the liver [4], although long-term administration of toxic elements Pb and Cd demonstrate the inhibition of selenoenzyme (GSH-Px) [5]. Effect of anorganic selenium on peroxidase activity was different in relation to copper effect. Decreasing of protein synthesis conditioned by prolonged intoxication resulted in decreased possibility of selenium incorporation in selenoproteins which led to accumulation of selenium in the tissue. Accumulation of selenium wasn't activate enzym peroxidase, but on the contrary inhibited its activity, perhaps by reason of impossibility to recognize selenium as foreign element because it was included in normal protein structure. Negative interaction between selenium and nutrients has been reported in the literature. Namely, high dietary selenium reduces the activity of some antioxidant enzymes [6]. Decrease of peroxidase activity caused H_2O_2-induced oxidative damage, and explained toxic effect of selenium manifesting during longer contamination, even with the lower doses.

Reference

1. Mäder M, Münch P, Bopp M. Regulation und Bedeutung der Peroxidase-Musteränderungen in sprossdifferenzieren den Kallus Kulturen von *Nicotiana tabacum L. Planta* 1975; 123: 257-265.
2. Bradford MM. A rapid and sensitive method for the quantitation of microgram quantities of protein utilizing the principle of protein-dye binding. *Anal Biochem* 1976; 72: 248-254.
3. Cai L, Koropatnick J, Cherian MG. Metallothionein protects DNA from copper-induced but not iron-induced cleavage in vitro. *Chemico-Biol Interactions* 1995; 96: 143-155.
4. Eaton DL, Stacey NH, Wong K-L, Klassen CD. Dose-response effect of various metal ioms on rat liver metallothionein, glutathione, heme oxigenase and cytochrome p-450. *Toxicol Appl Pharmacol* 1980; 66: 134-142.
5. Eybl V, Caisova D, Koutensky J. The influence of cadmium and lead on the activity of two selenoenzymes (GSH-Px and 5'DI-I), thyroid status and trace element levels in rats. In: Collery P, Brätter P, de Brätter VN, Khassanova L, Etienne JC, eds. *Metal Ions in Biology and Medicine*. Paris: John Libbey Eurotext, 1998: 534-538.
6. Albrecht R, Pelissier MA, Boisset M. Excessive dietary selenium decreases the vitamin A storage and the enzymatic antioxidant defense in the liver of rats. *Toxicol Lett* 1994; 70: 291-297.

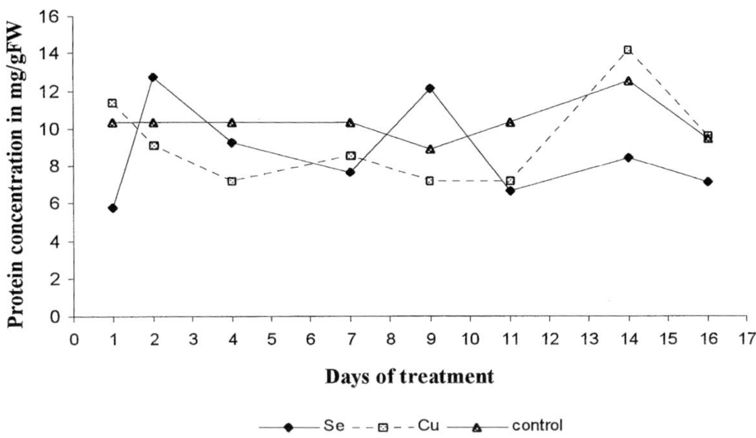

Figure I. Comparative relation of protein concentration in the liver of control and treated carp

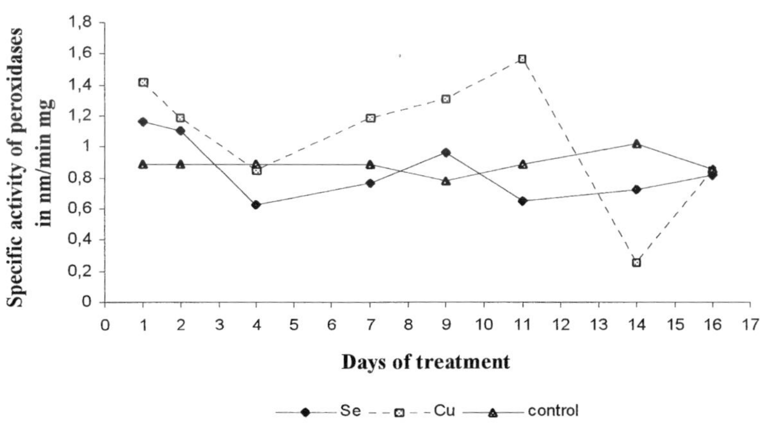

Figure II. Comparative relation of peroxidase activity in the liver of control and treated carp

Metal Ions in Biology and Medicine; vol 6. Eds. J.A. Centeno, Ph. Collery, G. Vernet, R.B. Finkelman, H. Gibb, J.C. Etienne. John Libbey Eurotext, Paris © 2000, pp. 264-266.

Are the characteristics of the newborn child (NC) related to the concentration of selenium in the mother?

Pérez Beriain R.M., García de Jalón A., Calvo Ruata M.L., Guirado F., Rebage V., Guerra M.

Servicio de Bioquímica Clínica, Sección de Nutrición y Metales, Hospital Universitario Miguel Servet, Calle Calamita n° 3, 50009 Zaragoza, Spain

INTRODUCTION

Selenium is one of approximately 90 stable elements in the earth's crust. Its atomic weight is 78.96 and its atomic number is 34. It was discovered by the Swedish chemist Berzelius, and for a long time was considered to be without any biological properties [1].

In 1957 Schwarz and Foltz established its importance as an essential nutrient in animals' diets [2]. Later, Rotruck *et al.* identified it in the active centre of the glutathione peroxidase enzyme [3]. This discovery clarified the relationship between selenium and vitamin E as antioxidant agents. Subsequently a W.H.O. team of experts declared selenium to be an essential nutrient, unable to substitute [4].

Pregnancy is a physiological condition which causes selenium deficiency owing to the removal of maternal selenium by the foetus [5,6].

AIMS

To establish the relationship between the serum concentrations of selenium in the mother and product of childbirth: the sex of the newborn child, weight and gestational age, as well as the type of childbirth (caesarean or vaginal).

MATERIALS AND METHODS

The serum concentration of selenium was determined in 265 women, who were aged between 17 and 46 (mean= 30.5 ± 4.9 years old), at the moment of childbirth, during the period from 29 September 1998 to 20 June 1999. The sex of the newborn child (NC) is known in 247 cases, the weight and gestational age in 264, and childbirth type is known in all of cases.

As a control group, we selected the serums of 63 healthy and not pregnant women who were aged between 17 and 44 (mean= 27.0 ± 6.9 years old).

The determination was carrried out by atomic absorption spectrophotometry (AAS) with a graphite camera and a Zeeman background corrector (*Perkin Elmer 4110 ZL*), using Pd $(NO_3)_2$ as matrix modifier.

Statistical calculations were carried out using SPSS statistics program. The statistical tests used, have been the Student T-test for equality of means, and the Mann-Whitney U - Wilcoxon rank Sum W test.

RESULTS AND CONCLUSIONS

In first time, we determined the selenium levels in 255 women at the moment of chilbirth, and we comparised that levels with the selenium levels of control group.

The results was:

	N	Mean (μg/l)	S.D.	C.I.(95%)
Mothers group	265	50.7	10.2	49.4 - 51.9
Control group	63	72.9	9.4	70.5 - 75.2

Table I.

The means comparison using the Student T-test gave a statistically significant difference with a $p<0.001$.

- **NC SEX.**

The distribution of selenium levels in the mothers according to NC sex was as follows:

	N	Mean (μg/l)	S.D.	C.I. (95%)
Mothers with female NC	111	50.9	11.2	48.7 - 53.0
Mother with male NC	136	51.1	9.4	49.4 - 52.7

Table II.

After carrying out a Student T-test for independent samples the difference was not significant.

We can conclude that the sex of the product of childbirth does not influence the mother´s selenium levels.

- **NC WEIGHT.**

The selenium levels in the mother according to NC weight are:

	N	Mean (μg/l)	S.D.	C.I. (95%)
Mothers with NC weight<2800g	43	53.5	7.9	51.0 - 55.9
Mothers with NC weight>2800g	221	50.2	10.5	48.7 - 51.6

Table III.

The Student T-test for independent samples determined a statistically significant difference with a $p=0.021$.

This may be due to the fact that the transfer of selenium from mother to child is produced the final moments of childbirth, which is when the NC gains the greatest percentage of weight.

- **GESTATIONAL AGE.**

According to gestational age, the results were:

	N	Mean (µg/l)	S.D.	C.I. (95%)
Mothers with premature NC	16	55.2	12.5	48.9 - 61.4
Mothers with term NC	238	50.5	10.0	49.2 - 51.7

Table IV.

The Mann-Whitney U - test shows that differences are not statistically significant.

Although the mean for mothers with premature N.C is greater that that for mothers whose NC were at term, the differences are not statistically significant due possibly to the small size of one of the samples.

- **CHILDBIRTH TYPE.**

Selenium levels are:

	N	Mean (µg/l)	S.D.	C.I. (95%)
Caesarean birth	10	56.8	12.0	49.2 - 64.3
Vaginal birth	255	50.4	10.1	49.1 - 51.6

Table V.

The Mann-Whitney U test shows a statistically significant difference with a p=0.054.

REFERENCES

1. Kieffer F. *Trace elements govern our health.* International Sandoz Gazzete. 1983.
2. Schwarz K, Foltz CM. *Selenium as an integral part of factor 3 against dietary necrotic liver degeneration.* J Am Chem Soc, 1957. 79 : 3292-3.
3. Rotruck et al. *Selenium Biochemical role as a component of glutathione peroxidase.* Science. 1973.179 : 588-90.
4. *Minor and trace elements in breast milk.* Report of a Joint WHO/IAEA. Collaborative Study. Geneva and Vienna. 1989.
5. Navarro M, Lopez H, Perez V, Lopez MC. *Serum selenium levels during normal pregnancy in healthy Spanish women.* Sci Total Environ. 1996 Jul 30; 186(3):237-42.
6. Odland JO, Nieboer E, Romanova N, Thomassen Y, Brox J, Lund E. *Concentrations of essential trace elements in maternal serum and the effect on birth weight and newborn body mass index in sub-artic and artic populations of Norway and Russia.* Acta Obstet Gynecol Scand. 1999 Aug; 78(7) : 605-14.

ACKNOWLEDGMENTS

This work has been supported by the Asociación para la Promoción de la Fundación Miguel Servet.

Metal Ions in Biology and Medicine; vol 6. Eds. J.A. Centeno, Ph. Collery, G. Vernet, R.B. Finkelman, H. Gibb, J.C. Etienne. John Libbey Eurotext, Paris © 2000, pp. 267-269.

Does hyposeleniaemia exist in newborn children (NC)?

Pérez Beriain R.M., García de Jalón A., Calvo Ruata M.L., Pérez Beriain T., Mayayo E., Bocos J.P.

Sección de Nutrición y Metales, Servicio de Bioquímica Clínica, Hospital Universitario Miguel Servet, C/ Calamita n° 3, 50009 Zaragoza, Spain

INTRODUCTION

Premature or lactational babies in their first months of life are population groups exposed to selenium deficiency, due to the small quantity of this element existing in their food (human milk and infant formulas) [1,2].

Older children´s most important source of selenium is from meat, fish and cereals. The values increase until they reach their maximum at the beginning of maturity (20 years old) [3].

It seems appropriate to divide the newborn population into subgroups by sex, gestational age, weight of the newborn child (NC).

If, in all those cases, the importance of selenium concentrations is due to the function this element plays in the elimination of free radicals, it is important to highlight its role as a necessary trace element to transform T4 into T3 (more active) [4].

AIMS

To study the influence of factors such as sex, gestational age and weight of NC on serum selenium levels.

MATERIALS AND METHODS

The blood selenium of 247 newborn children, born between June 1998 and June 1999, was analysed. The sex of 212 was recorded, as well as the gestational age of 218, the weight of 217 and the incidence of jaundice in 218.

The method used was atomic absorption spectrophotometry (AAS) using a graphite camera and Zeeman background corrector (*Perkin Elmer 4110 ZL*) and $Pd(NO_3)_2$ solution as matrix modifier.

The statistical analysis was carried out with the SPSS statistics program. The statistical test used, was the Student-T test.

RESULTS AND CONCLUSIONS

The determination of selenium in the 247 NC (fig. 1) shows concentrations of 31.2 +/- 16.8 µg/l which are more than 50% lower than serum selenium concentrations in adults.

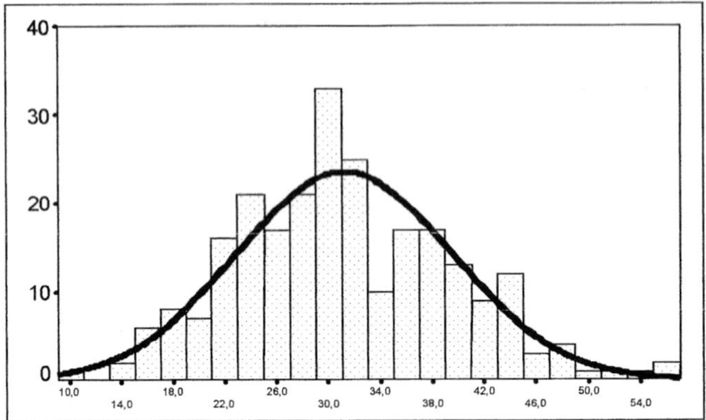

Figure 1. Distribution of selenium levels in newborn children.

Acoording to the different NC groups the results are:

1.-SEX: The following selenium concentrations were give according to sex:

	N	Mean (µg/l)	S.D.	C.I.(95%)
Male NC	105	29.9	7.7	28.4 - 31.4
Female NC	107	31.2	8.8	29.5 - 32.9

Table I.

The differences were not significant. We can conclude that NC sex does not influence selenium levels.

2.- WEIGHT: With regard to wight, selenium level distribution was:

	N	Mean (µg/l)	S.D.	C.I.(95%)
NC weighing <2500g	110	28.8	8.4	27.2 - 30.4
NC weighing >2500g	107	33.1	8.2	31.5 - 34.7

Table II.

The Student T for independent samples shows a statistically significant difference with a $p<0.001$.

3.- GESTATIONAL AGE: The results with regard to gestational age are:

	N	Mean (µg/l)	S.D.	C.I.(95%)
Premature NC	96	27.9	7.7	26.3 - 29.8
Term	122	33.2	7.8	31.8 - 34.6

Table III.

After carring out the means analysis with a student T for independent samples, we found a statistically significant difference with a $p<0.001$ (fig 2).

The premature NC show selenium levels lower than term NC.

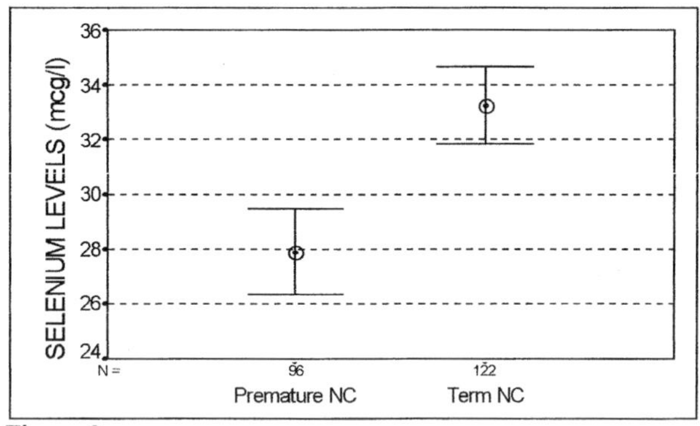

Figure 2.

4.- JAUNDICE: With regard to the incidence of jaundice, the results are:

	N	Mean (µg/l)	S.D.	C.I.(95%)
NC without jaundice	180	30.8	8.4	29.6 - 32.1
NC with jaundice	38	30.0	7.9	27.4- -32.6

Table IV.

The Student-T test for independent samples shows that the difference is not significant. Jaundice does not influence blood selenium level in newborn children.

52% of the NC in our study have a serum concentration of selenium lower than 30 µg/l, a level considered to be of risk in the literature. This could influence the activity of the 5′-desiodase, decreasing the T3 concentration and aggravating the endemic hypotyhroidism which exist in some districts of Aragon.

REFERENCES

1. Chandra RK. Trace elements in nutrition of children. Nestle Nutrition. Volume 8. Raven Press : New York, 1985.
2. Torres MA; Verdoy J, Alegria A, Barbera R, Farre R, Lagarda MJ. Selenium contents of human milk and infant formulas in Spain. Sci Total Environ. 1999 Apr 5; 228(2-3) : 185-92.
3. Denis A *et al. Los oligoelementos en pediatría*. Pediatrika 1988. VIII(1) : 13-23.
4. Kvecala J, Zamrazil V, Soutorove M. *Correlations between parameters of body selenium status and paripheral thyroid parameters in the low selenium region.* Analyst 1995 Vol. 120 nº 3 : 959-65.

ACKNOWLEDGMENTS

This work has been supported by the Asociación para la Promoción de la Fundación Miguel Servet.

Metal Ions in Biology and Medicine; vol 6. Eds. J.A. Centeno, Ph. Collery, G. Vernet, R.B. Finkelman, H. Gibb, J.C. Etienne. John Libbey Eurotext, Paris © 2000, pp. 270-272.

Selenium determination in human serum by zetaas: relevant analytical aspects

R. Sabé[1], R. Rubio[1], L. Garcia-Beltran[2]

[1] *Departament de Química Analítica, Universitat de Barcelona, Av. Diagonal, 647, 08028 Barcelona, Spain;* [2] *Servei de Bioquímica, Hospital General Universitari Vall d'Hebron, Pg. Vall d'Hebron, 119-129, 08035 Barcelona, Spain*

*to whom the correspondence should be addressed

Selenium is an essential element and it is usually determined in body fluids to assess nutritional status and possible toxic levels.

The most common technique for the determination of selenium in serum is atomic absorption spectrometry with electrothermal atomisation. Nevertheless there is controversy on the conditions of measurement, especially sample pre-treatment, furnace temperature programmes and chemical modifiers. The lack of control of these parameters has led to wide variation in the published data for assessing deficiency and toxicity.

Selenium measurement in serum by Zeeman-effect graphite furnace was optimised and the main quality parameters were established [1]. The detection limit was 2.6 μg Se l^{-1}. The accuracy in terms of recovery was evaluated by analysing two freeze-dried human serum reference materials; Seronorm™ Trace Elements, (Nycomed Pharma AS, Oslo, Norway) with a recommended value of 78 μg Se l^{-1} (analytical range from 75 to 84), and a Second-generation freeze-dried human serum, with a certified value of 1.05 μg Se g^{-1} dry weight, and a 95% confidence limits from 1.00 to 1.10, kindly supplied by Dr. R. Cornelis from the University of Ghent. The Seronorm™ selenium average content, from six independent replicates, was 81.5 μg Se l^{-1} with a relative standard deviation of 2.2%, while for the Second-generation freeze-dried human serum it was 1.07 μg Se g^{-1}, with a relative standard deviation of 2.1%.

In this paper the pre-analytical conditions such as the influence of blood collection devices for trace metal analysis and sample stability with time and temperature were studied. Two types of heparinised tubes, LH-Metall-Analytik S-Monovette (Sarstedt: polypropylene) and Na-Heparin Vacutainer-Hemogard (Becton Dickinson: glass), were tested to assess the influence of the material on the results. Aliquots from eleven donors, drawn into tubes of these two types, were analysed. After drawing, the samples were transferred to

polypropylene containers, kept at 4°C and analysed within 24 hours. No significant differences were observed ($p<0.05$).
Factors affecting stability were studied by analysing two plasma samples (15 ml each) from the same donor. Each plasma sample was divided into 22 aliquots. Eight aliquots were kept at 4°C and 14 at -20°C. The mean value obtained from two of the aliquots, kept at 4°C and analysed within two hours, was considered as the reference value. The remaining six aliquots at 4°C were analysed after 8, 24 and 48 hours. Longer periods at this temperature were not considered, since storage for more than 2 days at 4°C is not recommended. Aliquots stored at -20°C were analysed after 24 hours, 48 hours, 7 days, 15 days, 1 month, 2 months, 6 months and 1 year. Our results indicate that plasma samples stored at 4°C are stable for two days and those stored at -20°C are stable for a year, in terms of Se content.
Calibration methods using standard additions and external standard curve were studied and compared. Recent studies suggest that the external standard curve obtained by spiking a CRM [2] or by spiking a sample of the series to be analysed [3] could be used for selenium quantification in serum and plasma.
In the present study a series of plasma samples from subjects suffering from several pathologies were analysed by using both calibration methods. Differences in the slope were observed and consequently in the results if referred to an external curve. This pattern was then studied by analysing three groups of samples (Total Parenteral Nutrition (8 samples), cancer (6 samples) and healthy donors (29 samples)). Our results show that the two methods sometimes yield different Se content. Moreover, for the healthy donor group, 17% of the samples showed significant differences ($p<0.05$). Consequently, standard addition method is recommended.
Finally, reference levels of Se in serum in the area of Barcelona were established. A group of 58 healthy donors were analysed. The results from this study are reported on Table I.

Table I. Plasma selenium concentration in healthy population from the area of Barcelona.

	Age Range (years)	Mean ± sd ($\mu g\ l^{-1}$)	Range
Total (n=58)	39.0 ± 12.2	82.9 ± 20.0	
Males (n=31)	40.7 ± 12.7	81.7 ± 20.8	49.4-145.4
Females (n=27)	37.1 ± 11.5	84.3 ± 19.5	53.9-129.8

There were no significant differences by sex ($p<0.05$). Moreover, we report here data from patients under TPN (Total Parenteral Nutrition) (37 samples) and from patients with cancer (22 samples). The mean Se concentration was 66.4 ± 21.2 $\mu g\ l^{-1}$ (39.0-110.9) for TPN patients, and for patients with cancer, it was

64.9 ± 21.5 $\mu g\ l^{-1}$ (36.3-105.9). Significant differences in Se content were found, if compare that patients with healthy donors. However, no significant differences were found between the two pathologies.

The authors thank the DGICYT under Project 92-0541 for the financial support of this work.

[1] R. Sabé, R. Rubio and L. García-Beltrán, Anal. Chim. Acta 398 (1999) 279.
[2] M. Rükgauer, K. Uhland, E. Lindemann and J.D. Kruse-Jarres, Biomed. Tech. 41 (9) (1996) 236.
[3] M. Hoenig, Analusis 19 (1991) 41.

Metal Ions in Biology and Medicine; vol 6. Eds. J.A. Centeno, Ph. Collery, G. Vernet, R.B. Finkelman, H. Gibb, J.C. Etienne. John Libbey Eurotext, Paris © 2000, pp. 273-275.

Selenium in diet samples in Hungary

Ibolya Sziklai-László[1], M. Ágnes Cser[2], Pamela Snyder[3], Robert D. Snyder[3]

[1] KFKI Atomic Energy Research Institute, H-1525 Budapest, P.O. Box 49, Hungary; [2] Bethesda Children's Hospital, H-1146 Budapest, Bethesda Street 3, Hungary; [3] Thomas Jefferson University, Philadelphia, PA, 19107 USA

Abstract Selenium (Se) content of representative grain crops from several agricultural regions of Hungary and some basic nutrients such as, wheat and rye flours and different kinds of bread samples were measured by Instrumental Neutron Activation Analysis (INAA). The total, daily intake of Se was determined in healthy 8 to 17 years old American children residents in Hungary, employing the duplicate portion technique and results were compared to that of healthy Hungarian children.

Introduction. The dietary intake of Se in humans varies widely in different countries depending on the Se content of soil and its availability to plants. In order to stay in positive balance the North American adults need about 1μg of daily dietary Se per kg body weight (1). The recommended dietary allowance was calculated as 70 and 55 μg Se/day for adult males and females (2). The intake for European countries ranges from 30 to 60 μg Se/day (3), but requirements are not established yet. Low Se intakes have been found in neighboring countries (4,5,6). The Hungarian Food Composition Table (1995) does not contain the Se concentrations of the locally produced foods yet. There are only sporadic data on food Se contents and practically no data are available on basal or normative Se requirement in Hungary. The aim of the present study was to determine the Se intake of healthy American children living in Budapest, having different eating patterns from Hungarians, consuming not only locally grown food and compare results to that of healthy Hungarian children. In order to estimate the Se supply in Hungary representative grain crops and basic nutrients such as, wheat and rye flours, the main bread types consumed in Hungary were also analyzed for their Se content.

Materials and method Grain crops, flours and bread samples were homogenized and dried for 48 hours at 80 ^{0}C to constant weight. Diet samples were collected by using the duplicate-portion technique. The children and their parents were asked to weigh and record all food and drinks consumed over 3-day period (one week-end day). Samples were homogenized in a blender and suitable aliquots of the homogenate were lyophilized. After homogenization aliquots of the food samples were weighed in order to determine the conversion ratios from fresh to dry weight. For neutron irradiation sample masses of 100-200 mg from each were sealed in irradiation vials of high purity quartz (Suprasyl). Samples together with selenium standards (Merck) and reference materials were irradiated for 24 to 48 hours at a neutron flux density of $8x10^{13}$ $n.cm^{-2}.s^{-1}$ in the WWR-M type research reactor of the KFKI Atomic Energy Research Institute (Budapest, Hungary). For gamma spectroscopy measurements a CANBERRA Ge(Li) detector (with energy resolution of 1.82 keV and efficiency of 13.6% for the 1332.5 keV ^{60}Co line) and CANBERRA linear electronics were used. Gamma spectra evaluations were performed by the HYPERMET-PC program. Se content was estimated by measuring the gamma rays of ^{75}Se isotope. The accuracy of the Se determination by INAA was tested by co-analyses of NIST SRM 1567a Wheat Flour, 1548 Total Diet, NBS SRM 1568 Rice Flour and 1549 Non-Fat Milk Powder reference materials. The values found agreed very well with the certified value (coefficient of variation 4.5 %). Student's t-tests, linear regression analyses were carried out by Microsoft Excel 97.

Results Se contents were in wheat grains: 28±11 mcg/kg in barley: 43±10 mcg/kg, in oat: 39±6 mcg/kg, in rye: 47±9 mcg/kg, in rape: 18±5 mcg/kg in corn: 17±5 mcg/kg from main agricultural regions of Hungary. Some basic carbohydrate nutrients such as, wheat and rye flours (range 17-66 mcg/kg) and breads (15-68 mcg/kg) were also in lower range. Our results showed, that the average Se concentration of the diet was 144±45 mcg/kg (range 68-239, for dry weight) and 36±12 mcg/kg (range 15-61 for wet weight). Se levels of individual diets were the highest on weekend days, as high-protein ingredients (meat, fish or eggs) were included in the diet. The consumed daily diet varied from 1132 to 3142 (median: 1711) g/day wet weight, the dry mean material content was 446±125 g/day, representing 20 to 31% of the total weight. The dietary Se intake ranged from 26.8 to 99.7 mcg/day with a median of 55.6 mcg/day. Se intake in American boys was 71±19 mcg/day, higher than in girls (59±17 mcg/d), but the difference did not reach significance. Boys consumed 19 % more dry matter (504±194 g/d) than girls (424±84 g/day). The lowest intake of girls revealed to 26.8 mcg Se/day and that of boys to 37.9 mcg Se/day the highest reached 97.6 and 99.7 mcg Se/day respectively.

Discussion: The results of this study show that the locally produced grain crops varied greatly in their Se content and the mean concentrations are quite low, when compared to similar cereals grown in other European countries(7,8). Since concentrations of Se in the soils of the main agricultural regions of Hungary are very low, the low availability of Se for plants may explain the low Se content of the agricultural crops(9). The Se content of basic carbohydrate nutrients surveyed in the present study found to be low in comparison with corresponding data of other European countries(7,8). Selenium content of wheat from Hungary ranged from 12 to 47 mcg/kg with a mean value of 28±11 mcg/kg. Quantities of Se in wheat were all below 50 mcg/kg indicating to low soil Se supply in Hungary. Most of soil samples had less than 100 mcg/kg(9). Acidic to neutral pH conditions in soils promote low availability of Se for plants and this may explain the low Se content of the agricultural crops. Eating habits in Hungary do not give priority of food consumption with higher Se intake since white bread is more popular, than wholemeal, and cereal consumption is insignificant. Comparing the daily Se intake of American and Hungarian children, both in boys and girls the American children had significantly higher Se intake than the Hungarians, 71 mcg versus 45 in boys and 59 versus 39 mcg in girls. However differences in Se intake between boys and girls did not reach significance, boys tended to consume more Se similarly to observations made on male and female adults(4).

The daily caloric intakes were similar in both groups, but American children consumed more protein and carbohydrates. The Se intake of these children arises mostly from mixed food originated from other countries consumed more brown bread, meat and milk products, their higher protein intake resulted higher Se supply. Hungarians had higher fat intake, which was partly responsible for the lower Se intake. The dietary Se intake of the American children reached the Recommended Daily Allowance of the WHO(10) for children that are minimum of 50 mcg/day. However this was only 41 mcg/day in Hungarian children, especially in girls well below the recommended values. The main contributors of Se intake were eggs, pork and poultry. Hungarians consumed more white bread and pastas, fat and less fish and meat. Grain products with high Se content (cereals) were the most important dietary Se sources for the Americans, since grain products are the primary sources for Se in the infant and childhood diet(11). Americans consumed significantly more protein, first of all meat, known to be reach in Se and less fat, which has negligible Se content(11). In conclusion we could state, that locally produced food alone did not give enough Se supply. American children consumed more cereals of foreign origin, more brown bread, more milk and meat resulting a higher Se intake.

References

1. Levander O.A. Selenium requirements as discussed in the 1996 joint FAO/IAEA/WHO expert consultation on trace elem. in human nutr., Biomed Environ Sci 1997; 10:214-9.

2. National Research Council, Food and Nutrition Board: Recommended Dietary Allowances. 10th ed. Washington, D.C.: National Academy Press, 1989.

3. Robberecht H. J., Hendrix P., Van Cauwenbergh R., Deelstra H. A. Actual Daily Dietary Intake of Selenium in Belgium, using Duplicate portion sampling. Zeit. Lebensm. Unters. Fors. 1994; 192:251-254.

4. Klapec T., Mandic M.L., Grgic J., Primorac L., Ikic M., Lovric T., Grgic Z., Herceg Z... Daily dietary intake of selenium in eastern Croatia. Sci Total Environ 1998; 217:127-36.

5. Wasowicz W. Selenium in Eastern European countries. In: Proc. of the Fifth Int. Symp. on "Uses of Selenium and Tellurium". Carapella S.C., Oldfield J.E., Palmieri Y. (eds), selenium-Tellurium Development Assoc., 1994, 163-170, Belgium.

6. Kadrabová J., Madaric A., Ginter E. Determination of the daily selenium intake in Slovakia. Biol Trace elem Res, 1998; 61:3, 277-86.

7. Gissel-Nielsen, G., Selenium concentration in danish forage crops. Acta Agric. Scand. 1975; 25, 216-220.

8. Schulte W. Untersuchungen zum Selengehalt vo Futter- und Nahrungsmitteln in der Bundesrepublik Deutschland, Inaugural-Dissertation, 1988.

9. Gondi F., Pantó Gy., Fehér J., Bogye G., Alfthan G. Biol. Trace Elem. Res 1992; 35:299-306.

10. World Health Orgaization Geneva : Trace elements in human nutrition and health. Macmillan-Ceuterick, India-Belgium 1996

11. Pennington J.A.T., Schoen S.A. Contribution of food groups to estimates intakes of nutritional elements. Results from the FDA Total Diet Studies, 1982-1991. Internat. J.Vit. Nutr. Res. 1996; 342-349.

Metal Ions in Biology and Medicine; vol 6. Eds. J.A. Centeno, Ph. Collery, G. Vernet, R.B. Finkelman, H. Gibb, J.C. Etienne. John Libbey Eurotext, Paris © 2000, pp. 277-280.

Rhinotoxicity and olfactory uptake of metals

F. William Sunderman, Jr.

Department of Chemistry and Biochemistry, Middlebury College, Middlebury, VT 05753, USA

Abstract. Exposures of workers to inhalation of certain metal dusts or aerosols can injure the nasal mucosa and induce anosmia (*e.g.*, Ni, Cd) or cause septal perforation (e.g., Cr, As). Some metals (*e.g.*, Al, Cd, Co, Hg, Mn, Ni, Zn) can traverse the nose-brain barrier in experimental animals, passing along olfactory neurons from the nasal lumen to the olfactory bulbs. Carnosine (β-alanyl-L-histidine), a metal-binding peptide in olfactory neurons, may play a role in the rhinotoxicity and olfactory uptake of metals. Studies of nickel refinery workers show nickel compounds are carcinogenic for the nose and nasal sinuses.

Rhinotoxicity. Toxic effects of metals on the upper respiratory passages have long been recognized, owing to frequent mucosal irritation and nasal septal perforations in workers exposed to chromates, dichromates, arsenic trioxide, and arsenious acid, and by reports of anosmia in workers at nickel refineries and factories that produce nickel-cadmium batteries [1-6]. Rhinotoxicity of nickel also occurs in rats and mice, which show marked atrophy of the nasal epithelium after subchronic exposure to inhalation of $NiSO_4$ or nickel subsulfide (αNi_3S_2) [7,8]. Ni-induced atrophy of the nasal epithelium is a sensitive marker of Ni-toxicity [9]; it is attended by partial loss of sustentacular cells and bipolar olfactory receptor neurons, and diminished carnosine content of the olfactory bulbs [10]. Loss of olfactory neurons and anosmia have been reported in rodents following nasal instillation of $ZnSO_4$ [11-15]. $ZnSO_4$-induced anosmia can cause behavioral disturbances, such as impaired navigation in homing pigeons [16,17].

Nose-brain barrier. The barrier that impedes translocation of metals and other toxicants from the nasal lumen to the brain, has several components: (a) the physical barrier provided by nasal secretions, (b) the nasal mucociliary apparatus that clears particles, (b) tight junctions between olfactory neurons and sustentacular cells, (c) immunological defenses in the nasal mucosa, and (d) desquamation of epithelial cells, including olfactory receptor neurons, after toxicant exposures [18]. Olfactory receptor neurons are in direct contact with both the external environment and the brain [18]; unlike other neuronal cells, they regenerate from basal cells after damage [19]. Olfactory receptor neurons have dendritic knobs with receptor-bearing cilia or microvilli that project into the nasal lumen, and a single axon that traverses the cribriform plate into the ipsilateral olfactory bulb. Olfactory receptor neurons are connected via synapses in the olfactory bulb with the hypothalamus, hippocampus, olfactory tubercle, pyriform cortex, and other areas of the brain [18].

Neuronal transport of metals. Studies by autoradiography, radiometry, or atomic absorption spectrometry have shown that that certain metals (*e.g.*, Al, Cd, Co, Hg, Mn, Ni, Zn) are taken up from the nasal cavity into the olfactory epithelium and translocated via olfactory neurons to the olfactory bulb (Table 1) [20-34]. Some metals (*e.g.*, Mn, Ni) cross synapses in the olfactory bulb and migrate to distal nuclei of the brain. The axonal transport of metals can progress rapidly, within hours or a few days (*e.g.*, Mn), or slowly over days to weeks post-instillation (*e.g.*, Ni, Cd). The molecular mechanisms of metal uptake, transport, and toxicity in olfactory neurons are unknown. Indirect evidence points to carnosine (β-alanyl-L-histidine), a metal-binding peptide that is abundant in olfactory neurons, as a putative factor in the olfactory uptake and rhinotoxicity of metals [10,15,35-39]; metallothionein may also be involved [40]. Axonal transport of metals can likewise occur along the gustatory pathway. After intraglossal injection of $^{203}HgCl_2$ or $^{109}CdCl_2$ in rats, autoradiography demonstrated ^{203}Hg or ^{109}Cd in hypoglossal nuclei [41,42]. For more details on metal uptake via olfactory pathways, readers may consult reviews [43,44].

Table 1. Studies of metal uptake and translocation via olfactory pathways.

Metal	Species & compound	Route	Observations	References
Al	Rabbit, Al-lactate, $AlCl_3$	Nasal implants	Granulomas containing Al developed in olfactory bulbs and cerebral cortex following nasal implants of soluble Al salts in gelfoam pads.	Perl & Good [20]
Cd	Trout; pike, rat, $^{109}CdCl_2$	Intranasal application/ instillation	Autoradiography and γ-spectrometry showed high levels of ^{109}Cd in the ipsilateral olfactory bulb, but ^{109}Cd did not cross synapses to enter secondary olfactory neurons.	Tjälve *et al* [21, 22]; Gottofrey & Tjälve [23]
Cd	Rat, $^{109}CdCl_2$	Intranasal instillation	After unilateral exposure, ^{109}Cd levels in the ipsilateral olfactory bulb were ~40-times those in the contralateral olfactory bulb.	Hastings & Evans [24], Evans & Hastings [25]
Co	Rat, $^{57}CoCl_2$	Intranasal instillation	^{57}Co passed along olfactory neurons to the olfactory bulb; low level of ^{57}Co was seen in secondary olfactory neurons.	Persson *et al* [26]
Hg	Pike, $^{203}HgCl_2$	Intranasal application	^{203}Hg moved via olfactory neurons to ipsilateral olfactory bulb; transfer to secondary neurons was not observed.	Borg-Neczak & Tjälve 1996 [27]
Mn	Trout, pike, rat, $^{54}MnCl_2$	Intranasal application/ instillation	^{54}Mn rapidly traveled along the primary olfactory neurons, crossed the synapses in the olfactory bulb, and reached large areas of the brain (and also the spinal cord in rats).	Rouleau *et al* [28], Tjälve *et al* [22,29], Henriksson *et al* [30]
Mn	Rat; $MnCl_2$	Intranasal instillation	After one unilateral instillation, Mn reached peak levels in the ipsilateral olfactory bulb at 12 h and remained elevated for 3 days. After repeated treatments, Mn levels also became elevated in the ipsilateral striatum.	Gianutsos *et al* [31]
Ni	Rat, monkey, $^{63}NiSO_4$, ^{63}NiO	Inhalation	Acute inhalation of soluble $^{63}NiSO_4$ particles led to ^{63}Ni accumulation in olfactory bulbs at 2-20 wk postexposure. After inhalation of insoluble ^{63}NiO, no accumulation of ^{63}Ni was detected in the olfactory bulbs	Lewis *et al* [18]
Ni	Rat, pike, $^{63}NiCl_2$	Intranasal application/ instillation	^{63}Ni traveled by slow axonal transport in olfactory neurons to the olfactory bulb. ^{63}Ni was bound to particulate and soluble constituents in neuronal cytosol. Low levels of ^{63}Ni migrated to the olfactory peduncle and tubercle, and also to anterior parts of the cerebral hemispheres.	Henriksson *et al* [32] Tallkvist *et al* [33]
Zn	Rat; $^{65}ZnCl_2$	Stereotaxic injection in the brain	At 24 hr after ^{65}Zn injection into the olfactory bulb, ^{65}Zn was seen in the ipsilateral pyriform cortex and the amygdaloid nuclei, consistent with axonal transport of Zn.	Takeda *et al* [34]
Zn	Rat; $^{65}ZnCl_2$	Intranasal instillation	^{65}Zn passed via olfactory neurons to the olfactory bulb; low ^{65}Zn levels were found in secondary olfactory neurons.	Persson *et al* [26]

Nasal carcinogenesis. The propensity of nickel refinery workers to develop cancer of the nose and nasal sinuses has been known since 1932 [45]. The risks of sinonasal cancer are greatly increased in refinery workers exposed to soluble (*e.g.*, $NiSO_4$) or insoluble (*e.g.*, αNi_3S_2, NiO) nickel compounds, and in battery workers exposed to $Ni(OH)_2$ and CdO [46,47]. In 100 sinonasal cancers of Ni refinery workers, the diagnoses included squamous cell carcinoma (48%), anaplastic or undifferentiated carcinoma (39%), adenocarcinoma (6%), transitional cell carcinoma (3%), and other malignant tumors (4%) [48]. Nasal mucosal biopsies of nickel refinery workers frequently show preneoplastic lesions (*i.e.*, squamous or epidermoid metaplasia) with positive immunostaining reactions for keratin and involucrin [49]. Rhinoscopical examination of nickel-exposed workers reveals varying degrees of hyperplastic rhinitis, especially of the middle turbinates, with polypoid mucosa, distinct polyps, and/or localized thickening of the mucous membrane, suggestive of neoplasia [50]. Elevated nickel concentrations are found in biopsy specimens of nasal mucosa from active and retired workers; nickel is retained in the nose for years after cessation of nickel exposure, and slowly released with an estimated half-life of 3.5 years [51]. Since there is constant turn-over of nasal mucosa cells, the accumulated nickel probably resides in the underlying nasal stroma, although electron probe x-ray analysis has failed to disclose Ni-containing aggregates [52]. The prolonged tissue retention of nickel suggests the involvement of a nickel-binding ligand, such as carnosine, which could potentiate the carcinogenic effects of nickel [37].

References

1. Hine CH, Pinto SS, Nelson KW. Medical problems associated with arsenic exposure. *J Occup Med* 1977; 19:391-6.
2. Mancuso TF. Occupational cancer and other health hazards in a chromate plant. A medical appraisal. II. Clinical and toxicologic aspects. *Ind Med Surg* 1951; 20:393-407.
3. Tatarskaya AA. Occupational diseases of the upper respiratory tract in persons employed in electrolytic nickel refining departments. *Gig Trud Prof Zabol* 1960; 4:35-8.
4. Kucharin GM. Occupational disorders of the nose and nasal sinuses in workers in an electrolytic nickel refining plant. *Gig Trud Prof Zabol* 1970; 14:38-40.
5. Friberg L. Health hazards in the manufacture of alkaline accumulators with special reference to chronic cadmium poisoning. *Acta Med Scand* 1950; 138: suppl 240.
6. Adams RG, Crabtree N. Anosmia in alkaline battery workers. *Brit J Indust Med* 1961; 18:216-21.
7. Benson JM, Carpenter RL, Hahn FF, *et al.* Comparative inhalation toxicity of nickel subsulfide to F344/N rats and B6C3F1 mice exposed for 12 days. *Fund Appl Toxicol* 1987; 9:251-65.
8. Benson JM, Burt DG, Carpenter RL, *et al.* Comparative inhalation toxicity of nickel sulfate to F344/N rats and B6C3F1 mice exposed for 12 days. *Fund Appl Toxicol* 1988; 10:164-78.
9. Haber LT, Allen BC, Kimmel CA. Non-cancer risk assessment for nickel compounds: issues associated with dose-response modeling of inhalation and oral exposures. *Toxicol Sci* 1998; 43:213-29.
10. Evans JE, Miller ML, Andringa A, Hastings L. Behavioral, histological, and neurochemical effects of nickel(II) on the rat olfactory system. *Toxicol Appl Pharmacol* 1995; 130:209-20.
11. Smith CC. Changes in the olfactory mucosa and the olfactory nerves following intranasal treatment with one percent zinc sulfate. *Canad Med Assoc J* 1938; 39:138-40.
12. Edwards DA, Thompson ML, Burge KG. Olfactory bulb removal versus peripherally induced anosmia: differential effects on the aggressive behavior of male mice. *Behav Biol* 1972; 7:823-8.
13. Alberts J. Producing and interpreting experimental olfactory deficits. *Physiol Behav* 1974; 12:657-70.
14. Margolis FL, Roberts N, Ferriero D, Feldman J. Denervation in the primary olfactory pathway of mice: biochemical and morphological effects. *Brain Res* 1974; 81:469-83.
15. Harding JW, Getchell TV, Margolis FL. Denervation of the primary olfactory pathway in mice. V. Long-term effect of intranasal $ZnSO_4$ irrigation on behavior, biochemistry, and morphology. *Brain Res* 1978; 140:271-85.
16. Benvenuti S, Ioalè P, Gagliardo A, Bonadonna F. Effects of zinc sulphate-induced anosmia on homing behavior of pigeons. *Comp Biochem Physiol* 1992; 103A:519-26.
17. Benvenuti S, Gagliardo A. Homing behavior of pigeons subjected to unilateral zinc sulphate treatment of their olfactory mucosa. *J Exp Biol* 1996; 199:2531-5.
18. Lewis JL, Hahn FF, Dahl AR. Transport of inhaled toxicants to the central nervous system. Characteristics of a nose-brain barrier. In: Isaacson RL, Jensen KF, eds., *The Vulnerable Brain and Environmental Risks, vol. 3: Toxins in Air and Water*, New York: Plenum Press, 1994: 77-103.
19. Graziadei PP, Monti-Graziadei AG. Regeneration in the olfactory system of vertebrates. Amer J Otolaryngol 1983; 4:228-33.
20. Perl DP, Good PF. Uptake of aluminum into central nervous system along nasal-olfactory pathways. *Lancet* 1987; 1:1028.
21. Tjälve H, Gottofrey J, Björklund I. Tissue disposition of $^{109}Cd^{2+}$ in the brown trout (*Salmo trutta*) studied by autoradiography and impulse counting. *Toxicol Environ Chem* 1986; 12:31-45.
22. Tjälve H, Henriksson J, Tallkvist J, Larsson BS, Lindquist NG. Uptake of manganese and cadmium from the nasal mucosa into the central nervous system via olfactory pathways in rats. *Pharmacol Toxiol* 1996; 79:347-56.
23. Gottofrey J, Tjälve H. Axonal transport of cadmium in the olfactory nerve of the pike. *Pharmacol Toxicol* 1991; 69:242-52
24. Hastings L, Evans JE. Olfactory neurons as a route of entry for toxic agents into the CNS. *Neurotoxicology* 1991; 12:707-14.

25. Evans J, Hastings L. Accumulation of Cd(II) in the CNS depending on the route of administration: intraperitoneal, intratracheal, or intranasal. *Fund Appl Toxicol* 1992; 19:275-8.
26. Persson E, Henriksson J, Tjälve H. Uptake of cobalt and zinc from the nasal mucosa into the brain via olfactory pathways in rats. *J Trace Elem Exp Med* 1998; 11:450-1.
27. Borg-Neczak K, Tjälve H. Uptake of $^{203}Hg^{2+}$ in the olfactory system in pike. *Tox Lett* 1996; 84:107-12.
28. Rouleau C, Tjälve H, Gottofrey J, Pelletier E. Uptake, distribution and elimination of $^{54}Mn(II)$ in the brown trout (*Salmo trutta*). *Environ Toxicol Chem* 1995; 14:483-90.
29. Tjälve H, Mejàre C, Borg-Neczak K. Uptake and transport of manganese in primary and secondary olfactory neurons in pike. *Pharmacol Toxicol* 1995; 77:23-31.
30. Henriksson J, Tallkvist J, Tjälve J, Transport of manganese via the olfactory pathway in rats: dosage dependency of the uptake and subcellular distribution of the metal in the olfactory epithelium and the brain. *Toxicol Appl Pharmacol* 1999; 156:119-28.
31. Gianutsos G, Morrow GR, Morris JB. Accumulation of manganese in rat brain following intranasal administration. *Fund Appl Toxicol* 1997; 37:102-5.
32. Henriksson J, Tallkvist J, Tjälve H. Uptake of nickel into the brain via olfactory neurons in rats. *Toxicol Lett* 1997; 91:153-62.
33. Tallkvist J, Henriksson J, d'Argy R, Tjälve H. Transport and subcellular distribution of nickel in the olfactory system of pikes and rats. *Toxicol Sci* 1998; 43:196-203.
34. Takeda A, Ohnuma M, Sawashita J, Okada S. Zinc transport in the rat olfactory system. *Neurosci Lett* 1997; 225:69-71.
35. Margolis FL, Grillo M. Axoplasmic transport of carnosine (β-alanyl-L-histidine) in mouse olfactory pathway. *Neurochem Res* 1977; 2:507-519.
36. Biffo S, Grillo M, Margolis FL. Cellular localization of carnosine-like and anserine-like immunoreactivities in rodent and avian central nervous system. *Neuroscience* 1990; 35:637-51.
37. Datta AK, Shi X, Kasprzak KS. Effect of carnosine, homocarnosine, and anserine on hydroxylation of the guanine moiety in 2'-deoxyguanosine, DNA, and nucleohistone with hydrogen peroxide in the presence of nickel(II). *Carcinogenesis* 1993; 14: 417-22
38. Kanaki K, Kawashima S, Kashiwayanagi M, Kurihara K. Carnosine-induced inward currents in rat olfactory bulb neurons in cultured cells. *Neurosci Lett* 1997; 231:167-70.
39. Trombley PQ, Horning MS, Blakemore LJ. Carnosine modulates zinc and copper effects on amino acid receptors and synaptic transmission. *NeuroReport* 1998; 9:3503-7.
40. Shimada A, Irie M, Kojima S, Kobayashi K, Yamano Y, Umemura T. Immunohistochemical localization of metallothionein in the olfactory pathway of dogs. *J Vet Med Sci* 1996; 58:983-8.
41. Arvidson B. Retrograde axonal transport of cadmium in the rat hypoglossal nerve. *Neurosci Lett* 1985; 62:45-9.
42. Arvidson B. Retrograde axonal transport of mercury. *Exp Neurol* 1987; 98:198-203.
43. Arvidson B. A review of axonal transport of metals. *Toxicology* 1994; 88:1-14
44. Tjälve H, Henriksson J. Uptake of metals in the brain via olfactory pathways. *Neurotoxicology* 1999; 20:181-95.
45. Grenfell D, Samuel H. Cancer among Welsh nickel workers. *Lancet* 1932; 1:375.
46. Doll R, *et al.* Report of the International Committee on Nickel Carcinogenesis in Man. *Scand J Work Environ Health* 1990; 16:1-84.
47. Järup L, Bellander T, Hogstedt C, Spång G. Mortality and cancer incidence in Swedish battery workers exposed to nickel and cadmium. *Occup Environ Med* 1998; 55:755-759.
48. Sunderman FW Jr, Morgan LG, Andersen A, Ashley D, Forouhar FA. Histopathology of sinonasal and lung cancers in nickel refinery workers. *Ann Clin Lab Sci* 1989; 19:44-50.
49. Klein-Szanto AJP, Boysen M, Reith A. Keratin and involucrin in preneoplastic and neoplastic lesions. *Arch Pathol Lab Med* 1987; 111:1057-61.
50. Torjussen W. Rhinoscopical findings in nickel workers, with special emphasis on the influence of nickel exposure and smoking habits. *Acta Otolaryngol* 1979; 88:279-88.
51. Torjussen W, Andersson I. Nickel concentration in nasal mucosa, plasma, and urine in active and retired nickel workers. *Ann Clin Lab Sci* 1979; 9:289-98.
52. Torjussen W, Haug F-MS, Olsen A, Andersen I. Topochemistry of trace metals in nasal mucosa. Potentialities of some histochemical methods and energy dispersive x-ray microanalysis. *Acta Histochem* 1978; 63:11-25.

Metal Ions in Biology and Medicine; vol 6. Eds. J.A. Centeno, Ph. Collery, G. Vernet, R.B. Finkelman, H. Gibb, J.C. Etienne. John Libbey Eurotext, Paris © 2000, pp. 281-283.

Assessment of the environmental and health effects of manganese/MMT

Zayed J. and Fadlallah S.

TOXHUM (Human Toxicology Research Group) and Département de médecine du travail et d'hygiène du milieu, Université de Montréal, Faculté de médecine, C.P. 6128, Succ. Centre-ville, Montréal, Québec, Canada, H3C 3J7

Introduction

Methylcyclopentadienyl manganese tricarbonyl (MMT: $C_9H_7MnO_3$) is an organic derivative of manganese (Mn) used in Canadian gasoline since 1976 as an antiknock agent and to improve octane rating. In 1997, the Canadian federal government adopted a law (C-29) which banned both the interprovincial trade and the importation for commercial purposes of manganese-based substances, including MMT. However, the government reworded this law in July 1998, so that Mn-based fuel additives were not included in the restrictions. MMT is approved for use in several other countries as well. Nevertheless, these countries are not yet using MMT and they are waiting for strong evidence of the absence of effects on human health. Mainly based on the results of our research group, this paper presents some of the major concerns related to the use of MMT.

Environmental contamination and human exposure to MMT

Very few studies have determined the atmospheric concentrations of MMT. In 1979, a study conducted in Toronto revealed MMT concentrations in an underground parking garage ranging from 0.1 to 0.3 ng m^{-3} but MMT was not detected in ambient air on the streets of the city [Coe et al.,1980]. In a recent study, atmospheric concentration of MMT at selected outdoor sites in Montreal was assessed [Zayed et al.,1999a]. Results ranged from 1.8 ng m^{-3} to 25 ng m^{-3} (expressed as Mn). They are 18 to 83 times higher than those of Coe et al. [1980]. The highest values were obtained at a gas station (mean of 12 ng m^{-3}). Personal exposure to MMT was then measured for gas station attendants. Results vary between 0.3 and 10.8 ng m^{-3}, with a mean of 3.8 ng m^{-3}, which is similar to the level of the environmental contamination as established in the first study at the gas station. This reinforce the finding that MMT is obtained chiefly through evaporation.

MMT and NOx & CO emissions

A first study conducted by Lenane et al.[1994] using 48 cars found that, over a driving distance of 40,000 miles, the CO emissions were essentially the same for both the clear and the MMT-added gasoline, but the NOx emissions were significantly different. The amount of NOx emitted by the vehicles using MMT-added gasoline was

20% lower than the amount emitted by the vehicles using clear gasoline. Results obtained by Zayed et al. [1999b] revealed that CO emitted by the vehicles using MMT-added gasoline was twice the amount emitted by the vehicles using clear (MMT-free) gasoline. As for the NOx emission level, it was 18% higher for the vehicles using MMT-added gasoline than for the vehicles using clear gasoline. However, probably due to the small sample size, these differences are not statistically significant.

Qualitative and quantitative assessments of Mn emissions

The first study conducted on the combustion products of MMT provided qualitative data on the elemental composition of particles collected from a tailpipe and concluded that MMT leads to the formation of Mn oxides, mainly tetraoxide or hausmannite [Ter Harr et al., 1975]. In a recent car exhaust study Zayed et al. [1999c], conducted that Mn is emitted from the tailpipe primarily as a mixture of Mn phosphate and Mn sulfate with sizes ranging between 0.2 and 10 μm. On average, more than 99 % of the particles are in the respirable fraction (< 5 μm) and 86% are less than 1 μm. As far as human exposure is concerned, these results indicate that most of the Mn emitted at the tailpipe would eventually reach the alveolar region and be transferred to the bloodstream.

It has been suggested that one of the principal sources of environmental contamination and human exposure to inorganic Mn in the urban atmosphere would be the combustion of MMT in gasoline [Davis et al., 1988]. Since Montreal is one of the major Canadian cities with an important car fleet, the level of Mn contamination was assessed in relation to air pollutants, meteorological variables and traffic density. Variations in Mn air concentrations were significantly correlated in time with traffic density. In some micro-environments, air concentrations are equal or higher than the U.S.EPA reference concentration [Zayed et al.1999a].

Health effects concerns

The use of MMT has prompted numerous debates on the potential public health risk associated with Mn, which is the main substance emanating from the combustion of MMT. Many studies in occupational environments have shown that high atmospheric Mn concentrations have significant effects on human health. Most of the results focused on the relationship between Mn exposure by inhalation at very high concentrations and neurological signs and symptoms among working populations [Mergler et al., 1994]. Many neurodegenerative disorders similar to Parkinson's disease have been related to occupational exposure to Mn [Barbeau, 1984]. However, the extrapolation of these results to chronic exposure at low concentrations of Mn remains difficult.

Moreover, the toxicity studies present some limitations due to the fact that the onset of symptoms is insidious; its time–course is probably a function of exposure concentration and duration, as well as individual sensitivity. Due to predisposing factors, certain individuals may be more sensitive to different levels of environmental contamination and to adverse effects from exposure to Mn. These groups may include elderly and persons with liver disease [Silbergeled,1982].

Conclusion

There is still an important lack of adequate information and further studies are needed to provide successful implementation of evidence-based risk assessment approaches.

References

Barbeau A (1984): Manganese and extrapyramidal disorders (A critical review and tribute to Dr George C.Cotzias). *Neurotoxicology* 5:13-36.

Coe M, Cruz R, Van Loom JC (1980): Determination of methylcyclopentadienyl manganese tricarbonyl by gas chromatography-atomic absorption spectrometry at ng m^{-3} levels in air samples. *Anal.Chim.Acta* 120:171-176.

Davis DW, Hsiao K, Shikiya R (1988): Origins of manganese in air particulates in California. *JAPCA* 38:1152-1157.

Lenane DL, Fort BF, Ter Haar GL, Lynam DR, Pfeifer GD (1994): Emission results from a 48-car test evaluation of MMT performance additive. *Sci. Total Environ.* 146/147:245-251.

Mergler D, Huel G, Bowler R, Iregren A, Bélanger S, Baldwin M, Tardif R, Smargiassi A, Martin L (1994): Nervous system dysfunction among workers with long-term exposure to manganese. *Env. Res.* 64:151-180.

Silbergeld EK (1982): Current status of neurotoxicology, basic and applied. *Trends in Neurosciences* 5:291-294.

Ter Haar GL, Griffing ME, Brandt M, Oberding DG, Kapron M (1975): Methylcyclopentadienyl manganese tricarbonyl as an antiknock: composition and fate of manganese exhaust products. *JAPCA* 25:858-860.

Zayed J, Pitre J, Rivard M, Loranger S (1999a): Evaluation of pollutant emissions related to the use of methylcyclopentadienyl manganese tricarbonyl (MMT) in gasoline. *Water, Air & Soil Pollut* 109:137-145.

Zayed J, Thibeault C, Gareau L, Kennedy G (1999b): Airborne manganese particulates and methylcyclopentadienyl manganese tricarbonyl (MMT) at selected outdoor sites in Montreal. *Neurotoxicology* 20:151-160.

Zayed J, Hong B, L'espérance G (1999c): Characterization of manganese-containing particles collected from the exhaust emissions of automobiles running with MMT additive. *Environ.Sci.Technol.* 33:3341-3346.

Metal Ions in Biology and Medicine; vol 6. Eds. J.A. Centeno, Ph. Collery, G. Vernet, R.B. Finkelman, H. Gibb, J.C. Etienne. John Libbey Eurotext, Paris © 2000, pp. 284-286.

No kinetic interaction between absorbed mercury and silver in mice after low dose exposure

Jesper B. Nielsen[1] and Per Hultman[2]

[1] Department of Environmental Medicine, SDU, Odense University, DK-5000 Odense C, Denmark;
[2] Department of Health and Environment, Molecular and Immunological Pathology, Linköping University, S-581 85 Linköping, Sweden

Abstract
Exposure from amalgamated fillings is a combined exposure to mercury and silver. The potential kinetic interactions between these two metals may occur during absorption and during disposition and elimination. Interaction of absorbed metal is primarily between the ionic forms of mercury(II) and silver(I). Despite being divalent (mercury) and monovalent (silver), the detoxification of both metals has recently been demonstrated to depend on binding to identical seleno-proteins (1). The purpose of the present study was to evaluate the kinetic interactions of absorbed mercury and silver. Mercuric chloride was administered continuously through drinking water whereas silver nitrate was administered parenterally. Both metals were administered to mice at low dose levels relevant to the human exposure situation. Whole-body and organ depositions were monitored. The kidneys were the main organs for mercury deposition, whereas the dominating part of retained silver was deposited in the liver. Neither mercury nor silver kinetics were affected by simultaneous exposure to the other metal. The absence of kinetic interaction between mercury and silver at these low doses can, however, not exclude additive dynamic effects if both metals use identical mechanisms or targets organs.

Introduction
Experimental toxicological evaluations traditionally focus on toxic effects or the toxicokinetics of a single chemical. The exposure situations are, however, most often characterized by combined exposures to several chemicals among which some may have the potential for interactions. When interactions between chemicals have been studied, it is predominantly the synergistic or antagonistic effects on toxicity that is described, whereas changes in kinetics are less well studied. Exposure from amalgamated fillings is a combined exposure to metallic mercury and silver through inhalation and ionic mercury and silver through the gastrointestinal tract. As metallic mercury is oxidated to mercuric mercury almost immediately after absorption, interaction between the absorbed metals is primarily between the ionic forms of mercury(II) and silver(I). The purpose of the present experiments was to evaluate the kinetics of absorbed mercury and silver after simultaneous exposure of mice to well-characterized, low, and non-toxic doses of mercuric chloride and silver nitrate.

Materials & Methods

Female A.SW mice were kept in a well-controlled environment with free access to standard mouse pellets (<0.01 mg Hg/kg pellets) and water. Ag was administered ip and Hg orally. The different routes of exposure is acceptable as the focus is not on the absorptive process but on interaction between absorbed metals. Radioactive isotopes were used and whole-body retention was measured at regular intervals in live animals throughout the experimental period. Metal deposition was calculated and related to organ weight.

Experiment 1: $HgCl_2$ (1 mg/L) was administered through drinking water for 10 weeks. One group was given 6 ip injections of silver nitrate (25 µg $AgNO_3$/kg b.w.) at intervals of 3-4 days during the initial 3 weeks of mercury exposure. $HgCl_2$ was labelled with the gamma-emitting isotope ^{203}Hg ($^{203}HgCl_2$, Amersham, UK) to allow determination of deposition.

Experiment 2: $AgNO_3$ (9.1 µg; Merck) was administered to the mice as a single ip injection. One group was during the experimental period (two weeks) exposed to mercuric mercury through the drinking water (1mg/L). $AgNO_3$ was labelled with the gamma-emitting isotope ^{110}Ag ($^{110}AgNO_3$, Amersham, UK) to allow determination of deposition.

Results

All doses used in the present study were chosen sufficiently low to exclude toxicity but still allow valid quantitative measurements of Hg and Ag.

Experiment 1: Drinking water consumption and thus mercury intake (224 µg Hg) was not affected by simultaneous exposure to silver nitrate. The whole-body deposition of Hg in the two experimental groups was almost identical during the entire experimental period (table 1). There were no significant differences in target organ deposition of Hg between the group given $HgCl_2$ only, and the group supplemented with $AgNO_3$ (table 1). Thus, a hepatic deposition of 0.2 µg Hg/g was found, which was less than 10% of the mercury concentration measured in the kidneys. As the liver is considerable larger than the kidneys, the total hepatic deposition was, however, only 4 times less than the renal deposition of mercury. The concentration of mercury in the brain was 10% of the hepatic deposition (table 1).

Table 1. Whole-body and organ deposition of mercury in two groups of mice (n=8) after exposure to $HgCl_2$ or $HgCl_2$ plus $AgNO_3$ (medians with 25- and 75-percentiles).

	whole-body (µg Hg)	liver deposition (µg Hg/g)	kidney deposition (µg Hg/g)	brain deposition (µg Hg/g)
Hg	1.8 (1.5-2.1)	0.21 (0.19-0.23)	3.21 (2.51-4.17)	0.020 (0.015-0.021)
Hg+Ag	1.6 (1.5-1.8)	0.22 (0.22-0.24)	3.48 (2.64-4.05)	0.021 (0.018-0.035)

Experiment 2: The drinking water consumption was almost identical in the two experiments, thus assuring comparable daily $HgCl_2$ exposures. Whole-body elimination of a single dose of $AgNO_3$ was not affected by concomitant exposure to $HgCl_2$ (table 2). The whole-body retention of silver was characterized by a fast initial decline causing elimination of 70% of the administered dose within 24 hours after dosing. After 3 days, elimination of silver was stabilized with a whole-body elimination half-time of around 10 days. Organ deposition of

Ag in liver, kidneys, spleen and brain was likewise not affected by the exposure to $HgCl_2$ during the distribution and elimination phases of silver. The organ deposition of Ag was characterized by a two times higher concentration of Ag in the liver as compared to the concentration in the kidneys. The deposition of Ag in the brain was limited. Considering the weight of the target organs, calculations demonstrated that close to 30% of the whole-body retention of Ag at 2 weeks after a single intraperitoneal dose was found in the liver whereas only approximately 5% was deposited in the kidneys.

Table 2. Whole-body and organ deposition of Ag in two groups of mice (n=11) after exposure to $AgNO_3$ or $AgNO_3$ plus $HgCl_2$ (medians with 25- and 75-percentiles).

	whole-body (ng Ag)	liver deposition (ng Ag/g)	kidney deposition (ng Ag/g)	brain deposition (ng Ag/g)
Ag	464 (418-619)	165 (143-187)	88 (79-105)	4.9 (2.8-8.4)
Ag+Hg	464 (410-692)	148 (133-181)	95 (84-103)	3.8 (1.6-5.5)

Discussion

A whole-body steady state level for Hg close to 2/3 of the daily intake of $HgCl_2$ illustrates a low absorption and efficient elimination of absorbed Hg and explains that a steady state can be reached within 2-3 weeks of exposure. Absorption of orally administered $HgCl_2$ has previously been estimated around 15% (2). The kinetics of Ag was followed after a single ip. dose of $AgNO_3$. The initial decline in the fractional retention of Ag after ip. administration illustrates very fast elimination of Ag from the blood before more sustained target organ deposition in liver and kidneys. From these target organs, Ag is slowly eliminated with an apparent whole-body half-life close to 10 days. Considering the larger organ size, approximately five times more Ag was deposited in the liver than the kidneys. Comparable data on the distribution of Ag has been obtained previously after oral exposure to $AgNO_3$ (3). Despite being divalent (Hg) and monovalent (Ag), the detoxification of both metals depend on the binding to certain proteins and enzymes (1). The strongest influence on Hg kinetics would have been expected during the initial 3 weeks of $AgNO_3$ exposure. However, $AgNO_3$ did not change the kinetics of Hg nor did $AgNO_3$ cause increasing concentrations of Hg in target organs for Hg toxicity. In the second experiment, neither the elimination kinetics nor the tissue distribution of Ag were affected by the exposure to $HgCl_2$. Thus, at low, and for the human exposure situation relevant exposure levels, no kinetic interactions occurred between absorbed mercury and silver.

References

1. Sasakura C, Suzuki KT. Buiological interaction between transition metals (Ag, Cd and Hg), selenide/sulfide and selenoprotein P. J Inorg Biochem 1998; 71, 159-62.
2. Schoof R, Nielsen JB. Evaluations of methods for assessing the oral bioavailability of inorganic mercury in soil. Risk Analysis 1997; 17, 545-55.
3. Andersen O, Nielsen JB. Effects of simultaneous low-level dietary supplementation with inorganic and organic selenium on whole-body, blood and organ levels of toxic metals in mice. Environ Health Perspect 1994; 102, 321-4.

Metal Ions in Biology and Medicine; vol 6. Eds. J.A. Centeno, Ph. Collery, G. Vernet, R.B. Finkelman, H. Gibb, J.C. Etienne. John Libbey Eurotext, Paris © 2000, pp. 287-289.

On the mechanism of chromium(VI)-incuced toxicity: studies in human erythrocyte membranes

M.A.S. Fernandes[1], M.E.R. Santos[2], C.F.G.C. Geraldes[2], C.R. Oliveira[3], and M.C. Alpoim[2]

[1] Departamento de Zoologia, [2] Departamento de Bioquímica, [3] Serviço de Bioquímica da Faculdade de Medicina, Universidade de Coimbra, Coimbra, Portugal

The influence of several antioxidants and of the thiol group blocker N-ethylmaleide on Cr(VI)-induced humam erythrocytes membrane peroxidation was investigated. Deferoxamine, mannitol, ascorbate, α-tocopherol, 3(2)-tert-butyl-4-hydroxyanisole, salicylate, diphenylamine, and dimethylsulfoxide protect human erythrocyte membranes against Cr(VI)-induced peroxidation along a time period of 2 h. Glutathione significantly increased Cr(VI)-induced peroxidation, while it was not affected by sodium benzoate or N-ethylmaleimide. Addition of mannitol 90 min after the exposition of human erythrocyte membranes to Cr(VI) inhibited immediately the peroxidation, while addition of deferoxamine, SOD or CAT were without effect. The meaning of these results is discussed in terms of involvement of reactive oxygen species on the mechanism of Cr(VI)-induced toxicity.

Introduction

The toxic and carcinogenic effects of chromium have been attributed to Cr(VI) compounds, which readily cross the cell membranes, being reduced through reactive intermediates such as Cr(V) and Cr(IV) to Cr(III) by intracellular reductants [1]. These reactive chromium intermediates generate reactive oxygen species (ROS) via Fenton or Haber-Weiss type reactions [1] which can induce DNA damage and lipid peroxidation. Therefore the toxic and carcinogenic effects of Cr(VI) may be partially associated with the production of ROS [1]. The use of ROS scavenging agents may shed some light on the mechanism of Cr(VI)-induced toxicity and carcinogenesis [1]. To access the mechanism of Cr(VI)-induced toxicity the effects of radical scavengers (hydroxyl, peroxyl and alkoxyl), scavengers of superoxide anion and hydrogen peroxide, as well as the thiol group blocker N-ethylmaleimide (NEM) on Cr(VI)-induced human erythrocyte membranes peroxidation were studied.

Materials and Methods

Human erythrocyte membranes were prepared as described [2] and the peroxidation extent evaluated by measuring thiobarbituric acid-reactive substances (TBARS) [3], in membranes suspended (700 μM in phospholipid) in Hepes buffer (10 mM Hepes, 140 mM NaCl and 10 mM glucose) and untreated or treated for 2 h at 25°C with the antioxidants or NEM [4], before their exposition to 8 mM dichromate. The results correspond to the means±SD of at least three samples carried out in duplicate, and expressed as nmoles of malonaldehyde per milligram of protein (nmol MDA mg-1 protein). Statistical significance was set at p< 0.05.

Results

Mannitol, salicylate, dimethyl sulphoxide (DMSO) (Fig. 1 A), deferoxamine (DFO), 3(2)-*t*-butyl-4-hydroxyanisole (BHA), ascorbate, α-tocopherol succinate (Fig. 1 B) and diphenylamine (DFA) (Fig. 1 C) significantly decreased (p=0.0001) Cr(VI)-induced human erythrocyte membranes peroxidation, at peroxidation times ≥ 90 min, while sodium benzoate (Fig. 1 A) and NEM (results not shown) had no effect on it. In contrast, reduced glutathione (GSH) significantly increased (p=0.0001) Cr(VI)-induced peroxidation (Fig. 1 C). Addition of mannitol 90 min after the exposition of human erythrocyte membranes to Cr(VI) inhibited immediately membrane peroxidation (Fig. 1 A), while it was not affected by the addition of DFO (Fig. 1 B), superoxide dismutase (SOD) or catalase (CAT) (Fig. 1 D).

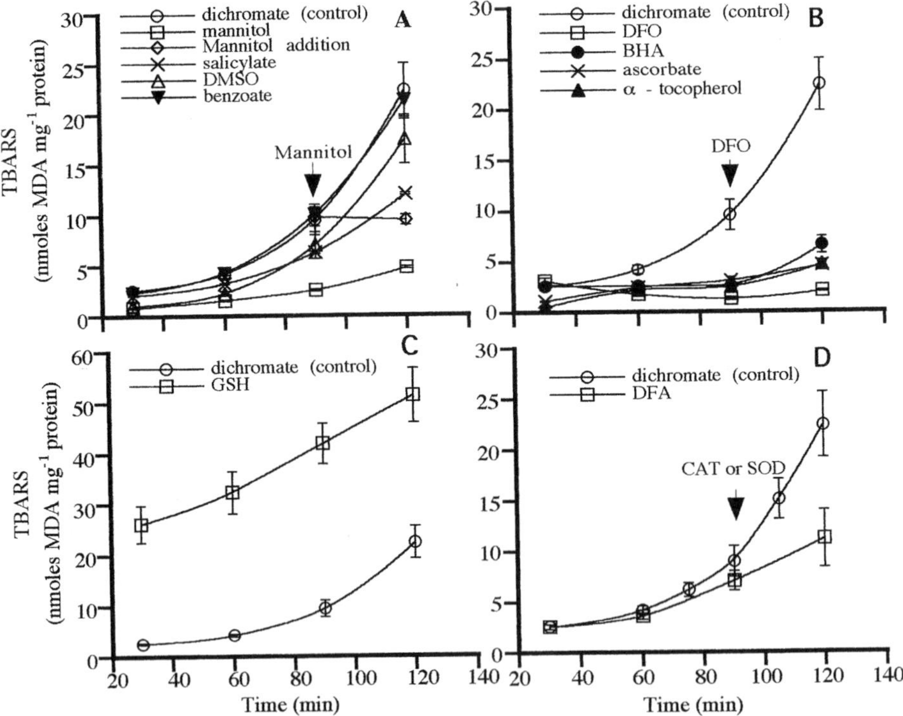

FIG. 1. Time dependent effects of mannitol (5 mM), salicylate (3 mM), benzoate (5 mM) and DMSO (18 mM) (**A**), DFO (4 mM), BHA (0.5 mM), ascorbate (3 mM) and α-tocopherol (10 μM) (**B**), GSH (5 mM) (**C**), and DFA (0.5 mM) (**D**) on 8 mM dichromate-induced human erythrocyte membranes peroxidation. The effects of mannitol (5 mM) (**A**), DFO (4 mM) (**B**), CAT (360 I. U.) and SOD (400 I.U.) (**D**) 90 min after exposition of human erythrocyte membranes to 8 mM dichromate are indicated by the arrows. Note: the Y axis of Fig. 1 C double that of Fig. 1 A, B and D.

Discussion and Conclusion

The protection of human erythrocyte membranes against Cr(VI)-induced peroxidation by mannitol, salicylate, and DMSO (hydroxyl radical scavengers) [5], DFO, ascorbate, α-tocopherol and BHA (peroxyl radicals scavengers) [5,6], and DFA (alkoxyl radical scavenger) [4] indicated that hydroxyl radicals [5,6], peroxyl radicals [4-6] and alkoxyl radicals are probably involved on the mechanism of Cr(VI)-induced toxicity.The greater protective effect of mannitol as compared to that of DFO, observed in human erythrocytes membranes after 90 min of exposition to Cr(VI), may be related to the fact that DFO scarcely penetrate intact human erythrocytes [7], while human erythrocyte membranes are completely permeable to mannitol [8].The potentiation of Cr(VI)-induced human erythrocyte membranes peroxidation by GSH, an efficient peroxyl radicals scavenger [6], is not surprising if we take into account that GSH is a potent Cr(VI)-reductant [1]. The lack of effects of SOD and CAT, superoxide anion and hydrogen peroxide scavengers respectively [9], to protect human erythrocyte membranes against Cr(VI)-induced peroxidation, 90 min after their exposition to Cr(VI), as well as the lack of effect of NEM indicated that superoxide anion, hydrogen peroxide and membrane thiol groups are not involved on the mechanism of Cr(VI)-induced membrane injury. In conclusion, hydroxyl, peroxyl and alkoxyl radicals, rather than superoxide anion, hydrogen peroxide and membrane thiol groups are involved on the mechanism of Cr(VI)-induced toxicity.

References

1. Shi X, Chiu A, Chen C T, Halliwell B, Castranova V, Vallyathan V. Reduction of chromium (VI) and its relantionship to carcinogenesis. *Journal Toxicology Environmental Health* , Part B 1999; 2: 87-104.

2. Fernandes M A S, Mota I M, Silva M T L, Oliveira C R, Geraldes C F G C, Alpoim M C. Human erythrocytes are protected against chromate induced peroxidation. *Ecotoxicology Environmental Safety* 1999; 43: 38-46.

3. Ernster L, Nordenbrand K. Microsomal lipid peroxidation. In: Colowick S P, Kaplan N O ed. *Methods in Enzymology*. New York: Academic Press, 1967; Vol. 10: 574-580.

4. Ohyashiki T, Kumada Y,Hatanaka N, Matsui K. Oxygen radical-induced inhibition of alkaline phosphatase activity in reconstituted membranes. *Archives Biochemistry Biophysics* 1994; 313:310-317.

5. Gassen M, Youdim M B H. Free radical scavengers: chemical concepts and clinical relevance.*Journal Neural Transmission Supplement* 1999; 56: 193-210.

6. Regoli F, Winston G W. Quantification of total oxidant scavenging capacity of antioxidants for peroxynitrite, peroxyl radicals, and hydroxyl radicals. *Toxicology Applied Pharmacology* 1999; 156: 96-105.

7. Ferrali M, Signorini C, Ciccoli L, Comporti M. Iron release and membrane damage in erythrocytes exposed to oxidizing agents, phenylhydrazine, divicine and isouramil. *Biochemical Journal* 1992; 285: 295-301.

8. Jung C Y, Carlson L M, Baltzer C J. Characteristics of the permeability barrier of human erythrocyte ghosts to non-electrolytes. *Biochemistry Biophysics Acta* 1973; 298: 101-107.

9. Yu B P. Cellular defenses against damage from reactive oxygen species. *Physiological Review* 1994; 74: 139-162.

Metal Ions in Biology and Medicine; vol 6. Eds. J.A. Centeno, Ph. Collery, G. Vernet, R.B. Finkelman, H. Gibb, J.C. Etienne. John Libbey Eurotext, Paris © 2000, pp. 290-292.

Bismuth Biokinetics and Nephrotoxicity after Acute Colloidal Bismuth Subcitrate Overdose in Rats

Berend T. Leussink[1], Anja Slikkerveer[1, 3], Walter J.J. Krauwinkel[3], Gijsbert B. van der Voet[1], Emile de Heer[2], Jan A. Bruijn[2], and Frederik A. de Wolff[1, 4]

[1] Toxicology Laboratory, and [2] Department of Pathology, Leiden University Medical Center, Leiden, The Netherlands; [3] Yamanouchi Europe BV Research Laboratories, Leiderdorp, The Netherlands; [4] Chair of Human Toxicology, Academic Medical Center, University of Amsterdam, Amsterdam, The Netherlands.

Introduction

Bismuth(Bi)-containing pharmaceuticals like colloidal bismuth subcitrate (CBS) are used in the treatment of peptic ulcers and in eradication of *Helicobacter pylori* infections of the stomach. Acute intentional overdose has been reported to result in reversible nephrotoxicity [1]. We are studying the mechanism of Bi nephrotoxicity in rats in order to elucidate the pathogenesis of this unusual effect. Previously, we found that a single large oral CBS dose (containing 3.0 mmol Bi/kg body weight) resulted in acute tubular necrosis which healed spontaneously in 10 days. Half this dose caused much less renal damage, whereas 0.75 mmol Bi per kg was shown to be the NOAED (the highest dose studied at which no observed adverse effects were found) [2].
In the study presented here we focus on the early development of Bi-induced renal damage in relation to the biokinetics in overdosed rats.

Methods

Forty female Wistars rats weighing 130 - 200 g (33 forming the treatment group; 7 controls) received either CBS (corresponding with 3.0 mmol Bi per kg body weight in 0.5 mL saline) or the vehicle by gavage. Animals from the treatment group were sacrificed at t = 1, 3, 6, 12, 24, or 48 h after dosing. Urine was collected between t=0-6, 6-12, 12-24, and 24-48 h, and blood samples were taken from the retro-orbital plexus at varying times after administration, and just before sacrifice by puncture of the abdominal aorta. Every left kidney was perfused with phosphate-buffered saline before freezing for cryostat sections and Bi analysis; every right kidney was fixed *in situ* with buffered formaldehyde solution and processed for paraffin sectioning and staining with periodic acid/Schiff (PAS). On the cryostat sections, a panleukocyte staining (CD45) was performed in order to evaluate the influx of inflammatory cells into the tubuli. Bi in blood, urine, and tissue was analysed with atomic absorption spectrometry as developed in our laboratory and described previously [3, 4]. Urinary glucose and protein, and plasma creatinine and urea were measured with a Hitachi 747 automatic clinical analyser.
Biokinetic analysis was performed with the NONMEM version V software program, using a one-compartment model with first order absorption kinetics, assuming instantaneous absorption and a lognormal distribution of the biokinetic parameters [5].

Statistical analysis was carried out with SPSS 7.5.2; values below the limit of detection (LOD) were set at the LOD itself. Parameters with a normal distribution were compared with Student's T-test; the Kruskal-Wallis one-way ANOVA and the Mann-Whitney U test were applied for parameters lacking a normal distribution. p-Values < 0.05 were considered to indicate statistical significance.

Results and Discussion

Five of the 33 Bi-treated rats died prematurely and were excluded from analysis. Results of the biokinetic population analysis are shown in Table 1. A rapid uptake with an absorption rate constant of 2.14 h^{-1} was calculated, corresponding with an absorption $t_{½}$ of 0.32 h. Elimination is slow: the apparent clearance of 2.28 $L.h^{-1}.kg^{-1}$ and a distribution volume of 65.7 $L.kg^{-1}$ correspond with an elimination $t_{½}$ of 16 h. The one-compartment model is probably too simple but proved to be the best fit. The blood levels (BiB) were significantly lower at t=1 h than at t=0.5 h and t=2 h, which may indicate two different distribution processes. This observation is in agreement with findings in humans [6]. Plasma creatinine and urea increased with a constant rate after t=1 h during the entire experimental period, indicating that most of the damage to the renal clearance function is induced during the first h of exposure. Glucosuria and proteinurea were also observed in the experimental but not in the control group.
Histological examination of the kidneys revealed cytoplasmic vacuolation of tubular cells at the cortico-medullary boundary from t=1 h onwards. Figure 1 shows that at t=3 h tubular necrosis had developed. At t=6 h, cytoplasmic vacuolation occurred in tubular cells in the cortex as well. At t=12 h, necrotic tubules appeared both in the cortex and the cortico-medullary boundary zone. The glomeruli, however, remained normal at all time points. An increase of PAS-positive grains in the tubular cytoplasm was seen as early as t=6 h. The number of interstitial leukocytes, demonstrated with panleukocyte staining, did not change before t=48 h after CBS. The damaged tubules in the cortico-medullary boundary zone (Figure 1) were identified as S3 segments of the proximal tubules [2]. The S3 segment seems to be most susceptible to Bi-induced damage because it necrotised before t=3 h after administration. In the S1/S2 segment, necrosis occured only between t=6 h and t=12 h after dosing, indicating less sensitivity for Bi. The tubular damage found in the present experiment is in agreement with the vacuolation and atrophy of the tubular cells as reported by others [7].
In conclusion, Bi-induced renal damage, as shown by biochemical and morphological observations, occurs concomittantly with rapid intestinal absorption of Bi from a CBS overdose. The long elimination $t_{½}$ may, at least partly, be explained by Bi-induced nephropathy.

References

1. Taylor EG, Klenerman P. Acute renal failure after colloidal bismuth subcitrate overdose. *Lancet* 1992; 340: 1298.

2. Leussink BT, Slikkerveer A, Engelbrecht MRW, De Heer E, Van der Voet GB, De Wolff FA, Bruijn JA. Colloidal bismuth subcitrate-induced nephrotoxicity: reversibility and morphology [abstract]. *J Am Soc Nephrol* 1997; 8: 604A.
3. Slikkerveer A, Helmich RB, Edelbroek PM, Van der Voet GB, De Wolff FA. Analysis if bismuth in serum and blood by electrothermal atomic absorption spectrometry using platinum as matrix modifier. *Clin Chim Acta* 1991; 201: 17-26.
4. Slikkerveer A, Helmich RB, De Wolff FA. Analysis of bismuth in tissue by electrothermal atomic absorption spectrometry. *Clin Chem* 1993; 39: 800-03.
5. Sheiner LB, Ludden TM. Population pharmacokinetics/dynamics. *Annu Rev Pharmacol Toxicol* 1992; 32: 185-209.
6. Hespe W, Staal HJM, Hall DWR. Bismuth absorption from the colloidal subcitrate. *Lancet* 1988; 2: 1258.
7. Szymanska JA, Chmielnicka J, Kaluzynski A, Papierz W. Influence of bismuth on the metabolism of endogenous metals in rats. *Biomed Environ Sci* 1993; 6: 134-44.

Table 1
Population values describing a one-compartment biokinetic model for Bi in blood (BiB) after a single high dose of CBS containing 3.0 mmol Bi per kg rat

	Typical value for the population	Precision (SD) of the typical value	Variation (%) in the population
Apparent clearance ($L.h^{-1}.kg^{-1}$)	2.28	0.8	103
Apparent V_D ($L.kg^{-1}$)	65.7	29.4	301
Apparent K_a (h^{-1})	2.14	0.321	38

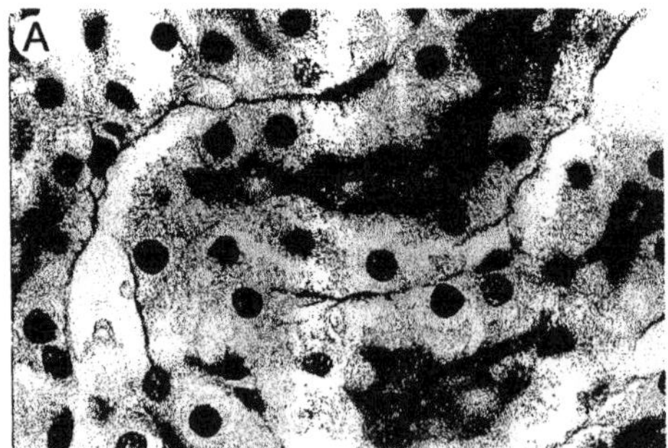

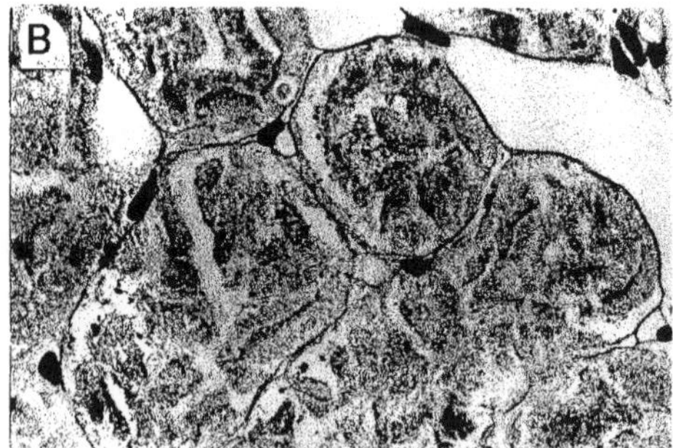

Figure 1. Changes in kidney morphology after CBS overdose. (A) S3 segments of the proximal tubule of a rat from the control group, and (B) S3 segments at t=3 h after administration. Vacuolation of the tubular epithelial cells occurs at t=1 h (not shown), whereas tubular necrosis is seen at t=3 h after dosing. Three-µm thick, paraffin-embedded, PAS-stained kidney sections. Magnification x600.

Metal Ions in Biology and Medicine; vol 6. Eds. J.A. Centeno, Ph. Collery, G. Vernet, R.B. Finkelman, H. Gibb, J.C. Etienne. John Libbey Eurotext, Paris © 2000, pp. 293-296.

Identification of a novel, cadmium-inducible, integral membrane protein from the nematode *Caenorhabditis elegans*

Vivian Hsiu-Chuan Liao and Jonathan Freedman

Nicholas School of the Environment, Duke University, Durham, NC 27708, USA

The transition metal cadmium is considered a serious occupational and environmental health threat. Cadmium has been classified as a type 1 human carcinogen [1] and it was ranked number 7 on the Agency for Toxic Substances and Disease Registry/Environmental Protection Agency "Top 20 Hazardous Substances Priority List" in 1997 [2]. It is continuously introduced into the atmosphere through the smelting of ores and the burning of fossil fuels [3]. Humans are continuously exposed to cadmium primarily via inhalation and the ingestion of cadmium-containing food [4]. The metal accumulates in liver, lung and kidney tissue and has a long retention time in the body [5, 6]. Toxicological responses of cadmium exposure include kidney damage, respiratory diseases, neurological disorders and lung, kidney, prostate, and testicular cancers [4, 7].

Following exposure to cadmium, cells respond by inducing the transcription of genes that encode a variety of defense and repair proteins. These include metallothionein, heme oxygenase, γ-glutamylcysteine synthetase, low and high molecular weight heat shock proteins, ubiquitin, superoxide dismutase, catalase, glutathione peroxidase, and glucose-6-phosphate dehydrogenase [8-14]. Cadmium affects gene expression by influencing signal transduction pathways, including those involving protein kinase C, cAMP-dependent protein kinase and calmodulin [15-17]. Thus, cadmium can modulate the activities of complex signal transduction pathways that in turn can influence the expression of a myriad of genes, many of which are not directly related to cellular defense and repair.

The reverse transcriptase-polymerase chain reaction protocol of differential display was used to identify new cadmium-responsive genes in the non-parasitic nematode *C. elegans* [18]. Fifty-three differentially expressed cDNA fragments that correspond to the products of thirty-two independent genes were identified [18]. One of these genes, designated *cdr-1* (cadmium responsive-1), encodes an mRNA whose steady-state level of expression increases >10-fold in response to cadmium exposure *in vivo*. The open reading frame of 831 base pairs encodes a 32-kDa protein. This protein does not share significant homology with eukaryotic proteins associated with stress responses [19]. However, CDR-1 has high levels of sequence identity to four predicted *C. elegans* proteins. This suggests that it is a member of a multi-gene family. Hydropathy analysis of the deduced amino acid sequence of CDR-1 indicates that it is an integral membrane protein, which contains two transmembrane spanning regions [20] (Fig. 1)

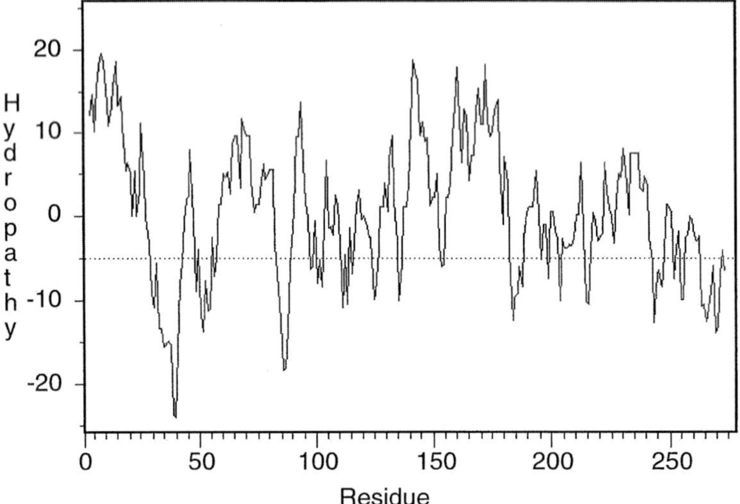

Figure 1. Hydrophobicity plot of CDR-1. Two transmembrane domains are located at amino acid residues 2 – 23 and 157 – 177.

The steady-state level of CDR-1 mRNA observed in cadmium-treated *C. elegans* is comparable to those of the two *C. elegans* metallothioneins. In addition, kinetic analysis reveals that the rate of *cdr-1* mRNA accumulation following cadmium exposure is similar to those of metallothionein. To investigate *cdr-1* transcription patterns *in vivo*, a combination of transgenic *C. elegans* that carry a *cdr-1/lacZ* reporter transgene and whole-mount *in situ* hybridization were used. When nematodes are exposed to cadmium, the *cdr-1* gene is transcribed exclusively in intestinal cells throughout all post-embryonic developmental stages (Fig. 2). In the absence of cadmium, *cdr-1* was not detected at any developmental stage or in any other cell type.

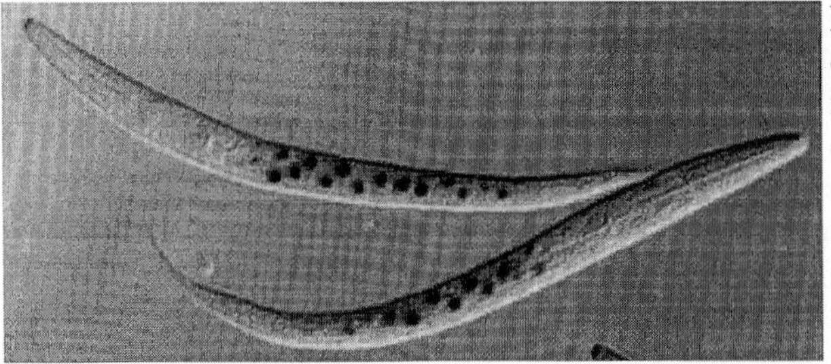

Figure 2 A strain of *C. elegans* that contains the *cdr-1/lacZ* transgene integrated into the genome were exposed to 100 µM $CdCl_2$ for 24 h and then stained for β-galactosidase activity [21, 22]. Two L1 larva are shown in which reporter transgene activity is observed in the intestinal cells.

These results indicate that *cdr-1* transcription is regulated in a cell-specific fashion. Consensus sequences for upstream regulatory elements that control intestinal cell specific transcription are present in the *cdr-1* promoter [23, 24].

Exposure of transgenic *C. elegans* to other stressors including metals (lead, mercury, copper, zinc), oxidative stress and heat shock did not induce *cdr-1* transcription. This result is unique for a metal/stress-inducible gene. Transcription of other stress response genes (e.g., metallothioneins, heat-shock proteins, glutathione peroxidase) is usually induced by multiple stressors; i.e., different transition metals, heat-shock and oxidative stress.

To determine the intracellular location of CDR-1, transgenic *C. elegans* were generated that expressed a CDR-1-green fluorescent protein [25] (GFP) fusion peptide under the control of the *cdr-1* promoter. In these nematodes, CDR-1-GFP will be regulated by the same factors that control the transcription of the endogenous gene. In the absence of cadmium, a low basal level of CDR-1-GFP expression was observed. Follow cadmium exposure, the level of CDR-1-GFP expression dramatically increased. The fusion protein was expressed exclusively in the intestinal cells, reproducing the results obtained with the *cdr-1/lacZ* transgene. CDR-1-GFP was observed in cytoplasmic, punctate structures, subsequently identified as lysosomes. Based on these results and the hydrophobicity profile, CDR-1 is likely to be a lysosomal integral membrane protein. This may be the first report of a cadmium-inducible or stress-response protein that is targeted to this organelle.

In conclusion, *cdr-1* represents in new class of cadmium-inducible genes. These genes encode lysosomal, integral membrane proteins. The function of CDR-1 and its relation to cadmium toxicity is still under investigation.

REFERENCES

[1] International Agency for Research on Cancer. Beryllium, Cadmium, Mercury and Exposures in the Glass Manufacturing Industry. Lyon: IARC, 1993.

[2] Fay RM, Mumtaz MM. Complex mixtures: hazard identification and risk assessment. *Food Chem Toxicol* 1996; 34: 1175-1176.

[3] Friberg L, Kjellstrom T, Nordberg GF. In: Friberg L, Nordberg GF, Vouk V, eds. Handbood of the Toxicology of Metals. Amsterdam: Elsevier/North-Holland, 1986: 130-237.

[4] Waalkes MP, Coogan TP, Barter RA. Toxicological principles of metal carcinogenesis with special emphasis on cadmium. *Crit Rev Toxicol* 1992; 22: 175-201.

[5] Aylett BJ. In: Webb M, ed. The Chemistry, Biochemistry and Biology of Cadmium. New York: Elsevier/North-Holland, 1979: 1-62.

[6] Bernard A, Lauwerys R. Cadmium in human population. *Experientia Suppl* 1986; 50: 114-123.

[7] Oberdorster G. Airborne cadmium and carcinogenesis of the respiratory tract. *Scand J Work Environ Health* 1986; 12: 523-537.

[8] Salovsky P, Shopova V, Dancheva V, Marev R. Changes in antioxidant lung protection after single intra-tracheal cadmium acetate instillation in rats. *Hum Exp Toxicol* 1992; 11: 217-222.
[9] Hamer DH. Metallothionein. *Ann Rev Biochem* 1986; 55: 913-951.
[10] Alam J, Shibahara S, Smith A. Transcriptional activation of the heme oxygenase gene by heme and cadmium in mouse hepatoma cells. *J Biol Chem* 1989; 264: 6371-6375.
[11] Hatcher EL, Chen Y, Kang YJ. Cadmium resistance in A549 cells correlates with elevated glutathione content but not antioxidant enzymatic activities. *Free Radic Biol Med* 1995; 19: 805-812.
[12] Wiegant FA, Souren JE, van Rijn J, van Wijk R. Stressor-specific induction of heat shock proteins in rat hepatoma cells. *Toxicology* 1994; 94: 143-159.
[13] Muller-Taubenberger A, Hagmann J, Noegel A, Gerisch G. Ubiquitin gene expression in *Dictyostelium* is induced by heat and cold shock, cadmium, and inhibitors of protein synthesis. *J Cell Sci* 1988; 90: 51-58.
[14] Kostic MM, Ognjanovic B, Dimitrijevic S, Zikic RV, Stajn A, Rosic GL, Zivkovic RV. Cadmium-induced changes of antioxidant and metabolic status in red blood cells of rats: *in vivo* effects. *Eur J Haematol* 1993; 51: 86-92.
[15] Beyersmann D, Hechtenberg S. Cadmium, gene regulation, and cellular signalling in mammalian cells. *Toxicol Appl Pharm* 1997; 144: 247-261.
[16 Wang Z, Templeton DM. Induction of *c-fos* proto-oncogene in mesangial cells by cadmium. *J Biol Chem* 1998; 273: 73-79.
[17] Templeton DM, Wang Z, Miralem T. Cadmium and calcium-dependent *c-fos* expression in mesangial cells. *Toxicol Lett* 1998; 95: 1-8.
[18] Liao VH, Freedman JH. Cadmium-regulated genes from the nematode *Caenorhabditis elegans*. Identification and cloning of new cadmium-responsive genes by differential display. *J Biol Chem* 1998; 273: 31962-31970.
[19] Altschul SF, Gish W, Miller W, Myers EW, Lipman DJ. Basic local alignment search tool. *J Mol Biol* 1990; 215: 403-410.
[20] Kyte J, Doolittle RF. A simple method for displaying the hydropathic character of a protein. *J Mol Biol* 1982; 157: 105-132.
[21] Mello C, Fire A. DNA transformation. *Methods Cell Biol* 1995; 48: 451-82.
[22] Fire A. Histochemical techniques for locating *Escherichia coli* beta-galactosidase activity in transgenic organisms. *Genet Anal Tech Appl* 1992; 9: 151-158.
[23] Fukushige T, Hawkins MG, McGhee JD. The GATA-factor *elt-2* is essential for formation of the *Caenorhabditis elegans* intestine. *Dev Biol* 1998; 198: 286-302.
[24] Moilanen LH, Fukushige T, Freedman JH. Regulation of metallothionein gene transcription. Identification of upstream regulatory elements and transcription factors responsible for cell-specific expression of the metallothionein genes from *Caenorhabditis elegans*. *J Biol Chem* 1999; 274: 29655-29665.
[25] Chalfie M, Tu Y, Euskirchen G, Ward WW, Prasher DC. Green fluorescent protein as a marker for gene expression. *Science* 1994; 263: 802-805.

Metal Ions in Biology and Medicine; vol 6. Eds. J.A. Centeno, Ph. Collery, G. Vernet, R.B. Finkelman, H. Gibb, J.C. Etienne. John Libbey Eurotext, Paris © 2000, pp. 297-299.

Joint toxicity of inorganic chemical mixtures: the role of dose ratios

Moiz Mumtaz[1], Hisham El-Masri[1], Din Chen[2], and Joel Pounds[3]

[1] Division of Toxicology, Agency for Toxic Substances and Disease Registry, Atlanta, GA, USA; [2] Pacific Biological Station, Nanaimo, BC, Canada; and [3] Pacific Northwest National Laboratory, Richland, WA, USA

INTRODUCTION: The exposure to environmental pollutants, through various media, is often to mixtures of chemicals. Humans are often concurrently exposed to multiple chemicals including toxic metals such as lead, cadmium, mercury, arsenic,and chromium. These are among the chemicals that the Agency for Toxic Substances and Disease Registry (ATSDR) has designated as priority chemicals found in the environment [1]. When such mixed exposures occur, the pharmacokinetics of the various chemicals and their contribution to the overall toxicity of the mixture are influenced by interactions of the mixture components. The modulation of this cascade of adverse effects is the consequence of multiple and complex interactions at sites of action, absorption, elimination, and storage. Some of the important organs affected by these chemicals are the liver, and the kidneys, and the nervous, hematological, and reproductive systems. It is often assumed that the interactive toxicity of a chemical mixture is consistent across mixing ratios. Because, information to draw such conclusions is limited, investigators need to conduct well-designed, relevant experiments that include the study of mechanisms, dose response, and magnitude of the interactions as they relate to toxicity of mixtures.

MATERIALS AND METHODS: Monkey kidney cells (LLC-MK2) in triplicate cultures in 12-well cluster dishes were treated with selected concentrations of $HgCl_2$, $CdCl_2$, or both metals for 20 hours. All experiments were conducted in D-MEM supplemented with 10% fetal bovine serum and antibiotic/antimycotic agent. The release of the soluble enzyme, lactate dehydrogenase (LDH), was measured kinetically and expressed as the fraction of the total LDH activity released for each culture. The fraction of LDH released (cytotoxicity) was transformed by the angle transformation, $\sin^{-1}(LDH)^{0.5}$, to normalize the variances, then analyzed by the statistical isobologram of Carter et al. [2]; and the linear models of null-interaction noninteraction of Kodell and Pounds [3] SAS v6.12 was used for data analysis. The Kodell and Pounds' linear models of null-interaction give two bench marks for comparison: dose/concentration additivity and response additivity which are predicted by the dose response curves of the individual mixture components. This approach explicitly addresses the lack of a completely general definition of additivity by using an Envelope of Additivity as the basis of comparison. The use of unspecified functions to describe the dose-response relations prevents this family from being limited to a few families of cure and surface shapes and provides flexibility to be generally applicable to many situations. The method is based on using the Box-Cox power transformation to derive the most suitable function of dose to be used in a linear response function obtained from a linear transformation.

The probability of a toxic response to a dose is estimated by separate regressions for each

$$P_{resp} = F_i\left(\alpha_i + \beta_i \frac{dose_i^{\lambda_i} - 1}{\lambda_i}\right)$$

toxicant by
where λ_1 and λ_2 are parameters to be estimated to provide the most suitable power

$$DA_{resp} = F_i\left(\alpha_1 + \beta_1 \frac{dose_1 + [(\beta_2/\beta_1)^{1/2} dose_2]^{\lambda_1} - 1}{\lambda_1}\right) - F_i\left(\alpha_2 + \beta_2 \frac{dose_2 + [(\beta_1/\beta_2)^{1/2} dose_1]^{\lambda_1} - 1}{\lambda_1}\right)$$

transformation of dose1 and dose2. Dose additivity is then predicted from

$$RA_{resp} = F_i\left(\alpha_1 + \beta_1 \frac{dose_1^{\lambda_1} - 1}{\lambda_1}\right) + F_i\left(\alpha_2 + \beta_2 \frac{dose_2^{\lambda_2} - 1}{\lambda_2}\right) - F_i\left(\alpha_1 + \beta_1 \frac{dose_1^{\lambda_1} - 1}{\lambda_1}\right) x\, F_i\left(\alpha_2 + \beta_2 \frac{dose_2^{\lambda_2} - 1}{\lambda_2}\right)$$

and response additivity is then predicted from,
RESULTS: The statistical isobole analysis identified all mixing ratios as synergistic except the 2:1 mixture (Table I, Pr>Chi). Kodell and Pounds' linear model nicely modeled the individual components (Figure 1). When each mixture was individually compared with the predicted models, the mixture is synergistic at 20:1 and 10:1 mixing ratios, response additive at 5:1, and within the envelope of additivity at 2:1. The model-predicted dose and response additivity is indicated by labeled solid lines, and the observed cytotoxic responses and the 95% confidence limits are shown for each mixing ratio (Panels B-F).

Table I. Summary of analysis by Statistical Isobologram

Data tested	$\beta_{12} \pm$ SE	Chi	Pr>Chi	Cd_{50}	Hg_{50}
all Hg:Cd mixtures	0.0088 ± .0014	3.7	.0001	19.5	35.9
20:1	0.0052 ± .0025	4.3	.0376	19.2	36.4
10:1	0.0182 ± .0021	78	.0001	19.3	36.2
5:1	0.0071 ± .0023	9.0	.0026	18.9	37.0
2:1	0.0070 ± .0042	2.9	.0910	18.9	37.1

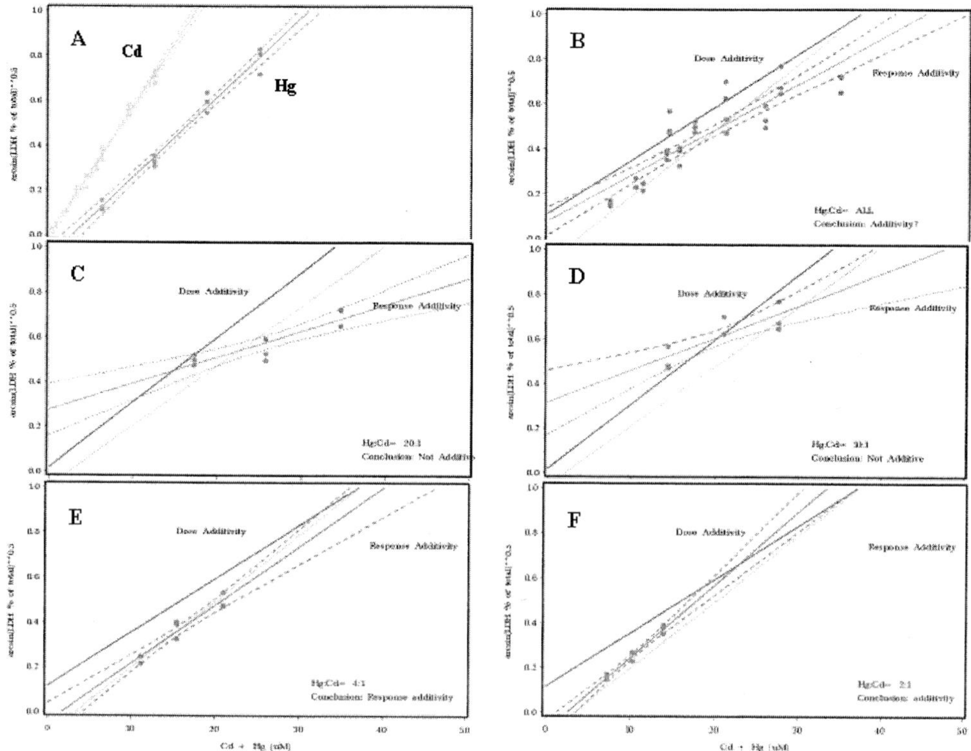

DISCUSSION AND CONCLUSION: The results of the two analyses are in general agreement that (a) the nature of the interaction is not identical at all mixing ratios, (b) the interaction is most synergistic at high Hg:Cd ratios, and (c) the interaction is additive when cells are exposed to a 2:1 ratio. The models used differ in their ability to provide (a) a clear comparison between the separate analyses and (b) graphic vs. statistical interpretation of the results. The results presented here support the conclusion that chemical interactions play a critical role in the expression of toxicity and that the type of interactions, namely, additivity to synergism, change as a function of dose. It is imperative that due consideration must be given to the mechanistic, biokinetic, and physiological factors affecting the joint toxicity. All the underlying assumptions should be critically evaluated when conducting joint toxicity of chemicals.

REFERENCES CITED

[1]De Rosa, CT, Johnson, BL, Fay, M., Hansen, H. and Mumtaz, M. Public Health Implications of Hazardous Waste Sites: Findings, Assessment and Research. European Conference in Combination Toxicol. Veldhoven, The Netherlands, October, 1995.

[2] Carter WH Jr, Gennings C, Staniswalis JG, Campbell ED and White KI Jr. A statistical approach to the construction and analytical analysis of isobolograms. J. Am. Coll. Toxicol. 7:963-973, 1988.

[3] Kodell RL and Pounds JG. Assessing the toxicity of mixtures of chemicals. In: Statistics in toxicology, (Krewski D and Franklin C, Eds). New York: Gordon and Breach, 1991.

Metal Ions in Biology and Medicine; vol 6. Eds. J.A. Centeno, Ph. Collery, G. Vernet, R.B. Finkelman, H. Gibb, J.C. Etienne. John Libbey Eurotext, Paris © 2000, pp. 300-302.

Variability in the development toxicity of aluminum in mice with the day of exposure

M.L. Albina, M. Bellés, D.J. Sánchez, J.L. Domingo and J. Corbella

Laboratory of Toxicology and Environmental Health, School of Medicine, "Rovira i Virgili" University, San Lorenzo 21, 43201 Reus, Spain

Aluminum (Al) exposure during pregnancy can induce embryo/fetal toxicity in mammals. Although it is well established that Al can be a developmental toxicant when administered parenterally [1,2], no evidence of maternal and embryo/fetal toxicity was observed when high doses of Al hydroxide were given orally to pregnant rats and mice during organogenesis [3,4]. However, recent studies have clearly demonstrated the importance not only of the route of Al exposure but also of the chemical form of the Al compound on the developmental toxicity of this element. Thus, oral administration of Al nitrate to pregnant rats on days 6-14 of gestation resulted in decreased fetal body weight and increased the number of external, internal and skeletal anomalies [5]. Moreover, signs of maternal and developmental toxicity were also found when Al hydroxide was given concurrently with citric acid to rats [6] or lactic acid to mice [7]. Both, citric and lactic acids, have shown to enhance the gastrointestinal Al absorption in experimental animals [8,9] and humans [10]. To extend the knowledge on the effects of Al during pregnancy, the aim of this study was to determine whether the day of exposure could modify the Al-induced maternal and developmental toxicity in mice.

Materials and Methods

Animals and chemicals. Virgin male and female Charles River CD1 mice, average weight of 26-31 g were purchased from Criffa (Barcelona, Spain). Following an acclimation period of one week, female mice were mated with males (2:1) overnight and examined the following morning for copulatory plugs. The day on which a vaginal plug was found was designated day 0 of gestation. Animals were assigned to experimental groups by stratified randomization so that body weights were equivalent across all groups on gestation day 0. Aluminum was administered as Al nitrate nonahydrate (E. Merck, Darmstadt, Germany). Solutions of Al nitrate were prepared in deionized water and the concentrations adjusted so that a 30-g mouse would receive a volume of 0.20 ml.

Experimental. Five groups of plug-positive females were given by gavage a single dose of 995 mg/kg of Al nitrate nonahydrate on one of the days 8-12 of gestation. This dose is one-fourth of the oral LD_{50} of Al nitrate nonahydrate in mice, 3981 mg/kg, previously reported [11]. Animals in the control group received deionized water by gavage. On gestation day 18, all animals were sacrificed under diethyl ether anesthesia and the number of early and late resorptions, as well as the number of dead and live fetuses was recorded. Each living fetus was weighed, and examined for externally visible abnormalities. Approximately one-half of the available fetuses were fixed in 95% ethanol, macerated in 1% KOH, stained with Alizarin red S, and examined for skeletal anomalies. The remaining fetuses were fixed in Bouin's fluid, sectioned, and evaluated for internal malformations and variations.

Results and Discussion

Aluminum nitrate nonahydrate administered orally to pregnant mice on one of the days 8-12 of gestation caused significant reductions (with the exception of day 11) in the number of live females with fetuses. The highest reductions were observed in the 8 (78.7%) and 12 (85.8%) day groups. While food consumption was only significantly diminished in the groups exposed to Al on day 12 of gestation, significant reductions in body weight gain, body weight at termination and gravid uterine weight were observed after Al administration on gestation days 8-12 (Figure I).

FIG. I. Maternal effects

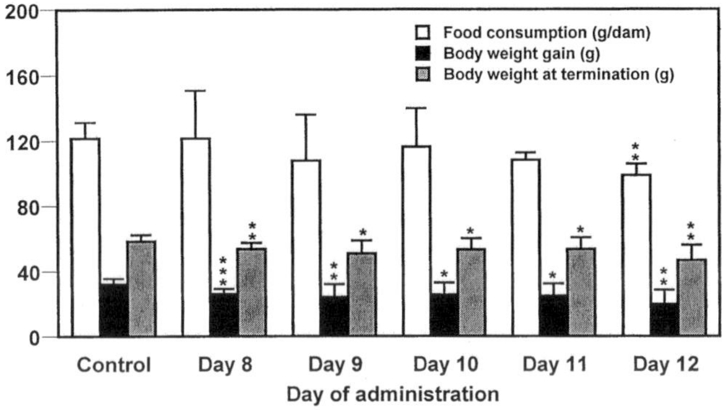

Results are expressed as mean values ± SD. *$P<0.05$,**$P<0.01$,***$P<0.001$: significantly different from control group.

No significant differences between Al-dosed groups and the control group were seen in the number of early and late resorptions, dead fetuses, and the sex ratio of live fetuses. However, body weight of live fetuses was significantly reduced in the Al-dosed groups. The highest reduction was noted on gestation day 12 (Figure II). Skeletal anomalies are shown in Figure III. The most common morphological defects associated with Al exposure were reduced ossification in a number of bones.

FIG. II. Fetal body weight (g)

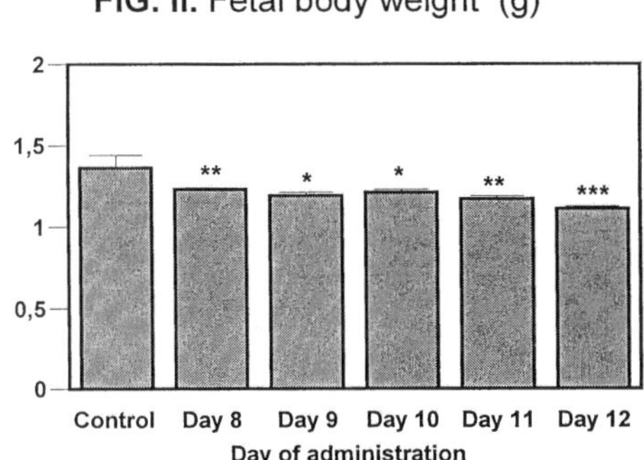

Results are expressed as mean values ± SD

FIG. III. Skeletal alterations

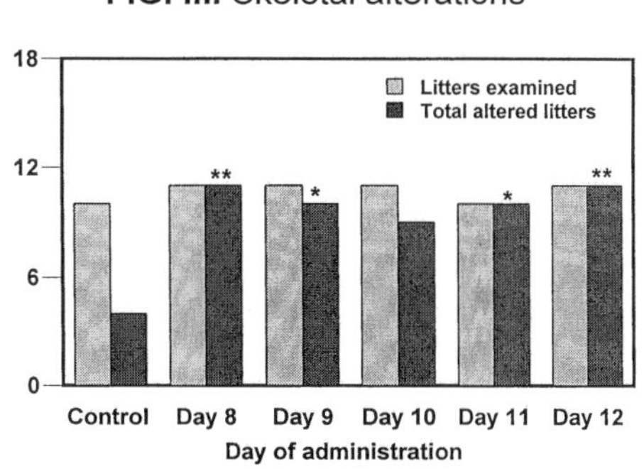

Results are expressed as mean values

*$P<0.05$,**$P<0.01$,***$P<0.001$: significantly different from control group.

The results show a pattern of Al-induced developmental toxicity similar to that found in previous studies [5,12,13,14]. Although no embryolethality was detected at any day of Al exposure, fetal body weight was significantly reduced in all the Al-treated groups, while the number of skeletal anomalies (mainly reduced or delayed ossification of a number of bones) was also higher in the Al-dosed groups than in the control group. According to these results, oral administration of a high Al dose (995 mg/kg of Al nitrate nonahydrate) would be able to cause developmental toxic effects in pregnant mice, with day 12 of gestation being the most sensitive time to produce these effects. However, it should be noted that this Al dose also induced concomitant maternal toxicity.

Acknowledgements

This work was supported the DGICYT, Ministry of Education, Spain, grant PM96-0030.

References

1. Domingo JL. Reproductive and developmental toxicity of aluminum: a review. *Neurotoxicol Teratol* 1995; 17:515-21.
2. Golub MS, Domingo JL. What we know and what we need to know about developmental aluminum toxicity. *J Toxicol Environ Health* 1996; 48:585-97.
3. Domingo JL. Developmental toxicity of metal chelating agents. *Reprod Toxicol* 1998; 12:499-10.
4. Gomez M, Bosque MA, Domingo JL, Llobet JM, Corbella J. Evaluation of the maternal and developmental toxicity of aluminum from high doses of aluminum hydroxide in rats. *Vet Hum Toxicol* 1990; 32:545-48.
5. Paternain JL, Domingo JL, Llobet JM, Corbella J. Embryotoxic and teratogenic effects of Al nitrate in rats upon oral administration. *Teratology* 1988; 38:253-57.
6. Gomez M, Domingo JL, Llobet JM. Developmental toxicity evaluation of oral aluminum in rats: Influence of citrate. *Neurotoxicol Teratol* 1991; 13:323-28.
7. Colomina MT, Gomez M, Domingo JL, Llobet JM, Corbella J. Concurrent ingestion of lactate and aluminum can result in developmental toxicity in mice. *Res Commun Chem Pathol Pharmacol* 1992; 77:95-06.
8. Partridge NA, Regnier FE, White JL, Hem SL. Influence of dietary constituents on intestinal absorption of aluminum. *Kidney Int* 1989; 35:1413-17.
9. Domingo JL, Gomez M, Llobet JM, Corbella J. Influence of some dietary constituents on aluminum absorption and retention in rats. *Kidney Int* 1991; 39:598-01.
10. Domingo JL, Gomez M, Llobet JM, Richart C. Effect of ascorbic acid on gastrointestinal aluminum absorption. *Lancet* 1991; 338:1467.
11. Llobet JM, Domingo JL, Gomez M, Tomas JM, Corbella J. Acute toxicity studies of aluminum compounds: antidotal efficacy of several chelating agents. *Pharmacol Toxicol* 1987; 60:280-83.
12. Golub MS, Gershwin ME, Donald JM, Negri S, Keen CL. Maternal and developmental toxicity of chronic aluminum exposure in mice. *Fundam Appl Toxicol* 1987; 8:346-57.
13. Bernuzzi V, Desor D, Lehr PR. Developmental alterations in offspring of female rats orally intoxicated by aluminum chloride or lactate during gestation. *Teratology* 1989; 40:21-27.
14. Muller G, Bernuzzi V, Desor D, Hutin MF, Burnel D, Lehr PR. Developmental alterations in offspring of female rats orally intoxicated by aluminum lactate at different gestation periods. *Teratology* 1990; 42:253-61.

Metal Ions in Biology and Medicine; vol 6. Eds. J.A. Centeno, Ph. Collery, G. Vernet, R.B. Finkelman, H. Gibb, J.C. Etienne. John Libbey Eurotext, Paris © 2000, pp. 303-305.

The current state of epidemic tea-induced fluorosis and its control countermeasures in Urumqi county Xinjiang

By Kang Ben, Lu Hua, He Hongchao

Urumqi County Sanitation and Antiepidemic Station, Urumqi, 830011, Xinjiang, China

Abstract:Urumqi county is the first area where tea-induced fluorosis is discovered and reported in Xinjiang.The essay states the current state of tea-induced fluorosis in Urumqi county,namely:the detectable rate of dental fluorosis for 6-8 school children is 33.3% and fluorosis of bone for adults is 16% ,mainly distributed among Kazak inhabitants in the pasture areas.The epidemic fluorosis among Kazak inhabitants is mainly attributable to the cheap-price brick tea ,its highest content of fluorine and their unique love for brick tea .The paper also advances problems occurred in the control work and its countermeasures.

Key Words: tea-induced fluorosis;epidemic state;control countermeasures; Urumqi county

Tea-induced fluorosis,as a new type of local epidemic fluorine disease in our country,is mainly distributed in ethnic minority regions with a traditional habit of drinking brick tea.In 1988,Wang Lian-fang and others first discovered and reported the tea-induced fluorosis of Kazak inhabitants at the Gaoyazi pasture in Urumqi county and then,Xie Wensheng and some others made a preliminary survey of other local areas,but lacking of systematic in-depth study .In order to get an accurate and systematic command of the distribution feature and character of tea-induced fluorosis,make a probe about the effect of tea-induced fluorosis upon ethnic minority masses'health and provide a scientific base for controlmeasures,we have chosen the typical townships and farms with a compact communityof ethnic minority as our survey spots ,with its findings shown as follows:

1.Current State

1.1 General Case:Urumqi county,which is located on the northern slope of the Mid Tianshan Mountains,at the southern edge of the Junggar Basin, has under its administration twenty-two townships(towns)farms,covering an area of 11,400 Sq.kilometers,including 50% of mountainous area and 33% of alluvial plain,with the gradient of the terrain being 2-3%. The pasture areas inhabited by ethnic minorityin compact community are mainly distributed at the southern upland or hilly land.The pasture inhabitants are dominated by Kazak nationality,who are mainly engaged in stock-breeding production and live a nomadic or semi-nomadic life.The settlements are mostly built on the low-hilly land with an altitude of 1500-1800 meters,with cool climate,around 3-month frost-free period and improper condition
for farm-crop growth. The economy ,relatively speaking ,lag behind ,with vast land and sparse population,without industrial pollution ;the fuel is dominated by timber, with fluorine content in drinking water being between 0.11-0.53mg/L ,without pollution of burning coal .Affected by traditional habits and confined by nomadic life,Kazak

inhabitants' diet pattern is monotonous ,whose staple food is nan(a kind of flour-baked food),meat and milk ,with little intake of vegetable ,melon and fruit .Milk-tea(brick tea mixed up with certain proportion of milk) is an essential tea for the nationality to drink every day .

1.2 State of Disease: A total number of 340 school children with ages rang ing from 8 to 10 has been checked .The detection has revealed 113 cases of dental fluorosis and 33.33% of detectable rate for dental fluorosis,whose rate is obviously higher than that(11-47%)of Han nationality .By having an X rays of 106 adults'forearms,shanks and pelvis who are 16 years and upward ,17 cases of fluorosis of bone has been detected ,belonging to minor ones,with ages ranging from 35to 70 years old .Of which ,5 cases are sclerotic type ,5 cases mixed type and 3cases areosis type ,with detectable rate of 16% .

1.3 Inhabitants'Brick Tea Consumption and Fluorine Intake in Brick Tea

Kazak inhabitants' brick-tea consumption is clearly higher than Han nation ality .Kazak people's per-capital daily consumption of brick tea is 24.4g while Han inhabitants'consumption is much lower than Kazak inhabitants',consuming 4.0g of tea a day,though they ,influenced by the local inhabitants ,also drink brick tea .The average fluorine intake in tea for Kazak nationality is 10.1mg/day while Han people is only 1.92mg/day .20 portions of pure tea at Kazak inhabitants' home have been examined ,with fluorine content being 1.2-6.1mg/L;20 portions of milk tea with fluorine content of 0.86-4.2mg/L;20 portions of milk with fluorine content of 0.15-0.46mg/L .33 portions of students' urine sample have been examined ,with urine fluorine of 0.31-3.25mg/L;20 portions of adults' urine sample with fluorine content of 0.64-7.2mg/L .Meanwhile ,a correlation analysis has been made about adults' daily tea-consumption and urine fluorine content,whose result bears a striking dependency relation with drinking tea($r=0.7238$ $P<0.01$).

2.Result Analysis

2.1 The tea-induced fluorosis in Urumqi county is mainly distributed among Kazak inhabitants in pasture areas with a traditional habit of drinking brick tea,with extensive popularity.The cheap-price and higher fluorine-content in brick tea as well as Kazak people's particular love for brick tea mainly result in an epidemic tea -induced flurosis among them .Meanwhile,it is also closely related to their environment ,resources ,economy and culture .

2.2 Xinjiang is a multi-national region with compact communities for ethnic minorities.The initial survey in the local region indicates that,apart from Kazak nationality ,Uygur ,Mongolian ,Tajik ethnic groups are also found to have suffered from epidemic tea-induced flurosis to different degrees .Therefore ,it can be expected that tea-induced flurosis probably covers quite a few ethnic-minority areas with a traditional habit of drinking brick tea in Xinjiang .

3.Problems and Countermeasures

3.1 The survey findings of Urumqi county and other local regions in Xinjiang have proven the presence of XJ tea-induced flurosis and made sure the sources of fluorine as well as access to fluorine intake ,however ,lacking comprehensive and systematic investigation about scope of epidemic tea-induced flurosis,its distribution area ,numbers of victim and harmful degree .At present ,the case is still in uncertain and indecisive state .Forces must be organized to undertake an investigation about tea-induced flurosis in a planned way .

3.2 The workers involved in prevention and treatment of endemic diseases fail to pay enough attention to the prevention and treatment of tea-induced flurosis so that the work remains at survey stage of epidemiology ,without systematicness.While tea-induced flurosis being monitored ,specialized research institutes of endemia and workers of prevention and treatment at grass-root units should be advocated and encouraged to make a study of crucial matters concerning its urgent solution and implementation of prevention and treatment measures and take comprehensive measures.

3.3 Hygiene publicity and health education seriously lag behind ,ethnic minority people with a habit of drinking brick tea lack enough knowledge about the harm of tea-induced flurosis ,have weak awareness of flurosis and fail to understand and accept the intervention measures .Especially lacking practical and efficient technique to get rid of flurosis by drinking tea up to now ,publicity and implementation of prevention and treatment measures to change milk tea ,strong-tea preparation and drinking habits can be effected .The black tea with low content of fluorine and similar tint,aroma and taste is chosen to substitute for brick tea;the boiling time is reduced and milk tea is blended instead of being boiled,which may well be practical and workable preventive measures to cut down the harm of tea-induced flurosis .

3.4 The root of tea-induced flurosis lies in the quality of raw tea .The target of fluroine in tea will be listed into the higiene standard for tea so as to control the fluroine content in raw tea and finished tea .The organizational and coordinating functions of all the relavant departments in reducing tea-fluorine content must be brought into full play so as to compel the producer to change the variety structure of brick tea and superior brick tea with lower fluorine content be vigorously developed .

3.5 Particular social groups ,special tea and tea-drinking habits are important factors to result in tea-induced flurosis .As a result ,nomadic production and life patterns will probably become a barrier in carrying out intervention .Along with social progress,economic development and realization of nomadic nationality's sedentary life manner,living customs and tea-drinking habit also probably follow a certain healthy bahavioural mode ,alleviate or even get rid of harmfrom tea-induced flurosis .

3.6 The domestic and international communication ought to be reinforced ,foreign technology introduced ,finance must be aided to study fluorine-alleviatingknow-how by drinking tea and push ahead its diffusion as well as practical application .

4.Reference Documents

(1) *China Tea-induced Flurosis and Current Research State ".China Journal of Endemia Prevention and Treatment ,1998,13(6):349-350 ,written by Jiang Ge.

(2)Xinjiang Kazak Inhabitants' Tea-drinking Habit and Flurosis.Endemia Bulletin ,1993,8(3).

Metal Ions in Biology and Medicine; vol 6. Eds. J.A. Centeno, Ph. Collery, G. Vernet, R.B. Finkelman, H. Gibb, J.C. Etienne. John Libbey Eurotext, Paris © 2000, pp. 307-309.

Increases in platinum metals in the UK and possible health effects

Margaret E. Farago, Emma J. Hutchinson, Niani Chandran and Peter R. Simpson

Environmental Geochemistry Research Group, The T H Huxley School of Environment, Earth Science and Engineering, Imperial College of Science Technology and Medicine, Royal School of Mines, London SW7 2BP, UK

That Pt in the environment has been increasing since the introduction of catalytic converters in Europe, has been reported by a number of authors. Studies of roadside dust and stream sediments in Sweden show an increase in Pt concentrations from 1984 to 1991 [1], [2]. Investigation of archive sewage sludge in Stuttgart, Germany [3] has revealed a large increase in Pt concentration since the introduction of catalysts in 1984. Zereini *et al* [4,5] have analysed soils near highways sampled between 1990 and 1994, their results show increases in Pt concentrations from 10 ng/g to 41 ng/g.

In this work [6], concentrations of Pt and Pd in soils and road dust sweepings collected in the cities of Birmingham and Nottingham in the UK in 1996 are shown in Table I. These are compared with values found by the analysis of archived samples collected in 1982 A marked increase in Pt concentration was observed for almost all soil

Table I. Platinum (ng/g) in garden soils (0-5 cm) and road dusts from Nottingham and Birmingham

Year	Sample	n	Range	Mean	Geomean
Nottingham					
1982	Soil	42	0.05-1.37	0.62	0.54
	Road dust	10	0.46-1.58	0.9	0.8
1996	Soil	42	0.19-1.33	0.8	0.75
1996	Road dust[a]	8	0.82-6.59	2.78	2.29
1998	Road dust[b]	20	7.3-297.8	96.8	69.5
Birmingham					
1982	Soil	57	0.09-4.13	0.64	0.46
1997	Soil	57	0.05-4.45	0.93	0.62
1997	Road dust	14	0.62-40.4	6.48	3.15

[a] Residential streets with low traffic densities [b] Includes major roads with high traffic densities

and road dust sampling sites in the 1996 survey compared with the 1982 survey in Nottingham. The differences were statistically significant at the 95% level (soil p = 0.00045, road dust p = 0.00058, Student's t test).

Platinum concentrations in Birmingham [6] show an increase between 1982 and 1997 for almost all sample sites. the change in platiunum concentration between the 1982 and 1997 surveys is significantly different at the 95% level (p = 0.0036).

Elevated concentrations of Pt were also observed in the city centre and in proximity to major roads in Nottingham, in both soils and road dusts, although the effect was much greater in road dusts. This supports the hypothesis that increased Pt concentrations are associated with increased traffic densities and that potential exposure is higher for residents of urban areas, particularly those living along busy roads.

Table II. Platinum ng/g in road dust from 4 road categories in Nottingham in 1998

Road category	n	Range	Mean	GM
Centre	4	96-234.5	168.5	160
A road	8	37-298	111	91
B road	2	39-80	60	56
Residential	6	7-86	42	30

The total emissions from vehicles equippped with catalysts it contaversial. Kummerer et al., [6] have suggested emission factorsof Pt from cars equipped with catalysts of 0.5-0.65 µg/km. Using the lower figure, the increases im emission of Pt can be calculated (Table III). However, newer estimates give the emissions as somewhat lower [7] (Table IV).

Table III. Total Emissions of Platinum by cars equipped with Vehicle Exhaust Catalysts (VEC) in the UK given in kg (Based on Statistical Data from the DOT).

	1993	1995	1997	1998
Number of Cars & Light Goods Vehicles	20.0×10^6	20.5×10^6	21.5×10^6	22.0×10^6
With VECs	1.9×10^6	6.0×10^6	10.5×10^6	12.9×10^6
% with VECs	9.5	29	49	59
km/car	15,000	15,000	15,000	15,000
Total km (VEC only)	2.85×10^{10}	9.00×10^{10}	1.56×10^{11}	1.94×10^{11}
Emission (µg/km)	0.5	0.5	0.5	0.5
Total Emission by cars (kg)	14.25	45.00	78.00	96.75

Table IV. Platinum emission factors for new catalysts for different test cycles (ng/km) [7]

Test cycle	Geometric mean	Arithmetic mean	25th Percentile	75th Percentile
US72 (urban)	29	37	14	57
80 km/hour (tunnel)	7	12	2	20
US72-EUDC (Extra urban cycle)	19	19	8	40
130 km/hr (motorway)	75	90	41	136

Platinum has been shown to be present in measurable concentrations in blood and urine samples from populations in the UK [8] and the possible health effects have been discussed.

References

[1] Wei C and Morrison GM (1994). Platinum analyses and speciation in urban gulleypots. *Anal Chim Acta.* 284: 587 - 592

[2] Wei C (1993). Chalmers Tekniska Hogskola, Doktorsavhandilngar n 934: 1 - 60.

[3] Helmers E, Mergel N and Barchet R. (1994). Platin in Klärschlammasche und an Gräsern. *Umweltwissenschaften und Schadstoff-Forschnung - Zeit Umweltchem. Ökotox.* 6 (3): 130-134.

[4] Zereini F, Zientek C and Urban H (1993). Konzentration und Verteilung von Platingruppenelementen (PGE) in Böden. UWFS - Z Umweltchem Ökotox. 5 (3): 130 - 134.

[5] Zereini F, Alt F, Rankenburg K, Beyer JM and Artelt S (1997c). Verteilung von PGE in den Umweltkompartimenten Boden, Schlamm, Straβenstaub, Straβenkehrgut und Wasser. Z Umweltchem Ökotox. 9 (4): 193 - 200.

[6] Hutchinson, E. J., Farago, M.E., and Simpson, P.R. 1999. Changes in platinum concentrations in soils and dusts from UK cities. In: Anthropogenic platinum emissions and their impact on man and environment. Alt, F., and Zereini, F. (eds). Springer Verlag, Berlin. pp 59-66.

[7]Artelt S, Kock H, Konig HP, Levsen K and Rosner G (1999). Engine dynamometer experiments: platinum emissions from differently aged three-way catalytic converters. *Atmospheric Environment.* 33: 3559-3567

[8] Farago ME, Kavanagh P, Blanks R, Kelly J, Kazantzis g, Thornton I, Simpson PR, Cook JM, Delves HT and Hall GEM (1998). Platinum concentrations in urban road dust and soil, and in blood and urine in the United Kingdom. *The Analyst.* 123: 451-454.

Metal Ions in Biology and Medicine; vol 6. Eds. J.A. Centeno, Ph. Collery, G. Vernet, R.B. Finkelman, H. Gibb, J.C. Etienne. John Libbey Eurotext, Paris © 2000, pp. 310-312.

Lead and other trace elements in osteoporosis

M. Bergomi[1], S. Rovesti[1], M. Ciaravolo[1], S. Gnudi[2], G. Vivoli[1]

[1] Department of Hygiene, Microbiology and Biostatistics, University of Modena and Reggio Emilia, Via Campi 287, 41100 Modena, Italy; [2] Internal Medicine, Istituti Ortopedici Rizzoli, Bologna, Italy

Abstract. Cu, Zn and Mn are essential for normal growth and development of skeleton in humans and animals, while their role in osteoporosis remains unsettled. Although it is well known that bone is the major organ of Pb deposition, it has only recently been considered a target of Pb toxic action. Pb has been found to affect bone function and has been implicated in the etiology of resorptive bone disease. To investigate the hypothesized relationship between Pb exposure and osteoporosis, we evaluated whether women with previous occupational Pb exposure are at higher risk of osteoporosis during the peri-menopausal period, and sought to elucidate the mechanisms by which Pb might influence bone metabolism. Bone mineral density and biochemical parameters of bone turnover were measured in occupational Pb exposed and control women. Preliminary results show a Pb mobilization in the post-menopausal period related to bone loss, an increased risk of osteoporosis, lower bone alkaline phosphatase activity and osteocalcin levels in Pb exposed compared to control women.

In addition to calcium, magnesium and fluoride, other minerals of nutritional and toxicological interest may play a role in osteoporotic disease [1-3].

There is evidence that copper (Cu), manganese (Mn) and zinc (Zn) are essential for normal growth and development of the skeleton both in humans and animals, but their involvement in osteoporosis remains unsettled. Animal studies have shown that long-term Cu and Mn dietary deficiencies significantly decrease bone mineral density and change bone crystal composition [2]. Osteoporosis-like symptoms have also been reported in Cu deficient preterm infants and children [4]. The osteopenia induced by estrogen deficiency was slightly more severe in low Cu diet animals [5]. Epidemiological studies in elderly humans yielded more conflicting results. Low serum Mn levels in osteoporotic women and low serum Cu levels in patients with femoral neck fractures have been observed, while other cross-sectional studies failed to detect any significant relationship between trace mineral levels in different biological matrixes and osteoporosis [2,6,7]. Hyperzincuria has frequently been detected in osteoporotic women. Elevated urinary but not plasmatic Zn levels, as well as the positive correlation between Zn excretion and bone resorption parameters however suggest that the Zn increased excretion in osteoporosis is dependent on bone resorption [8,9].

Although bone is the major organ of lead (Pb) storage and a potential internal source of exposure, particularly during periods of bone demineralization, only recently has been considered a potential target of Pb toxic action. Animal studies, cell culture experiments and clinical observations suggest that Pb may impair bone function. Lead may affect bone metabolism indirectly, by interaction with systemic regulators of bone function, and directly by altering the response of bone cells to hormonal regulation. Lead may also impair the ability of bone cells to synthesize or secrete components of bone matrix [10]. Further, lead may be implicated in osteoporosis, even if the literature data are few and conflicting [3,11,12].

Personal study. To gain insight into the relationship between Pb exposure and osteoporosis, we investigated women with previous occupational Pb exposure. Aim of the study was to establish whether chronic lead exposure increases the risk of osteoporosis during the peri-menopausal period, and elucidate the mechanisms by which Pb might influence bone metabolism. The subjects were selected according to criteria described elsewhere [12]; 46 exposed women (aged from 37 to 66 years), 14 in pre-menopausal and 32 in post-menopausal period, were recruited. Bone mineral density (BMD) and biological markers of lead exposure (Pb in blood and erythrocyte protoporphyrin) were measured in exposed women. A control group of 46 not occupationally lead exposed women comparable for age, menopausal status and body mass index was recruited and submitted to BMD evaluations. Bone mineral density was measured both at lumbar spine (L2–L4) and left hip (femoral neck). The prevalence of osteoporosis, estimated on the basis of BMD values at the two sites of measurement, was calculated according to WHO criteria, using the manufacturer's young normal range. In a subset of exposed and control women the following parameters of bone turnover were measured: hydroxyproline, calcium and phosphorus in urine; total alkaline phosphatase, bone alkaline phosphatase, ionized calcium, osteocalcin, parathormone, and 1,25 $(OH)_2$ Vitamin D in serum. Details of the analytical and statistical methods have been reported elsewhere [12].

According to our previous [12] and others' reports, biological indicators of Pb exposure show higher circulating Pb levels in post-menopausal than in pre-menopausal women (mean values 138.6 vs 127.6 μg/l), particularly in the recent menopause period (158.6 μg/l). In addition, Pb blood levels were significantly related to urinary hydroxyproline (r= 0.51; P= 0.011) in post-menopausal women. The BMD values of exposed and control women are shown in Table I.

Measurement sites	Menopausal status	Exposed women Mean ± SD	Control women Mean ± SD
Lumbar spine	Pre	0.954 ± 0.166*	1.070 ± 0.097*
	Post	0.987 ± 0.185	0.985 ± 0.133
	Peri	0.977 ± 0.179	1.011 ± 0.127
Femoral neck	Pre	0.824 ± 0.145	0.872 ± 0.034
	Post	0.820 ± 0.106	0.778 ± 0.101
	Peri	0.822 ± 0.118	0.807 ± 0.096

Table I. Bone mineral density (BMD) values (g/cm^2) measured at lumbar spine and femoral neck in lead exposed and control women grouped by menopausal status. *P= 0.034

In the pre-menopausal period the spinal BMD values of exposed women were significantly lower than those of controls, while no significant difference related to exposure condition was detected in post-menopausal women. The prevalence rate of osteoporosis was higher in exposed women than controls, particularly considering spinal measurements (19.6% vs 6.5% and 6.5% vs 4.3% for spinal and femoral measurements respectively), with a remarkable increase in osteoporosis risk (Table II).

Measurement sites	OR	IC 95%	P
Lumbar spine	3.49	0.94 -12.77	0.063
Femoral neck	1.53	0.29 - ∞	0.645

Table II. Odds Ratio (OR) of osteoporosis and 95% confidence intervals (IC 95%) in relation to Pb exposure calculated for lumbar spine and femoral neck BMD measurements.

Biochemical markers of bone turnover, bone alkaline phosphatase activity and osteocalcin levels in serum, were lower in post-menopausal women than control group (mean values 53.7 vs 80.6 U/l and 5.8 vs 7.1 ng/ml for bone alkaline phosphatase and osteocalcin respectively).
Data obtained to date do not rule out that long-term exposure to lead may affect bone function and increase the risk of post-menopausal osteoporosis. Future studies are required to establish the exact role of lead in the onset and progression of osteoporosis.

References

1. Okano T. Effects of essential trace elements on bone turnover—in relation to the osteoporosis. *Nippon Rinsho* 1996; 54: 148-54.
2. Saltman PD, Strause LG. The role of trace minerals in osteoporosis. *J Am Coll Nutr* 1993; 12: 384-9.
3. Silbergeld EK, Schwartz J, Mahaffey K. Lead and osteoporosis: mobilization of lead from bone in postmenopausal women. *Environ Res* 1988; 47: 79-94.
4. Uauy R, Olivares M, Gonzales M. Essentiality of copper in humans. *Am J Clin Nutr* 1998; 67: 952S-9S.
5. Yee CD, Kubena KS, Walker M, Champney TH, Sampson HW. The relationship of nutritional copper to the development of postmenopausal osteoporosis in rats. *Biol Trace Element Res* 1995; 48: 1-11.
6. Conlan D, Korula R, Tallentire D. Serum copper levels in elderly patients with femoral neck fractures. *Age and Aging* 1990; 19: 212-4.
7. Preisinger E, Leitner G, Alacamlioglu Y, Seidl G, Marktl W, Resch KL. Nutrition and osteoporosis: a nutritional analysis of women in postmenopause. *Wien Klin Wochenschr* 1995; 107: 418-22.
8. Herzberg M, Foldes J, Steinberg R, Menczel J. Zinc excretion in osteoporotic women. *J Bone Miner Res* 1990; 5: 251-7.
9. Relea P, Revilla M, Ripoll E, Arribas I, Villa LF, Rico H. Zinc, biochemical markers of nutrition, and type I osteoporosis. *Age and Aging* 1995; 24: 303-7.
10. Pounds J, Long G, Rosen J. Cellular and molecular toxicity of lead in bone. *Environ Health Perspect* 1991; 91: 17-32.
11. Adachi JD, Arlen D, Webber CE, Chettle DR, Beaumont LF, Gordon CL. Is there any associations between the presence of bone disease and cumulative exposure to lead? *Calcif Tissue Int* 1998; 63: 429-32.
12. Vivoli G, Bergomi M, Rovesti S, Borciani N, Gnudi S, Ripamonti C, Pratelli L, Buzzi M, Pizzoferrato A. Lead exposure and bone mineral density in perimenopausal women. In: Collery Ph, Brätter P, Negretti de Brätter V, Khassanova L, Etienne JC, eds. *Metal Ions in Biology and Medicine,* vol 5. Paris: John Libbey Eurotext, 1998: 669-74.

Metal Ions in Biology and Medicine; vol 6. Eds. J.A. Centeno, Ph. Collery, G. Vernet, R.B. Finkelman, H. Gibb, J.C. Etienne. John Libbey Eurotext, Paris © 2000, pp. 313-315.

Use of a modified cadmium pharmacokinetics model to validate urinary cadmium elimination as a biomarker of exposure

Harlal Choudhury[1], Terry Harvey[1], William C. Thayer[2], Tricia F. Lockwood[2], William M. Stiteler[2], Philip E. Goodrum[2], James M. Hassett[3] and Gary L. Diamond[2]

[1] *National Center for Environmental Assessment, U.S. EPA, Cincinnati, OH;* [2] *Syracuse Research Corporation, North Syracuse, NY;* [3] *State University of New York College of Environmental Science and Forestry*

We recently described a Cadmium Dietary Exposure Model (CDEM) for estimating exposures in risk estimates of U.S. populations (1). The methodology utilizes national survey data on food cadmium concentrations contained in the U.S. Food and Drug Administration Total Diet Studies (1982-1994)(2), and food consumption patterns derived from the Third National Health and Nutrition Examination Survey (NHANES III, 1988-1994)(3), to estimate demographically stratified dietary intakes in the U.S. population (U.S. DHHS, 1997; U.S. FDA, 1999). The arithmetic mean daily cadmium intake for the U.S. population (males and females combined) estimated by the CDEM is 21.5 µg/day (SD, 11.7; 5th-95th percentile range, 8.2-42.3). Here, we describe a comparison of model predictions with empirical observations of exposure biomarkers. Dietary exposures were translated into cadmium body burdens and their corresponding urinary cadmium excretion rates using a modification of the biokinetic model of Kjellström and Nordberg (1978) (KNM)(4).Urinary cadmium excretion predicted from the combined CDEM/KNM were compared to observations reported in NHANES III for non-smokers and subjects who had no reported history of employment in cadmium or metal-related industries (NSNO subset).

The CDEM/KNM estimates and empirical estimates of urinary cadmium in males and females are shown in Figure 1. Estimates for males based on the CDEM/KN compare reasonably well with the age-category means estimated from NHANES III, however, the model substantially under estimates observed urinary cadmium in females. Good agreement was achieved with the empirical estimates for females if a gastrointestinal absorption fraction of 0.1, rather than 0.5, was assumed for females.

In order to explore a possible mechanism for a higher cadmium absorption in females, we analyzed the iron status of the NSNO subset of the NHANES III. Subjects were classified into a *low iron* or *not low iron* categories based on their having a serum ferritin concentration less than or greater then 20 µg/L, respectively (5). The female group had a substantially higher incidence of low iron status than males and the difference appeared to be age-related, with the greatest gender difference occurring in the ages 17-59 years (females 29%, males 2.4%). A similar result was obtained when the criteria for the low iron category was transferrin saturation of less than 16% and erythrocyte protoporphyrin levels greater than 70 μg/dL (6). Based on estimates of the incidence of low iron status in females (29%) and males (2.4%) from the analysis of NHANES III data, and assuming that serum ferritin concentrations below 20 μg/L would be associated with a 4-fold higher bioavailability of cadmium compared to ferritin concentrations above 20 μg/L , based on (5), the ratio of the absorption fraction in females would be expected to be approximately two times that of males. This outcome is consistent with the reasonably good agreement between the CDEM/KNM predictions and the observed urinary cadmium excretion when an absorption fraction of 0.1 is assumed for females and a value of 0.05 is assumed for males (Figure 1).

The peak kidney cadmium burden that corresponds to the average dietary intakes in the U.S population estimated with the CDEM/KNM is approximately 5.1 mg (3.3-7.6, 5th-95th percentile range) in females and 3.5 mg in males (assuming absorption fractions of 0.1 and 0.05, respectively), and occurs at age 55 years. The latter estimates are within the range of measured kidney cadmium burdens in non-smokers without known occupational exposures to cadmium (7, 8).

REFERENCES

1. Lockwood TF, Choudhury H, Diamond GL, Goodrum, PE, Hassett JM, Stiteler WM. A cadmium dietary exposure model (CDEM) for use in risk assessment. *Toxicol. Sci.* 1998; 48:382.
2. U.S. DHHS. Third National Health and Nutrition Examination Survey, 1988-1994 (CD-ROM Series 11). Centers for Disease Control and Prevention, Department of Health and Human Services. 1997
3. U.S. FDA. Total Diet Studies. Market Baskets 91-3 through 97-1. U.S. Food and Drug Administration, Center for Food Safety and Nutrition, July 1999, http://vm.cfsan.fda.gov/~comm/tds-toc.html
4. Kjellström T, Nordberg GF. A kinetic model of cadmium metabolism in the human being. *Environ. Res.* 1978; 16: 248-269
5. Flanagan PR, McLellan, JS, Haist, Cherian MG., Chamberlain MJ, Valberg LS. Increased dietary cadmium absorption in mice and human subjects with iron deficiency. *Gastroenterology* 1978; 7: 841846.
6. Looker, A., Sempos CT, Johnson C, Yetley EA. Vitamin-mineral supplement use: Association with dietary intake and iron status of adults. *J. Am. Dietetic Assoc.* 1988; 88:808-814.
7. Ellis, K.J., Yuen K, Yasumura S, Cohn SH. Dose-response analysis of cadmium in man: body burden vs kidney dysfunction. *Environ. Res.* 1984; 33: 216-226.
8. Ellis, K., Cohn SH, Smith TJ. Cadmium inhalation exposure estimates: Their significance with respect to kidney and liver cadmium burden. *J. Toxicol. Environ. Health* 1985; 15:173-187.

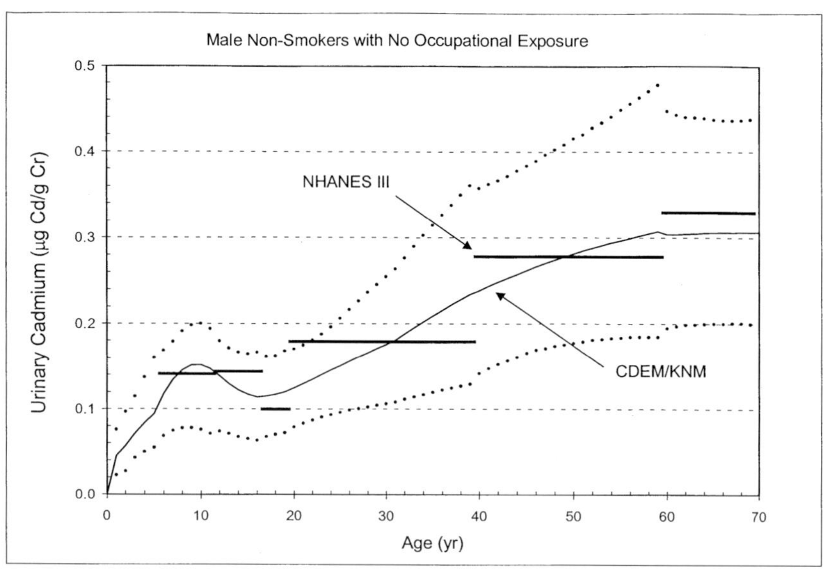

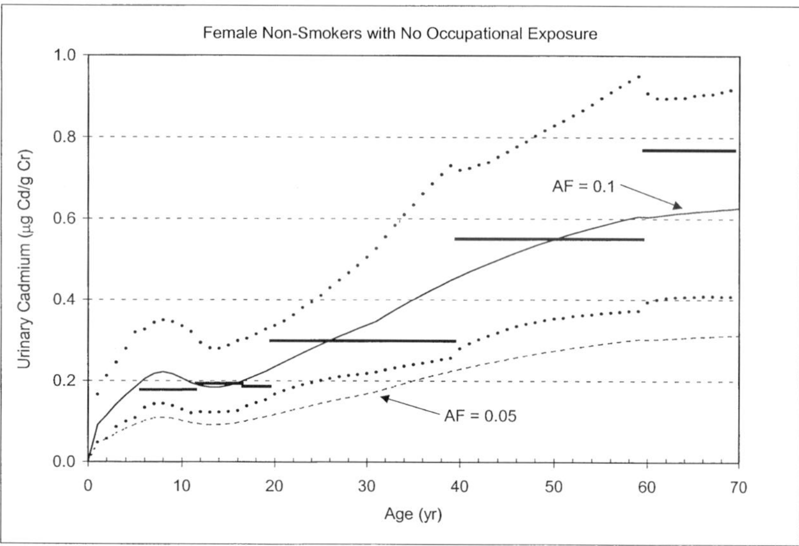

Figure 1. Comparison of Model Predictions and Observations of Urinary Cadmium Excretion in the U.S. Males (Top Panel) and Females (Bottom Panel). The horizontal bars represent the weighted age-category mean values obtained from the NSNO subset of the NHANES III. The curves show the central tendency (solid line) and 5th and 95th percentile predictions (dotted line) from the CDEM/KNM, assuming an absorption fraction of 0.05 in males or 0.1 in females. The lower curve in the plot for females (dashed line) are the predictions assuming a gastrointestinal absorption fraction of either 0.05.

Metal Ions in Biology and Medicine; vol 6. Eds. J.A. Centeno, Ph. Collery, G. Vernet, R.B. Finkelman, H. Gibb, J.C. Etienne. John Libbey Eurotext, Paris © 2000, pp. 316-318.

Comparison of airborne sampling method to biological monitoring of workers exposed to manganese

Deschamps F., Guillaumot M., Raux S.

Occupational Health Department, Faculté de Médecine, 51 rue Cognacq Jay, 51100 Reims, France

In 1981, a group of experts of the World Health Organisation (WHO) concluded that signs of adverse effects on the central nervous system may occur at manganese (Mn) concentrations in air ranging from 2000 to 5000 microgrammes/m3(1). However, on the basis of a wide variation in individual susceptibility, WHO suggests that the minimum effects level is probably below 1000 microgrammes/m3 (1). In 1979, the American Conference of Governmental Industrial Hygienists, proposed a threshold limit value for a time – weighted average (TLV – TWA) of 1000 microgrammes/m3 for Mn fumes, and in 1988, a TLV – TWA of 5000 microgrammes/m3 for Mn in inhalable dust. Actually, a TLV – TWA of 200 microgrammes/m3 is proposed for Mn in inhalable dust (2).

The aim of the present investigation was to assess, by airborne sampling method and biological monitoring, exposure of workers making enamels containing Mn and to detect effects on nervous system induced by this compound.

Subjects and methods

Workers exposed to Mn were chosen from a compagny making enamels. During the production process, the workers were exposed to airborne Mn dust, when intermediate products were mechanically transfered and when the final product was bagged. Job turnover within the plant was considerable, and exposure was regarded as the same for all workers. A questionnaire was filled during the annual medical examination for each subject with at least one year exposure to enamels. The questionnaire was used to measure the occurrence of symptoms from the central and peripheral nervous system, and included neuropsychological tests. A control group of workers, comparable for education and social background was chosen. The exposure to particles in the breathing zone of the workers was surveyed during the past year. The exposure levels to airborne Mn concentration in total dust were determined by personal and stationnary samplings. The analyses (WHATMAN filters) were performed by spectrophotometry. One sample of blood was taken from each exposed, and one third of the controls. Blood was taken from a cubital vein. A small volume of blood was washed through the needle before sampling. After a previous check of all the sampling materials for lack of metal contamination, a venous blood sample of 5 ml was collected immediately before the testing procedure, kept at 4°C, and analyzed immediately. Blood Mn was determined by atomic absorption spectrometry (PERKIN ELMER). The limit value was 220 nmol/liter.

Results

In a group of 138 workers exposed to Mn, the current exposure to airborne Mn (respirable Mn level) varied respectively for personal sampling (n = 15) and for stationary sampling (n = 15), from 10 to 293 microgrammes/m3, and from 10 to 45 microgrammes/m3. The mean values, amounted respectively 57,2 microgrammes/m3, ± 84,17 standard derivation (SD), and 12,93 ± 8 ,85 SD. Two levels concerning personal sampling were over 200 microgrammes/m3. The mean concentration of Mn in blood in the exposed group was 170,36 nmol/liter, SD ± 65,7, range 9 – 354 compared to 166 nmol/liter, SD ± 60,94, range 57 – 330 for the controls. Twenty five exposed workers had blood manganese levels over 220 nmol/liter. The exposed workers reported more symptoms like asthenia ($P < 0{,}05$), sleeps disturbance ($P < 0{,}004$), and headache ($P < 0{,}005$) but did not exhibited different performance concerning neuropsychological tests as compared with controls.

There was no significant correlation between the length of employment and the Mn contents in the blood. We observed no significant correlation between the Mn contents in the blood and the neurological findings.

Discussion

Our study concerning enamels workers shows a higher prevalence of disturbances of sleep among the workers exposed to Mn. Insomnia has also been noted in several other studies (3)(4)(5). Fatigue is one of prominent symptoms in our study and has been reported by others (4)(5).

These results indicate that the individual evaluation of the Mn exposure intensity remain difficult on the basis of Mn in blood. We do not find any relationship between lengh of employment and the concentration of Mn in blood. It should be realized that in view of the different pollution by Mn at various work places, duration of exposure is an inappropriate estimate of integrated exposures. Except for the study by HORIGUCHI et al (6), most of the other reports on occupational Mn exposure (7), failed to establish relationships between Mn in blood and the severity of Mn, induced neurological disorders. This was usually attributed to individual susceptibility to the disease and may also partly be due to the use of unreliable methods in the measurement of Mn in blood (8).

Finally, 2 of the 30 (6 %) of the air samplings were over the limits, in comparison to 25 of the 138 (18 %) blood manganese dosages.

In conclusion, this study confirms the observation that exposure to Mn respirable dust concentration below 300 microgrammes/m3 is not associated with impairment of central neural function, but only with mild clinical symptoms.

The present study indicates that the determination of Mn in blood is of limited value for the biological monitoring of workers exposed to Mn dust. But it is a more sensitive method than airborne sampling method to asses occupational exposure to Mn.

BIBLIOGRAPHY

(1) Organisation Mondiale de la Santé (OMS). Le manganèse. Genève : OMS, 1981. OMS critères d'hygiène de l'environnement n° 17.

(2) American Conference of Governmental Industrial Hygienists (A.C.G.I.H.). ABBE – 93 : threshold limit values for chemical substances and physical agents and biological exposure indices. Cincinnati, OH : A.C.G.I.H., 1992.

(3) Nelson K., GOLNICK J., KORN T., ANGLE C.
Manganese encephalpathy : utility of early magnetic resonance imaging. Br.J. Ind. Med., 1993 ; 50 : 510 – 513.

(4) MERGLER D., HUEL G., BOWLER R., IRE GREN A. BELANGER S., BALDWIN M. et al.
Nervous system dysfunction among workers with long term exposure to manganese. Environ. Res. 1994 ; 64 : 151 – 180.

(5) ROELS H., LAUWERYS R., BUCHET J.P., GENET P., JAWAD SARHAN M., HANOTIAU I. et al.
Epidemiological survey among workers exposed to manganese : effects on lung, central nervous system and some biological indices. Am. J. Ind. Med. 1987 ; 11 : 307 – 27.

(6) HORIGUCHI K., HORIGUCHI S., SHINA GAWA K., UTSUNOMIYA T., TSUYAMA Y.
On the significance of manganese contents in the whole blood and urine of manganese handlers. Osaka City Med. J. 1971 ; 16 : 29 – 37.

(7) SMYTH LT., RUTH R.C., WHITMAN NE, DUGAN T.
Clinical manganism and exposure to manganese in the production and processing of ferromanganese alloy. J. Occup. Med. 1973 ; 15 : 101 – 109.

(8) VALENTIN H., SCHIELE R.
Manganese. In ALESSION L., BERLIN A., ROI R., BONI M. (eds).
Human biological monitoring of industrial chemicals. Health and safety directorate, Commission of the European Communities, Luxembourg 1983 : 133 – 145.

Metal Ions in Biology and Medicine; vol 6. Eds. J.A. Centeno, Ph. Collery, G. Vernet, R.B. Finkelman, H. Gibb, J.C. Etienne. John Libbey Eurotext, Paris © 2000, pp. 319-321.

Influence of a soldier's status on the chromium level in their urine

M. Schlegel-Zawadzka[1], J. Bertrandt[2], A. Kłos[2], M. Krośniak[1]

[1] Department of Food Chemistry and Nutrition, Jagiellonian University, 9 Medyczna St., 30-688 Kraków, Poland; [2] Military Institute of Hygiene and Epidemiology, 4 Kozielska St., 01-163 Warsaw, Poland

Introduction

Chromium is involved in the metabolism of glucose and the mechanism of action of the pancreatic hormone, insulin. Its supplementation benefits all components of Syndrome X (obesity, dyslipidemias, insulin resistance and hyperinsulinemia as well as hypertension) [1].

Average intakes of chromium are between 20-40 µg Cr per day with some as low as 5 µg/1000/kcal [2]. Cr is poorly absorbed from the diet, typically 0.5%. Most chromium excretion is in the urine and faeces, although a small amount is excreted in the bile and in sweat. Table I presents an estimation of the intake and routes of loss of chromium [3].

Table I. Estimates of intake and routes of loss of chromium.

Intake		% of output in:			
µmol	mg	Urine	Faeces	Sweat	Hair/nails
2.9	0.15	46	53	0.7	0.4

The aim

The aim of this study was to examined the influence of two years constant conditions (feeding and environmental) on the chromium level in the urine in a group of young healthy soldiers.

Material and methods

The chromium level in the uremic samples was determined using a graphite furnace atomic absorption spectrometer (Perkin Elmer 5100 PC equipped with a 5100 ZL Zeeman Furnace Module). The analytical chromium wavelength was 357.9 nm. As urine control for measurement Seronorm™ Trace Elements (Nycomed Pharma, Oslo Norway) was used. Creatinine in urine was determined using the kinetic bioMerieux test without deproteinization. The complex formed by creatinine and picric acid in an alkaline medium is measured for one minute (France). Final results are given as chromium per gram of creatinine.

The group studied consisted of 50 male soldiers aged 20 years (av). They had lived for at least two years in an unpolluted area in Central Poland.

Results

The mean level±standard deviation of creatinine in the urine samples was 2.1±1.2 g/L. The chromium content in 4% of the samples (n=2) was above 1 µg/g creatinine. The mean level of chromium in the urine was 0,26±0,27 µg/g creatinine (range 0.00001-1.15 µg/g). The number of soldiers (n) according to the chromium concentration in their urine is presented in Figure 1.

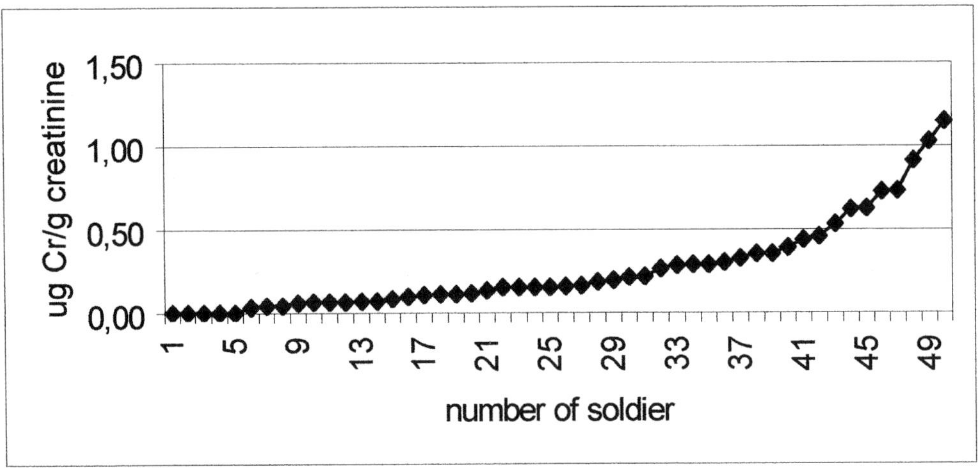

Figure 1. Chromium content in urine samples [µg/g creatinine].

Discussion

The serum chromium content does not represent the tissue chromium content, apart from a glucose tissue satiation.
Chromium absorbed is almost totally excreted in the urine - 0.5-1.5 µg daily and is in approximation equal to the amount absorbed from the daily diet [4]. The excretion of chromium in healthy people and in non-exposed to this element may be lower than 1 µg/day [5].

Nomiyama et al. determined the chromium in urine samples taken from 189 volunteers aged 10 from to 80 living in four different unpolluted areas of Japan. The chromium content was assayed with flame atomic absorption spectrometry. The average content was 0.47±0.42 µg/g creatinine (X+SE). Our results from a group of young male soldiers (all about 20 years old) are lower than the Japanese data [6]. According to Anderson et al., the degree of physical fitness affects urinary chromium loss [7]. The basal urinary excretion of subjects who exercise regularly was significantly lower than that of the sedentary control subjects 0.09±0.01 and 0.21±0.03 μg/day (mean±SE) respectively. Soldiers having routine daily exercise training and the same living conditions had essentially the same urine chromium excretion. Their chromium excretion is in the range treated as normal for non-exposed people.

Conclusions

The chromium content in urine samples show that living conditions do not influence the excretion of this element by soldiers. Its content is in a range, which is treated, as normal.

References

1. Preuss HG, Talpur N, Manohar V, Venkataramiah N, Anderson RA. Chromium and hypertension. *J Trace Elem Exp Med.* 1999; 12:125-130.
2. Stoecker BJ. Chromium absorption, safety, and toxicity. *J Trace Elem Exp Med.* 1999, 12:163-169.
3. Bender A, Bender A. E. Nutrition a reference book. Oxford University Press, 1997.
4. Anderson RA, Kozlovsky AS. Chromium intake, absorption and excretion of subjects consuming self-selected diets. *Am J Clin Nutr.* 1985, 41:1177.
5. Chromium. Environmental Health Criteria 61. WHO, Geneva 1988.
6. Nomiyama H, Yotoriyama M., Nomiyama K. Normal chromium levels in urine and blood of Japanese subjects determined by direct flames atomic absorption spectrophotometry, and valency of chromium in urine after exposure to hexavalent chromium. *Am Ind Hyg Assoc J.* 1980, 41:98-102.
7. Anderson RA, Bryden NA, Polansky MM, Deuster PA. Exercise effects on chromium excretion of trained and untrained men consuming a constant diet. *J Appl Physiol.* 1988, 64:249-252.

Metal Ions in Biology and Medicine; vol 6. Eds. J.A. Centeno, Ph. Collery, G. Vernet, R.B. Finkelman, H. Gibb, J.C. Etienne. John Libbey Eurotext, Paris © 2000, pp. 322-324.

Concentration and isotopic composition of uranium in blood, urine and semen

Shelly J. Hodge[1], John W. Ejnik[2], Katherine S. Squibb[3], Melissa A. McDiarmid[3], Larry D. Anderson[3] and Elena R. Morris

[1] Armed Forces Radiobiology Research Institute (AFRRI), 8901 Wisconsin Avenue, Bethesda, MD 20889-5603, USA; [2] Naval Drug Lab, Bldg. 38H, 320 B Bravo Street, Great Lakes, IL 60088, USA; [3] Department of Veterans Affairs/University of Maryland School of Medicine (VA/UMAB), 405 West Redwood Street, Baltimore, MD 21201, USA; [4] Department of Clinical Investigations/Walter Reed Army Medical Center, Building T-2, Room 208, 14th and Dahlia Street, North West Washington, District of Columbia 20307-5001, USA

ABSTRACT

Depleted uranium (DU) is produced by depleting natural uranium of ^{234}U and ^{235}U during the uranium enrichment process for nuclear fuel. Because of DU density, availability, and low cost, it has been incorporated into both projectiles and armor by the military. During the Persian Gulf War, soldiers may have inhaled, ingested, and/or experienced wound contamination by DU. Current interest in possible health effects resulting from exposure to DU has resulted in the need for an assay in which personnel can be screened for DU exposure.

Blood, urine and semen samples from individuals enrolled in the DU Follow-Up program at the Baltimore VA Medical Center were examined for uranium content. Samples were prepared by a series of dry-ashing steps at 450°C and wet-ashing with concentrated nitric acid and 30% hydrogen peroxide. When the ashing procedure was completed, samples were dissolved in 1 M nitric acid for analysis. Isotopic composition of uranium was determined by measuring the $^{235}U/^{238}U$ ratio, using an inductively coupled plasma mass spectrometer (ICP-MS).

Exposure to DU causes the amount of ^{235}U to decrease from about 0.7% (normal for natural uranium) to about 0.2% and the uranium concentration to increase above normal background levels. Since the detection limit of the ICP-MS is below levels of uranium typical in non-exposed cases, this assay can accurately determine whether the source of elevated uranium in an individual is from DU or natural uranium. Therefore, this assay can help answer whether DU exposure plays a role in illnesses associated with the Gulf War Syndrome.

Introduction Depleted uranium (DU) is used by the military primarily as armor and as kinetic energy penetrators to defeat armored vehicles. It is a byproduct of the enrichment process for reactor- and weapons-grade uranium (^{235}U). ^{235}U is reduced from 0.72% in natural uranium to 0.2% in DU. The remainder is ^{238}U (approximately 99.8%). The Persian Gulf War resulted in injuries by DU fragments. Fragments not immediately threatening the health of individuals were allowed to remain in place, based on standard treatment protocols designed for other metal shrapnel injuries. However, questions were soon raised as to whether this approach is appropriate for a metal with the unique radiological and toxicological properties of DU. Although DU emits less radiation than natural uranium, its chemical properties are, of course, essentially identical. These fragments dissolve slowly, and the DU is distributed to various parts of the body, especially kidney and bone [1]. Embedded fragments are unusual in that they are a long-lasting reservoir of DU that results in long-term exposures. Because of DU potential toxicity, there has been concern about long-term health effects in exposed personnel.

Experimental Fifty-two urine, 51 blood, and 38 semen samples were received blind from the VA/UMAB. Samples were placed in 40-mL acid-washed glass vials and heated at 120 °C until visibly dry, then at 300 °C for 6 h and 450 °C for 4 h (dry-ashing). Samples were then heated to just below boiling with 1 mL concentrated $HNO_{3\,(aq)}$ and 0.5 mL 30% $H_2O_{2\,(aq)}$ until dried (wet-ashing). Wet-ashing was repeated three times before samples were dry-ashed again (450 °C for 4 h), followed by wet-ashing three more times. The resulting white residue was dissolved in 1 M $HNO_{3\,(aq)}$ for analysis. Uranium measurements were obtained with ICP-MS employing operational parameters similar to those reported previously [2]. The instrument was calibrated with external standards of 500, 50, 5 and 1 ng/L of Normal Uranium in 1 M $HNO_{3\,(aq)}$. Ratios of ^{238}U to ^{235}U were obtained by isotopic analysis. Urine DU concentrations were expressed as μg DU/g creatinine.

Results and Discussion Of 52 urine samples analyzed, 12 were from individuals with embedded DU shrapnel, and 40 from individuals who may have been exposed via other routes, such as inhalation or ingestion - or not exposed to DU at all. Table I indicates that, of the 12 shrapnel-related samples, 10 contained significant amounts of DU. Concentrations of uranium measured using ICP-MS were consistent with concentrations measured in the same individuals using kinetic phosphorescence analysis (KPA) (Quanterra Inc.). Isotopic ratios obtained with the ICP-MS indicated a large percentage of the uranium was DU as opposed to natural uranium. The data also indicate that the more uranium present in the sample, the more of it was DU. The following equation was used to determine the percentage of DU.

$$\%DU = (0.72 - \%\,^{235}U \times 100)/(0.72 - 0.2) \qquad \text{[Equation 1]}$$

Equation I assumes natural uranium contains 0.72% ^{235}U and DU contains 0.2% ^{235}U. These percentages vary, so percent DU values calculated by this formula are approximate. When natural uranium levels contained more than 0.72% and no DU was present, negative numbers were obtained.

Uranium was also detected in blood and semen of some individuals and was more likely to be found in individuals with high uranium content in their urine. Accurate quantification of DU in semen and blood was not always possible due to insufficient or unavailable samples; so results are expressed qualitatively only. Four of 12 veterans with shrapnel had detectable semen concentrations of U, while 1 of 7 with no known shrapnel had detectable semen U. Three of 12 veterans with shrapnel had detectable blood concentrations of U, while 4 of 7 with no shrapnel had detectable blood U. In individuals without DU shrapnel injuries, isotopic measurements indicated that the uranium present was natural U, and not DU.

Shrapnel	Sample #	μg/g CR in [a]Urine U	%DU in Urine
Yes	7	39.166	98
Yes	50	31.781	97
Yes	26	4.285	92
Yes	1	3.423	92
Yes	47	3.000	91
Yes	10	2.772	82
Yes	44	1.572	82
Yes	34	1.120	78
Yes	41	1.062	71
Yes	25	1.000	70
Yes	20	0.015	
Yes	28	0.012	
No	30		
No	2		
No	3	0.044	-25
No	14	0.231	-130
No	39		
No	45	0.183	-87
No	52	0.004	-121

Table I. Summary of Data. (a) determined by KPA analysis.

References

1. Pellmar TC, Fuciarelli AF, Ejnik JW, Hamilton M, Hogan J, Strocko S, Emond C, Mottaz HM, Landauer MR. Distribution of uranium in rats implanted with depleted uranium pellets. *Toxicological Sciences* 1999; 49: 29-39.
2. Ejnik JW, Carmichael MM, Hamilton M, McDiarmid M, Squibb K, Boyd P, Tardiff W. Determination of the isotopic composition of uranium in urine by inductively coupled plasma mass spectrometry. *Health Phys.* 2000; 78 (2): 143-146.

Metal Ions in Biology and Medicine; vol 6. Eds. J.A. Centeno, Ph. Collery, G. Vernet, R.B. Finkelman, H. Gibb, J.C. Etienne. John Libbey Eurotext, Paris © 2000, pp. 325-327.

Correlation between blood lead and hair lead of men exposed environmentally and relationship between lead and essential metals in hair

Nowak Barbara[1], Chmielnicka Jadwiga[2]

[1] *Silesian University of Medicine, Department of Toxicology, 421-200 Sosnowiec, Jagiellońska 4, Poland;* [2] *University of Medical Academy, 90-145 Łódź Muszyńskiego 1, Poland*

ABSTRACT

The aim of this investigation was to evaluate the environmental exposure of Katowice District inhabitants in 1990-1997, as an area of high environmental exposure to lead on the basis of their concentrations in hair. The analysis of the elements listed above was carried out for 624 hair samples. Concentration of lead hair were determined using Atomic Absorption Spectroscopy. The results were calculated using the STATISTICA programme. Our major statistical analysis will focus on determining Analysis of R Spermana correlation between blood lead and hair lead for men environmentally exposed. We conclude that not only blood, but also the hair lead is a good marker of environmental exposure because hair lead influences significantly Ca and Fe as well as in blood.

INTRODUCTION

Association between blood lead and blood iron were investigated[i]. Another important metal in human organism is calcium which affects the toxicity of lead and may be substituted by lead[ii]. Iron deficiency increases absorption of lead[iii]. In the literature there is no data on the relationship between essential and toxic metals in adults' hair[iv]. Increasing lead concentration in hair lowers Fe and Ca concentrations, causing also changes in quantitative ratios between essential metals: Fe/Cu, Fe/Zn and Ca/Zn[v]. KATOWICE District is the most polluted region in Poland where Pb concentrations in soil and air are very high. Lead and Ca, Fe in human hair from inhabitants of two differently polluted regions in the south of Poland: KATOWICE and BESKID area were examined. The BESKID is an agricultural and forest mountain area.

MATERIALS AND METHODS

We took into consideration only healthy people, for whom health records were available. We selected only those samples where people were born and were living in the Katowice and Beskid area. Collecting of samples and analytical procedures for hair was carried out by Nowak and Kozłowski (1998)[vi].

RESULTS AND DISCUSSION

We used Spjotvoll/ Stoline test to investigate significance (ANOVA, $p<0.05$). We received essential differences in human hair (p. <0.05) for those two different polluted regions KATOWICE and BESKID for Pb [v], Fe (Fig.1) and Ca (Fig.2) for three age group (up to 15, 16-30 and above 30 years). We took into consideration our data in hair for Katowice inhabitants and for human blood in this region from Jakubowski (1991)[vii]. We obtained R Spermana, R=0.53 for p=0.09 (n=11). Measurement of blood lead and human hair lead was carried out simultaneously (in the same area) by Kasznia - Kocot et al. 1996)[viii], Zejda (1997)[ix], Chłopicka (1998)[x], Sp▯văčková (1997)[xi], Teresa (1997)[xii], Schuhmacher (1996)[xiii], Krause (1992)[xiv], Iyengar (1991)xv, Katz (1992)[xvi], Caroli (1994)[xvii], Jakubowski (1991), Nowak and Chmielnicka (in press)[v]

In the literature there is no data on the relationship between essential (Ca, Fe) and toxic metals (Pb) in adults' hair. The results indicate that hair of people living in differently polluted areas contains essentially different concentrations of essential metals (Fe, Ca) ($p<0.05$). For each investigated age group we observed lower Ca and Fe in the hair Fig.1, Fig.2 from people living in KATOWICE area compared with people living in BESKID area. We received from inhabitants of KATOWICE District higher lead hair than from people living in BESKID area ($p<0.05$)[v].

We conclude that not only blood, but also hair lead is good marker of environmental exposure. Hair lead similar as blood lead influenced to essential metals (Ca and Fe).

Fig.1.Categorized plot for variable Ca in human hair [μg/g]

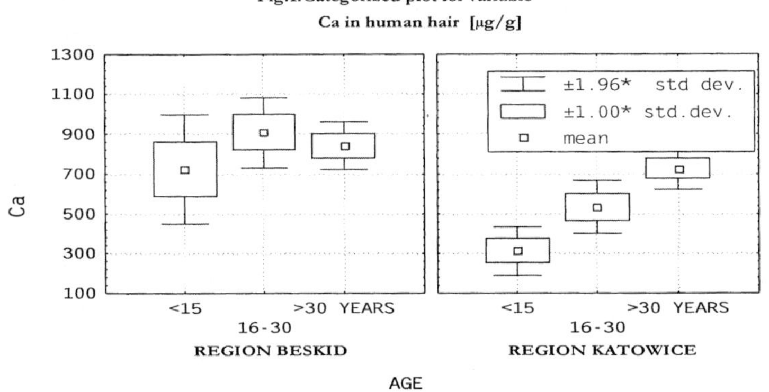

FIG.2. Categorized plot for variable Fe in human hair [μg/g]

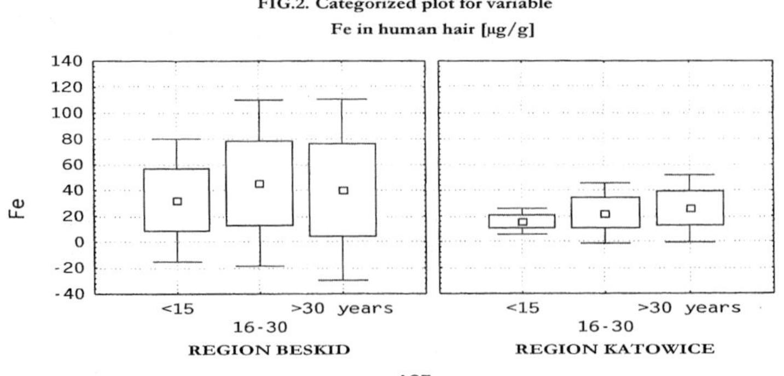

Acknowledgements

This paper was supported by grants KBN Silesian Medical School.

1 Wright.RO, Shannon .MW, Wright.RJ, Hu.H. Association between iron deficiency and low-level lead poisoning in an urban primary care clinic. Am. J. Public.Health,1999: 89(7):1049-53.
2. Goyer R.A, C.D. Klaassen, M.P. Wallkes , Metal Toxicology, Academic Press, Inc. 1995: 32-53.
3 Goyer, RA., Toxic and essential metal interactions, Annu, Rev, Nutr. 1997: 17: 37-50.
4 Cabeza J.M, Lead and zinc protoporfiryn in the blood of the child population in Austurias, Spain, Sci. Total Environ. 1991: 107: 91-98.
5 Nowak B, Chmielnicka J, Relationship of Lead and Cadmium on Essential Elements in Hair, Teeth and Nails of Men Exposed Environmentally", Ecotoxicol. Environ. Safety, 2000:i n press.
6 Nowak B., Koz?owski H., Heavy metals in hair and teeth: The correlation with metal concentration in the environment, Biol. Trace Elem. Res., 1998: 62: 213-228.
7 Jakubowski M., Ra?niewska G., Trzcinka-Ochocka M., Trojanowska B. St??enie kadmu i o?owiu we krwi oraz kadmu w moczu mieszka?ców trzech regionów Polski, Arch. Ochr. ?rodow.,1991: 3-4: 165-176
8 Kasznia -Kocot J., Zachwieja Z., Ch?opicka J., Kro?niak M., Zawarto?? wybranych mikroelementów i metali ci??kich we w?osach dzieci z Chorzowa, Pediatria Polska,1996: LXXI:1: 31-36
9 Zejda J.E., Grabecki J., Król B., Panasiuk Z., J?drzejczak A., Jarkowski M., Blood lead levels in urban children of Katowice voivodship, Poland: Results of the population -based biomonitoring and surveillance program, Eur. J. Publ. Hlth., 1997: 5: 2: 60-64
10 Ch?opickaJ. Z. Zachwieja, P. Zagrodzki, J.Frydrych, P.S?ota. M. Kro?niak., Lead and Cadmium in the hair and blood of children a highly industrial area in Poland, Biol. Trace Elem.Res. 1998: 62: 229-234
11 Spev??ková V., Kratzer K., Cejchanová M., Benes B., Determination of some metals in biological samples for monitoring purposes., Centr. Eur. J. Publ. Health, 1997: 5: 4: 177-179.
12 Teresa M., Vasconcelos S.D., Taveres Helena M.F.,) Trace element concentrations in blood and hair of young apprentices of a technical-professional school. Sci. Total Environ.1997: 205: 189-199.
13 Schuhmacher, M., Bells.M. Rico. A., Domingo, J.L., Corbella, J, Impact of reduction of lead in gasoline on the blood and hair lead levels in the population of Tarragona Province, Spain, 1990-1995, Sci. Total Environ.1996: 184: 203-209.
14 Krause C., Chutsch, Henke M., Leiske M., Schultz C., Schwarz E., Seifert B., Heavy metals in the Blood, urine and hair of a representative population sample in the Federal Republic of Germany 1985/86, Environmental Hygiene III, N.H. Seemayer W. Hadnagy (Eds.),1992: 159-162.
15 Iyengar G.V, Milestones in biological trace element Research, Sci. Total Environ.1991: 100: 1-15.
16 Katz S.A, Katz B.R., , Use hair analysis for evaluating mercury intoxication of the human body: a review, J. of Appiled Toxicol.,1992:.12 (2): 79-84
17Caroli S., Alimonti A., Coni E., Petrucci F., Senofonte O., Violante N., The assessment of reference values for elements in human biological tissues and fluids: A systematic review. Critical Rev. In Anal. Chem.,1994: 24(5&6): 363-398

Metal Ions in Biology and Medicine; vol 6. Eds. J.A. Centeno, Ph. Collery, G. Vernet, R.B. Finkelman, H. Gibb, J.C. Etienne. John Libbey Eurotext, Paris © 2000, pp. 328-330.

Comparison of blood lead levels in urban and rural Puerto Rican children

Ana B. Henríquez-Alberdeston[1, 2], René R. Dávila[3], Jose F. Rodriguez[4], Braulio Jiménez[1, 4], Carlos J. Rodríguez-Sierra[1, 2]

[1] *Center for Environmental and Toxicological Research,* [2] *Department of Environmental Health and* [3] *Department of Human Development-School of Public Health,* [4] *Department of Biochemistry-School of Medicine, Medical Sciences Campus, University of Puerto Rico*

Introduction

Blood lead levels have been steadily decreasing in the human population due mainly to the elimination of leaded-gasoline [1,2]. However, levels of lead in the environment are still high as to cause long term health effects in children (the population most at risk) [1]. Minority children from lower-income families, living in large metropolitan areas, or living in older housing are at high risk of lead poisoning [3, 4]. The United States Center for Disease Control and Prevention (CDC) has established that blood lead levels ≥ 10 μg/dL must result in intervention by the pertinent health institutions to identify the sources of contamination and reduce the risk to exposed children [1]. Puerto Rico has a large low-income Hispanic minority children population living in urban areas, where the prevalence of lead is uncertain due to the scarcity of data. The objective of this study was to compare blood lead levels in low-income children living in urban and rural Puerto Rico.

Methods

A total of 305 children among ages 1 to 7 years old participated in this study. These children attended a rural (n=153) and an urban (n=152) public health clinic. Parents agreed for their children to participate in the study and signed a consent form. Most of these children were Medicaid recipients of low socioeconomic status, putting then at greater risk for lead exposure than the general population. Lead blood levels were determined by graphite furnace atomic absorption spectrometry following CDC protocols [1]. CDC lead reference standards of bovine blood samples and laboratory bench spikes were analyzed along with children's blood samples. The analytical method has a limit of detection of 1.0 μg/L; linearity of 2.5-20 μg/L with a coefficient of variation between 2.4-4.1%. The general socio-demographic information from participants was obtained through a questionnaire and analyzed to determine if a correlation existed between lifestyle, health/nutrition, and socioeconomic level with children's blood lead levels (TableI). Descriptive statistics were calculated, and chi-square was performed to establish a relationship between children's lead blood levels and socio-demographic variables such as nutritional evaluation, specific habits, etc. The t-student test was used to measure differences in the average blood lead levels between urban and rural participants.

Results and Discussion

Blood lead levels were on average well below the threshold value recommended by CDC of 10μg/dL. The arithmetic mean and standard errors of whole blood lead levels were 3.15 ± 0.14 μg/dL and 2.78 ± 0.11 μg/dL for children attending the urban and rural health clinics, respectively. Observed differences in blood lead levels between children attending these two clinics was statistically significant ($p<0.05$). Children from the urban health clinic had blood lead levels ranging from 0.69 μg/dL to 13.50 μg/dL, while in children from the rural health clinic blood lead concentrations varied from 0.09 μg/dL to 10.70 μg/dL. Elevated blood lead levels (>10μg/dL) were only detected for two children (13.50 and 10.70μg/dL) attending the urban and rural health clinics, respectively. Higher levels of blood lead in urban children in comparison to rural children were associated with age of 3 years old, headaches, teeth discoloration and chewing toys frequently (Table I). It is doubtful that differences in teeth discoloration and headaches between the two children populations were due to lead exposure because these symptoms are commonly associated with blood lead levels >10μg/dL [1,2]. Children's toys could be a potential source of lead exposure, since the paint used to cover some toys could have significant levels of lead [5]. Although information on age was missing for 4 children of the urban clinic, 3 years old children seemed to contribute to the statistical difference observed between urban and rural children. A disadvantage of the study was that children were not sampled randomly. Therefore, the children in the study may not be representative of the Puerto Rican children population. In conclusion, these results show that Puerto Rican urban and rural children from low-income families that utilized these two public health clinics are not at high risk for lead poisoning.

Bibliography

1. Center for Disease Control and Prevention. *Preventing Lead Poisoning in Young Children. A Statement by the Centers for Disease Control,* 1991. Atlanta, Ga; US Dept of Health and Human Services, Public Health Service; 1991.
2. Veerula GR, Noah PK. Clinical manifestations of childhood lead poisoning. *J Tropic Med Hyg*. 1990; 93: 170-177.
3. Agency for Toxic Substances and Disease Registry. Toxicological profile for lead. Atlanta, Ga; US Dept of Health ad Human Services, Public Health Service; 1993.

4. Sargent JD, Brown MJ, Freeman JL, Bailey A, Goodman D, Freeman DH. Childhood lead poisoning in Massachussetts communities: its association with sociodemographic and housing characteristics. *Am J Public Health.* 1995;85:528-534.
5. Romieu I, Palazuelos E, Hernandez Avila M, Rios C, Munoz I, Jimenez C, Cahero G. Sources of lead in Mexico City. *Environ Health Perspect.* 1994;102:384-389.

Table I. Selected sociodemographic characteristics.

Characteristics	Arithmetic mean ± SE (μg/dL)		
	Rural clinic	Urban clinic	
Age (years)			P
1	2.76±0.33 (n=23)	3.14±0.23 (n=37)	0.36
2	3.10±0.39 (n=32)	3.07±0.20 (n=35)	0.94
3[a]	**2.42±0.19 (n=23)**	**3.21±0.25 (n=29)**	**0.02**
4	3.33±0.32 (n=31)	3.07±0.29 (n=23)	0.54
5	3.29±0.38 (n=26)	2.93±0.28 (n=13)	0.46
6	2.81±0.33 (n=11)	3.27±0.38 (n=9)	0.38
7	3.21±0.62 (n=7)	2.65±0.15 (n=2)	nd
Gender			
females	3.05 ± 0.26 (n= 69)	2.99±0.14 (n=65)	0.84
males	2.98±0.15 (n=84)	3.20±0.15 (n=83)	0.30
Habits			
hand-to-mouth activity	3.02±0.16 (n=103)	3.15±0.14 (n=92)	0.55
play w/ paint chips	3.16±0.32 (n=43)	3.12±0.17 (n=54)	0.92
chew toys frequently[b]	2.75±0.13 (n=74)	3.18±0.14 (n=78)	**0.02**
eat soil	2.88±0.15 (n=77)	2.91±0.16 (n=62)	0.89
Living			
near industrial site	2.83±0.29 (n=12)	3.49±0.36 (n=11)	0.17
near a high transit road	3.55±0.28 (n=56)	3.10±0.13 (n=79)	0.16
in a house > 40 y old	3.13±0.41(n=32)	3.07±0.22 (n=41)	0.91
Signs and Symptoms			
appetite loss	2.64±0.20 (n=36)	3.01±0.21(n=40)	0.20
constipation	3.07±0.30 (n=47)	3.15±0.22 (n=33)	0.84
stomach cramps	2.83±0.33 (n=31)	3.00±0.28 (n=25)	0.70
teeth discoloration[c]	2.52±0.28 (n=16)	3.41±0.38 (n=13)	**0.07**
irritability	2.79±0.24 (n=24)	3.43±0.29 (n=23)	0.10
frequent headaches[d]	2.34±0.30 (n=10)	3.22±0.35 (n=18)	**0.07**
learning problems	2.86±0.44 (n=14)	2.88±0.29 (n=10)	0.97
anemia	2.83±1.28 (n=18)	2.73±0.65 (n=17)	0.78

nd, is not determined; a and b are significant at $p<0.05$; c, and d are significant at $p<0.10$

Acknowledgments. Thanks to Lourdes Pérez for analysis by AAS, RCMI-G12RR03051, and CIDIC-MSC-UPR for financial support.

Metal Ions in Biology and Medicine; vol 6. Eds. J.A. Centeno, Ph. Collery, G. Vernet, R.B. Finkelman, H. Gibb, J.C. Etienne. John Libbey Eurotext, Paris © 2000, pp. 331-333.

Use of XAS for the elucidation of metal structure and function in biological molecules: applications to nickel biochemistry

Maroney M.J.

University of Massachusetts, Amnerst MA, USA

Nickel is a metal noted for both its deleterious effects on biological systems (*e.g.*, human carcinogenesis) and its essentiality to many organisms. The essentiality of Ni in bacteria, fungi, plants and invertebrates has long been recognized. Given the multiple functions for Ni now known in these organisms[*1,2*] and the response to low dietary intake of Ni, it has been strongly suggested that Ni has an essential function in higher animals, including humans.

Although no human Ni metalloenzymes are known, the impact of Ni biochemistry on humans is significant. These roles include infection by *Helicobacter pylori,* which has been associated with gastric ulcers and even with stomach cancer. This organism uses the ammonia produced by urease to modify the local pH, which allows the organism to survive in the stomach. Bacterial ureases also contribute to kidney and bladder stone formation and to pyelonephritis. The release of Ni to serum in response to myocardial infarction, unstable angina pectoris, cerebral stroke, and thermal burns[*3*]

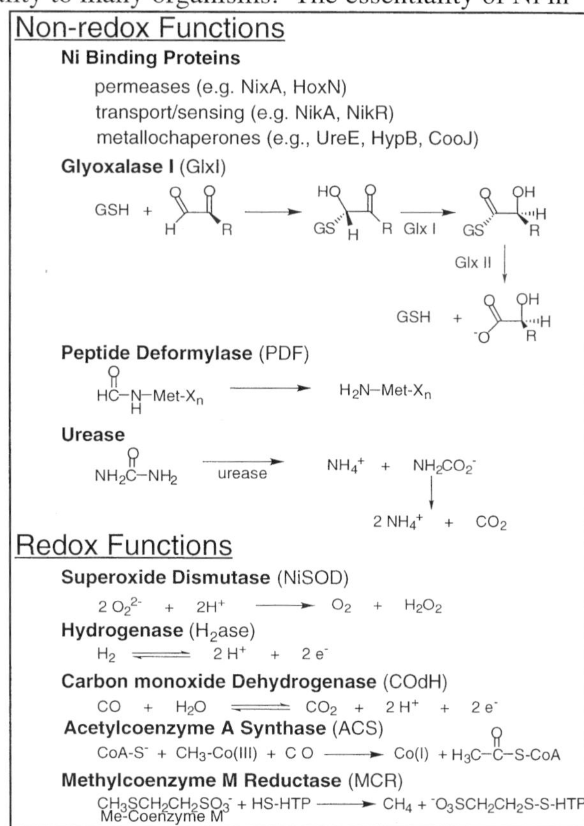

Figure 1. The biological roles of Ni enzymes and proteins.

suggest other possible roles for Ni in human metabolism yet to be discovered.

Specific biological roles for Ni were not known until the discovery that jackbean urease was a Ni enzyme (*ca.* 1975). Nickel is now associated with at least seven enzymatically catalyzed reactions, some of which are non-redox processes like hydrolysis and isomerization, and some of which are redox reactions (**Figure 1**)[*1,2*]. The role of Ni, a metal not noted for facile redox processes, in catalyzing biological redox reactions is poorly understood. Significant insight into the function of Ni in these enzymes can be obtained from the study of the structure of the Ni active sites and how the structure changes under catalytic conditions or when inhibitors are used. To do this, we have employed the analysis of x-ray absorption spectra, which offers the advantage that crystals are not required. Thus, one can obtain structural information regarding an active site metal from any state of an enzyme that can be freeze-trapped. Several trends in nickel metallobiochemistry emerge from the available crystal structures and XAS studies, including the presence of thiolate ligation of Ni in redox proteins, and polynuclear active sites.

One well-studied example of a Ni redox enzyme is hydrogenase (H_2ase). Structural data on a crystal containing a mixture of oxidized states of *Desulfovibrio gigas* H_2ase[*4*] show that the active site is composed of a Ni center ligated by four cysteine residues, two of which bridge to an Fe center (Ni – Fe = 2.9 Å) ligated by CN^- and CO ligands. A third bridge is formed by an O-donor ligand, which based on the Ni-O distance determined by XAS analysis (1.91(2) Å) is likely to be a hydroxo ligand. Data is also available from a crystal structure of *Desulfomicrobium baculatum* H_2ase that was completely reduced under H_2.[*5*] This enzyme has one selenocysteine ligand to Ni, lacks the O-bridging group and features a shorter Ni-Fe distance (2.5 Å). We have examined the structure of eight states of the H_2ase from *Chromatium vinosum*. K-edge energy analysis shows that the reduction of the enzyme and the formal redox state of the Ni atom are not correlated. Instead, the formal redox state of the Ni center appears to oscillate between Ni(III) in all of the epr active states and Ni(II) in all of the epr silent states. The short Ni-O bond that is a feature of oxidized enzyme (Forms A and B) and the unready epr silent intermediate (SI_u) is lost upon conversion to SI_r. This result establishes that this structural change is a feature of the reductive activation of the enzyme. A shortening of the Ni-Fe distance from 2.85(2) Å to 2.5 – 2.6 Å is also a feature of the reductive activation of the enzyme, and also occurs at the SI level. Thus, the change in the Ni-Fe distance appears to be associated with the loss of the O-bridging ligand, rather than with the presence of a bridging hydride. The difference in the Ni-S distances between terminal and bridging thiolate ligands are not larger than about 0.2 Å in *C. vinosum* H_2ase. Last, it is clear from multiple scattering analysis that exogenous CO (an inhibitor of the enzyme) binds linearly to the Ni center in the NiFe active site.

XAS also supports a dithiolato-bridged dinuclear structure for the Ni active site in *Streptomyces seoulensis* superoxide dismutase (NiSOD).[*6*] The analysis is consistent with five-coordinate Ni sites with a ligand environment composed of three S–donor ligands and two O/N-donor ligands (one of which must be an N-donor from the observation of N-hyperfine in the epr spectrum) in the oxidized enzyme. Dithionite reduction of the enzyme results in a planar Ni structure missing one of the O/N-donor ligands. Reduction by reaction with peroxide or by exposure to ^{60}Co radiation give distinct structures. These structures correspond to active enzyme samples and suggest a mechanism that does not involve the resting oxidized state of the enzyme.

In contrast to redox enzymes, Ni sites involved in catalyzing non-redox processes, or proteins that are involved in the acquisition, transport, and storage of Ni or in the assembly of Ni active sites, generally do not involve thiolate ligation. Recent examples include *E. coli* glyoxalase I, GlxI, the first example of an isomerase that is maximally activated by Ni.[*7*] *E. coli* GlxI is shown to bind two Ni atoms, although maximal activity has been observed with only one Ni^{2+} ion bound. In contrast with GlxI enzymes from other sources that are Zn enzymes, *E. coli* GlxI is not active with Zn bound. The structure of the Ni site is consistent with a $Ni(Glu)_2(His)_2$ site in the enzyme with the addition of two other O/N-donor ligands to form a six-coordinate active Ni site. The Zn-substituted enzyme has a spectrum consistent with a five-coordinate $Zn(Glu)_2(His)_2$ site with one additional O/N-donor ligand. These structures are compared with crystallographic data on the human GlxI, which contains Zn as the activating metal. The structures are consistent with the replacement of an active site Gln ligand in the human enzyme by a histidine in the *E. coli* GlxI.

NikR is a recently discovered Ni binding protein whose function is to repress the transcription of the periplasmic Ni transport system encoded by *nikA - E* in *E. coli* under high Ni concentrations (250 μM +).[*8*] The NikA-E proteins constitute an ATP-dependent Ni-specific transport system. Therefore, *nik* mutants that are defective in Ni transport are unable to synthesize any of the NiFe H_2ases found in *E. coli.* NikR belongs to the ribbon-helix-helix (β–α–α) family of DNA-binding transcription factors.[*9*] This structural motif is found in the N-terminal domain of *E. coli* NikR. The C-terminal region is associated with Ni-binding. Homologues of NikR have been identified in several other bacterial and archaeal genomes, implicating it in a general mechanism for Ni regulated DNA transcription. XAS results from NikR confirm the O/N ligand environment of the Ni center.

---

(1) Maroney, M. J.; Davidson, G.; Allan, C. B.; Figlar, J. The structure and function of nickel sites in metalloproteins.*Struct. Bonding* 1998; 92: 1-65.

(2) Maroney, M. J. Structure/function relationships in nickel metallobiochemistry.*Curr. Opin. Chem. Biol.* 1999; 3: 188-199.

(3) Leach, C. N.; Linden, J. V.; Hopfer, S. M.; Crisostomo, M. C.; Sunderman, F. W. Nickel concentrations in serum of patients with acute myocardial infarction or unstable angina pectoris.*Clinical Chemistry* 1985; 31: 556-560.

(4) Volbeda, A.; Garcin, E.; Piras, C.; de Lacey, A. L.; Fernandez, V. M.; Hatchikian, E. C.; Frey, M.; Fontecilla-Camps, J. C. Structure of the [NiFe] hydrogenase active site: Evidence for biologically uncommon Fe ligands.*J. Am. Chem. Soc.* 1996; 118: 12989-12996.

(5) Garcin, E.; Vernede, X.; Hatchikian, E. C.; Volbeda, A.; Frey, M.; Fontecilla-Camps, J. C. The crystal structure of a reduced [NiFeSe] hydrogenase provides an image of the activated catalytic center.*Structure* 1999; 7: 557-566.

(6) Choudhury, S. B.; Lee, J.-W.; Davidson, G.; Yim, Y.-I.; Bose, K.; Sharma, M. L.; Kang, S.-O.; Cabelli, D. E.; Maroney, M. J. Examination of the Nickel Site Structure and Reaction Mechanism in Streptomyces seoulensis Superoxide Dismutase.*Biochemistry* 1999; 38: 3744-3752.

(7) Clugston, S. L.; Barnard, J. F. J.; Kinach, R.; Miedema, D.; Ruman, R.; Daub, E.; Honek, J. F. Overproduction and Characterization of a Dimeric Non-Zinc Glyoxalase I from *Escherichia coli*: Evidence for Optimal Activation by Nickel Ions.*Biochemistry* 1998; 37: 8754-8763.

(8) De Pina, K.; Desjardin, V.; Mandrand-Berthelot, M. A.; Giordano, G.; Wu, L. F. Isolation and characterization of the nikR gene encoding a nickel-responsive regulator in Escherichia coli.*Journal of Bacteriology* 1999; 181: 670-674.

(9) Chivers, P. T.; Sauer, R. T. NikR is a ribbo-helix-helix DNA-binding protein.*Protein Science* 1999; in press.

Metal Ions in Biology and Medicine; vol 6. Eds. J.A. Centeno, Ph. Collery, G. Vernet, R.B. Finkelman, H. Gibb, J.C. Etienne. John Libbey Eurotext, Paris © 2000, pp. 334-338.

EPR spin labelling measurements of nuclear, chemical and biological agent-induced alterations of the insulin receptor in red blood cell membranes: a possible biomarker for dose assessment

Francesca C. Music, Jose A. Centeno, Ted L. Hadfield, Carmen M. Arroyo[1], Linda Steel-Goodwin[2], Richard E. Sweeney[3] and Alasdair J. Carmichael

Armed Forces Institute of Pathology, Washington, DC; [1] U.S. Army Medical Research Institute of Chemical Defense, Aberdeen Proving Ground, MD; [2] HQ USAF/SGXR Bolling AFB, DC; [3] RESECO, P.O. Box 2311, Upper Darby, PA

ABSTRACT

Background: Proliferation of radiological weapons, depleted uranium (DU) penetrators, and chemical warfare agents in the battlefield has increased the probability that military as well as civilian personnel will encounter local or widespread radiological and chemical hazards. The Department of Defense (DoD) must be able to identify and screen personnel who have been exposed to hazards, and determine the exposure rate of casualties. The need to develop biomarkers to detect radiation, vesicant or combined radiation/vesicant exposures that can be used in field scenarios is a high priority.
Technical Approach: Since 1991, the United States Army has increased the use of Electron Paramagnetic Resonance (EPR) technology in the study of defense mechanisms including drug interventions against chemical agents e.g. effects of sulfur mustard (HD) and the toxicological properties of DU [1-3]. Spin trapping has been used to evaluate antioxidant efficiency and properties of radioprotectors [4]. In addition, spin labeled protein techniques for studies of cell functionality have been performed to study the effects of radiation, mustards and high-energy explosives such as ammonium dinitramide [5]. We used EPR spin labeling to measure alterations induced by nuclear, chemical or biological (NBC) agents in the membrane-bound insulin receptor proteins of human red blood cells (RBCs). RBCs represent the majority of cells (3.8 - 5.8 million/mm^3) found in peripheral blood, and have multiple cell surface receptors and antigens. They are subject to many changes in structure and binding properties in different disease processes making them an ideal biological model for the effect of weapons of mass destruction (WMD). RBCs have receptors for insulin [6-7], therefore, the peptide hormone, insulin, was conjugated to the nitroxide reagent succinimidyl 2,2,5,5-tetramethyl-3-pyrroline-1-oxyl-3-carboxylate (TMPOC) to make the spin-labeled ligand for the insulin receptor. Cells from healthy human donors were exposed *in vitro* to gamma-radiation (^{60}Co, nuclear), sulfur mustard (HD, chemical) or a bacterial polysaccharide substance (biological). Experimental aliquots of the RBCs were exposed to various doses of the NBC agents and then allowed to react at a specific point-in-time after exposure with the spin-labeled insulin before measuring EPR spectra. All data points were normalized to the cell density of the experimental sample.
Results: The EPR dose response to gamma-radiation tended to increase between 0.5-Gy and 5.0-Gy, and then reversed to a decreasing trend at 10-Gy and 20-Gy. A steady decline in the relative EPR response across the range of HD concentrations tested was observed. Measurements were taken 24-48 hours post-exposure to HD. Furthermore, we applied these procedures to biological agents, in particular, biological toxin, however, they are not part of this work. A general observation could be made in that exposure for two hours to the bacterial polysaccharide yielded a completely random EPR response to the concentrations tested and no clear trend could be ascertained.
Summary: The EPR/spin labeling analytical technique for measuring alterations in RBC insulin receptors could be a useful alternative for assessing exposure doses of WMD casualties. These results and the limitations of EPR/spin labeling will be discussed in the context of a possible biomarker for NBC exposure assessment.

INTRODUCTION

EPR/Spin Labeling is concerned with the spatial distribution of paramagnetic centers (e.g. free radicals) in heterogeneous samples. Stable nitroxide free radicals can be used as reporter groups. Nitroxides are sensitive to molecular motion, polarity, structural order, and fluidity [7]. Specific changes in the nitroxide EPR spectra can be used for analyzing these parameters. Nitroxide free radicals are extensively used in molecular and cellular biology for purposes such as spin labeling. Nitroxides are also used for spin labeling drugs, thus allowing detection of the labeled compound by means of EPR spectroscopy [1-8]. In the present study, we used EPR/Spin Labeling to measure alterations induced by Nuclear, Biological, or Chemical (NBC) agents in the membrane-bound insulin receptor proteins of human red blood cells (RBCs).

Most cells contain insulin or insulin-like receptors, and these receptors have been reported to be affected by various metabolic disorders [7]. Since the first interaction NBC agents have with cells is at the cell membrane, insulin was the peptide hormone of choice for the NBC studies. Insulin requires zinc ions (Zn^{++}) to be an active hormone. Zinc ions are essential in the quaternary structure of insulin in solution [6]. In the presence of two Zn^{++}, the solutions of insulin are homogeneous forming hexamers with a molecular weight of 36,000. In the absence of the two Zn^{++}, the solutions of insulin become inhomogeneous in molecular weight. The Zn^{++} may be replaced by other divalent first row transition metal ions. Many of these (Mn^{++}, Cu^{++}, VO^{++}) display room temperature EPR signals, which may also be used as EPR markers in conjunction with spin labeling. For instance, VO^{++} has been used successfully as a spin probe for several metalloproteins. Similar to the isotropic three lines EPR spectrum of nitroxide spin labels which are susceptible to motion, the eight lines isotropic EPR of VO^{++} is very susceptible to motion becoming anisotropic when immobilized. For these reasons, insulin is the primary candidate to study the alterations of receptors and cell surface changes by NBC agents leading to a biomarker for WMD.

MATERIALS AND METHODS

Chemicals:

Nitroxide reagent succinimidyl 2,2,5,5-tetramethyl-3-pyrroline-1-oxyl-3-carboxylate (TMPOC; S-520) was purchased from Molecular Probes, Inc., Eugene, OR, USA.
Molecular Formula: $C_{13}H_{17}N_2O_5$
Molecular Weight: 281.29

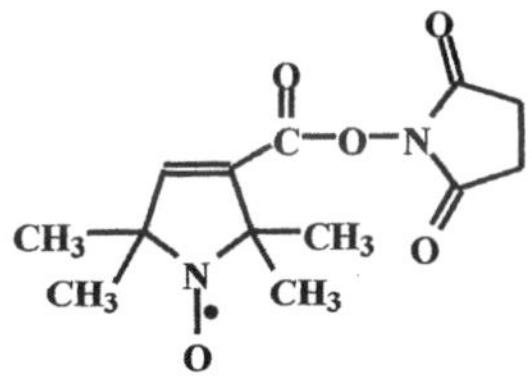

Scheme 1. Chemical formula of the spin label used in this study.

Insulin, zinc, porcine was obtained from CALBIOCHEM® Cat. No. 407693; CALBIOCHEM-NOVABIOCHEM CORP. La Jolla, CA, USA. The preparation of the spin-labeled ligand for the insulin receptor has a proprietary exclusive right to Dr. Alasdair J. Carmichael, Francesca C. Music, and Linda Steel-Goodwin.

PATENT: Application (June, 1998)

Title: "Spin Labeled Compounds as Magnetic Resonance Contrast Agents."

Inventors: Alasdair J. Carmichael, Francesca C. Music and Linda Steel-Goodwin.

The Armed Forces Radiobiology Research Institute's ^{60}Co-gamma facility was used for the radiation studies. The samples were ^{60}Co-gamma irradiated at a dose rate of one Gy/min. The HD exposures were performed in the US Army Medical Research Institute of Chemical Defense, Aberdeen Proving Ground. The HD concentration doses were 25 μM, 50 μM, 75 μM, 100 M, 150 μM, 200 μM, 250 μM, and 300 μM. Sulfur mustard (2,2'-dichlorodiethyl sulfide; HD) was acquired from the U. S. Army Edgewood Research, Development, and Engineering Center (Aberdeen Proving Ground, MD, USA). Bacterial polysaccharide was obtained from Sigma, St. Louis, MO, USA. The bacterial polysaccharide exposures were performed at the Armed Forces Institute of Pathology. All of the NBC exposures were conducted under surety programs for safety regulations established by each of the mentioned institutes.

Human Red Blood Cells:

Red blood cells were obtained from t the US Army, Walter Reed Army Medical Center, Department of Pathology. A sample from each donation had been tested by Food and Drug Administration-licensed kits and found negative for antibodies to human immunodeficiency virus and hepatitis C, and no reactive for hepatitis B surface antigen and all other FDA required tests. Tests for unexpected antibodies against red blood cell antigens were performed on samples from all donors. The results of these tests were negative.

EPR Instrumentation:

Three different Bruker, Inc. EPR units were used: two X-band (9.5 GHz) ESP 300 series: ESP 300 and ESP 300E with a TM rectangular standard resonance cavity with a 315-resonator mode, and the EMS 104 EPR analyzer. The EMS 104 is the world's first EPR analyzer that not only tunes and measures automatically, but also evaluates the spectrum and correlates the results with a calibration curve. Once the EMS 104 EPR instrument has been calibrated, measurement is a simple three-step procedure. The instrument setting for X-band measurements were central magnetic field: 347.7 mT; modulation frequency: 0.1-0.01 mT; microwave power: 39 mW; sweep time: 168 s; sweep width: 10.0 mT; time constant: 4 ms; receiver gain: 2×10^4 for the ESP 300. The ESM 104 lock-in detector was operated with a 50 kHz modulation variable from 1.6 μT to 1.6 mT.

Test procedures:

Control and exposed samples (1 mL volume RBCs) were spin-labeled by adding an excess of the spin-labeled insulin (A_{277}= 0.1370 – 0.1226; pH = 7.4) and rocked using a Speci-Mix from Barnstead/ Thermolyne, IA, USA. Following incubation and agitation for varying times, cells were centrifuged for approximately 30 minutes at 1000 rpm and the pellets were transferred to EPR quartz capillary sample tubes (i.d.= 1.0 mm; o.d.= 1.2 mm; 50 μL) Wilmad, NJ, USA. All EPR spectra were recorded within 1 minute of deposition in EPR quartz capillary tubes. The intensity of EPR spectra depends on the success of the labeling, amounts of material introduced in the EPR capillary tube and is specific to the RBC donor. Analysis of EPR spectra was performed by a well-established double integration procedure (Bruker, Inc. integration program). This analysis allows the evaluation of the dipolar broadening, $ÄH_D$, through spectral computation, which allows one to calculate the mean distance among the spin-label probe at the receptor surface of the cells. This parameter is the most relevant measurement to characterize the differences between labeled cells in the presence and absence of NBC perturbation, and for different times of incubation in RBCs. For statistical evaluation, the Student's T test was applied, group 1 vs. group 2 (n= 6-9); significance is $p < 0.05$.

RESULTS

Typical representations of the observed changes of the EPR spectra of the succinimidyl nitroxide labeled (TMPOC) of human RBCs in the control donor and exposed to 50 μM of sulfur mustard are illustrated in Figure 1 (*Panel A*).

A) Electron Paramagnetic Resonance (EPR) spectra of succinimidyl nitroxide (TMPOC) labeled insulin

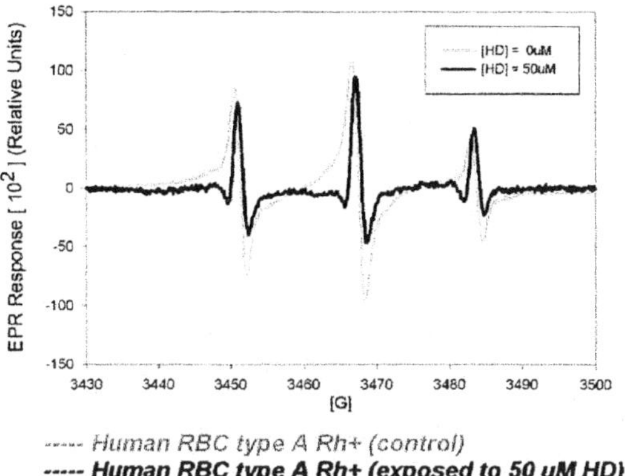

B) RBCs radiation dose response (within 24 hours after radiation)

C) Human RBC type O Rh⁺ (48 hours post-exposure)

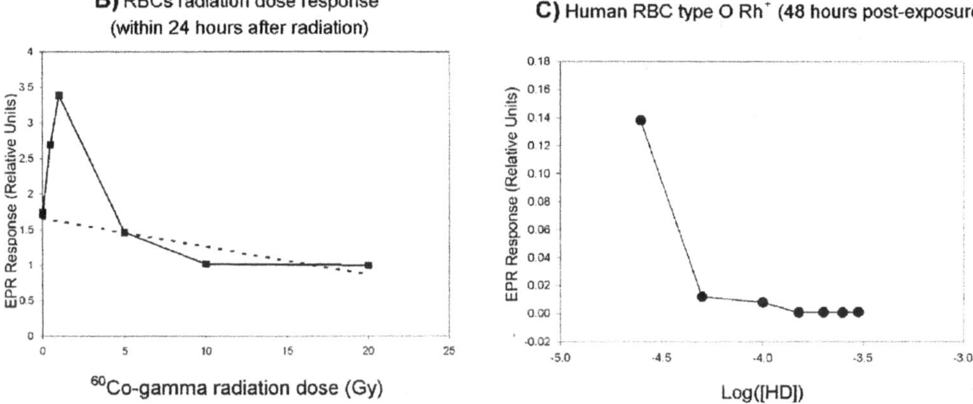

Figure 1. Panel A represents typical Electron Paramagnetic Resonance (EPR) spectra of succinimidyl nitroxide labeled (TMPOC). Panel B represents EPR response (relative units) among the spin-labeled insulin RBCs as a function of ^{60}Co-gamma dose-radiation the EPR response immediately after gamma exposure. Dose responses to ^{60}Co-gamma-radiation for five different donors tested twenty days after exposure are shown. Panel C illustrates representative data of the EPR response (relative units) among the spin-labeled insulin RBCs as a function of the range of HD concentrations tested.

For ^{60}Co-gamma radiation as illustrated in *Panel B* (measured immediately after radiation), the observed tendency for this particular donor is an increase in RBC insulin receptor affinity. This is measured by an increase in the intensity of the EPR for the bound nitroxide-labeled insulin. The increase occurs in the 0 to 5 Gy range and then decreases at higher radiation doses. The RBCs from the five different donors analyzed separately showed this tendency to some degree (data not shown). However, when the results of the five donors are averaged they show a continuous decrease from 0 to 20 Gy. This tendency is also shown in the dotted trend line in *Panel B*, which has a similar profile as the results obtained for the average of the five donors. The tendency of the insulin receptor affinity to initially increase for the five donors becomes more evident when measured 20 days after exposure to

^{60}Co-gamma radiation (data not shown). These results suggest that the insulin receptor becomes activated at low doses of radiation and thus has a higher affinity for the spin labeled insulin. The reverse is shown at higher radiation doses.

Panel C of Figure 1 shows a steady decline in the relative EPR response across the range of HD concentrations tested. Measurements were also taken 24-48 hours post-exposure to HD (data not shown). Exposure for 2 hours to the bacterial polysaccharide yielded a completely random EPR response to the concentrations tested and no clear trend could be ascertained.

DISCUSSION

TMPOC-insulin is a chemically non-reactive nitroxide. This spin probe can be used for analysis of membrane receptor fluidity and polarity, by analyzing line height ratios, dipolar broadening and hyperfine splitting constants [7]. The spin label TMPOC-insulin binds covalently to insulin receptors in the RBCs and allows measurement of the receptors/ RBCs mobility and polarity. Red blood cells comprise the majority of cells (3.8-5.8 million/mm^3) found in peripheral blood. These cells have many cell surface receptors and antigens. They are also subject to various changes in shape, binding properties and structure in different disease processes making them an ideal biological model for the effect of NBC interactions.

Our results clearly demonstrated that spin labeled-insulin penetrates into RBC insulin receptors. A major disadvantage of the labeling technique is that the nitroxide moiety changes the physicochemical properties of the labeled compounds [1]. In addition, the EPR spectra's parameters depend on the success of the labeling, amounts of material introduced in the EPR capillary tube, and are specific to the RBC donor. Further work is required to confirm these data on a dose-response basis and extend the proposed method to highly toxic agents and other cell lines. In this respect, the method appears promising for systematic investigation of cell response to a large variety of xenobiotics. The sensitivity of the spin label to the presence of free radicals allows detection of the initial steps yielding receptor activation or receptor damage.

ACKNOWLEDGMENT

We are grateful to Mr. David W. Kahler and Mr. Robert J. Schafer for providing assistance in EPR analysis and cell preparation.

REFERENCES

1. Arroyo CM. "Spin Trapping and Spin Labeling Studied Using EPR Spectroscopy". In: Magnetic Resonance Methods & Instrumentation, Encyclopedia of Spectroscopy & Spectrometry; Edited by John Lindon, George Tranter, and John Holmes, pp 1-9, 1999, Academic Press Ltd, London, UK, 1999: pp 1-9.
2. Gray B, Carmichael AJ. Kinetics of Superoxide Scavenging by Dismutase Enzymes and Manganese Mimics Determined by Electron Spin Resonance. Biochemical Journal 1992; 281: 795-802.
3. Hamilton MM, Ejnik JW, Carmichael AJ. Uranium reactions with hydrogen peroxide studied by EPR/spin trapping. Journal of the Chemical Society, Perkin Transactions 1997; 2: 2491-2492 1997.
4. Steel-Goodwin L, Carmichael AJ. Nitric Oxide and Smooth Muscle Relaxation in the Intestine. Chemical and Radiation Effects Measured by EPR/Spin Trapping. Radiation and the Gastrointestinal Tract (A. Dubois, G.L. King, and D.R. Livengood, Eds.). CRC Press 1994.
5. Steel-Goodwin L, Kuhlman KH, Miller C, Pace MD, Carmichael AJ. Effects of Reactive Oxygen and Nitrogen Species Induced by Ammonium Dinitramide Decomposition in Aqueous Solutions of DNA. Annals of Clinical and Laboratory Science 1997; 27: 236-245 1997.
6. MacDonald RS, Steel-Goodwin L, Smith RJ. Influence of dietary fiber on insulin receptors in rat intestinalmucosa. Ann Nutr Metab. 1991; 35(6): 328-38.
7. Faulkner-O'Brien LA, Beth AH, Papayannopoulos IA, Anjaneyulu PS, Staros JV. Preparation and Characterization of Spin-Labeled Derivatives of Epidermal Growth Factor (EGF) for Investigations of the Interactions of EGF with Its Receptor by Electron Paramagnetic Resonance Spectroscopy. Biochemistry. 1991; 30(37): 8976-85.
8. Sackmann E, Träuble T. Studies of the crystalline-liquid crystalline phase transition of lipid model membranes. I: Use of spin labels and optical probes as indicators of the phase transition. II: Analysis of electron spin resonance spectra of steroid labels incorporated into lipid membranes. III: Structure of a steroid-lecithin system above and below the lipid phase transition. J. Am. Chem. Soc. 1972; 94: 4482-99.

Metal Ions in Biology and Medicine; vol 6. Eds. J.A. Centeno, Ph. Collery, G. Vernet, R.B. Finkelman, H. Gibb, J.C. Etienne. John Libbey Eurotext, Paris © 2000, pp. 339-341.

Micro-pixe analysis of the testes and sperm of $CrCl_3$-treated mice

Graham Bench[1], Patrick Grant[1], Lucy M. Anderson[2], and Kazimierz S. Kasprzak[2]

[1] Lawrence Livermore National Laboratory, Livermore, CA 94550; [2] National Cancer Institute, FCRDC, Frederick, MD 21702

In order to unveil the mechanisms of transgenerational carcinogenesis following exposure of mice to $CrCl_3$ (Yu, W. *et al.*, *Toxicol. Appl. Pharmacol.* 1999; **158**: 161), chromium levels were followed in sperm and testes after intraperitoneal injection of 1 mmol $CrCl_3 \cdot 6H_2O$ (52 mg Cr)/kg body wt. to Swiss male mice. Animals were sacrificed 1, 3, 7, and 14 days after treatment. The reproductive organs were rapidly frozen in liquid nitrogen. Ten µm thick sections of testes and epididymides were prepared and freeze-dried. Sperm were teased from other epididymides after thawing, mounted on thin nylon membranes and subsequently freeze-dried. Individual sperm and 10 µm sections of testes and epididymides were analysed by Proton Induced X-ray Emission (microbeam PIXE; see below). Analysis of individual sperm from Cr-dosed animals revealed no sperm containing detectable levels of Cr (< 10 µg/g dry wt.) at any time point. Analysis of testicular sections from Cr-dosed animals revealed that Cr contents in regions containing seminiferous tubules were ~ 2 µg/g dry wt. in animals sacrificed at 3, 7, and 14 days with no significant differences in Cr concentration for the three sacrifice times. However, scans of regions containing the testicular envelope revealed Cr contents of up to 10 mg/g dry wt. Likewise, analysis of epididymal sections revealed that in the Cr-dosed animals the epididymal envelope had Cr contents of up to 70 mg/g dry wt., while regions in the center of the epididymides contained no detectable levels of Cr (< 2 µg/g dry wt.). Cr was not detected in any portion of testicular and epididymal sections from control animals. The trace amounts of Cr found in the seminiferous tubule regions may indicate a possibility of damaging effects of the metal on spermatogenesis. The highly concentrated extracellular Cr in connective tissue could be a source of diffusible reactive oxygen species that also could damage the sperm. Alternatively, the results may point to an indirect mechanism of transgenerational carcinogenesis by Cr.

Proton Induced X-ray Emission (Microbeam PIXE)

Microbeam PIXE is an x-ray fluorescence technique that typically uses 3 MeV energy proton beams focused to ~ 1 µm beam spot diameters to test microscopic specimens. It provides accurate quantification, simultaneous multi-element detection whilst maintaining down to part per million (by weight) or µg/g elemental sensitivity. The use of one method to quantify and localize numerous metals is particularly advantageous when comparing two or more processes related to metal concentrations. Moreover, the penetration depth of 3 MeV protons (~100 μm in biological material) allow microbeam PIXE to measure the total elemental contents within a cell or tissue section.

Incident protons interact primarily with atomic electrons in the specimen creating vacancies in inner shell orbitals. When a vacancy is filled by an outer shell electron, the excess energy resulting from the transition can be released as an x-ray photon whose energy is characteristic of the emitting atom. As the beam is scanned across the sample, x-ray energy spectra are stored for each beam location. Maps of element concentrations are generated from these data and x-ray spectra from locations corresponding to any region of interest can be extracted for quantitative analysis [1].

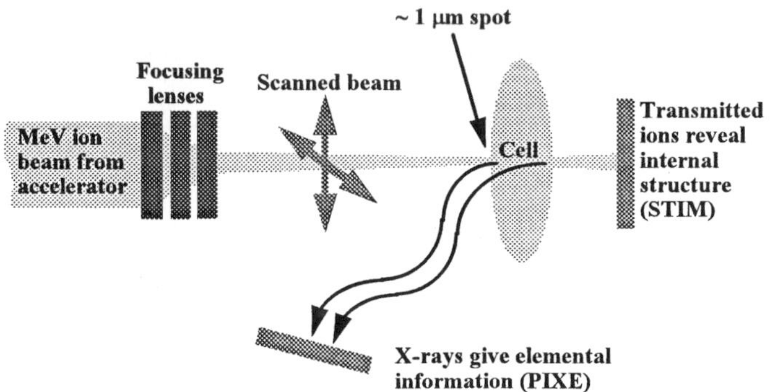

Figure 1: Schematic Outline of Nuclear Microprobe analysis.

Microbeam PIXE causes minimal alteration to the sample [2]. The MeV ion energies cause negligible sputtering of material from the specimen surface and very low radiation damage. The use of $\leq$ nA beam currents and a scanned beam minimizes thermal damage to the specimen. The Livermore nuclear microprobe system and spectrum analysis code [3] have been tested on a range of certified standards and have a quantitative accuracy of better than 95% for biological samples [3].

Scanning Transmission Ion Microscopy (STIM) [4], is also performed to complement microbeam PIXE data. With STIM the residual energy of protons after passing through the specimen is measured by detectors located behind the sample. Ion energy losses can be readily converted into specimen projected densities in order to obtain quantitative PIXE elemental concentrations [4].

Nuclear microscopy is one of a variety of particle and x-ray microprobe techniques that have been used for elemental localization studies in biological tissues that include electron probe x-ray analysis, x-ray induced x-ray fluorescence and secondary ion mass spectrometry. Each of these techniques has certain advantages and limitations when compared to the other methods. However, in general, only microbeam PIXE has the ability to make several quantitative measurements simultaneously at μg/g range sensitivity and micron scale spatial resolution while minimally affecting the specimen.

Sample preparation

Samples for PIXE analysis were prepared using previously described methods [5,6] to preserve elemental distributions as close as possible to those found "in-vivo". Frozen epididymides and testes were cryo-sectioned at -20^{0}C using stainless steel blades in a

Leica CM cryo-microtome to obtain 10 μm thick frozen hydrated sections that were mounted onto pre-cooled transparent nylon membranes stretched over a 15 mm diameter hole in a plastic support frame. The frozen hydrated sections were subsequently lyophilized under a vacuum of < 10^{-3} Torr for six hours. Once lyophilized all samples were stored in a clean, ultra-dry environment prior to PIXE analysis.

Sperm were isolated from selected epididymides by teasing apart each epididymis in 2 ml, 0.15 M ammonium acetate (Ameresco, OH), pH 7.4, aspirating the suspension to release the sperm and filtering it through a fine silk filter [6]. The suspension was centrifuged at 5,000 X g for 3 minutes. The sperm pellets were washed twice in 2 ml ammonium acetate, pH 7.4 and once in 2 ml water. Portions (1 to 2 μl) of the final aliquots containing sperm heads were mounted on nylon foils and freeze dried for PIXE analysis as previously described [6]. Optical studies revealed that the material deposited on the nylon foils was mainly comprised (> 95 %) of sperm heads.

Quantitative elemental imaging

Figure 2 illustrates the capability of PIXE to image elemental distributions and shows elemental maps obtained from an epididymal tissue section of a Cr dosed animal sacrificed 7 days after dosing. The color scale in each elemental map ranges from black through dark green to light green to white. The Cr content in the epididymal envelope is 7.0 ± 0.4 wt %. Cr is not present in the interior regions of the epididymal section above limits of detection.

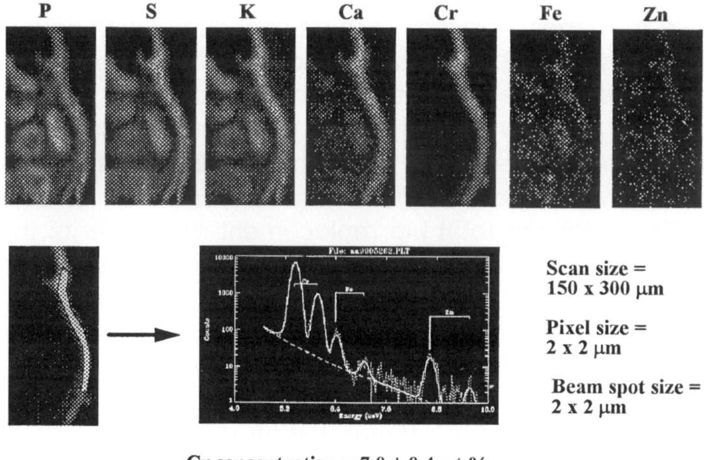

Figure 2: Elemental spatial maps in an epididymis from a Cr dosed animal

References

1. Antolak AJ, Bench GS, Morse DH. *Nucl Instr Meth* 1994; B85: 597.
2. Maenhaut W. *Scanning Microscopy* 1990; 4: 43.
3. Antolak AJ, Bench GS. *Nucl Instr Meth* 1994; B90: 596.
4. Lefevre HW, Schofield RMS, Bench GS, Legge GJF. *Nucl Instr Meth* 1991; B54: 363.
5. Mauthe RJ, Sideras-Haddad E, Turteltaub KW, Bench G. *J Pharm Biomed Anal* 1998; (4-5): 651.
6. Bench G, Corzett MH, Martinelli R, Balhorn R. *Cytometry* 1999; 35: 30.

Metal Ions in Biology and Medicine; vol 6. Eds. J.A. Centeno, Ph. Collery, G. Vernet, R.B. Finkelman, H. Gibb, J.C. Etienne. John Libbey Eurotext, Paris © 2000, pp. 342-344.

Serum chromium concentration in patients with cobalt – chromium total hip replacement components

Anastasia K. Skipor, M.S., Joshua J. Jacobs, M.D., Leslie M. Patterson, R.N. Wayne P. Paprosky, M.D., and Jorge O. Galante, M.D.

Department of Orthopedic Surgery, Rush Arthritis and Orthopedics Institute, Rush Presbyterian St. Luke's Medical Center, 1653 West Congress Parkway, Chicago IL 60612

Background: The introduction of newer orthopedic prosthetic designs, such as extensive porous surface coatings and modularity, that are intended for use in younger and more active patients have resulted in the increased recognition that metal release from these devices may be associated with adverse local and remote tissue responses [1, 2, 3] as a result of the known toxicities of the metal elements that comprise these implants. We have previously demonstrated that serum chromium (Cr) and titanium (Ti) levels were elevated in patients with well functioning joint replacements up to 36 months following surgery [4]. **Aims:** The aim of this study was to determine the concentration of Cr in serum in individuals with Cr-containing total hip replacement components that had been in situ for up to 60 months. This is a prospective, longitudinal, controlled study. **Methods:** Four groups of patients were studied. Classification was assigned on the basis of the composition and mode of fixation of the femoral stem. **Group 1** consisted of 15 patients with the hybrid total hip replacement. The femoral implant consisted of a modular cobalt alloy (Co-Cr) stem with a Co-Cr head. The implant was fixed to the femoral shaft with cement. The acetabular component consisted of a commercially pure titanium (cp Ti) acetabular shell with a diffusion bonded cp Ti fiber metal porous surface intended for cementless fixation. The acetabular component was secured to the pelvis with a varying number of Ti -6 aluminum -4 vanadium alloy (Ti-alloy) self tapping screws. A snap-fit ultra high molecular weight polyethylene liner served as a bearing surface. There were eight males and seven females with a mean age at surgery of 67 years (range 54 - 77 years). **Group 2** consisted of 17 patients implanted with a cementless Co-Cr femoral component with an extensively porous coated surface and a Ti-alloy acetabular component, both of which were inserted without cement. The acetabular component consisted of a cementless Ti-alloy shell with a beaded commercially pure titanium porous coating. It was secured to the pelvis with either three spikes or two screws both made of Ti-alloy. There were nine males and eight females with a mean age at surgery of 60 years (range 39 - 82 years). **Group 3** consisted of 18 patients with a modular femoral implant comprised of a cementless Ti-alloy stem onto which a cp Ti fiber metal porous surface was diffusion bonded on the proximal aspect of the device and a Co-Cr head. The acetabular component was identical to that in group 1. There were ten males and eight females with a mean age at surgery of 54 years (range 38 - 67 years). **Group 4** consisted of 17 contemporaneous controls without implants or systemic disease. There were eight males and seven females with a mean age at time = 0 of 58 years (range 35- 73 years). For all 4 groups serum was collected at pre-operative (or t = 0 for the controls) and at 12, 36 and 60 months post-operative. Serum Cr analysis was performed using electrothermal atomization atomic absorption spectrophotometry as previously described [4]. **Results:** Figure 1 shows the serum chromium values for all 4 groups. To provide a relative scale, the data are reported as the mean of each group at each time interval. Concentrations below the detection limit were assigned, by convention, a value of one-half the detection limit. Non-parametric

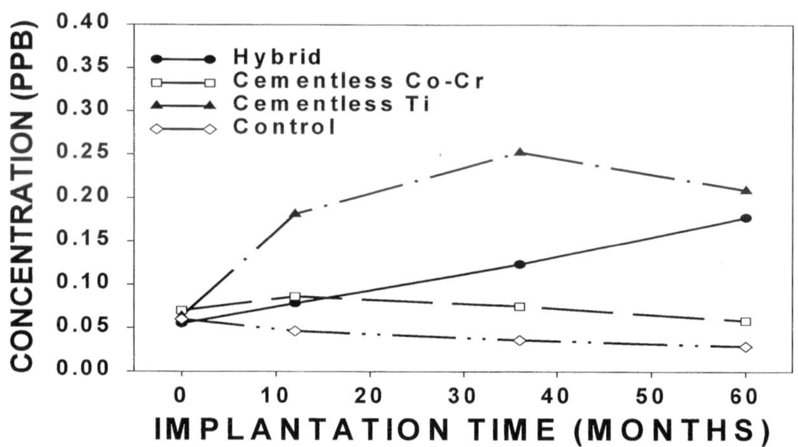

Figure 1: Serum chromium concentrations in ng/ml (ppb) as a function of time in the four groups studied.

statistical analyses were used for comparison due to the presence of left-censored data. Intergroup comparisons revealed that the 36 month serum Cr values were significantly elevated in all implant groups compared to controls ($p<0.006$) and the 60 month serum Cr values were significantly elevated in group 1 with respect to groups 2 and 4 ($p<0.001$) and in group 3 with respect to group 2 and 4 (p<0.000). Intragroup comparisons revealed that for group 1 concentrations at 60 months post-operative were significantly elevated compared to the pre-operative (p<0.007) and 12 month post-operative (p<0.035) values. For Group 2 the 36 month post-operative values were elevated compared to those of the 60 month post-operative (p<0.049) value and for group 3 the 12, 36 and 60 month post-operative values were statistically elevated compared to the pre-operative value (p<0.05). **Conclusions:** This study has shown significant elevations of Cr in serum in groups 1 and 3 at 60 months post-operatively in patients with well functioning total hip replacements. In addition, the finding that at 36 months post-operatively all three implant groups were elevated compared to controls as previously reported [4], is still valid in this study with slightly higher patient populations. We originally had hypothesized that patients with implants with extensively porous coatings inserted without cement, would have higher metal concentrations in their serum as a result of larger surfaces available for passive dissolution. The finding that the serum Cr concentration was the highest in the group with the cementless Ti stems (group 3), in comparison to the fully coated Co-alloy stems (group 2) or to the cemented Co-Cr stems (group 1), indicates that the dominant dissolution mechanism is active dissolution i.e. corrosion and wear, most likely due to the modularity of the femoral stems and not to passive dissolution due to the increased surface area as a result of porous coatings. The long termed toxicological risks, if any, are as yet not know.

References:

1) Merritt, K, Brown, SA. Biological effects of corrosion products from metal. In: Fraker, AC and Griffin, CD ed(s). *Corrosion and Degradation of Implant Materials. Second Symposium. ASTM STP 859.* Philadelphia: American Society of Testing and Materials, 1985:195-207.
2) Jacobs, JJ, Urban, RM, Gilbert, JL, Skipor, AK, Black, J, Jasty, M, Galante, JO. Local and distant products from modularity. *Clin Orthop* 1995;319:94-105.
3) Nyren, O, McLaughlin, JK, Gridley, G, Ekbon, A, Johnell, O, Fraumeni, JF Jr., Adami, HO. Cancer risk after hip replacement with metal implants: a population-based cohort study in Sweden. *J Nat Cancer Inst* 1995;87:28-33.
4) Jacobs, JJ, Skipor, AK, Patterson, LM, Hallab, NJ, Paprosky, WG, Black J, Galante, JO. Metal release in patients who have had a primary total hip arthroplasty. *J Bone and Joint Surg* 1998;80-A:1447-1458.

Metal Ions in Biology and Medicine; vol 6. Eds. J.A. Centeno, Ph. Collery, G. Vernet, R.B. Finkelman, H. Gibb, J.C. Etienne. John Libbey Eurotext, Paris © 2000, pp. 345-347.

Measurement of dental implant corrosion products and histologic correlation in peri-implant tissues

Elena R. Ladich[1], Leonor E. Martinez[1], Norca Torres[1], Gary L. Ellis[1], Alfonso E. Valenzuela[2], Florabel G. Mullick[1], Jose A. Centeno[1]*

[1] *Armed Forces Institute of Pathology, Department of Environmental and Toxicologic Pathology, 6825 16th Street NW, Washington D.C. 20306;* [2] *Hospital General De Tijuana, Av. Centenario 108521 Zona Rio, México*

Background: Metallic systems have been used in dentistry for more than one hundred years. Metallic materials utilized for the construction of dental implant restorations include a wide range of relatively pure metals and multicomponent alloys. While dental implants have been used successfully with few reported adverse biological effects; the clinical significance and long term effects of metal corrosion in the oral cavity have not been well documented.

Aims: The objective of this study was to determine local tissue concentrations of trace metals in peri-implant gingival biopsies and to correlate any significant histologic findings.

Experimental Methods: Twenty-one gingival biopsies from patients with metallic dental implants were received for analysis. The implants consisted of a variety of metal compounds and alloys. Toxic metal ion levels were obtained by two techniques, electrothermal atomic absorption spectrometry (EAAS) and optical emission spectrophotometry (OES). Concentrations of nickel, lead, and cobalt were measured by EAAS or OES from acid digested tissue samples, and calculated in parts per million (ppm). Mercury (Hg) levels were measured employing a technique based on cold-vapor generation. Nineteen of the twenty-one tissue samples were processed for light microscopy. The specimens were fixed in formalin and stained with hematoxylin and eosin.

Results: Increased levels of Ni, Co, Pb and Hg above published levels, were measured and varied with the type of implant used. Eighteen patients demonstrated increased concentrations of nickel, eight had elevated concentrations of lead, seventeen demonstrated increased levels of mercury, and five showed increased concentrations of cobalt. The range of values for the measured trace elements was as follows: Pb (0.4-53 ppm), Co (0.1-4.8 ppm), Ni (0.3-77 ppm), and Hg (0.03-5.0 ppm). Tissue sections were also examined using light microscopy. The most frequent diagnosis was chronic inflammation (14 biopsies). The inflammation ranged from mild to severe. Six of the fourteen showed superimposed acute inflammation. Osteomyelitis was seen in one specimen. Three specimens demonstrated fibrous tissue with hemorrhage, two of which additionally showed lipid like vacuoles. One specimen demonstrated partially necrotic squamous epithelium. Metastatic adenocarcinoma was identified in one specimen.

Conclusions: In summary, EAAS and OES are analytical techniques capable of identifying and demonstrating trace metals in local tissues surrounding endosseous dental implants. Increases above published reference values were identified for each metal analyzed and varied according to the metallic composition of the implant. Regarding tissue morphology, all of the peri-implant biopsies demonstrated histopathologic changes; chronic inflammation was the predominant histologic finding.

Introduction: Metallic materials utilized for the construction of dental implant restorations include a wide range of relatively pure metals and multicomponent alloys. Medical complications related to implanted metals include localized infection and implant failure.[1] Contact allergies associated with metallic dental implants have also been reported.[2] Metallic implants represent reservoirs of potentially toxic metals, which are released by corrosion or mechanical destruction. Potential adverse effects are related to the release of these metals which may give rise to local or systemic toxicologic effects. Currently, few studies exist concerning the interactions between dental implants and human tissues. No conclusive connections between metal concentrations and adverse medical outcomes have been established and investigations are still in the descriptive phase. The objective of this investigation was to determine local tissue concentrations of trace metals in peri-implant gingival biopsies and to describe any significant morphologic changes associated with the metal exposure.

Materials and Methods: Twenty-one gingival biopsies from patients with metallic dental implants were received for analysis. The patients were clinically identified as having diffuse pain in the vicinity of the implant, two of whom demonstrated local degradation of implanted material as well. The patients' ages ranged from 39 to 74-years-old. The duration of exposures to implanted materials ranged from three to twenty years. The metallic composition of the implants varied: eight consisted of a ceramic alloy composed of nickel, chromium, molybdenum, and beryllium, six were a nickel-chromium alloy, four were stainless steel, one titanium, one gold plated, and one aluminum.

Toxic metal ion levels were obtained by two techniques, electrothermal atomic absorption spectrometry (EAAS) (Perkin Elmer Analyst 800) and optical emission spectrophotometry (OES) (Perkin Elmer Optima 3000). Tissue specimens were dried under vacuum until a constant dry weight was obtained. The dry tissues were subsequently acid digested in a microwave digestion system (CEM MDS-2000). Quality control samples consisted of a blank reagent sample, spiked blank, NIST water and a control tissue spiked at certified levels for each of the elements of interest. Mercury (Hg) levels were measured employing a technique based on cold-vapor generation (CETAC M6000A).

Nineteen of the twenty-one tissue samples were processed for light microscopy. The specimens were fixed in formalin, embedded in paraffin and stained with hematoxylin and eosin.

Results: Increases above published reference values occurred in the tissue concentrations of the four metals analyzed (nickel, cobalt, lead, and mercury) and varied with the type of implant used. Eighteen patients demonstrated increased concentrations of nickel, eight had elevated concentrations of lead, seventeen demonstrated increased levels of mercury, and five showed increased concentrations of cobalt. Experimental results for the elements of interest are summarized in Table 1. Published reference values for similar types of samples are described in Table 1.[3]

Table 1. Metal Concentration of Peri-implant Gingival Tissues (ppm)

Element	Tissue	Measured	Ref. Values*
Co	gingival	0.1-4.8	1.11±0.27 (dentine)
Pb	gingival	0.4-53	0.46±0.25 (dentine)
Ni	gingival	0.3-77	<0.6 (tooth enamel)
Hg	gingival	0.03-5.0	<0.5 (whole tooth)

*Reference values obtained from Ref.(3).

Peri-implant biopsies were examined using light microscopy. The most frequent diagnosis was chronic inflammation (14 biopsies). The inflammation ranged from mild to severe. Six of the fourteen showed superimposed acute inflammation. Three specimens demonstrated fibrous tissue with hemorrhage, two of which additionally showed lipid like vacuoles. One specimen demonstrated partially necrotic squamous epithelium. Metastatic adenocarcinoma was identified in one specimen. Implant materials were not specifically demonstrated, although four specimens showed unidentified foreign material which in one case was suspected of being dental amalgam. None of the histologic changes represented a premalignant condition.

Discussion: In summary, EAAS and OES are analytical techniques capable of identifying and demonstrating trace metals in local tissues surrounding endosseous dental implants. Increased levels of Ni, Co, Pb and Hg above published reference values (for teeth) were identified and varied according to the metallic composition of the implant. Interpretation of these results is limited as a consensus has not yet been reached on reference values for metals in oral soft tissues.

Regarding tissue morphology, all of the peri-implant biopsies demonstrated histopathologic changes; chronic inflammation was the predominant histologic finding. None of the pathological changes were suggestive of precancerous states. One case of metastatic adenocarcinoma was identified, and felt not to be related to the implant. Currently, no reports exist in the literature of malignancy associated with dental implants.[4]

The potential adverse effects of dental implants on local or distant tissues are still not well understood. In the future, more detailed analytical and pathological correlative studies are needed to elucidate biological mechanisms of toxicologic effects related to metal exposure in the oral cavity.

References

1. Goodacre C, Kan J, Rungcharasseng K. Clinical complications of osseointegrated implants. *J Prosth Dent* 1999; 81: 537-52.
2. Marcusson J, Lindh G, Evengard B. Chronic fatigue syndrome and nickel allergy. *Contact dermatitis* 1999; 40: 269-72.
3. Tsalev D. *Atomic absorption spectrometry in occupational and environmental health practice. Determination of individual elements*. Boca Raton: CRC Press. 1984.
4. IARC (1999) *IARC monographs of the evaluation of carcinogenic risks to humans,* Vol.74, *Other data relevant to an evaluation of carcinogenicity and its mechanisms*, Lyon, 231-302.

Metal Ions in Biology and Medicine; vol 6. Eds. J.A. Centeno, Ph. Collery, G. Vernet, R.B. Finkelman, H. Gibb, J.C. Etienne. John Libbey Eurotext, Paris © 2000, pp. 348-350.

The application of chemical modification for the determination of manganese in whole blood and urine by electrothermal atomic absorption spectrometry

J.L. Burguera[1], M. Burguera[1], P. Carrero[1], F. Paredes[1], C. Rondón, E. Burguera P.[2]

[1] IVAIQUIM (Venezuelan Andean Institute for Chemical Research), Faculty of Sciences; [2] Department of Preventive and Social Odontology, Faculty of Odontology, University of Los Andes, P.O. Box 542, Mérida 5101-A, Venezuela

Abstract

The determination of manganese in the presence of some matrix modifiers, such as: Mg as $Mg(NO_3)_2$, Pd as $Pd(NO_3)_3$, Ni as $Ni(NO_3)_2$, Eu as Eu_2O_3 and Lu as Lu_2O_3 by electrothermal atomic absorption spectrometry (ETAAS) has been studied. The results obtained by atomization of aqueous manganese standard solutions by L'vov platform with deuterium background correction show that the atomic absorption signal was only increased an stabilized by Ni, Pd and Mg. Therefore, the efficiency of these modifiers was tested for the quantification of manganese in whole blood and urine. In either case, accurate results and good agreement with manganese certified whole blood and urine samples were found.

Introduction

Manganese was reported to be an essential trace metal in animals in the early 1930s. Although knowledge of the metabolism and enzymatic functions of manganese has increased, its significance in human is still not clearly defined. Therefore, the aim in the work described here was to study the effect of some potential modifiers which allows the development of a simple method for determination of manganese in whole blood (WB) and urine using ETAAS.

Materials and Methods

Collection of samples

10 mL of each blood sample was obtained between the hours of 8.00 to 10.00 am and was drawn from an antecubital vein using a vacutainer tube and adding 1µL of Triton X-100 per milliliter of whole blood. Each collected urine specimens were preserved by adding 2 µL of concentrated nitric acid per milliliter of urine and stored at 4 °C in acid-washed plastic tubes.

Procedure

To obtain maximum pyrolysis temperature, atomization temperature, and optimum mass of the modifier, 20 µL aliquots of sample (or aqueous manganese standards) and 10 µL of matrix modifier solution were injected sequentially into the

L'vov platform. The temperature program developed in this study and given in Table I was followed.

Table I. Furnace program for the determination of manganese in whole blood and urine

Step	T (°C)	Ramp time (s)	Hold tome (s)	Ar flow (mL/min)
Drying	120	10	10	300
Drying	600	5	5	300
Pyrolysis	T_{pyr} [a]	5	20	300
Atomization	2200	0	5	0
Cleaning	2600	1	3	300
Cooling	20	5	10	300

[a] T_{pyr} = Optimum pyrolysis temperature as indicated below.

Results and Discussion

The atomic absorption signal for manganese in aqueous solutions was increased and stabilized by 40 ng of Ni, 20 ng of Pd and 10 ng of Mg (Fig. 1); while lower sensitivities and a poorer stabilization of manganese were obtained with 40 ng of Eu and 40 ng of Lu. The best sensitivities and stabilization of manganese in WB and urine samples were observed in the presence of Ni and Pd, respectively.

The m_o observed for manganese in the absence of any modifier and Mg, Pd and Ni were of 2.6, 1.8, 2.0 and 1.5 pg, respectively. The detection limits of the analyte in the presence of Mg, Pd and Ni were respectively 0.8, 0.5 and 0.5 μg Mn/L and in either case the calibration curves were linear up to 6.0 μg Mn/L. Recovery studies were performed on pools of WB and urine samples. Regardless of the modifier under study, there was no loss of metal during the procedure, and the average recovery for the addition of 2 and 4 μg Mn/L in either sample were from 97.4 to 99.9 % (for WB) and from 95.0 to 102.0 (for urine), respectively. The accuracy of the procedure was further tested by determining manganese in 2 WB and urine certified samples. The results were in good agreement with the certified values (Table II). According to the results of this work, for the determination of manganese in WB and urine it is convenient to add Ni and Pd as matrix modifiers, respectively.

Applications

In the urine and WB of 30 "healthy" subjects under study concentrations of 0.72 ± 0.20 (range: < 0.50 - 1.60) and 13.71 ± 4.70 (range: 7.50 - 18.72) μg Mn/L were respectively detected. These values are in agreement with those previously published by other authors, e.g., Jarvisalo et al. (0.31 and 16.48 μg Mn/L in urine and WB, respectively) [1], and Milne et al. (10.9 μg Mn/L in WB) [2].

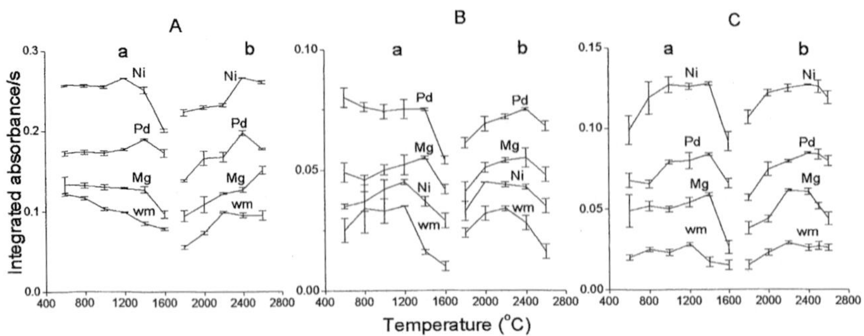

Fig. 1. (a) Pyrolysis and (b) atomization curves for: (A) 0.4 ng of Mn in an aqueous solution, (B) a urine sample and (C) a whole blood sample in the presence of 20, 20 and 10 ng of Ni, Pd and Mg, respectively. wm, with no modifier.

Table II. Certified Sample Analysis

Sample	Certified value (µg/L)	Modifier	Mn found (µg/L)
Urine (Seronorm, Batch 115)	22 ± 1	Ni	20.5 ± 1.4
		Mg	21.0 ± 1.2
		Pd	21.3 ± 1.2
Urine (NIST, SRM 2670; low levels)	30 ± 1	Ni	28.5 ± 1.7
		Mg	28.8 ± 1.6
		Pd	29.0 ± 1.6
WB (Seronorm, level 1)	9.0 ± 0.5	Ni	9.0 ± 0.2
		Mg	9.3 ± 0.5
		Pd	9.2 ± 0.4
WB (Seronorm, level 3)	15.0 ± 2.0	Ni	15.2 ± 0.6
		Mg	14.7 ± 0.7
		Pd	14.8 ± 0.6

References

1. Jarvisalo J, Olkinuora M, Kiilunen M, Kivisto H, Ristola P, Tossavainen A, Aitio A. Urinary and blood manganese in occupacionally nonexposed populations and in manual metal arc welders of mild steel. Int Arch Occup Environ Health 1992; 63: 495-501
2. Milne DB, Sims RL, Raiston NVC. Manganese content of the cellular components of blood. Clin Chem 1990; 36: 450-2.

Metal Ions in Biology and Medicine; vol 6. Eds. J.A. Centeno, Ph. Collery, G. Vernet, R.B. Finkelman, H. Gibb, J.C. Etienne. John Libbey Eurotext, Paris © 2000, pp. 351-353.

Non-invasive study of the *in vivo* distribution and migration of CO^{2+} in healthy Wistar rats. A feasibility study

Patrick Goethals and Anneke Volkaert

Institute for Nuclear Sciences, RUG, Proeftuinstraat 86, B-9000 Gent, Flanders, Belgium; e-mail: PatrickP.Goethals@rug.ac.be

Background. Long-lived radioisotopes become more and more important for the study of metabolism of toxic elements. Some of those elements have nuclides with interesting nuclear characteristics for studying non-invasively the in vivo behavior in animals using positron emission tomography (PET).

Aims. The accent was put on the non-invasive study of the in vivo distribution and metabolism of $^{55}Co^{2+}$ in normal Wistar rats.

Methods.

Synthesis

Carrier-free $^{55}Co^{2+}$ ($t_{1/2}$ = 17.53 h, $E_{\beta+max}$ = 1.50 MeV) was produced by proton irradiation (energy interval: 23-18 MeV, intensity 3-5 μA, duration 2 h) of a high purity Fe-foil. After dissolving the iron foil in HCl, $^{55}Co^{2+}$ was separated from the Fe-matrix by column chromatography [1,2]. The pH of the final isotonic solution ranged from 5 to 7. The whole procedure took about 5.5 hours (irradiation: 2 hours, cooling period: 1 hour, chemical purification: 2.5 hours). Traces of isopropyl ether were verified by GC-FID (Gas Chromatography with a Flame Ionization Detector).

Biodistribution studies in Wistar rats

Studies were performed on healthy male Wistar rats (n = 6, 270-350g). All animals were anaesthetized with sodium pentobarbital (Nembutal®, dose 40-60 mg kg^{-1}, intraperitonial). The right jugular vein catheterized for intravenous injection of ^{55}Co. The animals were secured in a holder in supine position in the gantry of the PET scanner (Siemens ECAT 915/31) with the positioning laser beam on the line nose-tail. Before tracer administration of the radiopharmaceutical, a ^{66}Ga transmission scan for attenuation correction was performed. 0.15-0.50 mCi (4.4 tot 18.5 MBq) of $^{55}Co^{2+}$ was administered intravenously over 30s for each experiment and a dynamic PET study (26 frames: 10×60s, 10×120s, 6×300s, total scanning period of 60 min) was started immediately. Images of all sequence frames were corrected for attenuation. Two rats were scanned with the PET camera in the same position 1 and 2 days after injection.

To facilitate the identification of hot spots of activity with organs and tissues, the transmission scan (Fig. 1 a), showing the contour of the body, is used as reference, besides our experience and knowledge obtained by dissection studies on small animals (Fig. 1b). Regions of interest (ROI's), corresponding with the real dimensions of the organs, were drawn automatically on the tomographic planes illustrating the dynamic profiles of activity in the heart, left kidney, liver, bladder, brain and muscular tissue.

Results.

Synthesis

About 5-8 mCi (185-300 MBq) of ^{55}Co with a non-radioactive carrier of less than 1 µg was produced routinely. Contamination of ^{56}Co ($t_{1/2}$ = 77.3 d) was less than 2% of total activity at the end of production. Quality control with GC-FID on a Porapack®Q-column showed that the isopropyl ether content was far below the toxic level.

Biodistribution studies in Wistar rats

The PET data, visualized in Fig. 1 to 2 of an animal, are representative for the whole group of Wistar rats (n = 6). The radioactivity distribution is visualized in the PET-views (Fig. 1 c & d) corresponding with coronal planes through the heart, liver, left kidney, brain, muscular tissue and the bladder, respectively at 60s and 30 min post injection. Fig. 2 illustrates the data corrected for blood pool activity for the liver, left kidney, brain, muscular tissue. It is clearly depicted that the highest activity is accumulated in the liver. The time-activity curves (Fig. 2) showed that $^{55}CoCl_2$ is rapidly cleared from the blood pool (heart).
At 10 min post injection, the blood pool activity levels decreased to less than 25% of the injected dose (I.D.). Simultaneously, besides a strong accumulation of the activity in the liver (30-50 % I.D. within 10 min), a continuous increase of the ^{55}Co-activity in the bladder took place (8 - 11 % I.D./ml within 1 hour). A low uptake was noticed in the brain (0.07 - 0.18 % I.D./ml) and in muscular tissue (0.07 - 0.11 % I.D./ml).
One day after injection highest activity concentration is still noticed in the liver while for the other organs and tissues the activity is strongly decreased.
*(DAR = $(\mu Ci/ml)_{organ}/(\mu Ci/ml)_{body}$)

Conclusion.

PET allows studying the biodistribution and the migration of $^{55}Co^{2+}$ in vivo in a non-invasive way. The advantage is that the number of animals can be seriously reduced in comparison to the earlier performed biodistribution studies (dissection).

References

1/ Lagunas-Solar M.C. and Jungerman J.A. (1979) Cyclotron production of carrier-free cobalt-55, a new positron-emitting label for Bleomycin *Int J Appl Radiat Isot* 30, 25-32
2/ Sharma H., Zweit J., Smith A.M. and Downey S. (1986) Production of cobalt-55, a short-lived, positron emitting radiolabel for Bleomycin *Appl Radiat Isot* 37, 105-109

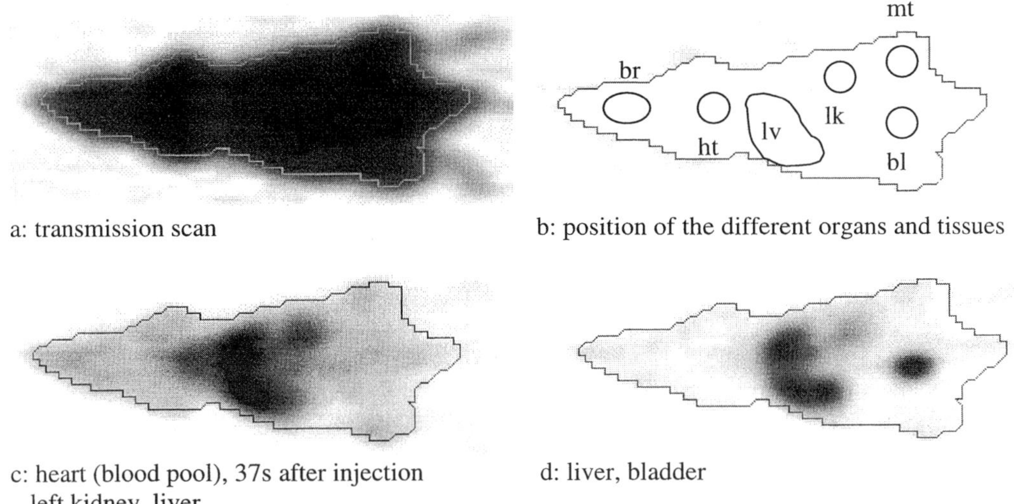

Fig. 1: Coronal PET views of a healthy Wistar rat injected with $^{55}CoCl_2$

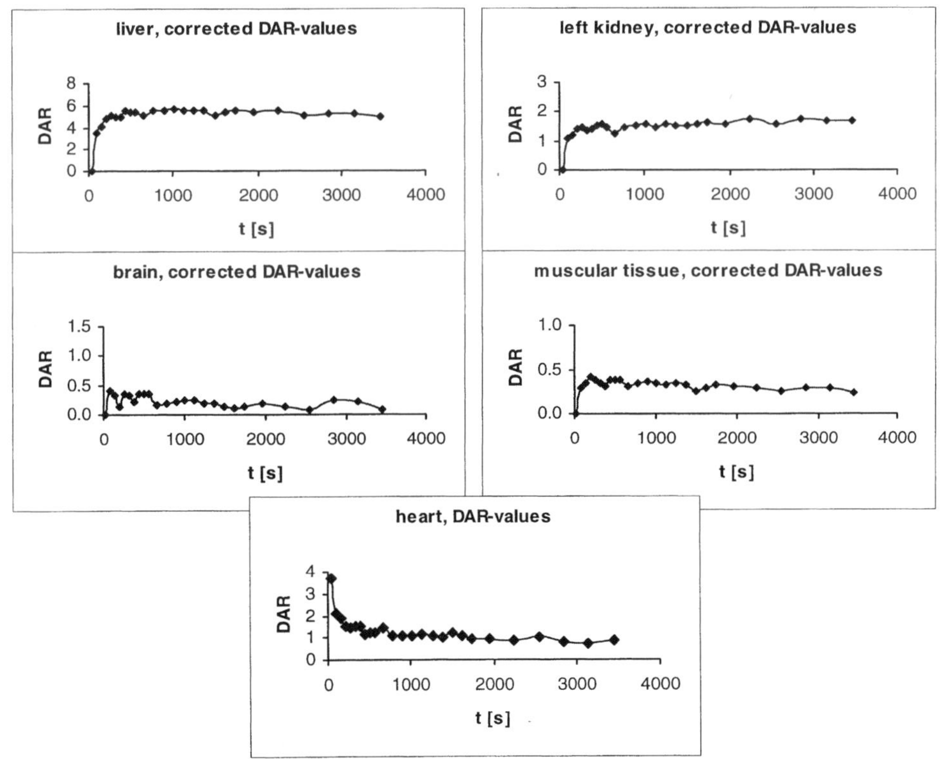

Fig. 2: Time-activity curves of liver, left kidney, brain, muscular tissue (corrected for blood pool activity) and heart (blood pool)

Metal Ions in Biology and Medicine; vol 6. Eds. J.A. Centeno, Ph. Collery, G. Vernet, R.B. Finkelman, H. Gibb, J.C. Etienne. John Libbey Eurotext, Paris © 2000, pp. 355-360.

Surface enhanced Raman spectroscopy study of the interaction of metal cations with DNA and its nitrogen bases

Nilka M. Rivera[1], Eduardo Goenaga[1], Samuel P. Hernández[1] and José A. Centeno[2]

[1] *Department of Chemistry, University of Puerto Rico-Mayagüez, PO Box 9019 Mayagüez, PR 00681-9019;* [2] *Department of Environmental and Toxicologic Pathology, Armed Forces Institute of Pathology, Washington, DC 20306-6000*

Abstract:

Interactions of metal cations: Li (I), K (I), Mg (II), Cd (II), Co (II), Ba (II), Pb (II), Fe (III), Cr (III) and Ru (III) with native calf thymus DNA (CT-DNA) and its constituent nitrogen bases: adenine (A), guanine (G), cytosine (C) and thymine (T) have been investigated using Raman Spectroscopy. In order to study nucleic acid concentration levels in the range of 10^{-3} M to 10^{-6} M, the signal enhancement technique applied at the sample level called Surface Enhanced Raman Scattering (SERS) was used. Metal cation concentration levels ranged from $1x10^{-1}$ M to $1x10^{-5}$ M. Main structural changes caused by cations consisted in selective attenuation of specific marker bands, disappearance and emergence of bands, and even complete disrupture of band structure of band structure of the biomolecules. Metal cations in the 3+ oxidation state were found to interact strongest with the molecules studied. In the case of 2+ cations, the order of the intensity perturbations to the vibrational structure of the molecules was:

Cd (II) ~ Co (II) > Ba (II) ~ Mg (II)

Metal cations in the 1+ oxidation state caused minimal perturbations to the SERS band structure of the molecules studied, but even these changes couid be detected.

Introduction:

Vibrational Spectroscopy has played a leading role in the study of biomolecules, both *in vitro* and *in vivo* investigations. Aside from the fundamental information conveyed by its various techniques, there are clear advantages that favor its preferential use over others. Among these are the ease sample preparations, sample recovery, little or no interference from the solvent (in the case of Raman Spectroscopy) and that the relevant information can be obtained from different physical states: diluted or concentrated solutions, hydrated fibers or films, and crystals.

The use of Raman Spectroscopy (RS) in nucleic acid research has been established for several years (1-3). Metal binding sites to nucleic acids can be assessed using vibrational spectroscopy. Conformational information can also be gained as well as changes induced by pathogenic and toxicologic agents. Direct evidence of complex formation to metal cations can also be studied. Structural perturbations induced by exogenous agents have also been established using various Raman techniques.

The focus of this investigation was to establish patterns in modification interactions of nucleic acids caused by metal cations. Oxidation state (cationic charge), chemical nature of metal (alkaline earth versus transition metal ions), and reactivity are among the main aspects considered. Surface Enhanced Raman Scattering (SERS) was used as a probe of the interactions due to the relatively low detection limit, allowing examining DNA concentrations as low as 10^{-6} M.

Materials and Methods:

Solutions of DNA (Sigma Chemicals Co.) were prepared dissolving 100 mg of Calf Thymus DNA in 10 mL of phosphate buffer (pH = 6.5), and stirring at 4°C for 24 hours. Dilutions by 1000 fold in buffer followed. The final concentration obtained calculated from the measure of UV-Vis spectra was approximately $4x10^{-5}$ M.

The metal salts solutions (Strem Chemicals) were prepared in deionized water at concentrations ranging between $2x10^{-1}$ M and $2x10^{-5}$ M. For the interactions, 500μL of DNA and 500 μL of the metal solution were mixed. Interactions were then incubated in a constant temperature bath at 37° C for the desired time.

In the SERS technique the use of a colloidal suspension is required. In this work silver hydrosols were prepared by reducing silver nitrate (Aldrich Chemical Co.) with a 1% sodium citrate (Aldrich) and stirring for about one hour (modifications of the method of Lee and Meisel).

For the preparation of samples for SERS spectroscopy, 100 µL of sodium perchlorate (Aldrich) 0.6 M were added to 800 µL of silver colloid. Then,100 µL of the interaction were added and analyzed using a Jobin/Ybon T64000 triple Raman spectrograph using 514.5 nm (argon ion) laser (70 m W of radiant power at sample). The data were obtained at 0, 24, 48 and 72 hours after the interaction.

Results:

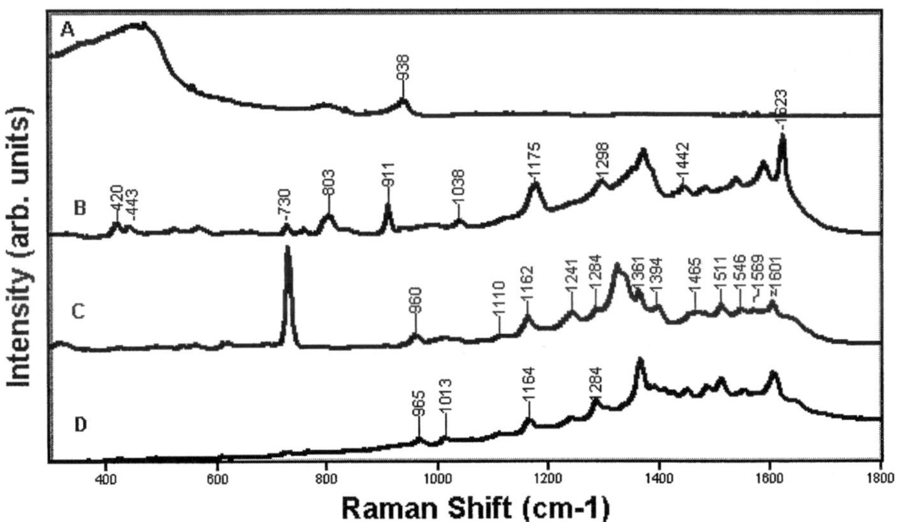

Figure 1: Comparison of DNA with the interaction with different metals: (A) DNA – Ru(III) 10^{-1} M after 48 hours of interaction, (B) DNA – Cd(II) 10^{-4} M after 72 hours of interaction, (C) DNA –Li(I) 10^{-5} M after 24 hours of interaction, (D) DNA without interaction.

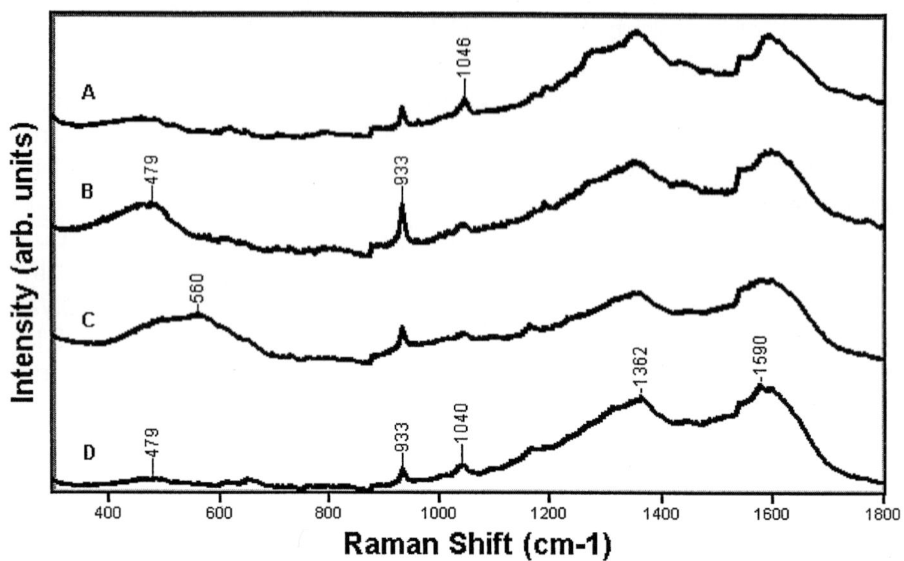

Figure 2: DNA - Cr (24 hours after the interaction). (A) Cr 10^{-1} M, (B) Cr 10^{-2} M, (C) Cr 10^{-3} M, (D) Cr 10^{-5} M.

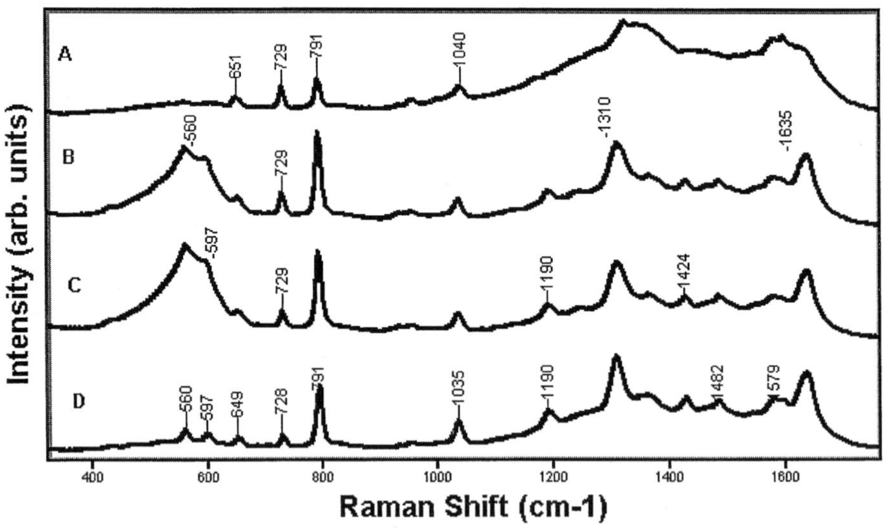

Figure 3: Cytosine-Cr (48 hours after the interaction). (A) Cr 10^{-2} M, (B) Cr 10^{-3} M, (C) Cr 10^{-4} M, (D) Cr 10^{-5} M.

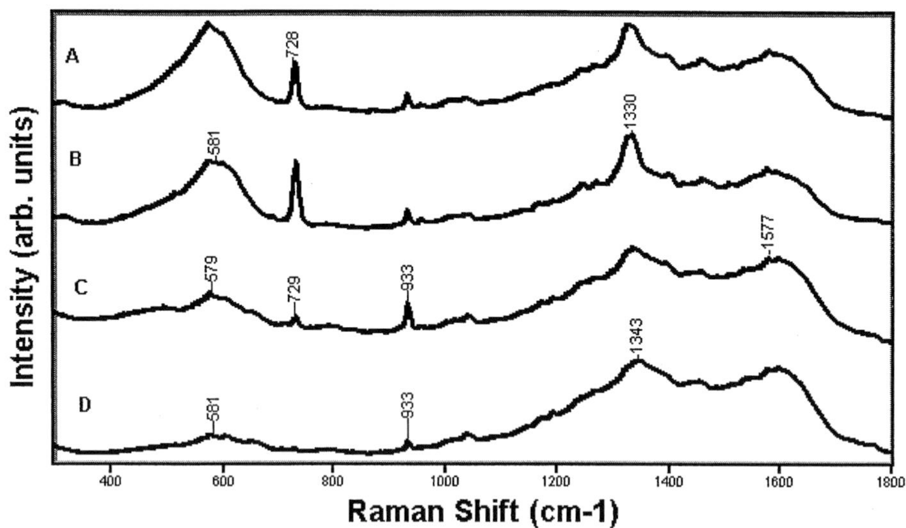

Figure 4: Thymine – Cr 10^{-3} M. (A) 0 hours after the interaction, (B) 24 hours after the interaction, (C) 48 hours after the interaction, (D) 72 hours after the interaction.

Discussion:

The SERS spectra of DNA – Ru (III), DNA –Cd (II) and DNA – Li (I) are shown in Fig. 1. These spectra illustrate many of the changes brought about to DNA by metal cations. The interaction of 3+ metal ions with DNA can be so strong that it often leads to total disruption of SERS band structure of the macromolecule as in Fig. 1-A [DNA-Ru(III)]. The only signals remaining after the interaction are due to internal polyatomic anions that serve as wavelength markers: ClO_4^- (~935 cm^{-1}) and NO_3^- (1038 –1040 cm^{-1}). The second type of interaction detected is that of metal ion – DNA complex formation as can be depicted from the emergence of two new bands (420 and 443 cm^{-1}) as part of the interaction of Cd^{2+} (10^{-4} M) with DNA after 72 hours of incubation. Finally, even 1+ metal cation can alter DNA conformation by selectively exposing adenine base residues so that they may be in closer contact to the colloidal silver surface. This can be concluded by observing the selective enhancement of adenine signals: 730 cm^{-1} (ring breathing mode) and 1325 cm^{-1} (indicative of base unstaking) of DNA – Li (I) at 1 x 10^{-5} M metal ion concentration.

Chromium (III) was found to affect most DNA and its bases. A DNA-Cr complex was found to form instantaneously. The complex detected was also evidenced by UV-Vis spectroscopy. Fig. 2 shows the metal ion concentration dependence. The optimum complex formation range is 10:1 to 100:1 (M-DNA) and is almost unnoticeable a 1:1 molar ratio (<1:100 metal to base pairs ratio). The complex band structure is very broad (>150 cm^{-1}) suggesting intermolecular, no-symmetrical nature and its, formation was also detected prominently with cytosine and thymine. Adenine showed the presence of the slight complex at 560 cm^{-1} and guanine at 556 cm^{-1} indicating the marked preference for pyrimidines for complex formation. Fig. 3 shows the dependence of the Cr (3+) complex with cytosine on the metal concentration (10^{-2} –10^{-5} M). At 10^{-1} M concentration level, the anionic strength is so high that the complex does not bind to the silver surface. The DNA – Cr^{3+} is so prominent that it can be detected even at 10^{-5} M Cr^{3+} concentration levels.

For a 100:1 molar ratio (~1:1 ion to base pairs ratio) the complex between Cr^{3+} and pyrimidines seems to form instantaneously (~0 hours). Fig. 4 shows the temporal evolution of the thymine – Cr^{3+} complex from its formation (Fig. 4-A) to its near disappearance at 72 hours (Fig. 4-D).

References:

1. Duguid J., Bloomfield V.A., Benevides J., Thomas G.; *Biophys. J.* 1992; 65:1916-1928.
2. Kornilova S. V., Kapinos L., Tomkova A., Mishkovskii P., Blagoi Y.P., Bolbukh T.V.; *Biophysics* 1994; 39:407-420.
3. Langlais M., Tajmir-Riahi H.A., Savoir R.; *Biopolymers* 1990; 30:743-752.
4. Lee P.C. and Meisel D.; *J. Phys. Chem.* 1982; 86: 3391-3395.
5. Séquaris J.M., Fritz J., Lewinsky H., Koglin E.; *J. Colloid. Inter. Sci.* 1985; 105: 417-425.
6. Sánchez-Cortés S. and García-Ramos J.V.; *J. Raman Sprectroscopy* 1998; 29: 365-371.
7. Hackl E., Kornilova S.V., Kapinos L., Andrashchenko V., Grigoviev D., Galkin V. and Blagoi Y.; *J. Mol. Struct.* 1997; 408-409: 229-232.

Metal Ions in Biology and Medicine; vol 6. Eds. J.A. Centeno, Ph. Collery, G. Vernet, R.B. Finkelman, H. Gibb, J.C. Etienne. John Libbey Eurotext, Paris © 2000, pp. 361-363.

DNA structural transitions under Cu^{2+} ions action in aqueous solution: role of Cu^{2+} ions interaction with DAN bases

Elene V. Hackl, Yurij P. Blagoi

Institute for Low Temperature Physics and Engineering, National Academy of Sciences of Ukraine, 47 Lenin Ave., 310164 Kharkov, Ukraine; e-mail: e_hackl@usa.net

In [1] we have shown that on the DNA interaction with Cu^{2+} ions in aqueous solution with relatively high DNA concentration IR spectrum of DNA is changed. This appears in shifts of absorption bands of DNA phosphate groups and bases as well as in strong increase (~3-3.5 times) of the absorption band intensities. Absorption band shifts we explained by Cu^{2+} ions binding to DNA (directly or through water molecules) while the strong increase of intensities of IR absorption bands of DNA complexes with Cu^{2+} ions, on the basis of comparison of the IR spectra of DNA-Cu^{2+} and DNA-Tb^{3+} complexes and light scattering data, we associated with DNA transition into compact form under Cu^{2+} ions action (for details, see [2, 3]).

It is known that electrostatic repulsion of negatively charged phosphate groups is one of the main barriers preventing from DNA condensation [4]. In order to DNA chains may approach it is necessary to neutralize 89-90% of the total charge on DNA phosphates [5]. But in [4, 6] it was shown that in the case of DNA interaction with divalent metal ions the necessary degree of neutralization is not reached. At the same time in [7], when studying Mn^{2+}-induced DNA condensation, it was found that DNA condensation may be induced by Mt^{2+} but in this case the condensation mechanism is not primarily electrostatic, but depends on destabilization of the DNA secondary structure due to Mn^{2+} ions binding to the DNA bases. To verify whether the DNA condensation under the Cu^{2+} ions action shown by us in [1-3] depends on interaction of these ions with DNA bases leading to destabilization of DNA structure, in the present work we studied Cu^{2+} interaction with polyphosphates as a DNA model system containing no bases.

Materials and method

In the work the polyphosphates $Na_{n+2}P_nO_{3n+1}$ ("Sigma", type 65) with average chain length of 65±5 P were used. Polyphosphates were dissolved in cacodylate buffer ($[Na^+]$ = 5×10^{-3} M, pH 7). The polymer concentration in solution was in the range of 16±2 mg/ml.

Infrared spectra of polyphosphate complexes with Cu^{2+} ions in aqueous solution were recorded by the infrared spectrophotometer UR-20 (Karl Zeiss, Jena) in the region 1000-1400 cm^{-1}. To take spectra the special CaF_2 cuvettes with path length of 50 μm were used. The cuvettes were thermostated at 27 ± 0.1 ^{0}C. In detail method was described in [2].

Results and discussion

As it was mentioned in Introduction, DNA interaction with Cu^{2+} ions in aqueous solution results in increasing the intensities of IR absorption bands of DNA phosphate groups and bases. Fig. 1 (curves 1,2) shows the dependencies of relative increase of intensities of bands at 1090 (symmetrical vibrations of phosphate groups) and 1680 cm^{-1} (C_6=O of guanine, C_4=O of thymine) for DNA-Cu^{2+} complexes [2].

To test whether the Cu^{2+} ions interaction with DNA bases may be responsible for the strong increase of absorption band intensities observed in IR spectra of DNA-Cu^{2+} complexes, in the present work we studied Cu^{2+} ions interaction with polyphosphates in aqueous solution. The IR spectra of polyphosphates (pP) and pP complexes with Cu^{2+} ions in the wide range of copper concentrations were recorded. At the absence of divalent metal ions the pP IR spectrum has 3 main absorption bands at 1053 cm^{-1} (vibrations of the C-O-P sugar-phosphate backbone), 1090 cm^{-1} (ν_S - symmetrical vibrations of phosphate groups) and 1270 cm^{-1} (ν_{aS} - antisymmetrical vibrations of phosphate groups). Cu^{2+} ion addition to pP leads to weak broading of all absorption bands (Fig. 2) and to their shift on 3-6 cm^{-1} to higher frequencies. At Cu^{2+} ions concentration rise the band integral intensity at 1053 cm^{-1} is changed strongest of all (Fig. 2). At the same time its peak intensity does not increase (the band integral intensity was calculated as the area of an absorption band). Thus increase of the band area at 1053 cm^{-1} observed is due to broadering of this band. At further rise of the Cu^{2+} concentration (up to 4×10^{-2} M) the peak intensity of the band at 1053 cm^{-1} decreases and the band is degenerated into a shoulder. This evidences the pP aggregation and sedimentation in complexes with high Cu^{2+} ion concentrations (when forming the DNA complexes with high Cu^{2+} ion concentrations DNA aggregation and partial precipitation were observed too [3]). Changes in the IR spectra of pP-Cu^{2+} complexes evidence the Cu^{2+} ions binding to phosphate groups of pP.

From Fig. 1, which shows the dependencies of relative changes of peak intensities of the absorption bands ν_S and ν_{aS} for pP complexes with Cu^{2+} ions on the total copper ion concentration in solution (curves 3, 4), it follows that, on the contrary to the DNA-Cu^{2+} complexes spectra, in the IR spectra of pP complexes with Cu^{2+} ions the increase of absorption band ν_S and ν_{aS} intensities at Cu^{2+} ion binding are not observed. On the contrary, at Cu^{2+} ions concentration higher than 4×10^{-2} M decrease of intensities of these bands occurs accompanied, as in spectra of DNA complexes with high Cu^{2+} ion concentrations, by significant broading of the absorption bands and by increase of background scattering. Such changes evidence the strong aggregation and precipitation of pP in complexes with high Cu^{2+} ion concentrations as it was noted above.

It should be noted that in the IR spectra of pP complexes with Ca^{2+} ions in aqueous solutions the increase of absorption band intensities was observed, at that the maximum intensity increase (1.5-1.6 times) was practically equal in the cases of pP and DNA complexes with Ca^{2+} ions (this question in detail is discussed in [Hackl et.al., manuscript in preparation]). Increase of intensities of the absorption bands was also observed in the IR spectra of Cu^{2+} ion complexes with single-chain poly(I) recorded at the experimental conditions analogous to those of the present work [Grigoriev et.al., submit.]. It was shown that Cu^{2+} ions interact both with the poly(I) phosphate groups and bases, first of all with C_6=O of inosine. This binding caused destabilization of the polymer and the helicity degree decrease down to the transition into the coil conformation.

Thus the comparison of modifications of the DNA and pP IR spectra on biopolymer interaction with Cu^{2+} ions in aqueous solutions permits to suppose that strong increase of intensities of absorption bands of DNA phosphate groups and bases in the IR spectra of DNA-Cu^{2+} complexes may be caused by Cu^{2+} ions interaction with DNA bases. Probably, partial DNA destabilization taken place as a result of such interaction facilitates the DNA compactisation under divalent copper ion action in aqueous solution.

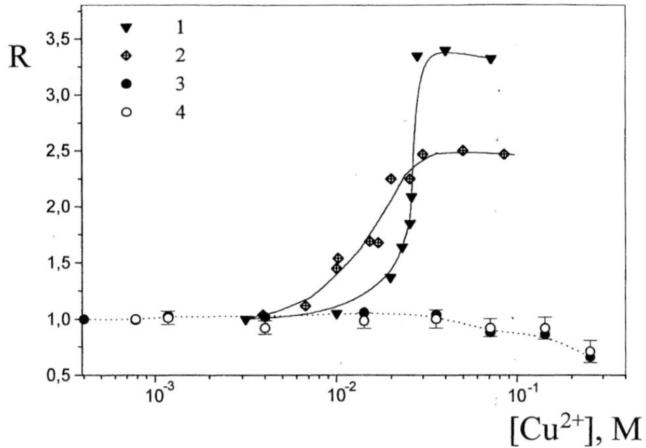

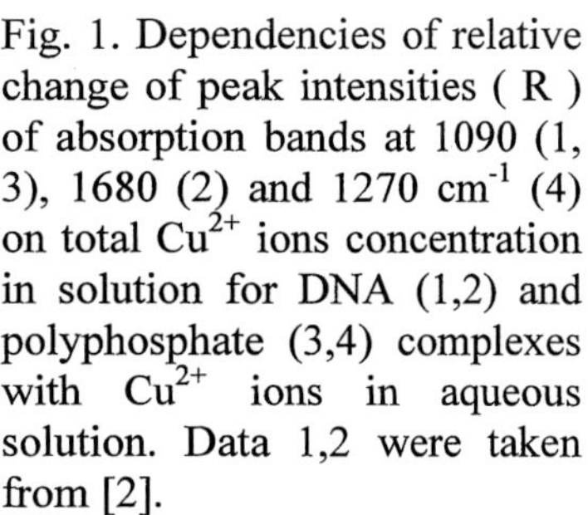

Fig. 1. Dependencies of relative change of peak intensities (R) of absorption bands at 1090 (1, 3), 1680 (2) and 1270 cm^{-1} (4) on total Cu^{2+} ions concentration in solution for DNA (1,2) and polyphosphate (3,4) complexes with Cu^{2+} ions in aqueous solution. Data 1,2 were taken from [2].
$R=D_i/D_0$, where D_0 is the optical density at maximum of absorption band at given frequency for DNA/polyphosphate without Cu^{2+} ions, D_i is the same value for DNA/polyphosphate complex with Cu^{2+}.

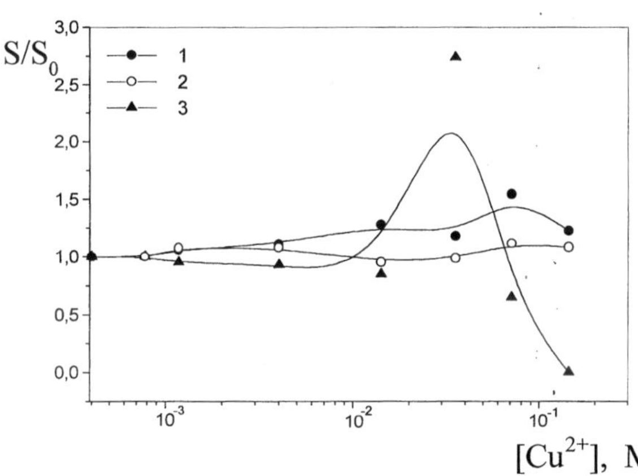

Fig. 2. Dependencies of relative change of integral intensities of absorption bands at 1090 (1), 1270 (2) and 1053 cm^{-1} (3) on total Cu^{2+} ion concentration in solution for polyphosphate complexes with Cu^{2+} ions in aqueous solution.
S_o is the integral intensity of an absorption band in IR spectrum of polyphosphates without Cu^{2+} ions, S is the same value for polyphosphate complexes with Cu^{2+}.

References

1. Hackl E, Kornilova S, Kapinos L, et.al. Study of Ca^{2+}, Mn^{2+}, Cu^{2+} ion binding to DNA in solutions by means of IR-spectroscopy. *J Mol Struct* 1997; 408 / 409: 229-32.
2. Kornilova S, Hackl E, Kapinos L, et.al. DNA interaction with biologically active metal ions. Cooperativity of metal ion binding at DNA compactization. *Acta Biochim Polon* 1998; 45: 107-17.
3. Hackl E, Kornilova S, Blagoi Yu. DNA compactisation in Cu^{2+} ions presence in aqueous and aqueous-alcohol solutions. *Visnyk problem biol i med* 1998; 8: 41-51.
4. Bloomfield V. DNA condensation by multivalent cations. *Biopolymers* 1998; 44: 269-82.
5. Wilson R, Bloomfield V. Counterion-induced condesation of deoxyribonucleic acid. A light-scattering study. *Biochemistry* 1979; 18: 2192-96.
6. Ma Ch, Bloomfield V. Gel electrophoresis measurement of counterion condensation on DNA. *Biopolymers* 1995; 35: 211-16.
7. Ma Ch, Bloomfield V. Condensation of supercoiled DNA induced by $MnCl_2$. *Biophys J* 1994; 67: 1678-81.

Metal Ions in Biology and Medicine; vol 6. Eds. J.A. Centeno, Ph. Collery, G. Vernet, R.B. Finkelman, H. Gibb, J.C. Etienne. John Libbey Eurotext, Paris © 2000, pp. 364-366.

Interactions of metal cations with monomers, dimers, triplexes and tetrads of nucleic acid bases: new findings from realiable theoretical ab initio studies

Jerzy Leszczynski

The Computational Center for Molecular Structure and Interactions, Department of Chemistry, Jackson State University, Jackson, MS 39217, USA

Metal ions are of the greatest biological importance because of their involvement in many natural processes. Their interactions with nucleic acids might cause heavy-metal toxicity in our environment, but on the other hand, interactions with metals provide for the application of cisplatin and its derivatives as anticancer agents. The structure and functions of nucleic acids are significantly affected by metal cations. There are two major sites of metal ion coordinations in nucleic acids. The metal cations are usually located around the phosphate groups and stabilize the DNA double helix by electrostatic interactions with a negatively charged sugar-phosphate backbone. However, in addition they can also interact with Nucleic Acid Bases (NAB). Such interactions are vital for stabilizing the triple and quadruple helices of DNA and the ribose-base stacking in Z-DNA. The recent computational studies could reveal details of the interactions of metal cations with NABs. Our recent comprehensive quantum mechanical studies allow for a number of factors which are responsible for the structures of interacting systems, their stabilization, and properties to be addressed.

All calculations were performed using reliable ab initio methods. This is only level of theory adequate for studying such systems since interactions between cations and base pairs cannot be studied by means of empirical potentials because of the importance of huge charge-transfer and polarization effects. The calculations were carried out at the MP2/6-31G*//HF/6-31G* level; relativistic pseudopotentials were used to describe the cations. Also Density Functional Theory (DFT) methods were applied to larger metal-guanine tetrad systems. An important step in revealing the details of interactions between DNA fragments and the metal cations was a study of complexes between the Watson-Crick AT and GC base pairs and various metal cations. All calculations were performed assuming planar symmetry of the complexes, and the cations were allowed to interact with the nitrogen N7 of adenine in the AT pair and with the N7 and O6 of guanine in the GC pair. The selected locations of the cations are known to be active sites in the DNA major groove.

The optimized geometries clearly indicate the nature of interactions in these systems. The three body systems can be considered as a combination of strongly bonded metal cation-purine base complexes and two weakly bonded subsystems: the metal cation-pyrimidine base and purine-pyrimidine bases. The optimized molecular parameters for the M...G and M...A subsystems are virtually the same as for the corresponding isolated metal cation-base pairs; the largest differences (decreased by 0.08 Å) was predicted for the Ba^{2+}-N7 distance in the complex with GC. The metal ion has significant influence on the hydrogen bonds. In the GC complexes the O...H(N2) bond lengths are reduced (up to 0.3 Å for the divalent ions) in comparison with the isolated GC pair. The central H...N1 bond remains virtually unchanged while the H...O6 hydrogen bond, which is closest to the metal ion coordination site, shows significant lengthening (up to 0.65 Å for the Zn^{2+} and Mg^{2+} complexes). The predicted changes are quite dissimilar for the M...AT complex. The bond distance of that closest to the metal site H...N6 hydrogen bond is decreased (up to 0.35 Å for the Zn^{2+} and Mg^{2+} complexes). The second H...N1 bond is lengthened (by as much as 0.18 Å for the Zn^{2+} complex).

There are a number of factors, which are responsible for the different changes in the molecular parameters of the GC and AT pairs interacting with the metal ions. The most obvious one is a shift of electron density from the N7 atom of the AT pair towards the metal cation, which would alter the charge densities of the atoms involved in the hydrogen bonds. On the other hand, the cation interacting with the GC pair increases the electron density around the O6 of guanine. However such changes could not explain all variations in the bond distances. An additional factor, the direct electrostatic repulsion between the metal cation and the closest hydrogen atom from cytosine, does also contribute to the predicted trends. The consequences of metal ion base pair interactions could be altered by involvement of a polar solvent (water). The presence of a solvent could be crucial for the ionic systems, and many previously predicted effects might be profoundly exaggerated. Such interactions have been studied for the M-GC complexes.

The investigated systems were constructed from divalent metal ions, solvated by a water shell. Five water molecules were used to achieve the most likely coordination numbers of six or seven. The cations were placed initially near the N7 atom of guanine. The molecular geometry of the complex was optimized without any symmetry constraints. For all studied cations (except Ba^{2+}) the GC (WC) pair adopts a planar geometry. The bulky barium atom causes significant nonplanarity (buckling) of the GC pair and is shifted away (by ca 0.5 Å) from the guanine plane. The inclusion of the water shell preserves direct interactions of the Mg^{2+} and group IIB metals with the O6 atom of guanine, contrary to the direct involvement in the metal bonding of the O6 site which has been observed for nonsolvated M-GC complexes. The larger ions, Ca^{2+}, Sr^{2+} and Ba^{2+} are coordinated to both the N7 and O6 sites. The cation-base distances are in agreement for the unsolvated cations, and except for the Mg^{2+} complex, the M-N7 distances are shorter than those between M-O(water). The most profound effect of the hydrated cation on the base pair geometry is an elongation (compared to the optimized GC geometry) by about 0.30- 0.35 Å of the O6(G)...N4(C) hydrogen bond distance. Since similar elongation for the unsolvated cations is more notable (up to 0.55 Å) such a difference can be attributed to the screening effect of the water shell around the cations.

The mechanism of autitumor activity of the *cis*-$[Pt(NH_3)_2Cl_2]$ drug is one of the most intriguing problems of molecular biology. Our recent calculations show that the *cis*-$[Pt(NH_3)_2]^{2+}$ binding to the N7 and O6 sites of guanine of the GC base pair causes significant changes in the interaction between guanine and cytosine compared to the Watson-Crick H-bonding pattern. Two local minima are predicted for the *cis*-$[Pt(NH_3)_2GC]^{2+}$ complex, which are associated with the stablization of cytosine at the N1-H and N2-H sites of guanine. The first minimum corresponds to the bifurcated H-bonding of the N1-H and N2-H sites towards the O6 site of cytosine (cisplatin-1). The second one corresponds to the H-bonding between the N1-H and N2-H sites of guanine and the N3 and O2 sites of cytosine, respectively (cisplatin-2). For both cisplatin-1 and cisplatin-2 the binding energy of cytosine at guanine is significantly larger (by about 11 Kcal/mol) compared to the GC pair. Our analysis of the electrostatic potential at the O6, N1-H and N2-H sites of the free guanine and *cis*-$[Pt(NH_3)_2G]^{2+}$ allows for a qualitative explanation of the effect of the *cis*-$[Pt(NH_3)_2]^{2+}$ coordination on the H-bonding interaction between cytosine and guanine.

Purine-purine-pyrimidine (Pu.PuPy) DNA triplexes are formed by binding a purine-rich oligonucleotide to the purine strand of a DNA duplex. The third strand assumes an antiparallel orientation with respect to the purine strand of the duplex and the purine bases are associated by reverse Hoogsteen hydrogen bonding. Formation of Pu.PuPy triplexes requires the presence of multivalent cations. These may be organic cations such as spermidene or metal cations. Cations may contribute to the stabilization of triplexes by screening the negative charges of phosphate groups on polynucleotide strands. However, divalent metal cations may affect triplex formation by direct binding to DNA bases. Our calculations lead to several conclusions concerning the possible mechanism of the metal-assisted stablization of Pu.PuPy triplexes: (i) the different role of the cations in stabilizing A.AT and G.GC triplexes correlates with the stronger binding of zinc to bases, compared to magnesium. This indicates that a binding of a cation to the N7 position of purine is essential for the triplex stabilization (ii) a strong enhancement of the purine-purine base pair stability (due to cation binding) is predicted for the GGC triplet, (iii) no enhancement of base pairing has been found for the A.AT triplet. Here, even a destabilizing effect can be expected from the possible activitation (pyramidalization) of the third-strand adenine amino group (iv) the apparent lack of the metal-induced base pairing enhancement in the A.AT systems suggests that a different mechanism may be responsible for the stability of the triplexes containing both the G.GC and A.AT base triplets.

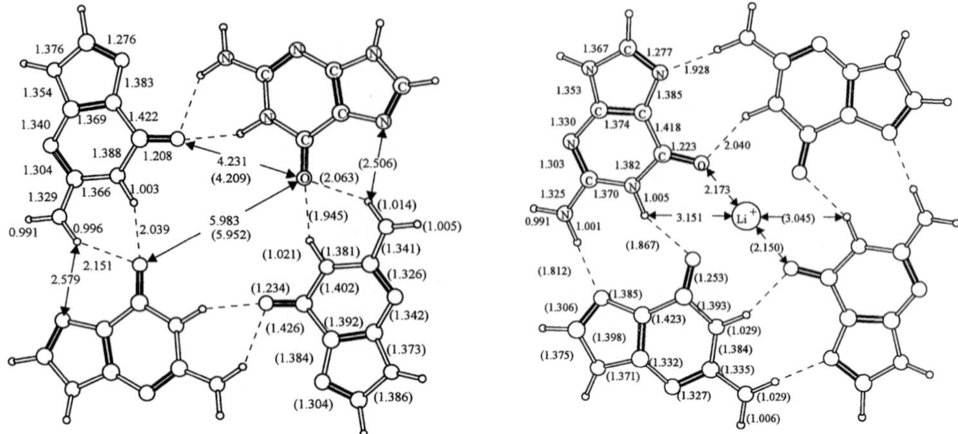

Our recent *ab initio* study of the molecular structure of the G-tetrad (left figure) without the presence of cations has shown that instead of the normal four-stranded Hoogsten-bonded G-tetrad structure, the G-tetrad is stablized by bifurcated hydrogen bonds. To understand how the different types of cation influence the structure of the G-tetraplex, it is necessary to investigate their interactions with the G-tetrad. The comprehensive study of the interaction between metal ions and G-tetrads enable us to address the following issues: Our results confirm the conclusion of Hud et al. that the ion selectivity exhibited by the guanine tetraplexes in water solutions is dominated by relative free energies of hydration. The lower relaxation energy and the smallest geometric distortion of the K^+-G-tetrad in the co-planar form combined with the 26.0 Kcal/mol increase in the K^+-G-tetrads interaction energy in the "sandwich" form enables us to conclude that the potassium cation should be located in the cavity formed by two successive guanine tetrads. The experimental results suggest that there is no such preference for the sodium cation G-tetraplex. Since both the "optimal fit" theory and the "enhanced inner hydrogen bonding" assumption fail to explain the ion selectivity exhibited in the co-planar cation guanine tetrad complexes, the origin of the preferred coordination of K^+ over Na^+ in between two successive guanine tetrads is the ability of K^+ to strengthen the octacoordination-oxygen interactions.

In conclusion, the ab initio technique is especially useful for studies of complexes between DNA components and various metal cations. Our recent studies reveal specific differences between various cations and the large effects of the solvation shell on the metal-base binding and on the base pairing. Based on theoretical results, we predict the enhancement of hydrogen bonding for DNA bases interacting with metal cations. Following those theoretical findings, such base-pairing enhancement has been very recently detected by structural studies and reported by Lippert's group. The results of our calculations allow for the unique interaction of cisplatin with the guanine-cytosine base pair and the bond-pattern alteration in the guanine tetrad by Li+, Na+ and K+ ions to be explained.

Thanks are to financial support from NSF Grant 9805465 and by the ONR Grant N00014-98-1-0592.

Pelmenschikov A., Zilberberg I., Leszczynski J., Famulari A., Sironi M., Raimondi M., *Chem Phys Lett* 1999; 314: 496-500.

Sponer J., Sabat M., Burda J.V., Leszczynski J., Hobza P., *J Phys Chem B* 1999; 103: 2528-34.

Gu J., Leszczynski J., Bansal M., *ChemPhysLett* 1999; 311: 209-14.

Metal Ions in Biology and Medicine; vol 6. Eds. J.A. Centeno, Ph. Collery, G. Vernet, R.B. Finkelman, H. Gibb, J.C. Etienne. John Libbey Eurotext, Paris © 2000, pp. 367-369.

Elucidation of metal binding sites for Ca(II), Mg(II) and Mn(II) in nucleic acid bases using a novel spectrophotometric method

B. Barzami[1], D.S. Shamloo[1], H. Farsam[2], H. Naderimanesh[3], and Sh. Nafisi[4]

[1] Department of Biochemistry, Tehran Medical Sciences University, P.O. Box, 14155-5399 Tehran Iran; [2] Department of Pharmaceutical Chemistry, Faculty of Pharmacy, Tehran Medical Sciences University, Tehran Iran; [3] Department of Biochemistry, Faculty of Basic Science, Tarbiat Modaress University, Tehran, Iran; [4] Department of Chemistry, Azad University, Tehran, Iran

Abstract:
We have employed a novel spectrophotometric method to estimate the sites of metal bindings to some nucleic acid bases using Mg(II), Ca(II) and Mn(II) ions. Several binding characteristics were established both for metal ions and bases. Purine derivatives such as theophylline, theobromine and caffeine were studied as well as some nucleotide bases. The results from purine derivatives were correlated with 13C NMR and FTIR. The data obtained from spectrophotometric method reaveled that the metal ions interacted with specific sites on the nucleotide bases. It was shown that the affinity of Mg(II),Ca(II) and Mn(II) to purines are stronger compared to pyrimidines. The order of binding strengths was shown to be Mn>Ca>Mg for initial ligand formation with the rings. The sites of binding were estimated to be mainly at (C_6=O), N7, Nl and partly with (C_2=0) and N_9 at pH=2.5-3.5 .

Introduction:
The importance of metal ions in cellular processes in general and in nucleic acids in particular,i.e. In synthesis, cleavage, and the stability of DNA has been investigated(1). The use of compound such as cisplatin that enhances the process of apoptosis is known to be via binding to N7 position of guanine ring (2,3). The binding of K^+,Na^+, and Li^+ to nucleotide in gaseous phase revealed that a common trend exists between the three metals. The metal ions form a bidentate ligand with N7 and amino group of adenine. In DNA, the hydrated cation of Mg(II), Ca(II) and Zn(II) were shown to form ligands with N7 of guanine in an octahedral fashion. Ca(II) forms ligand with N7, (C_6=O) of guanin(4). Zn(II) compared could form stronger binding with the organic bases(5). The factors affecting metal ligand binding in nucleic acid bases could be the basicity of sites, steric conditions, the metal ionic parameters, the substituent positioned at neighboring and additionally the kind of metal ions characteristics.(6). In this report we used a novel spectrophotometric method to estimate the metal binding sites in nucleic acid bases. This method was first devised for proteins as well as small molecules such as coenzymes and small peptides (7-9).

Experimental:
All the materials other than nucleic acid bases were purchased from Sigma Chemical Co. (Saint Louis Mo.) and Merck Nucleotide bases were from Pharma Waldhoff Germany, UV 160 recording spectrophotometer Shimadzu throughout experiments. 13C NMR was done using Bruker- DRX 500 AVANCE. 512 scans in 26 minutes. All the UV readings were at 260 and 270 nm. Solutions pH ranged from 2.5-3.5 using buffers with constant ionic strength of 0.1M. In l3C NMR the exact conditions were maintained except that D_2O was partly included in solutions, keeping all the concentrations and pH's constant .
IR measurements were done using infra red spectra recorded on a Bomem MB-100 Fourier Transform Infra red spectrophotometer equipped with a nitrogen cooled HgCdTe detector and a KBr beam splitter. Solution spectra were taken using AgBr windows with resolutions 2-4 cm^{-1} and 20 scans. H_2O subtraction is carried with a high efficiency as it was shown by the flat baseline near 2200 cm^{-1} where the water contribution mode is located (10) .

Results and discussions:
The amplitudes of d(dA)dpH vs pH where dA is the change in absorbance due to metal and dpH is the change in pH is shown in Fig(1) for nucleotides and derivatives at pH's 2.5-3.5 where the main bands with metal ions appeared. The height
of bars represent the intensity of interactions of metal ions with bases at pH's between 2.5 and 3.5. All the metal ions under study showed interactions at specific pH's. We undertook the analysis of the main bands appeared initially at this range of pH and tried to correlate the data with 13C NMR to substantiate our

findings. The initial analysis of data was specified for nucleotide derivatives Theophylline, Theobromine and Caffeine. The following tables depict the results for such studies.

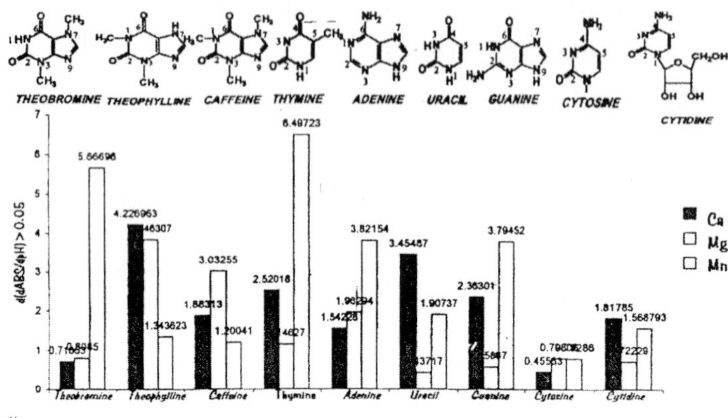

(fig 1)

Table I: Amplitudes of peaks of d(dA)/dpH as a means to evaluate the strength of binding between the metal ions and nucleotide derivatives.

Nucleotide derivatives	Ca(II)	Mg(II)	Mn(II)
Thephylline	4.2	3.8	1.3
Theobromine	0.7	0.8	5.6
Caffeine	1.9	3.0	1.2

Table I I: 13C NMR shifts produced by metal ion interactions with nucleotide derivatives.

Ring atoms	R_1	R_2	C_8	C_4	C_5	C_2	C_6	R_2
Theophylline–Ca	0	-5	-2.3	+1.1	+2.3	-4	-2.1	0
Theophylline–Mg	0	-7	-2.0	+2	+3	-1.9	-3.5	0
Caffeine + Ca	0	+2	-1.8	+1	0	-1.7	-2.2	0
Caffeine+ Mg	0	-2	-1.9	0	-4	-2.3	-2.6	0

From the data shown , the downfield shifts in 13C NMR that are represented by negative values are stronger in (C_6=O) and C_8 for Theophylline bonded to Mg(II). The C_8 shift may be a metal binding interaction with N_7 or N_1 .Due to paramagnetic quality of Mn(II) and the strong interference of noise with the resonance peaks, we were unable to use Mn(II) in 13C NMR experiments. From the UV data alone the interaction of Ca(II) and Mg(II) with theobromine was far less significant for Mg and Ca but showed a strong band for Mn(II). This may point to the fact that in the structure of theobromine the position at (C_6=O), N_1 and (C_2=O) are available in pyrimidine ring for Mn to bind freely with at least two ligand to the three adjacent eletron donating atoms (C_6=O). N_1, (C_2=O). It is noteworthy to mention that both the amplitudes of interactions as obtained from UV experiments and the chemical shifts obtained from 13C NMR show that possibly (C_6=O) is more reactive than (C_2=O) with the metal ions under study. Our results with nucleotide bases such as guanine, adenine, thymine, uracil and cytosine, could show this structure reactivity relationship. Although the 13C NMR was used as a second tool to confirm further our results, but several conclusions could be drawn independently from using the spectrophotometric method for these compounds. For example the trends of reactivity of the rings with Mn(II) are in compounds where the three components of the ring are available: (C6=O), N3, (C2=O) in purines and (C4=O), N3, (C2=O) in pyrimidines (Table 2).

The strong absorption band at 1669 cm^{-1} in the IR spectrum of caffeine could be assigned to the exocyclic stretching vibrations. Minor spectral changes were observed for this band in the spectra of metal-caffeine complexes.The absorption band at 1980 cm^{-1} could be assigned to the exocyclic (C6=O) stretching vibrations. The major spectral changes for this band was in the order of Mn>Mg>Ca. Other spectral changes were at 1620-1650 cm^{-1}, that was assigned to the change in hydrogen bond network due to the interactions with metals at imidazole ring with the metal ions under study. Comparing the results obtained from IR spectra and 13C NMR with the parameter d(dA)/pH calculated from spectral changes in ultraviolet absorption bands, it can be concluded that the results obtained correlated closely both in the site and the strength of metal bindings.

Table 3

Compound	Amplitude for Mn(II) interaction	Amplitude for Mg(II) interaction	Ratio of amplitudes Mn/Mg
Thymine	6.5	1.1	5.9
Uracil	1.9	0.4	4.7
Guanine	3.8	0.6	6.5
Theobromine	5.6	0.8	7.1

Furthermore a direct relationship was observed between the strength of binding of metal ions to bases (Table 3) as could be obtained from the amplitudes of d(dA)dpH. Some metal parameters such as melting point, boiling point vaporization, and heat of atomization showed to contain similar order of increasing quantity as their binding capacity to nucleotide bases (Mn>Ca>Mg). All the metal ion bonds with purines were significantly stronger than with pyrimidines as shown in the following table:

Table 3

Bases	Absolute value of bonding Mg(II)	Within row % Interaction Mg(II)	Absolute value of bonding Ca(II)	Within row % Interaction Ca(II)	Absolute value of bonding Mn(II)	Within row % Interaction Mn(II)
Purines	10.2	27.7	10.7	29	15.8	43
Pyrimidines	2.3	13.2	6.4	35.7	9.2	51.6

The presence of methyl group on the ring was shown to be favorable for stronger bindings. In conclusion we hope to continue this line of studies with the hopes that more information could be obtained regarding the nature of these bindings and quantitative informations regarding the bond strengths.

Acknowledgement:

We thank Pharma Waldhoff for their kind donation of nucleotide bases. We also thank Mr. Hamid Reza Bijanzadeh expert cooperation for preparation of 13C NMR Scans. Dr. Hamid Reza Zamaniazadeh for making the FTIR available, Miss Zamani for FTIR scan preparationsand Mr. Ali Shamsaie for his kind assistance in preparing the manuscript.

Refereces:

1-Goodman & Gilman, In: The Pharmacological Basis of Therapeutics ,8th ed.,1992

2- Saenger W, In: Principles of nucleic acid structures, pp 105-113 (1983)

3- Takahara P M, Rosenweig A C, Fradrick C A & Lippard S, Nature, 1995, 377, pp 649-652

4- Sponer J, Burda J V, Sabat M, Leszczynski J and Hobza P, J. Phys. Chem. A., 1998, 102 ,pp 5951

5- Cerado B A, Wesdemiotis C, J. Am. Chem. Soc., 1996, 118, pp 11884-11892

6- Lippert B, J. Chem. Soc., Dalton Trans., 1997, pp. 3971-3976

7- Farzami B, In:Protein Structure Function Relationship (Editors: Z H Zaidi, Smith P), Plenum Press, 1996

8- Farzami B, Moosavi A A and Naderi G A, Int. J. Biol. Macromolec., 1994, 16,4,181.

9- Farzami B, Kuimov,A N, Kochetov G A, In: Metal Ions in Biology and Medicine (Editors:Ph Col Poirier, N A Littlefield, J C Etienne, Th Theophanides), John Libbey Eurotext, Paris,399-404.

10- Aiex S, and P Dupuis, Inorg. Chem Acta , 1988,157,271-281.

Metal Ions in Biology and Medicine; vol 6. Eds. J.A. Centeno, Ph. Collery, G. Vernet, R.B. Finkelman, H. Gibb, J.C. Etienne. John Libbey Eurotext, Paris © 2000, pp. 370-372.

Mg(II) and Mn(II) complexes of cytosine and 1-methyl-cytosine: vibrational spectra

J. Anastassopoulou[1], T. Theophanides[1], B. Sombret[2], J.-P. Huvaine[2] and P. Legrand[2]

[1] *National Technical University of Athens, Radiation Chemistry and Biospectroscopy, Zografou Campus, 15780 Zografou, Greece;* [2] *University of Science and Technology, Chemistry Department, Lille, Villeneuve d'Ascq, France*

Abstract

We have studied the FT-Raman spectra of Mg(II) and Mn(II) complexes with the nucleic bases cytosine and 1-Methyl cytosine. The spectra have been analyzed in relation to their crystal structures that have been resolved recently. The Raman spectra reveal interesting differences in the vibrational frequencies of the nucleic bases linked to the life metals (Mg,Mn), as well as in the frequencies of the coordinated water. The spectra are indicative of the presence of supramolecular assemblies and extended hydrogen bonding in the systems. The Raman spectra of the solid materials, as well as the aqueous solutions of the materials will be presented and discussed.

Introduction

The investigation of Mg(II) and Mn(II) complexes with nucleic bases cytosine and 1-Methyl cytosine is of great importance, because these are life metals. The new Metal-base complexes have been prepared in biological conditions in water and their aquo complexes have been compared as far as the chemical compounds they form in water and which can be isolated from water solutions[1]. In particular, their vibrtional spectra will be analyzed and compared[2]. The crystal structure of Mg(II) aquo complex has been reported previously[3]. It was found that the hexaaquo complex displays a hydrogen bonding network and stabilizes a supramolecular assembly containing octahedral $[Mg(H_2O)_6]^{2+}$ units surrounded by six 1-Methyl-cytosine molecules, which are linked to the water molecules of coordination water by hydrogen bonding.

In this report we have studied the Fourier Transform Raman spectra of both complexes and the spectral analysis shows the extended hydrogen bonding that takes place in these compounds, which stabilizes the supramolecular assemblies.

Materials and Methods

The $Mg(ClO_4)_2$ and $Mn(ClO_4)_2$ salts and the nucleic bases cytosine (cyt) and 1-methyl cytosine (1-Mecyt) were purchased from Sigma. Mixing the salt and the nucleic base in water in 1:1 ratio we performed the preparation of the complexes. The chemical compounds were formed in solution and then were left the solution for a long time to form crystals, which were collected and studied.

The Fourier Transform Raman spectra were recorded with a Brucker FT-Raman spectrophotometer. The resolution was 4 cm^{-1}, with 200 accumulations in the 4000-700 cm^{-1} region applying surface analysis 50 μm.

Results and Discussion

The FT-Raman spectra for Mn(II) are given in Table 1. The spectra of both complexes show changes in some of the frequencies of the bases. In addition, the vibrations of the coordinated and crystal water are very strong and show strong hydrogen bonding with very large bands in the region of 3600-3200 cm^{-1}.

Table 1. FT-Raman spectral data of Mn(II) complexes with the nucleic bases cytosine and 1-Methyl cytosine and tentative assignments

Mn –1-Mecyt	Mn-cyt	cyt	1-Mecyt	assignments
3630	3622			Free νO-H
	3536		3541	νO-H H-b
3452	3459		3404	νN-H
3330	3366		3315	νH_2O H-b
3222	3213	3180	3224	νNH_2 H-b
3101			3091	νCH aromatic
1655	1669	1655	1655	νC=O
	1632			δH_2O
1609	1616	1607	1625	νC=C
1535	1521	1520	1528	δNH_2
1504	1506	1505	1489	νC=N
1440	1461	1468	1435	νC=N
1425	1425		1421	$\delta asCH_3$+ νC=N
1384	1364	1340	1381	δsCH_3
1331	1309			
1272	1291	1260	1294	$\nu C\text{-}NH_2$
	1243		1242	νC-N + νC-C
1220	1220	1225		νC-C+νC-N
1105	1087			νClO_4^-
973	998		989	νC-O
962	966			νC-C
932	931			
793	811	810	785	ring breathing
720	795		727	out-of-plane-NH_2

We observe slight changes in the carbonyl group due to hydrogen bonding. The $-NH_2$ group also is forming strong hydrogen bonding which slightly perturbs the double carbon-nitrogen bonds. The ring breathing mode also is slightly perturbed. However, the strong changes are shown only in the absorption of water in the complexes formed.

The magnesium complexes show similar trends in the spectra, indicating that the complexes are isostructural.

Referencies

1. Theophanides T, Interactions des Acides Nucleiques avec les Metaux, *Can. J. Spectr.*, 1981: **26**, 165-179.
2. Theophanides T, Vibrational Spectroscopy of Metal Nucleic Acids Systems, in *Infrared and Raman Spectra of Biological Molecules*, 1979 (ed. T. Theophanides), D. Reidel Publishing Co, Dodrecht, Holland, p. 205-223
3. Geday M A, De Munno G, Medaglia M, Anastasopoulou J & Theophanides T, Supramolecular assemblies containing Nucleic Bases and Magnesium (II) Hexahydrate Ions, *Angewante Chemie, Int. Ed. Engl.*, 1997: **36**, 511-513.

Metal Ions in Biology and Medicine; vol 6. Eds. J.A. Centeno, Ph. Collery, G. Vernet, R.B. Finkelman, H. Gibb, J.C. Etienne. John Libbey Eurotext, Paris © 2000, pp. 373-378.

Surface-enhanced Raman scattering study of the interaction of carboplatin with glycine, serine, cysteine, cystine and methionine

Wilmer Carrión, Samuel P. Hernández, Mayra E. Cádiz and Carmen A. Vega

Department of Chemistry, University of Puerto Rico-Mayagüez, P.O. Box 9019, Mayagüez, Puerto Rico, 00681-9019

Abstract:

Carboplatin is a platinum compound widely used in cancer chemotherapy. The characterization of its complexes with sulfur rich molecules is relevant in clinical aspects such as toxicity and circumvention of resistance. Reaction mixtures of carboplatin with the sulfur-containing molecules cysteine, cystine and methionine were prepared at a 1:1 molar ratio in PIPES buffer, pH 6.5. Different samples were incubated at 37 °C for 24 and 48 h. Reaction mixtures with glycine and serine were also prepared for comparison purposes. The surface-enhanced Raman spectrum of carboplatin and those of its reaction products were taken over silver colloids. Changes with incubation time of the Pt-N stretching band at 542 cm^{-1} suggest binding of serine and glycine through their NH_2 moiety. The strong intensity of this band with serine, when compared to glycine, suggests a contribution from the Pt-O stretching. When carboplatin was incubated with cysteine, cystine, and methionine, bands in the 344-359 cm^{-1} and 439 -535 cm^{-1} regions were observed, which were assigned to Pt-S and Pt-N stretching frequencies, respectively. This suggests chelation of Pt via both S and N atoms. The changes observed for the Raman bands with variations in incubation time evidenced the formation of adducts between carboplatin and all the molecules studied at pH = 6.5.

Introduction:

Cisplatin [*cis*-$PtCl_2(NH_3)_2$]and carboplatin [$Pt(NH_3)_2$(CBDA-*O,O'*)] are platinum(II) compounds used for the treatment a variety of cancers [1]. Although platinum(II) drugs exert their anti-tumor activity by cross-linking DNA, blocking its replication and transcription, it has been suggested that the interaction of these drugs with sulfur-rich molecules might be implicated in the inactivation the drugs, nephrotoxicity, and the mechanism for acquired resistance. In the case of carboplatin, sulfur amino acids have been proposed as potential nucleophiles in the activation of the slowly hydrolyzing complex [2]. Complexes of platinum(II) with amino acids of various stoichiometries and formulae have been reported [3]. In an effort to provide further insight into the binding of carboplatin to amino acids, we have used Surface Enhanced Raman Spectroscopy (SERS) to follow these interactions with variations in incubation time.

Materials and Methods:

Carboplatin was a gift from Bristol Myers Squibb Co. Stock solutions (2.0 mM) of glycine, serine, cysteine, methionine, and carboplatin were dissolved in 10 mM PIPES buffer, pH 6.5. Reaction mixtures with equimolar amounts were prepared by combining 5.0mL of each. These 10 samples were incubated at 37 °C for 24 h and 48 h. SERS analyses of these reaction mixtures were performed over silver colloids at the end of each time period. Each sample was prepared by 100 µL of sodium perchlorate (Aldrich), 800 µL of the colloid, and 100 µL of the reaction mixture. SERS spectra of both carboplatin and each amino acid were also recorded. Silver colloids were prepared according to the method of Lee and Meisel [4]. The spectra were taken on a Jobin-Ybon T64000 triple Raman spectrograph using a 514.5 nm argon ion laser and CCD detector.

Results:

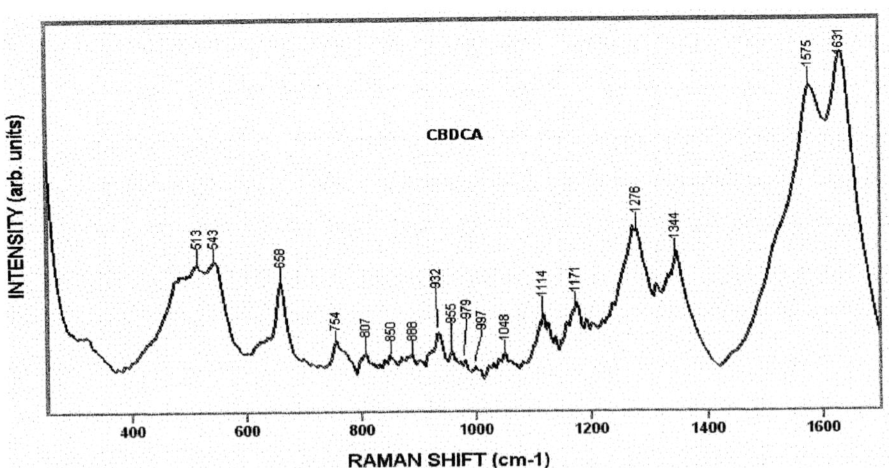

Figure 1. SERS spectra of carboplatin, [CBDCA]

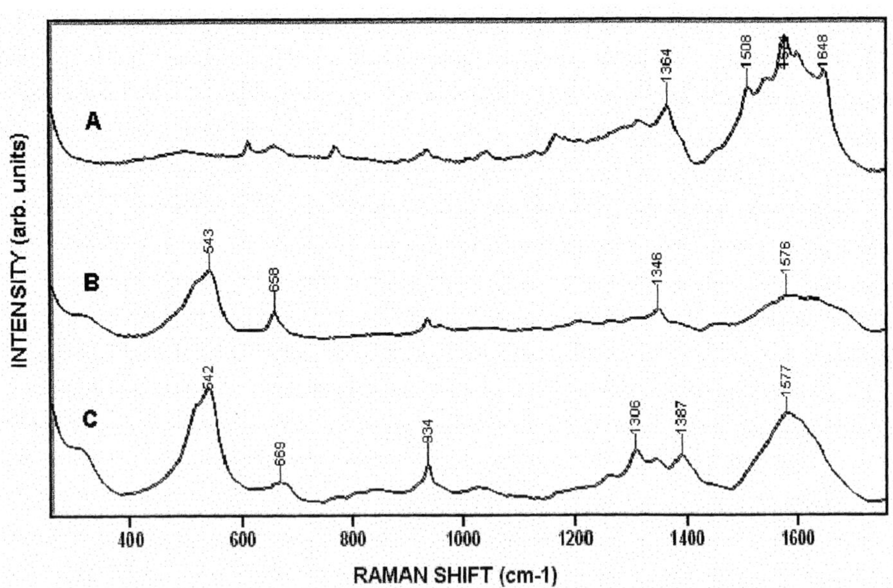

Figure 2. SERS spectra of glycine in free form (A), 24 hours of interaction with carboplatin (B), 48 hours of interaction with carboplatin (C).

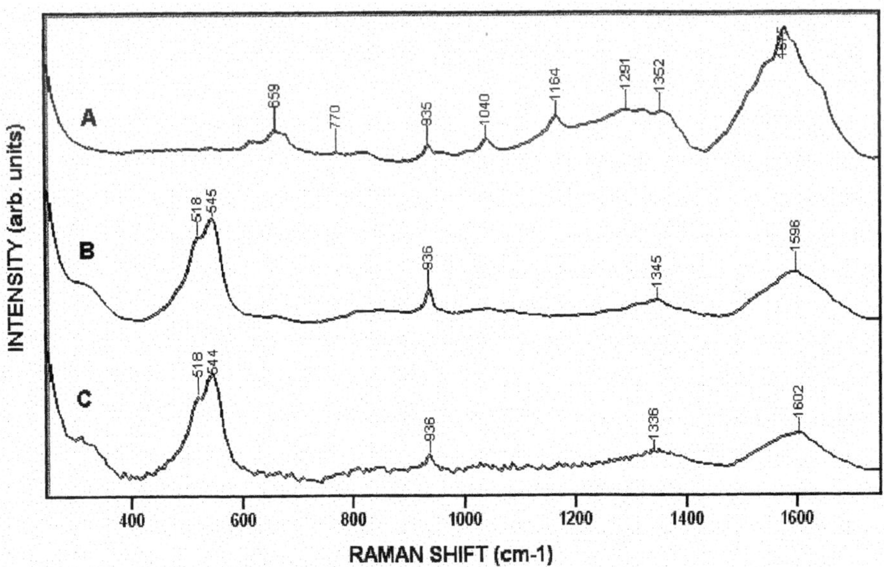

Figure 3. SERS spectra of serine in free form (A), 24 hours of interaction with carboplatin (B), 48 hours of interaction with carboplatin (C).

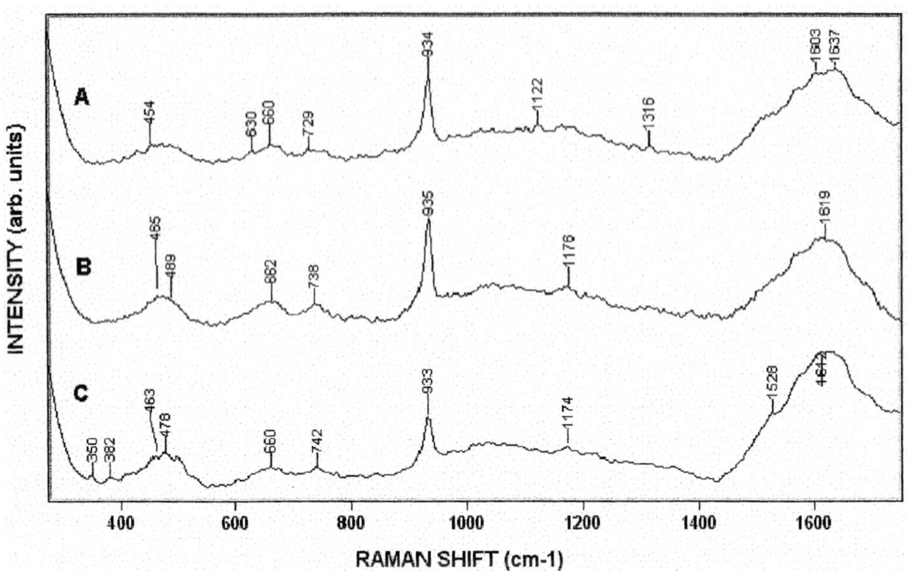

Figure 4. SERS spectra of cysteine in free form (A), 24 hours of interaction with carboplatin (B), 48 hours of interaction with carboplatin (C).

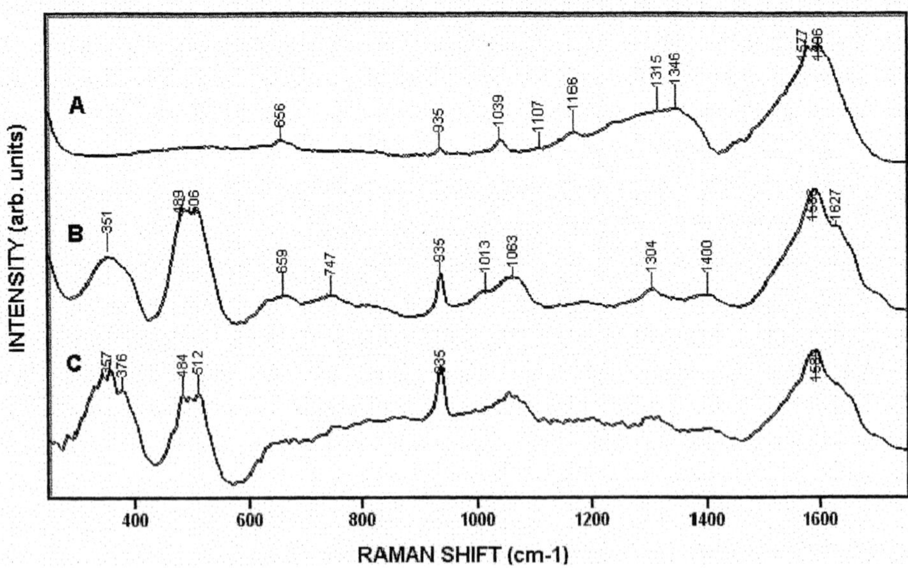

Figure 5. SERS spectra of cystine in free form (A), 24 hours of interaction with carboplatin (B), 48 hours of interaction with carboplatin (C).

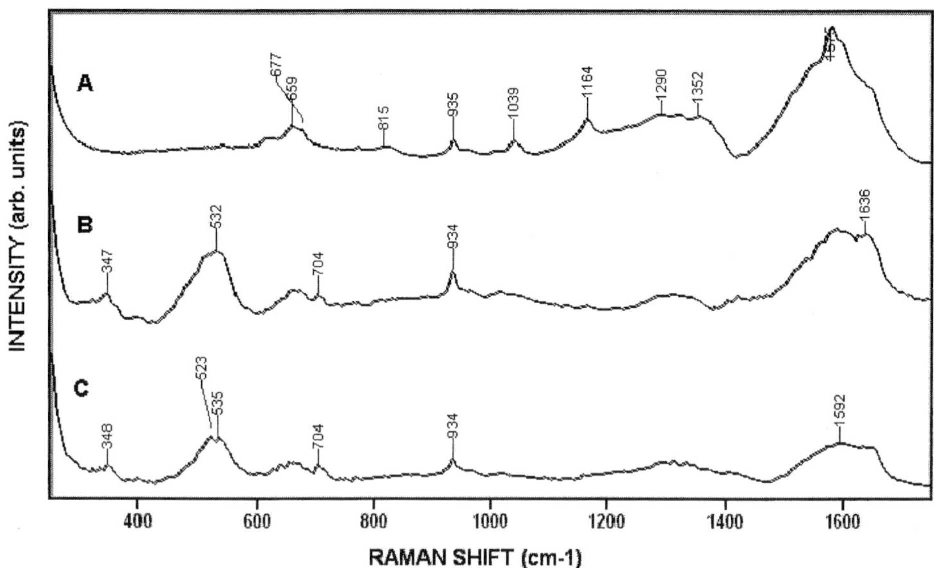

Figure 6. SERS spectra of methionine in free form (A), 24 hours of interaction with carboplatin (B), 48 hours of interaction with carboplatin (C).

Discussion:

Figure 1 shows the SERS spectrum of carboplatin. The bands at 1631 cm^{-1} and 1575 cm^{-1} are assigned to the C=O, and NH_3 stretching, respectively. The NH_3 bending appears at 1344 cm^{-1} and 1276 cm^{-1}. The characteristic Pt-NH_3 stretching bands are observed at 543 cm^{-1} and 512 cm^{-1} [5]. The SERS spectra of glycine and its complexes are shown in Figure 2. The more intense bands in the free glycine spectrum are those in the 1627 cm^{-1} - 1508 cm^{-1} region (COO^- and NH_3 stretching). After 24 h of incubation with carboplatin, noticeable changes are observed around 1350 cm^{-1} (C-O stretching). After 48 hours, changes in intensity and shifts of the bands in the 1306-1387 cm^{-1} region are evident. The relative intensity of the broad band at 543 cm^{-1}, compared with the band at 1577 cm^{-1}, suggests an overlap of the Pt-NH_3 stretching bands with Pt-N or Pt-O stretching bands of glycine complexes [3]. The spectra of serine and those of its interactions with carboplatin are shown in Figure 3. Serine bands were tentatively assigned as follows: 1604 cm^{-1} (C=O stretching); 1552 cm^{-1} and 1510 cm^{-1} (NH_3 stretching), 1291 cm^{-1}(C-OH bending); 1040- and 1010 cm^{-1} (out of phase CCO^- stretching) and 965 cm^{-1} (in-phase stretching of COO^-) [5]. After incubation with carboplatin, the more intense bands of the spectra are those at 518 cm^{-1} and 545 cm^{-1}, related to Pt-O and Pt-N stretching. These changes are consistent with the formation of a Pt complex with serine through both nitrogen and oxygen atoms.

Figure 4 shows the SERS spectra of cysteine and its complexes. A tentative assignment of bands is the following: 1637 cm^{-1}(COO^- stretching), 1506-1572 cm^{-1} region (NH_3 deformation), 728 cm^{-1} and 662 cm^{-1} (C-S stretching) [5]. The most significant changes in the spectra of the cysteine complexes are the shift of the C-S stretching band from 728 cm^{-1} to 740 cm^{-1}, and the presence of a Pt-S stretching band at 351 cm^{-1}. The formation of a new band at 478 cm^{-1} also suggests Pt-N binding, and a bidentate behavior for cysteine. The SERS spectra of cystine and of its complexes are shown in figure 5. Cystine has COO^- stretching, NH_3^+ stretching and the NH_3^+ wagging frequencies at 1596 cm^{-1}, 1579 cm^{-1} and 1038 cm^{-1}, respectively. At 24 h, very strong bands appeared at 351 cm^{-1} and 512 cm^{-1}, corresponding to Pt-S and Pt-N stretchings, respectively. The spectrum for the 48 h interaction is almost similar to the one for 24h, except for a considerable increase in intensity in the Pt-S band. These results also suggest a bidentate mode of binding of cystine to Pt. Figure 6 shows the SERS spectra of methionine and its complexes. Methionine shows characteristic C=O and NH_3^+ stretching bands at 1696 cm^{-1} and 1545 cm^{-1}, respectively. When methionine is incubated with carboplatin, bands appeared at 347 cm^{-1} and 541 cm^{-1}, which can be assigned to Pt-S and Pt-N bonds, respectively. This is consistent with a bidentate interaction of methionine with platinum.

One can conclude from these experiments that, under mildly acidic conditions, carboplatin is able to bind to all the studied amino acids. A bidentate mode of binding seems to take place with serine, cysteine, cystine, and methionine.

References:

1. Pil P, Lippard SJ. Cisplatin and related drugs. *Encyclopedia of Cancer* 1997; 1 : 392-410.

2. Frey U, Ranford JD, Sadler PJ. Ring-opening reactions of the anticancer drug carboplatin: NMR characterization of cis-[Pt(NH_3)$_2$(CBDCA-*O*)(5'-GMP-*N7*)] in solution. *Inorg Chem* 1993; 32 : 1333-1340.

3. Iakovidis A, Hadjiliadis N. Complex compounds of platinum(II) and (IV) with amino acids, peptides and their derivatives. *Coord Chem Rev* 1994; 135/136 : 17-63.

4. Lee PC, and Meisel D. Adsorption and surface-enhanced Raman of dyes on silver and gold sols. *J Phys Chem* 1982; 86: 3391-3395.

5. Nakamoto K. Infrared and Raman Spectra of Inorganic and Coordination Compounds: Applications in Coordination, Organometallic, and Bioinorganic Chemistry. 5th ed, 1997, John Wiley & Sons.

Metal Ions in Biology and Medicine; vol 6. Eds. J.A. Centeno, Ph. Collery, G. Vernet, R.B. Finkelman, H. Gibb, J.C. Etienne. John Libbey Eurotext, Paris © 2000, pp. 379-381.

Thermodynamic and kinetic parameter changes in chymotrysin and trypsin due to Ca(II) ligation

Bijan Farzami[1], Sakineh Kazemi Noureini and Hossain Naderimanesh[2]

[1] *Department of Biochemistry, Tehran Medical Sciences University, P.O. Box 14155-5399 Tehran Iran; and [2] Department of Biochemistry, Faculty of Basic Sciences, Tabriat Modaress University*

Abstract:
The thermal and urea denaturation techniques were used to elucidate the thermal stability of trypsin and chymotrypsin and the effect of Ca(II) ion was evaluated to estimate stabilities of these enzyme,. It was found that Ca(II) ion could enhance thermal stability of trypsin by 2 °C and of chymotypsin by 1.7°C . Thus the free energy and enthalpy of denaturation were found to be enhanced by 17.8 and 172 Kj/mole in chymotrypsin respectively. The heat capacity was found to be unaffected, but the entropy of denaturation was slightly enhanced by the effect of Ca(II). The stabilities of both proteins were enhanced by the effect of Ca(II) ion determined spectrophotometrically and in urea denaturation experiments. Thus [Dl/2] for trypsin in the absence of Ca(II) ion was 5.5M. and in presence of Ca(II) was 6.0 M. These values for chymotrypsin were found to be 5.8 M. and 6.3M. respectively. The corresponding results obtained from urea denaturation using PAGE were 5.2 M. and 6.2 M.. for trypsin and 5.2 M. and 6.5 M. for chymotrypsin.

Introduction:
Conformational stabilities of globular proteins are commonly evaluated by quantities such as free energy of denatuaration (ΔG den.), ligand binding energy and catalytic activity. and in many instances a retrospective relationship exists in such determinations. Serine proteases seem to be suitable models for studying the relationship between different parameters such as energy and cooperativity, conformational stability, folding, catalytic activity, and ligand binding(1). The Ca(II) binding sites in serine proteases is generally Asp. Glu. Val. The X-ray crystallographic studies had indicated that the Ca(II) binding site of trypsin forms hexacoordinated ligands with Ca(II) in an octaherral structure through Glu 70, Asn 72, Val 75, Glu 80 and two water molecules (2). The Ca(II) binding locus is at least 10 °A away form the catalytic site(3). In this report the effect of Ca(II) ligand on the conformational stability of enzyme was tested. The comparisons between these two enzymes could distinguish similarities as well as differences relating to their chemical and evolutional entities. (4). To this effect a non ionic denaturant, urea was used. This compound could disrupt hydrogen bonds and enhance stability of polar and apolar groups. It could reduce the hydrophobic interactions to the extent of 30% (5). The non-ionic additives could lower protein stability because they are repelled by polar groups on the protein surface, but due to their interactions with the nonpolar surfaces that are opened to the solvent, could reduce the folding stability of proteins (6). Furthermore, kinetic parameters obtained from binding studies of trypsin and chymotrypsin to inhibitors revealed changes toward higher stabilities with Ca(II) ligand.

Experimental
Heat denaturation:
UV differential spectrophotometric technique was used by employing Gilford spectrophotometer instrument equipped with a thermostat and an automatic temperature control. The temperature rate increase was maintained at one degree centigrade per minute. The differential UV absorption was measured for the solutions of enzyme with or without Ca (II) against 0.5 M tris or acetate buffer at pH=6 and temperature change of 32-84°C.
Urea denaturation analysis using UV spectrophotometric techniques:
In this method buffers containing 0.1 M tris acetate (pH=5) and variable concentrations of urea from 3 to 8 M were prepared, The samples prepared having 8.54×10^{-4} M. trypsin or 3.27 micro molar chymotrypsin with or without Ca(II)(0.02 M) in the above buffers. All samples were incubated at 4 °C in dark for 24 hrs. and were read at 297 nm. This absroption is mainly due to indole rings. All the tests were run in quadruplicates.
Kinetic analysis using specific protease inhibitors:
The proteolytic enzymes were first depleted of Ca(ll) by using sephadex G50 column to strip off the Ca(II) at pH 3.5. The enzyme obtained was incubated partly for at least 15 minutes with about 100 fold Ca(II) at pH=7.5 . The inhibition was carried out using several concentrations of inhibitors in each run. Aliquots

were then used to estimate the inhibition rate Constants.The substrates used in these experiments were PNPA, CBZ-Ala-PNA, and inhibitors were PMSF. TPCK and TLCK.

Results:

The results obtained from thermal denaturation indicates that Ca (II) could cause an increase in thermal stabilization of these two enzymes by 2°C in trypsin and 1.7°C in chymotrypsin. (Table l). ΔG(den.) in different temperatures shows the effect of Ca(II) in thermal stabilities of each of the enzymes.
The estimated values are depicted in the following table:

	Trypsin No Ca(II)	Trypsin +Ca(II)	Chymotrypsin -Ca(II)	Chymotrypsin +Ca(II)
TmK	333	335	327.3	328.8
ΔS 25 (KJ/mole)	1.52	2.03	1.43	1.9
ΔHm (KJ/mole)	508	680	463.5	625.37
ΔG 25(KJ/mole)	33	51.28	24	44
ΔCp (KJ/mole)	11.5	12.7	12.9	12.4
ΔHm (KJ/mole)	----	172	----	161.9
ΔΔG den(KJ/mole)	----	17.8	----	20

The results obtained from spectrophotometric method in different urea concentration indicated that Ca(II) the stability of the proteins by increasing Dl/2 by one unit of urea concentration. The primary experiments in this laboratory shows that the normal electrophoresis of these proteins in urea concentration gradient on polyacrylamide gel indicates that the folding of these two proteins are fast and reversible and the mechanism of their foldings obeys a two state trend. This type of mechanism was first suggested for these enzymes by Privalov (1979). Similar results were obtained in trypsinogen by Bulaj (1994). The results showing the enhancement of stability by Ca(II) correlated well in urea denaturation experiment, thermal denaturation and electrophoresis using urea concentration gradient. Furthermore the kinetic behavior of protein changed towards the specific inhibitors of the enzymes when they were associated with Ca(II). From inhibition rate constant ki and the inhibitory constant Ki, the ratio for ki/Ki was determined for Ca(II) associated enzymes and their free forms.The results showed that the enzymes were more protected against the action of inhibitors when they were associated with Ca(II).

Table2

Enzyme	Inhibitor	Substrate	pH	ki(min)	Ki.10^{-5} M	ki/Ki
trypsin + Ca	PMSF	PNPA	8.1	1.89	86	22
trypsin	PMSF	PNPA	8.1	1.54	4	3.82
trypsin + Ca	TLCK	PNPA	8.1	0.8	9.2	0.87
trypsin	TLCK	PNPA	8.1	0.57	2.7	2.11
Chymotrypsin +Ca(II)	TPCK	PNPA	8.15	1.25	5.2	2.40
chymotrypsin	TPCK	PNPA	8.15	0.97	1.2	8.1

The kinetic data, although can not be fully regarded as a corroborative means to the thermodynamic data presented in this report but the resistance towards inhibition caused by Ca(II) could be indicative of a conformation induced by the metal that is more compact than its free form. This conformation would possibly affect the binding site of the enzyme in such a way that although it would enhance the rate for its substrate to about 4 times, but could not be accomodative to an inhibitor that is not fully specific as the substrate.

Acknowledgement:

We thank Mr. Ali Shamsaie for his kind assistance in preparing the manuscript.

Reference:

1. Bode W J, Mol. Biol., 1979, 127: 57-374
2. Glusker J P, Advances in protein chemistry, USA Academic Press,1991, PP: 3-66
3. a: Adebodun F, Jordan, F. Biochemistry,1989, 28, 7524
   b: Adebodun F, Jordan, F. J. Cell. Biochem,1989, 40:249-260
4. Neuzath H et al, Science,1960, 158: 1638-1644
5. Doig A J and Williams D H, J. Mol. Biol.,1993, 217, 389-398
6. Creighlon T E, Proteins (2nd ed.),1993, PP. 293-296

Abbreviations:

PMSF; Phenylmethyl Sulfonyl Floride, TLCK; Tosyl Lysine Chloromethyl ketone, TPCK; Tosyl Phenyl Alanine Chloromethyl Ketone, PNPA; Para Nitro Phenyl Acetate

Metal Ions in Biology and Medicine; vol 6. Eds. J.A. Centeno, Ph. Collery, G. Vernet, R.B. Finkelman, H. Gibb, J.C. Etienne. John Libbey Eurotext, Paris © 2000, pp. 382-385.

Defective role of glycated albumin in transporting Ca(II) in diabetic sera: an evidence obtained by equilibrilum dialysis binding studies and microtitration

Bijan Farzami[1], Soudabeh Banazadeh[1], Shahab Eldin Sadr[2], Hamid Reza Pazoki Toroudi[2]

[1] *Department of Biochemistry, Tehran Medical Sciences University P.O. Box 14155-5399;* [2] *Department of Physiology, TehranMedical Sciences University Tehran, Iran*

Abstract:
Equilibrium dialysis showed that both glycated BSA or HSA could bind more freely to Ca(II) than their nonglycated forms. Albumin purified from diabetic sera showed similar trends. Microtitration of glycated albumin revealed that glycation occurs at pH ranges where lysyl residues are most dissociating (pH 9-11). Ca(II) affinity with glycated albumin was enhanced compared to normal albumin at pH ranges where aspartate and glutamate residues are most prone to bind to Ca(II) (pH=2.5-5.5). These results point to the fact that nonenzymatic glycation of albumin could alter spatial conformation of albumin in such a way that Ca(II) could gain more access to the interior parts of the molecule as could be evidenced by the two independent methods.

1- Introduction:

There are some evidences that glycation may contribute to alteration of function in some proteins such as albumine in diabetis(1). This protein which comprises about 60% of plasma proteins, has its main role in transporting an unusually broad spectrum of ligands (2,3). Some of the bindings may be with endogenous (e. g bilirubin, tryptophan, fatty acids and Ca(II))(4,5) and some with exogenous, e.g. drugs and dye substances (6,7). In present study we used an equilibrium technique to study the changes in molecular affinity of glycated albumin relative to normal albumin. We also report apparent binding properties of albumin extracted from human normal serum and that of diabetics. Further we indentified both the sites of glycation and observed an increase in Ca(II) binding sites in glycated form of albumin .This increase could be due to changes in molecular parameters caused by glycation.

2. Experimental

2.1 Purifucation of HSA:
Human serum albumin was purified from fresh normal serum and diabetic serum according to Mc Menammy (1971), HSA was defatted by the acid charcoal treatment, (Chen, 1967(9)).

2.2 Equilibrium dialysis with Ca(II):
The purified HAS and the HAS obtained from diabetic sera from the first stage, were adjusted for 0.25 g/100 ml with HEPES buffer (0.05 M. pH=7.4). The final Ca(II) concentrations in dialysis compartments were 45, 35, 25,15,5 mM. Each dialysis sector contained 23 ml of solution. The dialysis was carried out against similar concentrations of HEPES buffer on a mixing rotator for 48 hours.

2.3 Ca(II) selective electrode:
The content of dialysis compartments were analyzed for free Ca(II) selective electrode (Philipps; sensitivity, $0.04\text{-}4\times10^{-4}$ *ppm).* The ionic strength was adjusted in all samples with saturated KCl in dialysis solutions. After proper calibration of instrument with $CaCl_2$ standards equipped with the instrument, the free Ca(II) was measured in all the dialyzed samples.

2.4 Atomic absorption spectroscopy:
Shimadzu AA-680 equipped with GFA-48X Flameless graphite furance atomic absorption was used in all determinations The samples were deproteinated by a solution of 10% trichloroacetic acid. After calibration of instrument with standard solution of calcium chloride, the measurements were carried out. Thus the bound and free calcium ions were measured in the supernatant constituting the total calcuim ion. Strontium chloride was used in all solutions to avoid the errors caused by phosphate and sulphate (10).

2.5 Preparation of glycosylated BSA:
Bovine serum albumin was obtained from Sigma chemical Co (Saint Louis Mo., USA). 25ml of a solution of 2% albumin was prepared. 12.5 ml was spared and to the rest, 0.25g of glucose monohydrate (Merck)

was added. The solution was then filtered through 0.2 μm thick filter in strict sterile condition. The filtrate was sealed in a sterile tube and this was kept under strict sterile condition for further use. These processes were also applied for the 12.5ml of 2% albumin solution that did not contain glucose. Both preparations were kept at 37°C for 160 hrs (one week) in dark and sterile condition (11). Contents were then transferred to dialysis bags and dialyzed against distilled water for 24 hrs. These solutions were used for equilibrium dialysis.

2.6 Normal and glycated albumin titration:
The design of a titration method for polyelectrolytes such as proteins that have more than 60 ionizable groups for every 20 KD molecular weight is cumbersome and subject to variations. Nevertheless we used equal protein concentration and glycated albumin (0.05%) in an unbuffered solution containing 50mM KCl and compared the trend of titration in each specimen. The autotitration assembly equipped with autoburette and a pH-meter (Radiometer Coppenhagen, Denmark, model RTS 822). In titration, the solution pH was adjusted to pH=3. All the solutions contained equal concentrations of KCl (0.05M) for maintenance of constant ionic strength.

2.7 SDS-PAG Electrophoresis (discontinuous dissociating):
The Lamaeli method (12) was used for identifying the extent of albumin purity in all stages of purification. The peaks were compared to the peaks obtained from the standard BSA and HSA.

2.8 Albumin assay using bromocresol green (BCG):
At pH=4.2 a complex formed between albumin and BCG identified at 628nm could be applied to solutions with concentrations between 1-6 g/dl (13).

3. Results:

3.1 Results from equilibrium dialysis of BSA and its glycated form:
Binding constants were evaluated using parameter ν, introduced by Scatchard (14). ν, is defined as the moles of bound ligand to the total moles of albumin used. For the first approximation, if only the primary equivalent sites were considered the equation could be used as:

$$\nu = \frac{nK_a [A]}{1 + K_a [A]}$$

The reciprocal of which gives the Klotz equation:

$$\frac{1}{\nu} = \frac{1}{n} + \frac{1}{nK_a} \times \frac{1}{[A]}$$

Both Scatchard and Klotz equation were used to estimate the nK values for bindings of Ca(II) to albumin and its glycated form. The values of bound Ca(II) were determined from the subtraction of total Ca(II) found from atomic absorption spectrometry experiment and the free Ca(II) was determined by calcium electrode. When the values of 1/v were plotted against free 1/Ca, the slope gave the estimate of nK (Fig1). Since the concentrations of Ca(II) were several time larger than albumin, some nonspecific binding resulted in high values of n. Nevertheless the ratios of nK for normal albumin to that of glycated albumin could give a more reasonable index regarding the change in the affinities of Ca(II) towards albumin compared to normals. Similar treatment was carried out for human serum albumin and its glycated form.

3.2 Results obtained from albumin titration:
The quantity rH^+ is defined as the equivalence of dissociated H^+ in the process of titration to the total moles of solution for each one unit change in the value of pH. To account for the number of equivalences of H^+, the titrant used for the supporting electrolyte (KCl 40mM) is subtracted from the volume of titrant used to titrate the protein solution. Thus the rH + quantity was plotted against pH for equal concentrations of normal BSA (BSA-N) and the glycated BSA(BSA-G). Similarly these plots were repeated for solutions of BSA and their glycated form in the presence of Ca(II) ion. The quantity of rH^+ was similarly measured

for solution of normal human albumin and its glycated form (HAS-G), rH^+ values were plotted against pH in pH ranges of 3-11.5 (Fig2).

4. Discussion:

4.1 Equilibrium Dialysis:

The effect of glycation on binding of calcium ion to albumin: The purified albumin from pooled sera of normal and diabetic subjects were studied. The results obtained from equilibrium dialysis (Klotz plots, Figl) clearly indicate that Ca(II) ion could bind more to HSA-G than to HSA. These results were similarly obtained with BSA. The increase in Ca(II) glycated albumin could be significant in that it may effect the free and bound Ca(II) ion of serum. It is known that 6% of total calcium is bound to citrate and phosphate or other complexing anions. The remaining Ca(II) ion is almost free form or bound to albumin (15). Studies indicated that in diabetic patients (IDDM) the ionized form of Ca(II) ions remains constant or decrease slightly (16) while the total Ca(II) ion show an increase. Thus the ratio of Ca(II)/Ca(T) falls (17). This effect could either be due to an increase in bond Ca(II) to albumin or to other complexing anions or both. Our results indicates that glycated albumin could bind Ca(II) almost 20% more compared to normal albumin which may be instrumental in some pathogenesis of the disease .

4.2 Albumin titration:

The study of ionization properties of albumin in the presence of a ligand covalently bound to the molecule understanding of ligand sites of interaction. This could be seen from the plots of rH^+. For HSA-N compared to HAS-G(Fig.2), the higher values of rH^+ in pH ranges between 9-11 indicate the sites of glycation at lysyl residues. Similar result was obtained for BSA-N compared to BSN-G. In HSA titration, although the value of rH + was lower initially for HSN-N, but it reached the rH^+ value for HSN-G around pH=10 and surpassed that above pH=10. When the changes in rH^+ quantity was studied in solutions containing Ca(II) either with BSN-N or BSN-G as well as HSA-N and HAS-G, less protons were to be released in the initial portion of titration curves for glycated forms of albumin. This was perhaps due to change in molecular conformation of glycated albumin and thus made the titrable groups of aspartate and glutamate more available for Ca(Il) ion binding and resulted in lesser number of titrable groups. Although in titration where Ca(II) ion was omitted, the trend was almost reversed for both types of albumin which again indicate larger number of titrable groups i.e. aspartate and glutamate are available in the more open structure of glycated albumin. This result correlates well with the result obtained from equilibrium dialysis.

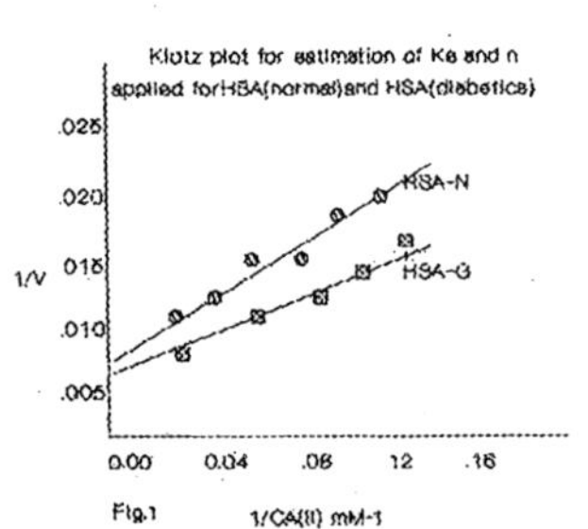

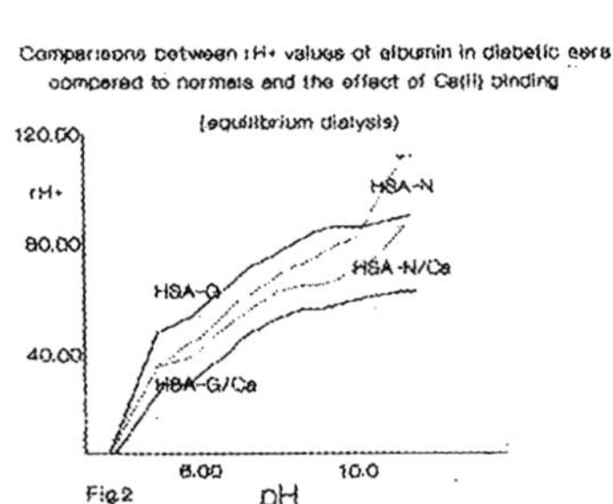

Acknowledgement:

We thank Mr. Ali Shamsaie for his kind assistance in preparing the manuscript.

References:

1. Shaklai N, Garlick R L and Bunn H F, J. Biol. Chem., 1984, 259, 3812-3817.
2. Brown J R and Shockley P in: Lipid-Protein Interaction (Jost P C and Griffith O H), pp. 26-68, John Wiley and Sons, New York.
3. Zakim D, Biophysical Chemistry, 1992, 42, 197-188
4. Minchiotti L,Galliano M, Zapprri M C and Tenni R, Eur. J. Biochem, 1993, 214, 437- 444

5. Noy N, Meredith S C, Biochem. J., 1991, 276,569-575
6. Tonsgard, H. J. and Kragh- Hansen, V. (1981) Pharmacol. Rev. 33, 17-52
7. Nishijo J, Morita N, Asda S, Niakae H and IwamotoE, Chem. Pharm. Bull, 1985, 33, 2648-2653
8. McMenammy R H et al, J. Biol. Chem, 1971, 246,4744
9. Chen R F, J. Biol. Chem. , 1967, 242:173.
10. Sunderman W, American Journai of Clinical Pathology, 1965, 43, 302
11. Shaklain N, J. Biol. Chem., 1984, 259,3812
12. Hames B D and Rickwood D, Gel electrophoresis of proteins: A practical approach, 1990
13. Silverman L M,Aminoacid and proteins(Determination of HSA by BCG), Text book of Clinical chemistry ,Narhert W. Tietz (editors), 1986
14. Ulrich Kragh Hansen and Henric Varam, Clinical Chemistry, 1993, 39,202-208
15. Granner D K, Hormones that regulates calcium metabolism,Harper's Biochemistry, 1992, p. 515
16. McNair P, European Journal of Clinimal Investigation, 1983, 13:267
17. Sarva A, 36:212(1990)

Metal Ions in Biology and Medicine; vol 6. Eds. J.A. Centeno, Ph. Collery, G. Vernet, R.B. Finkelman, H. Gibb, J.C. Etienne. John Libbey Eurotext, Paris © 2000, pp. 386-388.

High resolution ICP-MS connected directly with HPLC for the study of metal-transferrin binding in aluminum and iron

Megumi Hamano Nagaoka, Takashi Yamada and Tamio Maitani*

National Institute of Health Sciences, Kamiyoga 1-18-1, Setagaya, Tokyo 158-8501, Japan

SUMMARY

HPLC connected with high-resolution ICP-MS (HPLC/HR-ICP-MS) was applied to study the chemical state of Al and Fe bound to human serum transferrin *in vitro* and *in vivo*. HPLC/HR-ICP-MS chromatograms detected by ^{27}Al and ^{56}Fe levels were obtained without polyatomic isotope interference. This method seems effective for investigating the binding of metal and biological materials from the metal side.

INTRODUCTION

Accumulation of Al in the body causes several adverse effects[1]. The chemical state of a metal in blood is one of the most dominant factors for the tissue distribution of the metal. Serum Al is bound to transferrin (Tf). Tf has two metal-binding sites (N-lobe site and C-lobe site) and microheterogeneity in the number of sialic acids. Moreover, the number of carbohydrate chains in Tf decreases in patients with carbohydrate-deficient glycoprotein syndrome and in alcohol abusers[2,3]. Thus, the chemical state of a metal in Tf is not uniform. In this study, differentiation of the chemical states of Al and Fe bound to Tf was attempted by HPLC connected directly with high-resolution ICP-MS (HPLC/HR-ICP-MS) as the metal detection method.

MATERIALS AND METHODS

Reagents

Human serum apo-Tf and sialidase were purchased from Sigma

(St. Louis, MO) and used without further purification. Desferrioxamine (DFO) was obtained from Ciba-Geigy Japan (Takarazuka). Other chemicals were of reagent grade. All laboratory ware used were immersed in about 2 M HNO_3 at least for overnight and rinsed with water. Throughout the experiment, ultra-pure water (> 18 MΩcm), which was prepared with a Milli-Q SP Reagent Water System (Millipore, Bedford, MA), was used to avoid contamination from various ions.

Sample preparation

Apo-Tf was dissolved in 10 mM Tris-HCl (pH 7.5) containing 25 mM $NaHCO_3$. Fe^{3+}-citrate complex was prepared from equimolar proportions of ferric chloride and sodium citrate. The Fe-citrate solution was added to apo-Tf solution, and the mixed solution was allowed to stand for 24 h to complete the metal-Tf binding. Al-Tf complex was prepared with aluminum chloride in the same manner.

HPLC/HR-ICP-MS

An HPLC apparatus (LC-10Ai, Shimadzu, Kyoto, Japan) equipped with an anion-exchange column (MonoQ HR 5/5 (5 mm i.d. x 50 mm), Pharmacia, Uppsala, Sweden) and connected directly with an HR-ICP-MS machine (ELEMENT, Finnigan MAT, Bremen, Germany) was used. A 100-μl sample (0.2 mg apo-Tf in *in vitro* study) was applied to the system. Solvent used for gradient elution at a flow rate of 1 $ml min^{-1}$: solvent A (50 mM Tris-HCl (pH 7.4) and B (A + 0.25 M ammonium acetate). Gradient conditions: 0-7 min, linear gradient from 0 to 12% solvent B; 7-20 min, 12%; 20-40 min, linear gradient from 12 to 22%; 40-50 min, 22%. The eluate was transferred to a UV detector (280 nm) and then introduced to a Meinhard nebulizer of the HR-ICP-MS machine. The levels of Al (m/z 26.982) and Fe (m/z 55.957) were monitored continuously in the medium resolution mode ($m/\Delta m$=3000).

RESULTS AND DISCUSSION

Fe-Tf solution was applied to the system, and the eluate was monitored with UV absorption and ^{56}Fe level. Commercial apo-Tf contained a small amount of Fe. When the Fe/Tf molar ratio was below 1, all possible Fe-Tf forms, *i.e.* Fe_N-Tf (N-lobe site is occupied, 38 min), Fe_C-Tf (C-lobe site occupied, 22 min), and Fe_2-Tf (both sites occupied, 27 min), and apo-Tf (34 min) were detected. Peak assignments were performed based on the relative peak area of Fe-peak to UV-peak and the results of DFO-experiment[4]. In the stepwise addition of Fe, the peak areas of Fe_N-Tf and Fe_2-Tf increased successively with Fe-addition up to the Fe/Tf molar ratio of 1, while the peak area of Fe_C-Tf did not increase so much beyond the apo-Tf level. These results may suggest that if one site is first occupied by Fe ion another site is readily occupied to form Fe_2-Tf. This seems rational, because Tf receptor binds Fe_2-Tf most tightly.

When Al was added to apo-Tf solution stepwise, Al was detected as Al_N-Tf (38 min) and Al_N,Fe_C-Tf or Al_2-Tf (27 min). Since Tf could not be saturated with Al completely even by adding an excess amount of Al, the assignment of the latter peak to Al_N,Fe_C-Tf seems more possible.

To study the influence of decrease in the number of sialic acids on Fe-Tf binding, apo-Tf was treated with sialidase. Asialo-Tf produced eluted faster than the native Tf. When Fe was added to the asialo-(apo)-Tf solution stepwise, three Fe-peaks, *i.e.* two monoferric- and Fe_2-asialo-Tf, were still detected. Compared with native Tf, the changes in Fe-binding ability were not observed in asialo-Tf.

Sera from healthy persons without any metal spikes were subjected to the system. Al and Fe were detected as two and three major peaks, respectively. The peaks were assigned based on the experimental results of apo-Tf *in vitro*. Thus, the chemical states of Al and Fe bound to Tf could be clarified *in vitro* and *in vivo* with HPLC/HR-ICP-MS system without any polyatomic isotope interference.

REFERENCES

1. Jeffery EH. Biochemical mechanisms of aluminum toxicity. In: Goyer RA, Cherian MG, eds. *Toxicology of metals. Biochemical aspects*. Berlin: Springer-Verlag, 1995: 139-161.
2. Jaeken J, van Eijk HG, van der Heul C, Corbeel L, Eeckels R, Eggermont E. Sialic acid-deficient serum and cerebrospinal fluid transferrin in a newly recognized genetic syndrome. *Clin Chim Acta* 1984; 144: 245-247.
3. Stibler H. Carbohydrate-deficient transferrin in serum: a new marker of potentially harmful alcohol consumption reviewed. *Clin Chem* 1991; 37: 2029-2037.
4. Folajtar DA, Chasteen ND. Measurement of nonsynergistic anion binding to transferrin by EPR difference spectroscopy. *J Am Chem Soc* 1982; 104: 5775-5780.

Metal Ions in Biology and Medicine; vol 6. Eds. J.A. Centeno, Ph. Collery, G. Vernet, R.B. Finkelman, H. Gibb, J.C. Etienne. John Libbey Eurotext, Paris © 2000, pp. 389-393.

Electrothermal atomic absorption spectrometry for the determination of molybdenum in urine

C. Rondón, M.E. Roa, J.L. Burguera, M. Burguera, P. Carrero, M. Gallignani and M.R. Brunetto

IVAIQUIM (Venezuelan Andean Institute for Chemical Research), Faculty of Sciences, University of Los Andes, P.O. Box 542, Mérida 5101-A, Venezuela

Abstract

A comparison of the molybdenum determination in urine by electrothermal atomic absorption spectrometry (ETAAS) with Zeeman-effect background correction by using Pd + Mg (as magnesium nitrate) and Lu (as Lu_2O_3) as chemical modifiers was carried out. The pyrolysis and atomization curves, the amount of modifier and the calibration from a series of molybdenum standard solutions were studied by introducing the urine samples directly into the graphite furnace. The limits of detection and quantification respectively were 0.4 and 0.2 µg/L, and 11.4 and 0.6 µg/L for the determination of molybdenum in the presence of Pd + Mg and Lu. The characteristic masses (m_o) were 6.71 and 5.45 pg of molybdenum for Pd + Mg and Lu, respectively. Both modifiers have been applied to the study of the amount of molybdenum in human urine samples. The molybdenum levels found lie between 15 and 33 µg/L. However, these values were higher in the urine from the same subjects after an over-supply of molybdenum.

Introduction

Molybdenum is indispensable for the functioning of several human enzymes, e.g., for xanthine oxidase, aldehyde oxidase and sulfite oxidase. The detection of these enzymes and of genetically caused deficiency of the Mo cofactor in children as well as the occurrence of Mo-deficiency symptoms after molybdenum-free parenteral nutrition led to the detection of Mo essentiality [1]. Molybdenum is also potentially toxic. Therefore, concern is centered too over possible consequences of excessive exposure or ingestion [1,2]. It still remains unknown which tissue best reflects the nutritional status and/or eventual toxic exposure to this element. In particular, to the best knowledge of the authors, no systematic studies on urine Mo levels in general population or in exposed workers have been carried out. This fact could be likely due to the remarkably few papers which described the determination of molybdenum in urine. The determination of Mo in undigested human urine by electrothermal atomic absorption spectrometry (ETAAS) using Triton X-100 and chemical modification (Pd + Mg, Pd + hydroxylamine hydrochloride and barium difluoride, hydrogen peroxide + nitric acid) has been published [3,4]. Inductively coupled plasma mass spectrometry (ICP) has been applied for the determination of molybdenum in urine using preconcentration with a poly(dithiocarbamate) chelating resin [5]. The sensitive radiochemical neutron activation analysis and ICP- mass spectrometry (ICP-MS) [2] have been applied for Mo determination in urine. In this paper, the stabilization of molybdenum by palladium plus magnesium and lutetium as chemical modifiers was studied, showing the advantages and disadvantages of each one. Finally, the ETAAS procedure was tested for precision and accuracy

Materials and Methods

All reagents were of analytical grade, unless otherwise stated. Nitric acid was Suprapur grade from Merck. Distilled deionized water was used for the aqueous solutions. The solutions of the different modifiers were prepared as previously described [6].

Untreated urine samples were obtained from 25 healthy persons, 25-51 years old, before 9 a.m. and about two hours later after receiving an over-supply of 100 µg of molybdenum each (as sodium molybdate). The urine samples were collected in 100 mL polystyrene flasks pre-cleaned with nitric acid with polypropylene lids. Measurements were conducted the same day of sample collection. The persons lived in the Merida City, Venezuela. A Varian SpectrAA atomic absorption spectrometer with Zeeman-effect background correction was used. A hollow-cathode lamp operated at 7 mA was used and absorbances were measured at 313.3 nm with a slit width of 0.5 nm. Peak area integration was used for quantitative evaluation and pyrolytic coated graphite tubes were employed. The average absorbance values of three injections were obtained in all cases.

To obtain maximum pyrolysis temperature, atomization temperature, and optimum mass of the modifier, 20 µL of sample (or aqueous molybdenum standards) and 10 µL of matrix modifier solution were injected sequentially in the platform of the atomizer. The temperature program developed in this study and given in Table I was followed. Three drying steps were included in order to minimize the splattering of samples within the atomizer and therefore to avoid losses of the analyte. The atomization stage was carried out at 2800 °C and a cleaning step was also necessary to avoid memory effects or cross-contamination problems due to the reaction of the analyte with the pyrolytic coating of the graphite atomizer to form thermally stable molybdenum carbides at temperatures about 2200 °C [7]. The lifetime of the tubes was limited to 70 firings when the atomization and cleaning temperatures of 2800 °C were used for 2 s each. Higher temperatures were avoided in order to avoid a rapid deterioration of the atomizer.

Table I Furnace program for the determination of molybdenum in urine

Step	Temperature (°C)	Ramp time (s)	Hold time (s)	Ar flow (L/min)
Drying	85	5	0	3.0
Drying	95	40	0	3.0
Drying	120	10	0	3.0
Pyrolysis	1000	5	3	3.0
Atomization	2800	2	2	0
Cleaning	2800	2	2	3.0
Cooling	20	5	10	3.0

Results and Discussion

Firstly, a comprehensive comparison was made between the performances of molybdenum in the absence and presence of 0.01, 0.1, 0.5, 1.0, 5.0 and 10 µg of various potential chemical modifiers, such as Sm, Tb, Eu, Tm, Ho, Lu, Pd, Mg and Pg + Mg [6]. The integrated absorbance of molybdenum in the presence of either amount of Sm, Tb, Eu, Tm, Ho, Lu, Pd and Mg was similar to that obtained in the absence of modifier, except after the addition of Lu and Pd + Mg. In all cases, The integrated absorbance signals showed imperceptible background signals for molybdenum determination in aqueous solutions and a good separation of the atomization and background signals of molybdenum from urine samples indicating that the matrix interference was almost eliminated following the furnace program given in Table I and using the Zeeman-effect background correction (Fig. 1). It seems to be that the Zeeman-effect background corrector offers additional advantages over the deuterium-arc background corrector, with which relatively high background signals are obtained [3,4].

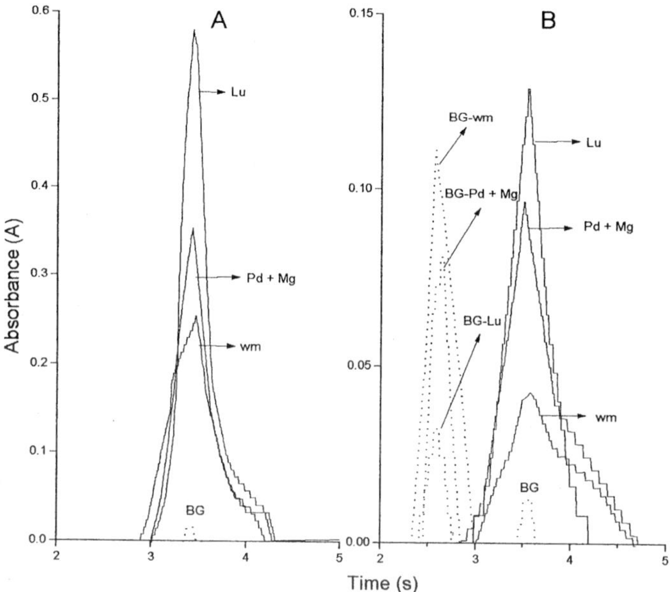

Fig. 1. Signal shapes for analyte signal and background (BG) in the absence of modifier and presence of Lu and Pd + Mg. (A) From aqueous standards; (B) from urine samples.

Analytical Figures of Merit

The addition of Pd (5 μg) + Mg (0.5 μg) or Lu (5 μg) improved the optimum pyrolysis temperature, the sensitivity and reproducibility of the molybdenum signals from aqueous and real samples with respect to those obtained in the absence of modifier (Fig. 2).

For that reason, these modifiers were further tested for the determination of molybdenum in real samples. The m_o when the integrated absorbance was measured for molybdenum were of 10.60 (without the addition of any modifier), 6.71 (in the presence of Pd + Mg) and 5.45 pg (in the presence of Lu). The limits of detection (3σ) were: 1.0 (20 pg), 0.4 (8 pg) and 0.2 (4 pg) μg/L in the presence of Pd + Mg and Lu, respectively. The method is quantitative and is applied over the ranges 3.3-200.0 , 11.4 - 200.0 and 0.6 - 120 of molybdenum in the absence and in the presence of Pd + Mg and Lu, respectively.

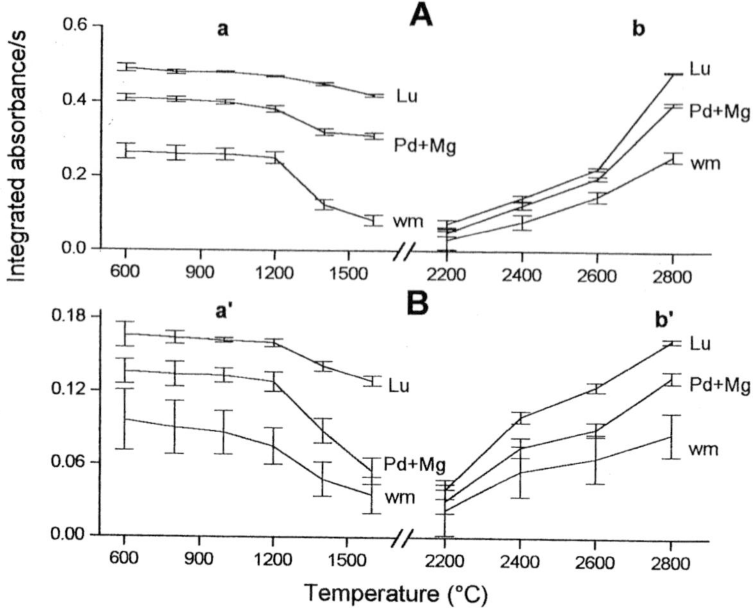

Fig. 2. Pyrolysis and atomization curves for 0.6 ng of Mo in an aqueous standard solution (A) and urine samples (B) in the presence of Pd + Mg and Lu modifiers. The pyrolysis curves (a and a') reflect atomization at 2800 °C, and the atomization curves (b and b') reflect the pyrolysis at 1000 °C.

However, the precision for the determination of molybdenum at concentrations of twice the detection limit and in the middle of the linear range, respectively were of 26.9 and 4.2 (in the absence of any modifier), 8.9 and 3.1 (in the presence of Pd + Mg), and 5.0 and 1.2 (in the presence of Lu) % relative standard deviation (three measurements).

To the best knowledge of the authors, there is not in the market certified reference material for molybdenum in urine samples. Therefore, the reliability of the method was checked by using both chemical modifiers (Pd + Mg and Lu). The analytical recoveries for 5, 10 and 30 µg/L of molybdenum added to a urine sample were investigated in the presence of the modifiers Pd + Mg and Lu. The results are given in Table 2. In all cases, the calibration graph with aqueous solutions was used. The recoveries values obtained, including those with Pd + Mg (from 104 to 106%) were acceptable. When Lu was added the recovery was about 100%.

Table 2 Recovery studies[a]

Mo added (μg/L)	Recovery (%)	
	Pd + Mg	Lu
5	106	99
10	104	100
30	104	100

[a]The endogenous Mo value in the urine sample was of 23.0 μg/L.

Application

The levels of molybdenum in the urine specimens of 25 subjects taken before and after receiving a parenteral dose of the analyte were evaluated. The molybdenum in urine was normally below 30 μg/L (mean 27 ± 5 and range from 15 to 33 μg/L). However, these values were higher in the urine from the same subjects after an over-supply of 100 μg of molybdenum (mean 60 ± 12 and range from 45 to 73 μg/L).

References

1. Holzinger S, Anke M, Röhrig B, Gonzalez D. Molydenum Intake of Adults in Germany and Mexico, Analyst 1998, 123: 447-450 and references therein.
2. Iversen BS, Menné C, White MA, Kristiansen J, Christensen JM, Sabbioni E. Inductively Coupled Plasma Mass Spectrometric Determination of Molybdenum in Urine from a Danish Population. Analyst 1998, 123: 81-85.
3. Calvo CP, Barrera PB, Barrera AB. Determination of Molybdenum in Human Urine by Electrothermal Atomization Atomic Absorption Spectrometry. Anal. Chim. Acta 1995, 310: 189-198.
4. Campillo N, Viñas P, López-García I, Hernández-Córdoba. Determination of Molybdenum, Chromium and Aluminium in Human Urine by Electrothermal Atomic Absorption Spectrometry Using Fast-programme Methodology. Talanta 1999, 48: 905-912.
5. Barnes RM, Fodor P, Inagaki K, Fodor M. Determination of Trace Elements in Urine Using Inductively Coupled Plasma Spectroscoy with a Poly(dithiocarbamate) Chelating Resin. Spectrochim. Acta 1983, 38B: 245-257.
6. Burguera JL, Burguera M, Rondon CE, Burguera E. Determination of Lead in Whole Blood and Urine be Electrothermal Atomic Absorption Spectrometry Using Various Chemical Modifiers. At. Spectrosc. 1997, 18: 109-113.
7. Slavin W, Graphite Furnace AAS. A Source Book, Perkin-Elmer, Norwalk, CT, 1984.

Metal Ions in Biology and Medicine; vol 6. Eds. J.A. Centeno, Ph. Collery, G. Vernet, R.B. Finkelman, H. Gibb, J.C. Etienne. John Libbey Eurotext, Paris © 2000, pp. 394-396.

Single cell gel/comet assay applied to DNA damage in *Nassarius tegula* and *Musculista senhousia*, San Diego Bay, California

Miguel P. Sastre[1], Scott Steinert[2] and Rebecca Streib-Montee[2]

[1] *Department of Biology, University of Puerto Rico, Humacao, PR 00791;* [2] *Spawar System Center, 53475 Strothe Road, San Diego, CA 92152-6310*

ABSTRACT

The objective of this research is to assess the single cell gel electrophosesis or comet assay to measure levels of DNA damage in different cell types of the Welk *Nassarius tegula* and the Mussel *Musculista senhousia*. Copper chloride exposure experiments indicate muscle cells of *N. tegula* exposed for 24 hours showed significant levels of DNA damage at 20-200 ppb, while at 96 hours significant levels of damage were observed at 100-200 ppb. In *M. senhousia* germ cells significant levels of damage were detected after 96 hours at 100-200 ppb. Significant levels of DNA damage were observed in somatic cells at 100-200 ppb both at 24 and 96 hours. After exposing *M. senhousia* for 3 weeks in a culture system to different concentrations of mixed sediments from a reference station and from Pier 4, US Naval Station, San Diego, significant damage was observed in *M. senhousia* mantle cells at 75 and 100% Pier 4. Results indicate *M. senhousia* could be used potentially as a bioindicator species to assess DNA damage caused by pollutants in San Diego Bay.

INTRODUCTION

The Asian Mussel, *Musculista senhousia* [1] lives in intertidal and subtidal soft sediments of bays and estuaries. The Western Mud Welk *Nassarius tegula*, lives on intertidal and subtidal sand and mud. There are well established polulations of both species in San Diego Bay. The single cell gel electrophosesis (SCGE)/ comet assay has been used succesfully for assesing DNA damage and repair [2, 3]. Cells are embedded in agarose gel and placed in a microscope slide, the cells are lysed, and the liberated DNA electrophoresed. When the DNA contains strand breaks, it moves from the "nucleus" to the anode. Cells with increased DNA damage display longer migration of DNA towards the anode and greater fluorescent intensity. The objective of this study is to evaluate the SCGE alkaline assay for measuring pollution-induced DNA damage in different cell types of *M. senhousia* and *N. tegula* in San Diego Bay, California.

MATERIALS AND METHODS

The SCGE assay was performed according to the technique described by Steinert [3]. In the sediment exposure experiment tail length and tail extent moment (tail length × tail fluorescence intensity) were measured and analyzed using a Komet® Image Analysis System software.

Duplicate 0, 20, 100 and 200 ppb Cu dilutions were prepared from a $CuCl_2$ stock and placed in plastic bags. *M. senhousia* and *N. tegula* were placed in separate bags. The comet assay was performed at 0, 24 and 96 h on three *M. senhousia* and on pooled hemolymph from four *N. tegula.*

Sediment exposure experiments were performed in a culture system intaking seawater from San Diego Bay. *N. tegula* and *M. senhousia* were collected from control sites in San Diego. Sediments were sampled from Pier 4, San Diego, a site having high concentratons of copper and PAH's; and from a control site. Sediments from both sites were mixed to make 0, 25, 50, 75 and 100% Pier 4 sediment. Twelve *M. senhousia* and *N. tegula* were exposed to each sediment concentration. After 3 weeks the comet assay was performed in 3 mussels and 4 gastropods from each tray.

RESULTS

Muscle cells of *N. tegula* exposed for 24 h to $CuCl_2$ showed significant levels of DNA damage at all concentrations. At 96 h significant levels of damage were observed at 100-200 ppb. Both at 24 and 96 h significant DNA damage was observed in hemocytes at 100-200 ppb (Figure 1). In germ cells of *M. senhousia* exposed for 96 h to $CuCl_2$ significant levels of damage were detected at 100-200 ppb. Both at 24 and 96 hours significant levels damage were observed in somatic cells from 100-200 ppb (Figure 2). No significant differences were observed in *N. tegula* muscle or hemocyte cells exposed to different concentrations of contaminated sediment. After exposing *M. senhousia* to the different sediment concentrations no significant treatment effect was observed in hemocytes if length of DNA migration was used to measure damage. When analyzing the same cells using tail extent moment a significant damage was observed at 75 and 100% Pier 4 sediment (Figure 3).

REFERENCES

1. **Crooks JA.** The population ecology of an exotic mussel, *Musculista senhousia,* in a southern California bay. *Estuaries* 1996; 19 : 42-50.
2. **Nascimbeni B, Philips MD, Croom DK, Andrews PW, Tice RR.** Evaluation of DNA damage in golden mice *(Ochrotomys nutalli)* inhabiting a hazardous waste site. *Environ. Molec. Mutagen* 1991; 17 : 55.
3. **Steinert SA, Streib-Montee R, Leather JM, Chadwick DB.** DNA damage in mussels at sites in San Diego Bay. *Mutation Res.* 1998; 399 : 65-85.

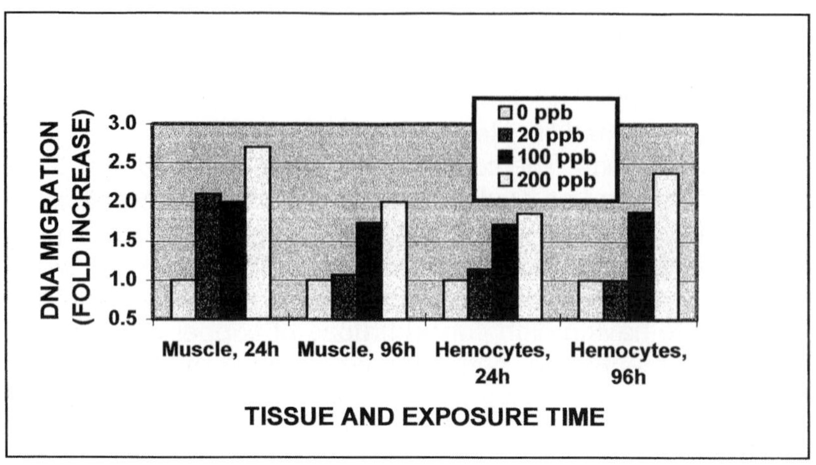

Figure 1. DNA damage in *N. tegula* cell types at different concentrations of copper chloride

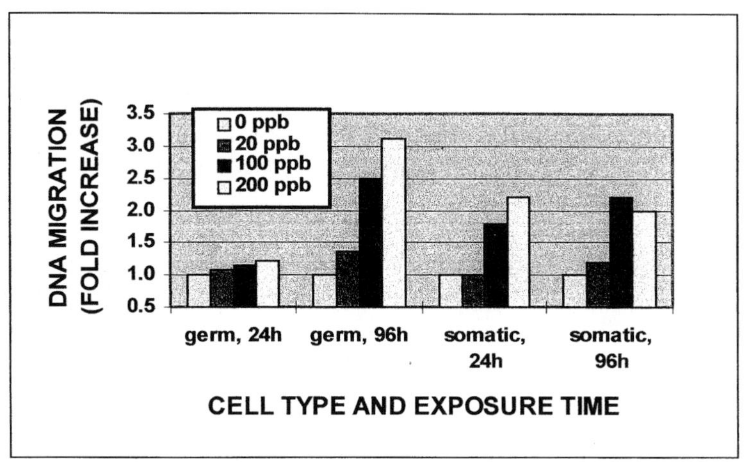

Figure 2. DNA damage in *M. senhousia* cell types at different concentration of copper chloride

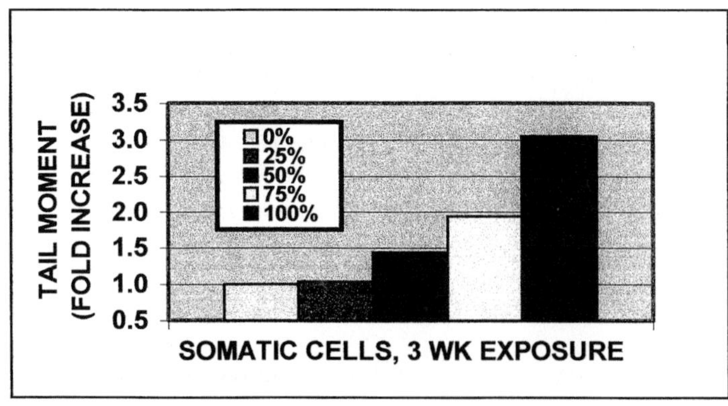

Figure 3. DNA damage in *M. senhousia* after exposure to different concentrations of contaminated sediment

Metal Ions in Biology and Medicine; vol 6. Eds. J.A. Centeno, Ph. Collery, G. Vernet, R.B. Finkelman, H. Gibb, J.C. Etienne. John Libbey Eurotext, Paris © 2000, pp. 397-400.

Achievements of the "European commission network on trace element speciation in occupational health and hygiene, food and environment"

R. Cornelis[1]*, C. Camara[2], L. Ebdon[3], L. Pitts[3], B. Sperling[4], R. Morabito[5], O.F.X. Donard[6], H. Crews[7], E.H. Larsen[8], B. Neidhart[9], F. Ariese[10], E. Rosenberg[11], O. Berrouiguet[12], G.M. Morrison[13], G. Cordier[14], F. Adams[15], I. Schoeters[16], J. Marshall[17], B. Stojanik[18], A. Ekvall[19], Ph. Quevauviller[20]

[1] Laboratory for Analytical Chemistry, University of Gent, Proeftuinstraat 86, B-9000 Gent, Belgium; [2] Universidad Complutense, Lab. de Químíca Analítica, Ciudad Universitaria, E-28040 Madrid, Spain; [3] University of Plymouth, Drake Circus, UK-PL4 8AA Plymouth Devon, Great Britain; [4] Bodenseewerk Perkin Elmer GmbH, Alte Nussdorfer Strasse, D-88662 Ueberlingen, Germany; [5] ENEA CRE Casaccia, Divisione Chimica Ambientale, S.P. Anguillarese 301, I-00100 Roma, Italy; [6] Université de Pau, Lab. de Chimie BioInorganique et Environnement, Hélioparc, F-6400 Pau, France; [7] MAFF CSL Food Science Lab., Central Science Laboratory, Sand Hutton, York Y041 1LZ, UK; [8] National Food Agency, Inst. of Food Chem. & Nutrition, Moerkhoej Bygade 19, DK-2860 Soeborg, Denmark; [9] GKSS Research Centre, Institute for Physical and Chemical Analysis, D-21502 Geesthacht, Germany; [10] Vrije Universiteit Amsterdam/IVM, De Boelelaan 1115, NL-1081 HV Amsterdam, The Netherlands; [11] Institut für Analytische Chemie, Getreidemarkt 9, A-1060 Wien, Austria; [12] Prolabo, 54, rue Roger Salengro, F-94126 Fontenay-Sous-Bois Cedex, France; [13] Department of Sanitary Engineering, Chalmers University of Technology, S-412 96 Göteborg, Sweden; [14] Rhône Poulenc, CRIT/C, 62 avenue des Frères Perret 85, F-69192 Saint-Fons, France; [15] University of Antwerp, Dept. of Chemistry, Universiteitsplein 1, B-2610 Antwerpen, Belgium; [16] Eurométaux, 12 avenue de Broqueville, B-1150 Brussel, Belgium; [17] ICI, PO Box 90, Wilton, Middlesbrough, TS90 8JE Cleveland, Great Britain; [18] Degussa AG, POB 13 45, Rodenbacher Chaussee 4, D-63403 Hanau, Germany; [19] Sveriges Provnings-och Forskinsinsitut, Brinellgatan 4, Boras, S-510 15 Alvsborgslan, Sweden; [20] DG XII, Competitive and Sustainable Growth, Montoyerstraat 75, 1049 Brussels, Belgium

Introduction

Information involving trace element content in different matrices is of everyday use in all aspects of life, be it related to environment, food, health or trade. This information is, however, most of the time limited to the total metal content and does not take into account the chemical form in which the trace element is present. This considerably limits the assessment of the impact of the trace element species in many areas. As a result both beneficial and toxic issues are overlooked resulting in inappropriate legislative actions.The thematic network «Speciation 21"has been creating a link between scientists in analytical chemistry working in speciation method development for the chemical speciation of trace elements, and potential users from industry and of legislative agencies, in the field of environment, food and occupational health and hygiene. This link materialized through a set of 9 meetings, 2 newsletters, 2 publications [1,2], a www-page (hhtp://www.speciation21.plymouth.ac.uk) and a book [3] about the state of the art and future perspectives in the field. This project was funded by the Commission of the European Community (DGXII -Standards, Measurement and Testing Programme. Contract no. SMT4-CT97-7509) for a duration of two and a half years, starting date October 1997. During these meetings a cross-fertilization of ideas between industrial, legislative and academic circles took place. It vitalized the interest in speciation of trace elements, broadened the mind of all delegates and proved to be productive in initiating new research areas. This is expected to show up in multi-disciplinary projects to be implemented within the Fifth Framework Programme. Once the analytical methodology for the measurement of the trace element species has been optimised, the importance of trace element speciation will grow enormously. The network will also have instrumental in promoting the dissemination of knowledge throughout the Member States. The following paragraphs give the essence of the «Speciation 21 « campaign in medicine and occupational health, food, and environmental sciences. A very important issue in all fields appeared to be risk assessment related to the chemical speciation of the elements.

Medicine and ccupational health and hygiene

Enhanced knowledge is needed about the chemical forms in which the trace elements are present in the human body. This is a real challenge to determine the pathways the species are following and to learn their subsequent action in target organs. The greatest problem faced in this area is species analysis within the cells, which has to be made without disturbing the cell in any way, since the act of disturbance will cause the cell's behaviour to alter.

A key focus in the area of occupational health and hygiene concerns the topochemical and morphological characterisation of environmental and industrial particulate samples [4]. Developments will allow us to gauge the impact of the species present on the surface of the particulate. It is impossible to gather the same information by conventional chemical means, since dissolution of the surface could well involve dissolution of the substrate thus invalidating the findings for the surface chemistry. Characterisation of the surface layer of metal aerosols encountered in the workplace of the metal industry is of primary concern, because these are the species that are liable to interact with cells, membranes and alveolar fluid of the respiratory tract. Typical particulates encountered in the ambient air in the metal industry consist of conglomerates or chains of up to a dozen particles. Silicates are major constituents of these aerosols. The chemical bonding of, e.g., the Cr(VI)-species to matrix components, such as those silicates, may be most relevant to allow an explanation of the diverging degrees of bioavailability and toxicity of Cr(VI) carrying particulates.Other elements of major concern for occupational health and hygiene are nickel, chromium, arsenic, platinum, gallium and indium. What is needed are new tests for exposure threshold values in metallurgy based on the study of metal species.

Food sciences

Involvement in speciation of trace elements in food has different objectives. The essentiality of some trace elements in food, including food supplementation is considered to be of prime concern. The distinction between toxic and non-toxic forms of some trace elements is the second matter of interest [5].

The specific form of the element must be viewed in relation to bioavailability from soil to

plant or animal, and from supplement to man. The element selenium is a good illustration of this. The bioavailability of selenium to humans is strongly dependent on the biological source of the elements, e.g. pea meal (low) versus selenised yeast (high). Distinction between toxic and non-toxic forms of the trace element is the second matter of interest and arsenic is one of the best examples. Inorganic arsenic compounds are toxic (arsenate, arsenite, arsine). There appears to be no toxicity related to organoarsenic compounds, such as the arseno-sugars. Study of the transformation between the inorganic and organic forms will help to clarify the pathways followed by this element in living systems. Regulations for arsenic in drinking water are becoming very strict. The recommendation by WHO has been lowered from 50 μg/L to 10 μg/L, a goal that will be extremely hard to achieve. In fish products, the average concentration of arsenic is relatively high, but only a small percentage is present as inorganic arsenic, with the main species being the non-toxic arsenobetaine. Consequently, consumers are not at risk from excessive intake of As in fish. Legislation of As on the basis of speciation is, therefore, required for the correct evaluation of the quality of fish and fish derivatives.
Other poignant topics are the migration of Ni and Cr from food contact materials. There is lack of information on the species in normal diet and on the effects in individuals that are sensitised and non-sensitised as well as on the dose needed for adverse effects.

Environmental sciences

The determination of «chemical forms of elements» forms the basis for understanding the bio-geochemical cycle of contaminants in the terrestrial and aquatic ecosystems and for detecting possible harmful substances which might be toxic to biota and human. This became very evident in couple of historical case studies. In the year 1952 a most serious epidemic of methylmercury poisoning occurred in the fish eating population of Minamata in Japan. This was the result of evacuation of mercury used as a catalyst in a polymer producing plant. Micro-organisms in the water methylated the Hg^{2+}. As methylmercury is very soluble in fat, it accumulates in aquatic plants and animals, such as fish. The concentration of methylmercury increases with ascending order of the food chain. Eventually a substantial number of the fish-eating population died or underwent severe injury.
A second historiacl example is that of the high mortality of oysters in the Arcachon Bay in the 80's due to organotin contamination.Whereas inorganic tincompounds are inoffensive, extremely small concentrations of organotincompunds appeared to be detrimental for the reproductive system of the oysters. The effects of organotin compounds in the aquatic environment continues to preoccupy environmentalists, industrialists, legislators and researchers. This case is an excellent example of how problems caused by the use of these very effective products continue to catch them all in the same spider's web. The chemical industry brought on the market the tributyltin (TBT) anti-fouling products, which were then enthusiastically applied by most ship owners on the hulls of their vessels. Some years later the adverse ecological effects due to organotin pollution became apparent, giving rise to successive legislation. In the meantime researchers in analytical chemistry developed methods to measure the residues in various matrices. Robust, validated methods with affordable instrumentation became a first priority, and is still of great concern to standardisation organisations and instrument developers. Reference materials, such as sediments, mussel tissue and water etc., certified for their content of TBT's became a

necessity. The analytical achievements should, however, evolve together with better documented knowledge about acceptable background levels. As the analytical performance in measuring TBT's is improving steadily, the ecotoxicology, human toxicology and risk assessment of these products can be studied more thoroughly. Considering the very long half-life of the products under anaerobic conditions, even with no further input of TBT when a world-wide ban is imposed, it may take another 150 years for natural processes to remove the material from sediments. It looks like the European Community will deal with the TBT issue for many years to come.
Besides organotin compounds, speciation of arsenic, chromium, mercury, and platinum in environmental studies, as well as the speciation of trace elements in the waste management industry are very hot topics . In each case the effects of long term low level exposure, a more profound study of bio- and geo-transformation, an improvement in the quality of the analytical results and the integration of basic science into the formation of control measures are leading motives to set specific goals in speciation analysis.

Further reading about speciation of trace elements can be found in special issue of journals [6, 7]. Succesful speciation projects within the EU are described in [8].

References

1. R. Cornelis, C. Cámara, L. Ebdon, L. Pitts, B. Welz, R. Morabito, O. Donard, H. Crews, E.H. Larsen, B. Neidhart, F. Ariese, E. Rosenberg, D. Mathé, G. M. Morrison, G. Cordier, F. Adams, P. Van Doren, J. Marshall, B. Stojanik, A. Ekvall, Ph. Quevauviller, Introduction to the EU-network on trace element speciation: preparing for the 21st century *Fresenius J Anal Chem* 363 1999; 363: 435- 438.
2. R. Cornelis, C. Camara, L. Ebdon, L. Pitts, B. Sperling, R. Morabito, O.F.X. Donard, H. Crews, E.H. Larsen, B. Neidhart, F. Ariese, E. Rosenberg, O. Berrouiguet, G. M. Morrison, G. Cordier, F. Adams, B. Dero, J. Marshall, B. Stojanik, A. Ekvall, Ph. Quevauviller, The EU-network on trace element speciation in full swing. *TrAC* 2000; 19 (Feb-March issue)
3. Trace Element Species for environment, food & health», Edts R. Cornelis, H. Crews, O. Donnard , L. Ebdon, Ph. Quevauviller. to be published in 2000 by the Royal Society for Chemistry, UK
4. H.M. Ortner, P. Hoffmann, F.J. Stadermann, S. Weinburuch, M. Wentzel, Chemical characterization of environmental and industrial particulate samples, *Analyst* 1998; 123: 833-842.
5. H.M. Crews, Speciation of trace elements in foods, with special references to cadmium and selenium: is it necessary? Spectrochim Acta, Part B Atomic Spectroscopy.1998; 155: 213-219.
6. O.F.X. Donard, J.A. Caruso, Edts, Speciation - The opportunity and the future. complete issue *of Spectrochim Acta, Part B Atomic Spectroscopy,* 1998; 53B: 155 - 378.
7. The *Analyst*. 1998; 123: 765 - 1161.
8. Ph. Quevauviller, Method performance studies for speciation analysis. The Royal Society for Chemistry, Cambridge, UK, 1998

Metal Ions in Biology and Medicine; vol 6. Eds. J.A. Centeno, Ph. Collery, G. Vernet, R.B. Finkelman, H. Gibb, J.C. Etienne. John Libbey Eurotext, Paris © 2000, pp. 401-405.

QSARs for metals — fact or fiction?

John D. Walker[1] and James P. Hickey[2]

[1] TSCA Interagency Testing Committee (ITC), U.S. Environmental Protection Agency (7401), 401 M Street SW, Washington, DC 20460; [2] U.S. Geological Survey, Great Lakes Service Center, 1451 Green Road, Ann Arbor, MI 48105

Abstract. Structural approaches have been used to classify inorganic chemicals, including metals. Can these approaches be used to develop Quantitative Structure Activity Relationships (QSARs) for metals? Will current and future regulatory programs to categorize and screen inorganic chemicals, including metals, for persistence, bioconcentration and toxicity provide sufficient incentives and resources to develop QSARs for metals? What are the limitations and uncertainties of using QSARs for inorganics and metals? What research needs to be conducted to reduce or eliminate these limitations and uncertainties? Will regulatory agencies accept estimates of persistence, bioconcentration and toxicity of metals based on QSARs? Are QSARs for metals fact or fiction? Inorganic chemists, biochemists, toxicologists, pathologists, ecologists and others who have studied and are studying the persistence, bioconcentration and toxicity of metals need to begin answering these questions, if QSARs for metals have any chance of being considered by the regulatory community.

Introduction. Quantitative Structure Activity Relationships (QSARs) have been used for over a century to predict partitioning and specific toxicities of selected organic chemicals. The potential to develop QSARs for predicting persistence, bioconcentration and aquatic toxicity of organic chemicals has provided the incentive for biannual workshops on QSARs in the environmental sciences (Kaiser, 1984, 1986; Turner et al., 1988; Hermens and Opperhuizen, 1991; Devillers and Karcher, 1995; Chen and Schüürmann, 1997; Walker 2000a-e).

Classifying Metals. Inorganic compounds have been classified according to at least 6 schemes, generally based on the electronic structure of the atom:

1. Valence orbitals and characteristic "inner" orbitals (Cotton and Wilkinson 1980; Greenwood and Earnshaw 1980);
2. Crystal Field Theory (Hoeschele, et al. 1991);
3. Kinetic Reactivity/Lability (Hoeschele, et al. 1991);
4. Metal Complex Thermodynamic Stability (Hoeschele, et al. 1991);
5. Hard and Soft Acid and Base Theory theory (Pearson 1963, 1966, 1987, 1993; Vouk 1979);
6. Lewis acidity (metal ions), basicity (ligands) /Softness index (Jones and Vaughn 1978;Williams and Turner 1981).

Only the last scheme appears to relate to SARs.

SARs for Metals. A few basic SARs for metals have been developed (Khangarot and Ray 1989; Newman and McCloskey 1996; Tarata et al. 1998; Lewis et al. 1999). Existing correlations strongly indicate that metal ion toxicity is a function of electron attraction strength, and mode of toxic action is related to the strength of covalent binding with cellular electron-rich sulfhydryl, imidazole, and carboxyl groups (e.g., Somers 1960; Biesinger and Christensen 1972; Hoeschele et al., 1991). All SAR efforts have confirmed this hypothesis, since the highest linear correlations for acute toxicity make use of one to two parameters relating to metal ion characteristics such as electronegativity, ionization potential, and/or the «hardness/softness» of the metal atom involved. A reasonably complete compilation of successful parameters have been discussed by Hickey (1996). At this time, Linear Solvation Energy Relationship holds promise to develop QSARs for metal-containing compounds (Hickey, 2000).

References

Biesinger, K. and G.M. Christensen. 1972. Effects of various metals on survival, growth, reproduction, and metabolism of *Daphnia magna*. J. Fish. Res. Board Can. 29:1691-1700.

Chen, F. and G. Schüürmann (Eds). 1997. Quantitative Structure-Activity Relationships (QSAR) in Environmental Sciences-VII. SETAC Press, Pensacola, Florida. 470 p. [ISBN 1-880611-23-6].

Cotton, F.A. and G. Wilkinson. 1980. Advanced Inorganic Chemistry: A comprehensive text. 4th Ed. New York, NY: Wiley-Interscience Publishers, John Wiley & Sons.

Devillers, J. (Editor-in-Chief) and Karcher (Guest Editor). 1995. *SAR and QSAR in Environmental Research* 3 (3, 4):167-324; 4(1 -4):1-252.

Greenwood, N.N. and A. Earnshaw. 1980. Chemistry of the Elements. New York. Pergammon Press.

Hermens, J.L.M. and A. Opperhuizen (Eds). 1991. QSAR in Environmental Toxicology - IV. Elsevier, The Netherlands. 705p. [ISBN 0-444-89471-3].

Hickey, J.P. 1996. Quantum Chemical Parameters: What do I use when? Chapter 22 In: Techniques in Aquatic Toxicology, G. Ostrander, Ed. CRC Press/Lewis Publishers, Boca Raton, FL.

Hickey, J.P. 2000. Estimation of main group and heavy metal environmental behavior using the Linear Solvation Energy Relationship I: Aqueous solubility and bioconcentration., In: Handbook on QSARs for Predicting Environmental Fate of Chemicals. J.D. Walker (Ed) Pensacola, FL: SETAC Press.

Hoeschele, D., J. E. Turner, and M. W. England. 1991. Inorganic concepts relevant to metal binding, activity, and toxicity in a biological system. In: QSAR In Environmental Toxiciology – IV, Joop L.M. Hermens, Anton Opperhuizen, Eds. Elsivier, New York, NY. Pp. 477-492.

Jones, M.M. and W.K. Vaughn. 1978. HSAB theory and acute metal ion toxicity and detoxification processes. J. Inorg. Nucl. Chem. 40:2081-2088.

Kaiser, K.L.E. (Ed.). 1984. QSAR in Environmental Toxicology. D. Reidel Publ. Co., Dordrecht, The Netherlands. 406p. [ISBN 90-277-1776-1].

Kaiser, K.L.E. (Ed.). 1986. QSAR in Environmental Toxicology - II. D. Reidel Publ. Co., Dordrecht, The Netherlands. 465p. [ISBN 90-277-2555-1].

Khangarot, B.S. and P.K. Ray. 1989. Investigation of correlation between physicochemical properties of metals and their toxicity to the water flea *Daphnia magna* Straus. Ecotoxicol. Environ. Safety 18:109-120.

Lewis, D.F.V., M. Dobrota, M.G. Taylor, D.V.Parke, 1999. Metal toxicity in two rodent species and redox potential: evaluation of quantitative structure-activity relationships. Environ. Toxicol. Chem. 18:2199-2204.

Newman, M.C. and J.T. McCloskey. 1996. Predicting relative toxicity and interactions of divalent metal ions: Microtox bioluminescence assay. Environ. Toxicol. Chem. 15:275-281.

Pearson, R.G. 1963. Hard and soft acids and bases. J. Amer. Chem. Soc. 85:3533-3539.

Pearson, R.G. 1966. Acids and Bases. Science 151:172-177.

Pearson, R.G. 1987. Recent advances in the concept of hard and soft acids and bases. J. Chem. Educ. 64:561-567.

Pearson, R.G. 1993. The principle of maximum hardness. Accounts Chem. Res. 26:250-255.

Somers, E. 1960. Fungitoxicity of metal ions. Nature 187:427-428.

C.P. Tatara, M.C. Newman, J.T. McCloskey, and P.L. Williams. 1998. Use of ion characteristics to predict relative metal toxicity of mono-, di-, and trivalent metal ions: *Caenorhabditis elegans* LC50, Aquat. Toxicol. 42:255-269.

Turner, J.E., M.W. England, T.W. Schultz and N.J. Kwaak. (Eds.). 1988. Proceedings 3rd International Workshop on Quantitative Structure-Activity Relationships (QSAR) in Environmental Toxicology [CONF-880520-9DE88013180].p.228. NTIS, Springfield, VA.

Vouk, V. 1979. General chemistry of metals. In: L. Friberg, G.F. Nordberg, and V.B. Vouk, eds., Handbook on the Toxicology of Metals, Elsvier, Amsterdam, pp. 15-30.

Walker, J.D. (Editor). 2000a. Handbook on QSARs for Pollution Prevention, Toxicity Screening, Risk Assessment and WWW Applications. Pensacola, FL: SETAC Press.

Walker, J.D. (Editor). 2000b. Handbook on QSARs for Predicting Endocrine Disruption Potentials of Chemicals. Pensacola, FL: SETAC Press.

Walker, J.D. (Editor). 2000c. Handbook on QSARs for Predicting Effects of Chemicals on Environmental-Human Health Interactions. Pensacola, FL: SETAC Press.

Walker, J.D. (Editor). 2000d. Handbook on QSARs for Predicting Environmental Fate of Chemicals. Pensacola, FL: SETAC Press.

Walker, J.D. (Editor). 2000e. Handbook on QSARs for Predicting Ecological Effects of Chemicals. Pensacola, FL: SETAC Press.

Williams, M.W. and J.E. Turner. 1981. Comments on softness parameters and metal ion toxicity. J. Inorg. Nucl. Chem. 43:1689-1691.

Metal Ions in Biology and Medicine; vol 6. Eds. J.A. Centeno, Ph. Collery, G. Vernet, R.B. Finkelman, H. Gibb, J.C. Etienne. John Libbey Eurotext, Paris © 2000, pp. 406-409.

Speciation of metalloproteins in blood cells

A. Raab[1], P. Brätter[1], M. Rükgauer[2], J.D. Kruse-Jarres[2]

[1] *Hahn-Meitner-Institut Berlin, Department of Trace Element Research for Health and Nutrition, Glienicker Str. 100, D-14109 Berlin Germany;* [2] *Katharinenhospital Institut für Klinische Chemie und Laboratoriumsmedizin, Kriegsbergerstr. 60, D-70174 Stuttgart Germany*

Abstract

We studied the binding pattern of trace elements in the different types of blood cells obtained from healthy donors and sepsis patients. After separation of the cells by gradient centrifugation, speciation of the metalloproteins in the cell-lysate was carried out using size exclusion chromatography (SEC) for protein separation and ICP-MS for the simultaneous detection of the elements Cu, Cd, Fe, Mn, Pb, Se and Zn in the eluted protein fractions. The SEC/ICP-MS combination was optimized with respect to the column material, buffer solution and flow rate. Significant expression of a Zn-containing protein, presumably thionein, was found in the white blood cells. In erythrocytes and thrombocytes the metalloprotein Cu/Zn-SOD was identified. Variation in the metalloprotein pattern of human blood cells are discussed with respect to inflammation conditions (Sepsis).

Introduction

According to the individual biological functions of erythrocytes, thrombocytes, granulocytes and lymphocytes it is assumed that they have a characteristic cytoplasmic metalloprotein composition. Erythrocytes are responsible for the transport of oxygen, thrombocytes are part of the coagulation system and lymphocytes as well as granulocytes belong to the immune system, respectively. Among the metalloproteins the metallothioneins (MT) have multifunctional properties including their possible role in cell proliferation, differentiation and apoptosis.Granulocytes contain various metalloproteins including alkaline phosphatase (Zn), catalase (Fe), Zn-containing metalloproteases. Erythrocytes contain a large amount of antioxidative enzymes including Cu/Zn-superoxid dismutase, Fe-containing catalase and Se-containing glutathione peroxidase. These enzymes are essential for the survival of the cell. In erythrocytes oxygen radicals are produced accidental, in granulocytes they are produced during the phagocytosis as part of the bacteriocidity.

The aim of this work was to study the variation of the metalloprotein pattern of human blood cells with respect to inflammation.

Methods

Blood was collected using Li-heparinized tubes. Latest 2 h after sampling the plasma was removed. The separation of the blood cells was carried out using density gradient centrifugation. The thrombocytes were separated from the other cells using HistoDenz™ (Sigma, Germany) as separation medium. The remaining

cells were resuspended and centrifuged in a density gradient using Polymorphprep™ (Nycomed Pharma AS, Norway) as separation medium. The uppermost zone contains the lymphocytes, they were cleaned using Lymphoprep™ (Nycomed Pharma AS, Norway). The second -granulocyte containing- zone was cleaned from erythrocytes if necessary. The erythrocytes in the pellet were washed with 0.9 % NaCl. The separated cells were diluted in buffer and stored deep frozen (-20°C) until speciation analysis. Purity of the cell fractions was controlled with a cell counter.
Before the injection into the chromatographic column the cell lysate was thawed and centrifuged for 60 min at 36000 g to remove the larger particles of cell membranes. The chromatographic separation was carried out on a Superdex 75J (1*30 cm) column (Pharmacia, Sweden) using a 20 mM TRIS [(Tris-(hydroxymethyl-)aminomethan] buffer at pH 7.4. The flow rate was 1 ml/min at ambient temperature. The outlet of the column was connected to an UV-monitor. The absorption was measured at 280 nm. The eluat was introduced into the nebulizer (Cross-Flow) of the inductively coupled plasma mass spectrometer (ICP-MS, Elan 6000 Sciex Perkin Elmer). Between the UV-monitor and the nebulizer a T-piece was used to mix the eluat of the column with a internal standard solution (10 ppb Rh, Ce, Ir in 1 % HNO_3, flow 0.1 ml/min).

Results and Discussion

Erythrocytes

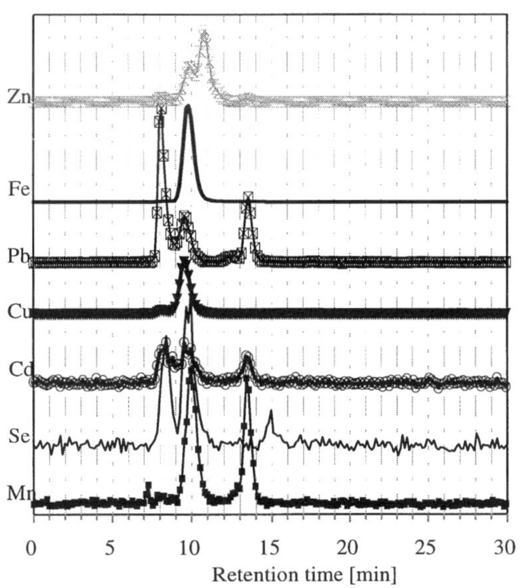

Fig. 1: Elution profiles of elements in erythrocyte lysate of a healthy person, Superdex 75 20 mM TRIS pH 7.4

The distribution pattern of the elements Mn, Se, Cd, Pb, Cu, Zn and Fe in erythrocyte lysate of a healthy person is shown in Fig. 1. The one iron signal belongs to hemoglobin, the iron-containing enzyme catalase is not visible. Different Zn-containing proteins were identified by means of their enzymatic activities in the separated fractions. At a retention time (RT) of 7 min elutes delta aminolevulinate dehydratase, which is also a lead-binding protein. The Zn-signal at RT=10 min is associated with Cu/Zn superoxid dismutase. It is the main Cu-containing enzyme in erythrocytes.

The main Zn-signal at RT=11 min belongs to carbonic anhydrase I and

II. Selenium elutes in 2 fractions at RT=7.5 and RT=10
The selenoenzyme glutathione peroxidase was identified in the fraction eluted at RT=7.5 min by means of the enzymatic activity, the other signal remains unidentified. The same applies for the Mn, Cd and two of the Pb-signals.

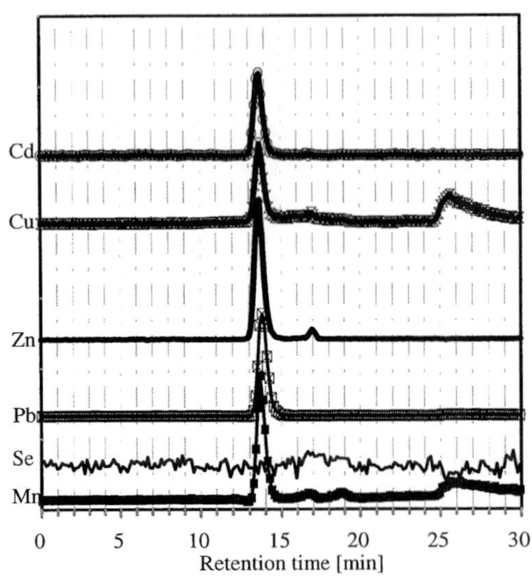

Fig. 2: Elution profiles of elements in granulocyte lysate of a healthy person, Superdex 75 20 mM TRIS pH 7.4

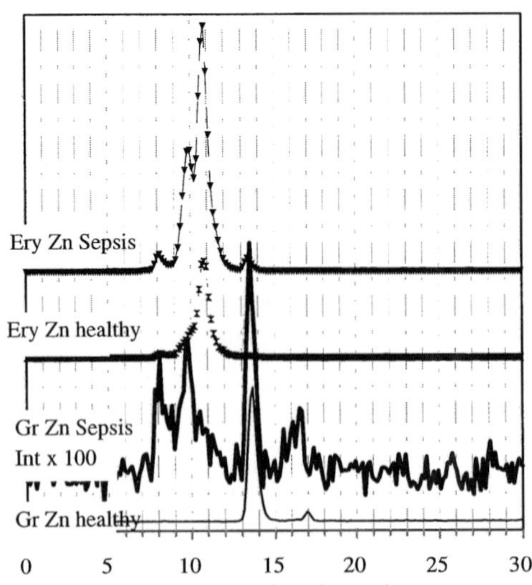

Fig. 3: Zinc pattern in granulocytes (Gr) and erythrocytes (ery) of a healthy person and a sepsis patient

Granulocytes

The distribution pattern of the elements Mn, Se, Cd, Pb, Cu and Zn in granulocytes lysate of a healthy person is shown in Fig. 2. Due to the low iron content of granulocytes it was not possible to detect Fe-containing proteins. Granulocytes contain predominantly metalloproteins with a molecular mass range below 12 kDa. Probably the signals found are associated with metallo-proteinases (Zn-containing) and metallothionein (coelution of Zn, Cu and Cd). In addition to the main signal at RT=13.5 min, there are two smaller signals for Zn and Cu at RT=16 and RT=17 min. Granulocytes do not contain enough glutathione peroxidase to produce a Se signal.

Lymphocytes and thrombocytes were also separated and chromatographed (pattern not shown here). In contrast to granulocytes and lymphocytes thrombocytes contain a large amount of the Se-dependent glutathione peroxidase. Their metalloproteins elute in the RT range 5 to 15 min.

We studied the distribution pattern of Mn, Cu, Cd, Pb, Zn and Se in erythrocyte and granulocyte lysate of postoperative sepsis patients in comparison to that of healthy people. Presumably connected with the pathological status of postoperative sepsis the separation of the different blood cell types by means of density gradient centrifugation was more difficult. During the first days of a sepsis episode a left shift of the white blood cells could be observed. In this period the release of neutrophil granulocytes from the bone marrow is intensified.

The granulocytes obtained from a sepsis patient contain much less metalloproteins than expected (Fig. 3-5). Compared to a healthy control the intensity of the Zn signal at RT=13.5 min from the sepsis patient (not substituted with zinc) is more than one order of magnitude lower.

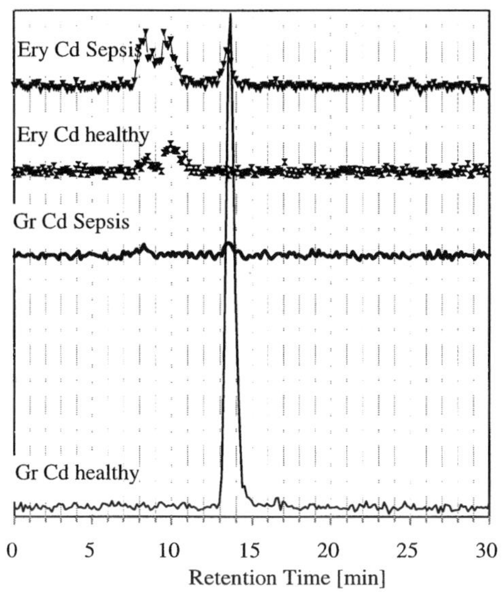

Fig. 4: Cadmium pattern in granulocytes (Gr) and erythrocytes (ery) of a healthy person and a sepsis patient

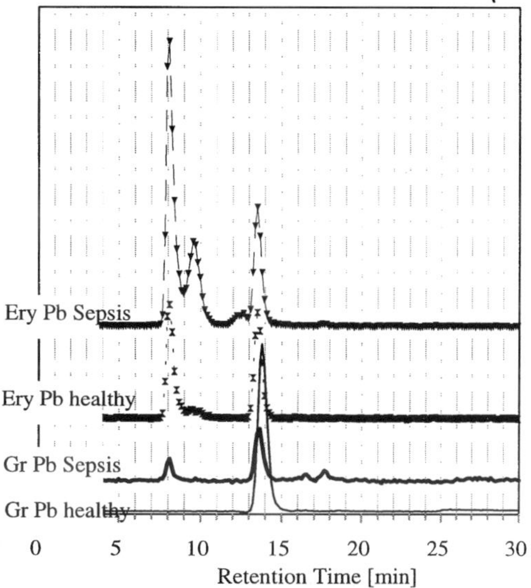

Fig. 5: Lead pattern in granulocytes (Gr) and erythrocytes (ery) of a healthy person and a sepsis patient

As observed for zinc, during the sepsis episode the concentration of Cd and Pb in granulocytes decrease. It is suggested that the low metalloprotein content of granulocytes is caused by the high proliferation rate and the quick turn over during a sepsis episode. The elution profiles of metalloproteins in erythrocytes from a sepsis patient show more signals than that of a healthy person (Fig. 3-5). As mentioned before, however, this might be due to the difficulties in the complete separation of the different cell types.

Metal Ions in Biology and Medicine; vol 6. Eds. J.A. Centeno, Ph. Collery, G. Vernet, R.B. Finkelman, H. Gibb, J.C. Etienne. John Libbey Eurotext, Paris © 2000, pp. 410-412.

Metalloid and metal speciation in a microelectronic research center

N. Proust[1], M. Guindo[1], R. Herzog[1], D. Thénot[1], J.P. Buchet[2], O. Donard[3], C. Pecheyran[3], M.P. Pavageau[3]

[1] *Thomson CSF LCR, 91404 Orsay cedex, France; nicole.proust@lcr.thomson-csf.fr; tel : 33 (0)1 69 33 92 52, fax : 33 (0)1 69 33 08 66;* [2] *Catholic University of Louvain, 1200 Bruxelles, Belgium,* [3] *CNRS EP 132, 64000 Pau, France*

In Thomson CSF Corporate Research Center a significant part of our activities is devoted to semiconductors such as gallium arsenide (GaAs), and related compounds (GaInAsP, GaInP...). Semiconductor deposition is done by various chemical vapor methods such as Metal Organic Chemical Vapor Deposition (MOCVD), Chemical Beam Epitaxy (CBE) and Molecular Beam Epitaxy (MBE). Arsenic and phosphorous precursors are mineral (As, AsH_3, PH_3) or organometallic (tertiarybutylarsine TBA, trisdimethylaminoarsine DMAA and tertiarybutylphosphine TBP) compounds. Gallium and indium sources are metalorganics.

In order to assess risks and to preserve health at work, measurements of toxic gases emitted during semiconductor processing and deposition reactor maintenance was done and arsine, phosphine, TBA and TBP were first measured with a chemically impregnated paper tape monitor. But unfortunately if there is a mixture of these molecules the detector will give a global answer as speciation is impossible.

In order to solve this problem we tried a new method of air sampling and analysis [1], presently under development, based on cryo-sampling, gas chromatography and ICP MS allowing speciation. This powerful technique devoted till now to ecotoxicology has been investigated here. It allows simultaneous determination of volatile metal and metalloïd compounds in air. Determining the nature and the concentration of each pollutant is of extreme importance in order to make a full assessment of the toxicological risk at the work stations as toxicity is very dependant on the molecule. We report mainly on preliminary As (fig. 1 and 2) and P (fig. 3 and 4) qualitative results obtained during semiconductor processing or maintenance. Speciation or identification of various As and P gaseous chemicals (mineral and metalorganic species) in ambiant air can be done, unexpected and unknown species are observed too.

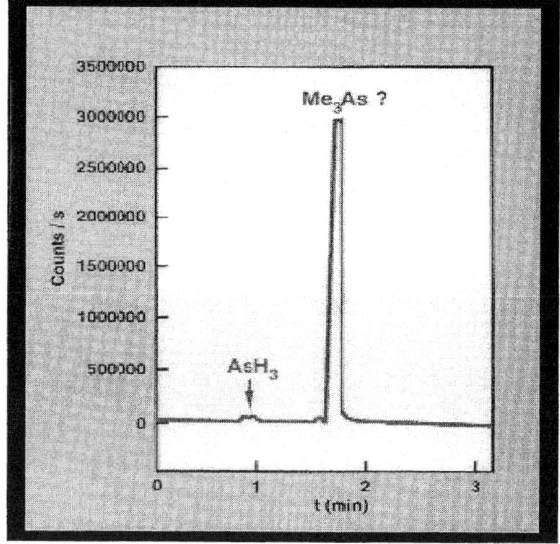

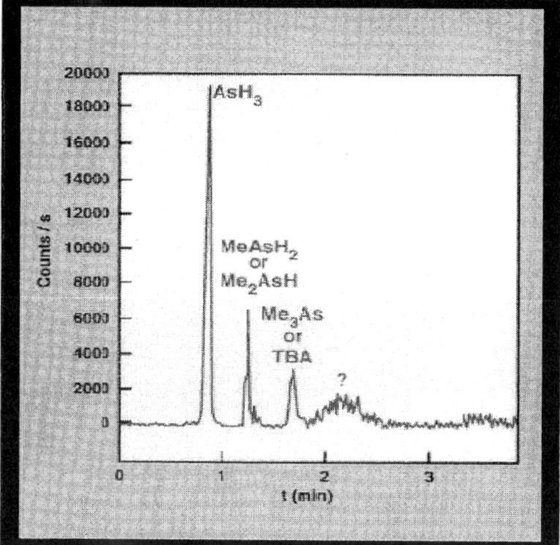

Figure 1 : CBE. Arsenic species in air over dirty mineral oil, pump on DMAA duct.

Figure 2 : CBE. Arsenic species in air over dirty mineral oil on TBA duct.

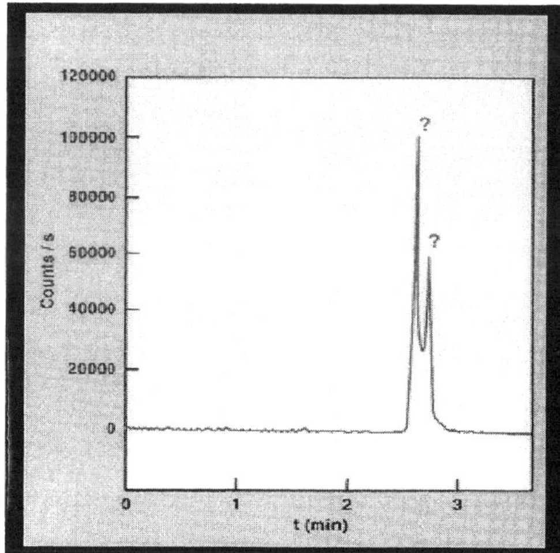

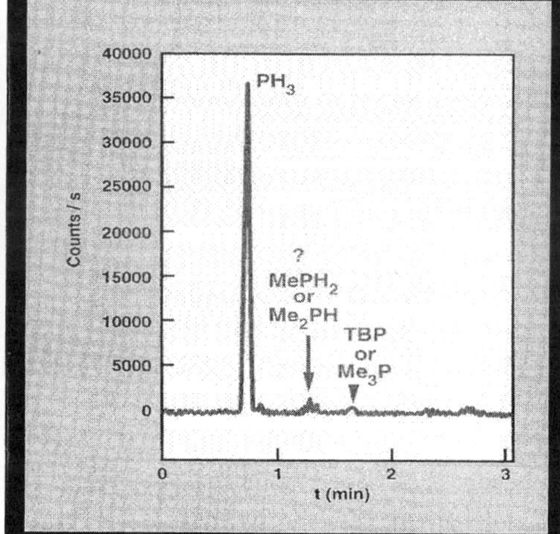

Figure 3 : MOCVD trap. Phosphorous species in air. (MDA 7100 < 3 ppb PH_3)

Figure 4 : CBE. Phosphorous species in air over dirty mineral oil, pump on TBP duct.

Biological monitoring based on arsenic speciation in urine is used to assess the potential absorption of As by semiconductor operators. Arsenic speciation is done in urine and

three metabolites As_{in} (inorganic As compounds, valence +3 and +5), MMA (Mono Methyl Arsonic acid), DMA (Di Methyl Arsinic acid) related to inorganic arsenic exposure are measured. Consumption of water containing arsenic, of seafood have to be avoided in order to suppress interferences which are making the analytical results not relevant and confusing. There is a relationship between exposure and metabolite excretion in urine and for industrial purposes a Biological Exposure Indice (BEI) has been proposed [2]. People are generally considered as non exposed to mineral arsenic if the sum (As_{in} + MMA + DMA) is in the range of 10µg As/g creatinine. In case of exposure, a 50 µg/m^3 TWA concentration will induced approximately an arsenic excretion of 50 µg/g creatinine and a 10 µg/m^3 a level of 30 µg/g creatinine.
For metabolite determination, urinary analysis is performed by hydride-cryogenic–atomic absorption which is a well qualified and reproducible technique. A comparison between a recent J.P Buchet's study on non exposed people and our results [3] has been done, the level of exposure in our research center seems to be low.

In conclusion in Thomson CSF Corporate Research Center there are potential expositions variable in duration and intensity to different As and P based chemicals, some are well qualified but others, possible during maintenance operations need to be characterized in detail at each work station, consequently analytical speciation has to be encouraged and developed as it is a powerful tool to assess risks more accurately.
As people are generally well protected by adequate protective equipment and requested to follow special work procedures the level of mineral As exposure seems to be low as it is shown by urinary results.

References

[1]Pecheyran C, Quetel C. R, Martin Lecuyer F and Donard O.F.X. Simultaneous determination of volatile metal (Pb, Hg, Sn, In, Ga) and non-metal species (Se, P, As) in different atmospheres by cryofocusing and detection by ICP/MS. Anal.Chem.1998,vol 70, p2639-2645.

[2] Lauwerys R.R and Hoet P, Industrial chemical exposure. Guidelines for biological monitoring, Lewis, 1993.

[3] Proust N, Guindo Nignan M, Thénot D, Herzog R, J.P. Buchet JP, Donard O, Pecheyran C. Arsenic speciation : exposure and associated biometrology in a microelectronic research center . Invited paper at SSA conference, San Diego, 1999.

Metal Ions in Biology and Medicine; vol 6. Eds. J.A. Centeno, Ph. Collery, G. Vernet, R.B. Finkelman, H. Gibb, J.C. Etienne. John Libbey Eurotext, Paris © 2000, pp. 413-415.

Risk posed by platinum-group metals as a consequence of the adoption of catalytic converters for automotive traction

S. Caroli[1], F. Petrucci[1], A. Alimonti[1], B. Bocca[1], F. Forastiere[2]

[1] *Istituto Superiore di Sanità, Viale Regina Elena 299, 00161 Rome, Italy;* [2] *Osservatorio Epidemiologico Regione Lazio, Via S. Costanza 53, 00198 Rome, Italy*

Introduction

In most industrialized countries new cars are nowadays equipped with catalytic converters to abate the emission of aromatic hydrocarbons, CO and NO_x. Such converters exist in a number of versions, although they basically consist of a monolithic honeycomb support made of cordierite (a phase of 2 $MgO \cdot 2\ Al_2O_3 \cdot 5\ SiO_2$), on which the so-called washcoat is supported. This last contains the active metals Pd, Pt and Rh in various combinations, or even alone, along with oxides of rare-earth elements acting as stabilizers. By general acknowledgement, the thermal and mechanical conditions under which such devices work (including abrasion effects and hot-temperature chemical reactions with oil fumes) can cause significant release of the Pt-group metals (PGMs) to the environment and eventually affect human health (1). The total extent of the emission, its composition in terms of relative concentrations of the three metals and the average size of the emitted particles strongly depend on the catalyst type and traffic conditions. This is still a highly controversial issue in that the estimated release of, *e.g.*, Pt is reported to range from a few ng km^{-1} to several $\mu g\ km^{-1}$ when the car has a speed of 50-100 km h^{-1}, although the age of the catalyst may in part account for such discrepancies. Palladium, Pt and Rh can play a role as sensitizers in the etiology of allergenic pathologies such as asthma, conjunctivitis, dermatitis, rhinitis and urticaria (2). Moreover, Pt is also a well-know cytotoxic agent and for this reason it is widely used in several anticancer drugs (*e.g.*, Cisplatin and Carboplatin) for the treatment of a number of malignancies (3). Beyond applications targeted to tumoral cells, however, chronic exposure to this metal can severely impact on living organisms. In this context, due consideration being given to the still keen lack of reliable experimental data on the levels of Pd, Pt and Rh in biological fluids, an investigation was carried out to quantify the concentration of such elements in the urine of a group of 316 schoolboys from the urban and the suburban area of Rome. The relevant findings are reported hereafter.

Experimental

Young subjects (age 6-10 years) attending primary schools in Rome and its outskirts were selected to represent both heavy- (H), intermediate- (I) and low-traffic (L) zones of the metropolitan area of the capital (seven schools in total). Informed consent of parents was obtained. For each subject a questionnaire was filled in at the moment of urine sampling in order to gain basic information on the life style, dietary habits and health conditions. In order to include in the study only those subjects with no specific pathologies. As the collection of 24-h urine samples was impracticable, it was decided to sample only morning urine under the responsibility of the school health care personnel specifically instructed to the task. For each subject, the element concentrations were ratioed to those of creatinine. These normalized figures provide complete information on the total daily excretion of Pd, Pt and Rh. The risk of chemical contamination of the urine samples at any stage of the collection and storage was carefully minimized by adopting strict procedures. This is all the more crucial given the extremely low amounts expected for the analytes of interest. To this end, carefully decontaminated high-density polyethylene screw-cap vials (Falcon®, Becton Dickinson, Lincon Park, NJ, USA) were employed. Immediately after sampling, each vial was labeled with the subject's name and a reference number coinciding with that on the relevant questionnaire and frozen at - 0 °C for subsequent delivery to the analytical laboratories of the Istituto Superiore di Sanità (Italian National Institute of Health). The total number of subjects eventually available was 316. All further operations were performed in a Class-100 clean room (Tamco, Rome, Italy). From each vial an aliquot of 5 ml urine was subsampled, poured into another chemically decontaminated polyethylene tube of the same type and added with 2.0 ml of 30 % high-purity H_2O_2 (Suprapur® grade, Merck, Darmstadt, Germany) and 1.0 ml of 65 % high-purity HNO_3 (Suprapur® grade, Merck). The specimens were subsequently UV-irradiated for 90 min at a distance of 15 cm from an Hg lamp (power 500 W) (Helios Italquartz, Milan, Italy). Clear and homogeneous solutions could be obtained upon completion of this treatment. A final 1:20 dilution of these solutions was carried out by means of high-purity water. Blank solutions were also set up by following the same procedure and by replacing the 5 ml urine sample with 5 ml high-purity water. Calibrants were prepared daily by dilution of stock solutions of 1000 mg l^{-1} of Pd (SPEX, Edison, NJ), of 1000 mg l^{-1} of Pt (PE Pure, Perkin-Elmer, Norwalk, CT, USA) and of 100 mg l^{-1} of Rh (Plasmachem, Farmingdale, NJ, USA). Magnetic sector high-resolution inductively-coupled plasma mass spectrometry (HR-ICP-MS) was resorted to for the analytical determinations as by this technique the Pt-group metals can be quantified in urine significantly below the ng l^{-1} level (8). The detection is more than adequate to the specific needs posed by this study. Nonetheless, some serious problems still remain as regards mass interferences caused by isobaric and multiple ions. Such interferences (*e.g.*, those of $^{206}Pb^{2+}$ on ^{103}Rh and of $^{40}Ar^{66}Zn$ on ^{106}Pd) not always can be solved by even the highest mass resolution ($m/\Delta m$) afforded by the spectrometer, *i. e.*, 7500. Appropriate mass correction equations must be thus developed to achieve accurate analytical signals. All experimental data were subject to basic statistical treatment to calculate means, medians, geometric means, standard deviations and quartiles. More refined treatments were applied to identify specific trends as a function of location, age and gender.

Results and Discussion

Table I reports the overall figures of merit obtained after pooling the data of the seven schools. The statistical treatment, based on the SIDRIA programme, revealed a clear difference between the subjects pertaining to urban areas (Rome, Frosinone and Latina/Anagni) as compared to those of a more rural site (Allumiere). This pattern correlates well with the intensity of traffic in the various zones of concern. From a general viewpoint the data obtained support to a certain extent the assumption that the overall exposure to PGMs is rather uniform over large areas with a more or less pronounced (but not dramatic) dependence on the intensity of local traffic. Not surprisingly, this can be assumed to be the consequence of the long-range transportation of finer particles of car exhaust fumes once these are released to the atmosphere. What can be concluded from this investigation is that: *i*) by urine analysis the environmental exposure of individuals to PGMs can be easily monitored; *ii*) PGMs can be reliably quantified in urine by HR-ICP-MS, although there is still room for improvement in the analytical approach; *iii*) the decision-maker should carefully deal with the problem of environmental dispersion of PGMs for their potentially serious consequences.

References

1. Lustig S., *Platinum in the Environment.* UTZ Verlag, München, 1997.
2. Dayan A. D. (Ed.), *Immunotoxicity of Metals and Immunotoxicology.* New York: Plenum Press, 1990.
3. Dominici C., Petrucci F., Caroli S., Alimonti A., Clerico A. & Castello M. A., A Pharmacokinetic Study of High-dose Continuous Infusion Cisplatin in Children with Solid Tumors, *J. Clin. Oncol.* 1989; 7: 100-107.
4. Krachler M., Alimonti A., Petrucci F., Irgolić K. J., Forestiere F., Caroli S., Analitical Problems in the Determination of Platinum-group Metals in Urine by Quadrupole and Magnetic Sector Field Inductively Coupled Plasma Mass Spectrometry, *Anal. Chim. Acta* 1998; 363: 1-10.

Table I

Overall concentrations and relevant statistical data for Pt-group metals in urine of children (pool of the seven schools, all values in ng g^{-1} creatinine).

Normalized concentration	Pd	Pt	Rh
± standard deviation	7.5 ± 5.4	0.9 ± 1.1	8.5 ± 8.0
Normalized media	6.5	0.6	6.0
Normalized range	0.1 - 36.6	<LoD* - 9.5	0.4 - 50.0
25 % quartile	3.4	0.2	3.1
75 % quartile	10.1	1.2	10.6

LoD = Limit of Detection

Metal Ions in Biology and Medicine; vol 6. Eds. J.A. Centeno, Ph. Collery, G. Vernet, R.B. Finkelman, H. Gibb, J.C. Etienne. John Libbey Eurotext, Paris © 2000, pp. 416-418.

Speciation of antimony in environmental specimens by HPLC-ICP-MS and HPLC-HG-AAS

Michael Krachler and Hendrik Emons

Research Centre Juelich, Institute of Applied Physical Chemistry, D-52425 Juelich, Germany

During recent years, the environmental concern about antimony (Sb) has grown considerably because anthropogenic emission has resulted in an increasing concentration of Sb in the environment. Potential harmful effects of inorganic and organic Sb compounds on organisms have motivated the US Environmental Protection Agency (EPA) and the German Research Community (DFG) to list Sb and its compounds as priority pollutants. However, the knowledge about the potential harmful effects of this metal is still scarce and needs to be further elucidated.
This study was undertaken to provide more relevant data on total Sb concentrations in environmental matrices from terrestrial and limnic ecosystems and first insights into Sb speciation in environmental and biological specimens.

Experimental

Ultra trace determinations of Sb were carried out by flow injection hydride generation atomic absorption spectrometry (FI-HG-AAS) after open vessel digestion of the samples with adequate mixtures of nitric, perchloric, hydrofluoric, and sulfuric acids [1-4]. For speciation studies, the three Sb species Sb(III), Sb(V), and trimethyl antimonydichloride (TMSb) were separated by high performance liquid chromatography coupled on-line either to HG-AAS or inductively coupled plasma mass spectrometry using an ultrasonic nebulizer with membrane desolvation (USN-ICP-MS), respectively. Two different anion exchange columns (Dionex AS14, ION-120) were employed for all chromatographic separations [5].

Results and Discussion

Detection limits based on FI-HG-AAS amount to 10 ng/L for total Sb concentrations in extracts of plant matrices. These detection limits are sufficiently low to adequately monitor trace concentrations of Sb even in unexposed specimens [1-3]. Environmental concentrations of Sb ranged from 2 ng/g in pigeon eggs to 589 ng/g in elder leaves collected beside a motorway [1-3]. Antimony concentrations in elder leaves from Germany were closely correlated with car traffic: maximum Sb concentrations of 589 ng/g were found directly beside a motorway, 207 ng/g in a distance of 50 m from the motorway and 153 ng/g in a close residential area. Interestingly, elder leaves from Argentina showed only about 4 ng Sb/g (Fig. 1).

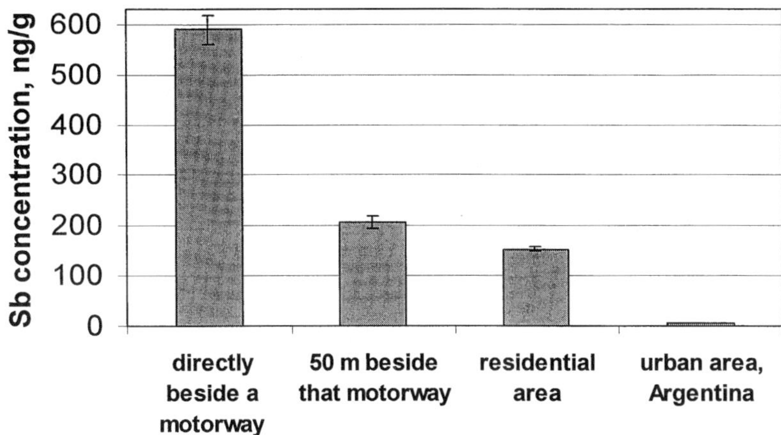

Fig. 1: Concentrations of Sb in virgin elder leaves from different sampling sites.

Chromatographic parameters for the separation of Sb(III), Sb(V), and TMSb were investigated throughout. Instrumental parameters for the HPLC-HG-AAS- and HPLC-ICP-MS-setup were optimized in dependence of the species. Finally, Sb(III) and Sb(V) were separated with a Dionex AS14 column using 1.25 mM EDTA at pH 4.7 as eluent. The ION-120 anion exchange column with 2 mM NH_4HCO_3 and 1 mM tartaric acid at pH 8.5 served as separation medium for TMSb and Sb(V).
Detection limits for each of the three Sb species were about 1 µg/L when HG-AAS was employed as element-specific detector, whereas detection limits for HPLC-ICP-MS were found to be two orders of magnitude lower as pointed out in Table 1.

Table 1: Detection limits (µg/L) for Sb(III), Sb(V), and TMSb using HPLC coupled to HG-AAS and ICP-MS as element-specific detectors.

	Sb(III)	Sb(V)	TMSb
HPLC-HG-AAS	0.7	1.0	0.4
HPLC-ICP-MS	0.014	0.012	0.009

The developed chromatographic procedures were applied to the determination of Sb compounds in tap water. As total concentrations of Sb are expected to be very low (< 1 µg/L), HPLC-ICP-MS was employed for that purpose. Fig. 2 summarizes the results of those investigations. Sb(V) could be identified as major Sb compound in tap water, with traces of Sb(III) being present. No TMSb, as somehow expected, could be found in tap water.

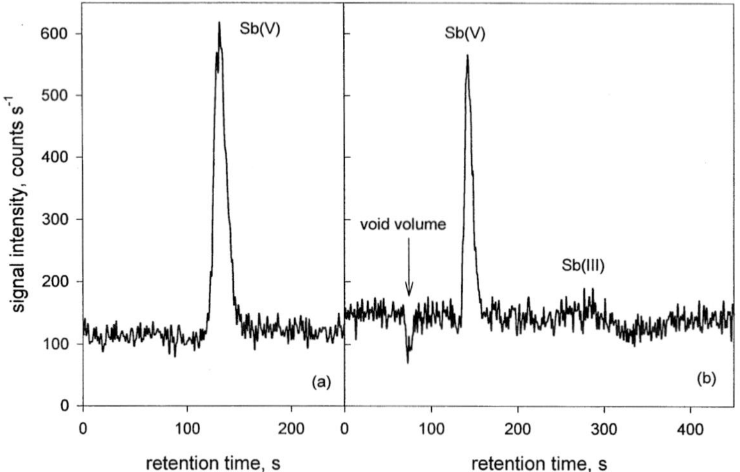

Fig. 2: Determination of Sb compounds in tap water using HPLC-ICP-MS. Results reveal that about 100 ng Sb(V)/L are present in that sample, traces of Sb(III), and no TMSb: (a) Separation of TMSb and Sb(V), (b) Separation of Sb(V) and Sb(III).

Conclusions: The analytical procedures developed are well suited for the trace determination and speciation of Sb in specimens of different provenience, thus shedding more light on the fate of Sb in biota.

This study was financially supported by the European Community through the Research Program TMR, EU contract No. FMBICT982889.

References:

[1] Krachler, M., Burow, M., Emons, H., *Analyst*, 1999, **124**, 777.
[2] Krachler, M., Burow, M., Emons, H., *Analyst*, 1999, **124**, 923.
[3] Krachler, M., Burow, M., Emons, H., *J Environ Monitoring*, 1999, **1**, 477.
[4] Krachler, M., Emons, H., *Analyst*, 2000, submitted.
[5] Krachler, M., Emons, H., *J Anal At Spectrom*, 2000, in press.

Metal Ions in Biology and Medicine; vol 6. Eds. J.A. Centeno, Ph. Collery, G. Vernet, R.B. Finkelman, H. Gibb, J.C. Etienne. John Libbey Eurotext, Paris © 2000, pp. 419-421.

Speciation of selenium by HPLC-ICP MS: application to mechanisms underlying metabolism

K.T. Suzuki*, Y. Kobayashi, Y. Shiobara and Y. Ogra

Faculty of Pharmaceutical Sciences, Chiba University, Chiba 263-8522, Japan. Fax/Phone: 81-43-290-2891; e-mail: ktsuzuki@p.chiba-u.ac.jp

Selenium (Se) is a micronutrient essential for health, and also it is highly toxic when present in excess. Both the organic and inorganic forms of Se can be utilized as nutritional sources, the former being selenocysteinyl (SeCys) and selenomethionyl (SeMet) residues, and the latter being selenite and selenate. The metabolic pathway for Se depends on its chemical form and the route of administration. Selenate is reduced to selenite and then to the hypothetical key intermediate selenide (H_2Se), which is then either utilized for the synthesis of selenoproteins or excreted after being methylated [1,2]. As a change in the chemical form of Se is reflected in the metabolic pathway, the chemical species of Se has to be determined to understand the mechanism.

A hyphenated technique, i.e., the combination of gel filtration by HPLC and simultaneous multi-element specific detection by mass spectrometry with ionization by inductively coupled argon plasma (ICP MS), has been applied to a Se speciation [2]. Both endogenous and exogenous Se (enriched tracer) in biological samples such as plasma/serum, urine, and the soluble fractions of the liver and other organs were separated on a gel filtration HPLC column, and Se in the eluate was determined using an ICP MS as an element-specific detector at m/e = 77 or 78 for endogenous Se and m/e = 82 for exogenous Se. The enriched Se (^{82}Se) used as a tracer in the present study is much more easily detectable than naturally occurring endogenous ^{77}Se or ^{78}Se because of the detection of the enriched isotope (97 % enriched ^{82}Se) by MS.

Selenite enriched with a stable isotope was used to trace the metabolic fate of exogenous Se [3]. ^{82}Se-Selenite injected intravenously into rats was shown to be taken up rapidly by red blood cells, reduced to selenide by glutathione, and then released into the plasma [4], where selenide binds selectively to albumin [5]. The ^{82}Se bound to albumin is taken up by the liver, where the labeled Se is detected as two distinct peaks, A and B. The peak A material is transformed to the peak B one in vivo with time, and also on methylation with methyl iodide in vitro. The peak B material is identical with the major urinary metabolite of Se but not identical with the trimethylselenonium ion. These results suggest that ^{82}Se taken up by the liver is either utilized for the synthesis of selenoproteins or metabolized to methylated urinary products. Among selenoproteins, the labeled Se was efficiently and rapidly incorporated into selenoprotein P (Sel P) and then excreted into the plasma [6]. However, the labeled Se was not detected in the forms of possible intermediates between the form transferred from albumin to the liver and that incorporated into Sel P. On the other hand, the labeled Se was shown to be detected in the forms of the two distinct Se peak, peaks A and B materials, the former being methylated to the latter, the major urinary metabolite.

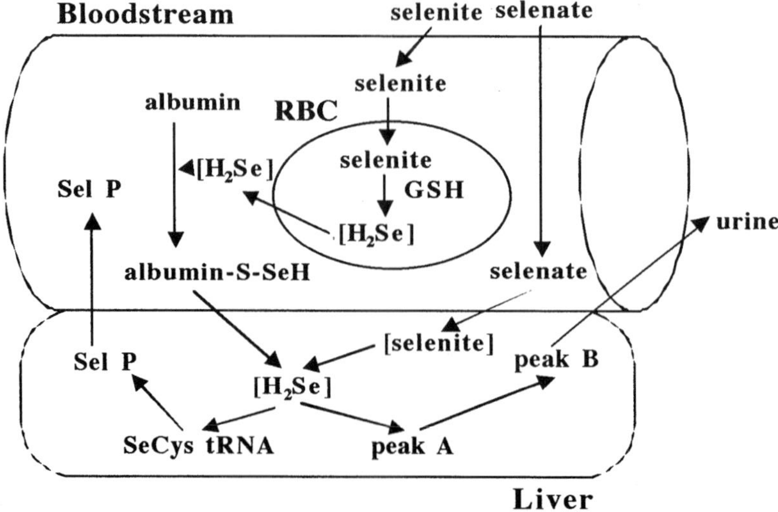

Figure 1. Schematic presentation of the metabolic pathways for selenite and selenate injected intravenously into rats.

^{82}Se-Selenate was injected intravenously into rats. Contrary to selenite, selenate was present in the plasma in the form of selenate without being taken up by RBCs until it disappeared from the bloodstream, and then was taken up directly by the liver. Once the ^{82}Se appeared in the liver, it was detected in the forms of the peak A and B materials in the liver as in the case of selenite [7]. The labeled Se disappeared from the peak corresponding to selenate in the plasma with time, and then started to be detected in the plasma as Sel p, a selenoprotein synthesized in the liver, suggesting that selenate is reduced to selenite during or immediately after the uptake by the liver, and then utilized for the synthesis of selenoproteins, similarly to selenite, and is incorporated most efficiently into Sel P, which is excreted into the plasma. Selenate was transformed much slowly than selenite to the peak B material on incubation in the liver homogenate in vitro. These results suggest that selenate is taken up directly by the liver and reduced during or immediately after the uptake, and that the reduction from selenate to selenite is the rate-limiting step. The chemical forms of the peak A and B materials are under investigation.

Selenite in the bloodstream is more efficiently taken up by RBCs than filtered by the glomerulus, transformed to selenide in RBC, transported to the plasma, and then transferred to the liver in a form bound to albumin, while selenate is thought to be taken up directly by the liver or filtered by the glomerulus. As a result, although some selenate was excreted directly into the urine right after the injection, selenite was not, suggesting that selenite is much more efficiently utilized by the body when injected intravenously. Our preliminary data showed that approximately one-fifth of the dose of selenite relative to selenate gave the same amounts of the peak B material, as the major urinary metabolite, and plasma Sel P, as the major selenoprotein synthesized in the liver, suggesting that the effective dose of Se for parenteral nutrition is approximately selenite = 1/5 of selenate. Although the metabolic pathways for Se injected intravenously in the forms of selenite and selenate are quite different in the bloodstream until they are taken up by the liver and transformed to the assumed common intermediate, selenide, those after the intermediate selenide seem to be identical.

References

1. K.T. Suzuki and Y. Ogra, Speciation of biological trace elements by HPLC-ICP MS: Application to elucidation of the mechanisms underlying the interaction between mercury and selenium (in Japanese). Biomed. Res. Trace Elements, 10, 95-102 (1999).
2. R. Lobinski, J. Edmonds, K.T. Suzuki and P. Uden, Species-selective analysis for selenium compounds in biological materials. Pure Appl. Chem. in press.
3. K.T. Suzuki, Simultaneous speciation of endogenous and exogenous elements by HPLC/ICP-MS with enriched stable isotopes. Tohoku J. Exp. Med., 178, 27-35 (1996).
4. K.T. Suzuki, Y. Shiobara, M. Itoh and M. Ohmichi, Selective uptake of selenite by red blood cells. Analyst, 123, 63-67 (1998).
5. Y. Shiobara and K.T. Suzuki, Binding of selenium (administered as selenite) to albumin after efflux from red blood cells. J. Chromatogr. B, 710, 49-56 (1998).
6. K.T. Suzuki, K. Ishiwata and Y. Ogra, Incorporation of selenium into selenoprotein P and extracellular glutathione peroxidase: HPLC-ICP MS data with enriched selenite. Analyst, 124, 1749-1753 (1999).
7. Y. Shiobara, Y. Ogra and K.T. Suzuki, Speciation of metabolites of selenate in rats by HPLC-ICP MS. Analyst, 124, 1237-1242 (1999).

Metal Ions in Biology and Medicine; vol 6. Eds. J.A. Centeno, Ph. Collery, G. Vernet, R.B. Finkelman, H. Gibb, J.C. Etienne. John Libbey Eurotext, Paris © 2000, pp. 422-424.

Distribution of silicon in body fluids and infant formula and its preliminary speciation

Stanislaw Lugowski[1], Dennis Smith[1], Hanna Bonek[1], John Semple[2], Walter Peters[3]

[1] IBBME, University of Toronto, 170 College Street, M5S 3E3 Toronto; [2] Women's College Hospital, 76 Greenville Street, M5S 1B2 Toronto; [3] Wellesley Hospital, 160 Wellesley Street, M4Y 1J3 Toronto

ABSTRACT

The controversies associated with silicone gel breast implants have been a driving force for biological silicon research. Similar considerations apply to the resolution of issues related to silicones and silicon compounds in situations such as renal dialysis, neurological diseases and adverse environmental exposures. Although silicon is considered to be an essential trace element in the broad sense of that term, biological studies on silicon are still at an early stage. Our goal was to measure silicon in whole blood, plasma, breast milk and infant formula and their methyl iso butyl ketone (MIBK) extracts. The analytical techniques used in our work are described in our publications [1], [2]. Procedures include very careful sample collection, sample preparation under Class 100 conditions and graphite furnace atomic absorption spectrophotometric determination of silicon with Ca matrix modifier. In our measurements ca 35 % of blood Si was found in plasma. The extractable species of Si from blood, plasma, breast milk and formula are 0.3 to 16% of total Si.

INTRODUCTION

Our previous studies [1] on Si and silicone levels in body tissues and fluids in women with implants and matched controls have found Si values in low ppb (ng/ml) range. The data indicate an overlap between implanted and non-implanted women with values in blood, for example, ranging from 30 – 300 ng/ml. In some study groups statistical differences between mean have been observed, in others there was no significant difference. In this context it should be noted that there are a variety of sources of polydimethyl siloxanes in the everyday diet, in medications and devices because of their anti-foaming and wetting characteristics, for example, indigestion tablets, fruit juices, cooking oil, injection syringes, and blood oxygenators as well as environmental sources. Preliminary studies indicate part of the silicon species is extractable by solvents such as n-heptane and MIBK.

Carlisle and others [3] asserted that Si was an essential trace element required for the metabolism of higher animals and was involved in several important metabolic processes. However none of the aspects of its involvement in these processes is understood [4]. Because no mechanism for direct action of

Si on biological functions has yet been demonstrated bioinorganic explanations have been proposed to explain essentiality [5] especially through interactions with other biometals [4], [5].

Little is known about the nutritional requirements or metabolism of silicon. Si and silicone levels (in body fat for example [6]) may be influenced by diet and water intake. High levels of Si have been associated with nephropathy, hepatic and bone diseases [7], [8] and the frequency of spontaneous abortion [9]. In this context, although most studies and reviews have found no association between auto-immune and connective tissue diseases, breast implants and Si/silicone levels the possibility of, as yet, recognized effects is still acknowledged [10].

Our analytical GFAAS methodologies together with improved sample collection and preparation in a Class 100 laboratory have yielded reliable data. One limitation in Si analysis of biological tissues up to the present has been absence of a Standard Reference Material (SRM) with a biological matrix [11]. We have undertaken an international initiative in collaboration with National Institute of Standards and Technology (NIST) to develop an SRM with certified Si content.

Distribution and speciation study of silicon/silicone in body fluids can help in understanding the role of Si in the human organism as well as silicone degradation in the human body. Our goal in this work was to measure silicon in whole blood, plasma, breast milk and infant formula and their MIBK extracts.

MATERIALS AND METHODS

Blood and breast milk were collected from the implant and control patients using our contamination-free approach described elsewhere [1]. Plasma was separated from the part of the blood sample. MIBK extraction from whole blood, plasma, breast milk and infant formula was performed. GFAAS measurements of elemental Si in water based and organic solvent samples were completed. Conditions of these measurements were described elsewhere [1].

RESULTS

Results of the measurements of elemental silicon in blood, plasma, breast milk, infant formula and their MIBK extracts are presented in the Table below. Values are expressed in ng/ml

Concentration of Si	Whole Blood	Plasma	Breast Milk	Formula
Total	79.2 (n=159)	56.7 (n=131)	24.7 (n=40)	2930 (n=23)
Extractable	5.82 (n=116)	7.84 (n=99)	3.96 (n=30)	8.83 (n=17)

DISCUSSION

The extractable species of Si from blood, plasma, breast milk and formula are 0.3 to 16% of total Si. The identification of these silicones compounds using FTIR was not satisfactory because the detection limit of silicones for identification in MIBK was at the level of 50 µg/ml, whereas the concentration found in our extracts was much lower. The identification of these extractable silicon compounds using other techniques is currently under investigation. It is interesting that infant formula contains much more Si than breast milk. Speciation of the silicon compounds and its distribution in body fluids is of paramount value to understand Si metabolism and for proper assessment of the sequelae to silicone implants in the human body.

REFERENCES

1. Lugowski S, Smith DC, Bonek H, Lugowski J, Peters W ,Semple J, Analysis of silicon and silicone in human tissue with special reference to silicone gel breast implants. *Trace Elem. Med. Biol.*, 2000 ; in press .
2. Peters W, Smith DC, Lugowski S, McHugh A, MacDonald P ,Baines C, Silicon and silicone levels in patients with silicone implants, M. Potter and N.R. Rose, Editors. in *Immunology of silicones*. Berlin. Springer: 1996. p. 39-48.
3. Carlisle EM, Silicon as an essential trace element in animal nutrition, D. Evered and M. O'Connor, Editors. in *Silicon Biochemistry*. Chichester. John Willey & Sons: 1986. p. 123-136.
4. Parry R, Plowman D, Delves HT, Roberts NB, Birchall JD, Bellia JP, Davenport A, Ahmad R, Fahal I ,Altmann P, Silicon and aluminium interactions in haemodialysis patients. *Nephrol. Dial. Transplant.*, 1998 ; 13 : p. 1759-1762.
5. Exley C, Silicon in life: A bioinorganic solution to bioorganic essentiality. *Journal of Inorganic Biochemistry*, 1998 ; 69 : p. 139-144.
6. Barnard JJ, Todd EL, Wilson WG, Mielcarek R ,Rohrich RJ, Distribution of organosilicon polymers in augmentation mammaplasties at autopsy. *Plast. Reconstr. Surg.*, 1997 ; 100(1) : p. 197-205.
7. Roberts NB ,Williams P, Silicon measurement in serum and urine by direct current plasma emission spectrometry. *Clin. Chem.*, 1990 ; 36 : p. 1460-1465.
8. Hokosawa S ,Yoshida O, Silicon transfer during haemodialysis. *Int. Urol. Nephrol.*, 1990 ; 22 : p. 373-378.
9. Aschengrau A, Zierler S ,Cohen A, Quality of community drinking water and the occurrence of spontaneous abortion. *Arch. Environ. Health*, 1989 ; 44 : p. 283-290.
10. Cook RR, Hoshaw ,Perkins LL, Failure of silicone gel breast implants, analysis of literature data for 1652 explanted prosthses. *Plast. Reconstr. Surg.*, 1998 ; 101 : p. 1162.
11. Lugowski SJ, Smith DC, Lugowski JZ, Peters W ,Semple J, A review of silicon and silicone determination in tissue and body fluids - a need for standard reference materials. *Fresenius J. Anal. Chem.*, 1998 ; 360 : p. 486-488.

Metal Ions in Biology and Medicine; vol 6. Eds. J.A. Centeno, Ph. Collery, G. Vernet, R.B. Finkelman, H. Gibb, J.C. Etienne. John Libbey Eurotext, Paris © 2000, pp. 425-429.

Speciation of vanadium in serum, urine and tissues of Wistar rats

Koen De Cremer and Rita Cornelis

Laboratory for Analytical Chemistry, Ghent University, Proeftuinstraat 86, 9000 Ghent, Belgium

Introduction

During the past twenty years the trace element vanadium has received a lot of attention from researchers because of its biochemical actions in the body (e.g. insulin-like or anticarcinogenic characteristics, interaction with ATP-ases,...) [1-3]. Therefore speciation of vanadium has become important. Earlier studies of vanadium speciation using HPLC (High Pressure Liquid Chromatography) suffered from a not quantitative recovery of vanadium from the gelfiltration column [4-5]. After testing different columns [6] we found that a Superose 12 column gives the best results in relation to vanadium recovery and resolution of the different protein peaks. For this experiment we used a ^{48}V-tracer that we injected during one week into 5 male Wistar rats. The aim of the experiment was to look for the different vanadium-protein complexes in serum, urine and tissues with this selected column and to compare our results with the previous reports. Besides a total recovery of the vanadium, a better resolution for the protein peaks and the traditional vanadium-transferrin and vanadium-ferritin peaks, we found two other peaks. The first of this peaks is the low-molecular bound vanadium and the broad peak at the end is the unbound vanadium peak.

Materials and Methods

Five male Wistar rats were injected during 1 week with ^{48}V-tracer. On Monday (start) and Friday (end) they received a 20 µCi dose, on Tuesday there was no injection and Wednesday and Thursday they received 2 µCi. One hour after the last injection, the rats were anaesthetized and blood and urine were collected using the Venoject system preventing possible oxidation of vanadium complexes. Afterwards, the rats were dissected and the tissues (spleen, kidney, testes, liver and lung) were cleaned and homogenized using an Evelyn-Potter homogenizer. A Purifier 10XT chromatography system with a Superose 12 HR gelfiltration column (Amersham Pharmacia Biotech) was used. As elution buffer we used 10 mM hepes + 0.15 M NaCl at pH 7.3 with a 0.5 ml/min flowrate. All the chromatographic separations were done in a cleanroom (class 100). For serum and urine the samples were kept under argon blanket to prevent possible oxidation[7] of vanadium complexes. All tubes and buffers were flushed with argon prior to use.

Results and Discussion

In the chromatogram of 1:1 diluted rat serum (fig. 1) we find one [A] narrow ^{48}V peak (12-13 ml) and a second [B] broad peak at the end (26-35 ml). The first peak elutes together with a

UV-absorbing signal while the second does not. The first peak corresponds to the transferrin and albumin regio in the chromatogram. Out of anion-exchange experiments (not shown) it is obvious that vanadium in serum binds to transferrin and not to albumin. The second peak comprises not bound (`free`) vanadium.

The chromatogram of rat urine (fig. 2) shows one ^{48}V peak in the region of 16-19 ml [C] and a small one [D] around 30 ml. Both peaks do not fully overlap with a UV-absorbing peak. The 16-19 ml region corresponds with the total volume of the Superose 12 column. Surprisingly there are a lot of peaks (UV absorbing and ^{48}V) that elute after this total volume. In case of proteins this delay is mainly due to hydrophobic interactions. For the retention of the second ^{48}V peak another mechanism is involved. In urine vanadium seems mainly bound to low molecular ligands (16-19 ml). Identification of this ligands is currently being studied.

In the chromatograms of the different tissues (only spleen is shown, fig. 3) 4 major vanadium peaks can be observed. The first small peak [E] around 9 ml elutes in the ferritin region. The second vanadium peak [F] at 12-13 ml elutes in the transferrin region. The third [G] vanadium peak (16-18 ml) is vanadium bound to low molecular ligands and the last broad vanadium peak [H] around 31 ml consists of free vanadium. In the chromatograms of kidney, testes, lung and liver also four vanadium peaks are present.

Out of these chromatograms we see that vanadium can interact with different biological ligands in serum, urine and tissues of rats. Due to the 100% recovery of the vanadium from the Superose 12 column we are able to detect a peak of `free` vanadium at an elution volume around 30 ml. In other reports this broad peak could not be detetected because of adsorption phenomema on the previously used columns being the reason of a not quantitative recovery. It is also beneficial that this free vanadium elutes such a long time after the total volume (19-20 ml) of the column. In this way the free vanadium is separated from the low molecular weight complexes which elute in the total volume of the column. The reason of the retarded elution of the free vanadium is now being studied. The vanadium peak at 16-19 ml is believed to comprise different low-molecular vanadium complexes so further investigation is planned to separate this peak into more components.

Acknowledgement

The authors wish to thank Dr. K. Strijckmans for irradiating the 48-vanadium tracer and L. Mees for the technical assistance. KDC is grant holder of the Flemish Institute for the promotion of Scientific-Technological Research in Industry (IWT)

References

1. Cam MC, Li WM, McNeill JH. Partial Preservation of Pancreatic β-Cells by Vanadium: Evidence for Long-Term Amelioration of Diabetes. *Metabolism* 1997; 46 : 769-778.
2. Fujimoto S, Fujii K, Yasui H, Matsushita R, Takada J, Sakurai H. Long-Term Acting and Orally Active Vanadyl-Methylpicolinate Complex with Hypoglycemic Activity in Streptozotocin-Induced Diabetic Rats. *J Clin Biochem Nutr* 1997; 23 : 113-129.
3. Chatterjee M, Bishayee A. Vanadium- A New Tool for Cancer. Prevention. In: Nriagu JO, ed. *Vanadium in the Environment Part Two Health Effects*. New York : John Wiley & Sons, 1998 : 347-390.
4. Chasteen ND, Lord EM, Thompson HJ, Grady JK. Vanadium Complexes of Transferrin and Ferritin in the Rat. *Biochim Biophys Acta* 1986; 884 : 84-92
5. Sabbioni E, Marafante E. Metabolic Patterns of Vanadium in the Rat. *Bioinorganic Chemistry* 1978; 9 : 389-407.
6. De Cremer K, Cornelis R. Gelfiltration and Anion-Exchange Chromatography for the Separation of Vanadium Binding Proteins in Plasma of Rats, Rabbits and Humans. In : *Proceedings TEMA 10*. New York : Kluwer Academic/Plenum Press, 2000 (in press).
7. Chasteen ND, Grady JK, Holloway CE. Characterization of the Binding, Kinetics and Redox Stability of Vanadium(IV) and Vanadium(V) Protein Complexes in Serum. *Inorg Chem* 1986; 25 : 2754-2765

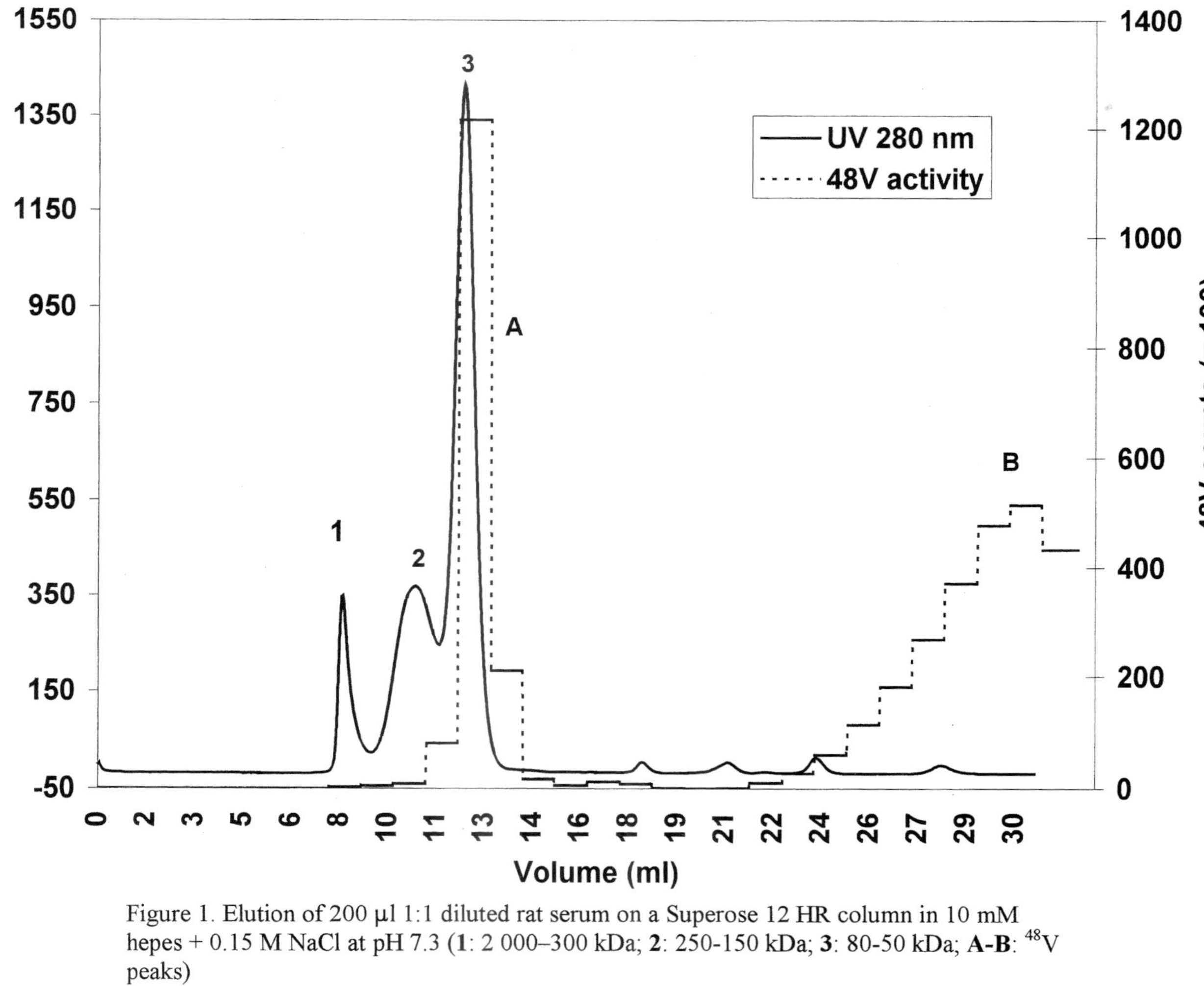

Figure 1. Elution of 200 µl 1:1 diluted rat serum on a Superose 12 HR column in 10 mM hepes + 0.15 M NaCl at pH 7.3 (**1**: 2 000–300 kDa; **2**: 250-150 kDa; **3**: 80-50 kDa; **A-B**: ^{48}V peaks)

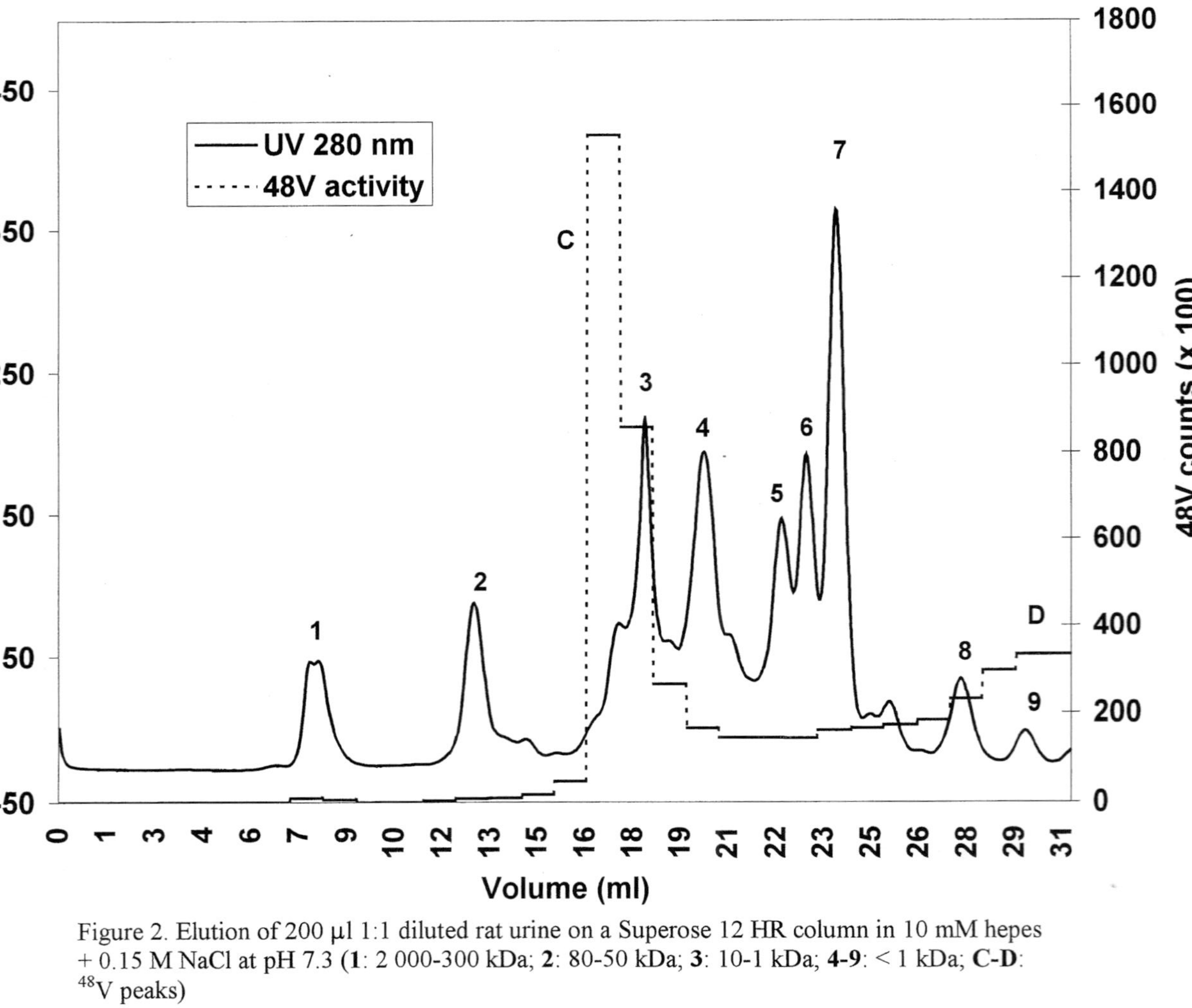

Figure 2. Elution of 200 µl 1:1 diluted rat urine on a Superose 12 HR column in 10 mM hepes + 0.15 M NaCl at pH 7.3 (**1**: 2 000-300 kDa; **2**: 80-50 kDa; **3**: 10-1 kDa; **4-9**: < 1 kDa; **C-D**: ^{48}V peaks)

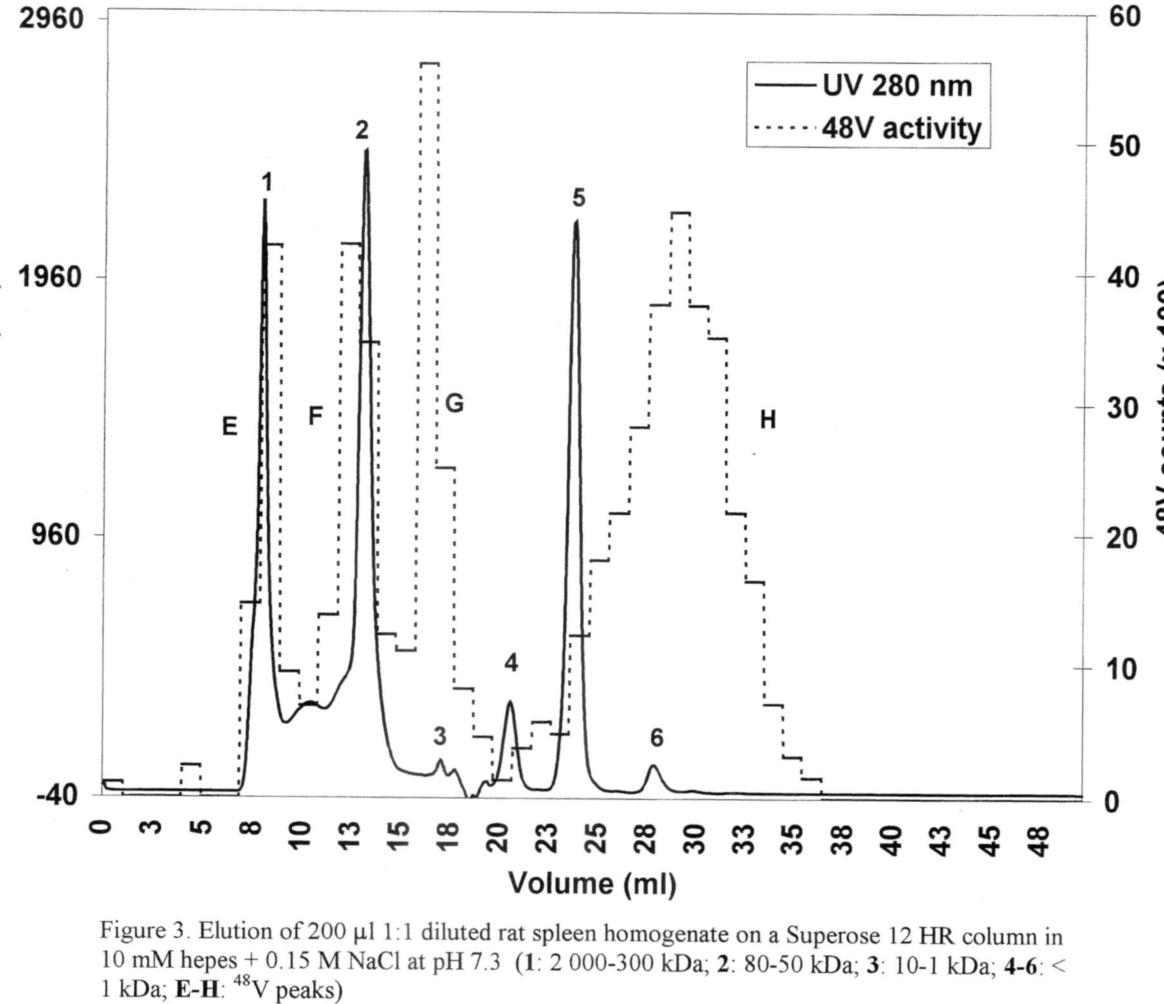

Figure 3. Elution of 200 µl 1:1 diluted rat spleen homogenate on a Superose 12 HR column in 10 mM hepes + 0.15 M NaCl at pH 7.3 (**1**: 2 000-300 kDa; **2**: 80-50 kDa; **3**: 10-1 kDa; **4-6**: < 1 kDa; **E-H**: ^{48}V peaks)

Metal Ions in Biology and Medicine; vol 6. Eds. J.A. Centeno, Ph. Collery, G. Vernet, R.B. Finkelman, H. Gibb, J.C. Etienne. John Libbey Eurotext, Paris © 2000, pp. 430-432.

Speciation of metallothioneins in animal and human samples from nanoliter volumes

Andreas Prange[1], Dirk Schaumlöffel[1], Andrea N. Richarz[2] and Peter Brätter[2]

[1] *GKSS Research Center, Institute for Physical and Chemical Analysis, Max-Planck-Str., D-21502 Geesthacht, Germany;* [2] *Hahn-Meitner-Institut Berlin, Glienicker Straße 100, D-14109 Berlin, Germany*

Abstract

A new approach using element speciation analysis for biochemical diagnostics is described. This involves the application of a newly developed coupling of capillary electrophoresis (CE) with inductively- coupled plasma - sector field mass spectrometry (ICP - SFMS) to the analysis of animal and human cytosols. Isoforms of metallothioneins are separated from 100 μL sample volumes via CE and the elements Cu, Zn, Cd and Pb are detected using ICP - SFMS.

Introduction

Metal-proteins have manifold functions in animal and human organisms. Of current interest are metal-proteins showing anti - oxidative properties, such as e.g. metallothioneins (MT's), which act as inhibitors to the formation of free radicals. A sensitive and specific determination of metallothioneins in small sample volumes from animal or human samples is therefore an important prerequisite for an extension of clinical-diagnostic as well as therapeutic methods of approach.

There is a lack of microanalysis procedures for element speciation in biomedical diagnostics, e.g. metal binding proteins such as metallothioneins in brain diseases. The aim of this contribution is therefore the development of an analytical procedure for the speciation of metallothioneins in human cytosols from small sample volumes.

Several approaches for coupling a chromatographic method with a metal - specific detector for speciation analysis have been described in the literature, such as reverse phase chromatography (RPC), ion exchange chromatography (IC), size exclusion chromatography (SEC) and capillary electrophoresis (CE) each coupled to inductively coupled mass spectrometry (ICP-MS) [1]. Our approach was to combine CE, which has excellent separation capability and permits the use of small sample volumes, with ICP-Sector Field Mass spectrometry for its high detection power.

Experimental

For a successful coupling of CE with ICP-MS the design of the interface is of prime importance. The CE / ICP-MS interface (CEI-100, CETAC Technologies) used here overcomes the major drawback of laminar flow inside the CE capillary and preserves the high resolving power of CE [2,3].

The conditions for the separation of the metallo-proteins in metallothionein standard solutions with respect to buffer concentrations and pH-values were optimized for the use of capillary electrophoresis. Furthermore the ICP-MS detection was compared to UV detection.

The extraction of cytosols is the first step in the analytical procedure. Tissue samples from human brain are homogenized in buffer solution, and ultracentrifugated. The supernatant is defatted and the cytosol pre-treatment with respect to matrix reduction is optimized for CE separation before injection into the column. Isoforms of metallothioneins are separated from 22 nL injection volumes via CE and the elements Cu, Zn, Cd and Pb are detected using ICP - SFMS.

Results and Discussion

The CE separation of a metallothionein isoform detected by ICP-MS is comparable to UV, but ICP-MS detection is much more sensitive and provides more information than UV detection. Because of the element-specific capabilities of ICP-MS, it can be noted which metal belongs to which isoform.

The buffer at the physiological pH of 7.4 is a good compromise. At high pH the separation is worse but fast. Although the separation at pH 6.9 is better, the migration time is longer and because of the deviation of the physiological pH, the native metal - protein relations could be changed. The buffer concentration of 20 mmol / L is deemed to be optimal; at higher concentrations, joule heating occurs, which leads to a worse separation.

The optimized separation method was applied to human brain cytosols. The electropherogram of the pure defatted cytosol shows the much longer migration times of the MT's than the MT's in standard solutions. For matrix reduction, to decrease the migration times, several methods were tested: dilution, heat de-naturation and acetonitrile precipitation. In comparison, the simple dilution of the sample is not very effective, heat denaturation lead to unidentified changes in the sample. Acetonitrile precipitation is deemed to be the best sample pre-treatment. The migration times of the MT's are comparable to standard solutions and no changes occur.

The electropherograms of the cytosols are detected at the element mass of Cu, Zn, Cd, and Pb. At the copper signal, 5 peaks can be observed, where 3 peaks are identified as MT1, MT2 and MT3 by spike experiments and comparison of migration times between standards and sample.

The analytical procedure developed was also used for comparative studies of brain samples taken from patients with Alzheimer's disease and healthy people with respect to the distribution of MT1, MT2 and MT 3 and the relation of the binding of copper and zinc to these MT isoforms (Fig. 1),.

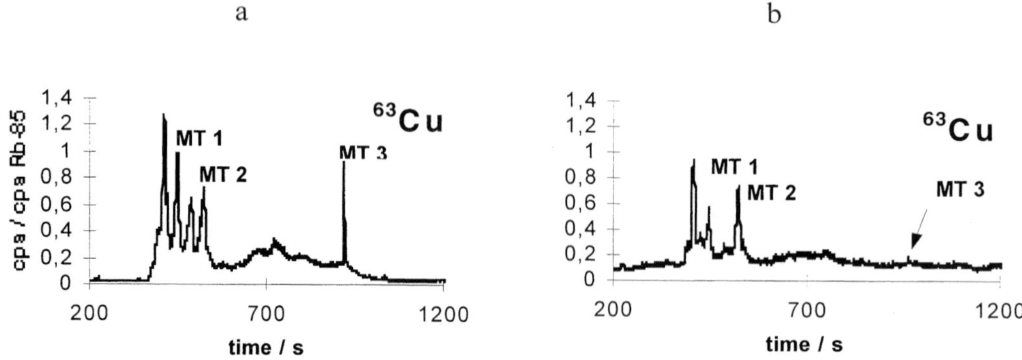

Fig. 1: Comparison of Cu-MT in human brain from healthy people (a) and patients with Alzheimer's disease (b)

Literature

(1) Lobinski R (1998) Elemental Speciation and Coupled Techniques. Applied Spectroscopy **51**, 260A

(2) Schaumlöffel D and Prange A (1999) A new interface for combining capillary electrophoresis with inductively coupled plasma - mass spectrometry. Fresenius J. Anal. Chem. **364** , 452 – 456

(3) Prange A and Schaumlöffel D (1999) Determination of element species at trace levels using Capillary Electrophoresis – Inductively Coupled Plasma - Sector Field Mass Spectrometry. J. Anal. At. Spectrom. **14**, 1329 -1332

Metal Ions in Biology and Medicine; vol 6. Eds. J.A. Centeno, Ph. Collery, G. Vernet, R.B. Finkelman, H. Gibb, J.C. Etienne. John Libbey Eurotext, Paris © 2000, pp. 433-435.

Voltammetric speciation of nickel subsulfide in mixtures and commercial nickel sulfides

John L. Wong, Min Tian, and Yanan He

Department of Chemistry, University of Louisville, Louisville, Kentucky, USA 40292

Abstract. The CPEV technique for Ni_3S_2 subspeciation was calibrated with known mixtures of Ni_3S_2 with NiS or NiS_2 and applied to the analysis of an industrial Ni_3S_2 and heazlewoodite. Voltammetric analysis of four commercial "NiS" samples revealed their differences from synthetic NiS and were identified to be mainly Ni_3S_2 by CPEV.

Introduction. Nickel subsulfide, Ni_3S_2, the most potent carcinogen among nickel compounds, poses an environmental health problem. We have reported carbon paste electrode voltammetry (CPEV) for specific determination of Ni_3S_2 in the solid state [1]. Herein we report its validation with known mixtures of Ni_3S_2 and analysis of commercial Ni_3S_2 and NiS.

Materials and Methods. The sample sources are as follows: Ni_3S_2 (99.7%) from Aldrich Chemical Co., Ni_3S_2 from International Nickel Co. (INCO) of Canada, an industrial standard, NiS from Alfa Chemical Co. and Strem Chemical Co., NiS_2 (99%) from Alfa, heazlewoodite (Australia mines) from Mineralogical Research Co. (California), and a reference ash SRM 1633b from NIST. A synthetic sample of NiS was prepared according to a reported procedure [2]. The electrochemical cell consisting of CPE in 1 M NaOAc-0.5 M HOAc (pH 5.0) was described [1].

Results and Discussion. Binary mixtures of Aldrich Ni_3S_2 with either synthetic NiS or NiS_2 were made in weight ratios of 7 : 3 and 3 : 7. The determinations of Ni_3S_2 in these mixtures are shown in Table I. From linear regression analysis of the anodic peak currents, the recoveries of Ni_3S_2 in % (R^2) were found to be satisfactory: 104.7 (0.975), 108.4 (0.944), 102.4 (0.985), and 108.2 (0.995).

In Table 2 are compared the cyclic voltammetric behavior of 4 NiS commercial samples (Com 1 – 4) with reference Ni_3S_2 and NiS. In the potential scan range of –0.8 V to 0.6 V, the mean E_{pa} –0.04 V, E_{pc} –0.48 V, i_{pa} / i_{pc} 2.13 of NiS Com 1 – 4 resembled those of Aldrich Ni_3S_2 but were distinctly different from the synthetic NiS. However, it should be noted that these differences became obscure in the scan range of −1.0 V to 1.0 V due to extensive redox reactions. In terms of the open circuit potential, a sample characteristic, the mean value of −0.28 V for NiS Com 1 – 4 was similar to Ni_3S_2 −0.29 V, but unlike the synthetic NiS 0.15 V. Nickel analysis (HF-aqua regia digestion followed by adsorptive stripping voltammetry of nickel dimethylglyoximate) was also performed. For NiS Com 1 – 4, Ni % theory 64.67, the % found were: 62.28±1.45, 61.81±1.17, 62.38±2.17, and 61.27±2.52. When the latter sample was pre-washed with CS_2, the Ni % was raised to 70.08±0.80, indicating sulfur was a contaminant in the bulk Ni_3S_2.

In Table III, Ni_3S_2 was quantitatively determined in 5 samples. CPEV analysis of INCO Ni_3S_2 showed 82.2 wt%. For heazlewoodite, after a prior treatment of CPE at −0.3 V for 20 s to resolve the broad anodic peak for Ni_3S_2, it was found to contain 26.3 wt% of Ni_3S_2. This content was determined to be 29.0 wt% by means of nickel chemical analysis. For the commercial NiS samples, the characteristic anodic peak of Ni_3S_2 was revealed by CPEV, which was quantitated by spiking with Aldrich Ni_3S_2. The Ni_3S_2 determined in these samples ranged from 80.2 to 70.5 wt%.

References

1. Wong JL, Liu AH, Tian M, Jin WR. Subspeciation of sulfidic nickel in particulate. Determination of Ni_3S_2, NiS, NiS_2 in reference and fly ash samples by carbon paste electrode voltammetry. Fresen J Anal Chem 1999; 363: 571-72.
2. Grau J, Akinc M. Synthesis of nickel sulfide by homogeneous precipitation from acidic solutions of thioacetamide. J Am Ceram Soc 1996; 79: 1073-82.

Table I. Determination of Ni_3S_2 in Mixtures with NiS or NiS_2 by CPEV[a]

Ni_3S_2:NiS_x Wt ratio	Ni_3S_2 Wt in CPE μg	NiS Wt in CPE μg	NiS_2 Wt in CPE μg	Ni_3S_2 Found by CPEV μg	R^2 Linear coeff.	Recovery %
7:3	364.6	156.3		338.5	0.975	104.7
3:7	156.3	364.6		138.9	0.944	108.4
7:3	364.6		156.3	373.6	0.985	102.4
3:7	153.3		364.6	169.1	0.995	108.2

[a]CPEV conditions: E_a=−0.6V, t_a=120 s, E_i=−0.6 V, E_h=0.6 V, ν=50 mV/s in 1 M HOAc-NaOAc (pH 5.0).

Table II. Anodic and cathodic peak potential, peak current ratios, and nickel analysis of commercial NiS and reference materials

Samples	Ni Anal[a]	Potential Scan From −0.8 V to 0.6 V			Potential Scan From −1 V to 1 V			Open Circuit Potential
		Anodic	Cathodic		Anodic	Cathodic		
	%	E_{pa}, V	E_{pc}, V	i_{pa}/i_{pc}	E_{pa}, V	E_{pc}, V	i_{pa}/i_{pc}	V
NiS Com-1	62.28±1.45	−0.08	−0.50	1.50	−0.05	−0.59	0.05	−0.26
NiS Com-2	61.81±1.17	−0.07	−0.46	1.00	−0.05	−0.59	0.02	−0.27
NiS Com-3	62.38±2.17	0.00	−0.47	3.55	−0.04	−0.58	0.08	−0.28
NiS Com-4	61.27±2.52	0.00	−0.48	2.13	−0.04	−0.58	0.04	−0.29
Ni_3S_2(Aldrich)	71.00±1.27	−0.04	−0.49	1.65	−0.05	−0.57	0.03	−0.29
Synthetic NiS	63.60±0.72	N.D.	−0.50	0.00	N.D.	−0.50	0.00	0.15

[a]sample digested in HF-aqua regia; Ni^{2+} determined as Ni-dimethylglyoximate by ASV. Ni % theory: NiS 64.67, Ni_3S_2 73.30. For quality assurance, SRM 1633b Ni %, theory 120±2.0 μg/g, found 118±1.29 μg/g

Table III. Ni_3S_2 found in commercial nickel sulfides by regression analysis of anodic peak currents[a]

	INCO Ni_3S_2	Heazlewoodite	NiS Com-1	NiS Com-2	NiS Com-3
R^2	0.983	0.991	0.976	0.996	0.986
Slope, mA/mg	0.026	0.023	0.003	0.003	0.004
Y intercept, mA	0.016	0.012	0.020	0.016	0.024
Ni_3S_2, % (N=4)	82.2±1.21	26.3±0.28	80.2±1.51	70.1±0.95	70.5±1.91

[a]after 4 increments of Ni_3S_2 7.5 mg each

Metal Ions in Biology and Medicine; vol 6. Eds. J.A. Centeno, Ph. Collery, G. Vernet, R.B. Finkelman, H. Gibb, J.C. Etienne. John Libbey Eurotext, Paris © 2000, pp. 437-439.

Zinc, neurotransmission and the mechanism of antidepressant action

Gabriel Nowak

Institute of Pharmacology, Polish Academy of Sciences, Smetna 12, 31-343 Kraków, Poland; Laboratory of Radioligand Research, Collegium Medicum, Jagiellonian University, 30-688 Kraków, Poland

Abstract

Zinc is a trace metal which plays a fundamental role in a wide range of biochemical processes in living organisms. Zinc is an important factor for physiological function of the mammalian nervous system. In the central nervous system, zinc modulates predominantly the excitatory amino acid neurotransmission (glutamatergic) system.

We have demonstrated previously that chronic antidepressant treatment, which is required for clinical improvement, reduced the reactivity/function of the glutamate/NMDA receptor complex.

Cerebral cortex. Chronic antidepressant treatment "down-regulated" (reduced density/affinity) of the cortical (but not hippocampal) NMDA receptors measured by radioligand-receptor binding methods. Moreover, chronic imipramine treatment increased the ability of zinc ion to modulate the NMDA receptor complex by increasing the potency of zinc to inhibit [^{3}H]MK801 binding to the NMDA receptor in the cerebral cortex but not in the hippocampus. It is known that zinc inhibits activation of the NMDA receptor complex. Thus, these data are in agreement with reported antidepressant- induced reduction of the NMDA receptor function.

Hippocampus. Our data demonstrated that chronic treatment with antidepressant drugs (imipramine or citalopram) increased (by 20%) the hippocampus/brain region ratio of zinc concentration, which may indicate redistribution of the rat brain zinc. On the other hand, electroconvulsive shocks induced robust increase (by 30%) of zinc concentration in the hippocampus (with slight a 11-15% effect in the rest of brain). In spite of the lack of alterations in the hippocampal NMDA receptors (measured by receptor binding methods), inhibitory effect of the increased hippocampal zinc concentration induced by chronic antidepressant treatment, may be responsible for functional reduction in the activity of that receptor complex also in the hippocampus.

These data indicate a critical and complex role of the interaction between zinc and NMDA receptor in the mechanism of antidepressant treatment and strongly support the glutamate hypothesis of the mechanism of antidepressant action.

Depression is a psychiatric disorder with high morbidity and mortality (leading to a significant percentage of suffering humans to commit suicide).The World Health Organization estimates that depression is now the fourth most important cause of human disability-adjusted life years, and predicts that it will be the second by the year 2020. Clinically effective antidepressant therapy include drugs with a remarkable structural diversity as well as non-pharmacological interventions such as electroconvulsive shock [3]. These treatments produce a variety of acute *in vivo and in vitro* effects that have not been casually related to antidepressant efficacy. Moreover, chronic antidepressant treatment, which is required for clinical improvement across therapies, has not been demonstrated to produce consistent changes in any single described transmitter system [6]. Recent reports, however, suggest adaptations in the glutamatergic receptors as a common target for various antidepressant therapies [6, 7]. This adaptation concerns the NMDA receptor [6, 7], the ionotropic type of glutamate receptor, which is sensitive to modulation by zinc ion [2].

Zinc is a trace metal which plays a fundamental role in a wide range of biochemical processes in living organisms. Zinc is an essential component of various proteins and is an important modulator in the mammalian central nervous system (CNS) [1]. In the CNS, zinc is found at high concentrations in the telencephalon, mainly in hippocampal neurons. Zinc exhibits both neurotoxic and neuroprotective effects (depending on the concentrations) and is distributed in three pools: protein-bound, free and vesicular form. The protein-bound pool (mostly enzyme proteins) represents more than 80% of the whole brain zinc. Free ionic zinc is present in the cytosol and interstitial fluid and is quickly bound after release. The vesicular zinc pool comprises about 15% of the brain zinc contents. This zinc pool is mostly localized in hippocampal and cortical neurons [1]. The neurons possess mechanisms for zinc uptake and storage in synaptic terminals and for stimulation of zinc ion release along with neurotransmitters [1, 2]. In the CNS, zinc modulates predominantly the excitatory amino acid neurotransmission (glutamatergic) system [2].

Recent results demonstrate that chronic electroconvulsive shock (ECS) treatment induce a robust increase of zinc concentrations in the hippocampus with a similar, although less significant effect in the cortex and cerebellum [5, 9]. Repeated administration of imipramine or citalopram induces a 20% increase of the hippocampal/brain region ratio of zinc [5]. The latter findings may indicate a significant "redistribution" of the brain zinc pool following antidepressant treatments. These partially common effects of ECS and antidepressant drugs on brain zinc concentrations might be related to their differences in clinical efficacy [3]. While chronic antidepressant treatment affects the NMDA receptor complex only in the cerebral cortex (measured by *in vitro* radioligand binding) [6], the electrophysiological results (measured *in vivo*) demonstrate a reduced function of hippocampal NMDA receptors [8]. Thus, it it possible that the electrophysiological *in vivo* measurements reflect the inhibitory effects of increased zinc concentrations induced by chronic antidepressant treatment, in particular, by ECS. Moreover, chronic antidepressant treatment induced reductions in the NMDA receptor subunit mRNA levels in both cerebral cortex and hippocampus [7]. Summary of the chronic antidepressant-induced alterations is demonstrated in Table 1. Finally, function of the NMDA receptor is diminished following chronic antidepressant treatment, as demonstrated in behavioral experiments (Popik et al., submitted), and in cerebellar granule cell culture [4].

Table 1. Chronic antidepressant-induced alterations in the rodent brain

parameter	cortex	hippocampus
NMDA receptor (binding)	↓	↔
NMDA receptor subunits mRNA	↓	↓
NMDA receptor function	?	↓
Zn concentration	↔	↑
Zn affinity to NMDA receptor	↑	↔

↑ increase, ↓ decrease, ↔ no alterations

The effects of antidepressant treatment on blood zinc concentrations in laboratory animals are unclear [5]. Yoshikawa et al. [10] reported that a single administration of imipramine increased duodenal zinc absorption. Therefore, more studies are needed to examine whether antidepressants may increase serum zinc concentrations. Moreover, preliminary results obtained in our laboratory indicate that zinc exhibits antidepressant-like effect in the "forced swim test" (behavioral despair test) in rats, a test with high predictivity of antidepressant efficacy in human depression.

The above data indicate a significant and complex role of zinc homeostasis in the mechanism of antidepressant treatment and strongly support the glutamate/NMDA hypothesis of the mechanism of antidepressant action.

References

1. Frederickson CJ. Neurobiology of zinc and zinc-containing neurons. *Int Rev Neurobiol* 1989; 31:145-238.
2. Harrison NL, Gibbons SJ. Zn^{2+}: an endogenous modulator of ligand- and voltage-gated ion channels. *Neurophamacology* 1994; 33:935-952.
3. Hollister LE, Csernansky JG. Clinical Pharmacology of Psychotherapeutic Drugs. 3rd edn. New York, Churchill Livingston, 1990.
4. Nonaka S, Hough CJ, Chuang DM. Chronic lithium treatment robustly protects neurons in the central nervous system against excitotoxicity by inhibiting N-methyl-D-aspartae receptor-mediated calcium influx. *Proc Natl Acad Sci USA* 1998, 95:2642-2647.
5. Nowak G, Schlegel-Zawadzka M. Alterations in serum and brain trace element levels after antidepressant treatment. Part I. Zinc. *Biol Trace Elem Res* 1999; 67:85-92.
6. Skolnick P, Layer RT, Popik P, Nowak G, Paul IA, Trullas R. Adaptation of N-methyl-D-aspartate (NMDA) receptors following antidepressant treatment: implications for the pharmacotherapy of depression. *Pharmacopsychiatry* 1996; 29:23-26.
7. Skolnick P. Antidepressants for the new millennium. *Eur J Pharmacol* 1999; 375:31-40.
8. Steward C, Jeffrey K, Reid I. LTP-like synaptic efficacy changes following electroconvulsive stimulation. *NeuroReport* 1994; 5:1041-1044.
9. Vaidya VA, Siuciak JA, Du F, Duman RS. Hippocampal mossy fiber sprouting induced by chronic electroconvulsive seizures. *Neuroscience* 1999; 89:157-166.
10. Yoshikawa T, Ikeda M, Tomita H, Kida A, Kubo T, Ishikawa K, Takeuchi S. Drug influence on intestinal zinc absorption. *Chem Abstr* 1997; 126:90.

Metal Ions in Biology and Medicine; vol 6. Eds. J.A. Centeno, Ph. Collery, G. Vernet, R.B. Finkelman, H. Gibb, J.C. Etienne. John Libbey Eurotext, Paris © 2000, pp. 440-442.

Brain manganese and neural function

Naoki Sotogaku, Atsushi Takeda, Shioji Ishiwatari, and Naoto Oku

Department of Radiochemistry, School of Pharmaceutical Sciences, University of Shizuoka, 52-1 Yada, Shizuoka 422-8526, Japan

Manganese (Mn) is an essential trace metal required for the development and function of the brain. This metal is a necessary component of glutamine synthetase and mitochondrial superoxide dismutase. Mn deficiency leads to an increased seizure susceptibility in animals, suggesting that Mn may be associated with protection from seizure in humans. On the other hand, chronic exposure to Mn damages several central neurotransmitter systems in the brain. Especially, Mn intoxication results in extrapyramidal symptoms related to alterations of the dopamine functions in the basal ganglia, probably due to a selective increase of Mn concentration in this area. Moreover, in patients with chronic liver failure and patients receiving long-term parenteral nutrition, some CNS disorders were also ascribed to Mn toxicity.

In attempts to clarify the actions of Mn both as a nutrient and a toxicant to the brain, several researchers have studied Mn uptake in the brain and suggested that Mn is transported into the brain across the blood-brain barrier. Moreover, the blood-CSF barrier may be also involved in Mn transport into the brain. In human brain, the concentration of Mn appears to increase with growth after birth, suggesting that Mn may have a special function in the brain development. However, it is difficult to analyze the utilization of endogenous Mn in the brain parenchyma because of its low level.

To study Mn transport in the neural circuit of rat brain, ^{54}Mn distribution in the brain was analyzed by autoradiography after intracerebral injection of $^{54}MnCl_2$. One day after injection into the striatum, ^{54}Mn was highly distributed in the thalamus, hypothalamus and substantia nigra. The ^{54}Mn distributed in the substantia nigra was inhibited by the pretreatment with colchicine (45 μg) into the medial forebrain bundle, suggesting that Mn is subjected to axonal transport in the striato-nigra and/or nigro-striatal pathways. In the case of ^{54}Mn injection into the olfactory bulb, ^{54}Mn was transported along the olfactory tract; ^{54}Mn was distributed in the piriform and amygdala areas (the primary olfactory cortex) and entorhinal area (the secondary olfactory cortex). These results suggest that Mn is subject to widespread axonal transport in the neural circuits. Moreover, Mn may be released from the terminals of the mitral cells (the secondary olfactory neuron) to the synaptic clefts, taken up by the piriform and amygdala neurons (the third olfactory neuron), and transported to the entorhinal area. In the present study, ^{54}Mn release from presynaptic neuron terminals during stimulation with high K^+ was studied using in vivo microdialysis to examine the possibility that Mn may be associated with synaptic neurotransmission.

Two hours after injection of $^{54}MnCl_2$ into the amygdala of rats, the amygdala was perfused for 60 min with Ringer's solution and perfused for 30 min with 100 mM KCl in Ringer's solution. ^{54}Mn levels in the perfusate were increased by stimulation with high K^+. The levels of neurotransmitters, e.g., glutamate and GABA, in the perfusate was increased by the stimulation. Twenty-four hours after the injection, ^{54}Mn levels in the perfusate were also increased by stimulation with high K^+. To clarify whether the increase of ^{54}Mn levels in the perfusate is associated with neuronal action, the amygdala was perfused with 1 μM tetorodotoxin, a Na^+ channel blocker, in Ringer's solution. The increase of ^{54}Mn levels in the perfusate by high K^+ was inhibited by the addition of tetorodotoxin. Therefore, Mn may be released during neuronal action in the amygdala. These results indicate the possibility that Mn may be involved in synaptic signaling functions in the amygdala.

To examine ^{54}Mn release from neuron terminals in other brain regions, the substantia nigra was perfused 2 h after injection of $^{54}MnCl_2$ into the substantia nigra of rats. ^{54}Mn levels in the perfusate were not appreciably increased by stimulation with high K^+, suggesting that Mn is scarcely released from neuron terminals in the substantia nigra. It is likely that Mn may be released from the terminals of a subclass of neuron.

In conclusion, the present data suggest that Mn may be involved in processes dynamically coupled to the electrophysiological activity of neuronal axons. This finding may be important for understanding of neural signaling processes.

Metal Ions in Biology and Medicine; vol 6. Eds. J.A. Centeno, Ph. Collery, G. Vernet, R.B. Finkelman, H. Gibb, J.C. Etienne. John Libbey Eurotext, Paris © 2000, pp. 443-446.

Aluminium neurotoxicity: implications in neurodegenerative diseases

Paolo Zatta

CNR Center on Metalloproteins, University of Padova, Department of Biology, 351231 Padova, Italy.
www.bio.unipd.it/~zatta/aluminum.html

In spite of its abundance in the biosphere, aluminum (Al) is only scarsely accumulated in living organisms. Nevertheless, the neurotoxic effects of Al in experimental animals has first documented over a century ago. Interest in Al toxicology was recently revived due to its identification as an etiological factor in a range of pathologies related to dialysis treatment of uremic subjects , including dialysis dementia, non iron-dependent microcytic anemia, and osteomalacia (1). Furthermore, about thirty years ago it was hypothesized that Al could be relevant to the etiopathogenesis of Alzheimer's disease (AD) as well as other neurodegenerative diseases (for a review see ref. 2). The etiopathogenic connection between Al and AD is to date only phenomenological in character. Thus, the *vexata questio* remains an ongoing topic of research in many laboratories, with an abundant flow of experimental data supporting the possibility that, if not an etiological factor, Al could at least represent an important co-factor able to aggravate the course of AD.

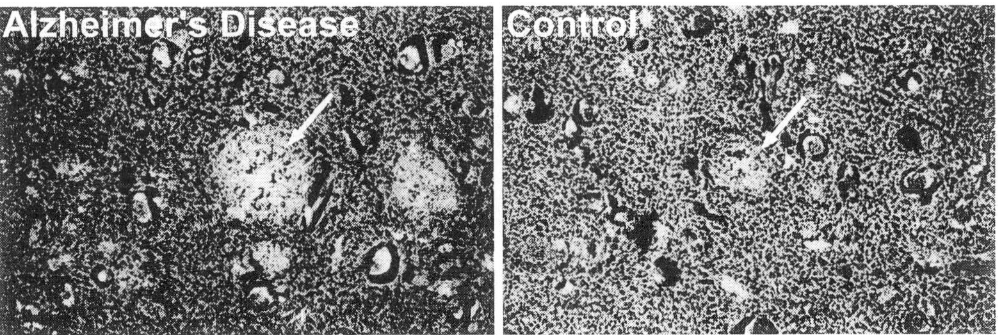

Fig. 1. Morin staining (3) identifies Al^{3+} by forming a yellow fluorescent complex (Morin-Al). In AD, Al accumulation is particularly evident in the *core* of the senile plaques not observed in the age-matched control .

It is now well established that an abnormal accumulation of Al occurs in the anatomopathological features characteristic of AD such as senile plaques (SP) and neurofibrillary tangles (NFT) (2). A clear example of Al accumulation in SP from an AD brain with respect to an age-matched control is reported in Fig. 1. It remains to be established whether this represents an epiphenomenon or play a role in disease induction. However, it is noteworthy that Al is able to compromise several metabolic pathways observed to be altered in AD.
For example, Table 1 reports findings made in our laboratory regarding the effects of Al on enzymatic activities and biophysical properties of the plasma membrane that might be relevant to AD.

TABLE I

Some effects produced by Al(III) on various biological targets observed in our laboratory

1. Inhibition of trypsin and α-chymotrypsin activities
2. Activation of Acetylcholinesterase and $Na^{+}K^{+}$ATPase
3. Modification of Krebs cycle metabolism
4. Alteration of lysosomal proton pump activity
5. Alteration in permeability of the blood-brain barrier
6. Alteration of the biophysical properties of cell membranes
7. Modification of mitochondrial Ca^{2+} flux
8. Inhibition of Ca^{2+}/Mg^{2+}-ATPase activity
9. Inhibition of E.R. Ca^{2+} flux
10. Interference with the VDAC channel opening
11. Neurogenic effect on neuroblastoma cells
12. Prooxidant action on lipid peroxidation
13. Activation of Monoamine oxidase B
14. Inhibition of Dopamine β-Hydroxylase

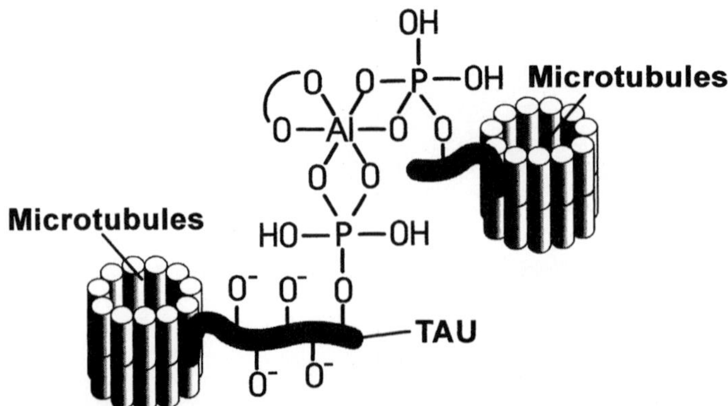

Fig.2: Hypothetical interaction between Al^{3+} and the phosphate groups of the hyperphosphorylated Tau proteins in AD brain tissue.

Besides the presence of abundant SP and NFT, another important pathological characteristic of AD is the hyperphosphorylation of tau proteins associated with the neurofilaments. We have hypothesized that in AD, Al could strongly bind to the phosphate residues associated with the hyperphosphorylated tau proteins, resulting in the formation of highly insoluble compounds potentially interfering with axonal transport, neuronal metabolism and eventually compromising the survival of neurons (4) (Fig. 2). This hypothesis was recently verified in *in vitro* and *in vivo* models (5, 6), reinforcing once again the possibility that Al could be a relevant co-factor in AD pathogenesis.
Another important aspect is that Al can, in particular conditions, cross the blood-brain barrier (BBB) (7) and accumulate inside neurons. An individual sensitivity to Al, linked to genetic predisposition, might potentiate this phenomenon and lead to AD. In this connection, it is noteworthy that although chronic dialysis patients may accumulate more Al in their brain tissue than that detected in AD brains, only few such patients develop AD; furthermore, dialysis encephalopathy (DE) caused by excess accumulation of Al can be reversed eliminating the source of Al contamination in dialysis fluids. In contrast to DE, Al is not distributed in all brain areas in AD, but is present at elevated concentration only focally in SP and NFT. In conclusion, in my opinion, Al *per se* is not the primary etiopathogenic factor in AD, but rather, for reasons yet to be discovered, acts as a cofactor in those individuals (*Al phenotypes?*) particularly sensitive to its accumulation, and thus aggravates a disease state induced by other events .

References

1. Zatta PF and Alfrey AC. *Aluminium Toxicity in Infants' Health and Disease.* Singapore, World Scientific Publ. 1995.
2. Zatta PF. Controversial aspects of aluminum accumulation and subcompartmentation in Alzheimer's disease. *Trace Elem Med* 1993; 10: 120-128.
3. De Boni U, Scott JW and Crapper DR. Intracellular aluminum binding.: a histochemical study. *Histochemistry* 1974; 40: 31-37
4. Zatta PF. Aluminum binds to the hyperphosphorylated Tau in Alzheimer's disease: A hypothesis. *Med. Hypoth*1995; 44: 169-172
5. Trojanowski JQ and Lee VM-Y. Phosphorylation of neuronal cytoskeleton proteins in Alzheimer's disease and Lewy body dementia. 1994; *Ann NY Acad Sci* 747: 92-109
6. Shin R-W. Interaction of aluminum with paired helical filament tau is involved in neurifibrillary pathology of Alzheimer's disease. *Gerontol.* 1997; 43: 16-23
7. Banks AW, Kastin WJ. The blood-brain barrier in aluminum toxicity and Alzheimer's disease. In: Zatta PF and Nicolini M, eds. *Non-neuronal cells in Alzheimer's disease.*Singapore: World Sc,1995:1-12.

Metal Ions in Biology and Medicine; vol 6. Eds. J.A. Centeno, Ph. Collery, G. Vernet, R.B. Finkelman, H. Gibb, J.C. Etienne. John Libbey Eurotext, Paris © 2000, pp. 447-449.

Intrahippocampal microinfusion of Pb^{+2} impairs spatial discrimination learning on the holeboard task

Adrínel Vásquez and Sandra Peña de Ortiz

University of Puerto Rico, Rio Piedras Campus, Department of Biology, P.O. Box 002360 Rio Piedras, Puerto Rico 00931-2360

Exposure to Pb^{+2} results in various cognitive and behavioral dysfunctions in humans and other animals. We report here that intrahippocampal microinfusion of Pb^{+2} acetate strongly impairs long-term memory while short-term memory is mostly unaffected in a hippocampal-dependent learning task. These results suggest that Pb^{+2} directly or indirectly interferes with the genetic regulatory events that are known to be essential for long-term memory in the brain.

Introduction: Pb^{+2} is a toxic heavy metal which is ubiquitous in nature and which is a contaminant in various environmental sources [1]. The nervous system is an important target organ for Pb^{+2} toxicity resulting in physiological, behavioral, and/or cognitive dysfunction [1-4]. The effects of Pb^{+2} toxicity in adults, which in humans is most commonly caused by acute or chronic occupational exposure, are still unclear. It is important to determine the mechanisms by which Pb^{+2} interferes with neuronal function so that treatment and/or preventive strategies may be designed to avoid the neurobehavioral and cognitive effects of this toxic heavy metal. A number of reports suggest that at least part of the effects of Pb^{+2} are due to its disruption of normal Ca^{+2} signaling in neurons [5]. In fact, recent studies showed that Pb^{+2} blocks the N-methyl-D-aspartate (NMDA) gated Ca^{+2} channel, known as the NMDA receptor [6] and which has been shown to play a pivotal role in learning and memory [7]. We are interested in characterizing the effects of Pb^{+2} in the adult brain at the molecular level. Our experiments target the rat hippocampus because of the known role of this brain structure in learning and memory processes in vertebrates. Here we report the results from the initial stage of our study which aims at determining the effects of intrahippocampal administration of Pb^{+2} in the acquisition and retention of the holeboard task for spatial discrimination learning. Additional studies aimed at characterizing the mechanisms by which Pb^{+2} causes its effects at a molecular level will be presented at the meeting. As a whole these studies will provide important information about the molecular mechanisms of Pb^{+2} neurotoxicity that are related to the cognitive impairment that is commonly seen after environmental and occupational exposure to Pb^{+2}.

Methods: Bilateral cannulas were surgically implanted over the CA1 region of the hippocampus of adult male rats (275-300g) using brain coordinates previously described [8]. Following a recovery period of 4 days rats entered a food restriction and habituation period to prepare them for training in the holeboard spatial discrimination task as described before [9]. This task is a hippocampal dependent spatial task in which animals learn to discriminate between relevant (baited) and irrelevant (non-baited) holes within a 16 hole arena [9]. Starting on Day 1 of training, rats received intrahippocampal microinfusions of 1 nmol Pb^{+2} or Na^{+} acetate 20 min prior to each session. Rats received a 5 trial session per day for at least four days. Training was done on alternate days to avoid tissue damage from repeated intracerebral microinfusions. Following acquisition, the rats were allowed to rest for 7 days after which they were subject to a retention test that consisted of 5 training trials. The behavioral parameters utilized to evaluate learning of the task included searching time, total errors (reference errors + working errors), and the reference memory ratio (RMR) which is calculated with the following formula (visits and revisits to baited holes ÷ total hole visits). All data were analyzed with one way analysis of variance (ANOVA) and Student's t-tests.

Discussion: Figure 1 shows the effects of intrahippocampal Pb^{+2} on spatial discrimination learning. Animals receiving Na^{+} acetate microinfusions developed spatial learning as indicated by statistically significant decreases in searching time, total errors, and RMR ($p < .0001$, $p < .0001$, and $p < .0001$, respectively). Moreover, these animals showed robust long-term memory on the retention test given 7 days after acquisition training. Statistical analysis of the behavioral data of Day 1 through Day 3 of training indicated that Pb^{+2} had little or no effect on early acquisition of the holeboard task. In contrast, analysis of the data for Day 4 of acquisition showed that 1 nmol Pb^{+2} acetate resulted in significant differences in total errors ($p < .05$) and searching time ($p < .05$) when compared to animals receiving Na^{+}acetate. These results indicate that Pb^{+2} affects the late stages of learning acquisition and suggest that Pb^{+2} might have a specific effect on long-term memory. This hypothesis is supported by the results of the retention test which showed significant impairment of long-term spatial memory 7 days after the end of acquisition training ($p < .005$ and $p < .0005$ for total errors and RMR, respectively). Since long-term memory, but not for short-term memory, requires new gene transcription and protein synthesis [10] we propose that the Pb^{+2}-induced impairment in long-term memory is due to abnormal regulation of gene expression. Future studies will address this hypothesis using cDNA microarrays and will study the molecular mechanisms involved in the proposed Pb^{+2}-dependent impairments in learning-induced gene expression.

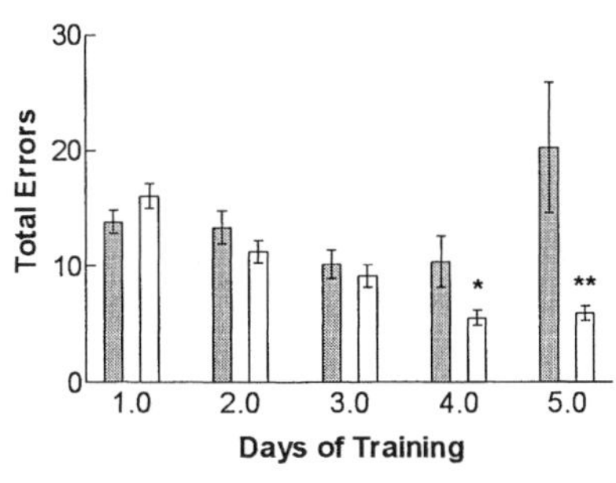

Figure1: Effects of intrahippocampal Pb^{+2} on spatial discrimination learning. The graph shows the effects of 1 nmol Pb^{+2} acetate (grey bars) and 1 nmol Na^{+} acetate (white bars) on acquisition for Day 1 to Day 4 of training in the holeboard task. Animals were allowed to rest for 7 days before they received a retention test on Day 5 of training. Results show the significant effects of Pb^{+2} on total errors for Day 4 ($p < .05$) and Day 5 ($p < .005$)

References:

1. Gerson B. Lead. *Clinics in Lab Med* 1990;10:441-457.
2. Alfano D and Petit T. Behavioral effects of postnatal lead exposure: Possible relationship to hippocampal dysfunction. *Neural Biol* 1981; 32:319-333.
3. Audesirk G. Effects of lead exposure on the physiology of neurons. *Prog Neurobiol* 1985; 24:199-231.
4. Bonithon-Kopp C, Huel G, Moreau T, and Wendling, R. Prenatal exposure to lead and cadmium and psychomotor development of the child at 6 years. *Neurobehav Toxicol Teratol* 1986;8:307-310.
5. Bressler JP, and Goldstein GW. Mechanisms of lead neurotoxicity. *Biochem Pharmacol* 1991;41:479-484.
6. Alkondon M, Costa A, Radhakrishnan V, Aronstan RS, and Albuquerque EX. Selective blockade of NMDA-activated channel currents may be implicated in learning deficits caused by lead. *FEBS* 1990; 261:124-130.
7. Bannerman DM, Good MA, Butcher SP, Ramsay M, & Morris RG. Distinct components of spatial learning revealed by prior training and NMDA receptor blockade. *Nature* 1995; 378:182-6.
8. Jett DA, Kuhlmann AC, and Guilarte TR. Intrahippocampal administration of lead (Pb) impairs performance of rats in the Morris water maze. *Pharmacol Biochem Behav* 1996; 57: 263-269.
9. Peña de Ortiz, Maldonado-Vlaar, CS, Carrasquillo Y. Hippocampal expression of the Orphan Nuclear Receptor Gene *hzf-3/nurr1* during spatial discrimination learning. *Neurobiol Learn Mem - In Press*
10. Bourtchuladze R, Frenguelli B, Cioffi D, Blendy J, Schutz G, Silva AJ. Deficient long-term memory in mice with a targeted mutation of the cAMP-responsive element-binding protein. *Cell* 1994; 79:59-68.

Metal Ions in Biology and Medicine; vol 6. Eds. J.A. Centeno, Ph. Collery, G. Vernet, R.B. Finkelman, H. Gibb, J.C. Etienne. John Libbey Eurotext, Paris © 2000, pp. 450-452.

Enhanced levels of zinc in drinking water adversely affect spatial learning in rats

Jane M. Flinn[1], Jessica Morvan[1], Jennifer Magaha[1], Lorraine Krause[1], Kathleen Navarrete[1], Blair F. Jones[2]

[1] *George Mason University, MS 3F5, 4400 University Drive, Fairfax, VA 22030-4444;* [2] *United States Geological Survey*

Abstract

Rats were raised on normal lab water enhanced with 10ppm $ZnCO_3$, both pre-and post-natally. Spatial memory was tested over a 10 day period using the Morris Water Maze. At 3 months, the $ZnCO_3$ group was significantly slower than the tap water controls between days 3 and 7 ($F(1,43)=6.06$, $p<.018$). At 9 months, the $ZnCO_3$ group was slower overall ($F(1,40)=8.28$, $p<.006$). These data suggest that long-term ingestion of zinc at concentrations similar to those known to occur in natural waters can have adverse effects on memory.

Zinc in the environment

Zinc is the most abundant and the most soluble of the transition metals in natural systems. High Zn concentrations in the natural environment are related to mountainous areas and igneous rocks, major fracture systems in carbonate rocks, or metalliferous shales. The highest levels of zinc in the natural environment are found in sulfide ores and in waters of major mining areas. While lead is declining in stream and reservoir sediments following the introduction of unleaded gasoline, gradual increases in zinc suggest a continued contaminant source to the environment [1]. The most likely association is with automotive materials, including the presence of zinc in tires. Increased zinc is associated with the organics derived from sewage treatment plants or volatile emissions from power generation. Rice [2] found Zn and Cu well correlated with population density or total urban land use. Concentrations exceeding the level for adverse effects to aquatic biota were widespread in urban areas.

Standards for drinking water quality for zinc have been based on aesthetic characteristics [3]. The current standard of 5 mg/l solute zinc is the threshold for astringent taste. Deleterious effects of zinc have been reported at 40 mg/l, but gastrointestinal stress requires levels of 200mg/l or more. Zinc concentrations at treatment plants in the U.S. were below 5 mg/l in 1979. However, in cities with soft, acidic water, Zn pickup occurs from the distribution system between plant and tap. In summary, zinc is ubiquitous in the geohydrologic environment and, under favorable conditions, can be quite mobile.

Potential role of excess zinc in learning and memory

The fourth most abundant intercellular metal, zinc is a biologically essential trace metal that is found in over 200 enzymes and proteins. Within the central nervous system zinc is found in its highest levels in the hippocampus, the amygdala, the striatum and the neocortex [4]. Zinc is co-localized in vesicles with glutamate. It acts as a neuromodulator and has an inhibitory effect on the NMDA type glutamate receptor [5], [6]. The NMDA receptor is thought to play an important role in learning and memory; impairments of memory are seen following its modification [7], [8].

The effect of zinc *deficiency* on memory has been well studied. Although there are few studies of the possibly adverse effects of high levels of zinc, Tsein, Huerta, & Tonegawa [9] and Turner and Soliman [10] found deficits in memory in rats following enhanced zinc-oxide in the food or oral administration of zinc-chloride by gavage. We have thus examined whether enhanced levels of zinc, similar to those seen in natural water, would affect spatial learning and memory in rats, if ingested for long periods of time.

Method

Sprague-Dawley rats were exposed to zinc-enriched water pre-and post-natally. Dams were raised on control or zinc enriched water (10 ppm $ZnCO_3$) for 10 days before being bred with males drinking normal lab water. Three male and three female pups were retained from each litter; the pups (and dams) were then maintained on the same type of water. The animals were tested in the Morris water maze at 3 and 9 months of age.

The Morris Water Maze is a shallow pool, approximately 6 feet in diameter, filled with milky, opaque water. There is a small platform just under the surface that the animals cannot see, but they can bump into while swimming. When an animal climbs onto the platform it is removed from the pool. It has been demonstrated that animals make use of spatial cues to remember position of the hidden platform.

Animals were placed in the pool and allowed to swim for a maximum of 4 minutes. They were given one trial per day for a period of 10 days. The amount of time the animals took to find the platform was recorded by an observer blind to the condition of the animal.

Figures

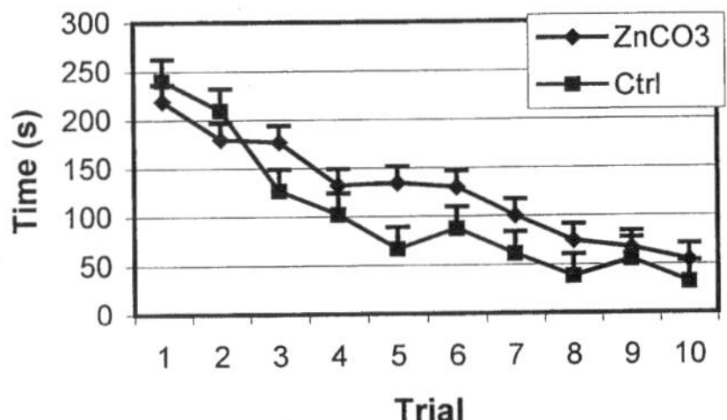

Figure 1: Females at 90 days. After pre-natal zinc exposure, and 90 days of zinc in their drinking water, the zinc exposed animals take more time to find the hidden platform using spatial cues. Differences are significant between trials 3-6.

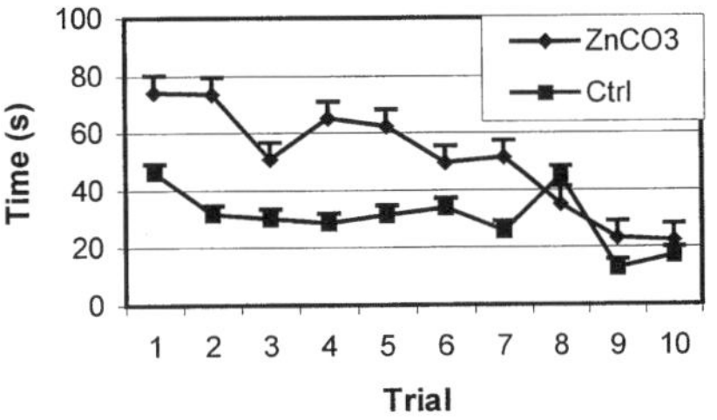

Figure 2: Females at 9 months. After 9 months of ingesting zinc-enriched water, the deficit in spatial ability among the female animals becomes more clear. Differences are significant between trials 1-7.

Results

The data was analyzed by repeated measures analysis of variance (RMANOVA). The analyses showed that at 3 months the $ZnCO_3$ group were slower than the control group between 3 and 7 days ($F(1,43) = 6.06$, $p<.018$). There was no significant difference between males and females. At 9 months the $ZnCO_3$ group was slower than the controls overall ($F(1,40)$ 8.28, $p<.006$) and there was a trend for the females to be slower than the males ($F(1,40) = 2.80$, $p<.1$). The lighter females drank equivalent amounts of water to the males, so they received more zinc per gram of body weight. The data for the females is shown for 3 and 9 months in figures 1 and 2.

Conclusion

The rats raised on elevated levels of zinc were slower to remember where the platform was located than the controls, although at both 3 and 9 months the groups were similar in performance by the eighth day. These data show that long-term ingestion of water containing enhanced levels of zinc likely to be found in natural waters can have adverse effects on memory.

References

1. Callender, E. and P.C. Van Metre, *Where the rubber meets the road—A source for zinc in the environment?*, . 1999, National Wetlands Research Center.
2. Rice, K.C., *Trace element concentrations in streambed sediment across the conterminous U.S.* Environmental Science & Technology, 1999. 33: p. 2499-2504.
3. Committee on Medical and Biologic Effects of Environmental Pollutants, D.o.M.S., National Research Council, *Zinc*, . 1979, National Research Council. p. 249-271.
4. Frederickson, C.J., *et al.*, *A quinoline fluorescence method for visualizing and assaying the histochemically reactive zinc (bouton zinc) in the brain.* J Neurosci Methods, 1987. 20(2): p. 91-103.
5. Peters, S., J. Koh, and D.W. Choi, *Zinc selectively blocks the action of N-methyl-D-aspartate on cortical neurons.* Science, 1987. 236(4801): p. 589-93.
6. Westbrook, G.L. and M.L. Mayer, *Micromolar concentrations of Zn2+ antagonize NMDA and GABA responses of hippocampal neurons.* Nature, 1987. 328(6131): p. 640-3.
7. Davis, S., S.P. Butcher, and R.G. Morris, *The NMDA receptor antagonist D-2-amino-5-phosphonopentanoate (D-AP5) impairs spatial learning and LTP in vivo at intracerebral concentrations comparable to those that block LTP in vitro.* J Neurosci, 1992. 12(1): p. 21-34.
8. Tsien, J.Z., P.T. Huerta, and S. Tonegawa, *The essential role of hippocampal CA1 NMDA receptor-dependent synaptic plasticity in spatial memory [see comments].* Cell, 1996. 87(7): p. 1327-38.
9. Komiskey, H.L., X.F. Chen, and D. Sarpong. *823.20: Memory in male rats impaired by subchronic zinc oxide.* in *Annual Meeting of the Society for Neuroscience.* 1997. New Orleans, LA.
10. Turner, T.Y. and M.R.I. Soliman. *386.7: The effect of zinc on brain dopamine (D2) receptor binding kinetics in rats.* in *Annual Meeting for the Society for Neuroscience.* 1999. Miami, FL.

Metal Ions in Biology and Medicine; vol 6. Eds. J.A. Centeno, Ph. Collery, G. Vernet, R.B. Finkelman, H. Gibb, J.C. Etienne. John Libbey Eurotext, Paris © 2000, pp. 453-455.

Neurodevelopmental toxicity of lanthanum in mice

Wayne Briner[1], Robert Rycek, Alison Moellenberndt, Kimberly Dannull

Department of Psychology, University of Nebraska-Kearney, Kearney, NE 68849, USA

Introduction.

La is a rare earth metal that is of interest to toxicologists for two reasons. First, use of La in industrial and manufacturing settings has expanded and La is a spin-off metal of the nuclear industry. Greater use of La in industry increases the chances of accidental exposure, both acute and chronic. La is also of interest because it is used extensively as a Ca^{2+} channel blocker. A variety of other biological activities have been noted including inhibition of Ca^{2+} binding to synaptosomal membranes, inhibition of Ca2+ dependent neurotransmitter release, and altered neurotransmitter receptor response [1].

Studies on the developmental toxicity of La have found reductions in the number of successful pregnancies and average litter sizes from a single injection of $LaCl_3$ (44mg/kg) in mice. No gross abnormalities were described [2]. Others have demonstrated opening of the cephalic neural tube in rat embryos exposed to La [3]. Preliminary work in this laboratory has shown a significant lag in neuromuscular development, when rats were exposed to 175mg/kg of La as a single SC dose during neural tube formation [4]. We have undertaken this study to provide a description of the neurodevelopmental toxicity of La.

Materials and Methods.

Female Swiss-Webster mice were housed under standard laboratory conditions. The mice were exposed to $LaCl_3$ in distilled drinking water under one of four doses (0, 125, 250, 500mg/L). Access to food and water was ad-lib. The mice were exposed for 14 days and then mated. Exposure to La continued through gestation, parturition, and the postnatal period for the dams and pups until sacrifice.

Developmental Assessment. Behavioral and neurologic assessments were made from age 4 - 20 days including the development of swimming behavior, ear and eye opening and weight gain.

Neurological Assessment. Between 30-32 days of age the animals were assessed with a modified version of a Functional observational battery [5].

Brain Chemistry. At 59-60 days of age the animals were euthenized with chloroform weighed, and had brains removed which were weighed and frozen. Lipid, protein and La content of the brains were determined as described below.

For analysis the brains were homogenized and protein concentration determined using the coomassie blue method. La content of the tissue was determined by placing the homogenate in acetate buffer (pH 3.1) to which was added arsenazo III. Transmission was read at 652nM and the tissue concentrations calculated from known standards [6].

Results.

La exposure did not appear to have a noticeable effect on the health of the dams. The spontaneous death rate was not higher, water intake and food consumption, while not formally assessed, did not appear to be different between the groups. The general health and constitution of the animals did not differ between the groups.

Gender distribution did not differ between the groups ($X^2(3)=4.44$, $p=.22$). Litter size did not differ significantly between the groups ($F(3,32)=0.33$, $p=.8$) nor did the mortality rate of the pups due to cannibalism or death of unknown cause ($F(3,32)=0.77$, $p=.52$).

Developmental Assessment. Weight gain did not differ amongst the treatment groups although there was a non-significant trend for the 250 and 500 mg/L La exposed groups to gain weight less readily than the other groups.

Eye and ear opening appeared to be delayed for the 125 and 250mg/L groups but accelerated for the 500mg/L group. This was apparent at 13 and 14 days post-natally (X^2 analysis $p<.05$ for all tests).

Swimming development was borderline significant for post-natal days 6 through 14 ($F(3,72)=2.90$, $p=.06$) with statistically significant effects for the 250 mg/L ($p=.02$) and 500 mg/L groups ($p=.03$).

Neurological Assessment (30-32 days of age). Tail Pinch response was significantly different with the 125 mg/L La group showing more freezing behavior. The 500 mg/L group demonstrated more turning toward site or walking away ($X^2(9)=35.20$, $p<.0001$).

For the Touch Response the 125 and 250 mg/L La exposed groups demonstrated more jerking toward the object. The 500 mg/L group reacted by turning toward object or walking away more often than controls ($X^2(9)=61.11$, $p<.0001$).

For the Visual Placing Response proportionately more mice in the 500mg/L group displayed early vigorous extension or placing before vibrissae contact. The 125 and 250 mg/L groups displayed placing after slight vibrissae contact more frequently ($X^2(9)=26.38$, $p=.002$).

Reactivity level was also significantly different with the 125 and 250 mg/L La groups displaying more aggressive behavior ($X^2(9)=28.03$, $p=.001$).

Brain Studies (59-60 days). The brain weight of the litters differed between groups with the 500mg/L group being significantly smaller than the control group ($F(3,31)=5.11$, $p=.006$). Brain La, protein, and lipid content did not differ between treatment groups. There was a statistically significant correlation between brain La and protein content ($r(19)=0.49$, $p<.05$).

Discussion.

Pre- and post- natal La exposure in mice appears to have a variety of developmental and behavioral effects. Developmental lags are seen in eye and ear development as well as the neuromuscular development of the animals.

As development progressed differences continued to persist. Given that final body weight did not differ between the groups it can be argued that the behavioral differences seen were due to the effects of La exposure and not a general developmental lag. The groups exposed to 125 and 250 mg/L of La displayed more freezing, jerking and aggressive behaviors that the control groups. This might better be described as a general hyperreactivity to intruding stimuli. Another explanation is that these animals exhibit impaired learning, as demonstrated by poor habituation. La is well known to interfere with neurotransmitter release and response [1], both necessary for normal memory formation. La has also been shown to interfere with short duration memory formation in mice [7] and memory retrieval in chicks [8].

The group exposed to 500 mg/L La produced several paradoxes. Eye and ear development for this group seemed accelerated, although they did lag in swimming development. Their adult responses to testing were similar to the control group and with regard to tail pinch, touch and placing response seemed to be more "normal" than the control group. We suggest two possible explanations for this. High dose La exposure may have selectively killed the more susceptible embryos in-utero. This would account for our informal observation of less frequent litters for this group. These less susceptible offspring would be more resistant to the postnatal effects of La and show fewer overall effects than the other two groups (125 & 250 mg/L). The second explanation may be a pharmacologic effect of La on growth and hormonal systems. For example, La can promote neurite formation and increases cell adhesion.

One interesting finding was the correlation between brain La and protein content. This argues that brain La is protein bound, presumably in a cellular store such as the endoplasmic reticulum, a suggestion supported by analysis of La's subcellular site of action [9].

Acknowledgments. This work was supported by the Whitehall Foundation.

References

[1]. Das T, Sharma A., Talukder G. Effects of lanthanum on cellular systems, a review. *Biol Trace Elem Res* 1988; 18: 201-228.

[2]. Abramczuk JW. The effects of lanthanum chloride on pregnancy in mice and on preimplantation mouse embryos in vitro. *Toxicol.* 1985; 34: 315-20.

[3]. Smedley MJ, Stanisstreet M. Calcium and neurulation in mammalian embryos. *J Embryol Exp Morphol* 1985; 89: 1-14.

[4]. Wadkins T, Benz J, Briner W. The effect of lanthanum administration during neural tube formation on the emergence of swimming behavior. In: Collery P, Bratter P, de Bratter V, Khassanova L, Etienne J, eds. *Metal ions in biology and medicine,* Paris: John Libby EuroPress, 1998:168-171.

[5]. O'Donoghue JL. Clinical neurologic indicies of toxicity in animals. *Env Health Perspect* 1996; 104, Suppl 2: 323-330.

[6]. Fernandez-Gavarron F, Brand JG, Rabinowitz JL. A simple spectrophotometric assay for micromolar amounts of lanthanum in the presence of Ca and phosphate. *J Bone Min Res* 1987; 2: 421-425.

[7]. Mizumori SJ, Sakai DH, Rosenzweig MR, Bennett EL, Wittreich P. Investigations into the neuropharmacological basis of temporal stages of memory formation in mice trained in an active avoidance task. *Behav Brain Res* 1987; 23: 239-50.

[8]. Summers MJ, Crowe, SF, Ng KT. Administration of lanthanum chloride following a reminder induces a transient loss of memory retrieval in day-old chicks. *Cogn Brain Res* 1996; 4: 109-19.

[9]. Provan SD, Miyamoto MD. Subcellular mechanism and site of action of ionic lanthanum at the motor nerve terminal. *Neuroreport* 1992; 3: 101-4.

Metal Ions in Biology and Medicine; vol 6. Eds. J.A. Centeno, Ph. Collery, G. Vernet, R.B. Finkelman, H. Gibb, J.C. Etienne. John Libbey Eurotext, Paris © 2000, pp. 456-458.

Zinc exerts an antidepressant–like effect in behavioural despair test in rats

Gabriel Nowak

Institute of Pharmacology, Polish Academy of Sciences, Smetna 12, 31-343 Kraków, Poland; Laboratory of Radioligand Research, Collegium Medicum, Jagiellonian University, 30-688 Kraków, Poland

INRODUCTION

Antidepressant therapy includes drugs with a remarkable structural diversity as well as nonpharmacological interventions. Most of the drugs are monoamine based, affecting the inhibition of reuptake/metabolism of noradrenaline, serotonin, or dopamine (Hollister and Csernansky, 1990). Recent studies indicate antidepressant-like properties of antagonists of the glutamate-NMDA receptor complex (Skolnick et al. 1996). Since zinc is an inhibitor of the NMDA receptor complex, in the present study we examined the effect of zinc in the forced swim test in rats, a test with high predicivity of antidepressant efficacy in human depression (Porsolt et al. 1978).

MATERIALS AND METHODS

The experiments were carried out on male Wistar rats (220-250g) housed in groups of 4 with free access to food and water. Zinc ($ZnSO_4$) was administered i.p. 3 times: 24, 5 and 1h before the test in doses of 0.5, 1, 5, 30 or 100 mg/kg and in doses of 0.5 and 1 mg/kg together with imipramine (5 mg/kg).

The studies were carried out according to the method of Porsolt (1978). The rats were placed individually in cylindrical tanks (height 40 cm, diameter 18cm) containing water at temp. 25 °C. After 15 min. they were removed to a drying room (30°C) for 30 min. Twenty-four hours after the pretest session, rats were replaced in the cylinders and the total duration of immobility during this test was measured for 5 min. The test was started 1h after the last dose of zinc.

RESULTS

Zinc (Zn) dose dependently reduced the immobility time, and reached statistical significance by the dose of 100 mg/kg (Fig.1). Imipramine (IMI) at dose of 5 mg/kg had no effect (Fig.2), while 30 mg/kg significantly reduced the immobility time (Fig.1). Joint administration of IMI (5 mg/kg) and zinc (0.5 or 1 mg/kg) caused a significant decrease in the immobility time (Fig.2).

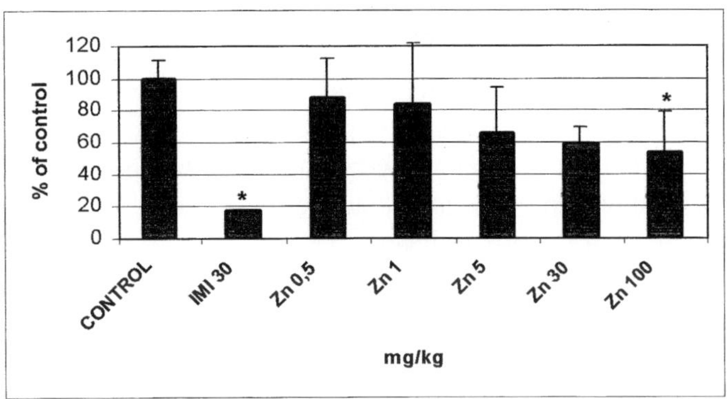

Fig.1. The effect of zinc (0,5, 1, 5, 30, 100 mg/kg) and IMI (30 mg/kg) i.p. on the immobility time of rats. Zinc and IMI were given three times (24, 5, 1h) before the test. * $p < 0.05$ vs control.

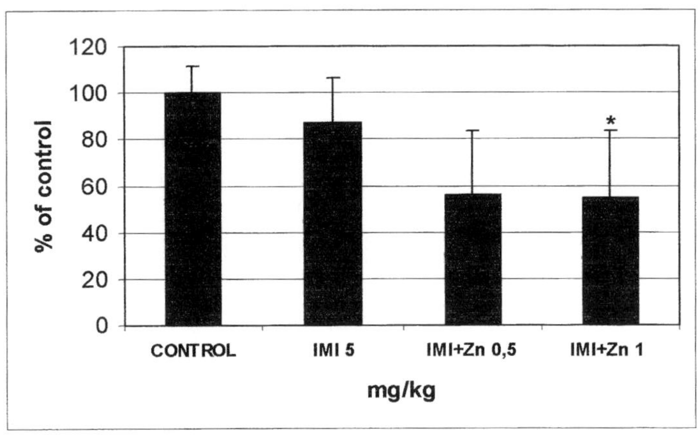

Fig. 2. The effect of joint administration of IMI (5mg/kg) and zinc (0.5 and 1mg/kg) on the immobility time. IMI and zinc were given three times (24, 5 and 1h) before the test. * $p< 0.05$ vs control.

DISCUSSION

The NMDA receptor complex consists of calcium channel with multiple, allosterically coupled recognition sites for glutamate, glycine, polyamines, channel blockers, magnesium and zinc (Skolnick et al.1996). Recent studies indicate antidepressant-like properties of antagonists of the glutamate-NMDA receptor complex (Maj et al.1992; Skolnick et al.1996; Skolnick 1999). Zinc is one of a very potent inhibitors of the NMDA receptor complex (Harrison and Gibbons, 1994). The present results indicate that zinc exhibits antidepressant-like properties in the forced swim test. Moreover, ineffective doses of zinc together with ineffective dose of imipramine exerted a significant antidepressant-like effect. It might be speculated that zinc supplementation may enhance the antidepressant therapy in human depression. If such supplementation of antidepressant treatment by zinc lowers the effective doses of antidepressant drugs also in humans, the unwanted side effects might be diminished and the costs of antidepressant therapy reduced.

REFERENCES

- Harrison NL, Gibbons SJ. Zn^{2+}: an endogenous modulator of ligand- and voltage-gated ion channels. *Neurophamacology* 1994; 33:935-952.
- Hollister LE, Csernansky JG. Clinical Pharmacology of Psychotherapeutic Drugs. 3rd edn. New York, Churchill Livingston, 1990.
- Maj J, Rogóż Z, Skuza G, Sowińska H. Effects of MK-801 and antidepressant drugs in the forced swimming test in rats. *Eur Neuropsychopharmacology*, 1992, 2: 37-41
- Porsolt RD., Anton G., Deniel M., Jalfre M.: Behavioral despair in rats: a new model sensitive to antidepressant treatments. *Eur J Pharmacol* 1978; 47: 379-391.
- Skolnick P, Layer RT, Popik P, Nowak G, Paul IA, Trullas R. Adaptation of N-methyl-D-aspartate (NMDA) receptors following antidepressant treatment: implications for the pharmacotherapy of depression. *Pharmacopsychiatry* 1996; 29:23-26.
- Skolnick P. Antidepressants for the new millennium. *Eur J Pharmacol* 1999; 375:31-40.

Metal Ions in Biology and Medicine; vol 6. Eds. J.A. Centeno, Ph. Collery, G. Vernet, R.B. Finkelman, H. Gibb, J.C. Etienne. John Libbey Eurotext, Paris © 2000, pp. 459-461.

Effects of depleted uranium on development of the mouse

Wayne Briner[1] and Kevin Byrd

Department of Psychology, University of Nebraska-Kearney, Kearney, NE 68849, USA

Introduction

Uranium is a heavy metal with toxic potential outside of its radioactivity. Depleted uranium (DU) use by the military is escalating with uranium entering the environment in increasing amounts. Previous studies in mice have found that uranium is a reproductive toxin producing fetal death, smaller pups, and fewer litters at 25 or 50 mg/kg of uranium acetate (oral administration) depending on length and timing of exposure [1, 2]. Skeletal malformations have been found in mouse pups when pregnant dams were exposed to 25 - 50 mg/kg of uranium acetate [3]. Injections of as little as 0.5 mg/kg of uranium acetate can produce discernable effects on pregnant mice or their offspring [4]. To our knowledge, no work has been done on the neurodevelopmental effects of DU. The purpose of this pilot study is to provide an initial description of the neurodevelopmental effects of depleted uranium exposure in mice.

Methods

Female Swiss-Webster mice, housed under standard laboratory conditions, were exposed to 0, 19, 37, or 75 mg/L of uranium acetate in drinking water for two weeks, then mated. Exposure of dams and pups continued until sacrifice. Access to food and water was ad-lib. Mice were assessed using the Fox Developmental Scale [5] until age 21 days. At 21 days of age the pups were assessed with a Functional Observation Battery [6] after-which the brains were removed for study.

Results

DU exposure did not appear to have a noticeable effect on the health of the dams. The spontaneous death rate was not higher, water intake and food consumption, while not formally assessed, did not appear to be different between the groups. The general health and constitution of the animals did not differ between the groups. No gross malformations were noted in the pups.

The uranium-exposed mouse pups developed on a number of behavioral indicies more quickly that the control groups. This included righting reflexes (all DU exposed groups, 6 & 7 post-natal days of age), forelimb placing and grasping (all DU groups, most pronounced for 75 mg/L group, aged 4 - 7 post-natal days of age), and swimming development (all DU groups, aged 11 - 13 post-natal days of age). Hindlimb placing was at first accelerated for the DU exposed groups (5 – 6 post-natal days of age) but latter delayed (8 post-natal days of age). Weight gain was also accelerated for DU exposed animals.

At 21 days of age post-natal the DU exposed mouse pups differed from control on the Functional Observation Battery with fewer spontaneous vocalizations (esp. 19 and 75 mg/L groups) and demonstrated more freezing and jerking behavior for the Touch Response test (all DU exposed groups). There was also a trend for the DU exposed animals to differ in their responses to the Tail Pinch test, to display more vigorous responses to the Arousal test, and to display either more quiet responses or more aggressive behavior in the Reactivity test.

Uranium exposed mouse pups had significantly higher body and brain weights at the time of sacrifice (37 and 75 mg/L groups). However, the brain as a percentage of body weight was smaller in the uranium exposed groups (37 & 75 mg/L groups).

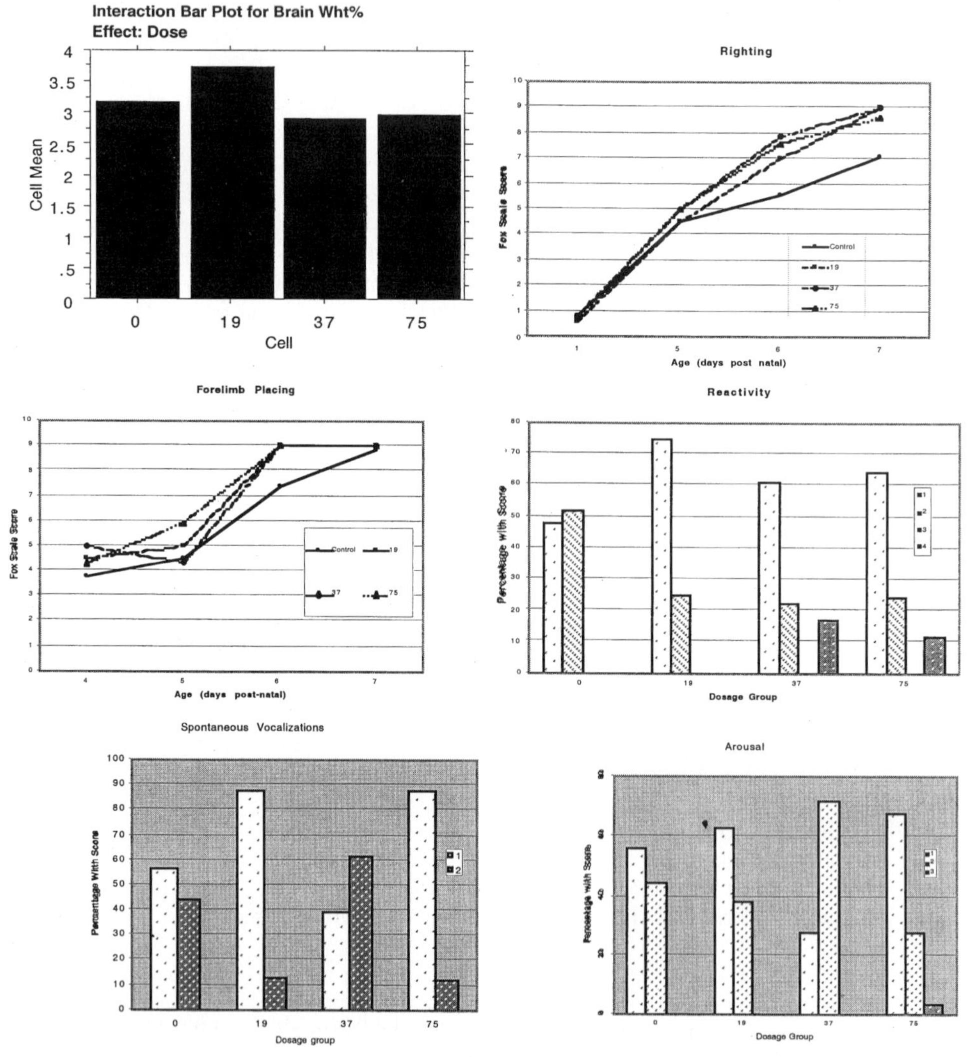

Discussion

The accelerated development reported here is not consistent with the findings reported by others, where uranium either had little effect or adverse effects on mouse fetal development [1, 2, 3, 4]. However, accelerated development caused by a compound administered during growth is not unheard of. In some instances growth hormone level is increased in treated animals because of pharmacologic effects of the compound in question. These findings might also be the result of strain differences or dosing and exposure differences.

Accelerated development is not necessarily beneficial to the animal and may mask adverse effects of DU exposure. DU exposed mouse pups demonstrate less vocalization, more freezing, altered arousal, and reactivity that is either diminished or excessive at 21 days of age. These argue that DU affects the animal's ability to regulate its response to the environment, perhaps through inability to habituate or alterations in emotional state. That these abnormal behavioral findings are due to DU exposure, and not an extraneous variable, is supported by the small brain sizes (as percentage of body weight) seen in DU exposed pups. This study raises the possibility that DU exposure can produce subtle alterations in brain structure or function that produce alterations in behavioral development at doses far lower than those needed to produce blatantly toxic effects. It has been suggested that lead and DU have approximate toxicities. While this remains to be seen, lead is a well-known behavioral teratogen, and our findings suggest that DU may also be. This study will be expanded to a larger dose range and sample size.

Acknowledgements

This study was supported by the Whitehall Foundation.

References

[1]. Domingo JL, Ortega A, Paternain JL, Corbella J. Evaluation of the perinatal and postnatal effects of uranium in mice upon oral administration. *Archv Environ Health* 1989; 44: 395-398.

[2]. Paternain JL, Domingo JL, Ortega A, Llobet JM. The effects of uranium on reproduction, gestation, and postnatal survival in mice. *Ecotoxi Environ Safety* 1989; 17: 291-296.

[3]. Domingo JL, Paternain JL, Llobet JM, Corbella J. The developmental toxicity of uranium in mice. *Toxicol* 1989; 55: 143-152.

[4]. Bosque MA., Domingo JL, Llobet JM, Corbella J. (1993). Embryotoxicity and teratogenicity of uranium in mice following subcutaneous administration of uranyl acetate. *Biol Trace Elem Res* 1993; 36: 109-118.

[5]. Fox WM. Reflex-ontogeny and behavioral development of the mouse. *Anim Behav* 1965; 13: 234-241.

[6]. O'Donoghue JL. Clinical neurologic indicies of toxicity in animals. *Env. Health Perspect.* 1996; 104 Suppl 2: 323-330.

Metal Ions in Biology and Medicine; vol 6. Eds. J.A. Centeno, Ph. Collery, G. Vernet, R.B. Finkelman, H. Gibb, J.C. Etienne. John Libbey Eurotext, Paris © 2000, pp. 462-465.

Biochemical and histological survey of young Wistar rats exposed to lead acetate

Nemmiche S.[1], Aoues A.[2]

[1] Institute of Biology, University of Mostaganem B.P. 227, 27000 Mostaganem; [2] Institute of Biology, University of Oran Es-Sénia, 31000 Oran

ABSTRACT :

Lead exposure from environmental and occupational sources still remains a serious health concern..The consequences of lead poisoning were first described approximately 2000 years ago. Today, concern exists about the health effects attributable to low level lead exposure in both children and adults. Many of the adverse health effects of low level environmental lead exposure appear to be mediated through the central and peripheral nervous systems and involve cognitive as well as neurotoxicity dependent upon age, route of administration, and dose. Lead must be absorbed and transported to target organs like brain, liver, and bone, before susceptible cells can be harmed. An animal model using rats was developed to initiate investigations on the nervous system, and reproduction system. The object of this study was to find alterations of the neurochemical parameters during developmental and detect histopathological lesions related to chemical dose treatment.

Young male and female Wistar rats (3 weeks of age) were given to experiments with drinking water and intravenous groups. Lead acetate was dissolved to give drinking water concentrations of 100, 250, 500, 1000, or 2000 ppm lead and intravenously at doses of 0.02, 0.2, and 2.0 mg Pb / kg BW. Some of the most profound effect of lead intoxication are found in the function of the central nervous system, which seems to be particularly vulnerable during development.

Key Words: Lead exposure, histopathology, brain, liver, rat.

I. INTRODUCTION

The persistence of the lead in the environment continues to be a contest for the public health, and attract the attention of countries further. Although it has been recognized since a long time that an exhibition to high level can produce a delay mental permanent and other cognitive deficits. The very extended problems with the lead, some manners come back to the more modern history, of its use in paintings, gases, etc., who has for result an omnipresent incorporation of this poisonous element in dusts, soils, food, and water, misleading a rife exhibition of the general population. Increasing concern and conscience, as considerable problem of the public health, particularly for children, incited a decline finally in the use of the lead, but didn't eliminate problems. If one now knows that it initiates effects with the lower levels that have ever been given previously account. It also remains a problem of the public health because strategies that aims to decrease the bodily load in lead, as the therapy of chelation is currently controversial.

II. Materials & Methods: The young rats of Wistar stump (Iffa Credo, France), aged of weaned three weeks and distributed in the individual cages, have been used. To do our survey, one kept five increasing doses of acetate of the lead 3-hydrates going of 100 to 2000ppm managed by oral way (water of drink) with a length of eight-week treatment [1]. Dose 100 ppm [2]; doses 250, 500, and 1000 ppm [1]; dose 2000 ppm [3]. For the intravenous way, three doses have been kept [4]: 0.02, 0.2, 2 mg Pb / kg body weight respectively, for a length of four week treatment. Parameters of the middle are controlled carefully (light/dark: 12/12, T°: 22±1°C, humidity: 70±10%, food ad libitum).

- Toxicological survey: The dosage of the lead is done on the following organs: brain, liver, kidneys, and bones by techniques of the authors [5, 3, 4, 6, 7]. The technical Lowry [8] do the total protein dosage. The technical WeckBerker [9] achieve the dosage of the reduced glutathion (GSH), and the dosage of the neurochemicals parameters (choline acetyltransferase activity (CAT) and glutamate decarboxylase: GAD) by techniques of the authors [10, 11].
- Histological survey: It is achieved on the following organs: brain, liver, kidneys, and male gonads (testicles) by the following coloration techniques [12]: Hémalun-Eosine method, Rhodizonate method, Mallory and Parker's, purple of Cresyl, and blue of the strong Luxol.

III. Results and discussions:

Toxicological Survey:

From data of dosage, it comes out again that the rate of the lead increases with the quantity of the lead brought by the water of drink. The mean of the blood lead, liver, brain, kidneys, and bone increases with the level of doses managed, with the meaningful interrelationship coefficients, that it is for groups treaties by oral way or those by intravenous way, and an interrelationship measures dose - answer superior for the IV way with regard to the oral way. The concentration of the cloth lead after an intravenous administration increases a linear way, proportionally with the dose, except lead of bone. This last represents cloth that can be the better used to characterize the accumulation of the lead relatively following an intravenous administration of weak level (0.02 to 0.2 mg Pb/kg of body weight), and to doses between 0.2 and 2.0 mg Pb/kg of body weight. Some similar results have been found by Hamilton [2] for those treaties by oral way, nevertheless for shares treated by intravenous injection one records a likeness more to least comparable to results of [13] that finds a PbS (blood lead) of 31 and 521 μg/dl respectively for a dose of 1 and 100 mg Pb/kg, on the other hand for the Pbcer (lead of brain), he gets 150 and 2700ng/g respectively. In a survey [14] on the system central monoamine (postnatal effect of the Pb), following an exhibition to the Pb (injection intrapéritoneal measures out 1 and 8 mg of Pb acetate/kg), they found to the PND21 (postnatal 21st day) a Pbcer of 351±17 ng/g to a dose of 1mg Pb/kg, and 1312±97 ng/g to a dose of 8mg Pb/kg. And to the PND51, they record the 1/3 of the Pbcer rate to the PND21, either 110±5 ng/g (for dose 1mg Pb/kg) and 434±26 ng/g (for dose 8mg Pb/Kg).

Whereas our results of the PbCer dosage by intravenous way were 200±40 ng/g and 900±80 ng/g for doses 0.02 and 0.2 mg Pb/kg, and 1600±50 ng/g to a dose of 2 Pb/kg , and those treaties by oral way by a strong person measure out 2000ppm one got a mean of 1400±20 ng/g. Freeman and *al* [5] record a PbS of 1740 µg Pb/l, and a PbOs of 294µg/g to a dose of 2mg/kg of which we found equal respectively to 1200 µg/l and 260 µg/g in ours experimentation. However other [6] who studied the toxicity of the Pb on rats F344, do some PbS find to the experimental doses of 10, 30, and 100ppm of acetate of the Pb in the food: 16±1.7, 31.8 ±3.8, and 84.8±8.9 µg/dl respectively; PbOs of 20, 100, and 260 µg/g; and of the PbCer of 0.1, 0.2 to 0.3, and 0.6 to 0.7 µg/g. Whereas Kala and Jadhav [15] working with doses of 25, 50, and 5000ppm (acetate of the Pb in the water of drink) on rats long Evans aged of 31 days find, after 90 days of treatment, a middle rate of PbS respectively of 13, 15, and 49 µg/dl. All these results gotten by different authors differ because of the effect of stump, the effect of age, the length and the way of the treatment, periods of taking for dosage (blood), etc. The rate of the GSH increased meaningfully ($P < 0.05$) with regard to the witness, one record a multiplication respectively by a factor of 1.78, 2.11, and 4.22 for groups IV1, IV2, and IV3. And it is interrelated ($r=0.94$) meaningfully ($P < 0.05$) with the level of doses. The rate of the CAT and GAD decrease respectively of 40% and 25% in the hippocampal region (PND28).

Histological Survey:

The effect of the lead on the hepatic tissue of the rat, we notice on intracellular modification translating themselves by a nuclear hypertrophy that entails a modification in report nucléocytoplasmic, and a frequency of mitotic divisions' superior to those of witnesses. Observations that can be sign of the development of a possible tumorale process, that must be to verify by the dosage of scorers' oncogèneses. The examination of the cerebral structure of rats doesn't reveal a difference between groups treaties to the lead and the no treaties, on the other hand tissular structure in hippocampale is well distinct, where one observes a light change to the level of gyrus dentate of the corner of Ammon more to the pronounced compared to witnesses. The renal lesions are characterized by a nuclear enlarging curbed in the renal tubeless, and in the external medulla. Cores rounded irregularly, having appearance polyhedral rather than the typical circular of a slightly oval shape. The renal lesions translate the existence of a nephrite interstitial subaiguë. The histological exam of testicular cuts doesn't show any sign of change of the spermatogenesis process.

Conclusion: Of after the gotten results, it comes out again in the first place that the lead accumulates mainly in bones where it is going to constitute an important reservoir like source of poisoning for the fetus via the umbilical cord, on the other hand the increase of the rate of the GSH reveals an intense hepatic metabolic activity well to face of it this xenobiotic: the lead, whose effects are well visible on cuts histologic. Let's add to it the preferential accumulation of the lead in hippocampal region. Thus, the exhibition to the lead during the prenatal period entails some neurological changes incontestably. Therefore strategies of struggle must be undertaken with more required, because some medicines chelateuses are potentially tératogènesis at less at the animal, the treatment of the saturnism will be above all preventive.

REFERENCES

1. Hamilton J. D., O'Flaherty E., Ross R., Shukla R., Gartside P. Structural Equation modeling and nested ANOVA: Effects of lead exposure on maternal and fetal growth in rats. Environm. Res. , 1994 ; 64:53-64

2. Khalil-Manesh F., Gonick H. C., Weiler E. W. J. Effect of chelation treatment with dimercaptosuccinic acid on lead-related blood pressure changes. Environ. Res. , 1994 ; 65:86-99.

3. Bielarczyk H., Tomsing J. L., Suszkiw J. B. Perinatal low-level lead exposure and the septo-hippocampal cholinergic system: selective reduction of muscarinic receptors and cholineacetyltransferase in the rat septum. Brain Research. 1994 ; 643:211-217.

4. Freeman G. B., Johnson J. D., Liao S. C., Feder P. I., Davis A. O., Ruby M. V., Schoof R. A., Chaney R. L., and Bergstrom P. D. Absolute bioavailability of lead acetae and mining waste lead in rats. Toxicology, 1994 ; 91:151-163.

5. Mindak W. Determination of lead in table wines by graphite furnace atomic absorption spectrometry. J. AOAC Intern., 1994 ; 77(4) : 1023-1030.

6. Dieter Michael P., Matthews H. B., Jeffcoat R. A., Moseman R. F. Comparaison of lead bioavailability in F344 rats fed lead acetate, lead oxide, lead sulfide, or lead ore concentrate from Skagway, Alaska. J. Toxicol. Environ. Health 1993 ; 39:79-93.

7. Gil Fernando, Maria L. Pérez. Microwave oven digestion procedure for atomic absorption spectrometry analysis of bone and teeth. Clinica Chimica 1993 ; 221:23-31

8. Lowry OH, Rosenbron G. H., Farr A. L., and Randall R. J. 1951. Protein measurement with folin phenol reagent.In: *Protein methods.* Daniel M. Bollag & Stuart J. Edelstein, ed. Wiley-Liss, Inc, NY, 1991.

9. Weckberker G., Cory J. G. Ribonucleotide reductase activity and growth glutathione depleted mouseleukemia L1210 cells in vitro. Can. Letters 1988 ; 40:257-264.

10. Jeltsch H., Cassel J. C., Neufang B., Kelche C., Hertting G., Jackisch R., and WillB. The effects of intrahippocampal raphe and/or septal grafts in rats with fimbria-fornix lesions depend on the origin of the grafted tissue and the behavioral task used. Neuroscience 1994 ; 63(1):19-39.

11. Fonnum F., A rapid radiochemical method for the determination of choline acetyl transferase. J. Neurchem., 1975 ; 24:407-409.

12. Culling C. F. A., Allison R. T. and W. T. Barr. Cellular pathology technique 4éme éd., Butterworths & Co. LTD, 642p, 1988.

13. Singh AK. Neurotoxicity in rats chronically exposed to lead ingestion: measurement of intracellular concentrations of free calcium and lead ions in resting or depolarized brain slices. Neurotoxicology .1995 ; 16(1) :133-8.

14. Luthman J., Lindqvist E., Gerhardt GA., Olson L., Hoffer BH. . Alterations in central monoamine systems after postnatal lead acetate treatment in rats. Environ. Res., 1994 ; 65(1) : 100-18.

15. Kala SV., Jadhav AL. Region-specific alterations in dopamine and serotonin metabolism in brains of rats exposed to low levels of lead. Neurotoxicology 1995 ; 16(2):297-308.

Metal Ions in Biology and Medicine; vol 6. Eds. J.A. Centeno, Ph. Collery, G. Vernet, R.B. Finkelman, H. Gibb, J.C. Etienne. John Libbey Eurotext, Paris © 2000, pp. 466-468.

Cadmium intoxication as a new agent in the ethiology of hearing loss

Hasan U. Ozcaglar[1], Bulent V. Ag rd r[1], Oktay Dinc[1], Gulsen Oner[2], Alper Derin[1], Sevilay Kl çarslan

[1] *Akdeniz University, Faculty of Medicine Departments of Ear Nose and Throath, and* [2] *Physiology, 070070 Kampus-Antalya, Turkey*

ABSTRACT

The significant alterations in the analysis of ABR and DPOAE were observed in rats subjected to 5 and 15 ppmCdCl2 containing drinking water for 30 days.Cochlear hair cells seemed more vulnarable than kidney tubule cells to cadmium toxiicity.

Keywords. cadmium toxicity, auditory changes,hearing loss

INTRODUCTION

Cadmium (Cd) is a major environmental and occupational hazard because of its widespread use in industry and subsequent release into environment. The results of epidemiological studies have revealed that Cd is the most toxic heavy metal to humans and accumulated cadmium exerts toxic effects on many biological systems. However, since 70% of ultra filtered Cd is taken up largely by the proximal tubules of the kidney. It is accumulated mainly in the kidney cortex resulting in tubule lesion after severe exposure [1].

There are many functional similarities between inner ear and renal tubular cells [2,3]. Both cells have abundant carbonic anhydrase activity [2,3]. Inhibition of this zinc dependent enzyme increases urinary bicarbonate excretion as well as changing the chloride content of the pery and endolymph [2,3] results in impairment of hearing quality [2,3]. Some autoimmune diseases which affect kidney functions also lead to change in hearing [4]. The presence of hearing loss in patients with kidney failure gives another proof for the functional similarity of tubular and inner ear cells [5].

High frequency of hearing loss in residents of industrialized countries[6] suggests the possible deteriorative effect of toxic environmental agents on hearing.Although reviewing the literature showed the presence of many functional similarities between renal tubular and inner ear cells, [2,3] the hazardous effect of nephrotoxic heavy metals such as cadmium on hearing has not been studied yet. In order to determine the effect of Cd on hearing , this experimental study was carried out in rats.

MATERIAL AND METHODS

48 Male albino rats weighing 180±25 g were used in this experiment. All animals divided into three equal groups were fed normal rat chow. While the

control rats drank tap water, the rats in the second and third group received 5 and 15 ppm $CdCl_2$ containing drinking water for 30 days.

On day 29 all rats were put on metabolic cage to measure daily urine output, water and food intake. On 30th day ,6 animals from each group were used for the measurement of kidney functions and blood pressure according to the methods used in our previous study [7].

10 animals from each group were anesthetized and they were examined and confirmed to have normal tympanic membranes . Then Auditory Brainstem Response (ABR) and Distortion Product Otoacustic Emission(DPOAE) recordings were made by the methods described previously [5,6,8]. Under the surgical microscope(OPM 99 Zeiss),the middle ear ossicles were removed and then a bone sample from cochlear labyrinth was taken. The ossicles of 5 animals were pooled and cadmium content of the blood ,tissues and the pools of ear bones was measured by the method described before[7]. One-way ANOVA test was used for the statistical evaluations of the data. The results were expressed as Mean ±SD. $P<0.05$ was accepted as statistically important.

RESULTS:

Table shows that dose dependent cadmium accumulation in renal cortex was associated with both blood pressure elevation and findings of nephrotoxicity. Cd induced functional changes in the third group were found to be statistically important when they were compared with control values ($p<0.01$), whereas the effect of 5 ppm $CdCl_2$ containing water was most obviously seen on hearing

Cadmium accumulation in ear ossicles and labyrinth was accompanied by some abnormalities in ABR waves in cadmium-exposed rats. In response to click stimuli the mean latency of wave I of ABR prolonged significantly but the latencies of waves III and V did not differ in any of three groups. The interpeak latency of I-III was shortened because of the significant delay in the wave I latency in both cadmium-exposed groups ($p<0.01$).DPOAE traces indicated obvious hair cell dysfunction in both treated groups.

DISCUSS ON

These results clearly demonstrated that 15-ppm $CdCl_2$ produced significant impairment in kidney functions, but were unaltered in 5 ppm$CdCl_2$ subjected animals. Our results also showed that first time in literature ,cadmium causes dose dependently hearing loss in rats. Analysis of ABR waves suggested that cadmium dependent impairment was localized mainly on cochlea without affecting central auditory pathways. Prolonged latencies of wave I and shortage in the interpeak of wave I-III intervals [5,8] supported the sensitivity of cochlea against cadmium

The mechanism by which cadmium impairs hearing is not known. But the similarities between proximal tubular and ear epithelial cells can partly involve in this co-impairment. Both cells have abundant amount of zinc dependent carbonic anhydrase enzyme activity which catalysis H^+ and HCO_3 production [2,3]. Cadmium by replacing zinc ion in this enzyme may change the ionic composition of endo and perilymp and causes hearing loss. The results of Sterkers et al [3] showing the close relationship between hearing and changes in electrolyte contents of perilymph in carbonic anhydrase inhibited rats seems to support our hypothetical explanation. If this hypothesis is true, cadmium mediated inhibition of carbonic anhydrase by disturbing the dynamic equilibrium of electrolytes will decrease the high sensitivity of hair cells against sound stimuli [2]. Our DPOAE results indicating the impairment of outer hair cell functions support this hypothesis. Gaborjan et al reported that Cd affected cochlea by changing dopamine uptake[9]. Despite the lack of obvious nephrotoxicity findings in rats subjected to 5 ppm Cd ,the presence of significant abnormalities in ABR waves shows that hearing system is more sensitive to cadmium toxicity than the kidney. However further studies are needed.

		Control	5 ppm cadmium	15 ppm cadmium
GFR(μl/min)		507.16±53.8(n=11)	419.85±38.27(n=5)	225.64±08.32(n=6)*
Blood pressure	Systolic	84.3±4.23(n=7)	102.7±73.41(n=10)*	118.83±25.2(n=6)*
	Diastolic	62.43±4.15(n=7)	69.96±55.11(n=10)	91.83±65.2(n=6)*
Tissue Cd Dry Wt	Renal Cortex μg/g.	1.386±0.28(n=7)	1.745±581.0(n=10)	2.101±403.0(n=9)*
	Ear ossicles (Pg/ear)	2.08	1.775±70.0	3.935
	Labyrinth (ng/g.)	64.5	66	108.5
ABR Results	I .Wave	1.335±0.31(n=20)	1.642±250.0(n=20)*	1.74±880.0(n=20)*
	III .Wave	3.0.38±0.361(n=20)	3.014±872.0(n=20)	3.2±8391.0(n=20)
	V. Wave	4.712±0.352(n=20)	4.539±683.0(n=20)	4.918±974.0(n=20)
	I-III interval	1.709±0.332(n=20)	1.460±0.062(n=20)*	1.3960±0.209(n=20
	III-V interval	1.719±0.245(n=20)	1.753±0.419(n=20)	1.655±0.360(n=20)
	I-V interval	3.433±0.186(n=20)	2.974±805.0(n=20)	3.218±934.0(n=20)

Table : The effects of cadmium on studied parameters.

References

1. Dobson, .: "Environmental health criteria for cadmium-environmental aspects" World Health Organisation, Environmental Health Criteria, Geneva, 1992
2. Sterkers, O., Eveleyne, F., Amiel, C.; "Production of inner ear fluids" Physiol Rew, 1988, 68,(4), 1083-1128.
3. Sterkers, O., Eveleyne, Clavde, A.; "How are inner ear fluids formed ?" NIPS, 1987,(2)176-179.
4. Johnson, L.G., Arenberg,K.; "Cochlea abnormalities in Alport's Syndrome" Arch Otolaryngol,1981, (107), 340-34
5. Özça lar, H.Ü., Dinç, O., Fi enk, F., K l nçarslan, S.;"Auditory Evoked Potantials of chronic renal failure patients before and after hemodialysis" Proceedings of the XV. World Congress of ORL Head-Neck Surgery, stanbul 1993, (1), 391-394.
6. Oeken,J:"Topodiagnostic assesment of occupational noise-induced hearing loss using DPOAE compared to the S S test".Eur Arc Otolaryngol :1999, 256:115-121.
7. Öner, G., entürk, Ü., Uysal, N.;"Role of cadmium induced lipid peroxisation in kidney response to atrial natriouretic hormone" Nephron,1996, 72:257-262.
8. Özgirgin, N., Vural, O.;"Gürültüye ba l i itme kay pl kobaylarda beyinsap uyar lm cevap odyometrisi, ERA" Otolaringoloji ve Stomatoloji Dergisi, 1987, 67-
9. Gaborjan A, Lendvai B,Vizi, ES: "Neurochemical evidence of dopamine release by lateral olivococlear efferents and its presynaptic modulation in guinea-pig cochlear. Neuroscience 1999, 90(1):131-8

Metal Ions in Biology and Medicine; vol 6. Eds. J.A. Centeno, Ph. Collery, G. Vernet, R.B. Finkelman, H. Gibb, J.C. Etienne. John Libbey Eurotext, Paris © 2000, pp. 469-471.

Hypocholesterolemic effect of aspirin in copper deficiency in rats may be due to its antioxidant properties

Meira Fields[1], Charles G. Lewis[1] and Isabelle Bureau[2]

[1] *Beltsville Human Nutrition Research Center, Nutrient Requirements and Functions Laboratory, U.S. Department of Agriculture, ARS, Beltsville, Maryland 20705, USA;* [2] *Joseph Fourier University, La Tronche, France*

Address all correspondence to: Dr. Meira Fields, USDA, ARS, BHNRC, NRFL; Bldg. 307, Rm. 330, BARC-East; Beltsville, MD 20705-2350; telephone: 301-504-9412; fax: 301-504-9062; email: **fields@307.bhnrc.usda.gov**

Introduction

During the last decade, it became apparent that reactive oxygen species and free radicals are involved in the pathogenesis of many chronic degenerative diseases such as cardiovascular disease, diabetes, cancer, neurodegenerative diseases and aging. Oxidative stress has been implicated as an important etiological factor in atherosclerosis and vascular dysfunction (1). Atherosclerosis, the principle cause of cardiovascular disease, is the leading cause of death in Western societies.

It is well established that a high level of blood cholesterol is a risk factor for heart disease. We have recently reported that oxidative stress caused by inadequate consumption of dietary copper is responsible for raising blood cholesterol (2). If oxidative stress and reactive oxygen species are involved in cardiovascular disease, then antioxidants should be effective in preventing its occurrence.

Aspirin, widely used as an analgesic-antipyretic agent, may reduce and prevent the risk of cardiovascular disease due to its antithrombotic potential (3, 4). It has been reported to reduce blood cholesterol levels in rats (5). We therefore suggested that its effect on blood cholesterol in rats may be due to its antioxidant properties. This study was conducted to determine whether the hypocholesterolemic properties of aspirin in rats are due to its antioxidant capabilities.

Materials and Methods

Weanling male Sprague-Dawley rats were randomly divided into 4 dietary groups. Half of the rats were fed a copper-adequate diet (6.0 μgCu/g); and the other half a copper-deficient diet (0.8 μgCu/g). Half the rats consumed aspirin (acetylsalicylic acid) (2.84 g/kg) diet. This study was terminated after 5 weeks due to the untimely death of one copper-deficient rat fed aspirin. Post-mortem examination revealed clotted blood in the chest cavity due to a ruptured heart in the area of the apex.

Table 1: Liver copper, SOD and lipid peroxidation and plasma cholesterol

	Liver Copper (μg/g wet wt)	SOD (u/g)	LPO (μmol/g)	Cholesterol (mg/dl)
Copper adequate				
no aspirin	3.5 ± 0.4	796 ± 46	30 ± 5	127 ± 4
+ aspirin	4.2 ± 0.2	1042 ± 65	37 ± 7	110 ± 4
Copper-deficient				
no aspirin	1.1 ± 0.1	156 ± 12	98 ± 12	173 ± 4
+ aspirin	1.6 ± 0.3	140 ± 19	54 ± 16	148 ± 6
ANOVA				
Cu	S	S	S	S
Aspirin	S	S	NS	S
CuxAspirin	NS	S	S	NS

SOD = Superoxide dismutase LPO = lipid peroxidation

Results

All rats which consumed the copper-deficient diet became copper deficient based on liver copper concentration and liver SOD activity. All copper-deficient rats exhibited oxidative stress as assessed by hepatic lipid peroxidation. Copper deficiency resulted in high levels of blood cholesterol. Aspirin administration reduced blood cholesterol in all rats. The reduced blood cholesterol in copper-deficient rats given aspirin was associated with a reduction of lipid peroxidation.

Discussion

The present study was designed to determine whether prevention of oxidative stress will be effective in reducing levels of blood cholesterol, a risk factor metabolite associated with heart disease. Oxidative stress was induced by consumption of a diet inadequate in copper. The consumption of a copper-deficient diet resulted in a suppressed activity of SOD, a major antioxidant enzyme which plays an important role in the defensive mechanism against reactive oxygen species. The significant reduction of SOD activity in copper-deficient rats was accompanied by an increased oxidative stress assessed by liver lipid peroxidation. In addition, copper deficiency was also associated with elevated levels of blood cholesterol. The consumption of aspirin reduced blood cholesterol in all rats. A greater reduction was noted in copper-deficient rats receiving aspirin. The mechanism responsible for hypocholesterolemic effect of aspirin is not fully understood. Recently, aspirin has been proposed to possess antioxidant properties (6). Based on data presented herein, it is suggested that when antioxidant protection is compromised, aspirin can function as an antioxidant. This suggestion is supported by a reduction in lipid peroxidation by aspirin in copper-deficient rats.

References

1. Steinberg D, Parthasarathy S, Carew TE, Khoo JC, Witztum JL. Beyond cholesterol: Modifications of low-density lipoprotein that increase its atherogenicity. N. Engl. J. Med. 1989; 320:915-924.

2. Fields M, Lewis CG. Hepatic iron overload may contribute to hypertriglyceridemia and hypercholesterolemia in copper-deficient rats. Metabolism 1997; 46:377-381.

3. Hammond EC, Garfinkel L. Aspirin and coronary heart disease: Findings of a prospective study. Br. Med. J. 1975; 2:269-271.

4. Fuster V, Dyken ML, Vokanas PS, Hennekens C. Aspirin as a therapeutic agent in cardiovascular disease. Special Writing Group. Circulation 1993; 87:659-675.

5. Klevay LM. Aspirin hypocholesterolemia associated with increased microsomal copper in liver. Nutr. Res. 1986; 6:12-8-1292.

6. Oberle S, Polte T, Abate A, Podhaisky HP, Schröder H. Aspirin increases ferritin synthesis in endothelial cells. A novel antioxidant pathway. Cir. Res. 1998; 82:1016-1020.

Metal Ions in Biology and Medicine; vol 6. Eds. J.A. Centeno, Ph. Collery, G. Vernet, R.B. Finkelman, H. Gibb, J.C. Etienne. John Libbey Eurotext, Paris © 2000, pp. 472-474.

Proinflammatory neuropeptides in magnesium deficiency

W.B. Weglicki, J.H. Kramer, I.T. Mak, B.F. Dickens, A.M. Komarov and T.M. Phillips

Dept. of Physiology and Experimental Medicine, George Washington University Medical Center, Washington, DC

Animal models of Mg-deficiency and oxidative stress: Diminished dietary Mg intake may have an increased long-term medical risk,[1] severe dietary Mg-deficiency has been reported to cause diverse pathology in animal models. Feeding rats the MgD_9 (9% of RDA levels) diet for three weeks resulted in a 50% loss of RBC glutathione; most of the decrease occurred during the second week.[2] The loss of RBC glutathione, a key cellular antioxidant, resulted in the red cells becoming more sensitive to an applied oxidative stress. We demonstrated that this glutathione can be preserved if the animals were supplemented with variety of antioxidant nutrients and antioxidant drugs.[2] This suggested that glutathione loss is caused by increased oxidation. Mg-deficiency was associated with reduced tolerance towards postischemic stress, as indicated by greater mechanical dysfunction, enhanced tissue injury, and greatly elevated free radical production and oxidative injury in MgD_9 hearts compared to Mg-sufficient group.[3] Treatment *in vivo* with antioxidants such as Vit. E prevented much of the Mg-deficiency induced loss of myocardial tolerance to I/R stress.[3, 4, 5]

Severe Mg-deficiency Cardiomyopathy and the neuropeptide/cytokine response: While investigating the potential mechanisms responsible for the onset of cardiomyopathy during Mg-deficiency, we discovered that elevated circulating levels of numerous inflammatory mediators occur early after initiating the diet. The most significant finding was elevated serum levels of neuropeptides, including substance P [6] which has pro-inflammatory properties. Since calcitonin gene-related peptide (CGRP) is also elevated, the early neuropeptide release may arise from sensory-motor neuron fibers. Since the rise in these neuropeptides preceded increases that were observed for other circulating mediators (NO•, PGE_2, T-cell-derived interferon-γ, mast cell-derived histamine, IL-1, IL-6, and TNFα), we hypothesized that substance P may be inducing many of these other inflammatory events which eventually promote the cardiomyopathy seen later on in this model. The rise in substance P (and CGRP) which occurs between day 2 and day 10 was followed by an increase in circulating white blood cell numbers and histamine levels (which peaks on day 11 and is reduced by day 14). When Mg-deficient rats were treated with a specific substance P receptor blocker, we observed marked attenuation of these elevations in histamine, PGE_2, TNFα,[6, 7] and the oxidative-induced loss of blood glutathione[7]. In the mouse, significant

substance P elevations occurred in the plasma during the first week of Mg-deficiency, and promoted increased sensitivity of T-lymphocytes toward substance P.[8] In addition, T-lymphocytes isolated from Mg-deficient mice responded differently with respect to their cytokine production when challenged with substance P. The increased sensitization and increased substance P receptor expression further supports the role of substance P in the activation of T-lymphocytes. Furthermore, Mg-deficiency results in endogenous activation of neutrophils[9] as indicated by enhanced *ex vivo* superoxide anion generation in freshly isolated neutrophils. We hypothesized that MgD_9-induced release of substance P initiated a cascade of inflammatory/pro-oxidant events leading to the cardiomyopathic characteristics associated with longer-term (> 3 wks) severe dietary Mg restriction. As expected, treatment of rats with the NK-1 receptor antagonist CP-96,345 caused a dramatic reduction in PGE_2 release at the end of the first week, and histamine release during weeks two and three of the diet. These findings suggest that substance P does modulate these later inflammatory processes. Postischemic hearts from L-703,606 treated MgD_9 rats exhibited a dose-dependent improvement ($p<0.05$) in recovery of cardiac work.
Our findings indicate that ***substance P receptor blockade is inhibiting in vivo inflammatory responses observed only in the Mg-deficient animal, and suggests that substance P plays a crucial role in the reduced myocardial tolerance to reperfusion injury observed during Mg-deficiency.***
Evidence of NO• Production: We became interested in the possibility that enhanced NO• production *in vivo* occurs during Mg-deficiency. Our studies showed an elevation in NO• production during severe Mg-deficiency,[9, 10] as measured by serum nitrate and nitrosohemoglobin (formed by the interaction of NO• and heme), both of which were blocked by a relatively low dose of the NOS inhibitor, L-NAME. This increase in NO• coincided with the elevation of circulating substance P. We also demonstrated that inhibition of NO• synthase (with L-NAME) attenuated depletion of RBC glutathione during Mg-deficiency, suggesting a cytotoxic role for NO• during Mg-deficiency. In conclusion, our recent research has shown that treatment with substance P receptor blockers, nitric oxide synthase inhibitor, and antioxidants can ameliorate most of the cardiovascular injury observed in animal models of dietary Mg-restriction – ***in spite of persisting hypomagnesemia***. These observations, along with the induction of inflammatory mediators, indicate that the central and peripheral nervous systems are involved in a systemic neurogenic inflammatory response.

Literature Cited

1. Seelig MS: Consequences of magnesium deficiency on the enhancement of stress reactions; Preventive and therapeutic implications. *J.Am.Coll.Nutr.* 1994;13:429-446
2. Mak IT, Stafford RE, Weglicki WB: Loss of red cell glutathione during Mg deficiency: prevention by vitamin E, D-propranolol, and chloroquine. *Am.J.Physiol.* 1994;267:C1366-C1370
3. Kramer JH, Misík V, Weglicki WB: Magnesium-deficiency potentiates free radical production associated with postischemic injury to rat hearts: vitamin E affords protection. *Free Radical Biol.Med.* 1994;16(6):713-723
4. Kramer JH, Phillips TM, Weglicki WB: Magnesium-deficiency enhanced postischemic myocardial injury is reduced by substance P receptor blockade. *J.Mol.Cell.Cardiol.* 1997;29:97-110
5. Weglicki WB, Phillips TM, Mak IT, Cassidy MM, Dickens BF, Stafford RE, Kramer JH: Cytokines, neuropeptides, and reperfusion injury during magnesium deficiency. *Ann.N.Y.Acad.Scien.* 1994;723:246-257
6. Weglicki WB, Phillips TM: Pathobiology of magnesium deficiency: a cytokine/neurogenic inflammation hypothesis. *Am.J.Physiol.* 1992;263:R734-R737
7. Weglicki WB, Mak IT, Stafford RE, Dickens BF, Cassidy MM, Phillips TM: Neurogenic peptides and the cardiomyopathy of Mg-deficiency: Effects of substance P-receptor inhibition. *Mol.Cell.Biochem.* 1994;130:103-109
8. Weglicki WB, Dickens BF, Wagner TL, Chmielinska JJ, Phillips TM: Immunoregulation by neuropeptides in magnesium deficiency: *Ex vivo* effect of enhanced substance P production on circulating T lymphocytes from Mg-deficient mice. *Magnesium Res.* 1996;9:3-11
9. Mak IT, Dickens BF, Komarov AM, Phillips TM, Weglicki WB: Activation of the neutrophil and loss of plasma glutathione during Mg-deficiency---modulation effect by NOS inhibition. *Mol.Cell.Biochem.* 1997; 176:35-39
10. Mak, I. T., Komarov, A. M., Wagner, T. L., Stafford, R. E., Dickens, B. F., and Weglicki, W. B. Effect of dietary Mg-deficiency on nitric oxide (NO) production and the role of NO in mediating oxidative depletion of glutathione in red cells. *Am.J.Physiol.* 271:C385-C390 1996

Metal Ions in Biology and Medicine; vol 6. Eds. J.A. Centeno, Ph. Collery, G. Vernet, R.B. Finkelman, H. Gibb, J.C. Etienne. John Libbey Eurotext, Paris © 2000, pp. 475-477.

Influence of heavy metals (especially lead) on lipid metabolism and the oxidation-reduction status of the organism

E. Dynerowicz-Bal, J. Antonowicz-Juchniewicz, A. Skoczyńska, R. Andrzejak

Department of Internal and Occupational Diseases, Wrocław Medical University, ul. Pasteura 4, 50-367 Wrocław, Poland

Introduction

Recent studies have shown that metals, like iron and copper, but also lead, undergo redox cycling, deplete glutathione and protein-bound sulfhydryl groups, resulting in the production of reactive oxygen species or impairment of antioxidant defence of the organism. As a consequence, enhanced lipid peroxidation and DNA damage occur [1].

Material and methods

The health state of a group of 80 workers of the Non-Ferrous Metal Institute in Legnica, Poland (occupationally exposed to lead, copper and zinc) was evaluated in 1998, with special attention to the concentrations of trace elements in blood, the parameters of lipid metabolism and the oxidation-reduction status of the organism. The following parameters were determined: blood lead level, serum manganese, copper, zinc, calcium, magnesium levels, free erythrocyte protoporphyrin (FEP) concentration, serum total cholesterol, HDL- and LDL-cholesterol, triglycerides (TG), lipid peroxides (LPO), serum nitric oxide (NO), and serum total antioxidant status (TAS).

Results

The mean levels of Pb in blood of the workers did not exceed the highest concentrations allowable for occupational hazard. However, they could be subdivided into two clear groups: below (subgroup 1) and above 300 μg/l (subgroup 2). The level of FEP, lead overload indicator, was low in subgroup 1, but elevated in subgroup 2 (Table I). Also the levels of copper and iron, the elements which can provide protection against lead toxicity, were significantly increased in workers in subgroup 2.

The lipid metabolism disorders were not found in the majority of the workers examined; though the mean levels of triglycerides were statistically higher in subgroup 2.

Taking into account the serum NO level and serum TAS level, neither the evidence of the excessive rise in the free radicals formation nor the increase of antioxidative defence were noticed in the workers examined. But it must be stressed that, though no difference in TAS was observed, significantly higher levels of NO were found in the higher lead group.

Table I
The mean values of parameters in two subgroups divided according to the blood lead levels

Parameter	Subgroup 1 (Pb<300 μg/l) n=39	Subgroup 2 (Pb≥300 μg/l) n=41	Level of confidence (p)
Mn_s (μg/l)	2.2 ± 1.46	2.46 ± 1.58	-
Cu_s (μg/dl)	117.6 ± 14.23	123.91 ± 9.11	p<0.03
Zn_s (μg/dl)	117.71 ± 19.01	120.63 ± 17.89	-
Ca_s (μg/ml)	101.87 ± 5.93	101.6 ± 5.15	-
Mg_s (μg/ml)	20.05 ± 1.74	20.06 ± 1.91	-
Fe_s (μg/dl)	113.98 ± 32.3	133.46 ± 35.42	p<0.012
FEP (μg/100 ml E)	29.12 ± 16.0	74.53 ± 101.91	p<0.007
TAS (mmol/l)	1.44 ± 0.12	1.48 ± 0.12	-
NO (mmol/l)	2.74 ± 1.05	3.61 ± 2.23	p<0.03
Cholesterol (mg%)	195.28 ± 31.62	204.17 ± 41.28	-
LDL (mg%)	118.13 ± 29.71	112.36 ± 39.45	-
HDL (mg%)	55.86 ± 12.95	56.62 ± 13.03	-
TG (mg%)	110.25 ± 59.72	185.66 ±128.77	p<0.001
LPO (nmol/ml)	1.02 ± 0.24	1.07 ± 0.42	-

Lower index s at the element symbol denotes the given element's serum level.

In addition to the positive correlation between blood Pb levels and FEP, significant correlation among blood Pb levels, serum Cu and TG were found. Blood Pb level did not affect TAS or lipid metabolism parameters (except of TG). However, as shown in Table II, significant positive correlation were detected between FEP in erythrocytes and serum Mg and Mn, as well as between lipid metabolism parameters and TAS or NO.

Table II
Significant correlation between blood and serum parameters (level of confidence p<0.05)

Pb	-	Cu	=	+0.23	FEP	-	Mg	=	+0.33
Pb	-	FEP	=	+0.4	TAS	-	Cholesterol	=	+0.27
Pb	-	TG	=	+0.31	TAS	-	TG	=	+0.31
FEP	-	Mn	=	+0.26	NO	-	TG	=	+0.42

Discussion

Both mean blood Pb and serum trace elements (Ca, Mg, Mn, Zn) levels were within the range for persons occupationally exposed to lead. This finding confirms the presence of equilibrium between pro- and antioxidant agents. Furthermore, the values of TAS are within the normal range, which supports the above observations.

The significant elevation of Cu serum levels in workers with the higher blood Pb level confirms the protective role of this element against lead toxicity [1, 2].

The increased serum Fe level in the same group of workers can be explained not only by the degradation of heme due to lead exposure [2], but also by the production of NO, which is the strong tissue oxidant, capable of releasing iron from proteins [3].

Prolonged lead exposure results in lipid metabolism disturbances [1, 4]. Our data support this notion, by demonstrating a positive correlation between blood Pb level and serum TG level. Lipid metabolism parameters correlate also with TAS and NO, which can be associated with the physiological response to oxidative stress, resulting from Pb exposure.

We find it very interesting, that the elevation of Pb level is accompanied by the statistically significant increase of serum NO level, especially while we did not see a proof for increased lipid peroxidation (lack of correlation between Pb and LPO), which has been proposed as the main mechanism of lead toxicity [1]. It can be explained by the relatively low mean blood lead levels in our study, in contrast to lead poisoning cases described in the literature. Therefore, the increase of NO level could be the first stage of the toxic oxidative reaction, harmful to the tissues and resulting from exposure to lead at occupationally accepted concentrations.

References:

1. Stohs SJ, Bagchi D. Oxidative mechanisms in the toxicity of metal ions. Free Radical Biol. Med. 18, 321-336, 1995
2. Antonowicz J, Andrzejak R, Smolik R. Influence of heavy metal mixtures on erythrocyte metabolism. Int. Arch. Occup. Environ. Health 62, 195-198, 1990
3. Halliwell B. The role of oxygen radicals in human disease, with particular reference to the vascular system. Haemostasis 23 (suppl. 1), 118-126, 1993
4. Ito Y, Niiya Y, Kuriata H. Serum lipid peroxide level and blood superoxide dismutase activity in workers with occupational exposure to lead. Int. Arch. Occup. Environ. Health. 56, 119, 1985.

Metal Ions in Biology and Medicine; vol 6. Eds. J.A. Centeno, Ph. Collery, G. Vernet, R.B. Finkelman, H. Gibb, J.C. Etienne. John Libbey Eurotext, Paris © 2000, pp. 478-480.

Mn^{2+} protects and Zn^{2+} has no effects on Fe^{2+} and Fe^{2+}/Al^{3+}-induced oxidative stress in human platelets

R.P. Pedrosa[1], M.C. Alpoim[1], M.T.C.F. Brito[1], M.A.S. Fernandes[2] and C.R. Oliveira[3]

[1] *Departamento de Bioquímica,* [2] *Departamento de Zoologia,* [3] *Serviço de Bioquímica, Universidade de Coimbra, Coimbra, Portugal*

Abstract: In order to understand the deleterious effects of Fe^{2+}, Al^{3+}, Zn^{2+} and Mn^{2+} on neurodegenerative processes, namely Alzheimer's and Parkinson's diseases, we studied the effects of these metals on the susceptibility of human platelets to lipid peroxidation, reactive oxygen species generation and membrane fluidity. Our results show that Mn^{2+} protects human platelets from Fe^{2+} and Fe^{2+}/Al^{3+}- induced membrane oxidative degradation as evaluated by the probes cis-parinaric acid and 2', 7'-dichlorofluorescin diacetate, while Zn^{2+} has apparently no effect.

Introduction

Recently attention has focused on the involvement of oxidative stress in the pathogenesis of neurodegenerative disorders including Alzheimer's (AD) and Parkinson's (PD) diseases [1,2]. Disruption of metal homeostasis, namely Fe^{2+}, Al^{3+} and Zn^{2+} in multiple regions of AD brains [3,4], and Mn^{2+} in neurological disorders similar to parkinsonism [5], supports the oxidative stress hypothesis of this diseases. In particular, Fe^{2+} is known to generate highly reactive hydroxyl radicals via Fenton-reaction and/or the Haber-Weiss cycle [6,7], and Al^{3+} stimulates lipid peroxidation, and reactive oxygen species (ROS) generation induced by Fe^{2+}[8].

To evaluate the involvement of metals-induced oxidative damage in neurodegeneration, platelets were used as a model of neuronal cells. For such propose, we investigate the effects of Zn^{2+} and Mn^{2+} on Fe^{2+} and Fe^{2+}/Al^{3+}-induced membrane oxidative damage, ROS generation and membrane fluidity on human platelets of healthy elderly individuals.

Experimental Procedures

Platelets isolation - Platelets were isolated as previously described [9]. Phospholipids were extracted following Bligh's procedure [10] and the phospholipid contents was evaluated according to Fiske and Subarrow as modified by Bartlett [11].

Lipid peroxidation - The probe cis-parinaric acid (PnA) was used to measure the oxidative membrane damage [12]. The time dependence loss of PnA fluorescence was monitored in a Perkin-Elmer LS 50 B spectrophotometer, with excitation wavelength 323 nm (slit=5) and emission wavelength 413 nm (slit=10). The rate of fluorescence of PnA (0.5μM) was measured before and after the addition of the metal ions.

ROS generation - The probe 2', 7'-dichlorofluorescin diacetate (DCFH) was used to measure the cytoplasmatic ROS generation [13]. The cells suspension ($6x10^6$/ml) was incubate with 5μM

DCFH-DA at 37°C for 20 min. After loading the cells suspension was centrifuged at 14000 rpm for 10 s, and the pellet was ressuspended in 2ml of Hepes buffer. The fluorescence was monitored on a Spex, 1681, fluorometer, with excitation wavelength at 502 nm (slit=1.5), and emission wavelength 550 nm (slit=6). The solution of the different metal ions was added 80 s after beginning to monitor the fluorescence.

Membrane fluidity - The membrane order of platelets was evaluated by fluorescence using the probe TMA-DPH, in a Perkin-Elmer LS 50B spectrophotometer, as described [14].

Results

Lipid peroxidation

The incubation of human platelets with different Fe^{2+} concentrations leads to a Fe^{2+} concentration dependent membrane oxidative degradation, as evaluated by the Fe^{2+} concentration dependent increase in the fluorescence decay rate of PnA. Zn^{2+} also promotes an increase in the fluorescence decay rate of PnA. However, this effect decreases with increasing Zn^{2+} concentrations. Mn^{2+} alone had no effect on PnA decay rate (data not shown).

The Fe^{2+}-induced human platelets membrane oxidative damage is substantially reduced when human platelets were pretreated with Zn^{2+} or Mn^{2+} before the addition of Fe^{2+}(Fig.1), while Al^{3+} (200µM) potentiates Fe^{2+}-induced injury (data not shown). Zn^{2+} and Mn^{2+} also protects human platelets from Fe^{2+}/Al^{3+}-induced membrane oxidative damage, (data not shown).

ROS generation

Incubation of human platelets with Fe^{2+} leads to a concentration dependent increase in cytosilic ROS generation, as evaluated by the increase in the rate of DCFH oxidation. In contrast incubation of human platelets with Mn^{2+} leads to a reduction of ROS levels in cytosol, while Zn^{2+} had no effect on it (data not shown). Pretreatment of human platelets with Mn^{2+} leads to a pronounced reduction on Fe^{2+}-induced cytosolic ROS levels, while Zn^{2+} pretreatment had no effect on it (Fig.2).

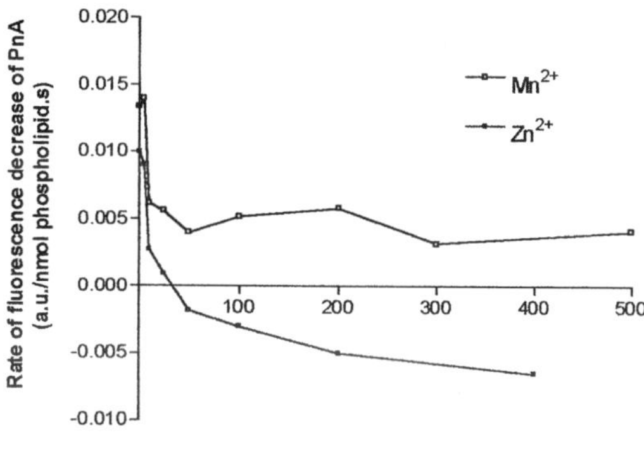

Fig. 1. A representative experiment of the effect of different concentrations of Zn^{2+} and Mn^{2+} on PnA fluorescence decay rate induced by Fe^{2+} (50 µM). Experiments were carried out using a platelet suspension (100 µl of a 0.2 O.D. suspension) pretreated with different Zn^{2+} and Mn^{2+} concentrations, and PnA (0.5 µM) in 2 ml of Hepes buffer pH 7.4 (10 mM hepes, 144 mM NaCl, 5 mM KCl and 4.6 mM glucose) at 37°C in a termostated cuvette under stirring. Fe^{2+} (50 µM) was added 180 s. after the addition of PnA and PnA fluorescence decay rate was measured for 5 min.

Membrane fluidity

Incubation of human platelets with Fe^{2+}, Al^{3+}, Zn^{2+} and Mn^{2+} has no effect on membrane fluidity as evaluated by the probe TMA-DPH. Also, the addition of Fe^{2+} or Fe^{2+}/Al^{3+} to Zn^{2+} or Mn^{2+}

pretreated cells had no effect on membrane fluidity(data not shown).

Discussion

Fe^{2+} induces human platelets membrane oxidative damage and an increase in cytoplasmatic ROS generation. The dependence of membrane oxidative degradation with Fe^{2+} concentration finds its support on the increase generation of ROS with increasing Fe^{2+}concentrations, because ROS are known to induce lipid and protein peroxidation [1].

Mn^{2+} decreases the endogenous cytosolic ROS levels in human platelets, inhibits Fe^{2+}-induced ROS generation in human platelets and also protects human platelets from Fe^{2+}-induced membrane oxidative damage. This protective effect may probably be explained by Mn^{2+} ability to act as chain-breaker, suppressing ROS generation thus inhibiting lipid peroxidation.

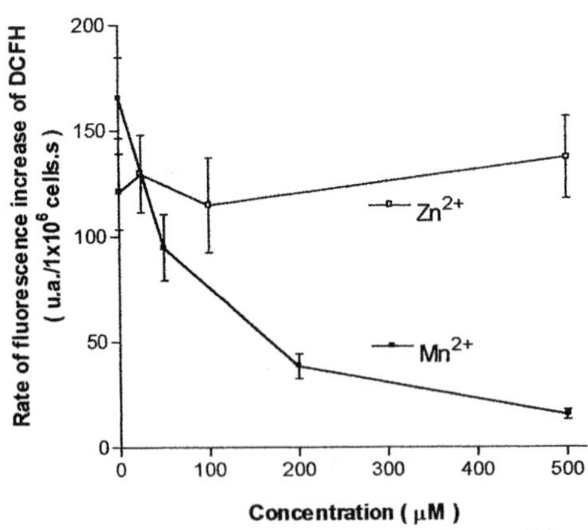

Fig. 2. ROS generation on the cytoplasm of human platelets induced by 50 µM of Fe^{2+} on the presence of different concentrations of Zn^{2+} and Mn^{2+}. Experiments were carried out by addition of 50 µM Fe^{2+} to platelets suspensions ($6x10^6$ cel./ml), pretreated with different Mn^{2+} or Zn^{2+} concentrations. DCFH concentration was 5 µM in a final volume of 2 ml. The results correspond to the mean ± SD of at least three experiments carried out in triplicate.

Zn^{2+} apparently protects human platelets from Fe^{2+}-induced membrane oxidative damage. However, Zn^{2+} has no effect on endogenous ROS levels and on the levels of Fe^{2+}-induced ROS generation. Thus, Zn^{2+} effects may probably be the result of Zn^{2+}-induced changes in membrane structure organisation, leading either to probe self quenching or a decrease in membrane accessibility to Fe^{2+}. However, Zn^{2+} had no effect on platelets membrane fluidity, using membrane probe TMA-DPH, thus apparently showing that membrane organisation remained unaffected. More studies will be needed to elucidate the role of Zn^{2+}.

In conclusion Mn^{2+} protects and Zn^{2+} has no effects on Fe^{2+} and Fe^{2+}/Al^{3+}-induced oxidative stress in human platelets.

References

1- Beni G, and Moretti A. *Neurobiol. Ageing* 1995; 16: 661-674.

2-Schapira AHV. *Neuropathol. Appl. Neurobiol.*1995; 21: 3-9.

3-Andras E, Farkas É, Scheiber H, Réffy A, and Bezúr L. *Arch. of Gerontol. and Geriatrics* 1995; 21: 89-97.

4-Crapper DR, Krishnan SS, and Dalton AJ. *Science*1973; 180: 511-513.

5 Barbeau A. *Neurotoxicology* 1984; 5: 13-36.

6-Gerlach M, Ben-Shachar D, Riederer P, and Youdin MBH. *J. Neurochem.* 1994; 63: 793-807.

7-Halliwell B. *J. Neurochem.* 1992; 59: 1609-1623.

8-Bondy SC, and Kirsteen S. *Mol. Chem. Neuropathol.* 1996; 27: 185-194.

9-Marinho C, Januário C, Matias F, Cunha L, and Oliveira CR. *Med. Sci. Res.* 1990; 18: 567-568.

10-Bligh EG, and Dyer WJ. *Can J. Biochem.Physiol.* 1959; 37: 911-917.

11-Bartlett G R. *J. Biol. Chem.* 1959; 234: 466-468.

12-Fernandes R, Pereira P, Ramalho JS, Mota MC, and Oliveira CR. *Current Eye Research* 1995; 395-402.

13-Royall JA, and Ischiropoulos H. *Arch. Biochem. Byophys.*1993; 302: 348-355.

14-Rego AC, and Oliveira C R. *Arch. Biochem. Byophys.* 1995; 321: 127-136.

Metal Ions in Biology and Medicine; vol 6. Eds. J.A. Centeno, Ph. Collery, G. Vernet, R.B. Finkelman, H. Gibb, J.C. Etienne. John Libbey Eurotext, Paris © 2000, pp. 481-483.

The role of free radicals in copper mediated toxicity in hepatocytes

N.T. Watt, G.S. Evans and M.S. Tanner

University Division of Child Health, Stephenson Wing, Children's Hospital, Sheffield UK

Background. Copper (Cu) is an essential micronutrient in which a pivotal balance must be maintained between adequacy and excess. The one electron difference between the two valencies of Cu allows it to participate in redox cycling reactions and act as a catalyst in Fenton chemistry. Significant evidence documents the ability of Cu-catalysed radicals to damage cellular macromolecules in vitro [1] which could contribute to the pathology of the hepatic copper toxicoses; Wilson's disease and Indian Childhood Cirrhosis. Although Cu exposure alone has been shown to be insufficient to induce cirrhosis in a rat model [2], radical damage maybe particularly significant in the presence of additional redox active agents.

Aims

- To determine whether an additional redox active agent can synergise with copper to potentiate the damage caused by copper alone in a model system of immortalised HepG2 hepatocytes.

- To investigate whether anti-oxidant compounds can attenuate this level of injury.

Methods. HepG2 cells were cultured in 1%-FCS-containing media supplemented with copper in the range 0 - 1000μM alone, or in combination with 125μM ascorbic acid (AA) or 1mM DMSO for periods of exposure up to 72 hours. Following exposure, the effect on cell number was determined by staining with 5μM propidium iodide (P.I.). The amount of oxidative activity occurring within the cells was measured using 100μM dihydrodichlorofluorescein diacetate. Viable and non-viable cells were identified by double fluorochrome staining using Hoescht 33342 and P.I.. Discrimination between apoptotic and necrotic cells was made on the basis of nuclear morphology.

Results

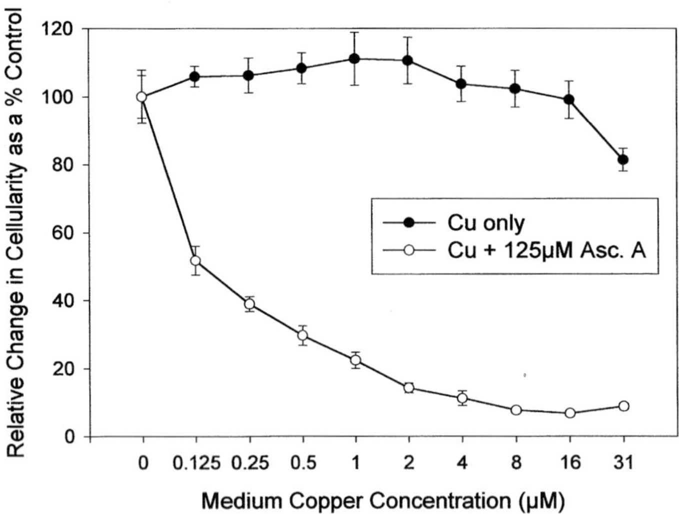

Fig 1 Effect of Copper Exposure either Alone (●) or in the Presence of 125μM Ascorbic Acid (○).

Significant reductions in cell number were observed following exposure to 63μM Cu for 48 hours ($p<0.05$). The inclusion of 125μM AA caused significant reduction in cell number at Cu concentrations as low as 125nM ($p<0.001$), increasing the rate of both apoptosis and necrosis (See fig 1 & 2). 1mM DMSO was cytoprotective at all Cu concentrations investigated ($p<0.001$) reducing the incidence of necrosis. Increases in oxidative activity were recorded at all Cu concentrations ($p<0.001$) which were further elevated upon addition of 125µM AA ($p<0.001$). 1mM DMSO inhibited any increase in oxidative activity until concentrations of 125µM Cu were achieved.

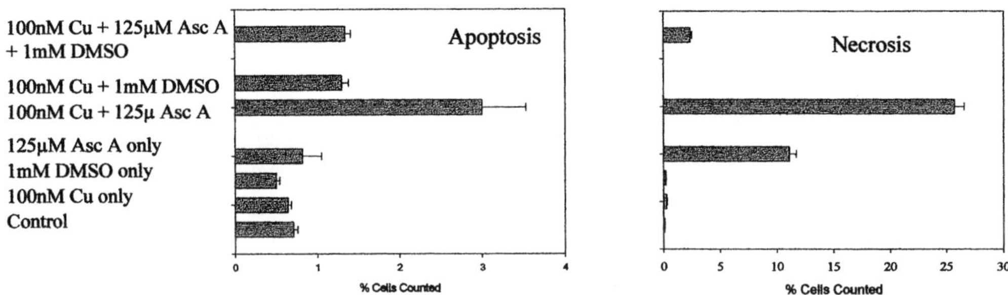

Fig 2 Quantitation of Hoescht 33342 & P.I. Staining for cell viability following treatment for 48 hours.

Conclusions. Cu and AA are an extremely potent combination inducing necrosis at Cu concentrations as low as 125nM in cultured hepatocytes. The inclusion of DMSO was cytoprotective in this model implicating a role for hydroxyl radicals in copper cytotoxicity. These data suggest that the inherent redox status of the individual may influence disease expression and also indicates a role for anti-oxidant therapy in the treatment of these disorders.

References

Halliwell B & Gutteridge J. Free Radicals in Biology and Medicine. Oxford: Clarendon Press, 1993

Morris P, O'Neill D, Tanner M Synergistic liver toxicity of copper and retrorsine in the rat. *J Hepatol.* 1994; 21:735-742.

Metal Ions in Biology and Medicine; vol 6. Eds. J.A. Centeno, Ph. Collery, G. Vernet, R.B. Finkelman, H. Gibb, J.C. Etienne. John Libbey Eurotext, Paris © 2000, pp. 484-486.

Role of metals ions in oxidative stress in Alzheimer disease

I. Manso[1], C. Díez[1], R. Fernández[2] and M.C. Martín Mateo[1]

[1] *Biochemistry Dpt.,* [2] *Neurology Unit., University Hospital of Valladolid, Spain*

Abstract

Alzheimer's disease is the most common form of adult dementia onset. The neurotoxic trace elements are relacioned with oxidative stress. Alzheimer's patients are found to have high mercury, copper and aluminium concentrations in their brains; moreover, these metals are known to be able to generate free radicals that interact with nerve cells leading to death. Hemolysis percentage is determined in a control groups of healthy subjects and Alzheimer's patients having treated their red blood cells "in vitro" with copper, mercury and aluminium. In a paralleled way inhibitory effect of some aminoacides such as cysteine, thourine and albumin is studied. Mercury, copper and aluminium are shown to be able to induce hemolysis because of generating free radicals which lead lipids peroxidation destroying plasmatic membrane. Aluminium needs a relatively high concentration to reach 100% hemolysis at the end of the period. Mercury, on the other hand, is the strongest hemolyzant metal, since small concentrations (0.017 mM) lead to 100% hemolysis in a short period of time. When donors′ red blood cells were incubated in buffer barbital and mercury (0.05 mM) differences between donors′ cells and those Alzheimer patients performance were more significant. It doesn't happen the same when red blood cells are incubated with aluminium. Concentration development is also studied for oxihemoglobin, desoxihemoglobin and metahemoglobin along the time. It is shown, for all hemolyzant metals, that oxihemoglobin concentration decreases while metahemoglobin concentration increases during hemolysis process.

Introduction

In 1973 it was suggested that aluminium could be a neurotoxic agent in Alzheimer's disease as a result of having noticed aluminium high levels in those patients' brains[1]. Nowadays this metal is supposed to alter the hematoencephalic wall. Mercury at low blood concentrations is toxic besides to inhibit a great amount of enzymes of the hexose monophosphate shunt and to produce oxygenated free radicals[2], it was found to induce hemolysis in red cells since it reacts very quickly with sulfhydryl groups of their membranes. Copper hemolyzant effect occurs in two phases[3]: a prelytic induction phase in which a minimal amount of hemolysis occurs, followed by a lytic, rapid hemolysis phase, to account for the prelytic period, the normal cell protective mechanisms are initially assumed operable, but gradually fail over the prelytic period. This lead to a rapid hemolysis phase. Our organism possesses molecules which let it protect from damages coming from free radicals generated by those metals and in this way cysteine acts inhibiting hemolysis produced by mercury and copper. Albumin is aluminium specific inhibitor.

Materials and methods

A group of 15 patients with early Alzheimer disease was studied, togheter with a control group of 18 donors blood.

Blood samples were treated with equal volumes of citrate buffer (40 mM), sodium chloride (155 mM) and sodium phosphate (20 mM). The samples were centrifuged to separate the RBC and then were washed with barbital buffer pH 7.4 . The erythrocyte solution of final volume 6 ml was adjusted to a 1.5 % haematocrit and was incubated for 6 hr at 37°C in the presence of each hemolyzant metals and the inhibitors.

Percentage hemolysis was determined from spectrophotometric readings at 410 nm.

Red blood cells mixture is washed with fresh buffer and in the same way percentages of Oxy, desoxy and metaheglobin are calculated with the lecture at 560, 576 and 630 nm[4].

Results

Cooper hemolyzant effects are shown in fig. 1. Those that Aluminium in fig. 2. And Mercury results in fig.3.

In these charts we can observe these metals effect in donors and patients´blood. Likewise enhibitor effect is described.

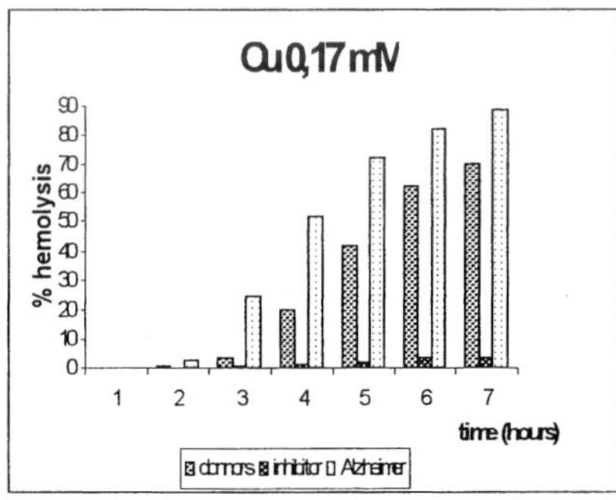

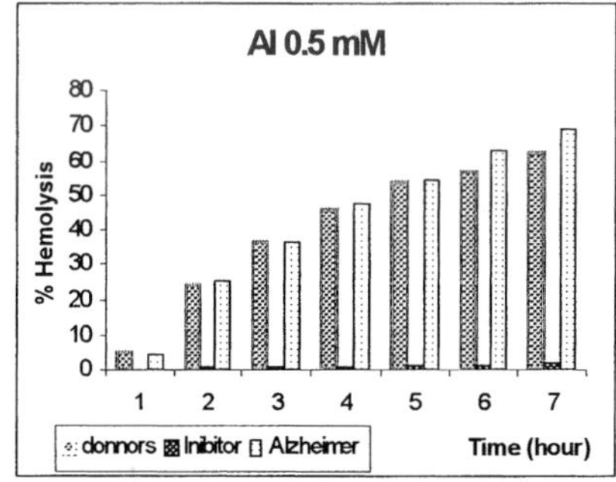

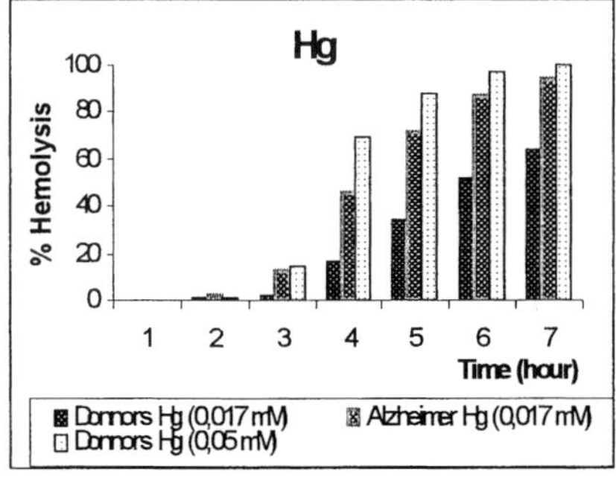

Fig. 1 Hemolysis induced by Cu 0.017 mM in barbital buffer. (Donnors, Inibitor aminoacid and Alzheimer).

Fig. 2 Hemolysis induced by Al 0.5 mM in barbital buffer.

Fig. 3 Hemolysis induced by Hg in donors and patients´ bloood.

Discussion

Hemolysis induced by Cu (0.017 mM) in buffer barbital reaches 70.2% after 6 hours incubation. We could observed this metal acted such as it was expected (prelytic period and lytic period).

Cisteine inhibitor effect is shown in 0.33 mM concentration where hemolysis hardly ever reaches 4% after six hours. In Alzheimer's patients hemolysis is higher than in donors with the same metal concentration (88.43%).

For aluminium is needed 0.5 mM concentration to have got 62.1% hemolysis after six hours incubation in buffer barbital. Albumin acts as this metal hemolysis inhibitor at 1.33 mM concentration; in this case hemolysis just reaches 1.8%. Differences are hardly observed in hemolysis produced by this metal in patients and donors.

Mercury is the most hemolizant metal since with 0.05 mM concentration it can be able to produce 100% hemolysis after six hours, cisteine is still able to inhibe hemolysis at 0.33 mM concentration. Thourine also acts as mercury hemolysis inhibitor but less effective. It is necessary to have 3.33 mM concentration to inhibe hemolysis, reaching 22.1% when a low mercury concentration is used (0.017 mM). Important differences in hemolysis are observed between patients (93.3%) and donors (63.7%). These differences are hardly unobserved at higher concentrations.

References

[1]Gisbert Calabuig, J.A. (1998) Medicina Legal y Toxicología. 5° Edición. Ed. Masson, S.A.

[2]Barnes G., Frieden E., (1973): Trace Metal Ion Induced Hemolysis. Biochem. Biophiys. Acta.;302:457-458

[3]Caffrey J.M., Asok Dasmahapatra JR. Smit H.A., Hede K. Frieden E. (1986) The effect of Copper Ion on Glutation and Hemolisys in Rabbit Erythrocytes. Biological Trace Elements Research, vol. 11: 19-27

[4]Benesch RF., Benesch R., Yung S., (1973): Equations for the Spectrophotometric Analysis of Haemoglobin Mixtures. Analytical Biochemistry 55: 245-248

Metal Ions in Biology and Medicine; vol 6. Eds. J.A. Centeno, Ph. Collery, G. Vernet, R.B. Finkelman, H. Gibb, J.C. Etienne. John Libbey Eurotext, Paris © 2000, pp. 487-489.

Membrane oxidative damage induced by Fe^{2+} and Fe^{2+}/Al^{3+} is more pronounced in Alzheimer's than in age-matched controls

R.P. Pedrosa[1], M.A.S. Fernandes[2], M.C. Alpoim[1], M.T.C.F. Brito[1], I. Santana[3] and C.R. Oliveira[4]

[1] *Departamento de Bioquímica,* [2] *Departamento de Zoologia,* [3] *Serviço de Neurologia H.U.C.,* [4] *Serviço de Bioquímica, Universidade de Coimbra, Coimbra, Portugal*

Abstract: In this study we evaluate the effects of Fe^{2+} and Fe^{2+}/Al^{3+} on the susceptibility of human platelets of Alzheimer's disease (AD) and age-matched controls to lipid peroxidation, reactive oxygen species generation and membrane fluidity. Our studies demonstrate that Fe^{2+}-induced membrane oxidative damage, is more pronounced in AD than in age-matched controls. Al^{3+} stimulated membrane oxidative degradation induced by Fe^{2+} is also, substantially greater in AD than in age-matched controls. In contrast, the reactive oxygen species generation induced by Fe^{2+} and Fe^{2+}/Al^{3+}, is similar in AD and age-matched controls.

Introduction

Alzheimer's disease (AD), a progressive neurodegenerative disorder is the fourth leading cause of death in the western countries. Although the ethiology and pathogenesis of AD are not known, the oxidative stress hypothesis has gained considerable momentum [1,2]. The abnormal release of metals ions, namely Fe^{2+}, Al^{3+}, Zn^{2+} and Cu^{2+} in certain AD brain areas enhance the oxidative stress hypothesis in AD pathogenesis [3,4]. It is known that Fe^{2+} plays an important role as a catalyst for reactive oxygen species (ROS) generation, via Fenton-reaction and/or the Haber-Weiss cycle [5,6], and Al^{3+} stimulates lipid peroxidation, induced by Fe^{2+}[7].

In order to elucidate the role of metal ions in neurodegeneration, we evaluate the implications of Al^{3+} and Fe^{2+} on the cellular oxidative status, using as neuronal model human platelets from AD and age-matched controls. For such propose we studied the effects of Fe^{2+}, Al^{3+} and Fe^{2+}/Al^{3+} on the susceptibility of human platelets of AD and age-matched controls to lipid peroxidation, ROS generation and membrane fluidity.

Experimental Procedures

Platelets isolation - Platelets were isolated as previously described [8]. Phospholipids were extracted following Bligh's procedure [9] and the phospholipid contents was evaluated according to Fiske and Subarrow as modified by Bartlett [10].

Lipid peroxidation - The probe cis-parinaric acid (PnA) was used to measure the membrane oxidative damage [11]. The time dependence loss of PnA fluorescence was monitored in a Perkin-Elmer LS 50 B spectrophotometer, with excitation wavelength 323 nm (slit=5) and emission wavelength 413 nm (slit=10). The rate of PnA (0.5μM) was measured before and after the addition of metal ions.

ROS generation - The probe 2', 7'-dichlorofluorescin diacetate (DCFH) was used to measure the cytoplasmatic ROS generation [12]. The cells suspension ($6x10^6$/ml) was incubate with 5μM DCFH-

DA at 37ºC for 20 min. After loading the cells suspension was centrifuged at 14000 rpm for 10 s, and the pellet was ressuspended in 2 ml of Hepes buffer. The fluorescence was monitored on a Spex, 1681, fluorometer, with excitation wavelength at 502 nm (slit=1.5), and emission wavelength 550 nm (slit=6). The solution of the different metal ions was added 80 s after beginning to monitor the fluorescence.

Membrane fluidity - The membrane order of platelets was evaluated by fluorescence using the probe TMA-DPH, in a Perkin-Elmer LS 50B spectrophotometer, as described [13].

Results

Lipid peroxidation

The incubation of human platelets from AD and age-matched controls with different Fe^{2+} concentrations leads to a Fe^{2+} concentration dependent membrane oxidative degradation, as evaluated by the Fe^{2+} concentration dependent increase in the fluorescence decay rate of PnA. However,. this effect is substantially greater in AD than in age-matched controls (Fig.1). Al^{3+} alone had no effect on PnA decay rate but, Al^{3+} pretreatment of human platelets substantially stimulates Fe^{2+}-induced membrane oxidative damage. However this effect is substantially greater in AD than in age-matched controls (data not shown).

ROS generation

The incubation of human platelets from AD and age-matched controls with Fe^{2+} show a Fe^{2+} concentration dependent increase in ROS generation, as evaluated by the increase in the rate of DCFH oxidation. However, this effect was similar in AD and age-matched controls (Fig.2). Al^{3+} alone had no effect on ROS generation both in AD and age-matched controls platelets, but Al^{3+} pretreatment of human platelets potentiates Fe^{2+}-induced ROS generation both in AD and age-matched controls. However, the levels of Fe^{2+}-induced ROS generation, on Al^{3+} pretreated platelets were similar in AD and age-matched controls (data not shown).

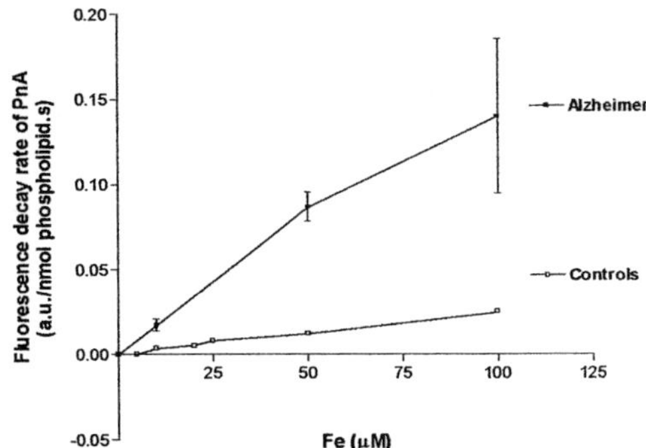

Fig. 1. The effect of different Fe^{2+} concentrations on the fluorescence decay rate of PnA. Experiments were carried out by addition of different concentrations of Fe^{2+} to platelet suspensions (100 μl of a 2 O.D. suspension) from AD patients and age-matched controls, in Hepes buffer pH 7.4 (10 mM hepes, 144 mM NaCl, 5 mM KCl and 4.6 mM glucose), at 37° C in a termostated cuvette under stirring. PnA concentration was 0.5 μM. The results correspond to the mean +/- SD of at least three experiments carried out in triplicate.

Membrane fluidity

Incubation of human platelets with either Al^{3+} or Fe^{2+} has no effect on membrane fluidity, as evaluated by the probe TMA-DPH. Also, Fe^{2+} addition to Al^{3+}-pretreated human platelets has no effect on membrane fluidity.

Discussion

The dependence of membrane oxidative degradation with Fe^{2+} concentration finds its support on the increase generation of ROS with increasing Fe^{2+}concentrations. However, in spite of the effect of Fe^{2+}-induced membrane oxidative degradation being substantially greater in AD than in control platelets, the Fe^{2+}-induced ROS generation, was similar in AD and age-matched controls. Therefore, the greater effect of Fe^{2+}-induced membrane oxidative degradation in AD than in controls will be probably related with differences in membrane composition of AD platelets and controls, in spite of no differences in membrane fluidity were observed between AD and controls, using the core probe TMA-DPH.

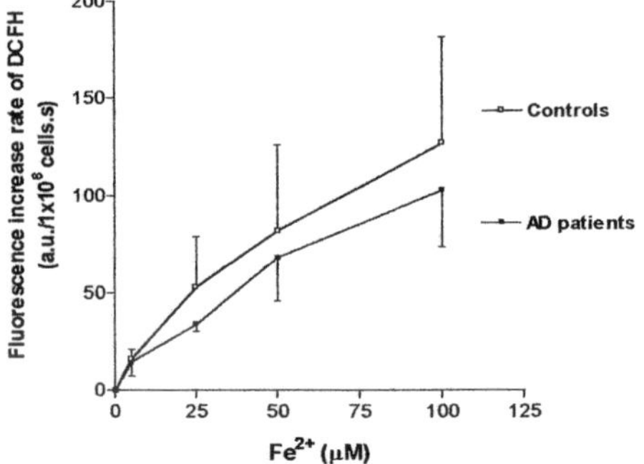

Fig. 2. The effect of different Fe^{2+} concentrations on ROS generation on the cytoplasm of platelets from AD patients and age-matched controls. Experiments were carried out using a platelet suspension ($6x10^6$ cells/ml) in Hepes buffer pH 7.4 (10 mM hepes, 144 mM NaCl, 5 mM KCl and 4.6 mM glucose). DCFH-DA concentration was 5 μM. The results correspond to the mean +/- SD of at least three experiments carried out in triplicate.

Al^{3+} potentiates Fe^{2+}-induced human platelets membrane oxidative degradation and ROS generation both in AD patients and in age-matched controls. This findings found support in literature since Al^{3+} is know to stimulate Fe^{2+}-induced lipid peroxidation. This effect is usually related with the capacity of Al^{3+} to increase membrane lipid packing enhancing the propagation of lipid peroxidation chain reactions [14]. The effect of Al^{3+} on Fe^{2+}-induced membrane degradation is more pronounced in AD than in control platelets, but there are no statistically difference in the ROS levels induced by Fe^{2+} in Al^{3+} pretreated platelets from AD and controls. This results also indicate that the difference between AD and controls in membrane susceptibility to oxidative degradation is probably related with differences in membrane composition, in spite of the fact that no differences in membrane fluidity were observed. Given that, further studies will be necessary to elucidate the differences between AD and controls in membrane susceptibility to Fe^{2+}-induced oxidative degradation.

References

1- Beni G, and Moretti A. *Neurobiol. Ageing* 1995; 16: 661-674.

2-Schapira AHV. *Neuropathol. Appl. Neurobiol.*1995; 21: 3-9.

3-Andras E, Farkas É, Scheiber H, Réffy A, and Bezúr L. *Arch. of Gerontol. and Geriatrics* 1995; 21: 89-97.

4-Crapper DR, Krishnan SS, and Dalton AJ. *Science*1973; 180: 511-513.

5-Gerlach M, Ben-Shachar D, Riederer P, and Youdin MBH. *J. Neurochem.* 1994; 63: 793-807.

6-Halliwell B. *J. Neurochem.* 1992; 59: 1609-1623.

7-Bondy SC, and Kirsteen S. *Mol. Chem. Neuropathol.* 1996; 27: 185-194.

8-Marinho C, Januário C, Matias F, Cunha L, and Oliveira CR. *Med. Sci. Res.* 1990; 18: 567-568.

9-Bligh EG, and Dyer WJ. *Can J. Biochem.Physiol.* 1959; 37: 911-917.

10-Bartlett G R. *J. Biol. Chem.* 1959; 234: 466-468.

11-Fernandes R, Pereira P, Ramalho JS, Mota MC, and Oliveira CR. *Current Eye Research* 1995; 395-402.

12-Royall JA, and Ischiropoulos H. *Arch. Biochem. Byophys.*1993; 302: 348-355.

13-Rego AC, and Oliveira C R. *Arch. Biochem. Byophys.* 1995; 321: 127-136.

14- Oteiza PI. *Arch. Biochem. Biophys* 1994; 308: 374-379.

Metal Ions in Biology and Medicine; vol 6. Eds. J.A. Centeno, Ph. Collery, G. Vernet, R.B. Finkelman, H. Gibb, J.C. Etienne. John Libbey Eurotext, Paris © 2000, pp. 490-494.

Fe^{2+} induced hydroxil radicals effects on the plasma membrane of *Escherichia coli* K-12 cells

A. Yu. Ivanov[1, 5], A.V. Gavrjushkin[2], L.A. Khassanova[3, 5], Ph. Collery[5], C. Choisy[5], J.C. Etienne[5], Z.M. Khassanova[4, 5]

[1] *Institute of Cell Biophysics, Russian Academy of Sciences, 142292 Pushchino, Russia;* [2] *State Research Institute of Applied Microbiology, 142279 Obolensk, Russia;* [3] *Department of Environmental Protection of Bashkir State University, 32, Frunze Street, 450072 Ufa, Russia;* [4] *Department of Botany of Bashkir State Pedagogical University, 3a, October Revolution Street, 450025 Ufa, Russia;* [5] *Institut International de Recherche sur les Ions Métalliques, 45, rue Cognacq Jay, Centre Hospitalier Régional Universitaire, 51092 Reims cedex, France*

ABSTRACT

A method of electro-orientational spectroscopy (EO) was used to study the toxic effect of hydroxyl radicals ($OH^\cdot$), generated by decomposition of H_2O_2 by Fe^{2+} ions (Fenton's reaction) on the barrier properties of the plasma membrane (PM) of *Escherichia coli* K-12 cells. The data of EO spectroscopy suggest that only in the case of cells pre-incubation with Fe^{2+} ions in constant concentration maintained in the system by ascorbate (ASC) or dithiothreitol (DTT) the addition of H_2O_2 led to the changes of barrier properties and damages of cell PM. PM damages by $OH^\cdot$ radicals depend on the concentration of Fe^{2+} and H_2O_2, incubation temperature and the substance used to restore Fe^{2+}. Considerable decrease of $OH^\cdot$ radicals toxic effect on the cell PM in thiolic restorer (DTT) presence suggests that the primary target of hydroxyl radicals is SH-groups of membrane proteins.

INTRODUCTION

Free radicals such as super oxide and hydroxyl are well known toxic agents. Their effects lead to protein modification (Van der Zee et al., 1985; Richards et al., 1988), peroxide oxidation of lipids (Vladimirov et al., 1972; Van der Zee et al., 1985), derangement of ionic homeostasis, membrane depolarization and reduction of cell membrane potential (Deuticke et al., 1987; Richards et al., 1988). However the role of divalent metal ions as Fe^{2+}, Cu^{2+}, Co^{2+} in the $OH^\cdot$ radicals toxicity for barrier properties of PM is not completely clear. The aim of our investigation was to study the PM barrier properties of *E. coli* K-12 cells under the influence of $OH^\cdot$ radicals generated by decomposition of H_2O_2 by Fe^{2+} ions (Fenton's reaction).

MATERIALS AND METHODS

Escherichia coli K-12 cells were grown in shaken flasks (150 rpm) at 37^0C in M9 medium with 0.1% yeast extract for 5 h, which corresponded to the exponential growth phase. Cells were twice washed with distilled water, recovered by low speed centrifugation and kept at 4^0C during the experimental period (2-4 h) at the concentration of 10^{10} cells/ml. Cell suspension in distilled water (electric conductivity not more than 0.00013 Sm/m and pH 6.0-6.2) at concentration $5 \cdot 10^7$ cells/ml was prepared. Fe^{2+} required concentration was added to the suspension and *E. coli* K 12 cells were pre-incubated at room temperature for 15 min. Then ascorbate (ASC) or dithiothreitol (DTT), hydrogen peroxide (H_2O_2) were added successively to the cell suspension for 60 min at 37°C or 20° C. Freshly prepared basic 0.01 M solution of bivalent iron sulfate, 0.1 M solution of ascorbic acid with KOH (pH 7.5), 0.1 M solution of

DTT and 3% H_2O_2 were used. All measurements were taken at pH 5.0 and specific electric conductivity 0.0022 Sm/m. The required pH were prepared by adding 0.01 N HCl and electric conductivity was standardized by adding 0.01 M NaCl. The pH of the medium was monitored continuously using with an ionometer «pH-340» (Russia), electric conductivity was measured with a conductometer «OK-102/1» («Radelkis», Hungary). Cell electro-orientational (EO) spectra were registered by determining the relative changes of the cell suspension optical density in a uniform field of alternating electrical current with an intensity of 80 V/cm and a fixed frequency ranging from 0.5 MHz to 10 MHz (Miroshnikov et al., 1986). Cell PM damages were judged by the EO spectra shifts from the high frequency area to the low frequency area, calculated as the cell EO-effect value: $\Delta\beta/\beta o = (\beta c-\beta o)/\beta o$ (Ivanov et al., 1997; Khassanova et al., 1998). All the measurements were taken at room temperature.

RESULTS AND DISCUSSION

EO spectra of *E. coli* K-12 cells, both intact and pre-incubated with various Fe^{2+} concentrations, and then treated with 150 μM H_2O_2 in 150 μM ASC presence are presented on the figure 1. EO spectra of H_2O_2 treated cells show decreases in absolute EO values at the increase of Fe^{2+} concentration. Cell pre-incubation with Fe^{2+} and H_2O_2 treatment in ASC presence testified PM damages.

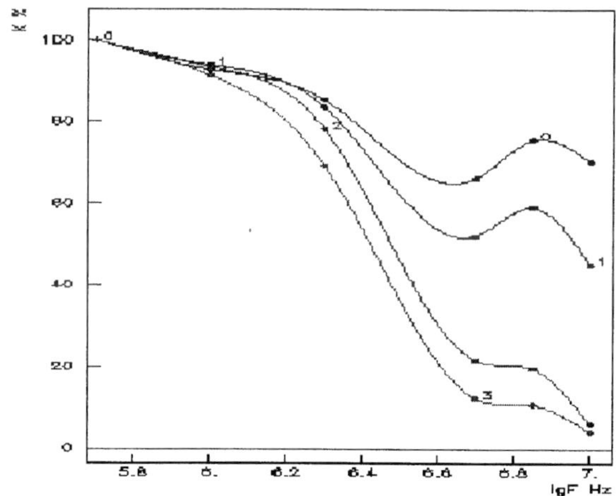

Fig.1. EO spectra of *E. coli* K-12 cells intact (0) and pre-incubated (1-3) with various Fe^{2+} concentrations (2.5, 5 and 10 μM) and then treated with 150 μM H_2O_2 in 150 μM ASC presence. $K = (\Delta D_i / \Delta D_o) \times 100\%$, where ΔD_i is the change in the optical density of the suspension upon the application of an electric field; ΔD_o is the same for the cell suspension incubated in standard measuring medium at a frequency of 0.5 MHz.

It should be noted that the *E. coli* K-12 treatment with 150 μM H_2O_2 does not influence on the character of intact cell EO spectra, either in the presence of ASC or without it. Simultaneous cell incubation with Fe^{2+}, ASC and H_2O_2 does not change the character of EO spectra. The data of EO spectroscopy suggest that only in the case of cells pre-incubation with

Fe^{2+} ions in constant concentration maintained by ASC or DTT (150-500 μM) the addition of H_2O_2 leads to the changes of barrier properties and damages of cell PM.

Concentration dependencies of *E. coli* K-12 PM damages (parameter $\Delta\beta/\beta_o$) are shown on the figures 2 and 3. Only low Fe^{2+} concentrations (10 μM of Fe^{2+} is maximal) augment $\Delta\beta/\beta_o$ values. The further increase of Fe^{2+} concentration up to 25-50 μM does not intensify the toxic effect of H_2O_2. In contrast, the increase of H_2O_2 concentration leads to the rise of $\Delta\beta/\beta_o$ values characteristic for *E. coli* K-12 cells with fully damaged PM (70°C, 15 min). The degree of cell PM damages linearly depends on H_2O_2 concentration.

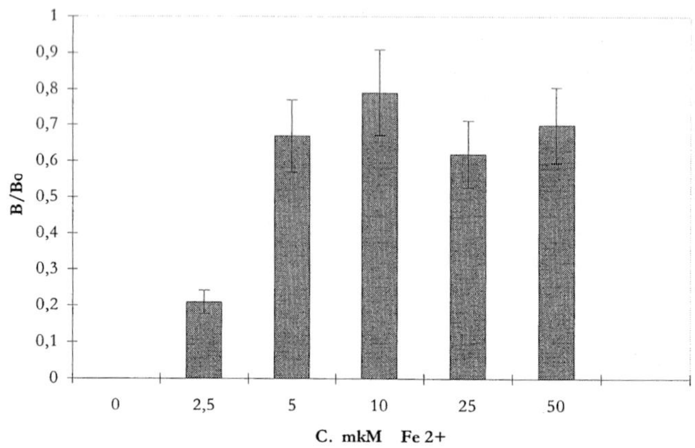

Fig.2. $\Delta\beta/\beta_o$ values of *E. coli* K-12 cells pre-incubated with various Fe^{2+} concentrations (2.5, 5, 10, 25 and 50 μM) and treated with 150 μM H_2O_2 in 150 μM ASC presence.

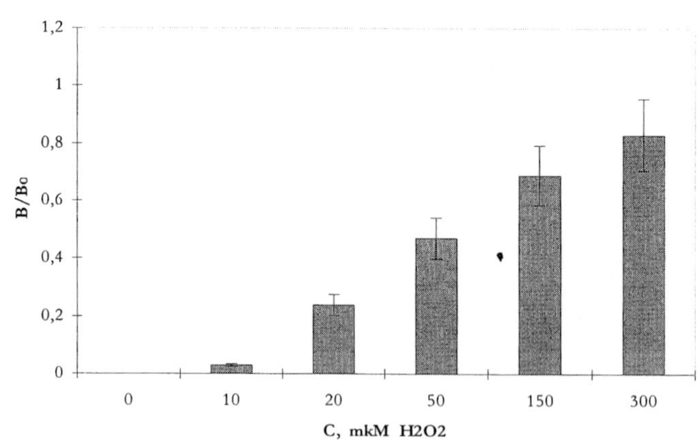

Fig.3. $\Delta\beta/\beta_o$ values of *E. coli* K-12 cells pre-incubated with 5 μM Fe^{2+} and treated with various H_2O_2 concentrations (10, 20, 50, 150 and 300 μM) in 150 μM ASC presence.

Thus, the PM damages by H_2O_2 depend on Fe^{2+} and H_2O_2 concentration. Earlier it was shown that there is a critical concentration of Fe^{2+} ions at which cell damages are maximal. Fe^{2+} ions can serve as pro-oxidants only at low concentrations (Vladimirov et al., 1972).

Also cell PM damages are dependent on the temperature of incubation media and the substance used to restore Fe^{2+} ions. The influence of incubation temperature on $\Delta\beta/\beta_o$ values of *E. coli* K-12 cells pre-incubated with Fe^{2+} and treated with various H_2O_2 concentrations in ASC presence as a restorer is shown on the figure 4.

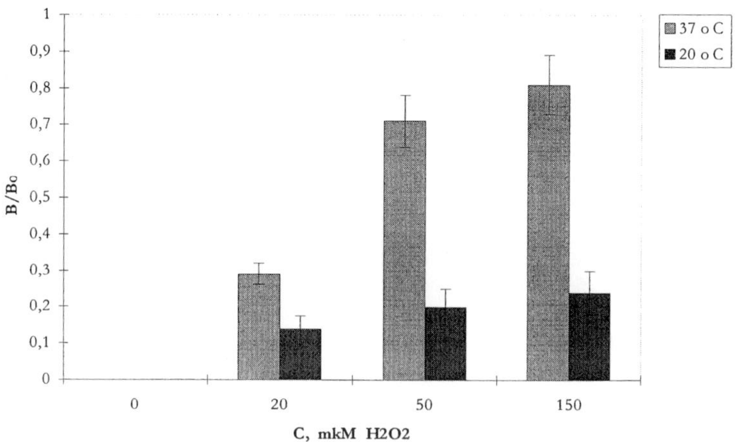

Fig.4. $\Delta\beta/\beta_o$ values of *E. coli* K-12 cells pre-incubated with 5 μM Fe^{2+} ions and treated with various H_2O_2 concentrations (20, 50, 150 μM) in 150 μM ASC presence at 37°C and 20°C.

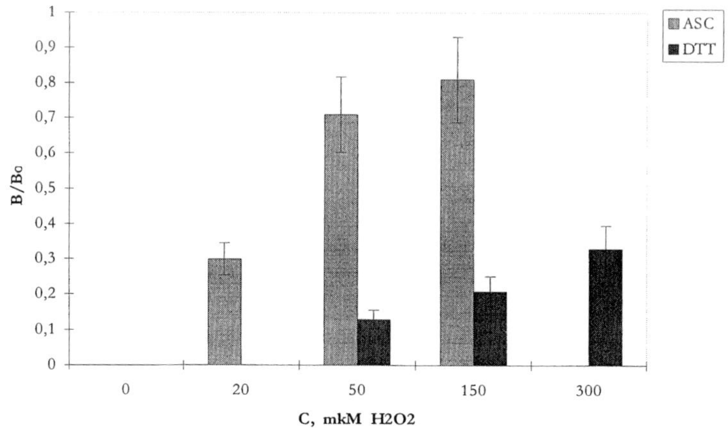

Fig.5. $\Delta\beta/\beta_o$ values of *E. coli* K-12 cells pre-incubated with 5 μM Fe^{2+} ions and treated with various H_2O_2 concentrations (20, 50, 150 μM) in 150 μM ASC presence, and with various H_2O_2 concentrations (50, 150, 300 μM) in 150 μM DTT presence.

Exposure of *E. coli* K-12 cells at 20°C instead of 37°C significantly decreases the toxic effect of OH˙ radicals on the cell PM. The temperature rise intensified OH˙radicals toxic effect and activated their interaction with biomolecules at 37° C (Prior, 1979). Comparative study of OH˙ radicals damaged effect on *E. coli* K-12 PM in the presence of thiolic (DTT) and nonthiolic (ASC) donors of electrons (figure 5) shows that the DTT utilization substantially decreased the toxic effect of OH˙ radicals on the barrier properties of *E. coli* K-12 PM. This fact suggests that the primary target of OH˙radical attack is SH-groups of membrane proteins.

REFERENCES

FOMCHENKOV V.M. et al. Electric characteristics of bacterial cells measured when the barrier function of cytoplasmic membrane is disordered. *Microbiologiya* (Moscow). 1986, 55: 754-759.

IVANOV A.Yu., FOMCHENKOV V.M. The damaging effect of surfactants on *Escherichia coli* cells as a function of the culture growth phase. *Microbiologiya* (Moscow). 1989, 58: 969-975.

IVANOV A.Yu. et al. Toxic effect of hydroxylated heavy metal ions on the plasma membrane of bacterial cells. *Microbiologiya* (Moscow). 1997, 66:588-594.

MIROSHNIKOV A.I., FOMCHENKOV V.M., IVANOV A.Yu. Electrophysical analysis and cell separation. Nauka (Moscow). 1986, 198 p.

PRIOR W.A. Free radicals in biology. Academic Press (New York, San Francisco, London). 1976, 1:17-19.

VLADIMIROV Yu. A., ARCHAKOV A.I. Peroxide oxidation of lipids in biological membranes. Nauka (Moscow). 1972, 252 p.

RICHARDS D.M.C., DEAN R.T., JESSUP W. Membrane proteins are critical targets in free radical mediated cytolysis. *Biochem. Biophys. Acta.* 1988, 946: 281-288.

DEUTICKE B., HELLER K.B., HAEST W.M. Progressive oxidative membrane damage in erythrocytes after pulse treatment with t-butylhydroperoxide. *Biochem. Biophys. Acta.* 1987, 899: 113-124.

VAN DER ZEE J., DUBBELMAN T.M.A.R., VAN STEVENINCK J. Peroxide-induced membrane damage in human erythrocytes. *Biochem. Biophys. Acta.* 1985, 818: 38-44.

Metal Ions in Biology and Medicine; vol 6. Eds. J.A. Centeno, Ph. Collery, G. Vernet, R.B. Finkelman, H. Gibb, J.C. Etienne. John Libbey Eurotext, Paris © 2000, pp. 495-497.

Mechanisms of action and cytotoxicity of a new vanadyl(IV)/aspirin complex in osteoblast-like cells

Susana B. Etcheverry[1, 2], Daniel A. Barrio[1], María S. Molinuevo[1], Ana M. Cortizo[1]

[1] Cátedra de Bioquímica Patológica, [2] CEQUINOR, Facultad de Ciencias Exactas, Universidad Nacional de La Plata, 47 y 115 (1900) La Plata, Argentina, Fax: +54 +221 453 0189, e-mail: etchever@nahuel.biol.unlp.edu.ar

Abstract

The effects of a new vanadyl(IV) complex with aspirin (VO/Aspirin) on osteoblast-like cells in culture were analyzed in this study. The vanadium compound exerted a biphasic effect on cell proliferation being toxic at high concentrations. VO/Aspirin as well as vanadyl(IV) cation elicited lipid peroxidation in the cells. The observed biological effects may be partially mediated through the inhibition of different cellular phosphatases.

Introduction

Our interest in the coordination chemistry of vanadium is based on its potential therapeutical applications. Vanadium regulates different metabolic processes such as glucose uptake and oxidation, lipid metabolism, and proliferative events [1]. Increasing evidence also suggests that vanadium causes toxic effects in living organisms [2].

Vanadium compounds inhibit the activity of protein tyrosine phosphatases , increasing the level of phosphorylated tyrosine residues in the cells [3,4]. In addition, a role for an oxidative stress has been suggested in the action of vanadium [5].

As part of a project devoted to the synthesis, characterization and bioactivity of vanadium derivatives, we have analysed the mechanism of action and cytotoxicity of a new vanadyl(IV)/Aspirin complex in osteoblast-like cells in culture .

Materials and methods

The complex $[VO(aspirin)ClH_2O]_2$ was prepared mixing aspirin and $VOCl_2$ in a 2/1 molar ratio in ethanol with constant stirring under nitrogen atmosphere (pH 3.5, 0°C) [6].

UMR106 osteosarcoma and MC3T3E1 non-transformed osteoblast-like cells were incubated with different doses of VO/Aspirin and VO at 37°C.

The effects of vanadium compounds on proliferation were assayed by the crystal violet technique [7] and their action on lipid peroxidation through the thiobarbituric reactive substances (TBARS) determination [8].

We have also studied the effects on neutral and alkaline phosphatase activities in the cytosolic and microsomal fractions of the osteoblast-like cells.

Results and discussion

In the cytosolic fraction both vanadium compounds inhibited the alkaline and neutral phosphatases with equal potency, in the range of 10 - 100 μM (Table I). In the microsomal fraction, the alkaline phosphatase activity was inhibited in a dose-response manner (10 - 100 μM), with a stronger effect of vanadyl cation than the complex. The neutral phosphatase activity was also inhibited in a dose response-manner but the VO/Aspirin complex showed a greater effect. For instance, 80% of inhbition was observed after incubation with 22 μM VO/aspirin or with 75 μM VO.

Table I. Effect of vanadium compounds in the inhibition constant Ki [μM] of phosphatase activity.

	Neutral Phosphatase		Alkaline Phosphatase	
	Cytosolic	Microsamal	Cytosolic	Microsomal
VO	> 100	> 100	80	45
VO/aspirin	> 100	> 100	80	75

Figure 1 shows the effect of vanadium derivatives on osteoblast proliferation. Both vanadium(IV) compounds exerted a biphasic effect on mitogenesis being toxic at high concentrations. In the tumorigenic UMR106 cells, VO/Aspirin was more potent in stimulating cell proliferation (5-10 μM) and more toxic than VO in the range of 50-100 μM). In the non-transformed MC3T3E1 cells, the complex was more potent than VO to inhibit cellular proliferation (25-100μM).

Figure 1.

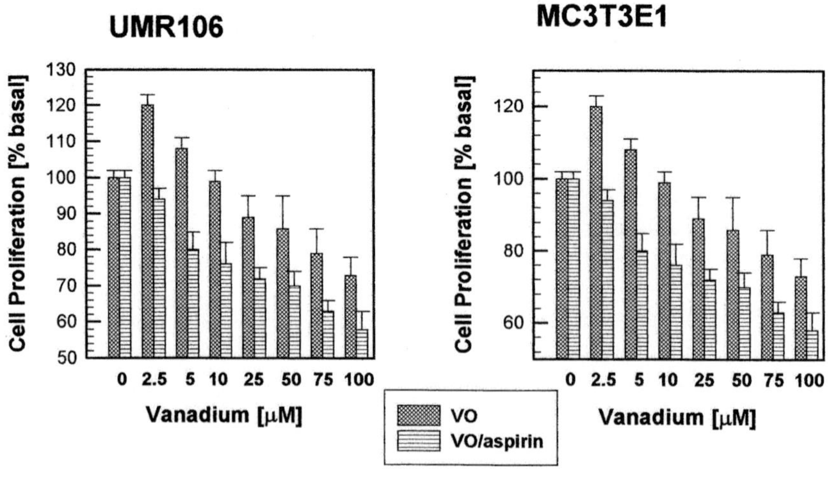

Evaluation of lipid peroxidation by TBARS showed that both vanadium(IV) derivatives produced lipid peroxidation in a dose-response manner.

In conclusion, the VO/aspirin complex was more potent than VO in stimulating cell growth at low doses but also showed more toxic effects at higher concentrations. These effects may be partially explained through the inhibition of neutral phosphatase in the particulate fraction and the induction of higher levels of lipid peroxidation.

Acknowledgements

This study was supported by grants from Universidad Nacional de La Plata, CICPBA, CONICET (PIP 1044/98) and Agencia Nacional de Promocion Cientifica (PICT 00375).
SBE is member of the Carrera del Investigador, CONICET, Argentina, and AMC is member of Carrera del Investigador, CICPBA, Argentina.

References

1. Etcheverry SB, Cortizo AM. Bioactivity of vanadium compounds on cells in culture. In: Nriagu J.O,ed. *Vanadium in the Environment.* New York::John Wiley & Sons, Inc. 1998: 359-394.

2. Domingo JL. Vanadium: A review of the reproductive and developmental toxicity. *Reprod Toxicol* 1996; 10: 175-182.

3. Gresser MJ, Tracey AS. Vanadate as phosphate analog in biochemistry. In: Chasteen ND, ed. *Vanadium in biological systems.* The Netherlands: Kluwer Academic Publishers, 1990: 63-69.

4. Sálice VC, Cortizo AM, Gómez Dumm CL, Etcheverry SB. Tyrosine phosphorylation and morphological transformation induced by four vanadium compounds on MC3T3E1 cells. *Mol Cel Biochem* 1999: 198: 119-128.

5. Krejsa CM, Schieven GL. Impact of oxidative stress on signal transduction control by phosphotyrosine phosphatases. *Environ Health Perspect* 1998: 106 Suppl.5: 1179-1184.

6. Etcheverry SB, Williams PAM, Barrio DA, Sálice VC, Ferrer EG, Cortizo AM. Synthesis, characterization and bioactivity of a new VO^{2+}/Aspirin Complex. *J Inorg Biochem (In press).*

7. Cortizo AM, Etcheverry SB. Vanadium derivatives act as growth factor mimetic compounds upon differentiation and proliferation of UMR 106 osteoblast-like cells. *Mol Cel Biochem* 1995:145: 97-102.

8. Ohkawa H, Ohishi N, Yagi K. Assay for lipid peroxides in animal tissues by thiobarbituric acid reaction. *Anal Biochem* 1979: 95: 351-358.

Metal Ions in Biology and Medicine; vol 6. Eds. J.A. Centeno, Ph. Collery, G. Vernet, R.B. Finkelman, H. Gibb, J.C. Etienne. John Libbey Eurotext, Paris © 2000, pp. 498-500.

Influence of antioxidants, metal-chelators, and thiol groups blocker on chromate-induced human erythrocytes injury

M.A.S. Fernandes[1], C.F.G.C. Geraldes[2], C.R. Oliveira[3], and M.C. Alpoim[2]

[1] Departamento de Zoologia, [2] Departamento de Bioquímica, [3] Serviço de Bioquímica da Faculdade de Medicina, Universidade de Coimbra, Coimbra, Portugal

The influence of vitamin E, vitamin C, salicylate, deferoxamine, and N-ethylmaleimide on Cr(VI)-induced human erythrocytes haemoglobin oxidation and peroxidation was investigated. Pretreatment of human erythrocytes with vitamin E, vitamin C, salicylate, and deferoxamine significantly increased Cr(VI)-induced human erythrocytes haemoglobin oxidation, while it was significantly decreased by pretreatment with N-ethylmaleimide. In contrast, pretreatment of human erythrocytes with deferoxamine immediately inhibited Cr(VI)-induced human erythrocytes peroxidation, while it was significantly increased by pretreatment with N-ethylmaleimide during the first 4 hours of cells exposition to Cr(VI). For time periods superior to 6 h pretreatment with N-ethylmaleimide significantly decreased Cr(VI)-induced human erythrocytes peroxidation. The results are discussed in terms of drug ability to interfer with the electron transfers between haemoglobin-Fe^{2+} and Cr(V) and consequently with reactive oxygen species generation.

Introduction

The toxic and carcinogenic effects of chromate (Cr(VI)) have been attributed to Cr(VI) compounds, which readily cross cell membranes and enter the cells being reduced, through reactive intermediates Cr(V), Cr(IV), to the more stable Cr(III) by intracellular reductants. This process generates reactive oxygen species (ROS) via Fenton or the Haber-Weiss type reactions. Because ROS can induce DNA damage and lipid peroxidation, the toxic and carcinogenic effects of Cr(VI) may be partially associated with the production ROS [1]. Previous studies showed that Cr(VI)-induced haemoglobin oxidation and membrane peroxidation in human erythrocytes [2,3], being suggested that Cr(VI) is cytotoxic to human erythrocytes. To attenuate or to prevent Cr(VI)-induced human erythrocytes injury, in the present study we tested the influence of antioxidants, namely vitamin E, vitamin C, and salicylate [4], as well as the influence of the metal-chelating agent deferoxamine [5], and that of the thiol groups blocker N-ethylmaleimide (NEM) [6,7] on Cr(VI)-induced human erythrocytes haemoglobin oxidation and peroxidation.

Materials and Methods

Human erythrocyte suspensions were prepared as previously described [3]. Human erythrocytes haemoglobin oxidation was measured according to the method of Martinek [8], in cells either untreated and pretreated, at 30°C for 2h, with α-tocopherol succinate (vitamine E, 20 μM), vitamin C

(1 mM), sodium salicylate (salicylate, 3 mM), deferoxamine (DFO, 4 mM) or NEM (1 mM) [9], after incubation with 4 mM dichromate along the time. The results were expressed as percentage (%) of haemoglobin oxidation. Human erythrocytes peroxidation was evaluated by measuring thiobarbituric acid-reactive substances (TBARS) [3], in cells either untreated or treated with DFO (4 mM) and NEM (1 mM) and incubated with 8 mM dichromate, and the results expressed as nmoles of malonaldehyde per million of cells (nmol MDA/10^6 cells). Statistical significance was set at $p < 0.05$.

Results

Pretreatment of human erythrocytes with vitamine E, vitamin C, salicylate, and DFO significantly increases (p=0.0001) dichromate-induced human eryhrocytes haemoglobin oxidation, while it was significantly decreased by pretreatment with NEM (p=0.0001) (Fig. 1 A). Pretreatment of human erythrocytes with DFO immediately inhibits Cr(VI)-induced human erythrocytes peroxidation (Fig.1 B). In contrast, pretreatment of human erythrocytes with NEM significantly increases (p=0.0001) Cr(VI)-induced human erythrocytes peroxidation during the first 4 h of erythrocytes exposition to Cr(VI), decreasing it significantly (p=0.0001) for exposition times above 6 h.

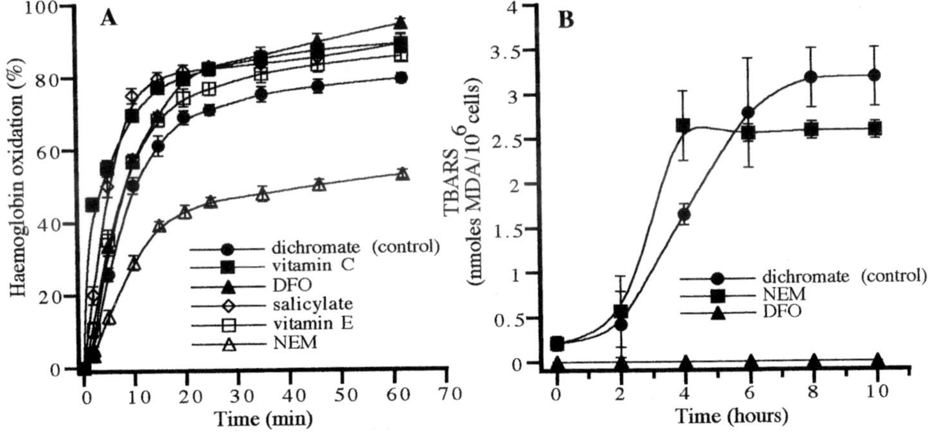

Fig. 1. Time dependent effects of vitamin E, vitamin C, salicylate, DFO and NEM on 4 mM dichromate-induced human erythrocytes haemoglobin oxidation (**A**), and time dependent effects of DFO and NEM on 8 mM dichromate-induced human erythrocytes peroxidation (**B**). Results correspond to means±SD of at least three samples carried out in duplicate.

Discussion and Conclusion

It was previously suggested that during the intracellular human erythrocytes Cr(VI) reduction to Cr(V) ROS are produced via the Haber-Weiss cycle or through a Fenton-like reaction and that Cr(VI)-induced human erythrocytes haemoglobin oxidation, due to the electron transfers between the haemoglobin-Fe^{2+} and Cr(V) intermediates, protects the cells against Cr(VI)-induced peroxidation [3].The finding showing that pretreament of human erythrocytes with vitamin E, vitamin C, salicylate and DFO potentiates Cr(VI)-induced haemoglobin oxidation, together with that showing that pretreatment of the cells with DFO prevents Cr(VI)-induced peroxidation, indicates that these drugs potentiate the electron transfers between the haemoglobin-Fe^{2+} and Cr(V), decreasing Cr(V)-mediated generation of ROS. The findings showing that pretreatment of human erythrocytes with NEM attenuates Cr(VI)-induced haemoglobin oxidation and potentiates Cr(VI)-induced peroxidation during the first 4 h of cells exposition to Cr(VI), indicates that NEM decreases the electron transfers between the haemoglobin-Fe^{2+} and Cr(V), thus increasing Cr(V) -mediated generation of ROS in cells exposed to Cr(VI) during this time period. However, in NEM pretreated cells exposed to Cr(VI) for time periods superior to 6 h Cr(VI)-induced peroxidation was attenuated. This may be achieved by decreasing the content of Cr(V) in human erythrocytes as a consequence of lowering Cr(VI)- reduction by intracellular thiol-reductants. In conclusion, vitamin E, vitamin C, salicylate, and DFO potentiates Cr(VI)-induced haemoglobin oxidation, while by contrast it is attenuated by NEM. However, Cr(VI)-induced peroxidation is prevented by pretreatment of human erythrocytes with DFO, while it is potentiated by NEM at least in the first 4 hours of exposition of human erythrocytes to Cr(VI).

References

1.Shi X, Chiu A, Chen C T, Halliwell B, Castranova V, Vallyathan V. Reduction of chromium (VI) and its relantionship to carcinogenesis. *J. Toxicol Environ.Health* Part B 1999; 2: 87-104.

2. Alpoim M C, Geraldes C F, Oliveira C R, Lima M C. Molecular mechanisms of chromium toxicity: oxidation of hemoglobin. *Biochem Soc Trans* 1995; 23: 241-242.

3. Fernandes M A S, Mota I M, Silva M T L, Oliveira C R, Geraldes C F G C, Alpoim M C. Human erythrocytes are protected against chromate induced peroxidation. *Ecotoxicol Environ Safety* 1999; 43: 38-46.

4. Gassen M, Youdim M B H.Free radical scavengers: chemical concepts and clinical relevance. *J Neural Transm Suppl* 1999; 56:193-210.

5. Romero R A, Salgado O, Elejalde L E, Rodriguez-Iturbe B, Tahán J. E. Changes of metal concentrations in blood and peritoneal dialysate during long-term desferrioxamine B therapy. *Transplan-Proc* 1996; 28: 3387-3389.

6. Snyder L M, Fortier N L, Leb L, McKenney J, Trainor J, Sheerin H, Mohands N.The role of membrane protein sulfhydryl groups in hydrogen peroxide-mediated membrane damage in human erythrocytes. *Biochem Biophys Acta* 1988; 937: 229-240.

7. Sullivan T G, Baysal E, Stern A. Inhibition of hemin-induced hemolysis by desferrioxamine: binding of hemin to red cell membranes and the effects of alteration of membrane sulfhydryl groups. *Biochem Biophys Acta* 1992; 1104: 38-44.

8. Martinek G. Spectrophotometric determination of abnormal hemoglobin pigments in blood. *Clin Chim Acta* 1965; 11: 146-158.

9. Ohyashiki T, Kumada Y,Hatanaka N, Matsui K. Oxygen radical-induced inhibition of alkaline phosphatase activity in reconstituted membranes. *Archives Biochemistry Biophysics* 1994; 313:310-317.

Metal Ions in Biology and Medicine; vol 6. Eds. J.A. Centeno, Ph. Collery, G. Vernet, R.B. Finkelman, H. Gibb, J.C. Etienne. John Libbey Eurotext, Paris © 2000, pp. 501-504.

Ionic magnesium and selenium in serum after a cycle-ergometric test in football-players

M. Guerra, A. Monje, R. Perez-Beriain[1], A. García de Jalón[1], J. Villanueva, A. Herrera and J.F. Escanero

[1] Biochemical Laboratory, Universitary Hospital "Miguel Servet", Department of Pharmacology and Physiology, Faculty of Medicine, University of Zaragoza, c/ Domingo Miral, s/n, 50009 Zaragoza, Spain

Introduction. Exercise causes an increase of free radicals in serum (1). Selenium (Se) is considered as an antioxidant metal and no variations of this element in serum have been reported after a cycle-ergometric test (2). By contrast, ionic magnesium (Mg^{++}) decreases after the test (3). On the other hand, magnesium (Mg) deficiency induces a vitamin E (another antioxidant agent) reduction in liver as well as oxidative stress (4). Status of Mg seems to affect indirectly the antioxidant capacity of serum, influencing the levels of the different modulatory factors (5). Taking into account these facts, this paper tries to analyze the possible variations in serum of total Mg (Mgt), Mg^{++} and Se, as a modulator of the oxidative stress, and their correlations after a cycle-ergometric test.

Material and Methods. *Subjects:* Fifteen male football-players with the following anthropometric characteristics were studied: age, 17.4 ± 0.3 years old; weight, 70.2 ± 5.23 Kg; height, 1.77 ± 0.50 m. The time spended training was 10 hours/week.

Cycle-ergometric test: It started with a warm-up of two minutes during which the athletes pedalled against a resistance of 25 W, at a rate of 50 pedal strokes/min and after the warm-up period the test began with a resistance of 50 W and the same rate pedalling, increasing the power every two minutes by 50 W until maximum power, considered as the point when the last stage was maintained for more than a minute, was reached. Throughout the test, the athletes were monitored to control heart rate and electrocardiographical pattern with an electròcardiograph monitor (Fukuda). The VO_{2max} was measured by a Jeager ergopneumo test. VO_{2max} ($ml.Kg^{-1}.min^{-1}$) values were 56.8 ± 3.68.

Sampling: Blood was taken at the beginning, at the end and 30 min after (recovery) the test and collected in heparine lithium tubes. Serum was separated and aliquots were frozen (-20º C) to Se determination.

Analytical procedures: Mgt was evaluated by atomic absorption spectrophotometry (Perkin-Elmer 4100 B). Mg^{++} was determined by selective electrode potentiometry (AVL 988-4 analyzer). Total serum Se was performed by Zeeman electrothermal atomic absorption spectrophotometry (Perkin-Elmer 4110 ZL). The following reagents were used: diluent solution, 0.2 % triton X-100 and nitric acid 0.2 % (v/v) in purified water by reverse osmosis; matrix modifier: a mixed solution of palladium nitrate 100 mg/L in diluent solution. Standards and samples (1/1) were treated with diluent solution. Se determination was made using peak area absorbances at 196.0 nm with a slit width of 2.0 nm and a reading time of 5 seconds. Biochemistry Laboratory is submitted to the External Quality Control of the French Society of Clinical Biology. Hematocrite was evaluated by centrifugation using a capillary micromethod. The variation values of basal hematocrite immediately after the exercise and 30 minutes after completion were used to calculate the percentage variation of plasma volume during the exercise, according to van Beaumont equation (6):

$$\% P= 100/100\text{-}Hcte_1 \times 100\ (Hcte_1\text{-}Hcte_2)/Hcte_2$$

Statistical treatment: Results were analyzed by means of Stat View programme, using a Macintosh computer.

Results. Serum values (mean ± standard deviation) of Mgt, Mg^{++} and Se, (before plasmatic volume correction) are presented throughout the periods of time analyzed in Table 1.

	Beginning	At the end	Recovery
Mgt (mmol/L)	0.750 ± 0.044	0.806 ± 0.086	0.736 ± 0.040[#]
Mg^{++} (mmol/L)	0.531 ± 0.034	0.512 ± 0.030	0.502 ± 0.028**
Se (µmol/L)	0.781 ± 0.089	0.781 ± 0.099	0.802 ± 0.054

**p<0.01, in relation to the beginning. #p<0.05, in relation to the end.

Total Mg and Mg^{++} in serum decreased significantly at the recovery of the exercise. Se had not significant variation neither at the end nor at the recovery in relation to the beginning.

The results (mean ± standard deviation) concerning to Mg^{++} and Se in serum (after correction) are presented for the different times analyzed in Table 2.

	Beginning	At the end	Recovery
Mg^{++} (mmol/L)	0.532 ± 0.034	0.452 ± 0.050**	0.503 ± 0.037** ##
Se (µmol/L)	0.781 ± 0.089	0.689 ± 0.072**	0.804 ± 0.073[##]

**p<0.01, in relation to the beginning. ##p<0.01, in relation to the end.

Ionic Mg after correction decreased significantly at the end of exercise and at the recovery. Serum Se decreased significantly only at the end of exercise.

Studies of correlation. The following correlations were found: a). Mg^{++} and Se levels in serum at the end of the exercise (-0.80) with a $r^2 = 0.64$ and a regression equation ($y = -1.81x + 1.61$); b). Mg^{++} at the beginning and Se after exercise (0.82), with a $r^2 = 0.67$ and a regression equation ($y = -2.24x + 1.97$), and c). Mg^{++} at the recovery and Se after exercise (0.87), with a $r^2 = 0.76$ and a regression equation ($y = -2.14x + 1.76$).

Discussion. Basal levels of Se found in this study for young sportsmen are lower than the average (0.952 ± 0.200 µmol/L) of a control group of 248 healthy men, with a wide range of ages (10-88 years old), from our Autonomic Community of Aragón (Spain).

The values of this control group are similar to another one from China with a proper ingestion of Se (7). Serum levels of Se of the young sportsmen tested in this study are also lower than the ones reported by other autors (8, 9, 10), including young people in good shape without competition training (1) and those from a German population (0.84 ± 0.20 µmol/L), where Se is considered to be low in soil an food (11).

The 46 % of young sportsmen of this study have the basal values of Se in serum under the limits (0.75 µmol/L) considered by Roussel et al (8) as a risk level to have a deficit. These decreases are in agreement with those reported by Fogelholm and Lahtinen (10) for sportsmen.

The results found after the cycle-ergometric test until exhaustion show a significant decrease of the serum Se after the plasma volumen correction. Laires et al (2) did not found these variations, probably due to the fact that they did not take into account the serum volumen correction in their results.

The decrease of serum Se, after a bout of exercise, could be explained by three hypothesis:

a). The increases of consumed O_2 volumen during the exercise arise the production of free radicals. Each 25 molecules of oxygen reduced by the citocrome oxidase produce one free radical (11).

b). The increases of the tumour necrosis factor (TNF) and others mediators produced during the exercise, probably due to priming effects, increase the generation of free radicals (12, 13).

c). The decreases of Mg increase the oxidative metabolism as well as the TNF-alpha and other citokines in serum (14). In exercise until exhaution an increase of Mg levels in serum have been reported (4).

All these effects can interact among them (prime effect) (15, 16). The study of the correlations shown in "Results" could confirm this interpretation.

In conclusion, after cycle-ergometric test, variations in the levels of serum Mg^{++} and Se are found. Decreased of Mg^{++} in serum have good correlation with the Se concentrations. These data may support that the Mg status variations have a relationship with Se status.

This paper has been supported by a grant PCM5094 of the Autonomous Government of Aragon (DGA)

References.

1. Tessier F, Hida H, Favier A, Marconnet P. Muscle GSH activity after prolonged exercise, training, and selenium supplementation. *Biol Trace Elements Res* 1995; 47: 279-85.

2. Monteiro CP, Varela A, Pinto M, Neves J, Felisberto GM, Vaz C, Bicho MP, Laires MJ. Effect of an aerobic training on magnesium, trace elements and antioxidant systems in a Down syndrome population. *Magnes Res* 1997; 10: 65-71.

3. Guerra M, Monje A, Vidal MD, Zapatero MD, Villanueva J, Aliaga C, Dominguez M, Herrera A, Escanero JF. In: Collery P, Corbella J, Domingo JL, Etiene JC, LLobet JM, eds. Total and ionic plasmatic magnesium assessment after a bicycle ergometric test *Metal Ions in Biology and Medicine*. Paris: John Libbey Eurotext, 1996; 4: 400-04.

4. Calviello G, Ricci P, Lauro L, Palozza P, Cittadini A. Mg deficiency induces mineral content changes and oxidative stress in rats. *Biochem Mol Biol Int* 1994; 32: 903-11.

5. Manuel B, Keenoy Y, Moorkens G, Meludu S, Vertommen J, Noë M, Leeuw I. In: Theophanides T, Anastassopoulou J, eds. Magnesium and oxidative stress status in patients with chronic fatigue. *Magnesium: Current Status and New Developments*. Dordrecht: Kluwer Academic Publishers, 1997: 99-104.
6. Van Beaumont W. Evaluation of hemoconcentration from haematocrit measurements. *J Appl Physiol* 1972; 32: 71-73.
7. Janghorbani M, Xia Y, Ha P, Whanger PD, Butler JA, Olesik JW, Daniels L. Metabolism of selenite in men with widely varying selenium status. *J Am Col Nutr* 1999; 18: 462-69.
8. Roussel AM, Arnaud J, Richard MJ, Faure H, Clauw F, Favier A. Antioxidant trace element status and related metalloenzymes in a French SU.VI.MAX subsample. In: Collery Ph, Brätter P, Negretti de Brätter V, Khassanova L, Etienne JC, eds. *Metal Ions in Biology and Medicine*. Paris: John Libbey Eurotext, 1998: 5: 390-94.
9. Roussel AM, Lachili B, Arnaud J, Richard MJ, Benlatréche C, Favier A. Oxidative stress and antioxidant trace element status in Algerian diabetic pregnat women. In: Collery Ph, Brätter P, Negretti de Brätter V, Khassanova L, Etienne JC, eds. *Metal Ions in Biology and Medicine*. Paris: John Libbey Eurotext, 1998: 5: 395-99.
10. Fogelholm GM, Lahtinen PK. Nutritional evaluation of a sailing crew during a transatlantic race. *Scand J Med Sci Sports* 1991; 1: 99-103.
11. Rükgauer M, Neugebauer R, Plecko T, Kruse-Jarres JD. The selenium-dependent antioxidative system. In: Collery Ph, Brätter P, Negretti de Brätter V, Khassanova L, Etienne JC, eds. *Metal Ions in Biology and Medicine*. Paris: John Libbey Eurotext, 1998; 5: 544-46.
12. Kanter MM. Free radicals, exercise and antioxidant supplementation. *Int J Sports Nutr* 1994; 4: 205-20.
13. Guerra M, Villanueva J, Ramos MJ, Borque L, Escanero JF. Tumor necrosis factor and acute phase proteins in plasma after a cycle-ergometer test on elite athletes. *2nd International Beckman Award* 1994; 2: 64-67.
14. Paubert-Braquet M, Hoford D, Klozt P, Guilbaud J, Braquet P. Tumor necrosis factor alpha 'primes' the platelet-activating factor-induced superoxide production by human neutrophils: possible involvent of G proteins. *J Lipid Mediat* 1990; 2: S1-14.
15. Weglicki WB, Phillips TM, Freeman AM. Magnesium deficiency elevates circulating levels of inflammatory cytokines and endothelin. *Mol Cell Biochem* 1992; 110: 169-73.
16. Chaudhri G, Clark IA. Reactive oxigen species facilitate the in vitro and in vivo lipopolysaccharide-induced release of tumor necrosis factor. *J Immunol* 1989; 143: 1290-94.
17. Meurer R, MacIntyre DE. Lack of effect of pertussis toxin on TNF alpha induced formation of reactive oxygen intermediates by human neutrophils. *Biochem Biophys Res Comm* 1989; 159: 763-69.

Metal Ions in Biology and Medicine; vol 6. Eds. J.A. Centeno, Ph. Collery, G. Vernet, R.B. Finkelman, H. Gibb, J.C. Etienne. John Libbey Eurotext, Paris © 2000, pp. 505-507.

Issues in environmental risk assessments of metals

Peter M. Chapman and Freiyue Wang

EVS Environment Consultants, 195 Pemberton Avenue, North Vancouver, B.C., Canada V7P 2R4; >pchapman@attglobal.net>

Ecological risk assessment (ERA) is a process that evaluates the potential for adverse ecological effects occurring as a result of exposure to contaminants or other stressors. ERA begins with hazard identification/problem formulation, progresses to effects and exposure assessment, and finishes with risk characterization (an estimate of the incidence and severity of any adverse effects likely to occur). Risk management initially sets the boundaries of the ERA and then uses its results for decision-making (Fig. 1):

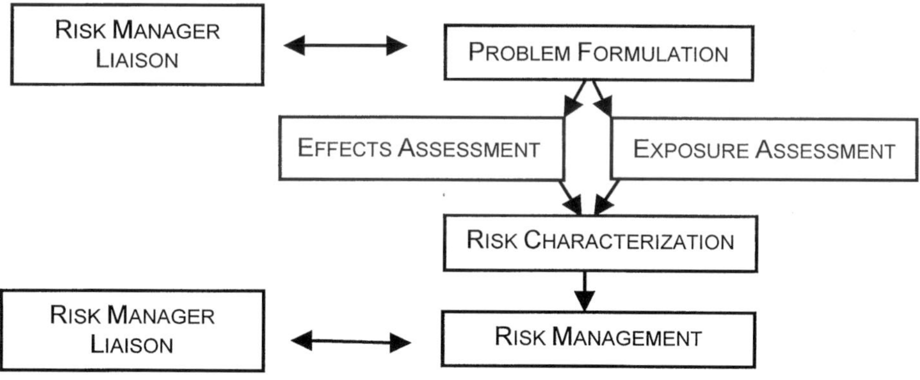

Figure 1: ERA Framework

Key information required for an ERA includes: the emissions, pathways and rates of movement of contaminants in the environment; and, information on the relationship between contaminant concentrations and the incidence and (or) severity of adverse effects. Because of specific properties and characteristics of metals in general and of certain metals in particular, a generalized ERA process applicable to organic substances is inappropriate for metals. First, metals are naturally occurring and can arise, sometimes in very high concentrations, from non-anthropogenic sources; organisms can and do adapt to a wide range of metal concentrations. Second, certain metals (e.g., copper, zinc) are essential for biotic health, which means there is an effect threshold for both deficiency and excess, and that standard body burden measurements can be misleading. Third, metals can occur in the environment in a variety of forms that are more or less available to biota but adverse biological effects can only occur if metals are or may become bioavailable. Fourth, bioavailability and hence the possibility of toxicity (metals must be bioavailable to be toxic, but bioavailability does not necessarily result in toxicity) are dependent on environmental biochemical conditions. Whereas environmental chemistry affects metal speciation and hence bioavailability, biotic factors affect actual uptake into tissues. ERAs involving metals must include the above four major considerations; other considerations vary depending on whether the ERA is for a site, a region, or is global in scope.

Regional or global hazard identification of metals cannot use persistence (P) or bioaccumulation (B) criteria because, unlike organics, they do not apply [1,2] and their discriminatory power is low [3]. Such classification exercises must rely on toxicity (T) determinations. Canada is determining the hazard of metals and metal substances (and other inorganics) in use in commerce primarily by: assessing solubility in water (≥ 1 mg/L), then the stability of the dissolved form, and finally the toxicity of either the parent compound or its dissociated components (≤ 1 mg/L) [3]. P and B criteria are not useful at any stage in an ERA of metals. However, what is useful in an ERA is information on transformations between bioavailable and non-bioavailable forms (including complexation) and to organometals. The latter can be treated similarly to organic substances in terms of B.

Regional or global risk assessment of metals should be based on metallo-regions, specifically a portion of the Earth's surface having common geological and biological characteristics. This concept combines both the ecological regional or watershed approach (physical, chemical and biological boundaries/stressors) with recognition of geological differences in natural metal concentrations in the environment.

Risk assessments at any level (site-specific, regional, global) progress from conservative (protective) assumptions to more realistic scenarios. Thus standard ecotoxicity testing under defined conditions, though not designed or intended to be environmentally realistic, is appropriate for problem formulation (Figure 1) but not for final risk characterization. The effects assessment portion of an ERA must be more ecologically realistic whether a screening or detailed level risk assessment is involved. The former will be less certain than the latter [4]. Increased ecological realism may involve laboratory testing reflecting site specific conditions (e.g., pH, water hardness, dissolved organic carbon [DOC], microcosms), and/or *in situ* testing (e.g., mesocosms). A key issue in this regard is bioavailability.

The exposure assessment of an ERA must distinguish bioavailable metals from non-bioavailable metals. The majority of metals present in the environment are not bioavailable due to binding to compounds. The Biotic Ligand Model (BLM) may provide a general model for bioavailability determinations. Regional and global ERAs can be improved by the appropriate use of normalizing factors (e.g., pH, water hardness, DOC). However, bioavailability remains highly site-specific. Thus site-specific ERA will be more certain than global ERA.

The final portion of an ERA, risk characterization, integrates the previous three steps (Fig. 1) to estimate the incidence and severity of any likely environmental effects. It also includes an uncertainty assessment of each component and of the overall ERA. The particular characteristics of metals need to be considered in both risk characterization and uncertainty assessment if the end product is to be realistic and useful.

References Cited

[1] Chapman PM, Allen HE, Godtfredsen K, Z'Graggen MN. Evaluation of BCFs as measures for classifying and regulating metals. *Environ Sci Technol* 1996; 30: 448-452.

[2] Chapman PM, Thornton I, Persoone G, Janssen C, Godtfredsen K, Z'Graggen MN. International harmonization related to persistence and bioavailability. *Human Ecol Risk Assess* 1996; 2: 393-404.

[3] IWG. Categorization of inorganic substances on the Domestic Substances List – Findings and recommendations of an expert workgroup. Environment Canada Advisory Group, Inorganics Working Group, Ottawa, ON, Canada. Environment Canada Technical Report. In Press.

[4] Hill RA, Chapman PM, Lawrence GS, Mann GS. Perspective: Level of detail in ecological risk assessments. *Mar Pollut Bull* In Press.

Metal Ions in Biology and Medicine; vol 6. Eds. J.A. Centeno, Ph. Collery, G. Vernet, R.B. Finkelman, H. Gibb, J.C. Etienne. John Libbey Eurotext, Paris © 2000, pp. 508-510.

Natural sources of metals to the environment

Robert G. Garrett

Geological Survey of Canada, 601 Booth St., Ottawa, Ontario K1A 0E8, Canada

All metals present in the environment, except those small quantities that have arrived extra-terrestrially, or have been created in nuclear reactions, have been present since the formation of the earth. As part of the natural biogeochemical cycle, metals are released from rocks by weathering processes, are cycled through various environmental compartments by biotic and abiotic processes, and ultimately find their fate in the oceans as sediments. Given sufficient geological time they become "rocks" again, tectonic processes form new land, and the cycle continues. With the advent of man, additional processes have become involved in the redistribution of metals between environmental compartments; and the rate of transfer between many compartments has increased significantly since the industrial revolution. However, the dominant control on the distribution of metals in the earth's surface layers remains the geochemistry of the parent rocks in all but the worst cases of industrial contamination.

A fundamental link exists between mineralogy and geochemistry. Trace metal background levels in rocks are controlled by the abundance of the common rock-forming minerals present. It is the availability of substitution sites (e.g., Al, Ca, Mg, Fe, Na, K) in mineral structures that permit trace element incorporation. The key controls of replacement are ionic charge and radius, and electronegativity. Thus Rb with similar ionic radius and electronegativty as K replaces it in K-rich feldspars, and levels of Rb are highest in K-feldspar rich rocks. The same relationship explains the similar behaviour of S and Se, which is evidenced in both the mineral and biological "kingdoms". Of particular interest are elements that pair differently, e.g., Cd with a similar ionic radius to Ca, but a similar electronegativity to Zn. This explains phenomena of both mineral and biological importance. In geology Cd commonly is regarded as a chalcophile element, it is associated with Zn in sulphide minerals due to its electronegativity. However, due to its similar ionic radius to Ca it is present in calcium phosphate, apatite; particularly those apatites that form certain sedimentary rock-phosphates mined for the production of agricultural fertilizers. In fertilizer manufacture, most of the Cd remains in the product, and thus, undesirably, Cd may be added to agricultural lands with the P required to encourage plant growth. In the biological realm, Cd can replace Ca in carboxyl-based, and Zn in sulphurhydryl-based, compounds, thus providing a pathway for Cd to enter biota in one form but then cause an effect through a different mechanism. Ionic and electronegativity relationships permit the prediction of many of the associations observed between elements in both rocks and their weathering products, i.e. soils, waters and newly deposited sediments. In addition to weathering, metals may be added to surface environments directly by volcanic activity through eruption, gaseous fumaroles and hot-spring activity; and through de-gassing along fractures and faults that provide suitable pathways from depth. For example, on June 14-15, 1991, it is estimated that Mt. Pinatubo ejected 3-5 km^3 of rock, equivalent to 10^4 M tonnes that contained some 100,000 tonnes of Pb and 800 tonnes of Hg [1].

A major challenge being addressed by geoscientists is the quantification of natural releases for comparison with anthropogenic releases. Whereas anthropogenic releases can be estimated relatively easily, such is not the case for natural releases [1]. For example, the recent discovery of marine hydrothermal vents off New Zealand, each of which is emitting some 1 kg/yr of Hg [2] was a new natural source that was only previously suspected. There are likely many thousands more of similar undiscovered vents.

The earth's surface is chemically inhomogeneous due to the diversity of igneous, metamorphic and sedimentary rocks, with varying mineralogies, that were formed by a variety of different processes from different source materials.

	Hg (ppb)	Cd (ppm)	As (ppm)	Ni (ppm)	Pb (ppm)	Cu (ppm)	Zn (ppm)
Continental Crust	80	0.2	1.7	61	13	50	81
Igneous Rocks							
Ultramafic	4	0.1	1	2000	1	10	50
Mafic	13	0.2	2	130	6	87	105
Intermediate	21	0.1	2	15	15	30	60
Felsic	39	0.1	1	5	19	10	39
Sedimentary Rocks							
Sandstone	57	0.02	1	3	14	15	16
Limestone	46	0.05	2	13	16	4	16
Shale	270	0.2	9	29	80	45	130
Black Shale		4	22	68	15	50	189

Table I. Some Average Trace Element Compositions of Common Rocks

Table I provides examples of the ranges, some up to two orders of magnitude, that occur for metals between rock types [3]. The actual ranges of individual values from these, and other, rocks are even larger. The erosion and weathering of bedrock provide the earth's surface that supports life; and interaction with rocks and their weathering products influences the chemistry of the water that is essential for life's continued existence. Geochemical maps depicting the distribution of trace elements at a wide range of scales, from local to continental, are prepared by industry, private and government institutions to support decision making for both economic development and public policy. The role of geochemical maps and data have been recognized internationally as an important tool for environmental and resource management [4]. Through the environment, the composition of diet is affected, and it has been long recognized that particular areas are characterized by endemic plant, animal or human health problems, from which developed the study of epidemiology. Geologically associated human health problems, both nutritional deficiencies (e.g., Zn, I, Se) and toxicity issues (e.g., Hg, As), and the role of geochemistry, are receiving increasing attention, as demonstrated by recent publications [e.g., 5, 6 & 7]. Thus a knowledge of the natural distribution of metals at the earth's surface, and the processes affecting their distribution and controlling the presence of bioavailable forms that can cause biotic effects, is essential if the problems of micronutrient deficiency and endemic disease are to be are addressed.

References:

1. Garrett RG. Geological sources of metals to the atmosphere. In Proceedings of the Workshop on the Atmospheric Transport and Fate of Metals in the Environment. Ottawa : Intl. Council on Metals and the Environment, 1999 : 71-84.

2. Stoffers P, Hannington M, Wright I, Herzig P, de Ronde C and Shipboard Scientific Party. Elemental mercury at submarine hydrothermal vents in the Bay of Plenty, Taupo volcanic zone, New Zealand. *Geology* 1999; 27 : 931-934.

3. Garrett RG. Natural processes influencing the distribution of metals at the earth's surface. In The Impact of Metals on the Environment. Stockholm : Royal Swedish Academy of Engineering Sciences (IVA), 1998 : 7-23.

4. Darnley AG, Björklund A, Bølviken B, Gustavsson N, Koval PV, Plant JA, Steenfelt a, Tauchid M and Xie Xuejing. A Global Geochemical Database for Environmental and Resource Management. Paris : UNESCO, Earth Sciences 19, 1995.

5. Combs GF Jr., Welch RM, Duxbury JM, Uphoff NT and Nesheim MC (Eds.). Food-Based Approaches to Preventing Micronutrient Malnutrition. Ithaca, NY : Cornell Intl. Institute for Food, Agriculture and Development, 1996.

6. Dissanayake CB and Chandrajith R. Medical geochemistry of tropical environments. *Earth-Science Reviews* 1999 : 219-258.

7. Appleton JD, Fuge R. and McCall GJH (Eds.). Environmental Geochemistry and Health. London : Geological Society Special Publication No. 113, 1996.

Metal Ions in Biology and Medicine; vol 6. Eds. J.A. Centeno, Ph. Collery, G. Vernet, R.B. Finkelman, H. Gibb, J.C. Etienne. John Libbey Eurotext, Paris © 2000, pp. 511-513.

The importance of metal speciation in environmental assessment

Herbert E. Allen

Department of Civil and Environmental Engineering, University of Delaware, Newark, DE 19716 USA; <allen@ce.udel.edu>

Trace metals in aquatic and soil systems exist in a number of different soluble and particulate forms that impact the effect of the metals on these ecosystems. Although assessment of metals in many regulatory programs is based on data for total metal concentrations, such values rarely correlate with effects. In water, sediment or soils it is not uncommon to find that for the same level of biological effect their is as much as a three order-of-magnitude change in metal concentration. Consequently, other means are needed for the prediction of risk.

Metal concentrations in natural waters are very low, typically at the μg/L level, and samples have frequently been subjected to contamination during collection and processing. Consequently, older data are of suspect quality. Over the past decade there has been more attention placed on using clean techniques in sampling and analysis. The use of clean rooms has become routine. Microwave digestion methods which samples are less subject to contamination from airborne particles are supplanting open vessel procedures. Sensitive analytical methods, less prone to interference - for example, ICP-MS – are being routinely used. These improvements have allowed the accurate determination of low concentrations of metals present in the environment.

Because bioavailability of metals depends on chemical form or speciation it is necessary that analytical methods be available to determine or predict the bioavailable fraction of metal [1, 2]. The free metal ion concentration has most commonly been related to biological effect. Voltammetric techniques have commonly been applied for chemical speciation of metals. Anodic stripping voltammetry is the most commonly used electrochemical technique but cathodic stripping voltammetry has also been applied to the analysis of copper, nickel, zinc and other metals. The methods provide differentiation of zinc associated with weak vis-à-vis stronger ligands and the results of titrations of samples with metal ion are expressed as complexation capacity.

Chemical equilibrium computer programs are useful for computing the distribution of species in samples containing defined total concentrations of metal and ligands, if appropriate stability constants are available. The description of metal complexation with natural organic matter (NOM) is much more complicated than is description of complexation with simple ligands. NOM is an unresolvable mixture of a very large number of compounds varying in their properties, including their ability to bind metal ions. Approaches proposed for the modeling of metal complexation by NOM and humic substances include gaussian distribution models and models having multiple discrete sites to account for the properties of NOM.

Water Quality Criteria used in the United States are instituted for the protection of aquatic life. These values are generated based on an assessment of acute and chronic bioassay tests conducted in either natural waters or in reconstituted laboratory test water. These criteria consider hardness as the only water quality parameter that is to be used in modification of the numeric values. In addition to hardness, pH and dissolved organic matter affect metal toxicity. Toxicity of a metal in water at some sites can be more than an order-of-magnitude different from that implied by the criteria. Site specific criteria modifications based on toxicity testing in site waters have been used to modify criteria to account for the changed bioavailability [2]. More recently the biotic ligand model (BLM) has been developed to allow toxicity to aquatic organisms to be predicted. The BLM accounts for speciation of metal ions in the water column and their interaction at receptor sites on an organism. Competition of protons, calcium ions and other cations for reaction with natural organic matter and with the biotic ligand sites are specifically addressed. The BLM relates the fraction of the receptor sites on the organism bound by the metal of concern to toxicity.

Total metal concentrations in sediment cover several orders of magnitude with no distinction of sediments that cause effects and those that do not except at low total metal concentrations. Non-toxic sediments can contain as much as 3 orders of magnitude more metal some sediments not exhibiting toxicity. In both sediment and soils, partitioning to the aqueous phase is a major determinant of exposure. If the partitioning is very strong, effects due to the metal would not be expected.

Sulfide present in sediment binds metal strongly resulting in its detoxification. Sulfide is determined by cold acid distillation (acid volatile sulfide, AVS). Potentially toxic metals that can displace iron in FeS, are cadmium, copper, lead, nickel and zinc. The SEM value is the sum of these metal concentrations on a µmol/g dry weight of sediment basis. It is determined as the concentrations of the metals solubilized in the acidification for AVS determination.. The SEM/AVS ratio is useful in prediction of those sediments for which toxicity will not be exhibited. Ratios less than one have not been found to be toxic to organisms. That is, there is not toxicity if the amount of sulfide available to bind metals exceeds the concentration of metals. It should be noted that it is the absence of toxicity that is predicted. No prediction of toxicity is provided by this procedure [3].

The partitioning of a metal between soil and soil solution is a primary determinant of the risk that a given concentration of metal poses. As with sediments, metal concentrations in soil can vary by more than three orders of magnitude, but the solid phase concentration is not reflective of either mobility or bioavailability. Partitioning of metals is highly dependant on pH. It is common knowledge that metal toxicity in soils can often be reduced by raising soil pH through liming. As with water, it is tempting to consider the concentration of the free metal ion to predict effects on plants in soils. Because the chemistry of soil is more complex than that of water, and due to the large influence that plants have on their environment, prediction of effects has not been possible to date. Use of partitioning models to predict metal ion activity has shown promise in providing better relationships to ecotoxicological factors than are obtained using total metal.

Assessment of potential impacts of metals in water, sediment and soils cannot be judged on the basis of their total concentration. Knowledge of metal speciation and of the total system chemistry is essential. In the absence of understanding of the environmental chemistry, regulatory bodies have tended to incorporate large safety factors into standards to ensure that the standards will provide at least the desired level of protection.

REFERENCES CITED

[1] Allen HE. The significance of trace metal speciation for water, sediment and soil quality standards. Sci Total Environ 1993; 134, Supplement Part 1 : 23-45.

[2] Allen HE, Hansen DJ. The importance of trace metal speciation to water quality criteria. Water Environ Res 1996; 68 : 42-54.

[3] Di Toro DM, Mahony JD, Hansen DJ, Scott KJ, Hicks MB, Mayr SM, Redmond MS. Toxicity of cadmium in sediments: The role of acid volatile sulfide. Environ Toxicol Chem 1990; 9 : 1487-1502.

Metal Ions in Biology and Medicine; vol 6. Eds. J.A. Centeno, Ph. Collery, G. Vernet, R.B. Finkelman, H. Gibb, J.C. Etienne. John Libbey Eurotext, Paris © 2000, pp. 514-516.

The challenges of hazard identification and classification of metals and insoluble metal substances

William Adams, Bruce Conard and Guy Ethier

Kennecott Utah Copper Corporation, Magna, UT 84044, Inco Limited, Toronto, Canada M5H 4B7, and International Council on Metals and the Environment, Ottawa, Canada K1P 6E6; <Adamsw@kennecott.com>

Procedures for aquatic hazard identification of organic and inorganic substances are currently being harmonized by member states of the OECD for the purpose of classifying commercial substances. One common theme in member country systems is the use of toxicity, persistence and bioaccumulation measurements to estimate aquatic hazard. It is recognized within the OECD and European Union systems that special attention must be given to metal elements and sparingly soluble metal-containing compounds. This recognition is based upon a common understanding that standard hazard testing procedures designed for soluble organic chemicals do not accommodate the special characteristics of sparingly soluble metals and metal compounds (SSMMCs).

Toxicity - It is recognized that the toxicity of a metal is due predominately to the free metal ion in solution. Most of the toxicity data available to date have been derived using soluble metal salts, where it is assumed that for such salts the dissolved metal ion is completely available. The toxicities of most dissolved metal salts to sensitive species lie in the range of 0.1 to 1000 ug/L (Table 1). In order to assess the acute aquatic toxicity of SSMMCs, the rate and extent of transformation of metal to a soluble ionic forms must be measured. Transformation of sparingly soluble metal substances to soluble forms is a function of several key factors including metal particle size and surface area, as well as ionic strength, and the pH of the test solution. A standard protocol for measuring transformation is currently being developed by the OECD. Initial results obtained using a draft protocol (under development by the OECD) indicate that unrealistically high concentrations of soluble metals (#0.45μm) which may exceed aquatic EC/LC_{50} values are obtained as compared to concentrations that occur in natural environments. The current protocol lacks naturally occurring complexing ligands and evaluation of the presence of colloids. Further development of this protocol is underway.

Table 1. Summary of acute and chronic toxicity data (US EPA water acute and chronic quality criteria values)

Metal (Soluble Salt)	Acute Toxicity, μg/L (CMC) [a]	Chronic Toxicity, μg/L (CCC) [a]
Iron	---	1000
Arsenic	340	150
Zinc	120	120
Aluminum	750	87
Chromium III	570	74
Nickel	470	52
Cobalt	706	42
Chromium VI	16	11
Copper	13	9
Selenium	20	5
Lead	65	2.5
Cadmium	4.3	2.2
Mercury	1.4	0.77
Silver	3.4	0.1

[a] CMC & CCC = acute and chronic water quality criteria values taken from US EPA water quality criteria documents [1].

Persistence - Measurements of persistence typically used for organic substances, providing an estimate of the persistency of exposure, (biodegradation/ CO_2 evolution) do not apply to metals. It is widely recognized that elements are non-degradable. Alternative measurements such as hydrolysis, complexation and precipitation are appropriate measures of persistency of exposure for metals. Complexation with dissolved organic carbon in surface waters and sulfide binding in sediments are key processes controlling metal exposure in aquatic ecosystems. There are significant differences in metal binding constants ranging across more than 20 orders of magnitude [2]. These properties point to differences in metal ion bioavailability and further indicate that persistency measures used for metals are unique from those for organic substances.

Bioaccumulation - The potential for organic chemicals to accumulate in ecosystem food chains is measured or estimated by log octanol-water partition coefficient (Kow) and is reported as a bioconcentration or bioaccumulation factor (BCF/BAF). Values above a factor of 1000 are often used to indicate concern. However this estimator of hazard is not appropriate for metal ions. BCFs and BAFs for metals cannot be estimated by log Kow, are inversely related to exposure concentration, and are not reliable predictors of concern for food chain accumulation. While a concern for bioaccumulation of a given metal in tissues of aquatic or terrestrial organisms might exist at a given site due to site-specific exposure conditions, BCFs and BAFs are not indicators of concern for hazard or secondary poisoning for metals and inorganic metal compounds. Further, recent literature reviews indicate that BCFs and BAFs are not useful for predicting chronic or long-term toxicity of metals to aquatic organisms [3].

In summary, approaches for assessing the hazard of metals are evolving, but at present, are not yet satisfactory. Our present understanding of how metals and metal compounds should be assessed for hazard includes the following: Toxicity should be assessed in terms of the potential for the test substance to undergo transformation to bioavailable metal ions. Persistence should be assessed in terms of potential for formation of soluble and insoluble metal complexes (including hydroxides, sulfide, carbonates, and binding to dissolved organic carbon and suspended solids) which act to reduce exposure. Potential for bioaccumulation should be assessed on a case by case basis in terms of biotransformation to organo-metallic substances and evidence of biomagnification

References Cited

[1] U.S. Environmental Protection Agency. National Recommended Water Quality Criteria, Federal Register, Vol. 63, No. 234, pp. 67548-67558.

[2] Allen, H., and Y. Lu. 2000. Persistence of Metals. Experts Workshop on Review of the State-of-the-Science Regarding PBT Concepts for Metals and Metal Compounds. January 19, 2000, Arlington, VA., Electric Power Research Institute. Special Technical Publication, workshop proceedings, Palo Alto, CA.

[3] Brix, K., and DeForest, D. 1999. Critical Review of the Use of Bioaccumulation Potential for Hazard Classification of Metals and Metal Compounds, Parametrix, Inc., Kirkland, WA.

Metal Ions in Biology and Medicine; vol 6. Eds. J.A. Centeno, Ph. Collery, G. Vernet, R.B. Finkelman, H. Gibb, J.C. Etienne. John Libbey Eurotext, Paris © 2000, pp. 517-520.

Calcium deficiency rickets in Bangladesh

G.F. Combs, Jr.[1], P.R. Fischer[2], N. Hassan[3], A. Daly[1], J.M. Duxbury[4], R.M. Welch[4, 5], C.A. Meisner[6], S. Haque[7] and the Bangladesh Rickets Prevention Consortion*

[1] *Division of Nutritional Sciences, Cornell University, Ithaca, NY, USA;* [2] *Mayo Clinic, Rochester, MN, USA;* [3] *Dhaka University, Dhaka, Bangladesh;* [4] *Dept. of Soil and Crop Sciences, Cornell University, Ithaca, NY, USA;* [5] *US Plant, Soil and Nutrition Laboratory, USDA, Ithaca, NY, USA;* [6] *International Wheat and Maize Improvement Center, Dhaka, Bangladesh;* [7] *Social Assistance and Rehabilitation for the Physically Vulnerable, Dhaka, Bangladesh**

ABSTRACT

Recent surveys have suggested that rickets may affect as much as a third of children in some parts of Bangladesh. A case-control evaluation of children in Chakaria thana, Cox's Bazaar District, showed that children showing signs of rickets had elevated serum levels of 1,25-dihydroxy-cholecalciferol (1,25-DHCC) but normal levels of 25-hydroxycholecalciferol (25-HCC). While there were some cases of hypophosphatemic rickets, most of these cases appeared to be due to primary deficiencies of calcium, which appeared not to be plentiful in the local food system.

INTRODUCTION

In the last 15 years, rickets, the impaired ossification of growing bone, has been identified in an estimated 4-9% of children of Chakaria thana, Cox's Bazaar District, in southeastern Bangladesh. Local clinical experience indicates that standard vitamin D therapy has not proved beneficial, suggesting that the disorder may due to primary calcium (Ca) deficiency as has been reported in some parts of Africa [1-7]. That the disease has emerged in Chakaria only within the last two decades suggests that changes in food habits and/or environmental exposures to Ca-antagonists may be factors in its etiology. This study was conducted to explore the etiology and characterize the clinical aspects of the Chakaria rickets.

*Institute of Mother and Child Nutrition, Dhaka, Bangladesh, UNICEF, Bangladesh, Dhaka, Bangladesh; Amis des Enfants du Monde, Paris, France; Bangladesh Rural Advancement Committee, Dhaka, Bangladesh, in addition to the authors' institutions.

MATERIALS AND METHODS

Clinical and biochemical evaluations were made on children identified as rachitic (14) or non-rachitic (13) by their respective families. Blood was obtained and physical and radiographic examinations were made. Samples of drinking water (tube well), cooking water (pond), and cooked and uncooked rice were collected from one household of a rachitic children and from two households without affected children. Samples of foods likely to be sources of Ca and other limiting nutrients were purchased from local markets. Water pH was measured at the point of sampling; samples were held frozen (blood) or at ambient temperature (water), or dried (food) prior to analysis. Samples were digested with nitric-perchloric acids and analyzed for 24 elements by inductively coupled plasma emission spectrometry (ICP).

RESULTS AND DISCUSSION

Rachitic children (9 males, 5 females) varied from 36-98 (mean 69) months of age; their mothers reported them being symptomatic since an average age of 24 (range 0-48) months. None reported other chronic illnesses, renal disease, or anticonvulsant use. Rachitic deformities included knock-knees (10), bowed legs (4), and sabre tibae (3). Ten of the 14 affected children had active rickets as determined by serum alkaline phosphatase (AP) activities >350 U/L 7 of 12 evaluated showed radiographic evidence of active rickets.

All children showed normal serum levels of Ca, P and 25-HCC; but those in the rachitic group has significantly greater serum activities of AP and concentrations of 1,25-DHCC than controls (Table 1). Two subjects in the rachitic group had serum 25-HCC levels and 9 of 13 subjects tested had serum 1,25-DHCC levels above the upper limit of "normal". Of the 10 children with active rickets, only two had serum 25-HCC levels <14 ng/mL, one of whom was hypophosphatemic. Three apparently unaffected children in the control group had physical findings consistent with rickets (each with beaded ribs, one also with widened wrists, and another also with knock-knees) without elevated AP activities; these findings would indicate healed rickets.

The concentrations of other minerals in serum or whole blood were similar for rickets cases and controls with the exception of P (serum: cases, 43 mg/l vs. controls, 52 mg/l, P>.05; whole blood: cases, 216 mg/l vs. controls, 235 mg/l, P>.05) (Table 1). The concentrations of all minerals, including potential antagonists of Ca-utilization, in whole blood (Table 2) and both pond and well water were within normal limits.

Rice, the major staple local food, was very low in Ca (36 mg/kg as eaten). All elements in other local foods were within normal ranges (e.g., rice, Fig. 1) with two exceptions: amaranth and shrimp each contained high concentrations of almost all elements (amaranth, mg/kg dry weight: Ca, 26,947; Al, 1455; Pb, 1.5; Sr, 129; Ba, 32; Cr, 9.8; V, 3; As, 0.2; shrimp, mg/kg dry weight: Ca, 37,278; Al, 209; Pb, 0.3; Sr, 322; Ba, 34; V, 0.5; As, 4.3).

Table 1. Values of parameters of bone health in rachitic and control children.

Group	Ca mg/dl	P mg/dl	Alk. Pase, units/l	25-HCC ng/ml	1,25-DHCC pg/ml
Controls	9.7±0.4	5.3±0.5	206± 51	25± 6	73±36
Rachitic	9.5±0.6	4.1±1.0	492±206	20±14	139±41
P value	N.S.	<0.003.	<0.0001	<0.008	<0.0005

Table 2. Whole blood concentrations of potential Ca-antagonists

Group	Al ng/ml	Zn mcg/ml	Cd mcg/ml	Sr mcg/ml	Pb mcg/ml	Ba mcg/ml	As mcg/ml
Controls	19.5±19.2	297.5±32.5	1.05±0.23	4.3±1.0	3.16±0.98	5.91±0.85	0.84±0.56
Rachitic	35.7±47.4	295.1±36.9	1.09±0.19	4.5±1.21	4.16±1.25	6.57±1.17	0.45±0.27
P value	N.S.	N.S.	N.S.	N.S.	N.S.	N.S.	N.S.

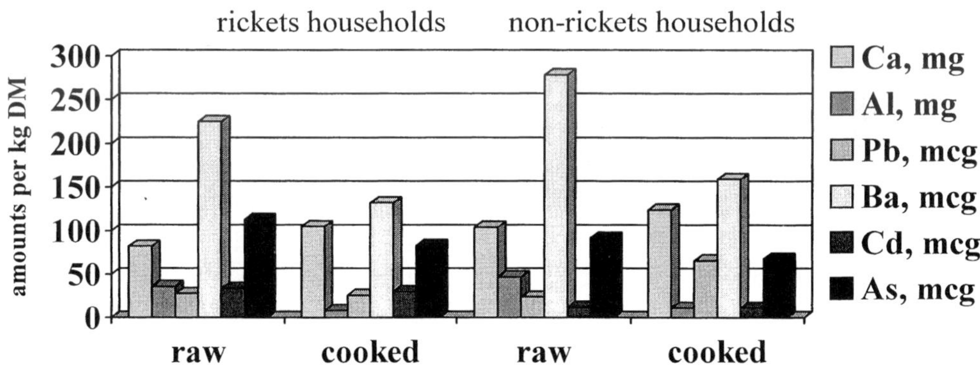

Figure 1. Ca and potential Ca-antagonists in rice

That most rachitic children did not show low serum 25-HCC levels indicated that active rickets in Chakaria is not necessarily associated with vitamin D deficiency. In fact, cases presented a picture consistent with calcium deficiency, as indicated by the up-regulation of 1,25-DHCC production, which has been described among children in other developing countries [1-7]. The findings of rachitic deformities and elevated serum 1,25-DHCC levels among some "unaffected" children further suggest that sub-clinical Ca deficiency may also be prevalent Chakaria, as might be expected. This cursory evaluation of local foods did not indicate wide exposure to known mineral antagonists of Ca utilization; instead, it suggested a food supply generally low in Ca. The emergence of rickets as a public health problem in Chakaria would appear to correspond to changes in local food systems: introduction of winter rice (requiring irrigation during the dry season); increased shrimp cultivation in flooded rice paddies; installation of deep (tube) wells to provide potable water; increased population size. It is possible that one or more of these changes has led to the de-diversification of diets around rice and other low-calcium foods.

REFERENCES

[1] Pettifor, J., Ross, P., Wang, J., Moodley, G., and Couper-Smith, J. Rickets in children of rural origin in South Africa: is low dietary calcium a factor? J. Pediatr. 1978, 92:320-324.

[2] Okonofua, F., Gill, D.S., Alabi, Z.O., Thomas, M., Bell, J.L., and Dandona, P. Rickets in Nigerian Children: a consequence of calcium malnutrition. Metab.1991, 40:209-213.

[3] Oginni, L.M., Worsfold, M., Oyelami, O.A., Sharp, C.A., Powell, D.E., and Davie, M.W.J. Etiology of rickets in Nigerian Children. J. Pediatr. 1996, 128:692-694.

[4] Thacher, T.D., Ighogboja, S.I., and Fischer, P.R. Rickets without vitamin D deficiency in Nigerian children. Ambulatory Child Health 1997, 3:56-64.

[5] Oginni, L.M., Sharp, C.A., Worsfold, M., Badru, O.S., Davie, M.W.J. Healing rickets after calcium supplementation. Lancet 1999, 353:296-297.

[6] Thacher, T.D., Glew, R.H., and Isichei, C.O. Rickets in Nigerian children: response to calcium supplementation. J. Trop. Pediatr. 1999, 45:202-207.

[7] Thacher, T.D., Fischer, P.R., Pettifor, J.D., Lawson, J.O., Isichei, C.O., Reading, J.C. and Chan, G.M. A comparison of calcium, vitamin D or both for nutritional rickets in Nigerian children. New Eng. J. Med. 1999, 341:563-568.

Metal Ions in Biology and Medicine; vol 6. Eds. J.A. Centeno, Ph. Collery, G. Vernet, R.B. Finkelman, H. Gibb, J.C. Etienne. John Libbey Eurotext, Paris © 2000, pp. 521-523.

Estimation of trace element supply in Austria

W. Pfannhauser, A. Sima, S. Heumann, U. Schaller, M. Wilplinger, I. Schönsleben

Institute of Bio- and Food Chemistry, Graz University of Technology, A-8010 Graz, Petersgasse 12/2, Austria

Different approaches to estimate the uptake of the trace elements Se, Cu, Mo, Zn, Cr, Ni were taken.
Market basket studies, summing up data from food analysis according to food consumption statistics (1), duplicate diet studies using 10 – 20 volunteer during a week (2,3) and a special investigation using only locally grown food were performed.

This special investigation included 10 different locations in Austria. A diet compiled by dieticians was purchased and cooked using exclusively food grown in a diameter of 10 km around the spot.
The aim was to look on local differences in supply related to geological conditions and to check if a sufficient supply by using Austrian food (preferably coming from organically grown products) can be guaranteed.

Tab 1 shows the uptake calculated from these investigation.

element	range [mg/d]	average [mg/d]
Zn	8,6 - 30,5	15,0
Mo	0,023 - 0,38	0,2
Ni	0,060 – 0,090	0,079
Cu	1,3 – 1,6	1,5
Cr	0,008 - 0,104	0,048

Selenium supply is under discussion in Austria.
There are signs indicating an undersupply.
Previous data on Selenium in human sera showed that in a part of Austria (4).
This was the reason to carry out various studies under different conditions.
All these studies showed a borderline intake in the Austrian population.

Tab.2 shows the results

Tab. 2 : Selenium supply in Austria

Study	average [µg/d]	range [µg/d]
Market basket study (1)	45,5	
Duplicate Diet Study (2) [1991]	35,5	15 – 118
Diet Study (3) [1996]	47,8	36,5 - 67,8

The data indicate that there are signs of lack in Austria regarding Selenium and Chromium (RDA 50 – 200 µg / day).

Tab. 3 Recommendation for Selenium intake

Recommendation	Daily uptake (µg/d)
Recommended Dietary Allowances	50 - 200
German Society of Nutrition (DGE)	20 - 100
WHO (5) [1996] :	
Normative minimale mean intake	
men	40
women	30

Whereas all other elements investigated seem to be in sufficient amount present in normal diets.

Literature

(1) Pfannhauser W
Versorgungsstatus mit dem essentiellen Spurenelement Selen in Österreich
Lebensmittelchemie 1994 ;48: 123

(2) Pfannhauser W
Das essentielle Spurenelement Selen : Bedeutung, Wirkung und Vorkommen in der Nahrung. III. Selenversorgung und Aufnahmedaten aus Österreich im Vergleich mit Daten aus anderen Ländern. Schlußfolgerungen.
Ernährung / nutrition 1992; 16: 642

(3) Wilplinger M, Sima A, Pfannhauser W

Selengehalt in der Nahrung und dessen Zusammenhang zum Gehalt im Boden
Lebensmittelchemie 1998 ; 52:93 – 95
(4) Tiran B, Tiran A, Petek W, Rossipal E, Wawschinek O,
Selenium status of healthy children and adults in Styria (Austria)
Investigation of a possible undersupply in the Styrian population
Trace Elements in Medicine,
1992 ; 9 : 75-79

(5) FAO / WHO Trace Elements in Human Nutrition
Geneva, 1996

Metal Ions in Biology and Medicine; vol 6. Eds. J.A. Centeno, Ph. Collery, G. Vernet, R.B. Finkelman, H. Gibb, J.C. Etienne. John Libbey Eurotext, Paris © 2000, pp. 525-527.

Marginal dietary pyridoxine and supplemental dietary homocystine and methionine affect the response of the rat to nickel deprivation

Forrest H. Nielsen, Katsuhiko Yokoi and Eric O. Uthus

United States Department of Agriculture, Agricultural Research Service, Grand Forks Human Nutrition Research Center, Grand Forks, North Dakota, USA 58202-9034

Although apparent deficiency signs have been described for several animal species, unequivocal acceptance of Ni as an essential nutrient awaits the definition of a specific biochemical function in higher animals [1]. In our laboratory, efforts to establish this hypothesized function have been directed towards identifying possible metabolic pathways that Ni affects. The efforts involving the use of nutritional stressors such as vitamin B_{12}, folic acid and pyridoxine (B_6) deficiency have suggested that Ni has a biochemical function associated with these three vitamins. Nutritional deficiency of each of these vitamins has been associated with an increase in circulating homocysteine. Thus, in an effort to obtain more clues for identifying an essential function for Ni in rats, an experiment was performed in which the reduced form of homocysteine, or homocystine (Hcy), and the in vivo precursor of homocysteine, methionine (Met) were used as nutritional stressors. Because B_6 is important in the metabolism of homocysteine, it was also included as a stressor. B_6 was chosen over folic acid and vitamin B_{12} because of the possibility that its more extensive role in metabolism would identify additional possibilities beyond sulfur amino acid and labile methyl metabolism where Ni is of nutritional importance.

MATERIALS AND METHODS. Male weanling Sprague-Dawley rats were randomly assigned to treatment groups of eight in a fully-crossed, 2 x 2 x 3 arrangement. The factors were, per kg of fresh diet, Ni supplements of 0 and 1 mg; B_6 supplements of 0 and 7.5 mg; and amino acid supplements of none, 10 g of Hcy and 10 g of Met. The dried skim milk-ground corn-corn oil basal diet contained about 8 ng of Ni, 1.8 mg of B_6 and 4.7 g of Met per kg. The rats were fed their respective diets for 10 weeks. At the 9th week urine excreted over a 20-hour period was collected. The 10th week rats were fasted overnight, weighed, anesthetized and exsanguinated via the abdominal vena cava. Plasma triglycerides (TG), pyridoxal 5'-phosphate (PLP), sulfate, alanine aminotransferase (ALT) and aspartate aminotransferease (AST), and urinary nitrate were determined by using standard published methods. Data were statistically compared by using the statistical packages SAS/STAT or SYSTAT.

TABLE I. Effects of Met, Hcy and B_6 on the response to Ni deprivation.

Dietary Supplements			Plasma				Urinary	
Ni	B_6	AA	PLP	ALT	AST	TG	Sulfate	Nitrate
mg/kg	mg/kg	g/kg	pmol/ml	U/l	U/l	mg/100mL	mM☞mol/20h	
0	0	None	255	13.6	53.6	70	0.141	2.41
0	7.5	None	700	18.4	55.8	65	0.106	2.82
1	0	None	178	7.0	42.3	66	0.104	2.45
1	7.5	None	585	17.8	49.7	70	0.131	1.96
0	0	10Met	254	9.8	39.3	77	0.147	2.80
0	7.5	10Met	550	16.3	51.6	90	0.128	3.11
1	0	10Met	296	9.8	41.8	65	0.157	2.13
1	7.5	10Met	710	18.6	53.8	47	0.158	2.51
0	0	10Hcy	298	8.9	38.1	82	0.210	2.55
0	7.5	10Hcy	801	18.0	46.3	102	0.099	2.06
1	0	10Hcy	325	10.1	41.5	66	0.156	2.31
1	7.5	10Hcy	766	23.9	60.8	59	0.140	2.07
Pooled SD			111	5.8	10.8	23	0.061	0.60
			Analysis of Variance - P Values					
Ni			0.99	0.75	0.72	0.0001	0.55	0.002
B_6			0.0001	0.0001	0.0001	0.83	0.01	0.87
AA			0.0002	0.53	0.33	0.25	0.30	0.04
Ni x B_6			0.90	0.07	0.25	0.09	0.05	0.45
Ni x AA			0.003	0.05	0.009	0.02	0.62	0.23
B_6 x AA			0.12	0.34	0.25	0.73	0.17	

						0.07
NixB_6 x AA	0.23	0.82	0.61	0.19	0.35	0.13

RESULTS. As shown in Table I, Ni deprivation affected the response of the rat to B_6 deficiency and Hcy and Met supplementation, or vice versa. As expected, the animals fed low B_6 had decreased concentrations of plasma PLP, ALT and AST. Dietary Ni affected the response of PLP in plasma to Met and Hcy supplementation. In the Ni-supplemented rats, both amino acids increased the PLP concentration in plasma. In the Ni-deficient rats, Met supplementation decreased the PLP concentration, and Hcy increased the PLP concentration. Dietary Ni also affected the response of ALT and AST in plasma to Met and Hcy. Both ALT and AST activities were decreased by Met or Hcy supplementation in Ni-deficient rats with the effect more marked in the B_6-deficient rats. In the Ni-supplemented rats, ALT activity was increased by amino acid supplementation. Amino acid supplementation did not have much effect on AST in Ni-supplemented, B_6-deficient rats, but Hcy supplementation apparently increased plasma AST activity in Ni-supplemented, B_6-adequate rats. Plasma TG concentrations also were affected by an interaction between Ni and amino acid supplementation. Nickel deficiency increased the plasma TG concentration. This increase was most evident in rats supplemented with Met or Hcy because the amino acid supplements increased plasma TG concentrations in the Ni-deficient rats, but in Ni-supplemented rats, the amino acid supplements decreased TG concentrations when B_6 was adequate, and did not markedly affect concentrations when B_6 was deficient. An interaction between Ni and B_6 affected plasma sulfate concentrations; they were increased by B_6 deficiency in Ni-deficient rats with the increase most marked when Hcy was supplemented to the diet. B_6 deficiency did not markedly affect plasma sulfate concentrations in Ni-supplemented rats. Urinary nitrate excretion was higher in Ni-deficient than Ni-supplemented rats; Hcy supplementation seemed to diminish this effect in B_6-adequate rats, and Met supplementation seemed to enhance this effect in B_6-deficient rats.

DISCUSSION. The findings show that rats fed Ni in amounts not much different than those found in natural diets respond differently than rats fed low amounts of Ni when fed diets high in sulfur amino acids and low in B_6. Thus, Ni most likely is of nutritional importance. The findings also indicate that Ni status can affect amino acid metabolism and lipid or energy metabolism, especially when nutritional stressors of the metabolism are present. Because the effects of the nutritional stressors varied with Ni status in the present study, possibly fruitful areas to further pursue with the objective of finding the mechanism/s through which Ni is physiologically active are indicated. For example, Met and Hcy supplementation had quite different effects in rats depending upon Ni status; this suggests that Ni has a role that, when lacking, results in a difference in the elimination of the excess of these two amino acids that can be catabolized in the same metabolic pathways. The major pathway of homocysteine catabolism involves the processes of decarboxylation and transamination. Methionine also can be used and resynthesized to form polyamines; this pathway involves transamination and decarboxylation. Interestingly, decarboxylation results in a large drop in free energy. Perhaps Ni is involved in a decarboxylation reaction which indirectly results in changed plasma TG concentrations. Determination of further transamination and decarboxylation end-products, and activities of enzymes involved in the their formation, in sulfur amino acid metabolism might indicate a possible site where Ni is biochemically important.

REFERENCES. 1. Nielsen FH. Ultratrace elements in nutrition: current knowledge and speculation. *J Trace Elem Exp Med* 1998; 11:251-274.

Metal Ions in Biology and Medicine; vol 6. Eds. J.A. Centeno, Ph. Collery, G. Vernet, R.B. Finkelman, H. Gibb, J.C. Etienne. John Libbey Eurotext, Paris © 2000, pp. 528-530.

Mechanism of citrate-enhanced intestinal absorption of aluminum and bismuth

A. Slikkerveer, G.B. van der Voet, F.A. de Wolff

Toxicology Laboratory, Leiden University Medical Center, P.O. Box 9600 – 2300, RC Leiden, The Netherlands.

Introduction

Bismuth compounds are used in the treatment of peptic ulcer and *Helicobacter pylori* infections. Bismuth is known as a neurotoxin as well as a nephrotoxin. The counter-ions of Bi have a strong influence on both intestinal absorption, distribution and development of toxicity.
Evaluation of the amount of Bi absorbed from the gastrointestinal tract and the factors influencing this process is necessary for assessment of the internal exposure of patients and the possible risks associated with the use of Bi compounds. Our earlier work demonstrated that citrate-containing Bi compounds were absorbed from the small intestine to a larger extent than Bi compounds not containing citrate (1). It was suggested that the presence of citrate in the small intestine might be a factor influencing Bi absorption as was demonstrated for aluminium (Al)(2, 3).
The present study was performed to further evaluate the effect of citrate on the intestinal absorption of Bi compounds as compared to Al using an *in vivo* perfusion model of rat small intestine (4). The mechanism of citrate-enhanced absorption was further studied by blocking the active transport route with 2,4-dinitrophenol (DNP) and passive transport with 2,4,6-triaminopyrimidine (TAP)(2,3).

Materials and Methods

Female Wistar Rats with body weights of 200-220 g were housed in climate chambers with rat chow and tap water *ad libitum*. The rats fasted 24 hrs before the start of the experiment with free access to water. An *in vivo* perfusion model of the rat small intestine was used in combination with systemic blood sampling from the left carotid artery using an *in situ* cannula (1-3). An isotonic Bi-containing medium was brought at 37 °C and recirculated through duodenum, ileum and jejunum at a perfusion rate of 10 ml/min. Samples of perfusate and blood were collected directly before the experiment and for 60 min at 15-min time intervals during the experiment and analyzed by electrothermal atomic absorption spectrometry (5). Disappearance of Bi from the perfusate was considered as measure for mucosal uptake, while appearance of Bi in the blood was a measure for the intestinal absorption.
Perfusions were performed with Al chloride as reference, Bi chloride, Bi citrate, Bi subsalicylate (BSS), colloidal Bi subcitrate (CBS) and ranitidine Bi citrate (RBC). One gram of elemental Bi for each compound was perfused for 60 min in absence and presence of 0.1 mol/L citrate. Perfusions were also performed with Al chloride and Bi chloride in the presence of citrate and the active transport blocker 2,4-dinitrophenol (DNP) and the passive transportblocker 2,4,6-triamino pyrimidine (TAP) 10 mmol/L. Four rats were perfused with each perfusate.

Results

The addition of citrate to the perfusate led to a dramatic increase in Bi absorption for all compounds tested (Figure 1). A significantly higher amount of

Bi was absorbed from all compounds with added citrate than from the compounds without added citrate; the highest absolute absorption levels were found for colloidal Bi subcitrate (CBS) and Bi subsalicylate (BSS), sequentially followed by Bi citrate, ranitidine Bi citrate (RBC) and Bi chloride.

The addition of DNP as well as TAP led tot a decrease in blood levels of Bi (BiB) after 60 min (Figure 2). The decrease in BiB by 82 ± 1% after perfusion with TAP was significant p=0.005 at both 30 and 60 min, while the addition of DNP resulted in a significant decrease 81% after 30 min, which disappeared after 60 min (52%) p=0.042 and 0.151, respectively.

Discussion

The presence of added citrate to CBS leads to the highest absolute Bi loading, followed sequentially by BSS, Bi citrate, RBC, BSN and Bi chloride. In relative terms, however, the sequence was different; the enhancement factor for intestinal absorption for the non citrate-containing compounds was much stronger than for the citrate-containing compounds. The chemical species produced by BSS are the strongest absorbable ones followed sequentially by those from BSN, Bi chloride, Bi citrate, RBC and CBS. Apparently their absolute quantity in the intestine seems the limiting factor for the loading proces.

Both TAP and DNP decreased the citrate-enhanced absorption of Bi, suggesting that the absorption proces involves both a passive and an active mechanism. In analogy with the absorbable Al-citrate complex the existence of an absorbable Bi-citrate complex is postulated.

Dietary citrate may, therefore, be a risk factor in patients on bismuth therapy.

References

1 Slikkerveer A, Helmich RB, Van der Voet GB, De Wolff FA. Absorption of bismuth from several bismuth compounds during in vivo perfusion of rat small intestine. *J Pharm Sci* 1995; 84: 512-515

2 Van der Voet GB, Van Ginkel MF, De Wolff FA. Intestinal absorption of aluminum in rats: stimulation by citric acid and inhibition by dinitrophenol. *Toxicol Appl Pharmacol* 1989; 99: 90-97

3 G.B. van der Voet. Intestinal absorption of aluminium. In: Chadwick D, Whelan J eds. *Aluminium in Biology and Medicine (Ciba Foundation Symposium 169)* Chichester: Wiley, 1992: 109-122 (ISBN 0 471 93413 5)

4 Van der Voet GB, De Wolff FA. A method of studying the intestinal absorption of aluminium in the rat. *Arch Toxicol* 1984; 55: 168-172

5 Slikkerveer A, Helmich RB, Edelbroek PM, Van der Voet GB, De Wolff FA. Analysis of bismuth in serum and blood by electrothermal atomic absorption spectrometry using platinum as matrix modifier. Clin Chim Acta 1991; 201: 17-26

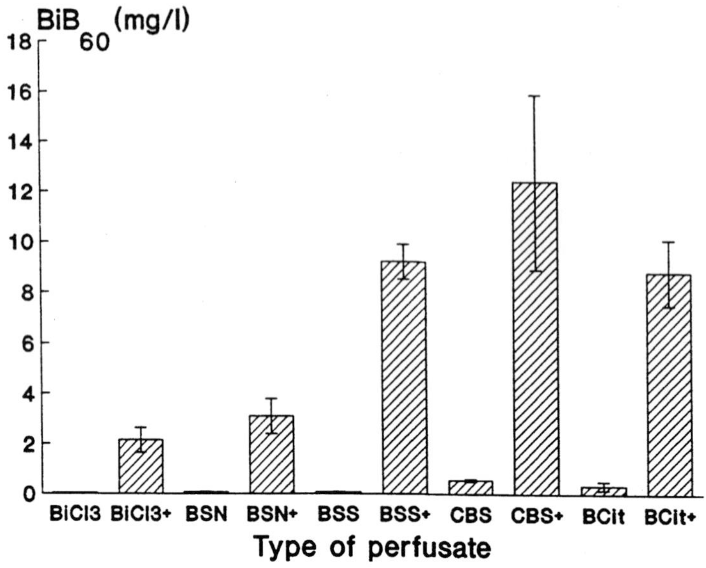

Figure 1
Effect of citrate on the concentration of Bi in blood (BiB_{60} for several Bi compounds (+ = 0.1 mol/L citrate). Mean ± SEM.

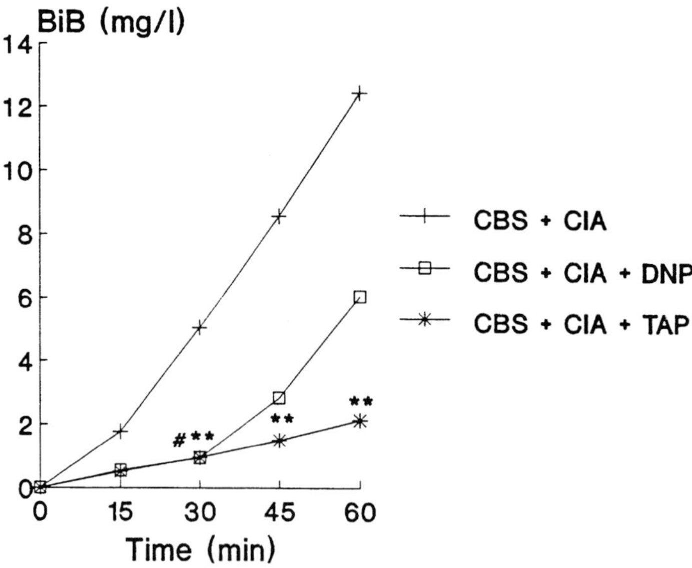

Figure 2
Effects of TAP and DNP on the absorption of Bi from CBS with added citrate (CBS+CIA) over a period of 60 min. TAP; **; $p<0.01$; DNP; #; $p<0.05$.

Metal Ions in Biology and Medicine; vol 6. Eds. J.A. Centeno, Ph. Collery, G. Vernet, R.B. Finkelman, H. Gibb, J.C. Etienne. John Libbey Eurotext, Paris © 2000, pp. 531-533.

Hydroponic cultivation of metal accumulating plants as a source of mineral nutrient supplements

Burt D. Ensley, Mark P. Elless, Michael J. Blaylock, Jianwei W. Huang and John R. Benemann

NuCycle Therapy, Inc., 1 Deer Park Drive, Suite M, Monmouth Junction, NJ 08852

The body requires major and minor minerals to maintain good health. Fresh fruits and vegetables are good sources of vitamins, but contain relatively low levels of essential minerals. Even vegetables believed to be high in mineral content usually do not provide adequate dietary concentrations when consumed in normal sized portions.

Screening studies have recently identified cultivars of Indian mustard (Brassica juncea), an edible plant, that accumulate large amounts of various elements in their above ground biomass under certain cultivation conditions. In some cases the trace element concentrations exceed 1% of the plant dry weight, and generally are over two orders of magnitude higher than typical mineral concentrations in conventional edible plants. These discoveries have raised for the first time the possibility that plants can be used as a concentrated form of essential mineral nutritional supplements. The form of the mineral in the plants can also offer a potential benefit, since the bioavailability, or amount of mineral taken up and utilized by the body, can be modified depending on the mineral source. Although plant components such as phytates can interfere with mineral uptake by the body, plants are generally considered to be superior sources of supplements.

The bioavailability of select minerals in the mineral enriched plant tissues was measured in vitro through two independent procedures. One involved a series of sequential extractions [1] that is used to assess bioavailability of trace metals in solid media [2]. The procedure uses increasingly stringent extractants to characterize the solubility (water soluble, acid soluble, reducible, oxidizable, residual) of trace elements in a given matrix. The second procedure utilizes simulated gastric fluid to predict the solubility of the metal in the stomach [3]. These analyses measure the solubilization of the minerals from the plant tissue but not absorption as defined for bioavailability [4]; however, minerals must be in a soluble form before taken up or used by the body.

The nutritional minerals Cr, Fe, Mn, Se, Zn accumulated by the Brassica plants were found to be easily solubilized by the sequential extraction procedure (Table 1). More than 80%, and in most cases 100% of the total mineral content in the enriched plants was solubilized by the sequential extraction method. Each of these five plant bound minerals was found to be much more soluble than those in an over-the-counter multivitamin tested in the same procedure, suggesting that a plant based source of these minerals produces a more available mineral form compared to the form of minerals found in popular commercial supplements.

Table 1. Solubility of Fe, Zn, Cr, Mn, and Se based on sequential extraction of trace mineral enriched B. juncea plants compared with a common trace element/multivitamin supplement.

Supplement	Metal	Water-Soluble	Acid-Soluble	Reducible	Oxidizable	Residual
-------------------% of total metal concentration-------------------						
B. juncea	Cr	76.95a	13.30a	3.06a	3.94a	2.74a
Multivitamin I		0.00b	0.00b	0.00b	0.00b	100.00b
B. juncea	Fe	47.85a	19.10a	16.91a	3.41a	12.71a
Multivitamin I		1.82b	0.10b	1.36b	0.21b	96.51b
B. juncea	Mn	87.14a	12.38a	0.28a	0.16a	0.04a
Multivitamin I		67.81a	15.31b	15.55b	0.73b	0.59b
B. juncea	Se	93.91a	3.63a	0.35a	1.84a	0.27a
Multivitamin I		0.00b	0.00b	100.00b	0.00b	0.00b
B. juncea	Zn	92.10a	7.41a	0.37a	0.06a	0.05a
Multivitamin I		3.73b	19.06b	64.96b	5.57b	6.68b

Results of the simulated gastric fluid digestion confirm the data obtained from the sequential extraction study. Simulated gastric fluid extracted 31% of the total Fe in the plant sample and 81%, 69%, 100%, and 100% of the total Cr, Mn, Se, and Zn, respectively. The high solubility of these metals in the enriched plant material produced RDI values significantly greater than those found in commercially available supplements.

Simulated intestinal fluid digestion studies showed that the solubility of the commercial supplements decreased in comparison to their behavior in the gastric fluid digestion whereas the metals within the enriched plant matter remained soluble. It is believed that the high pH of the intestinal fluid precipitates cationic metals that were soluble in the acidic simulated gastric fluid as oxyhydroxides, whereas cationic metals associated with the plant matter are apparently chelated with organic complexes which prevents their precipitation. Solubility of these metals in the enriched plant material produced soluble-based %RDI values significantly greater than those of commercially available supplements. The high total mineral concentrations in the plant biomass coupled with a high degree of solubility in both the simulated gastric and intestinal fluid supports the use of these plants as mineral supplements.

The low solubility displayed in this study of Cr, Fe, Mn, Se, and Zn in several leading nutritional supplements clearly shows a need for a supplement that supplies greater available levels of these minerals for absorption to attain the recommended daily intake (RDI), not only in total metal form, but in a soluble form. For example, the multivitamins tested in this study contain 100% of the RDI for Fe and Zn; however, only a maximum of 9% and 8% of the RDI for Fe and Zn, respectively, were solubilized by simulated gastric fluid. Because eventual absorption of the metals by the body requires the metals to be soluble, achieving the 100% RDI criterion by total metal content alone is insufficient to meet daily nutritional requirements.

Bioavailability requires solubility, absorption, and eventual metabolism by the body. Even though solubility in stomach acid is important for digestion of food intake, metals must remain soluble in the intestinal fluid before absorption can occur. Soluble ions, not solid precipitates, are required for absorption. The poor performance of the mineral-based supplements, particularly the multivitamins, in providing the metals in soluble form in the intestinal fluid simulant clearly shows that these supplements do not provide their metals in bioavailable form. The enriched plant matter can provide intestinal fluid soluble Cr, Mn, Se, and Zn at levels that exceed at least 50% of each metal's respective RDI in as little as 0.25 g of plant material, thereby providing a bioavailable source of these metals.

1. Ramos, L., Hernandez, L.M., and Gonzalez, M.J. Sequential extraction of copper, lead, cadmium, and zinc in soils from or near Donana National Park. Journal of Environmental Quality 1994. 23:50-57.
2. Berti, W., Cunningham, S.D., and Jacobs, L.W. Sequential chemical extraction of trace elements: Development and use in remediating contaminated soils. Proc. 3rd International Conference on Biogeochemistry of Trace Elements. 1995.
3. Glahn, R.P., Lai, C., Hsu, J., Thompson, J.F., Guo, M., and Van Campen, D.R. Decreased citrate improves iron availability from infant formula: application of an in-vitro digestion/Caca-2 cell culture model. Journal of Nutrition. 1998. 128:257-264.
4. Newman, M.C. and Jagoe, C.H. Ligands and the bioavailability of metals in aquatic environments. in Bioavailability: Physical, Chemical, and Biological Interactions, Hamelick, J.L., Landrum, P.F., Bergman, H.L., and Benson, W.H., eds. CRC Press, Lewis Publishers, Boca Raton, FL. 1994.Pages 39-61

Metal Ions in Biology and Medicine; vol 6. Eds. J.A. Centeno, Ph. Collery, G. Vernet, R.B. Finkelman, H. Gibb, J.C. Etienne. John Libbey Eurotext, Paris © 2000, pp. 534-536.

Activation of phagocytic cells and inflammatory response during experimental magnesium deficiency

Y. Rayssiguier, F. Bussière, C. Malpuech-Brugère, E. Rock, A. Mazur

Centre de Recherche en Nutrition Humaine, INRA, Unité Maladies Métaboliques et Micronutriments, Theix 63122 St-Genès-Champanelle, France

Abstract

Weanling male Wistar rats were fed either a Mg-deficient or control diet for 8 days. Mg deficiency results in polymorphonuclear neutrophil and macrophage activation, hyperreactivity of immune cells, excessive production of free radical, and inflammatory cytokines. The effect of various Mg concentrations on reactive oxygen species production was investigated in vitro. Increasing concentration of Mg was shown to attenuate neutrophils respiratory burst. These studies suggest the importance of the inflammatory response in experimental Mg deficiency. Moreover, pharmacological concentrations of Mg may have a beneficial anti-inflammatory effect.

Magnesium plays an essential role in fundamental cellular reactions and the importance of the immuno-inflammatory processes in the pathology of Mg deficiency has been recently reconsidered (1-2). In 1932, Kruse and coworkers (3) reported peripheral vasodilatation with hyperemia as a part of symptoms caused by Mg deficiency in rats. Thereafter many investigators have recognized the same symptoms in relation with degranulation of mast cells with a release of histamine and inflammatory mediators. This inflammatory response has been proposed to be responsible for oxidative damage in Mg deficiency but the underlying mechanism is unknown (4).

Weanling male Wistar rats were fed either a Mg-deficient diet or a control diet for 8 days. The present study confirms the occurrence of an inflammatory response in Mg deficiency (5) (peripheral vasodilatation, leucocytosis, increase in IL 6 plasma levels and rises in plasma levels of acute phase proteins).

When peritoneal cells were isolated by peritoneal washes with saline, the mean number of macrophages recovered in Mg-deficient animals was significantly higher than in control rats. To measure the respiratory burst of macrophages, chemiluminescence was monitored. Chemiluminescent activity of resident macrophages from Mg-deficient rats was higher than that of control rats. After in vitro phorbol myristate acetate (PMA) stimulation, chemiluminescent activity of macrophages from Mg-deficient rats was 4-fold higher as compared to cells from control rats, and superoxide generation was markedly increased in the same way. Together, these results indicate that in Mg-deficient rats, macrophages are metabolically stimulated (5).

Basal chemiluminescence activity or polymorphonuclear neutrophils (PMN) from Mg-deficient rats was 8-fold higher than that of cells from control rats. Moreover, superoxide anion production following PMA or opsonized zymosan activation was higher in neutrophils from Mg-deficient as compared to control rats. Thus, PMN from Mg-deficient rats are activated endogenously and are further stimulated by PMA or zymosan challenge. The inflammatory response in Mg-deficient rats suggested that Mg deficiency might be accompanied by the activation of inflammatory cells. Accordingly, Mg deficiency results in macrophage and neutrophil activation (6).

Since the cellular Mg content is tightly regulated and changes only slightly even when the extracellular concentration is drastically decreased, total intracellular Mg is probably unaffected in these experimental conditions. Thus, the effect of Mg deficiency may be induced by the reduction of the extracellular Mg^{2+} concentration. The effect of various Mg concentrations on reactive oxygen species production was investigated in vitro. Increasing concentration of Mg was shown to attenuate neutrophils respiratory burst. High levels of Mg (8 mM) as compared to physiological concentration (0.8 mM) reduced the superoxide anion production following zymosan activation by 50% in PMN from both control and deficient animals. Similar observations were made using human PMN following formyl-methionyl-leucyl-phenylalanine (fMLP) stimulated superoxide anion (6). Thus, experimental Mg deficiency results in activation of phagocytic cells and high concentrations of Mg inhibit the rate of superoxide anion formation. The pathophysiological response to the immune stress includes activation of several processes which are dependent on cytosolic Ca^{2+} elevation. Since Mg frequently acts as a natural Ca antagonist, additional studies are needed to determine if the proinflammatory effect of Mg deficiency is the consequence of a reduced extracellular $Mg^{2+}/Ca2^{+}$ antagonism resulting in increased intracellular free Ca^{2+} concentration.

These studies suggest the importance of the inflammatory response in Mg deficiency. There is ample evidence correlating Mg deficiency and cardiovascular diseases. Inflammatory may be of special importance since atherosclerosis starts as an inflammatory immunological disease. Defects in lipoprotein metabolism, inflammatory cell recruitement, macrophage activation, oxidative modification of lipoproteins, release of growth factors and cytokines that cause cell migration and proliferation have been described in the same experimental model (7).

References

1. Weglicki WB, Phillips TM. Pathobiology of magnesium deficiency: a cytokine/neurogenic inflammation hypothesis. *Am J Clin* 1992; 263: R734-R737.

2. Malpuech-Brugère C, Nowacki W, Rock E, Gueux E, Mazur A, Rayssiguier Y. Enhanced tumor necrosis factor α production following endotoxin challenge in rats is an early event during magnesium deficiency. *Biochim Biophys Acta* 1999; 1453: 35-40.

3. Kruse HD, Orent ER, McCollum EV. Studies on magnesium deficiency in animals. I. Symptomatology resulting from magnesium deprivation. *J Biol Chem* 1932; 96: 519-539.

4. Rayssiguier Y, Gueux E, Bussière L, Durlach J, Mazur A. Dietary magnesium affects susceptibility of lipoproteins and tissues to peroxidation in rats. *J Am Coll Nutr* 1993; 12: 133-137.

5. Malpuech-Brugère C, Nowacki W, Daveau M, Gueux E, Linard C, Rock E, Lebreton JP, Mazur A, Rayssiguier Y. Inflammatory response following acute magnesium deficiency in the rat. *Biochim Biophys Acta* 2000; in press.

6. Bussière F, Tridon A, Malpuech-Brugère C, Rock E, Mazur A, Rayssiguier Y. Effect of magnesium on the production of reactive oxygen species by neutrophils. (abstract). *Magnesium Res* 2000; in press.

7. Rayssiguier Y, Mazur A, Gueux E, Rock E. Magnesium deficiency affects lipid metabolism and atherosclerosis process by mechanism involving inflammation and oxidative stress. In: Halpern MJ, Durlach J eds, *Current Research in Magnesium*. London: John Libbey, 1996, 251-255.

Metal Ions in Biology and Medicine; vol 6. Eds. J.A. Centeno, Ph. Collery, G. Vernet, R.B. Finkelman, H. Gibb, J.C. Etienne. John Libbey Eurotext, Paris © 2000, pp. 537-539.

Screening of copper status in cattle and supplementation studies with coordination compounds

Eduardo Kremer[1], María H. Torre[1], Inés Viera[1], Gianella Facchin[1], Alicia Cuevas[1], Enrique J. Baran[2], Juan Bussi[3], Mauricio Ohanian[3], Julio Irigoyen[4], Teresita Porochin[4], Verónica DiDonato[4], Carlos Irigoyen[4], Juan Romero[4]

[1] *Química Inorgánica, Facultad de Química, Uruguay;* [2] *CEQUINOR, Facultad de Ciencias Exactas, UNLP, Argentina;* [3] *Instituto de Química, Facultad de Ingeniería;* [4] *Facultad de Veterinaria, Regional Norte; Universidad de la República, Uruguay*

Abstract

Several copper complexes with essential aminoacids were prepared and characterized. They were administered subcutaneously in a propilenglycol suspension to dairy cattle. CuPhe proved the most effective in copper supplementation.

Introduction

Copper is the third most abundant transition metal in mammals and a great number of metalloproteins containing this metal have already been identified. Research has shown that clinical signs of Cu deficiency seldom occur until the body's Cu reserves are depleted and a biochemical dysfunction has been created. In cattle, low weight, fertility and immunity, along with lack of pigmentation in fur and decrease of milk production are common signs of Cu deficiency [1]. Uruguay is a country where cattle production is economically important and is classified as copper deficient according to Mc Dowell and Conrad. So, copper supplementation becomes necessary. Coordination compounds of this metal can be appropriate sources to restore copper levels. In this work essential aminoacids were chosen as ligands because they are known to intervene in copper transport. Moreover, the resultant complexes have good thermodynamic stability. Field experiences with cattle were necessary to determine the activity of these compounds. Both studies of the complexes and field experiences made possible to get closer to determine structure-activity relationships (SAR).

Experimental Procedure

Copper complexes with glycine (CuGly), alanine (CuAla), valine (CuVal), leucine (CuLeu), isoleucine (CuIle) and phenylalanine (CuPhe) were synthesized as described in [2] using Sigma reagents.

They were characterized analytically, by means of copper dosification (iodometry) and elemental analysis of the other components, and structurally by means of IR spectroscopy using a Bomem FTIR (MB Series) with KBr pellets.

Lipophilicity tests were performed determining the partition coefficient of the complexes in physiological solution/n-octanol [3].
Injectables for cattle containing CuGly, CuVal and CuPhe were prepared as suspension in propilenglycol under aseptic conditions. The dose of copper in them was 100 mg Cu/ 5 mL and they were administered subcutaneously into the side of the neck. A total of nineteen animals of Holando breed (including an untreated control group) were used in field experiences.
The effect of parenteral copper supplementation was evaluated analyzing blood samples for Cu in serum and assessing corporal status monthly.
Blood serum was analyzed for total Cu using atomic absorption spectrometry on a Shimadzu AA6401 equipped with HCl CuL233 lamp and air/acethylene flame. The sample reference and serum are diluted 1/6 per cent 1-butanol. The mixture is nebulized directly in the flame. Calibration was performed by standard addition methods with copper reference solution (High Purity Standards, 1000 +/-3 μg/mL in 2% HNO_3)
Corporal status was assessed by veterinarians according to scale ranging from 1 to 5, and includes evaluation of muscular status and subcutaneous fat.

Results and discussion

The complexes synthesized responded to the following stoichiometries: $Cu(Gly)_2.H_2O$, $Cu(Ala)_2$, $Cu(Val)_2$, $Cu(Leu)_2$, $Cu(Ile)_2.H_2O$ and $Cu(Phe)_2$. Yield and purity were adequate to be used as injectables (yield > 90%, purity > 98.5%).
The spectra of all complexes showed coordination of copper to the N and O atoms of the aminoacids. The Cu-ligand vibrations were found in the expected spectral ranges, indicating the *cis* arrangement for CuGly and CuIle and *trans* for the rest of the complexes.
The result of the lipophilicity assays shows that this property increases with an increase in ligand complexity. LogK for CuGly, CuVal and CuPhe are –1.30, -1.10 and -0.09 respectively.
Field Experience 1.
Mean concentration of copper in serum ($[Cu]_{serum}$) was plotted against time (Figure 1) for cattle injected once at day 0 with different copper preparations. CuPhe seems to be adequate for copper supplementation: increases significantly $[Cu]_{serum}$ immediately after injection, taking and keeping it over that of the control group in the long term. CuVal seems to have no effect, there is no significant difference of $[Cu]_{serum}$ level reached with that of the control group. CuGly plot varies in the same way as that of the control group, but $[Cu]_{serum}$ level is way below that of the control group, most of the time under normal levels. So, efficiency in supplementation seems to be in direct relation with lipophilicity of the complexes.

Figure.1 Mean concentration of copper in serum ($[Cu]_{serum}$) versus time

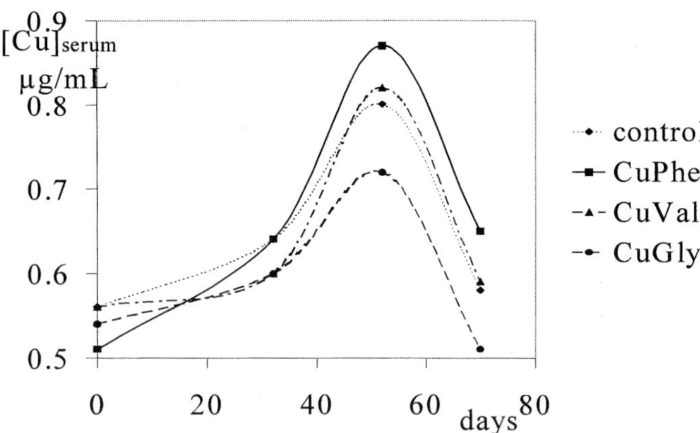

Field Experience 2.

Mean concentration of copper in serum and corporal status were reported against time for cattle injected once at day 0 and then again at day 75 with CuPhe. It can be observed in Table I that the treatment increases $[Cu]_{serum}$ and keeps it within normal values [1] for a good part of the year.

Table I. Mean concentration of copper in serum.

Days	0	34	47	62	75	123	160	204
$[Cu]_{serum}$ (μg/mL) treated	0.57	0.70	0.72	0.73	0.68	0.70	0.65	0.49
$[Cu]_{serum}$ (μg/mL) untreated	0.56	0.60	0.60	0.58	Died			
Corporal status treated	3.2	4.4						
Corporal status untreated	2.3	3.0						

In conclusion, CuPhe increases rapidly and effectively $[Cu]_{serum}$ in dairy cattle.

Acknowledgements

This work is part of a joint research project of Montevideo and Salto (Uruguay) and La Plata (Argentina), under the auspices of the two Universities. The Uruguayan group thanks also CONICYT (grant 3009) for support.

References

[1]Smart M E, Cymbaluk N F, Christensen D A. A review of copper status of cattle in Canada and recomendations for supplementation. *Can Vet J* 1992; 33 163-170.

[2]Szabó-Planka T. Metal ion coordination in policrystalline copper (II) complexes of α-aminoacids. *Acta Chim Hung* 1985; 120 (2) 143-151.

[3]Tortaro R M, Apella M C, Torre M H, Friet E, Viera I, Kremer E, Baran E J. Evaluation of Superoxide Dismutate-Like Activity in Some Copper (II) Complexes of Aminoacids. *Acta Farm Bonaerense* 1993; 12 (2) 73-78.

Metal Ions in Biology and Medicine; vol 6. Eds. J.A. Centeno, Ph. Collery, G. Vernet, R.B. Finkelman, H. Gibb, J.C. Etienne. John Libbey Eurotext, Paris © 2000, pp. 540-543.

Assessment of chromium (Cr) content in daily food rations used for alimentation of soldiers serving in air cavalry units in Poland

J. Bertrandt, A. Kłos, E. Stężycka

Military Institute of Hygiene and Epidemiology, 4 Kozielska St., 01-163 Warsaw, Poland

Introduction

Chromium occurs in nature mainly as trivalent chromium compounds, which are the most Cr indissoluble form, or as a Cr^{6+} which compounds reveals strong oxidising action. Chromium is one of microelements which delivery with food is necessary to keep a good health state. In human nutrition Cr has long been recognised as an essential trace element, required for normal metabolism of carbohydrates, proteins and lipids and as active component of glucose tolerance factor (GTF). Huge shortage of trivalent chromium among adults may be the reason of diabetes type II and other cardiovascular system disease occurrence [1]. It was found that trivalent chromium deficiency may create many disease symptoms as impaired glucose tolerance, fasting hyperglicemia, glycosuria, hypoglycemia, elevated circulating insulin, decreased insulin receptor number, decreased insulin binding, decreased lean body mass, elevated per cent body fat, abnormal nitrogen metabolism and many others [2]. Cr presence in the biological active form increases sensitivity of organism's cells on insulin at the some time decreases the level of insulin circulating in blood [3,4]. Positive influence of Cr^{3+} administration on glucose level decrease in blood of people suffering from diabetes was found [5]. Chromium plays very important part in lipid metabolism. Administration of chromium preparations to the people suffering from atherosclerosis causes increase of cholesterol in HDL [6] and decrease of triglyceride and whole cholesterol value in blood serum of people at advanced age [7,8,9]. Researches on chromium content in blood serum of people suffering from hyperlipidemia showed chromium low level analogous as among diabetics [10,11]. At present it is assumed that estimated safe and adequate daily dietary intake (ESADDI) of chromium for adults is 50 – 200 µg/d [12] but the normal intake by woman is 50 – 60% of 50 µg/d (25 –30 µg/d) [11]. The World Health Organisation has recommended a basal Cr intake needed to prevent pathologically relevant and clinically detectable signs of impaired function to be 25 µg/d and 23 µg daily to maintain a level of tissue storage [13]. Results of many researches on chromium intake together with food revealed its smaller content than ESADDI value. Cr intake with food in the USA and other countries is very low and makes 50 to 60% of minimum ESADDI value [14]. According to Anderson typical American diet delivers 33 µg Cr daily to men and 25 µg to women [1]. Chromium content in food rations used for alimentation of breast-feeding women was 41µg/d [15], whole new-borns' breast-fed got only 0.13 µg/d with mothers' milk [16]. Low Cr content with daily food rations was found also in England [17], Finland [18,19] and in Canada [20].

The aim of work

The aim of work was to estimate the chromium consumption in daily food ration used for alimentation of soldiers serving in the Polish Army air cavalry units.

Materials and methods

Chromium content was estimated in 50 daily food rations taken in winter, spring and autumn seasons. Assessment of Cr content was done after samples dry mineralisation in 550^0 C. Indication was done by atomic spectrometry absorption method on spectrophotometer Pye Unicam 9 directly from the solution got from the samples burn to ashes and dissolved in hydrochloric acid, using the background correction by deuteride lamp [21].

Results

It was found, that average chromium content in daily food ration was 220.0 ± 77.6 µg, and ranged from 120.7 µg to 319.4 µg. Differences in Cr depending on the season were found but there were not statistically significant relating to samples taken in winter and spring. The highest Cr content was indicated in food rations taken for examination in the winter season – 294.8 ± 96.5 µg and spring – 240.4 ± 59.9 µg while during autumn its content was lower and indicated 135.4 ± 66.0 µg.

Figure1 presents contents of chromium in daily food ration in different seasons of the year.

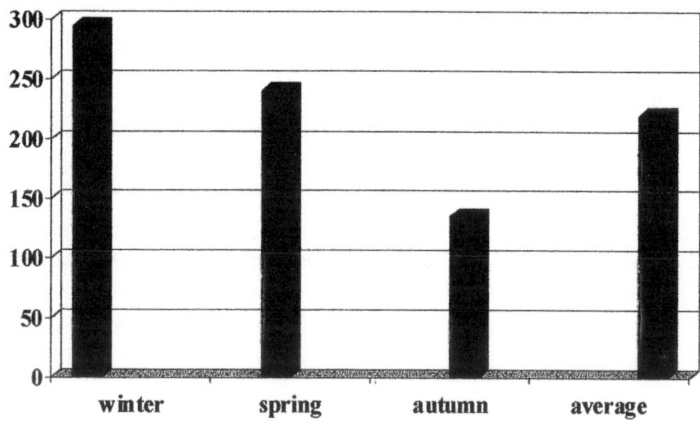

Figure 1. Content of chromium in daily food rations depends on year season (in µg).

Discussion

Available published figures show small chromium content in daily food rations used for human alimentation what does not meet the requirements for this trace element [1,15,16,17,18,20,19]. Results obtained during our researches indicate huge Cr content in food rations that are significantly higher than ESADDI value for adults. Results of our previous studies concerning chromium content in daily food rations, planned for consumption for people at advanced age, showed Cr intake of 118.5 µg together with meal [22]. Results of other investigations showed that requirements for chromium in children nutrition were met in the kindergartens in Warsaw [23]. Researches on Cr intake in food rations used for workers and non workers families alimentation performed in 5 big cities in Poland showed its content of 65 – 187 µg and were included in US National Academy of Science recommended norms of 50 – 200 µg [24]. Results of other studies, performed in Poland by Rutkowska at all, indicate high chromium intake with diet, often exceeding 100 µg [25]. Chromium content in food rations in Hungary is also comparatively high and indicates in average 100µg/d [26].

Chromium intake together with food differs very much and depends on product source of animal protein. Beef or liver includes high chromium content while fish low amounts.

Analysed food rations were typical for soldiers' nutrition and contained bigger amounts of meat and meat products in comparison to civilian diet. It may explain significantly higher Cr intake in food rations used for soldiers' nutrition.

Indicated the higher chromium contents in food rations taken for examination during winter and spring season should be related to significantly higher frequency of cooked, reach in meat and its products, with a high calorie content meals.

Analysing Cr content in daily food rations it should be taken into consideration that only the meals given for consumption were examined. Chromium presence in meals is a sum of its content in food products and contamination resulted from used of chromium plated kitchen utensils.

Compared to world-wide information results of our researches on chromium content show significantly higher content what is included in the recommended norms or is even higher but not twice more.

Conclusions

1. Huge range of obtained results of Cr content in meals shows great difference of its content in raw material and food products.
2. Food rations used for soldiers' serving in the Polish Army air cavalry units alimentation met the requirements for chromium intake and did not create any threat of to big content.

Acknowledgments

This study was supported by a Research Grant No 148/115C-TOO96 "Żywienie" from National Scientific Research Committee (KBN) in Poland

References

1. Anderson RA, Kozlovsky AS. Chromium intake, absorption and excretion of subjects consuming self-selected diets. *Am J. Clin Nutr* 1985; 41:1177-1183.
2. Anderson RA. Stress effects on chromium nutrition of humans and farm animals. In *Biotechnology in the Fed Industry. Proceedings of Alltech's Tenth Symposium.* Nottingham: Univ. Press, 1994: 267 – 274.
3. Mertz W. Chromium in human nutrition: a review. *J Nutr* 1993; 123:626–633.
4. Anderson RA. Chromium, glucose tolerance, diabetes and lipid metabolism. *J Advancement Med* 1995; 8:37-49.
5. Mossop RT. Effects of chromium (III) on fasting glucose, cholesterol and cholesterol HDL levels in diabetics. *Cent Afr J Med* 1983; 29:80-82.
6. Abraham AS, Brooks BA, Eylath U. The effects of chromium supplementation on serum glucose and lipids in patients with and without non-insulin-dependent diabetes. *Metabolism* 1992; 41:768-771.
7. Doisy RJ, Streeten DHP, Freiberg JM, Shneider AJ. Chromium metabolism in man and biochemical effects. In *Trace Elements in Human Health and Disease. Vol II. Essential and Toxic elements.* New York: Academic Press, 1976: 79-104.
8. Offenbacher EG, Pi-Sunyer FX. Beneficial effect of chromium-richyeast on glucose tolerance and blood lipids and elderly subjects. *Diabetes* 1980; 29:919-925.
9. Riales R, Albrink MJ. Effect of chromium chloride supplementation on glucose tolerance in serum lipids including high-density lipoprotein of adult men. *Am J Clin Nutr* 1981; 34:2670-2678.
10. Zima T, Mestek O, Tesar V, Tesarova P, Nemecek K, Zak A, Zeman M. Chromium levels in patients with internal diseases. *Biochem Mol Biol International* 1998; 46:365-374.

11.Ding W, Chai Z, Duan P, Feng W, Qian Q. Serum and urine chromium concentrations in elderly diabetics. *Biological Trace Element Research* 1998; 63:231-237.
12.National Research Council. *Recommended dietary allowances.* Washington. National Academy Press, 1989: 241-243.
13.World Health Organisation. Chromium. In *Trace Elements in Human Nutrition and Health.* Geneva. Macmillian Ceuterick Press, 1996: 155-160.
14.Anderson RA. Nutritional factors influencing the glucose/insulin system: chromium. *J Am Coll Nutr* 1997; 26 S35-S41.
15.Anderson RA, Bryden NA, Patterson KY, Veillon C, Andon MB, Moser-Veilon PB. Breast milk chromium and its association with chromium intake, chromium excretion, and serum chromium. *Am J Clin Nutr* 1993; 57:519-523.
16.Mohamedshah FY, Moser-Veilon PB, Yamini S, Douglass LW, Anderson RA, Veilon C. Distribution of the stable isotope of (^{53}Cr) in serum, urine and breast milk in lactating women. *Am J Clin Nutr* 1998; 67:1950-1955.
17.Bunker VW, Lawson MS, Delves HT, Clayton BE. The uptake and excretion of chromium by the elderly. *Am J Clin Nutr* 1984; 39:797-802.
18.Koivistoinen P. Mineral element composition of Finnish foods: N, K, Ca, Mg, P, S, Fe, Cu, Mn, Zn, Mo, Co, Ni, F, Se, Si, Rb, Al., B, Br, Hg, As, Cd, Pb and Ash. *Acta Agric Scand* 1980; 22:37-160.
19.Kumpulainen J, Vuori E. The low chromium content of Finnish diets compared to diets in other countries. *XII International Congress of Nutrition, Abstracts.* San Diego 1981:197.
20.Gibson RS, Scythes CA. Chromium Selenium and other trace element intakes of a selected sample of Canadian premenopausal women. *J Biol Trace Elem Res* 1984; 6:105-116.
21.Buliński R, Marzec Z. Badania zawartości niektórych pierwiastków śladowych w produktach spożywczych krajowego pochodzenia. Cz. II. Zawartość chromu i niklu w zbożach grochu i fasoli. *Chem Toksykol* 1983; 16:53.
22.Bertrandt J, Kłos A, Dębski B, Zalewski W. Chromium content of daily food rations used for alimentation of elders. *International Symposium on the Health Effects of Dietary Chromium, Abstracts.* Dedham 1998:19.
23. Bertrandt J, Kłos A, Dębski B, Zalewski W. Chromium content of daily food rations for children in kindergartens. *International Symposium on the Health Effects of Dietary Chromium, Abstracts.* Dedham 1998:20.
24.Marzec Z, Buliński R. Wartość odżywcza całodziennych racji pokarmowych odtwarzanych w kilku regionach kraju. Cz. VII. Ocena pobrania kobaltu, chromu, niklu i selenu. *Roczn PZH* 1992; XLIII:135-138.
25.Rutkowska U, Buliński R, Iwanow K, Marzec z, Kunachowicz H, Trzebska-Jeske I. Laboratoryjna ocena wartości odżywczej przecietnych całodziennych racji pokarmowych wybranych grup ludności w Polsce. *Roczn PZH* 1987; XXXVIII:121-125.
26.Lindner-Szotyori K, Gergely A. Uber die versorgung der Ungarischen Bevolkerung mit einigen wichtigen Spurenelementen. *Die Nachrung* 1980:24:829.

Metal Ions in Biology and Medicine; vol 6. Eds. J.A. Centeno, Ph. Collery, G. Vernet, R.B. Finkelman, H. Gibb, J.C. Etienne. John Libbey Eurotext, Paris © 2000, pp. 544-546.

Application of a metal-chelating protein, phosvitin to the establishment of safe food system

Masayuki Gotoh[1], Soichiro Nakamura[2], Yasuhide Gohya[1], and Tatuya Hobara[3]

[1] Department of Environmental Science, Ube College, Ube, Japan 755-8550; [2] Department of Living Science, Shimane University, Matsue, Japan 690-8504; [3] School of Medicine, Yamaguchi University, Ube, Japan 755-8505

ABSTRACT - A metal-chelating protein, egg yolk phosvitin was conjugated with galactomannan through a controlled Maillard reaction under the dry-heating at 60 °C in 79% relative humidity for one week. Antioxidant activity and antimicrobial effect against *Escherichia coli* were significantly enhanced by the covalent binding of the polysaccharide with an elevation of the emulsifying activity of the protein.

INTRODUCTION

Since food-poisoning frequently occurs throughout the year and causes serious results, harmless agents have been sought for natural compounds for food safety. In this study, a new type of macromolecular antioxidant with a wide antimicrobial effect was tried to produce from a metal-chelating protein, phosvitin, that has been identified as an iron carrier in egg yolk, with as much as 95% of iron in yolk bound to phosvitin due to high phospholylation properties. The iron binding strength is extremely strong, phosvitin could therefore be used as a potent natural antioxidant on the basis of its potential to inhibit metal-catalyzed lipid oxidation.

Besides, the polyanionic and chelating behavior of phosvitin could recall us that the natural protein has a potential of applying for a bacteriostatic agent such as EDTA. Phosvitin could cause the increase of permeability and loss of cellular constituents, resulting in inactivating, destroying genetic materials and finally killing bacteria.

This study reveals that phosvitin has a significant antimicrobiological action against *Escherichia coli*, in addition to antioxidant effect.

MATERIALS AND METHODS

Materials - Phosvitin was prepared from hen egg yolk according to the method of Mecham and Olcott[1)]. Galactomannan, a mannase hydrolysate of guar gum, was supplied from Taiyo Chemicals Co. (Japan). All chemicals used were analytical grade.

Preparation of phosvitin-galactomannan conjugate - Phosvitin was dissolved in water with galactomannan in the weight ratio of 1:3. Lyophilized mixture was incubated at 60 °C for one week under the relative humidity of 79%.

Antioxidative assay in model system- Celite was treated with nitrohydrochloric acid for 1 week, and subsequently washed with deionized water until disappearing chlorinity reaction. The purified celite used as a food model matrix was mixed in water with phosvitin samples and freeze-dried in a given weight ratio. The resulting powder was mixed with methyl linoleate in the weight ratio of 3:1. Four grams of the powder food model was put into a petri dish with diameter of 9 cm, incubated at 20 °C. Lipid oxidation in the model system was monitored by measuring peroxide value (POV).

Antibacterial Assay - Sample was added to the 10^6 cells/mL *Escherichia coli* K12 suspension to give a final protein concentration of 0.1%. Five mL of the suspension was incubated at 50 °C for 40 min. After a given incubating time, suspensions were immediately added to a sterile tube immersed in an ice bath. A 100 mL portion was spread over MacConkey agar (Difco, Detroit, MI) plates. The number of colonies formed after incubation at 35 °C for 24h was measured to calculate the survival ratio.

Measurement of Emulsifying Properties - An emulsion was prepared by homogenization of 1.0 mL of corn oil and 3 ml of a 0.1% sample solution, using an Ultra Turrax (Hansen & Co., West Germany) at 12,000 rpm for 1 min at 20 °C. A 100μL portion of emulsion was taken from the bottom of the test tube at a given standing time, and diluted with 5 ml of 0.1 % sodium dodecyl sulfate solution. The turbidity of diluted emulsion was then determined at 500 nm.

RESULTS AND DISCUSSION

Metal chelating behavior of phosvitin - Binding capacity of metal ions to phosvitin was assessed using atomic absorption spectrophotometry. 0.1% phosvitin indicated chelating effect of 91.8% for Fe^{3+}, 74.8% for Ca^{2+}, 48.4% for Mg^{2+} at pH 7.5, respectively. The chelating abilities were not deteriorated after conjugation with galactomannan.

Antioxidative activity of phosvitin-galactomannan conjugate - The inhibition effect of hosvitin-galactomannan conjugate on metal-induced lipid oxidation was investigated using Fe^{2+}-supplemented powdered model food system. The extent of lipid oxidation with higher concentration of Fe^{2+} was effectively inhibited by the conjugate (Fig.1). The antioxidant activity of the conjugate was 1.3-1.4 times stronger than that of the phosvitin-galactoman-

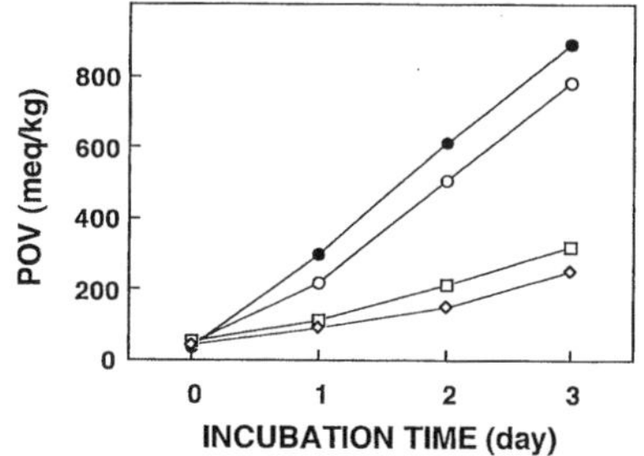

Fig.1. Antioxidative effect on Fe^{2+}-catalyzed oxidation in the power oil model system: (●)10mg/L Fe^{2+}; (○)1mg/L Fe^{2+}, both without phosvitin; (□)0.1% mixture with 1mg/L Fe^{2+}; (◇)0.1% conjugate with 1mg/L Fe^{2+}.

nan mixture. We hypothesize that the galactomannan segment of the phosvitin-galactomannan conjugate macromolecule assisted with the configuration of phosphoseryl residues of the phosvitin segment to interact with Fe^{2+} where chelation reaction occur in the microenvironment and thus contributed in part to reducing the initiation reaction of lipid peroxidation.

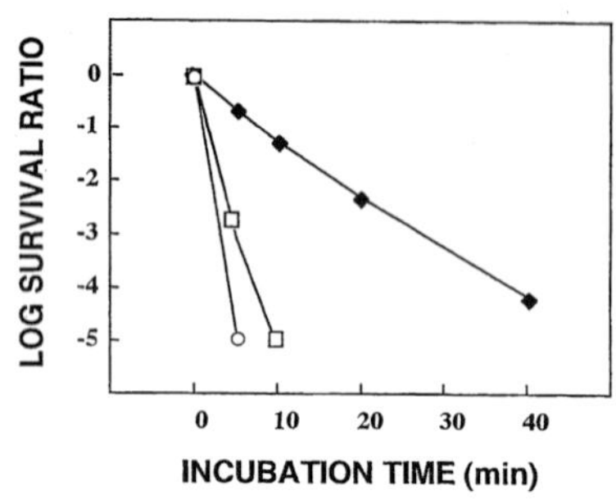

Fig.2. Bacterial effect against *E. coli* at 50°C: (◆) control; (□) 0.1% phosvitin-galactomannan mixture; (○) 0.1% phossvitin-galactomannan conjugate.

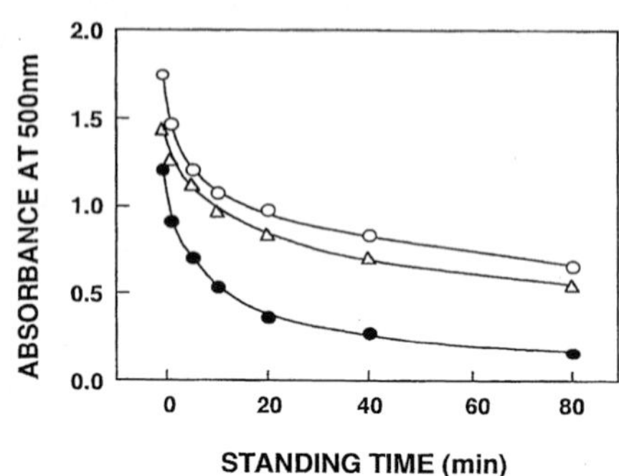

Fig.3. Emulsifying properties in 0.1M phosphate buffer, pH7.4: (●)0.1% mixture; (○)0.1% conjugate; (△)0.01% conjugate.

Bactericidal effect against *Escherichia coli* - Fig.2 shows antimicrobial effect of phosvitin-galactomannan conjugate against *Escherichia coli.* One million cells completely disappeared in 1 mL of L-broth coexisting with 0.1% phosvitin-galactomannan conjugate when incubated at 50 °C for 10 min, where 10 cells were survived with 0.1% phosvitin-galactomannan mixture. The potent bactericidal action at 50 °C was followed by cell disruption with the leakage of intracellular materials. Ca^{2+} ion displayed a protective effect against the bactericidal activity at 50 °C for 40min (data not shown). The conjugation of phosvitin with galactomannan significantly improved both emulsifying propeties (Fig.3).

The whole molecule of phosvitin would stay in the water-oil interface, thereby attracting more water molecules surrounding the oil droplets due to the hydrophilic property of the galactomannan moiety. As the same reason, a significant part of the bactericidal activity of phosvitin against *E. coli* may reside in the synergistic effect of the high metal-chelating ability and the high emulsifying activity.

REFERENCES

1) Mecham DK and Olcott HS. Phosvitin, the principal phosphoprotein of egg yolk. *J Am Chem Soc* 1993; 39: 647-650.

Metal Ions in Biology and Medicine; vol 6. Eds. J.A. Centeno, Ph. Collery, G. Vernet, R.B. Finkelman, H. Gibb, J.C. Etienne. John Libbey Eurotext, Paris © 2000, pp. 547-549.

Serum Mg, Zn and Se in selected Czech population

Hlúbik P., Opltová L., Vejvodová M., Chaloupka J.

Department of Hygiene, Purkyne Military Medical Academy, Trebesská 1575, 500 01 Hradec Králové, Czech Republic

We conducted an epidemiological study focused on monitoring topical health state in the members of Fire Rescue Service from selected areas of the Czech Republic. Altogether, there were 812 healthy volunteers chosen at random. The examination was focused on the evaluation of selected anthropometrical (body weight, body mass index - BMI, fat tissue percentage, waist circumference) and biochemical (glycemia, total- and HDL-cholesterol, triacylglycerols, uric acid and selected vitamins serum concentrations, serum AST, ALT and GMT activities) parameters of the nutritional status. The levels of magnesium (Mg), zinc (Zn) and selenium (Se) in serum were determined by atomic-absorption spectrophotometric method (AAS Unicam, GB). Serum which was mineralized in microwave processor (Milestone, Italy) provided selenium analysis.

Considering the wide range of monitored characteristics of topical health, the statement is focused on the evaluation of serum levels of Mg, Zn and Se, and their links to selected biochemical and anthropometrical parameters. The results of the study contribute to information about normal values of serum Mg, Zn and Se concentrations in Czech population. Their statistical evaluation is documented in table 1. The distribution of Mg, Zn and Se serum concentrations in examined population group approached normal distribution.

Table 1

Mg, Zn and Se serum concentrations								
	mean	sd	median	Q_3-Q_1/2	percentiles			
					5th	10th	90th	95th
Mg [mmol/l]	0,82	0,057	0,81	0,04	0,72	0,74	0,88	0,92
Zn [µmol/l]	18,25	2,54	18,00	1,56	14,74	15,25	21,00	21,75
Se [µmol/l]	0,80	0,14	0,80	0,11	0,56	0,60	1,01	1,10

In the monitored group, the average serum concentrations of Mg and Se show a tendency towards lower values of so-called physiological range, however, they correspond with other findings within the Czech population. The concentrations of Zn correspond with commonly used normal values.

The concept of the study made it possible to reveal relations between the serum Mg, Zn, Se levels and the age or biochemical and anthropometrical parameters which are generally used as risk indices of cardiovascular disease. The results of that statistical evaluation are documented in the form of correlation matrix (table 2). No statistically significant relations among the age of examined subjects and their serum Mg, Zn and Se concencentrations were proved (these findings were confirmed by analysis of variance, too). No statistically significant correlations were found among Mg serum concentrations and the other followed parameters. Statistically significant negative correlations were revealed for relations among Zn serum concentration and cholesterolemia- TCH ($p \leq 0,05$) and triacylglycerolemia- TAG ($p \leq 0,01$). Statistically significant ($p \leq 0,01$) negative correlation was proved among Se serum concentration and ascorbemia (vit.C).

Table 2

Correlation matrix

	age	BMI	waist	Mg	Zn	Se	TCH	TAG	vit. C
age	1,00								
BMI	0,265	1,00							
waist	0,356	0,844	1,00						
Mg	ns	ns	ns	1,00					
Zn	ns	ns	ns	ns	1,00				
Se	ns	ns	ns	ns	ns	1,00			
TCH	0,446	0,248	0,282	ns	-0,234	ns	1,00		
TAG	0,204	0,343	0,399	ns	-0,317	ns	0,419	1,00	
vit.C	-0,279	ns	ns	ns	ns	-0,271	-0,212	ns	1,00

Statistical significance of r : $p \leq 0,01$, $p \leq 0,05$, ns = no significance

No statistically significant difference between serum concentrations of followed elements in men and women was found.

High incidence of the obesity and overweight in examined population group prompted to evaluation of Mg, Zn and Se saturation in subjects classified to 4 BMI (body mass index) categories (table 3). The Mg, Zn and Se serum concentrations in subjects with normal BMI (20-25 kg/m^2) were compared with concentrations in category of overweight 1st grade (BMI 25,1-28 kg/m^2), overweight 2nd grade (28,1-30 kg/m^2) and the category of obesity (BMI over 30 kg/m^2) by analysis of variance. Mg concentrations showed the tendency to decrease with higher BMI, while by Zn and Se serum concentrations the tendency to increase in higher BMI categories was found. No statistical significance of these changes was proved.

Table 3

	Serum concentrations in BMI categories			
	normal	1stgrade overw.	2ndgrade overw.	obesity
Mg [mmol/l]	1,12	0,81	0,83	0,82
Zn [μmol/l]	18,0	18,4	18,4	18,3
Se [μmol/l]	0,81	0,80	0,84	0,88

In our view, the results of our study, especially lower Mg and Se serum levels, reflect the influence of the environmental conditions, life style and dietary habits of the Czech population.

Abstract.

The nutritional status of selected population - 812 members of Fire Rescue Service from Czech Republic was assessed. The results contribute to information about normal values of serum magnesium, zinc and selenium concentrations in Czech population. Mean serum concentration of Mg was 0,816 ± 0,057mmol/l, that of Zn was 18,25±2,54μmol/l and mean Se serum concentration was 0,802±0,14μmol/l. The distribution of Mg, Zn and Se serum levels in examined population group approached normal distribution.

In the monitored group, the average serum concentrations of Mg and Se showed a tendency towards lower values of so-called physiological range, however, they corresponded with other findings within the Czech population. The concentrations of Zn corresponded with commonly used normal values.

The concept of the study made it possible to reveal relations between the serum Mg, Zn, Se levels and the age or biochemical and anthropometrical parameters which are generally used as risk indices of cardiovascular disease. No statistically significant relations among the age of examined subjects and their serum Mg, Zn and Se concencentrations were proved. Statistically significant negative correlations were revealed for relations among Zn serum concentration and cholesterolemia ($p \leq 0,05$) and triacylglycerolemia ($p \leq 0,01$). Statistically significant ($p \leq 0,01$) negative correlation was proved among Se serum concentration and ascorbemia.

High incidence of the obesity and overweight in examined population group prompted to evaluation of Mg, Zn and Se saturation in subjects classified to 4 BMI (body mass index) categories. Mg concentrations showed the tendency to decrease with higher BMI, while by Zn and Se serum concentrations the tendency to increase in higher BMI categories was found. No statistical significance of these changes was proved.

Lower Mg and Se serum levels reflect the influence of the environmental conditions, life style and dietary habits of the Czech population.

Metal Ions in Biology and Medicine; vol 6. Eds. J.A. Centeno, Ph. Collery, G. Vernet, R.B. Finkelman, H. Gibb, J.C. Etienne. John Libbey Eurotext, Paris © 2000, pp. 550-553.

Effects of alchohol intake on mineral distribution in rats and on serum mineral levels in human

Tatsuya Hobara, Teruyo Aramaki, Masayuki Okuda, Masayuk Gotoh, Ichiro Kunitsugu and Chika Yamada

Department of Public Health Yamaguchi University School of Medicine 1144 Kogushi Ube 755-8505 Yamaguchi, Japan. e-mail: hobara@po.cc.yamaguchi-u.ac.jp

Introduction

There are many reports that indicate a correlation between mineral distribution in the organs, and the overall nutritional condition and occurrence of certain diseases in human beings 1-3). Alcohol intake has been speculated to affect the mineral distribution in the body.This is due to the negative impact of alcohol on the bodily systems, including disturbance of the process of intestinal mineral absorption, increse in the consumption of nutrients, and change in the metabolic function caused by hepatic disturbance. In this study, the authors investigated the effect of alcohol intake on mineral distribution (Ca, Mg, Fe, Mn, Zn, Cu and P) in the organs of rats. Moreover, we analized the mineral levels of serum in the alcoholic liver disease and the non-alcoholic liver disease in humans. We compared mineral levels in serum of rats and humans, and have found interesting phenomena regarding the mineral levels of organs.

Material and Method

1) Animals

Male Sprague-Dawley rats (200-240g) were obtained from Charles River Japan (SPF) and acclimatized in our own facility for 12 days before use.Ten animals were divided into two groups(5 rats per group).One group was fed a diet containing about 16% ethanol powder (Alcok-300,Sato Food Ind.Co.Ltd. JAPAN). Another group was fed a control diet, containing the same components without alcoholic powder. Rats were fed these diets at 6 weeks under conditions of controlled temperature (23 ± 2°C), humidity (60 ± 10%), lighting (light on; 7:00 A.M. to 7:00 P.M.) and ventilation (ventilated 13-15 times per hour).

2) Animal sampling

Blood was drawn from the vena cava superior of each rat. The animals were anesthetized by ether asphyxiation. Fifteen organs were then extracted :cerebrum, cerebellum, stomach, ileum, colon, liver, pancrease, kidney, spleen, heart, lung, uterus, ovary, muscle, bone.

3) Analysis

The metal content of blood, serum and above organs was analized using the Zeeman background-corrected flameless atomic absorption method using Hitachi Z-8100. (Ca, Mg, Fe, Mn, Zn, Cu). P was analized by the Spectrophotometer (Hitachi, U-2000). Serum AST, ALT and r-GTP were analized with Autoanalyzer (Hitachi 7250).

4) Statistical analysis

All data were presented as means ± SD. The data were compared by ANOVA and Newman-Keul's test. P values < 0.05 were regarded as ststistically significant.

Results

1) Animal experiments

With regard to food intake volume, significant differences were obseved between the alcoholic group and the control group ($p < 0.05$). On the otherhand, there were no significant differences in rate of increase in body and organs weight. The average levels of AST, ALT and r-GTP were 152.8, 26.0 and 7.2 units respectively, in control group. In comparison,those of alcoholic groups were 222.5, 50.2 and 2.3 units, respectively. Moreover, in the alcoholic group, histologic changes in the liver consisted of collagenous, deposit of lipid in the central lobular area, along with cellular swelling, but these changes were not observed in the control groups. Thus the alcoholic group of rats showed hepatic disturbance in the both the clinical examination and histological study.

2) Mineral concentration in the organs and blood

Figure 1 and 2 show the mineral concentration in blood and organs of the two groups. Ca concentration in the lungs of the alcoholic group was higher than that of the control group. On the other hand, concentration in the ovaries in the control group was higher than that of the alcoholic group.With respect to Mg concentration in the liver and kidney, the control group was higher than the alcoholic group, while the levels found in the ovary were the opposite. In P concentration, the alcoholic group was higher than the control group in the cerebrum, cerebellum, liver and bone. In Mn concentration, the alcoholic group was significant higher than the control group in the cerebrum, liver, kidney and bone. Although a Mn concentration was found in the ovary, muscle, serum and blood of the alcoholic group, none was detected by this method in the control groups. In Zn concentration of cerebellum, levels in the control group were higher than those of the alcoholic group. Cu concentration in the cerebrum and pancrease were higher in the alcoholic group than the control group.

3) Serum levels of AST, ALT and r-GTP in humans.

The avarage levels of AST, ALT and r-GTP were 203, 251 and 284 units respectively, in the case of alcholic liver disease.Those in cases of non-alcoholic liver disease were 173, 297 and 159 units,respectively.

4) Mineral concentrations of serum in humans and rats

Table 1 shows the mineral concentration of serum in humans and rats. There were higher concentrations of Ca, Fe and Zn found in the human serum of those with alcoholic and non-alcoholic hepatic disease than were found in the control group. There were no coefficient differences between the alcholic and non-alcoholic liver disease. Moreover, the serum concentration levels of Mn and P were signifficantly higher in cases of alcoholic liver disease than in non-alcoholic liver disease or in the control. The Mn levels in the serum exhibited a signifficant difference between the alcoholic group and the control group. In other minerals, Ca, Zn and Cu levels of alcoholic group tended to be higher than those of the control group.

Discussion

Drinking large quantities of alcohol produced many disturbances in the nutritional condition, the organs including liver and kidney, and the uptake of nutrients. A few cases were examined especially for the relationship between the concentration of mineral in organs and the alcohol intake. In these experments, the authors examined the causal relationship of the chronic alcoholic intake or the alcoholic liver disease with the movement of minerals in the organs. The volume of food consamption in alcoholic rats was higher than that of the control rats, but there were no differences between the alcoholic rats and control rats in the incresed rate of weight and organ. This phenomenons suggests that the alcohol intake decresed absorption of nutrients in the intestine and changed with the metabolization of nutriments. In this experiments, histological change were found in the liver of the alcoholic group and this picture was similar to the hepatic disturbance of tetrachloride. This appearence showed that the alcohol diets given rats in our experiments producted the hepatic disturbance. Serum levels of Ca, Fe, Mn and Zn, the alcoholic group was higher than that of the control group. These figures demonstrated a similar tendency in the effects of alcohol in rats and humans. With regard to the mineral concentration of rat's organs, Mg levels of liver and kidney in the control group were higher than those of alcoholic group. This showed that Mg intake of these organs was inhibited by the alcoholic intaked. On the other hand, the P levels of alcoholic group were higher than that of control group in all organs. This mineral had accumulation in the organs in order to aid in the absorption of alcohol. In Mn levels of the cerebrum, liver, kidney , bone and serum, the alcoholic group was higher than the control group rats. In human serum, this mineral was only high in cases of alcoholic hepatic disease. Krieger reported that the Mn levels in the blood and cerebrum were high in patients with hepatic encepharopathy 4-6).For this reason, it was supposed that Mn uptake rate was increased in the intestine by the alcohol consume and Mn excretion rate was decresed from the kidney by the hepatic disturbance. Moreover, the symptoms of hepatic encepharopathy resembled those of Mn toxicity. This phenomenon was presumed that the sourse of hepatic encephalopathy was not only the incresed of anmonium in blood, but also the accumulation of Mn in the lens nuclear. Moreover, Cu levels of the cerebrum in the alcoholic group increased and this appeared to further promot the above symptom.

References

1) Roggin GM, Iber F, Kater RM and Tobon F : Malabsorption in the chronic alcoholic. Johns Hopkins Med.J., 1969; 125: 321-330.
2) Mezey E : Intestinal function in chronic alcoholism. Ann. NY. Acad. 1975: 252 : 215-227.
3) Moon JO, Park SK and Nagano H : Hepatoprotective effect of Fe-TPEN on carbon tetrachloride induced liver injuries. Biol. Pharm. Bull., 1988 ; 21 : 284-288.
4) Krieger D. Krieger S., Jansen O., Gass P., Theilmann L., and Lichitnecker H : Manganese and c chronic hepatic encephalopathy. Lancet, 1995 : 346 : 270-274.
5) Schafter DF, Stephenson KV, Barak AJ andSorrell MF : Effects of ethanol on the transport of manganes by small intestine of the rat. J. Nutr. 1974 : 104 : 101-104.
6) Rodriguez MF, Gonzalez RE, Santolaria FF, Galindo ML, Hernandez TO et. al. : Zink, copper, manganese and iron in chronic alcoholic liver disease. Alcohol, 1977: 14 : 39-44.

Table1. Plasma mineral levels in rats fed on alcohol and control diets for 6weeks and serum mineral levels in humans with liver desease and controls.

	Plasma mineral levels in rats		serum mineral levels in humans		
			Liver diseases		Control
	Alcohol	Control	Alcoholic	non-Alcoholic	
	(n=5)	(n=5)	(n=18)	(n=10)	(n=20)
Ca (μg/ml)	102±18	90±10	114±10*	113±7*	103±16
Mg (μg/ml)	20.1±5.3	21.5±5.0	19.6±3.1	18.5±2.1	19.2±3.2
P (μg/ml)	77±23	84±21	117±21*	106±54	101±19
Fe (μg/ml)	1.08±0.44	0.76±0.58	2.46±1.09**	2.06±0.62*	1.60±0.48
Mn (μg/ml)	1.80±1.0*	trace	1.68±1.25**	0.83±0.80	0.60±0.60
Zn (μg/ml)	1.16±0.37	1.06±0.38	1.37±0.38**	1.18±0.43*	0.81±0.24
Cu (μg/ml)	1.08±0.19	0.85±0.09	0.89±0.24	0.95±0.49	0.75±0.19

Values are mean ±SD. *:Signifficantly different from the control group at $p<0.05$,
**:Signifficantly different from the control group at $p<0.01$.

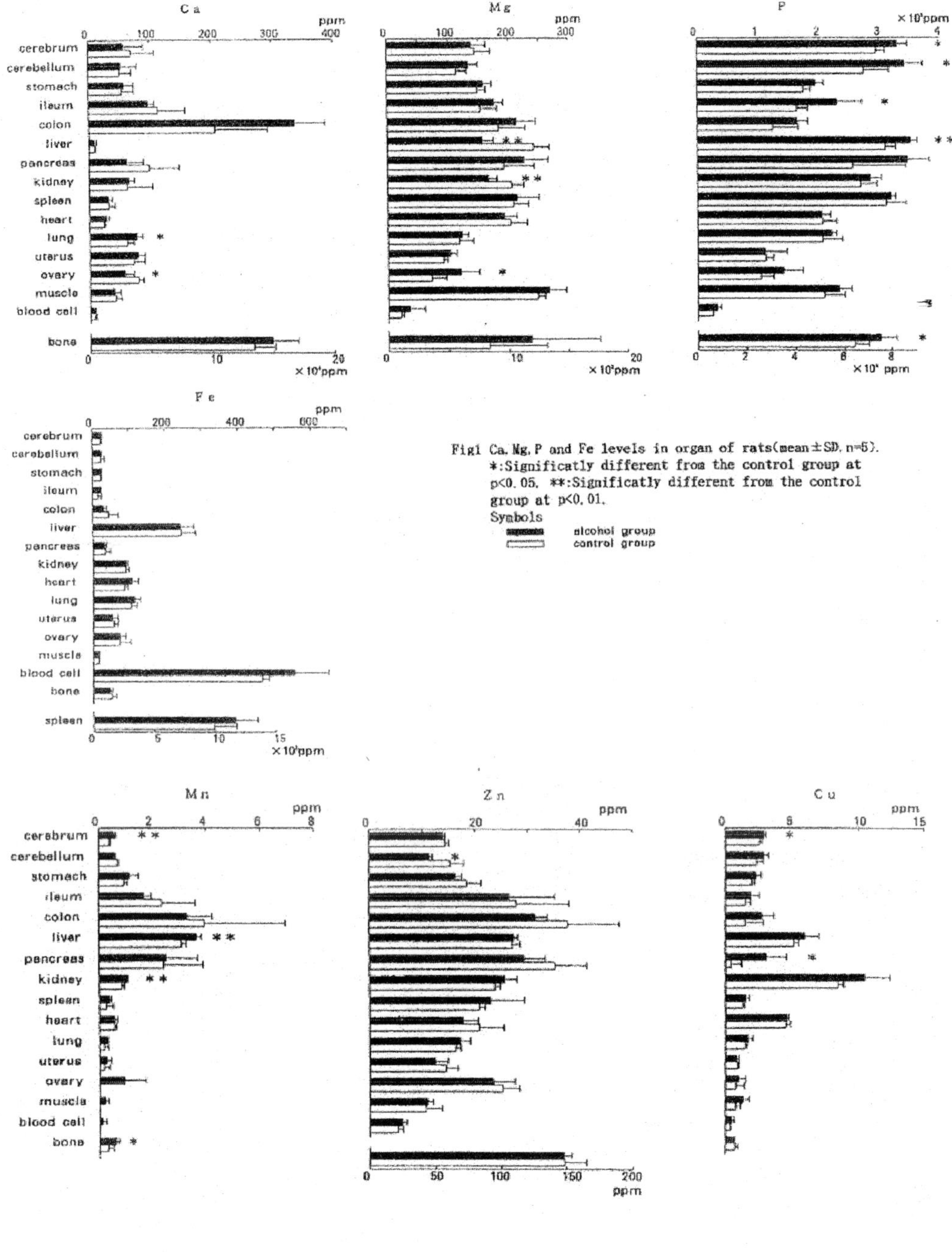

Fig1 Ca, Mg, P and Fe levels in organ of rats(mean±SD, n=5).
*:Significatly different from the control group at $p<0.05$. **:Significatly different from the control group at $p<0.01$.
Symbols
alcohol group
control group

Fig2 Mn, zn and Cu levels in organ of rats(mean±SD, n=5).
*:Significatly different from the control group at $p<0.05$. **:Significatly different from the control group at $p<0.01$.
Symbols
alcohol group
control group

Metal Ions in Biology and Medicine; vol 6. Eds. J.A. Centeno, Ph. Collery, G. Vernet, R.B. Finkelman, H. Gibb, J.C. Etienne. John Libbey Eurotext, Paris © 2000, pp. 554-557.

Assessment of some heavy metals in the human body, in the Eastern Romania area

Carmen Hura, I. Palamaru, B.A. Hura

Food Toxicology Laboratory, Institute of Public Health, Iassy, Romania

Abstract

Ever since humans have become aware that health is inseparably linked to an intact and healthy environment, the control and reduction of pollution have become the focus of worldwide concern. The aim of this study was the evaluation of the metals contents in the young body in relation with the intake some food. The study presents the results obtained in 1998-1999 period of some metals [Pb, Cd, Ni, Zn, Cu, Mn] in human body [urine] in relation with these in some food [milk, vegetables, daily diets] in the Eastern Romania area. The investigations was carried on urine from 100 children [1-10 years old] and 40 young [>11 years old] which living in Iassy, Bacau, Vrancea, Botosani districts. Atomic absorbtion spectrophotometry method was used for the determination of the metals content in human body and foods. In all analysed samples these metals were found. Generally, a wide variation between individual samples was observed. The mean metals levels in the young urine varied between 0.13 μg/l Mn and 1.73 μg/l Zn in Bacau district and 0.19 μg/l Mn and 0.74 μg/l Zn in Vrancea district. The results of the investigations of these metals in foods showed a significantly increased Cd and Pb contents in milk and daily diets.

Introduction

In the past years pollution of the environment by heavy metals of antropogenic origin has become a major threat to all living organisms including the man. This threat is aggravated by the ability of heavy metals to accumulate at the top of the ecological pyramid and their high mobility and persistence in ecosystems. Nowadays, the increased environmental levels of metals have been implicated in elevations in the concentrations of several elements in human body. Although current environmental levels of toxic metals rarely produce morbidity or death in the general population, the interest in biological effects from metal has increased during the last decades [1, 2].

The aim of this study was the evaluation of the metals contents in the human body in relation with the intake some food [3, 4].

Material and methods

The study presents the results obtained in 1997-1999 period of some metals [Pb, Cd, Zn, Cu, Mn, Ni] in human body (urine) in relation with these in some food (vegetables, milk, daily diets) in the Eastern Romania area. The investigations was carried on urine from 100 children (1-10 years old) and 40 young (> 11 years old) which living in Iassy, Bacau, Vrancea, Botosani districts. Atomic absorbtion spectrophotometry method was used from the determination of the metals content in human body and foods.

Results

In the Eastern Romania area in all analysed samples these metals were found. Generally, a wide variation between individual samples was observed.

Human body

The mean levels of heavy metals measured in urine samples in the some districts of Eastern Romania area are present in *Table I - V*.

Table I shows the mean levels of the metals [Zn, Cu, Mn] in spot urine samples from children of Iassy district in 1997 period. Mean values of Zn in urine varied between 0.7 μg/l [>11 years group] and 1.51 μg/l [6-10 years old group]. In this urine samples the Cd, Pb, Ni were not detected.

Table I – Mean levels of heavy metals in urine samples in Iassy district, 1997 (μg/l)

Age [years]	Nr. [samples]	Zn	Cu	Mn
< 5	3	1.22	0.08	1.00
6-10	15	1.51	0.22	0.25
>11	8	0.70	0.34	0.16

The mean levels of metals [Zn, Cu, Mn, Ni, Cd, Pb] in the spot urine samples in Bacau district (*Table II*) varied with slow values between the sex and the age.

Table II – Mean levels of heavy metals in urine samples in Bacau district, 1998, (μg/l)

Age [years]	Nr. [samples]	Zn	Cu	Mn	Ni	Cd	Pb
<5	13	1.78	0.14	0.14	0.08	0.18	0.14
6-10	5	1.96	0.49	0.06	-	0.24	0.10
>11	27	1.66	0.23	0.15	0.25	0.17	0.14

Table III presents the mean levels of metals in urine samples in Vrancea district analysed in 1998 period. The mean levels of Zn, Cu, Mn and Ni in the urine samples were slow. The mean levels of Cu varied between 0.39 μg/l (<5 years old group) and 0.25μg/l (6-10 years old group). The mean levels of Cd in urine varied between 0.17 μg/l (>11 years old group) and 0.29 μg/l (< 5 years old group).

Table III–Mean levels of heavy metals in urine samples in Vrancea district, 1998, (μg/l)

Age [years]	Nr. [samples]	Zn	Cu	Mn	Ni	Cd	Pb
<5	4	0.73	0.39	0.21	0.44	0.29	0.08
6-10	3	0.70	0.25	0.18	0.47	0.23	0.21
> 11	6	0.77	0.28	0.17	0.43	0.17	0.20

Table IV presents the mean levels of metals in urine samples, in Botosani district, in 1999 period. The mean levels of Zn and Cu in urine samples varied very low with the age and the sex. The mean concentrations of Cd and Pb varied between 0.1μg/l (>11years old group) and 0.18μg/l (<5 years old group) respectively 0.1μg/l (< 5 years old group) and 0.19μg/l (>11 years old group).

Table IV–Mean levels of heavy metals in urine samples in Botosani district, 1998 (μg/l)

Age [years]	Nr. [samples]	Zn	Cu	Mn	Ni	Cd	Pb
<5	12	1.42	0.33	0.14	0.42	0.18	0.10
6-10	2	1.65	0.6	0.33	0.11	0.11	0.12
>11	2	1.92	0.4	0.12	0.19	0.10	0.19

Table V indicates the results of mean levels of metals in urine samples in 1997-1999 period in four districts in Eastern Romania area. The mean levels of Zn and Cu in urine samples were found varying between 0.74μg/l (Vrancea) and 1.73 μg/l (Bacau) respectively 0.23 μg/l (Botosani) and 0.33 μg/l (Vrancea). The mean levels of Mn and Ni in urine samples varied between 0.13μg/l (Bacau, Botosani) and 0.21μg/l (Iassy) respectively 0.2μg/l (Bacau) and 0.47μg/l (Vrancea). The mean levels of Cd and Pb in spot urine samples varied between 0.14 μg/l (Botosani) and 0.21μg/l (Vrancea) respectively 0.11μg/l (Botosani) and 0.17μg/l (Vrancea).

Table V – Mean levels of heavy metals in urine samples in 1997-1999 period (μg/l)

District	Year	Nr	Zn	Cu	Mn	Ni	Cd	Pb
Iassy	1997	26	1.23±0.35	0.25±0.10	0.21±0.09	-	-	-
Bacau	1998	45	1.73±0.70	0.25±0.17	0.13±0.09	0.20±0.05	0.19±0.08	0.13±0.06
Vrancea	1998	13	0.74±0.40	0.33±0.13	0.19±0.06	0.47±0.15	0.21±0.09	0.17±0.08
Botosani	1999	16	1.5±0.60	0.23±0.10	0.13±0.06	0.39±0.20	0.14±0.08	0.11±0.05

Food

The results were distinguished the presence of the metals [Zn, Cu, Cd, Pb] in the analysed food [vegetables, milk, daily diets]. *Table VI* shows the mean levels of Zn, Cu, Cd and Pb in the vegetables, milk and daily diets analysed in1999 year in Iassy, Bacau, Vrancea and Botosani districts. In the vegetables, the mean levels of Zn, Cu, Cd and Pb were found in the admissible limits (MAL). In milk samples the mean levels of Zn and Cu were found in the admissible limits with the exception of Zn levels in milk of Botosani district, which was 13.24 mg/kg. The results of the investigations showed a significantly increased of Cd and Pb concentrations in the milk and the daily diets in all district with a mean levels of Cd varied between 0.01 mg/kg milk (Iassy) and 0.073 mg/kg milk (Vrancea). The mean levels of Pb in milk varied between 0.4 mg/kg (Bacau) and 0.6 mg/kg (Iassy, Botosani) these concentrations were higher than the maximum admissible limits in Romania [MAL= 0.1 mg/kg]. In daily diets the mean levels of these metals [Zn, Cu, Cd, Pb] varied from the district to the district (*Table VI*)

Table VI–Mean levels of metals in food in some districts in Eastern Romania area, 1999 (mg/kg)

District	Vegetables				Milk				Daily diet			
	Zn	Cu	Cd	Pb	Zn	Cu	Cd	Pb	Zn	Cu	Cd	Pb
Iassy	-	-	-	-	5.0	0.38	0.01	0.6	4.0	0.32	0.11	0.15
Bacau	1.47	0.09	0.04	0.5	1,76	0.08	0.06	0.4	1.97	0.22	0.06	0.35
Vrancea	5.27	2.4	0.14	0.45	5.0	0.35	0.07	0.43	3.6	0.3	0.13	0.6
Botosani	4.73	1.14	0.13	0.22	13.24	0.15	0.02	0.6	4.6	0.23	0.11	0.63
MAL	**15.0**	**5.0**	**0.1**	**0.5**	**5.0**	**0.5**	**0.01**	**0.1**	-	-	-	-

Conclusions

Determinations of these pollutants in human body and foods are important in clinical routine analysis and environmental monitoring for the prevention, control and reduction of pollution as well as for occupational health and epidemiological studies.

References

1. Folin M, Contiero E, Vaselli G.M. – trace element determination in humans. The use of blood and hair, *Biol.Trace Elem.Res.* 1991, 31; 147-158.
2. WHO – Biological Monitoring of Chemical Exposure in the Work Place, vol.1 and vol.2.
3. Hura C., Leanca M, Palamaru I – Chemical pollutants in daily diets, a risk for cancer disease. *Rev. Hygiene and Public Health,* 1995, nr.1, vol.45; 13-16.
4. Hura C. - Chemical Pollution of Food and Health, Iassy, Ed. Socom Hermes, 1997.

Metal Ions in Biology and Medicine; vol 6. Eds. J.A. Centeno, Ph. Collery, G. Vernet, R.B. Finkelman, H. Gibb, J.C. Etienne. John Libbey Eurotext, Paris © 2000, pp. 558-560.

Ferrous and ferric ions with phytate *in vitro*

Donald Oberleas

Food and Nutrition, Texas Tech University, Lubbock, TX and Gerber Products Company, Fremont, MI, USA

Ferric iron has been utilized in phytate analysis since 1913 [1]. Others have studied iron and phytate in vitro with buffering agents which confounded their data [2]. This is a study of ferrous and ferric ions and phytate at pHs from 1 to 7 in vitro without confounding buffer. Both 1:1 and 2:1 molar ratios of iron ions to phytate were studied.

Materials and Methods: One mL iron solution equaled 0.1 mmol of Fe and was dissolved in 0.1 mol/L HCl. Sodium phytate was prepared so 1 mL equaled 0.1 mmol phytate ion dissolved in 2.0 mol/L HCl. Concentrations of HCl of 2, 0.2, 0.02 mol/L and/or NaOH of 2, 0.2, 0.02, and 0.002 mol/L were used to adjust pH.

Experimental Design: Design was that both valence states (ferrous and ferric) were represented at every pH 1 - 7. The solubility of each component at Fe:phytate 1:1 and 2:1 molar ratios were studied.

Procedures: To each of 7 calibrated 50 mL centrifuge tubes was added 1.0 mL ferrous or ferric iron for 1:1 molar ratio or two mL for 2:1 molar ratio. One mL of 2 mol/L HCl was added to each tube. Water was added to 20 mL. Each solution was stirred with a small magnetic bar. All tubes were adjusted to a pH of 1 to 1.5 with 2 mol/L HCl. 1 mL of acidified phytate solution was always added last. Tube solutions were adjusted carefully to the appropriate pHs of 1, 2, 3, 4, 5, 6, and 7 with HCl or NaOH slowly and patiently to achieve the series of final pHs. Final volumes of 45 mL were necessary for the phytate containing (1:1 and 2:1) series. Tubes were capped and allowed to stand overnight to form a final equilibrium.
Tubes were centrifuged at 3500 rpm (~4300 g) for 20 minutes. Supernates were not soluble in acid, thus it was necessary to solubilize the solutes and precipitates with NaOH to effect solution with resulting formation of stable colloidal iron. The solutions were made to volume for iron analysis. Iron analysis was by ICP (Induction Coupled Plasma Spectrometry) (Leeman Labs., Inc., Lowell, MA) by a procedure standardized

in Gerber Product Company research laboratories. Appropriate standards were utilized to assure accuracy of the procedure.

Results: With 1:1 molar ratio of ferrous iron and phytate, at pH 1 the solute portion was without visible precipitate. At pHs 2 and 3 a small amount of murkiness formed with little precipitation. Only 4 - 9% of the ferrous iron was precipitated. Precipitate increased at pH 4, peaked at pH 5 with 78% of the iron precipitated, and decreased slightly at pH 6. At pH 7, white precipitate formed with 49% of the iron. With 1:1 ferric phytate solutions, a large white precipitate formed at pHs 1 - 4. At pH 1, 79% of the ferric iron precipitated. For pHs 2-4 this increased to 95% at pH 3. At pHs 3 and 4, the precipitates had a light rusty-brown character. At pH 5 and 6, a brown colloidal suspension formed without visible precipitation 37 and 29% of the ferric iron, respectively in the precipitate. At pH 7, a small brown precipitate formed in addition to the colloidal suspension with 55% of the ferric ion precipitated. Phytate was more difficult to quantify because of dilutions required to solubilize the precipitates and provide quantitative integrity, some of the sample phytate was below the detectable limit. For the ferrous:phytate (1:1) series, only pH 6 had more than 50% of the phyate in the precipitate. This agrees with the view that 2 or more cations must complex with a single phytate to form an insoluble complex. This was likewise true for ferric iron. The brown colloids and precipitates formed at pHs 5-7 contained no phytate. Phytate, at these pHs, was quantitatively recovered in the solute. The iron content of the precipitates is shown in Figure 1.

Figure 1. The amount of ferrous (right) and ferric (below) contained in the precipitate at each pH and at molar ratios of 1:1 as described in the procedure.

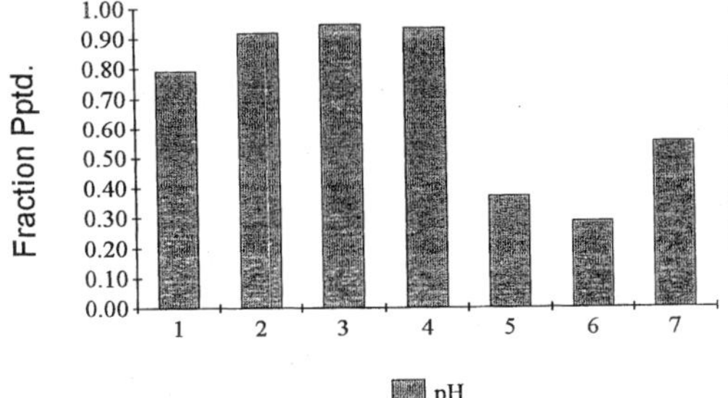

At 2:1 molar ratio, ferrous ion reacted similar to other divalent cations except over a slightly broader pH range. At pH 1, 40% of the ferrous iron was precipitated. This exceeded 90% at pHs 4 and 5 and declined at pHs 6 and 7 to 87 and 84% respectively. Phytate was detectable in the solutes of samples with pH of 1 and 2 and from the precipitates at pHs 2 through 7. All precipitates were white at all pHs. For ferric ion,

over 98% was in the precipitate at pHs 1 and 2. This declined from pH 3 to 7 with 72% of the ferric iron in the precipitate at pH 7. Phytate was undetectable in any solute from the ferric ion series. Phytate was detectable in slightly decreasing amounts in the precipitates as pH increased from 1 to 7. Visually, white precipitates were present at pHs 1-3 whereas pH 4 had a slightly brown cast and 5 to 7 was darker brown. This indicates that ferric iron complexes phytate at all pHs studied. Either gradual dissociation to form FeOH above pH 3 or hydroxylating and forming a light brown color in the precipitate while associated with the phytate complex. It is not possible to discern within the current experiment which may be occurring. Figure 2 shows the iron content of the various precipitates.

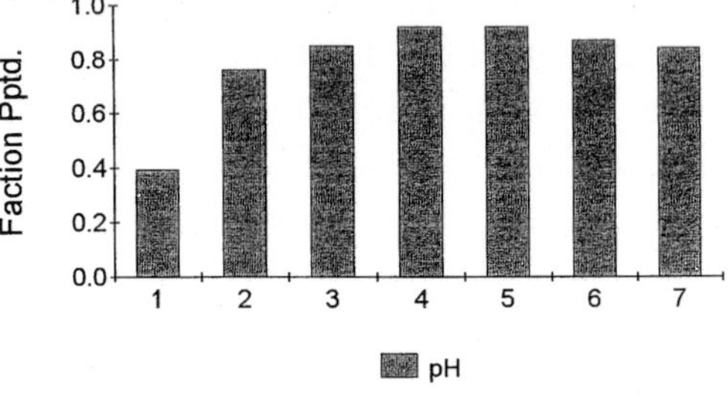

Figure 2. The fraction of ferrous (right) and ferric (below) ion contained in the precipitate at the various pHs and at 2:1 molar ratio as described in the procedure.

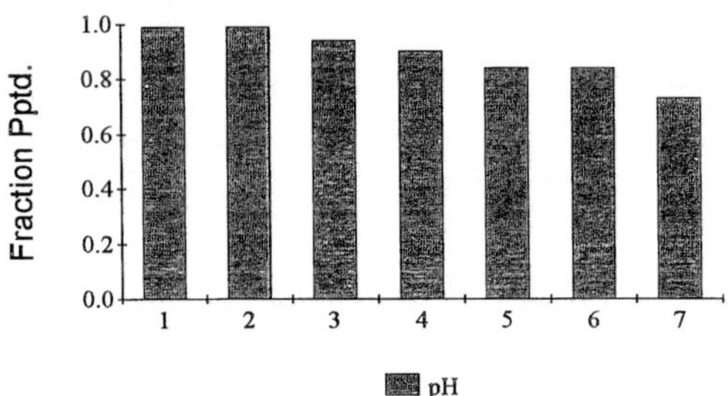

Conclusion: Ferrous and ferric ions react differently with phytate. Ferric ions would predominate in phytate complexes at lower pHs. At pHs 5 - 7 ferrous ion formed the more stable complex with more of the ferric ions forming hydroxides. Slight changes in the concentration of ferrous or ferric ions in the presence of phytate can alter the complexations formed. Both ferrous and ferric ions form complexes at lower pHs than cations studied previously. These complexes may change very little as the pH of the GI tract increases. Both ferrous and ferric ions may complex with phytate in the stomach.

References:

1. Heubner, W and Stadtler, H Uber eine Titrationmethode zur Bestimmung des Phytins. Biochem Z 1914; 64:422-37.

2. Graf, E and Eaton, JW Effects of phytate on mineral bioavailability in mice. J Nutr 1984; 114:1192-98.

The author wishes to thank Ms K. Strand, Gerber Products Company for the ICP iron analyses.

Metal Ions in Biology and Medicine; vol 6. Eds. J.A. Centeno, Ph. Collery, G. Vernet, R.B. Finkelman, H. Gibb, J.C. Etienne. John Libbey Eurotext, Paris © 2000, pp. 561-562.

The influence of different dietary magnesium levels on the metabolism of calcium, phosphorous and magnesium in growing rats

Shanfen Bao, Lin Zhao, Zhen Li Tao Cong

Trace Element Research Laboratory, 301 Hospital, Beijing, P.R. China

Abstract. 30 male Sprague Dawley rats were divided into three groups each of ten and housed in non-metal metabolic cages individually. The rats in the first group were fed Mg deficient diet (86 mg/kg), the rats in the second group were fed Mg adequate diet (548 mg/kg) while in the third group fed Mg excess diet (5402 mg/kg). All the diets were semi-synthetic containing Ca:3.7g/kg, P:4g/kg. After 25 days feeding and adaptation to the metabolic cages, the five–days period of metabolic experiment were carried on. The samples of feces and urine were collected respectively. At the end of the period, heparinized fasting blood samples were taken from the heart under light anesthesia .The femur and tibia were dissected, after being measured of weight, length and volume, stored together with kidney at -20°C until analysis for Ca, Mg and P. Results: there was no much influence on the apparent absorption of Ca (86%) at the Mg deficient or adequate Mg supplement , excess Mg in diet made this absorption of Ca decrease a little (83%), However, excess Mg increased urinary Ca excretion significantly and decreased the retention of Ca; Magnesium deficient diet increased the P excretion in urine obviously and reduced the retention of P in the body; With the increasing of Mg contents in diet, the Mg excretion in feces and urine increased significantly , that means the homeostasis of Mg is regulated by both intestine and kidney. With respect to the growing rats, either Mg deficiency or excess in diet are detrimental to the skeletal growth and development. Mg deficient diet caused calcium accumulation in kidney , probably involving in the pathogenesis of nephrolithiasis.

The aim of the present study is to observe the effect of different dietary magnesium on the apparent absorption of calcium and phosphorous in growing rats.

Materials and methods (omitted)

Results (omitted)

Discussion

In our previous studies[1,2], true Ca absorption in different dietary Ca sources was determined in ^{45}Ca labeled rats by isotope dilution technique Meantime, the apparent absorption was observed too. Ca absorption is different depending on the dietary Ca levels. The apparent absorption of Ca was about 83% and 94~98% when the Ca contents in diets were 4.3g/kg and 2.7g/kg respectively. The result of present study corresponded to previous studies, apparent absorption of Ca in three groups was about 86% when Ca contents in diets was 3.7g/kg.

Concerning the effect of magnesium supplement on calcium absorption, this study showed that magnesium deficient or supplement does not have obviously influence on the apparent absorption of calcium. The contents of Mg in diets of third group was nearly one order of magnitude higher than that of second group (5402 and 548 mg/g diet) and rats in third group developed light diarrhea, food intake decreased, in such excessive magnesium supplement state apparent absorption of calcium decreased only 3% (from 86% in second group to 83% in third group). So it is considerable that adequate Mg supplement has no influence on the absorption of calcium, However, excessive Mg increased the calcium excretion from urine, the reabsorption of calcium in kidney decreased and the retention of calcium in body was lower. Bergstra et al reported [3] increase magnesium in diet caused urinary calcium increase but the apparent absorption of calcium had no much changes . However, they had no observation on bone.

All the parameters of femur including weight, length, volume and density in rats receiving Mg adequate diet were superior to other two groups. There was the same trend in tibia of rats. It was obviously that from the results of elements analysis of femur and tibia the contents of Ca and P in rats receiving Mg adequate diets was higher than that in rats receiving both Mg deficient and excess diets. With the increase of Mg in diets the deposits of Mg in bone increased significantly.

The absorption of P was 94-93% when there was low or adequate Mg contents in diets, but when dietary Mg was excessive the metabolism of P was derangement and lots of P was excreted from feces causing a lower apparent absorption. These probably due to the large number of magnesium in the intestine, which combined with calcium and phosphate to form the insoluble complex of Mg-Ca-phosphate.

The calcium deposit in tissues especially in kidney was found in Mg deficient rats. For a long time , hypercalciuria is thought to be the cause of formation of calcium stone in kidney.[4]. It was also reported that either high phosphorus or low Mg diets induced calculus of kidney in rats, but the mechanism is not clear [5]. In this experiment we can see the homeostasis of P is regulated mainly by the kidney. In Mg deficient group less P was excreted from feces, lots of P was excreted from urine. Meanwhile Mg depletion decreased urinary Mg greatly. Lack of competition of Mg, phosphorous was more easily to combine with calcium and form insoluble Ca-Phosphate complex depositing in kidney.

Conclusion: Excessive magnesium in diets leads to a little descent of apparent absorption of calcium, decrease of calcium retention as the urinary calcium excretion increased. Magnesium deficient diets significantly increased phosphorous excretion in urine, consequently, decreased the retention of phosphorous. With respect to the growing rats, both Mg deficiency and excess in diet are detrimental to the skeletal growth and development. Mg deficient diet caused calcium accumulation in kidney , probably involving in the pathogenesis of nephrolithiasis.

References

1. Windisch W, Bao SF, Kirchgessner M. Isotope–dilution technique for determination of endogenous faecal excretion and true absorption of calcium in ^{45}Ca labelled rats. J Anim Physiol and Anim Nutr 1997; 77:189-197
2. Bao SF, Windisch W, Kirchgessner M Calcium bioavailability of different organic and inorganic dietary Ca sources (citrate, lactate, acetate, oyster-shell, eggshell,β-tri-Ca-phosphate) J Anim Physiol and Anim Nutr 1997; 78:154-160
3. Bergstra AE, Lemmens AG, Beynen AC. Dietary fructose vs. glucose stimulates nephrocalcinogesis in female rats. J Nutr 1993;132:1320-27
4. Hoek AC, Lemmens AG, Mullink JWMA, Beynen AC. Influence of dietary calcium phosphorous ratio on mineral excretion and nephrocalcinosis in female rats. J Nutr 1988 118:1210-16
5. Sterck JGH, Ritskes-Hoitinga J, Beynen AC. Inhibitory effect of high protein intake on nephrocalcinogenesis in female rats. British J Nutr 1992; 67:223-33

Metal Ions in Biology and Medicine; vol 6. Eds. J.A. Centeno, Ph. Collery, G. Vernet, R.B. Finkelman, H. Gibb, J.C. Etienne. John Libbey Eurotext, Paris © 2000, pp. 563-565.

Zinc and iron metabolism in chickens on a high zinc or high iron diet

Yoshimi Teraki[1], Yuka Okumura[2] and Akira Uchiumi[3]

[1] Isehara-Hinata Hospital, Isehara, Kanagawa 259-1101, Japan; [2] The Nippon Dental University School of Dentistry at Niigata, Niigata 951-8151, Japan; [3] National Institute of Material and Chemical Research, Tsukuba, Ibaraki 305-0003, Japan

Abstract: Young chickens maintained on a high zinc or iron diet from day 4 till day 60 of age exhibited a marked depression of weight gain and severe anorexia, and showed noticeably increased iron concentrations in serum and viscera. The increase in serum and tissue iron content might be a proximate cause of the severe anorexia and weight gain depression in the chickens.

Introduction

Excessive or deficient mineral intake is considered to bring about disorders in growing birds as well. It has been documented that excessive iron intake led to development of toxic symptoms including anorexia and weight gain depression in fowls[1]. This study was conducted to investigate effects of feeding on a diet of high zinc or iron content upon the growth of and development of chicks.

Materials and Methods

Fifteen White Leghorn chicks hatched in an automated incubator were divided into three groups and allocated to feeding on each of three different diets (standard, high zinc, and high iron; see Table 1 for respective zinc and iron content; Oriental Yeast Co., Ltd., Tokyo) from day 4 till day 60 of age. The flocks were observed for clinical signs daily during the feeding period, after which they were sacrificed/necropsied with blood and visceral tissue sampling. Elemental analysis of blood and tissues was performed with an atomic absorption photometer and an inductively coupled argon plasma emission spectrometer, and by fluorescent X-ray analysis.

Results

1. Weight gain and food intake

There was a marked suppression of growth of chicks maintained on a high zinc diet and those on a high iron diet. At 60 days of age their body weights were as low as about one-fourth (148.0±10.6 and 131.5±7.6 g, respectively) of those of controls (560±165 g) on a standard diet. The birds on the high mineral diets exhibited also a severe anorexia; their food intake at 35 days of study feeding was nearly three-fold less as compared with a control value.

2. Zinc content in blood and organs (Table 1)
The high zinc diet feeding produced a significant increase in serum zinc level and also noticeable increases in hepatic and pancreatic zinc levels, but no changes in zinc content in the kidneys, spleen or duodenum. The birds receiving the high iron diet showed a significant increase in pancreatic zinc content.

Table 1. Zinc concentration in blood and organs

	Standard diet group 60-day-old chickens (n=5) fed on diet containing 53.0 ppm Zn and 129.0 ppm Fe	High zinc diet group 60-day-old chickens (n=5) fed on diet containing136.0 ppm Zn and 374.0 ppm Fe	High iron diet group 60-day-old chickens (n=5) fed on diet containing 49.8 ppm Zn and 758.0 ppm Fe
Serum	26.5 ± 0.2 µg/dl	103.6 ± 6.8 µg/dl*	45.7 ± 0.4 µg/dl
Liver	40.0 ± 1.7 µg/g	118.0 ± 9.2 µg/g*	34.0 ± 1.6 µg/g
Kidney	27.0 ± 1.5 µg/g	29.0 ± 1.5 µg/g	27.0 ± 0.1 µg/g
Spleen	30.0 ± 0.7 µg/g	35.0 ± 2.5 µg/g	34.0 ± 1.4 µg/g
Pancreas	47.0 ± 2.9 µg/g	165.0 ± 7.6 µg/g*	115.0 ± 14.2 µg/g*
Duodenum	33.0 ± 2.0 µg/g	42.0 ± 5.6 µg/g	41.0 ± 4.2 µg/g

* Significantly different from control group ($p<0.01$) Mean ± S.E.

3. Iron content in blood and organs (Table 2)
Serum iron levels were significantly elevated 3- to 5-fold with the high zinc or high

Table 2. Iron concentration in blood and organs

	Standard diet group 60-day-old chickens (n=5) fed on diet containing 53.0 ppm Zn and 129.0 ppm Fe	High zinc diet group 60-day-old chickens (n=5) fed on diet containing 136.0 ppm Zn and 374.0 ppm Fe	High iron diet group 60-day-old chickens (n=5) fed on diet containing 49.8 ppm Zn and 758.0 ppm Fe
Serum	44.9 ± 6.5 µg/dl	140.6 ± 8.8 µg/dl*	297.7 ± 12.6 µg/dl*
Liver	353.0 ± 29.6 µg/g	271.0 ± 35.0 µg/g	1132.0 ± 39.5 µg/g*
Kidney	70.0 ± 2.2 µg/g	102.0 ± 5.8 µg/g*	117.0 ± 7.6 µg/g*
Spleen	103.0 ± 6.8 µg/g	222.0 ± 10.1 µg/g*	113.0 ± 6.3 µg/g*
Pancreas	19.0 ± 7.2 µg/g	19.0 ± 1.7 µg/g	91.3 ± 6.7 µg/g*
Duodenum	43.2 ± 6.0 µg/g	92.1 ± 4.6 µg/g*	141.0 ± 12.7 µg/g*

* Significantly different from control group ($p<0.01$) Mean ± S.E.

iron diet feeding. Significant increases in renal, splenic and duodenal iron content were also noted in both the high mineral diet groups. There was a 3.2-fold iron accumulation in the liver of birds on the high iron diet, compared with the controls. Tissue iron levels in the pancreas and liver were markedly increased in the high iron diet group, while the pancreatic iron was not elevated in the high zinc diet group displaying a high zinc content in this organ.

Discussion

This study examines the effects of excessive mineral intake, especially of zinc and iron, on the growth and development of chickens. Dinsmore et al.[2] have described that anorexia nervosa in humans is unlikely to be attributable to a decrease in serum zinc but appears to be associated with a significant elevation of serum ferritin seen in those patients possibly due to either increased iron stores or ferritin release from cellular breakdown. Borch-Iohnsen Schreiner et al.[3] reported that hypoxia in mice was ascribable to excessive iron accumulation since those animals exhibited a hepatic iron content three times as high as normal. It has also been documented that the upper limit of iron content in drinking water for broilers is 0.3 mg/L while weight loss and anorexia occurred with 3% iron in drinking water[1].

A study reported by Richter[4] indicated that massive hepatic siderosis did not result from high iron diet feeding but would be induced by various manipulations such as cyclic starvation combined with an iron-enriched diet in animals. The present results are considered to imply that the increased serum and tissue levels of iron in the chickens receiving high zinc or high iron diet were the contributory cause of anorexia and weight loss.

There have been many reports concerning relationship of anorexia with zinc deficiency[5] but articles dealing with the relationship to iron have been few. We previously documented increases in blood and tissue iron content, a marked growth retardation and anorexia observed in chickens maintained on a zinc deficient diet[6]. The finding was considered to imply that zinc deficiency brought about the increase in serum and tissue iron concentration. It is concluded that increased iron in blood and organs causes anorexia and growth disturbance in chickens as well.

References

1) Puls R. Mineral levels in animal health: Diagnostic data. 2nd Ed, p. 143. Sherpa International, Clearbrook, B.C. 1994.
2) Dinsmore WW, Alderdice JD, McKee CM, McMaster D, Adams C, Love AHG. Trace elements in anorexia nervosa. *Acta Pharmacol et Toxicol* 1986; 59: 159-62.
3) Borch-Iohnsen Schreiner B, Myhre K. Iron overload in hypoxic mice. *Acta Pharmacol et Toxicol* 1986; 59: 146-47.
4) Richter GW. The iron-loaded cell. The cytopathology of iron storage. A review. *Am J Pathol* 1978; 91: 363-96.
5) Akar N. Anorexia and zinc. *Lancet* 1984; 11: 874.
6) Teraki Y, Okumura Y, Uchiumi A. Effect of low zinc diet on growth of chicken. *Trace Metal Metabolism* 1986; 14: 41-44.

Metal Ions in Biology and Medicine; vol 6. Eds. J.A. Centeno, Ph. Collery, G. Vernet, R.B. Finkelman, H. Gibb, J.C. Etienne. John Libbey Eurotext, Paris © 2000, pp. 567-569.

Enhancement of the transferrin-independent uptake of gallium

Kathryn A. Morton, Cheryl A. Luttropp, Jean-Baptiste Roullet

Oregon Health Sciences University, Portland, Oregon, USA

ABSTRACT

Background: Stable and radioactive gallium (Ga) have utility for imaging and adjunctive chemotherapy. Although Ga binds to transferrin (Tf) and enter cells by the Tf receptor (TfR), evidence also supports Tf-independent mechanisms for uptake, which may be selectively regulable.
Aims: **(1)** to determine whether Tf is required for uptake of Ga *in vivo*; **(2)** to compare factors that regulate Tf-independent uptake of Ga; and **(3)** to find an effective, non-toxic method to selectively stimulate Ga uptake by tumors.
Methods: **(1)** Uptake of Ga-67 was compared in normal and congenitally hypotransferrinemic tumor-bearing mice. **(2)** A pair of cell lines was developed, one with no TfR (TfR-) and the other with constitutive over-expression of a transfected human TfR (TfR+). The uptake of Ga-67 was compared by the cells and by derivative tumors grown in mice. Factors that regulate Tf-independent uptake of Ga-67 were examined. **(3)** The effect of photo-degradation nifedipine (PDN) on Tf-independent Ga-67 uptake was identified and characterized.
Results: **(1)** While normal soft tissue activity is markedly depressed in the hypotransferrinemic mouse, uptake of Ga-67 by bones and at least some tumors is similar for normal and hypotransferrinemic mice. **(2)** The uptake of Ga-67 is 10-fold greater by tumors grown in nude mice from TfR+, than TfR-, cells. However, significant Tf-independent accumulation of Ga-67 occurs *in vitro* and *in vivo*. This can be stimulated by supra-physiologic levels of calcium and iron salts. **(3)** The nitroso-photo-derivative of nifedipine (nitrosipine) enhances Ga-67 uptake 1000-fold in tumor cells and 20-25-fold in non-transformed cells. Uptake of Fe2+ and Mn2+ are also driven by nitrosipine. Rate of metal uptake, but not total capacity, is greater at pH 6.5, than 7.4. Promotion of uptake requires Na+, but not Ca2+. Nitrosipine activity is observed at concentrations non-toxic to cells. In tumor-bearing mice, the tumor:normal tissue ratios of Ga-67 uptake are increased >15-fold by administration of nitrosipine.
Conclusions: The Tf-independent uptake of gallium may be increased in tumors and tumor cells by nitrosipine.

NARRATIVE

For 30 years, the tumor-imaging potential of Ga-67 has been recognized. Stable Ga has also been used as an adjunct to chemotherapy. The mechanism by which Ga accumulates in normal tissues and in regions of pathology remains controversial. If these factors could be better understood, efforts to improve and broaden the applicability of Ga for oncologic imaging and therapy might be possible. It is widely accepted that Ga, as an analog of iron, binds to circulating transferrin (Tf), and gains access to cells by means of the transferrin receptor (TfR). However, there is significant evidence that Tf-independent mechanisms of Ga uptake may also be important. This conflict is difficult to resolve because Tf and the TfR are ubiquitous *in vivo*.

To circumvent this problem *in vivo*, the distribution and uptake of Ga-67 were compared in hypotransferrinemic (HP) and normal Balb/C tumor-bearing mice(**1**). Uptake of Ga-67 by all normal soft tissues is markedly depressed in HP, compared to normal Balb/C, mice. Uptake of Ga-67 by bone and tumor is equivalent in both types of mice. The ratio of tumor:background activity is substantially higher in HP than in normal mice. These data suggest that Ga-67 uptake is Tf-mediated in normal soft tissues, but is Tf-independent in bone and in (at least some) tumors.

The relative importance of Tf-dependent and -independent mechanisms for Ga uptake, and factors that drive Tf-independent uptake, were investigated. For these studies, two transfected CHO cell lines were developed. One has no TfR. In the other, a transfected human TfR is over-expressed constitutively. Ga-67 uptake by these cells, and by derivative tumors grown in nude mice, was examined(**2**).

As has also been shown by others, over-expression of the TfR promotes uptake of a Ga-Tf complex, both *in vitro* and *in vivo*. However, the Tf-independent uptake of Ga-67 is nonetheless significant, even in the presence of Ga-Tf, and can be augmented to exceed Tf-mediated levels by increasing the extracellular concentration of Fe or Ca salts. This suggested a depolarization effect, as displayed by several types of ion channels, some of which are non-selective in their transport of metal cations. In testing the effect of various ion channel agonists and antagonists on the Tf-independent uptake of Ga-67, it was observed that photo-irradiated nifedipine produces a 1000-fold increase in Tf-independent uptake of Ga-67 by cells, an effect that is independent of expression of the TfR(**3**). No effect on Ga-67 uptake is produced by light-shielded nifedipine, nor by light-shielded or photo-irradiated nimodipine or BAY K 8644.

The active derivative in promoting Ga uptake has been isolated and characterized. It is the fully aromatic nitroso-derivative of nifedipine, called "nitrosipine". It is the major product produced with fluorescent irradiation. Nitrosipine is stable at room temperature in solid state or solution, and in acidic and neutralizing conditions that mimic those encountered in the normal GI tract. It is easily isolated and crystalized. Nitrosipine can easily be detected by HPCL in serum and displays some protein binding.

Nitrosipine does not alter the lipophillicity of Ga-67 citrate but a slight shift in the UV/vis spectrum of nitrosipine occurs when Ga-67 citrate is present in relatively high concentrations. Nitrosipine promotes uptake of Ga-67 at concentrations that are non-toxic to cultured cells. Nitrosipine is a weak calcium channel blocker but the mechanism of promotion of Ga-67 uptake is unrelated to either voltage-gated, adrenergic, cholinergic, receptor-mediated, or protein kinase C mediated calcium channel activity. Although nitrosipine may evolve small amounts of nitric oxide, the mechanism for Ga uptake is not mediated by nitric oxide. Nitrosipine also induces uptake of Fe and Mn cations (relative efficiency: Ga>Fe>Mn). Nitrosipine-induced cation tranport requires Na+ but not Ca+, is saturable, and is more rapid at pH 6.5 than 7.4.

Tumors and tumor cells may be more sensitive to stimulation of Ga-67 uptake by nitrosipine than normal cells and tissues. Nitrosipine promotes the uptake of Ga-67 by fibroblasts and keratinocytes, but by 10-100 fold less than in tumor cells. Early observations in tumor bearing mice suggest that nitrosipine enhances the tumor uptake of Ga-67 by >15 fold over that of normal tissues.

---

1 Sohn M-H, Jones BJ, Whiting JH, Jr, Datz FL, Lynch RE and Morton KA. Distribution of gallium-67 in normal and hypotransferrinemic tumor-bearing mice. J Nucl Med 34: 2135-2143, 1993.

2 Luttropp CA, Jackson JA, Jones BJ, Sohn, M-H, Lynch RE, and Morton KA. Uptake of gallium-67 in transfected cells and tumors absent or enriched in the transferrin receptor. J Nucl Med 39: 1405-1411, 1998.

3 Luttropp CA, Vu C, Morton KA. Photo-degraded nifedipine strongly mediates the transferrin-independent uptake of Ga-67 in cultured cells. J Nucl Med, 40:159-165, 1999.

Metal Ions in Biology and Medicine; vol 6. Eds. J.A. Centeno, Ph. Collery, G. Vernet, R.B. Finkelman, H. Gibb, J.C. Etienne. John Libbey Eurotext, Paris © 2000, pp. 570-572.

Schedule of administration of gallium compounds in cancer therapy

Philippe Collery[1], Bernard Desoize[2], Bijan Farzami[3], Jean-Pierre Perchellet[4], Lylia Khassanova[5], Hervé Millart[1], Bernhard Keppler[6], Jean-Claude Etienne[1]

[1] Institut International de Recherche sur les Ions Métalliques, Faculté des Sciences, Bâtiment 18, B.P. 1039, 51687 Reims cedex 2, France; [2] Faculté de Pharmacie, 51 rue Cognacq Jay, 51100 Reims, France; [3] Department of Biochemistry, Tehran Medical Sciences University, P.O. Box 14155-5399 Tehran, Iran; [4] Anticancer Drug Laboratory, Division of Biology, Kansas State University, Manhattan 66506-4901, USA; [5] Department of Environmental Protection of Bashkir State University, 32, Frunze Street, 450072 Ufa, Russia; [6] Institute of General and Inorganic Chemistry, Vienna University, Waehringer Str. 42, A-1090 Vienna, Austria

Introduction

Gallium (Ga) is the second metal ion, after platinum, to be used in cancer treatment. Even though the antitumour effects of Ga nitrate were demonstrated a long time ago, the best schedule of administration of Ga compounds still needs to be determined.

Molecular and cellular studies

There is a clear evidence that Ga exerts many effects at molecular and cellular levels (1,2,3). The main mechanism of action could be related with the antagonistic effects between Ga and essential metal ions like magnesium, iron, zinc and calcium. Ga metal ions interact with many key biomolecular targets as DNA, decreasing the enzyme activities of DNA polymerase, ribonucleotide reductase, Mg ATPase, tyrosine phosphatase, reducing the cell membrane permeability and the tubulin polymerisation. They decrease the cell viability or induce apoptosis and the effects depend on the dose but over all on the time of exposure.

Antitumor effects

A parenteral administration of Ga nitrate inhibits the tumour growth in transplanted tumour-bearing animals (4) and an oral administration of Ga chloride significantly decreases the tumour volume (5) by comparison with controls.

Ga compounds have thus been entered in clinical trials.

Ga nitrate has been investigated after a bolus intravenous infusion. It resulted in a high kidney uptake with a renal dose-limiting toxicity (6). The renal concentrations were found to be 130 higher than in the tumour (7). After an intravenous infusion of 700 mg/m2 with prehydratation every 2 weeks the most serious toxicities were renal impairment but also optic neuritis (8). Even though the mean C(max) are as high as 15.2 ± 3.1 µg/ml and the total Ga at the plateau at 1.9 µg/ml there was only one partial response among 21 non small cell lung cancer evaluable patients. A short infusion of gallium nitrate achieving these high peak plasma concentrations resulted in little efficacy in non small cell lung cancer patients and phase II trials failed to demonstrate an efficacy, except in refractory lymphomas (review in 9).

To reduce the toxicity, the continuous intravenous infusion over 5 to 7 days at doses ranging from 100 to 300mg/m2 was proposed (10). Plasma Ga concentrations higher than 1000 µg/l were noted (11). The phase II clinical studies showed promising effects in patients with refractory transitional cell carcinoma of the urothelium (12), or in refractory lymphomas (13). The next step was the combination of intravenous infusions of Ga nitrate with other cytotoxic agents, resulting in a high response rate in metastatic urothelial carcinoma but with severe toxicities and therefore without survival improvement (14-20).

On the other hand, the oral and daily administration of Ga chloride has also been proposed to reduce the renal toxicity, to increase the ratio of Ga uptake by the tumor and mainly to allow the more prolonged contact between the cancer cells and Ga (21). The high Ga tumour uptake observed in experimental was confirmed. Pharmacological studies showed that the plasma Ga concentrations vary according to the type of the tumour, the volume of the tumour, the presence or the absence of metastases. The optimal doses of Ga chloride was found to be of 400 mg. The increase to higher doses up to 1200 mg/24h did not increase the plasma Ga concentrations in lung cancer patients. The combination with cytotoxic agents has been proposed (22-23). It appeared again that the increase of the Ga chloride doses from 400 mg/24h to 1200 mg/24 did not increase the efficacy but induced a toxicity. When administered with cisplatinum, it was shown that even the platinum doses had to be adjusted in order to avoid the cumulative toxicity of this metal and to permit a long period of administration of both Ga chloride and cisplatinum. The long time of administration of Ga chloride could be a major condition to induce a tumour fibrosis, as observed in experimental conditions (24,25), and therefore to increase the survival in cancer patients. Other cytotoxic agents than cisplatinum, which has a cumulative renal toxicity, should be preferred in association with Ga chloride.

Schedule of administration of Ga compounds in combination with other cytotoxic agents

An important condition to increase the efficacy of Ga compounds when administered in cytotoxic agents, should be the schedule of administration. It was proven that a synergism could occur in vitro between Ga and taxol (26), gemcitabine (27) or vinorelbine (28). One important fact was demonstrated in a study comparing different modalities of exposure of Ga with taxol : Ga had to be administered before the exposure with taxol and not simultaneously in order to obtain the best synergistic effects.

Conclusion

The oral administration of Ga chloride allows a continuous cell exposure to the Ga metal ion. At doses of 400 mg/24h this treatment may be maintained during several months without toxicity. Other cytotoxic agents may be administered in combination with the aim of a synergism. All drugs should be administered at non toxic doses. The schedule of administration of Ga chloride in combination with other cytotoxic agents has still to be defined. According to in vitro studies, Ga chloride and the other anticancer drugs should not be administered simultaneously but alternatively (beginning of the treatment by an oral administration of Ga with an interruption of this Ga administration before the intravenous infusion of the other cytotoxic agents). A long period of time of administration of this combined therapy is required to take into account the delayed antitumor effects as well as the induction of a tumour fibrosis and therefore to improve the survival improvement .

References

1) Collery P. Gallium compounds in cancer therapy. In: Metal compounds in cancer therapy. Ed. S.P. Fricker. Chapman & Hall, London 1994, pp. 180-197.

2) Perchellet EM, Ladesich JB, Collery P, Perchellet JP. Microtubule-disrupting effects of gallium chloride in vitro. Anticancer Drugs 1999, 10: 477- 488.

3) Gogvadze V., Zhukova A., Ivanov A., Khassanova L., Khassanova Z., Collery P. The effect of gallium on the calcium retention capacity of rat liver mitochondria. in: Metal Ions in Biology and Medicine. Eds. Ph. Collery, Corbella J., Domingo J.L, Etienne J.C, Llobet J.M. John Libbey Eurotext. 1996, 4, 249-252.

4) Adamson R.H., Canellos G.P., Sieber S. M. Studies on the antitumor activity of gallium nitrate and other group IIIa metal salts. Cancer Chemother. Rep. 1975, 59: 599-610.
5) Collery P, Anghileri L.J., Morel M., Tran G., Rinjard P., Etienne J.C. Tumor growth inhibition by gallium chloride after oral administration in tumor-bearing mice. Eds. J. Anastassopoulou, Ph.Collery, J.C.Etienne, Th. Theophanides. Metal Ions in Biology and Medicine. John Libbey Eurotext, Paris. 1992, 2, 176-177.
6) Bedikian A.Y., Valdivieso M., Bodey G.P., Burgess M.A., Benjamin R.S.,Hall S., Freireich E.J. Phase I clinical studies with gallium nitrate. Cancer Treat. Rep. 1978 , 62: 1449-1453.
7) Hall S.W., Yeung K., Benjamin R.S., Stewart D., Valdivieso M., Bedikian A.Y., Loo T.L. Kinetics of gallium nitrate, a new anticancer agent. Clin. Pharmacol. Ther. 1979, 25: 82-87.
8) Webster LK, Olver IN, Stokes KH, Sephton RG, Hillcoat BL, Bishop JF. A pharmacokinetic and phase II study of gallium nitrate in patients with non-small cell lung cancer. Cancer Chemother Pharmacol 2000; 45: 55-58.
9) Collery P, Pechery C. Clinical experience with tumor-inhibiting gallium complexes. Metal complexes in cancer chemotherapy. Ed. B.K. Keppler. VCH, Weinheim 1993, pp.249-258.
10) Leyland-Jones B, Bhalla RB, Farag F, Williams L, Coonley CJ, Warrell RP Jr. Administration of gallium nitrate by continuous infusion: lack of chronic nephrotoxicity confirmed by studies of enzymuria and beta 2-microglobulinuria. Cancer Treat Rep 1983, 67: 941-942.
11) Warrell RP Jr, Skelos A, Alcock NW, Bockman RS. Gallium nitrate for acute treatment of cancer-related hypercalcemia : clinicopharmacological and dose response analysis. Cancer Res 1986, 46 : 4208 - 4812.
12) Seidman AD, Scher HI, Heinemann MH, Bajorin DF, Sternberg CN, Dershaw DD, Silverberg M, Bosl GJ. Continuous infusion gallium nitrate for patients with advanced refractory urothelial tract tumors. Cancer 1991, 68 : 2561-2565.
13) Warrell RP Jr, Coonley CJ, Straus DJ, Young CW. Treatment of patients with advanced malignant lymphoma using gallium nitrate administered as a seven-day continuous infusion. Cancer 1983, 51:1982-1987.
14) McCaffrey JA, Hilton S, Mazumdar M, Sadan S, Heineman M, Hirsch J, Kelly WK, Scher HI, Bajorin DF. Phase II randomized trial of gallium nitrate plus fluorouracil versus methotrexate, vinblastine, doxorubicin, and cisplatin in patients with advanced transitional-cell carcinoma. J Clin Oncol 1997,15: 2449-2255.
15) Chitambar CR, Zahir SA, Ritch PS, Anderson T. Evaluation of continuous-infusion gallium nitrate and hydroxyurea in combination for the treatment of refractory non-Hodgkin's lymphoma. Am J Clin Oncol 1997, 20:173-178.
16) Dreicer R, Propert KJ, Roth BJ, Einhorn LH, Loehrer PJ. Vinblastine, ifosfamide, and gallium nitrate-an active new regimen in patients with advanced carcinoma of the urothelium. A phase II trial of the Eastern Cooperative Oncology Group (E5892). Cancer 1997, 79:110-114.
17) Dreicer R, Lallas TA, Joyce JK, Anderson B, Sorosky JI, Buller RE .Vinblastine, ifosfamide, gallium nitrate, and filgrastim in platinum- and paclitaxel-resistant ovarian cancer: a phase II study. Am J Clin Oncol 1998, 21: 287-290.
18) Einhorn LH, Roth BJ, Ansari R, Dreicer R, Gonin R, Loehrer PJ . Phase II trial of vinblastine, ifosfamide, and gallium combination chemotherapy in metastatic urothelial carcinoma. J Clin Oncol 1994,12 : 2271-2276.
19) Sandler A, Fox S, Meyers T, Christou A, Weber G, Gonin R, Loehrer PJ, Einhorn LH, Dreicer R. Paclitaxel plus gallium nitrate and filgrastim in patients with refractory malignancies: a phase I trial. Am J Clin Oncol 1998, 21:180-184.
20) Warrell RP Jr, Danieu L, Coonley CJ, Atkins C. Salvage chemotherapy of advanced lymphoma with investigational drugs: mitoguazone, gallium nitrate, and etoposide. Cancer Treat Rep 1987, 71 : 47-51.
21) Collery P, Millart H, Lamiable D, Vistelle R, Rinjard P, Tran G, Gourdier B, Cossart C, Bouana JC, Pechery C, Etienne J.C, Choisy H, Dubois de Montreynaud J.M. Clinical pharmacology of gallium chloride after oral administration in lung cancer patients. Anticancer Res 1989, 9 : 353-356.
22) Collery P, Morel M, Desoize B, Millart H, Perdu D, Prevost A, Vallerand H, Pechery C, Choisy H, Etienne JC Combination chemotherapy with cisplatin, etoposide and gallium chloride for lung cancer: individual adaptation of doses. Anticancer Res 1991, 11:1529-1532.
23) Collery P, Millart H, Kleisbauer JP, Paillotin D, Robinet G, Durand A, Claeyssens S, Legendre JM, Leroy A, Rousseau A, Pechery C, Kochman S. Dose optimization of gallium chloride, orally administered, in combination with platinum compounds. Anticancer Res. 1994, 14, 2299- 2306.
24) Collery Ph, Millart H, Simoneau J.P, Pluot M, Halpern S, Pechery C, Choisy H, Etienne Jc. Experimental treatment of mammary carcinomas by Gallium chloride after oral administration : intratumor dosages of Gallium, anatomopathologic study and intracellular micro-analysis. Trace Elements in Medicine, 1984, 1, 159-161.
25) Collery Ph , Millart H , Pluot M, Anghileri Lj. Effects of gallium chloride oral administration on transplanted C3HBA mammary adenocarcinoma: Ga, Mg, Ca and Fe concentration and anatomopathological characteristics. Anticancer Res. 1986, 6 : 1085-1088.
26) Hata Y, Sandler A, Loehrer PJ, Sledge GW Jr, Weber G. Synergism of taxol and gallium nitrate in human breast carcinoma cells: schedule dependency. Oncol Res 1994, 6:19-24 .
27) Myette MS, Elford HL, Chitambar CR. Interaction of gallium nitrate with other inhibitors of ribonucleotide reductase: effects on the proliferation of human leukemic cells. Cancer Lett. 1998, 129:199-204.
28) Collery P, Lechenault F, Juvin E, Khassanova L, Vernet G, Cazabat A, Lebargy F. Synergistic effects between gallium chloride and vinorelbine on U937 malignant cell lines. In : Metal Ions in Biology and Medicine, Collery P, Brätter P, Negretti de Brätter V, Khassanova L, Etienne J.C. Eds. John Libbey Eurotext, Paris, 1998, 5, 588-593.

Metal Ions in Biology and Medicine; vol 6. Eds. J.A. Centeno, Ph. Collery, G. Vernet, R.B. Finkelman, H. Gibb, J.C. Etienne. John Libbey Eurotext, Paris © 2000, pp. 573-576.

Tris(8-quinolinolato)Ga(III) is active against unicellular and multicellular resistance

Bernard Desoize[1], Philippe Collery[2], Marie-Geneviève Akéli[1], Jean-Claude Etienne[2] and Bernhard Keppler[3]

[1] *Faculté de Pharmacie and* [2] *Centre Hospitalier Universitaire de Reims, rue Cognac-Jay, 51100 Reims, France;* [3] *Institute of General and Inorganic Chemistry, Vienna University, Waehringer Str. 42, A-1090 Vienna, Austria*

Introduction

Resistance to chemotherapy is a major problem. Unfortunately, the classical model used to study this resistance is cells growing as a monolayer on a plastic surface. A549 human cells (NSCLC) grown as spheroids may offer a more suitable alternative model. By analogy to solid tumours, spheroids develop gradients of nutrient diffusion, resulting in centralised populations of quiescent and hypoxic cells. Tumour spheroids are also characterised by a resistance to chemotherapy which is dependent on intercellular contacts. This has been described as "multicellular resistance", in contrast to "unicellular" resistance, such as MDR, observed when cells have no contacts with adjacent cells (1). This three-dimensional model provides conditions more similar to those found *in vivo* in laboratory animals and in patients than does the two-dimensional model. Several mechanisms of multicellular resistance have been described (1). In the present paper, the mechanism underlying the resistance observed in cells grown as spheroids is explored and search for drugs which could circumvent this type of resistance are investigated.

Tris(8-quinolinolato)Ga(III) or KP46 is a gallium (Ga) compound with better bioavailability than Ga chloride ($GaCl_3$) when administered orally (2). The activity of KP46, $GaCl_3$, Tb Cl3, etoposide, doxorubicin, cisplatin and vinblastine were compared in terms of the unicellular and multicellular resistance observed in cell culture models of the parent A549 cell line and of a resistant subline.

Materials and Methods

Cell lines: The human NSCLC line A549 was cultured in RPMI with Glutamax containing 10 % FCS. Resistance was developed by exposure to increasing concentrations of etoposide. Both cell lines were free of mycoplasma, as assessed by DNA staining with Hoechst 33258. Drugs were added to cells cultured as a monolayer after 24 h of incubation and cells were harvested after another 72 h. For spheroid formation, cells were seeded in 96-well plates coated with 2 % agarose (10,000 cells/well) and agitated for 4 h. After 96 h, drugs were added and cells harvested after a further 72 h-incubation.

Cytotoxicity assay: Cytotoxicity was assessed quantitatively by measuring the concentration of intracellular ATP (ATPlite-M ref. 60116941, Packard Instrumt). Drug doses that inhibited cell growth by 50 % (IC50) were calculated.

Results

The *in vitro* cytotoxicity of KP46 was much more potent than that of gallium or terbium chloride (table I).

Table I. *Comparison of IC50 (µmol/l) of metals against the parent A549 and resistant A549R cells, cultured as monolayer and spheroids.*

	KP46		GaCl3		Tb Cl3	
	A549	A549R	A549	A549R	A549	A549R
Monolayer	19.5±0.5	17.5±0.5	>100	>100	>100	>100
Spheroid	23.5±1.5	24.5±0.5	>100	>100	>100	>100

KP46 is less potent than the four established anticancer drugs tested. Nevertheless, the efficacy of KP46 on resistant cells and its MDR indices should be considered (table II).

Table II. *Comparison of IC50 (µmol/l) and of multidrug resistance (MDR) indices for cells grown as* ***monolayer***.

	Etoposide	Doxorubicine	Cisplatine	VLB	KP46
A549	3.2 ± 0.3	0.2 ± 0.1	3.0 ± 0.5	0.008 ± 0.001	19.5 ±0.5
A549 R	68.8±13.2	2.9 ± 0.3	8.8 ± 0.6	29±9.10-3	17.5 ±0.5
MDR indices	21.5	14.5	2.9	3.6	0.9

All compounds tested were less effective when cells were cultured as spheroids. Surprisingly, resistant cells have approximately the same sensitivity to the drugs as the parent cell line, i.e. the MDR indices are close to 1 (table III).

Table III. *Comparison of IC50 (µmol/l) and of* multidrug *resistance (MDR) indices for cells grown as* ***spheroids***.

	Etoposide	Doxorubicine	Cisplatine	VLB	KP46
A549	521 ± 80	7 ± 1	81 ± 15	53 ± 6	23.5 ±1.5
A549 R	765 ± 61	9 ± 4	50 ± 12	145 ± 3	24.5 ±0.5
MDR indices	1.5	1.3	0.6	2.7	1.04

When IC50 values for A549 cells cultured as a monolayer and as spheroids are compared, multicellular resistance (MCR) indices are very large for the conventional anticancer drugs, whereas that of KP46 resistance is close to 1 (table IV).

Table IV. *Comparison of IC50 (µmol/l) and of multicellular resistance (MCR) indices on A549 cells grown as a monolayer and as spheroids.*

	Etoposide	Doxorubicin	Cisplatin	VLB	KP46
Monolayer	3.2 ± 0.3	0.2 ± 0.1	3.0 ± 0.5	0.008 ± 0.001	19.5 ±0.5
Spheroids	521 ± 80	7 ± 1	81 ± 15	53 ± 6	23.5 ±1.5
MCR indices	163	35	27	6 625	1.2

The classical mechanisms of resistance are not relevant for the multicellular resistance model. In A549 and A549R cells, *mdr*1 expression was negative when cultured under either of the growth conditions; MRP was weakly expressed and LRP highly expressed when cells were cultured as a monolayer. When cultured as spheroids, MRP expression was higher, but LRP was only weakly expressed.

It could be asked whether KP46 exerts a purely cytotoxic effect, i.e. it does not act to reverse MDR and multicellular resistance. Alternatively, it could combine a cytotoxic effect and a reversal of MDR. The second hypothesis was tested by combining KP46 and vinblastine *in vitro*. No synergy was observed (table V) when the two compounds were added simultaneously.

Table V. *Cumulative toxicity of KP46 and vinblastine in A549 cells cultured as spheroids. IC50 values are expressed as percent of control.*

	0	KP46 (3 µmol/l)
0	100 %	79 %
vinblastine 0.01 µmol/l	70 %	78 %

In parallel experiments, vinblastine labelled with tritium was added to evaluate its incorporation into spheroids. It appeared that vinblastine incorporation was decreased in the presence of KP46 (table VI).

Table VI. *Incorporation of ^{3}H-vinblastine in A549 cells cultured as spheroids.*

	0	KP46 (3 µmol/l)
^{3}H-vinblastine (pmol/ml)	725	369
Proteins (µg/ml)	545	455
^{3}H-vinblastine (pmol/µg proteins)	1.3	0.81

Multicellular resistance could be partially due to a hypoxic core at the centre of spheroids. It is well-known that hypoxia increases the reduction potential of cells and induces glutathion-S-transferase. Since buthionine sulphoximine (BSO) decreases glutathione levels within cells, it also decreases cellular reduction potential. Thus, BSO should decrease the cytotoxic effect of xome drugs, while it could increase that of drugs, such as doxorubicin, which generate free radicals. Doxorubicin was used in this series of experiments as a positive control. BSO (10-20 µmol/l) increased doxorubicin (3 and 5 µmol/l) toxicity against A549 cells, but did not modify the cytotoxicity of KP46.

Cell aggregation was inhibited, with the purpose of reversing multicellular resistance, using either YIGSR (10-30 µmol/l), which is derived from the laminin β1 chain, or TGFβ1 (10 µmol/l), which increases expression of clusterin and induces rapid spreading of thyroid cells (3). The addition of either of these compounds inhibited A549 spheroid formation, but had no effect on KP46 toxicity against A549 cells.

The kinetics of KP46 and vinblastine cytotoxicity were also studied, i.e. drugs were added at days 0, 1, 2, 3 or 4, during the formation of spheroids, and cells were harvested after a further 3 days. It appeared that KP46 toxicity was decreased after 24 h of incubation (fig.1a) and reached a plateau as soon as 48 h, whereas vinblastine resistance appeared after 48 h, increasing steadily on a logarithmic scale until 96 h (fig.1b and c).

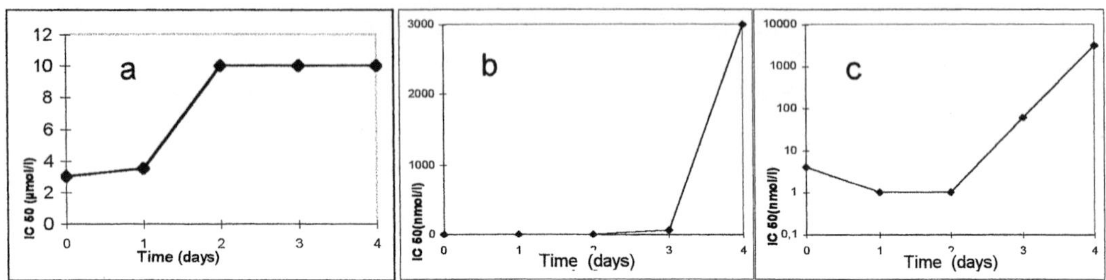

Figure 1. *Kinetics of the cytotoxicity of KP46 (a) and VLB, on a linear scale (b) and a logarithm scale (c), against A549 spheroids.*

Discussion - Conclusion

A549 and A549R cells are much less sensitive to anticancer drugs when cultivated as spheroids. The mechanism of action of KP46 is not well understood. KP46 has only weak activity against A549 cells cultured as a monolayer, compared to the four drugs which are currently used in the clinic. However, efficacy was comparable against A549R cells and against either cell line when cultured as spheroids. KP46 does not disaggregate spheroids and has no MDR-revertant activity per se. The degree of spheroid core hypoxia had no effect on KP46 activity. Since the kinetics of cell killing of KP46 and vinblastine were not comparable, it can be concluded that they do not have the same mechanism of action and that multicellular resistance occurs by different mechanisms for the two drugs.

Multicellular resistance could result from several mechanisms. In our model of sensitive and resistant cells lines, it was demonstrated that the classical mechanisms involving *mdr*1, MRP & LRP were not involved.

These results confirm that multicellular resistance is a complex phenomenon. Spheroids are considered to resemble *in vivo* metastatic nodules and are more representative of the tumorigenic phenotype than are cells in a monolayer culture. As a consequence, new drugs should be screened against such a model.

References

1. Desoize B, Gimonet D, Jardillier JC. Cell culture as spheroids : an approach to multicellular resistance. *Anticancer Res*, 1998 ; 18 : 4147-58.
2. Collery P, Domingo JL, Keppler BK. Preclinical toxicology and tissue distribution of a novel antitumour gallium compound: tris (8-quinolinolato) gallium (III). *Anticancer Res*1996 ; 16 : 687-92.
3. Wegrowski Y, Perreau C, Martiny L, Haye B, Maquart FX and Bellon G. Transforming growth factorβ1 up-regulates clusterin synthesis in thyroid epithelial cells. *Exp Cell Res* 1999 ; 247 : 475-83.

Metal Ions in Biology and Medicine; vol 6. Eds. J.A. Centeno, Ph. Collery, G. Vernet, R.B. Finkelman, H. Gibb, J.C. Etienne. John Libbey Eurotext, Paris © 2000, pp. 577-579.

Antitumor effects of a Vanadium (III) complex with cysteine on malignant cell lines and tumor bearing Wistar rats

R. Liasko[1], S. Karkabounas[1], Th. Kabanos[4], Ph. Collery[5], M. Malamas[2], Ch. Thomas[1], D. Stefanou[3] and A. Evangelou[1]

[1] *Lab. Exp Physiology,* [2] *Pharmacology and* [3] *Pathology, Faculty of Medicine, University of Ioannina, Greece;* [4] *Lab. of Inorganic Chemistry, Faculty of Chemistry, University of Ioannina, Greece, and* [5] *Centre Hospitalier Universitaire, Hôpital de la Maison Blanche, Reims, France*

ABSTRACT

BACKGROUND:Vanadium(V) is a trace metal possessing significant antitumor effects.Organic complexes of vanadium ,mainly of VIII, have not been widely investigated so far .AIM:In the present study effects of a newly synthesized V(III) complex with cysteine in HeLa cells line cultures and leiomyosarcoma-bearing Wistar rats ,in comparison to vanadyl sulfate, are investigated. METHODS: HeLa cells line cultures were incubated in the culture medium with 0,01 mM to 1mM concentrations of V as V(III)-cysteine complex and Vanadyl sulfate, for 24h. The viability of malignant cells was then determined by Trypan blue.

Male Wistar rats developed leiomyosarcomas due to s.c injection of 10.08 mg of Benzo(α)-pyrene(BaP), were divided into four groups(21 animals each) and treated , since tumor detection till death, by oral, daily administration of V(III)-cysteine and vanadyl sulfate at doses of 0,5 mg V/kg b.w and by cysteine 4.5 mg/kg b.w. The fourth group was used as a control group. *In vitro* estimation of total antioxidant capacity of both substances were performed by the Randox method. RESULTS: Vanadyl sulfate possess no antioxidant capacity, while V-cysteine posses a high one. Results in cells and animals, indicated that both vanadyl sulfate and V(III)-cysteine complex exerted antiproliferating effects on malignant HeLa cells, with V(III)-cysteine complex being more potent at high V concentrations(above 0,5 mM V). V(III)-cysteine complex exerted more potent antitumor effects than Vanadyl sulfate on tumor-bearing Wistar rats estimated by the survival time of animals in and the tumor growth rate in each group. A 17,5% remission of tumors developed, observed in of the animals treated by the complex .CONCLUSIONS: According to the above, V(III)-cysteine organic complex exerts more potent antitumor effects than the inorganic salt vanadyl sulfate ,both in malignant cell line cultures and tumor bearing animals, being also less toxic than the inorganic salt, in V treated animals. The high antioxidant capacity of the complex may explain some of its beneficial effects, in animals.

Introduction

Vanadium(V) is a trace metal possessing significant antitumor effects on experimental cancer and antiproliferative effects on malignant cell lines cultures(1)..We have recently synthesized V(III) complexes with aminoacids and peptides among which experimental investigation revealed that the V(III)-cysteine complex (VC) possess the most potent anticarcinogenic effects(2-3). In the present study comparison of the effects of Vanadium(III)-cysteine complex to the inorganic salt Vanadyl Sulfate(VS) on HeLa cell line cultures and tumor bearing Wistar rats are reported.

Materials and Methods

Total antioxidant capacity(TAC) of VC ,VS and cysteine solutions in tap water was estimated, *in vitro*,by the ABTS radical cation photometric assay(Randox) and results were expressed in mM of Trolox having antioxidant capacity equivalent to 1mM of the substance under investigation. HeLa cells cultured in DMEM with 10% fetal calf serum, were incubated for 24h with 0.01mM to 1mM of Vanadium as VS salt and VC complex. Antiproliferative effects of V compounds were estimated by the dye exclusion method with Trypan blue and cytometry.

Male Wistar rats , 3 months old, injected sc by 10.08 mg of Benzo(α)pyrene (BaP) and then randomized into four groups of 21 rats each, were also used for the study. One of the groups was used as control. Animals of the other groups (treatment groups), were administered with 0.5 mg V/ kg b.w/day orally, either as V(III)-cysteine complex or as Vanadyl Sulsfate. The fourth group was treated by cysteine at daily doses isomolar to cysteine complexing with V(4.5mg/kg b.w/day). Animals were followed-up till death, then autopsy and necrotomy were performed , tumors and vital organs weighted and submitted to histologic examination. Antitumor effects of the various schemas were evaluated by calculating the mean survival time, death rate, tumor growth rate and histology of the tumors of animals in each group. statistical evaluation of the results was performed by the t-student's test

Results

Total antioxidant capacity (TAC) and Lag time of substances tested was found as following (Table 1).

Table 1: TAC and lag time of the substances tested in relation to time from solution preparation.

Substances (in solution)	Time from preparation (min)	TAC (mM)- Lag Time (sec)
Cysteine	10	0.430 36.0
Cysteine	300	0.000 00.0
V(III)-cysteine	10	0.760 38.4
V(III)-cysteine	300	0.680 35.2
Vanadyl sulfate	10	0.000 00.0

VC complex possess a high total antioxidant capacity and lag time in water preparations which is not abolished 5 hours after solution preparation in contrast to VS which does not exhibit any antioxidant capacity. Estimation of antiproliferating effects of V compounds (VS and VC) revealed that VC complex exhibits significantly higher antiproliferative effects on HeLa cells than VS mainly at concentrations over 0.5 mM ($p<0.001$),(table 2).

Table 2: Number of surviving HeLa cells (mean ± SD) after 24h incubation, in relation to V concentration.

V conc (μM)	Vanadyl Sulfate	V(III)-cysteine complex	Significance (p)
00 (control)	75.6±10.6	75.6±10.6	---
10	67.4± 6.9	74.8± 7.9	NS
50	31.2± 1.8	31.7± 3.7	NS
500	23.4± 2.5	16.6± 3.7	<0.01
1000	6.0± 1.3	0.1± 0.1	<0.001

There was a significant prolongation of mean survival time of animals treated by VC(243±21 days) , VS (218±28 days)and Cysteine (220±31days) in comparison to control(172±19 days). Survival of animals treated by the VC complex was however significantly prolonged compared to that of the other groups of treatment ($p<0.01$). Tumor growth rate of the animals treated by the VC complex (0.7±0.3g/day) was also significantly lower than that of the other treatment and the control group(1.4±0.43g/day).Death rate curve revealed that animals' death initiation was significantly delayed in TR-VC group in comparison to the other groups of the study (initiation from the 28th week in TR-VC group and between the 21st and 22nd week in the other groups). There was also a 17.5% complete remission of tumor developed, revealed by autopsy in the TR-VC group . Histology revealed that BaP induced the development of soft tissue malignant tumors (leiomyosarcomas) at the site of injection. Metastases were also found in lungs of animals in all groups. No differences in the histological grade of tumors was found among groups.

Discussion

Results of our study revealed that both vanadyl sulfate and vanadium(III)-cysteine complex possess significant antitumor properties as it is evident by their effects on malignant cell lines(HeLa) and rats bearing and soft tissue malignant tumors which are considered resistance to chemotherapy and radiation. V(III)-cysteine complex exhibits however more potent effects than vanadyl sulfate as it is evident by the comparison of its actions on HeLa cells and experimental malignant tumors,being also as we have previously reported(3)less toxic than VS to rats. The latter may be due to its high antioxidant capacity which is not abolished for ours in water solution in contrast to vanadyl sulfate which possess no antioxidant capacity. Sulfhydryl derivatives of cysteine, not easily oxidized in solutions such as N-acetyl-cysteine have also been found to prevent cells from oxidative stress and or to enhance, depended on its concentration the free radical production of vanadium inorganic salts on malignant cells(4,5).

Antitumor effects of vanadium on cells and animal malignancies have so far attributed to a variety of biological effects of V, such as increased intracellular concentrations in malignant tumors(6), inhibition of DNA polymerases, nucleotid transferases and phoshotransferases in cells(7-8). The oxidizing effects of vanadium, induced through its participation to free radical reactions, taking place mainly in malignant cells, is also supported by a number of recent reports(9).In conclusion the V(III)-cysteine complex seems to exert more potent antiproliferative and antitumor effects than the inorganic salt vanadyl sulfate, being also less toxic. Experimental results as above may indicate the application of vanadium preparations in the treatment of human malignancies.

References

1.Djorgevitz C: Antitumor activity of vanadium compounds. In "Metal Ions in Biological Systems" H. Siegel and A Siegel (Eds), Marcel Dekker publ., NY USA, Vol. 31 pp 596-616,*1995.*

2.Evangelou A, Karkabounas S, Kalpouzos G, Malamas M, Liasko R, Stefanou D, Vlahos A, Cabanos T: Comparison of the therapeutic effects of two vanadium complexes administered at low concen-trations on BaP-induced malignant tumors in rats. *Cancer Lett 119:221-225,1997*

3. Liasko R, Cabanos Th, Karkabounas S, Malamas M, Tasiopoulos A, Stefanou D, Collery Ph and Evangelou A: Beneficial effects of a vanadium complex with cysteine administered at low doses on BaP-induced leimyosarcomas in Wistar rats. *Anticancer Res 18:3609-3614,1998.*

4. Huckle WR, Earp HS:Synergisitic activation of tyrosine phosphorylation by orthovanadate plus A23177 or aromatic 1,2-diols. *Biochem 33:1519-1525,1994*

5.Shi XL, Sun XY, Datal NS: Reaction of vanadium(V)with thiols generates vanadium(IV) abd thiyl radicals. *FEBS Lett 27:185-188,1990*

6.Iwai K, Kimora S, Ido T, Iwata R: Tumor uptake of vanadium-48 vanadyl chlorine E-6 sodium, as a tumor imaging agent in tumor bearing mice. *Nucl Med Biol 17:775-780,1980.*

7.Jandhyala BS, Hom GJ: Minireview; physiological and pharmacological effects of vanadium . *Life Sci 33:1325-1340,1983*

8.Kustin K, Macara JG: The new biochemistry of Vanadium. *Comments Inorg Chem 102:1-72,1982*

9. Cruz T, Morgan A, Min W: In vivo and in vitro antineoplastic effects of orthovanadate. *Moll Cell Biochem 153:161-166,1995*

Metal Ions in Biology and Medicine; vol 6. Eds. J.A. Centeno, Ph. Collery, G. Vernet, R.B. Finkelman, H. Gibb, J.C. Etienne. John Libbey Eurotext, Paris © 2000, pp. 580-584.

Kinetics and DNA-metal binding studies of titanocene antitumor agents

Carmen E. Rivera and Enrique Meléndez

University of Puerto Rico, Department of Chemistry, P.O. Box 9019, Mayaguez Puerto Rico 00681

ABSTRACT

UV-VIS titration methods were used to study the kinetic of ligand hydrolysis and interaction of titanocene complexes to calf thymus DNA. The kinetic data provided the half-life time ($t_{1/2}$) for each of the species. The half-life time is 1-3 hours, enough time to pursue the binding studies. The binding parameters have been obtained using Scatchard plots. The best fit was obtained when the exclusion sites is for 4. The binding constants (K) are in the order of 10^5, indicating strong affinity of titanocene complexes to DNA. The binding ability of the complexes was studied in presence of high concentration of NaCl.

INTRODUCTION

The potential use of metal complexes in chemotherapy has been well documented since 1969 when cis-diamminedichloroplatinum(II), cis-platin, showed to possess antitumor properties [1]. Subsequently, in the early seventies and eighties, platinum complexes became very popular antineoplastic agents with high efficacy against human testicular, ovarian, bladder, head and neck carcinomas [2,3]. However, the toxic side effects such as nephrotoxicity and myelotoxicity are the major drawbacks of these inorganic complexes for clinical applications [2,3]. The need of searching new compounds forced the researchers to look into new emerging areas, e.g. organometallic chemistry.

The antitumor activity of titanocene dichloride, Cp_2TiCl_2 (I), was reported for the first time in 1979 by Köpf-Maier and Köpf [4]. Other transition metal sandwich complexes of general formula Cp_2MX_2 (M = V, Nb, Mo; X = halides and pseudohalides) and $Cp_2Fe^+X^-$ have demonstrated antitumor activity [5-7] but among them, Cp_2TiCl_2 showed to be the most active [5,8-11]. Titanocene dichloride is active against colon, lung and breast cancers and is currently on clinical trials [12]. However, we envision that its activity could be improved by replacing the chloride by more active ligands. Therefore, part of our research efforts have been directed to prepare and chemically characterize modified titanocene derivatives in order to improve the antitumor activity of the parent complex, Cp_2TiCl_2.

One of the aspects of our research is to gain a better understanding on how the metal antitumor agents interact with biological macromolecules, in hope of unraveling the mechanism of action and possibly modify these species to attain the desired biological activity. Most antitumor agents act by interfering with molecular processes in the cell replication cycle [13]. Exist many covalent and non-covalent interactions by which an antitumor agent can get engaged and express its action. Cationic metal species could interact externally with phosphates, involving Metal-O(phosphate) coordination [14]. Furthermore, the metal can coordinate to the DNA bases forming Metal-N bonds or N-M-O chelates [14]. In addition, the complex can bear biologically active ligands that could interact separately expressing its activity or in cooperation with the metal exhibiting potentially synergism. In this regard, we have prepared and spectroscopically characterized titanocene derivatives, $[Cp_2TiL]Cl_2$ (L = 6-thioguanine (II), 6-thiopurine (III), 2-thiocytosine (IV), 2-thiouracil (V)) [15]. Now we are investigating the interaction of these complexes to Calf-thymus DNA. Since titanocene dichloride and thionucleobases are antitumor agents, if both interact in a concerted manner, the $[Cp_2TiL]Cl_2$ complexes, under appropriate conditions, could exhibit synergism [16-19]. Our initial interest is to determine the binding parameters of these complexes to DNA. Herein we report our findings.

Experimental

a) Complexes. The complexes, $[Cp_2TiL]Cl_2$, were prepared according to a published procedure [15]. Verification of their identity was accomplished by ^1H NMR and IR spectroscopies. The complexes are soluble in DMSO and DMSO/water solutions. DMSO solutions of 1 x10^{-3} M were prepared and used as stock solutions for the titration.

b) DNA. Calf-thymus DNA was obtained from Sigma Chemical Company either as solid polymer or in preweighed (2mg) ready to dissolve vials. For the polymer, 5mg/ml was dissolved in Tris buffer (pH=7.4) at 4° C for 72 hours. A portion of this solution was treated with a mixture of chloroform and isoamylic alcohol to remove any protein remaining. The resulting DNA solution was centrifuged and the DNA pellet isolated and redissolved in Tris buffer at pH of 7.4. It is important to observe that the native DNA showed the same performance as the purified one. The DNA concentration was determined spectrophotometrically using an ε_{260} of 6600 $M^{-1}cm^{-1}$. For the DNA solution containing NaCl, aliquots of concentrated solution of NaCl were added to the DNA solution adjusting the final concentration of NaCl to 01.M.

c) Methods. Spectrophotometric titrations were carried out at 25°C and a pH of 7.2-7.4. EDTA was not used in the DNA solutions since it formed a white precipitate, presumably a Ti-EDTA complex and created interference with the analysis. Spectrophotometric measurements were performed in a double beam Lambda BIO 20 Perkin Elmer spectrometer termostated at 25°C. The system is interfaced with a 586 Nokia Computer System and the spectral handling was carried out using WinLab Software. Titration solutions were prepared by adding to complex solution (1 mL of Ti 1 x 10^{-3} M) succesive amount of DNA (2-4 x 10^{-4}M) and completing to total volume of 10 mL with tris buffer. After one hour of rest time, the solutions were loaded in a 1.0 cm quartz cell and the spectra recorded, using the appropriate mixture of Tris and DMSO in the background to cancel out the solvent interference. The data were analyzed by a non-linear least squares procedure according to Mc Ghee and von Hippel formalism, to estimate the standard deviations on the binding constants [20].

Results

Titanocene dichloride as well as antimetabolites such as thiopurine and thiopyrimidines (thionucleobases) are known to interfere with DNA synthesis but certainly, their mechanism of action differ [8,13,21-23]. Thionucleobases act by interfereing with the biosynthesis of nucleic acids or proteins either by inhibiting an especific enzyme or by substituting for a metabolite thus rendering the key molecule functionally inoperable [13]. In general, the antimetabolites are cell cycle dependent agents. On the other hand, Cp_2TiCl_2 in water is known to form $Cp_2Ti(H_2O)_2^{2+}$ and this presumably coordinates through the oxygen of the phosphate and nitrogen of the nucleobase [24-28]. Therefore, the DNA titration is aimed at the understanding of the Ti-DNA binding equilibrium.

All the synthesized complexes used in this study are moderate stable in DMSO and DMSO/water solutions. We have determined the stability in DMSO and DMSO/water solutions. $Cp_2Ti(H_2O)_2^{2+}$ (in DMSO/water) or $Cp_2Ti(DMSO)_2^{2+}$ (in DMSO) have been determined to be the initial products of solvolysis. The half-life time, $t_{1/2}$, for the $[Cp_2TiL]Cl_2$ complexes is 1-3 hours for the thionucleobase loss and 7-41 hours for the Cp loss [15]. Therefore, the complexes have sufficient stability to perform the DNA titration. Figure 1 presents the structures of complexes under study [15]. All of them contain the Cp_2Ti^{2+} unit, the responsible for the DNA coordination, the variations are in the ligands.

The interaction of Ti complexes with increasing amount of Calf-thymus DNA yields an irreversible spectral changes characterized by hypochromism on the absorption bands of the complexes. However, each complex behaves different depending on the thionucleobase. The data was analyzed using the McGhee and von Hippel equation (1) based on the near neighbor exclusion model:

$$r/c = K(1-nr)[1-nr/1-(n-1)r]^{(n-1)} \quad (1)$$

where K = intrinsic binding constant

n = number of consecutive site made inaccessible by the binding a single drug compound.

r = ratio between the bound drug and DNA concentration

Figure 2 shows a typical Scatchard plot for a Ti-DNA ratio of 0-200%. A nonlinear least-squares fit was applied to the data. The best fit to the curve (data) was obtained when the exclusion site size (n) was 4. The intrinsic binding constants (K) were obtained from the intercept on the ordinate of the Scatchard plot (r/D_f). Table I collects all the intrinsic binding constants and exclusion site size for the complexes.

Table I. Intrinsic binding constants (K, M^{-1}) and exclusion sites (n) for titanocene derivatives.

Complex	K	[NaCl]	n
Cp_2TiCl_2	$2.61(8) \times 10^5$	-------	4
	$2.27(2) \times 10^5$	0.1 M	4
$[Cp_2Ti(2\text{-thiocytosine})]Cl_2$	$1.03(9) \times 10^5$	-------	4
	$3.1(1) \times 10^6$	0.1 M	4
$[Cp_2Ti(6\text{-thioguanine})]Cl_2$	$3.96(4) \times 10^5$	-------	4
	$6.84(2) \times 10^4$	0.1 M	4
$[Cp_2Ti(2\text{-thiouracil})]Cl_2$	$5.85(8) \times 10^5$	------	4
	$1.31(4) \times 10^5$	0.1 M	4
$[Cp_2Ti(6\text{-mercaptopurine})]Cl_2$	$7.91(1) \times 10^5$	------	4
	$3.64(9) \times 10^5$	0.1 M	4

The table shows that the number of exclusion sites is 4 for all the complexes. To have a baseline and point of comparison, binding interaction between Cp_2TiCl_2 and DNA was performed. From the series of complexes studied we can observe that Cp_2TiCl_2 showed the smallest binding constant and surprisingly is insensitive to the ionic strength. As we move along in the series of complexes, it can be noticed an enhancement in the binding constants. In general all complexes have a K in the 10^5 magnitude when no salt is added. The 2-thiouracil and 6-mercaptopurine complexes showed small dependence on ionic strength of the solutions. For the 6-thioguanine complex, the K value is lower by less than one order of magnitude, showing clearly dependence on ionic strength. In many cases, the ability of a drug to interact with DNA decreases as a result of an increase on the ionic strength [29,30]. More ions in solution make less accessible the possible binding sites in the DNA to drugs . On the other hand, the 2-thiocytosine complex showed an opposite behavior, an increase in the K by about one order of magnitude.

Discussion

Our Ti-DNA interaction studies by UV-VIS spectrophotometry revealed, for all the complexes examined, non-linear Schatchard plots and non-cooperative binding behaviors. This suggests that titanocene complexes make inaccessible more that one binding site in the DNA. This could be consistent with other research groups, which invokes Cp_2TiCl_2 involved in Ti-O (phosphate) and Ti-N (DNA base) coordinations. (24-28). However, with this data we can not elucidate these type of interactions.

The intrinsic binding constants (K) are very high (10^5) indicating a strong and stable DNA-Ti interaction as well as some apparent ligand dependency. However, the fact that thionucleobases are biologically active while the cell cycle is active and this is not the case for isolated DNA, suggests that this apparent enhancement in the binding constants may be attributed to the solubility that induce these ligands to titanocene in buffer conditions and not by the activity of the ligands. Of course, some hydrogen bonds could be invoked between DNA and thionucleobases that could enhance the binding interactions however, interaction studies of thionucleobases and Calf-thymus DNA produced no measurable effects on the UV-VIS spectra. Nevertheless, at this point we can not completely rule out this type of hydrogen bonding interaction.

To determine the binding ability of the complexes to DNA, the concentration of NaCl was adjusted to 0.1 M. This substantial change in ionic strength of the solution would evidence any change in the binding parameters. Surprisingly, the effect of NaCl on the K values has no predictable pattern. On the Cp_2TiCl_2, the presence of salt has no measurable effect and for $[Cp_2Ti(2\text{-thiouracil})]Cl_2$ and $[Cp_2Ti(6\text{-mercaptopurine})]Cl_2$ the effect is subtle. More dramatic effects are observed in $[Cp_2Ti(6\text{-thioguanine})]Cl_2$ and $[Cp_2Ti(2\text{-thiocytosine})]Cl_2$. For $[Cp_2Ti(6\text{-thioguanine})]Cl_2$ the binding interaction is discouraged while for $[Cp_2Ti(2\text{-thiocytosine})]Cl_2$ is encouraged. A clear explanation for this behavoir can not be provided at the present time and awaits for specificity studies using NMR spectroscopy. Finally, we have realized that in order to address the effect of the ligand on the antitumor activity of the titanocene complexes, an in vitro screening tests with tumor cell lines is needed. This area is currently under investigation [31].

Acknowledgements

The author are grateful to NIH-SCORE grant and the Department of Chemistry, University of Puerto Rico for financial support.

References

1. Rosenberg B, Camp LV, Trosko JE, Mansour VH (1969) Nature 222:385.
2. De Vita VT, Hellman S, Rosenberg SA (eds) (1985) Cancer, Principles and Practice of Oncology, Lippincott, Philadelphia.
3. Nicoloni M, (ed) (1988) Platinum and other metal coordination compounds in cancer chemotherapy. Nijhoff, Boston.
4. Köpf H, Köpf-Maier P (1979) Angew Chem Int Ed. Engl 18:47.
5. Köpf-Maier P, (1994) Eur J Clin Pharmacol 47:1.
6. Köpf-Maier P, Köpf H (1988) Structure and Bonding 70:103.
7. Köpf-Maier P, Köpf H (1987) Chem Rev 87:1137.
8. Chritodoulou C, Eliopoulos AG,Young LS, Hodgkins L, Ferry D, Kerr DJ (1998) Br J Cancer 77: 2088.
9. Vellena-Heinsen C, Friedrich M, Ertan AK, Farnhammer C, Schmidt W (1998) Anti-Cancer Drugs 9: 557.
10. Friedrich M, Villena-Heinsen C, Farnhammer C, Schmidt W, (1998) Eur J of Gynaecological Oncology 19:333.
11. Harstrick A, Schmoll HJ, Sass G, Poliwoda H, Rustmum Y, (1993) Eur J Cancer Part A, 29A:1000.
12. Berdel WE, Schmoll HJ, Scheulen ME, Korfel A, Knoche MF, Harstrick A, Bach F, Buumgart J, Sab G (1994) J Cancer Res Clin Oncol 120(supp):R172.
13. a. Ottenbrite RM, Butler GB (eds) (1984) Anticancer and Interferon Agents: Synthesis and Properties, Drug and Pharmaceutical Sciences vol 2, Marcel Dekker, NY.
    b.Foye WO (ed) (1995) Cancer Chemotherapeutic Agents, American Chemical Society, Washington, DC.
14. Tullius TD (ed) (1989) Metal-DNA Chemistry, ACS Symposium Series 402, American Chemical Society, Washington DC.
15. Meléndez E, Rivera C, Marrero M, Hernández E, Segal A (2000) Inorg Chim Acta (298/2): 178.
16. Sadler PJ (1991) Adv Inorg Chem 36: 9489.
17. Pasini A, Zunino F (1987) Angew Chem Int Ed 26: 615.
18. Sherman SE, Lippard SJ (1987) Chem Rev 87:1153.
19. Drewinko B, Dispasquale MA, Yang LY, Berlogie B, Trujillo JM (1985) Chem-Biol Interact 55:1.
20. McGhee JD, von Hippel PH (1974) J Mol Biol 86:469.
21. Köpf-Maier P, Köpf H (1980) Naturwissenschaften 67:415.
22. Köpf-Maier P, Wagner W, Köpf H (1981) Naturwissenschaften 68:272.
23. Köpf-Maier P (1982) J Cancer Res Clin Oncol 103:145.
24. Yang P, Guo M (1998) Met-Based Drugs 5:41.
25. Zhang Z, Yang P, Guo M, Wang H (1996) J Inorg Biochem 63: 183.
26. Zhang Z, Yang P, Guo M (1996) Transition Met Chem 21:322.
27. Mokdsi G, Harding MM (1998) J Organomet Chem 565:29.
28. Murray J H, Harding MM (1994) J Med Chem 37:1936.
29. Chaires J B, Priebe W, Graves D E, Burke T G (1993) J Am Chem Soc 115:5360.
30. Manning G S (1979) Acc Chem Res 12:443.
31. González F, Meléndez E unpublished results.

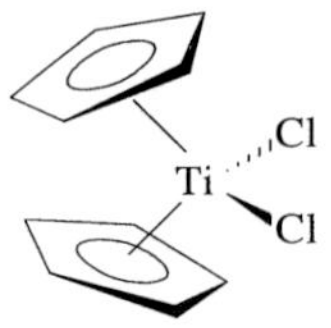

I

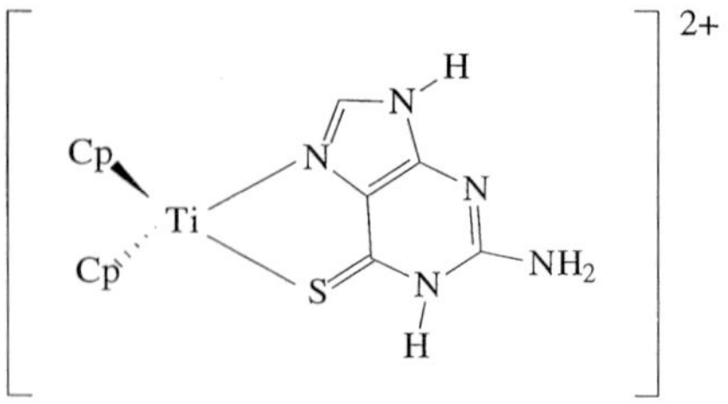

II

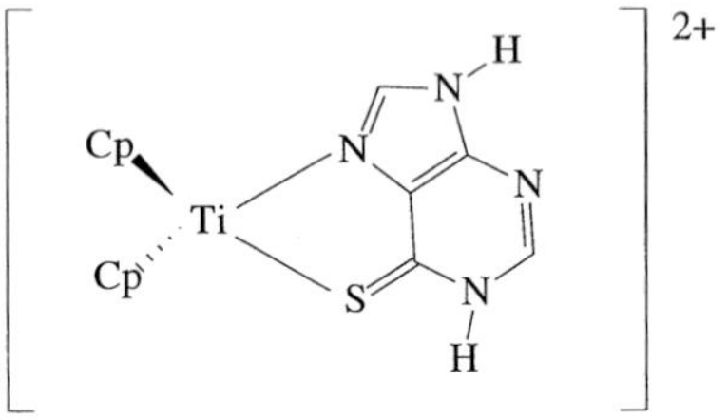

III

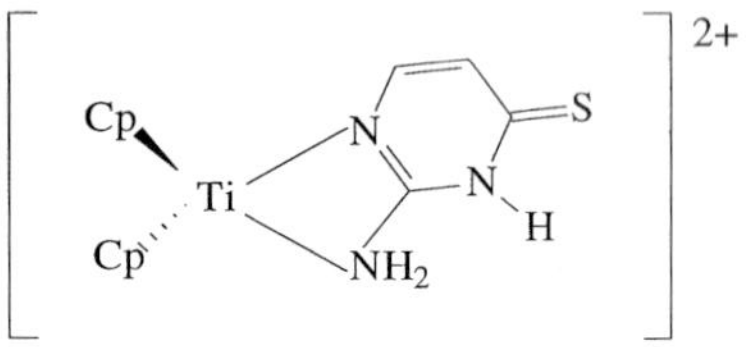

IV

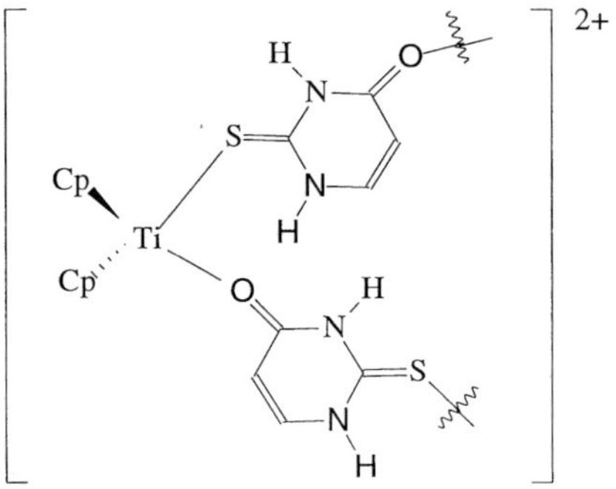

V

Figure 1. Structure of titanocene dichloride and titanocene derivatives.

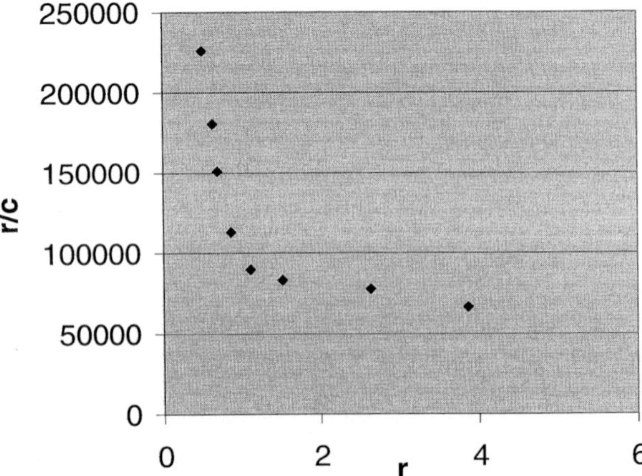

Figure 2. Scatchard plot of the binding of titanocene to calf thymus DNA.

Metal Ions in Biology and Medicine; vol 6. Eds. J.A. Centeno, Ph. Collery, G. Vernet, R.B. Finkelman, H. Gibb, J.C. Etienne. John Libbey Eurotext, Paris © 2000, pp. 585-587.

Copper valproate: vibrational spectrum, thermal behaviour and biological assays

Gloria E. Tobón Zapata[1], Osvaldo A.N. Baldini[2], Luis B. Blanch[2], Enrique J. Baran[3] and Susana B. Etcheverry[3]

[1] *Departamento de Farmacia, Facultad de Química Farmacéutica, Universidad de Antioquia, Medellín, Colombia;* [2] *Area de Diseño de Fármacos,* [3] *CEQUINOR (Centro de Química Inorgánica), Facultad de Ciencias Exactas, Universidad Nacional de La Plata, 47 y 115 (1900) La Plata, Argentina*

Introduction

Copper is an essential element for animals and plants [1] and under ionic form has great affinity for various biological molecules in the organism. Several diseases that affect the central nervous system (CNS) are accompanied by seizures and they are associated with alterations of copper metabolism [2]. Valproic acid (2-propilpentanoic acid) in the form of its sodium salt has wide spectrum of activity as an anticonvulsant drug. It has been previously shown [3] that copper (II) complexes of anticonvulsant and antiinflammatory ligands are more active and appropriated drugs than the parent ligands themselves. The aim of this study was the synthesis of the copper (II) complex of valproic acid, its physicochemical characterization and the evaluation of its anticonvulsant activity in a Swiss mice laboratory model.

Synthesis of $[Cu(C_7H_{15}COO)_2]_2$

The complex was obtained by slow addition of an aqueous copper(II) acetate solution to an ethanolic solution of valproic acid. The green-blue precipitate was washed several times with water and ethanol and purified by chromatography in a silica gel column (elution solvents: dichloromethane, dichloromethane-methanol (10:1) and methanol). Yield of the analytical pure complex = 55%.

Physicochemical properties

Vibrational spectrum: (IR). The strong band located at 1700 cm^{-1} in the spectrum of valproic acid is assigned to the C=O stretching vibration. In the complex, the very strong band at 1580 cm^{-1} corresponds to ν_{as} COO^- , whereas the corresponding symmetric mode is found as a medium intensity band at 1419 cm^{-1}. $\Delta\nu$ (ν_{as}-ν_s = 161 cm^{-1}) indicates coordination through a bidentate carboxilate group. The two weak bands at 481 and 414 cm^{-1} may be assigned to Cu-O vibrations [4].

*Thermal analysis.*It was carried out under an oxygen atmosphere. After a three step decomposition, CuO was identified as the final residue by IR spectroscopy. The total weight loss (77.0%) is in good agreement with the calculated value (77.3%). This thermogravimetric anlysis confirms the absence of coordinated water molecules.

Evaluation of $[Cu(C_7H_{15}COO)_2]_2$ as anticonvulsant agent

Pharmacological testing of $[Cu(C_7H_{15}COO)_2]_2$ was carried out through the guidlines of the Epilepsy Branch of the National Institute of Neurological Disorders and Stroke (NINDS) following the protocol adopted by the Antiepileptic Drug Development (ADD) Program [5]. The preliminary results (phase I) [6] obtained by the application of the Maximal Electroshock Seizures (MES) and the rotorod test can be seen in Table I. The phase I testing was done following intraperitoneal injection (IP) of drug suspensions in PEG400 (30%). These results indicate that copper valproate showed a low protection index. The 100 µmol/kg dose was ineffective to protect against the induced seizures. Doses of 200 and 300 µmol/kg protected 25% of animal sample 1 hr after IP injection. Unfortunately, these doses were toxic for the mice because they died between 48 and 72 hr after the administration of the drug. Finally, the 400 µmol/kg dose protected the 60% of the animals but all of them showed neurotoxicity signs in the rotorod test and died between 24-48 hours after the IP injection. Altogether, these results indicate that copper valproate protects Swiss mice against induced seizures at doses that are close to the lethal ones for the animals. Taking into account that copper valproate as a monodrug was not satisfactory, laboratory trials were undertaken to study the possible beneficial association between this drug and sodium valproate in order to obtain better anticonvulsant action with reduction of toxic effects. Results are shown in Figure I. As can be seen, the association of a constant dose (100 µmol/kg) of copper valproate with different doses of sodium valproate (250-1000 µmol/kg), showed again less protection than the sodium valproate used as monodrug. For doses lower than 750 µmol/kg, a low protection index (12,5%) was determined. The upper dose produced 25% of protection.

Copper valproate													
Time	30 min				1 hr			2 hr			4 hr		
Dose (µmol/kg)	100	200	300	400	100	200	300	100	200	300	100	200	300
MES	5/5	4/4	4/4	5/5	4/4	3/4	3/4		3/4	3/4		3/4	3/4
Rotorod test	3/5	1/4	1/4	5/5	0/4	0/4	0/4		0/4	1/4		0/4	0/4

Table I. Results from MES and rotorod tests.

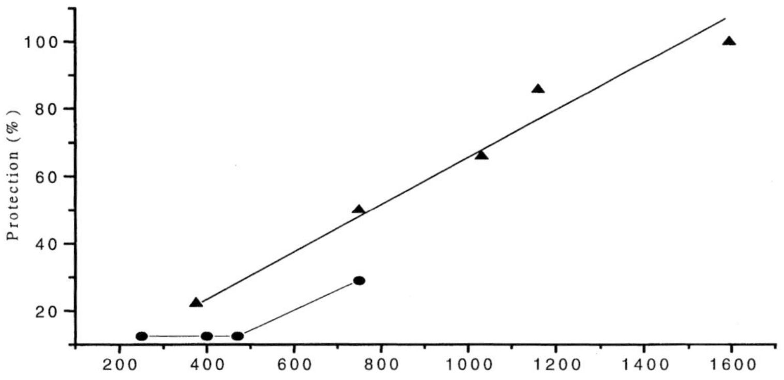

□ sodium valproate □Copper valproate ((100 µmol/kg) with different doses of sodium valproate.

Fig.1. Effect of the association of the copper complex with sodium valproate

Bibliography.

1- Danks DM, Disorders of copper transport. In: Scriver CR, Beaudet AL, Sly WS, Valle D., eds. *The Metabolic and Molecular Bases of Inherited Disease*. New York: McGraw-Hill, 1989: 1411-1431.

2- Kurkeci AE, Alpay F, Tanindi S, Gocay E, Ozcan O, Akin R, Isimer A, Sayal A. Plasma Trace Element, Plasma Gluthation Peroxidase, and Superoxide Dismutase Levels in Epileptic Children Receiving Antiepileptic drug therapy. *Epilepsia*. 1995; 36: 600-604.

3- Abuhijleh AL, Woods C. Syntesis, Characterization, and Oxidase Activities of Copper (II) Complexes of the Anticonvulsant Drug Valproate. *J Inorg Biochem* 1996; 64:55-67.

4- Nakamoto K. *Infrared and Raman Spectra of Inorganic and Coordination Compounds;* New York: John Wiley, & Sons, Inc. 1996.

5- a)Anticonvulsant Screening Proyect, Antiepileptic Drug Development Program; National Institute of Health, DHEW publ. (NIH), (USA), 1978: 78-1093.

b) Krall RL, Penry JK, White BG, Kupferbeg HJ, Swinyard EA., Antiepileptic Drug Development II. Anticonvulsant Drug Screening. *Epilepsia* 1978; 19: 409-428.

6- Porter RJ, Cereghino JJ, Gladding GD, Helssie BJ, Kupferberg HJ, Scotville B, White BG. Antiepileptic Drug Development Program. Cleveland *Clin. Q*. 1984; 51: 239-305.

Metal Ions in Biology and Medicine; vol 6. Eds. J.A. Centeno, Ph. Collery, G. Vernet, R.B. Finkelman, H. Gibb, J.C. Etienne. John Libbey Eurotext, Paris © 2000, pp. 588-590.

Chemopreventive potential of vanadium on dimethylhydrazine-induced rat colon cancer

Anjan Banerjee, Aditi Roy, Niharendu Bhusan Kanjilal, Uttam Bhattacharya and Malay Chatterjee*

Division of Biochemistry, Department of Pharmaceutical Technology, Jadavpur University, Calcutta 700 032, India

Abstract: The present study was aimed to determine whether the dose (0.5ppm) and form (ammonium monovanadate) of vanadium (V), effective in experimental hepatocarcinogenesis, can be extended to cancer of the colon as well. Male Sprague Dawley rats subjected to dimethylhydrazine (DMH)-injection (20mg/kg b.w./week, i.p., for 16 weeks) were administered V *ad libitum*, through drinking water, upto 32 weeks. Tumor incidence ($P<0.001$) and tumor multiplicity ($P<0.05$) were significantly reduced by V treatment as against DMH control values. GST activity remained depleted ($P<0.001$) with DMH treatment. V supplementation raised the enzyme activity by 6-fold in the colon and 4.7-fold in the liver of the DMH-induced rat. Data conclusively documents an anticarcinogenic potential of V in rat colon cancer.

Introduction: Under certain experimental conditions, DMH induces colon carcinomas in rats with great reproducibility and marked organ specificity [1]. Our laboratory has observed anticarcinogenic biological response of V against Dalton's lymphoma and chemical rat hepatocarcinogenesis model. Kingsnorth and his coworkers reported a no-effect of V on DMH-induced mice [2]. With GSTs having been acknowledged as preneoplastic markers [3], the present study was made to investigate chemopreventive efficacy of V (0.5ppm) by assessing GST activity (16 weeks) and tumor incidence/ multiplicity (32 weeks) in DMH-induced rat.

Materials and Method: Male Sprague Dawley rats (80-90g), purchased from Indian Institute of Chemical Biology, Calcutta 700 032, India, were maintained on a semipurified basal diet and water *ad libitum*. After an initial acclimatisation to standard laboratory conditions for 10 days, animals were assigned into experimental and control groups. **Group A** served as DMH (administered i.p. at 20mg/kg b.w., once a week, in 0.9% NaCl solution for 16 weeks) control animals. **Group B** animals represented the normal control group. **Group C** animals were subjected to both DMH and V (0.5ppm, as ammonium monovanadate, through drinking water) treatment, the latter being administered *ad libitum* till the end of the study at 32 weeks. **Group D** animals were V controls. They were not subjected to any DMH injection.
Interim sacrifice was performed at 16 weeks, from the day of DMH initiation, to evaluate GST enzyme activity. The terminal sacrifice was carried out at 32 weeks for morphometric analysis. Data for GST activity and tumor multiplicity were statistically analysed by Student's t-test. Fischer's exact probability test was performed for the tumor incidence study.
Results and Discussion: Results of the present study (table I) confirmed a positive role of V in experimental carcinogenesis. A decrease in colonic GST activity after DMH injection may implicate enhanced covalent binding of DMH metabolites to cellular DNA leading to neoplastic growth. Enhanced GST activity with V supplementation indicates an increased ability of organism to reactive carcinogenic metabolites and thereby reduce the risk of tumor induction [4]. This is evident with tumor incidence and tumor multiplicity studies made on the rat (table I). The use of V for the prevention and treat ment of cancer is thus in its infancy. Teasing out the details should be a great adventure to economically deal with a threatening, hostile environment.
Reference: 1.McLellan E.A. and Bird R.P. Effect of disulfiram on 1,2-dimethylhydrazine and azoxymethane-

induced aberrant crypt foci. Carcinogenesis 1991; 12: 969-972.
2.Chatterjee M. and Bishayee A. Vanadium-A new tool for cancer prevention. In: Jerome O Nriagu. Part II. Vanadium in the environment. New York: John Wiley & Sons.1998: 347-390.
3.Sato K. Glutathione transferases as markers of preneoplasia and neoplasia. Adv. Cancer Res. 1990; 52: 205-255.
4.Zeng G.Q., Kenney P.M. and Lam L.K.T. Myristicin-A potential cancer chemopreventive agent from parsley leaf oil. 1992; 40: 107-110.

Table I: Effect of V (0.5ppm) on GST activity and morphometry in DMH-induced rat colon cancer.

Group	GST activity in [a]		Colon [b] Tumor Incidence	Colon Tumor Multiplicity [c]		
	Colon	Liver		Adenoma	Carcinoma	All Neoplasia
A	0.35 ± 0.02 [d]	0.40 ± 0.03 [e]	100	4.7 ± 0.9	3.1 ± 1.4	7.9 ± 1.3
B	0.61 ± 0.20	0.84 ± 0.10	—	—	—	—
C	2.02 ± 0.12 [f]	1.88 ± 0.9 [f]	53.3 [g]	2.4 ± 0.9	1.3 ± 0.5	3.7 ± 1.1 [h]
D	0.65 ± 0.11	0.89 ± 0.19	—	—	—	—

[a]: Specific activity for GST is represented in terms of units/mg protein; [b]: Defines % tumor bearing rats; [c]: Defines mean tumor/ animal; [d]: Values represent mean S.E.; [e]: P<0.001 when compared against group B value; [f]: P<0.02 in comparison to group A; [g]: Significantly less than group A at P<0.01; [h]: Significantly less than group A at P<0.05 by Student's t-test.

Metal Ions in Biology and Medicine; vol 6. Eds. J.A. Centeno, Ph. Collery, G. Vernet, R.B. Finkelman, H. Gibb, J.C. Etienne. John Libbey Eurotext, Paris © 2000, pp. 591-593.

Cis-platinum (inosine)$_2$Cl$_2$ and CIS[Pt(NH$_3$)$_2$(ALA)](NO$_3$) toxicity and antitumor activity on benzo(a)pyrene treated Wistar rats

Kostas Charalabopoulos[1, 2], Vassiliki Papalimneou[2], Vicky Kalfakakou[1], Dimitris Hadjiliadis[3], Patra Vezyraki[1], Spiros Karkabounas[1], Dimitris Stefanou[4], Angelos Evangelou[1], Nick Hadjiliadis[5]

[1] Dept. of Physiology, Medical Faculty, University of Ioannina, 45110 Ioannina, Greece; [2] Charing Cross Hospital, Athens, Greece; [3] Duke University Medical Center, Durham, North Carolina, 27710, USA; [4] Dept. of Pathology, Medical Faculty, University of Ioannina, 45110 Ioannina, Greece; [5] Dept. of Inorganic Chemistry, University of Ioannina, Greece

ABSTRACT

Cancer chemotherapy based on metal complexes started at clinical level since the late seventies with the use of cis-platin. The drug is still in use today mainly against testicular and ovarian carcinomas, etc..We studied the toxicity and the antitumor effects of two Pt complexes, on sarcomas bearing wistar rats, 1) cis-Pt(ino)$_2$Cl$_2$, (ino=inosine) and 2) cis-[Pt(NH$_3$)$_2$(ala)](NO$_3$),ala=1-alanine, water soluble and stabile complexes.

70 male wistar rats were divided in to three main groups of 20 animals each and into two smaller groups of 5 animals each., aging three months, and weighting from 200-250 g. 10.08 mgr benzo(a)pyrene (BaP) was injected subcutaneously in each rat of the first three groups. About two weeks after BaP injection, 15 wistar rats died due to acute carcinogen toxicity.

Three new groups were reorganized of 15 animals each. The animals were not treated until 85th to 90th day. After tumor diagnosis, oral administration of 0.1 mgr/kgr of each Pt complex was used for the two of the three main groups until death. Discontinuation of drug administration was done when toxic effects were observed. At the two smaller groups (5 animals each) the Pt complexes were administrated in higher doses (0.2 mg/kg). Haematological parameters, temperature, weight, aminotransferases and electrocardiogram were measured.

The survival time for the group treated with cis-Pt (ino)$_2$Cl$_2$ was 272±18 days, with cis-[Pt(NH$_3$)$_2$(ala)] (NO$_3$) was 246±26 and the control group survival time was 195±22 days. Statistical analysis showed that the use of these complexes for the treatment of cancer was significant. Severe toxicity was not observed.

These above two Pt complexes have an effective antitumor activity without severe toxicity.

INTRODUCTION

Cancer chemotherapy based on metal complexes started at clinical level since the late seventies with the use of cis-DDP or cis-Platin (1). Cis-Platin is still in use today against testicular and bladder tumors, ovarian carcinomas, head and neck cancers, etc (2).
In order to mimic the simplest models of crosslinks of the type DNA-Pt-proteins and study the interactions between nucleosides and dipeptides when Pt is present, we have used two substances:

1) Cis-$Pt(ino)_2Cl_2$, ino=inosine and
2) Cis-$[Pt(NH_3)_2(ala)](NO_3)$, ala=alanine

We studied the toxicity and the antitumor effects of those two complexes on sarcomas bearing wistar rats.

MATERIAL AND METHODS

Seventy (70) male wistar rats were divided into three main groups of twenty (20) animals each and into two smaller groups of five (5) animals each.
The animals were three months old and their weight ranged from 200 g to 250 g.
10,08 mg benzo(a)pyrene (BaP) was injected subcutaneously in each rat of the first three groups. About two weeks after BaP injection, fifteen (15) wistar rats died because of acute carcinogen toxicity. Three new groups were reorganised of fifteen (15) animals each. The animals were not treated until 85th to 90th day. After tumor diagnosis, oral administration of 0,1 mg/Kg of each Pt complex was used for the two of the three main groups until death. Discontinuation of drug administration was done when toxic effects were observed.
At the two smaller groups (5 animals each) the Pt complexes were administrated in higher doses (0,2 mg/Kg). Hematological parameters, temperature, weight, aminotransferases and electrocardiogram were measured. Histological examination of tumor samples showed different types of sarcomas.

RESULTS

The survival time for the group treated with cis-$Pt(ino)_2Cl_2$ was 272±18 days, with cis-$[Pt(NH_3)_2(ala)]$ (NO_3) was 246±26 days and the control group survival time was 195±22 days.
Statistical analysis showed that the use of these complexes for the treatment of cancer was significant ($p<0,001$). Toxic effects included:

- One (1) animal died because of heart failure.
- Leucocyte count was decreased in 17%±5.
- Mild hemolysis and hematouria were observed.
- Mild weight loss.
- Elevated temperature in low levels after the 8th day of drug administration.
- Increase in serum levels of aminotransferases.
- Hair loss.
- Malaise, especially at the last administration days.

DISCUSSION

The antitumor mechanism of action of cis-Platin is attributed mainly to the formation of an intrastrand crosslink with desoxyribonucleic acid (DNA), involving the N_7 sites of two guanine residues (3,4,5,6). In an attempt to discover more metal based anticancer drugs with higher activity and lower toxicity, several hundreds of coordination and organometallic compounds were synthesized and tested (5,7).

Many organometallic complexes of Pt showed high antitumor activity in vitro in a wide variety of human tumors.

We studied, as previously described, the cis-$Pt(ino)_2Cl_2$ and cis-$[Pt(NH_3)_2(ala)]$ (NO_3) complexes.

Finally, we showed that these complexes have an effective antitumor activity without severe toxicity.

REFERENCES

1. Pestayko AW, Crooke ST, Carter SK. Cisplatin, current status and new developments. *New York: Academic Press*, 1980.
2. Barnard CFJ, Cleare MJ, Hydes PC. Second generation anticancer platinum compounds. *Chem Brit* 1986, 22:1001-04
3. Sherman SG, Lippard SJ. Struetural Aspects of platinum anticancer drug interactions with DNA. *Chem Rev* 1987; 87:1153-81.
4. Aletras V, Hadjiliadis D, Hadjiliadis N.On the mechanism of action of the antitumor drug cis-platin (cis-DDP) and its second generation derivatives. *Metal Based Drugs* 1995; 2:153-185.
5. Kepler BK. Metal complexes in cancer chemotherapy. Weinheim: Verlag Chemie, 1993.
6. Katsarou E, Charalabopoulos K, Hadjiliadis N Ternary complexes of cis-$(NH_3)_2$ Pt Cl_2 (cis-DDP) with guanosine (guo), cytidine (cyd) and the aminoacids glycine(gly), l- alanine (ala), l-2-aminobutyric acid (2-aba), l-norvaline (nval) and l- norleucine (nleu). *Metal Based Drugs* 1997, 2: 57-63.
7. Köpf- Maier P, Köpf H. Non- platinum group metal antitumor agents: History, current status and perspectives.*Chem Rev* 1987; 87:1137-1152.

Metal Ions in Biology and Medicine; vol 6. Eds. J.A. Centeno, Ph. Collery, G. Vernet, R.B. Finkelman, H. Gibb, J.C. Etienne. John Libbey Eurotext, Paris © 2000, pp. 594-596.

Element variation following chelation therapy in young and old aluminum-loaded rats

J.M. Esparza[1], M. Gómez[1], J.L. Domingo[1], J.M. Llobet[2] and J. Corbella[2]

[1] *Laboratory of Toxicology and Environmental Health, School of Medicine, "Rovira i Virgili" University, San Lorenzo 21, 43201 Reus; and* [2] *University of Barcelona, Barcelona, Spain*

Chelation therapy is the basis for the treatment of most acute and chronic metal accumulation and toxicity. Aluminum (Al)-selective chelation may be achieved by targeted chelator distribution or by the use of adjuvants with the chelating agent [1]. Although the trihydroxamic acid desferrioxamine (deferoxamine, DFO) has been shown to be effective for the treatment of Al overload, this drug suffers from a number of important disadvantages [2]. Recently, we compared in Al-loaded rats the relative efficacy of a series of 3-hydroxypyrid-4-ones on the urinary excretion and tissue distribution of Al [3,4]. The purpose of the present study was to assess the potential age-related changes on the metabolism of some essential elements, Calcium (Ca), Copper (Cu), Iron (Fe), Magnesium (Mg), Manganese (Mn) and Zinc (Zn) in a number of tissues of old and young Al-loaded rats following administration of the chelators.

Materials and Methods

<u>Animals and chemicals</u> Male Sprague-Dawley rats were obtained from Interfauna Ibérica (Barcelona, Spain). Young rats were 21 days of age upon arrival (70-80 g), while old rats were 18 months of age (720-780 g). Aluminum was administered as Al nitrate nonahydrate (E. Merck, Darmstadt, Germany). Deferoxamine (DFO) was purchased from Ciba (Barcelona, Spain). 1,2-Dimethyl-3-hydroxypyrid-4-one (deferiprone) and 1-(p-methylbenzyl)-2-ethyl-3-hydroxypyrid-4-one (MeBzEM) were a generous gift from Professor Mark M. Jones, Vanderbilt University (Nashville, TN, USA).

<u>Experimental</u> Fifty animals in each age group were given Al nitrate dissolved in drinking water at 50 mg Al/kg/day for 2 weeks. In order to enhance the gastrointestinal Al absorption, during this period citric acid (178 mg/kg/day) was also added to the Al solutions [5]. Subsequently, the doses of Al and citric acid were increased to 100 and 356 mg/kg/day, respectively, and administered in drinking water for 100 consecutive days. Chelation therapy was initiated 24 h after the end of Al exposure. Three groups of Al-loaded rats were given solutions of MeBzEM (oral), deferiprone (oral) and DFO (s.c.) for 5 days at doses of 0.89 mmol/kg. Two groups (young and old) of Al-loaded rats received a combined administration of deferiprone (oral) and DFO (s.c.) at 0.45 mmol/kg/day during 5 days. Two additional groups (young and old rats) received a s.c. injection

of 0.9% saline and deionized water by gavage (positive control groups), while two groups of young and old rats nonexposed to Al received the same treatment that the positive control groups (negative controls). Twenty-four hours after the last administration of the chelators, animals were anesthetized with diethyl ether and killed. Samples of the following tissues were collected: spleen, liver, kidney, bone (femur) and brain. The concentrations of Ca, Cu, Fe, Mg, Mn and Zn in these tissues were analyzed as described previously [6].

Results and Discussion

The tissue concentrations of Ca, Cu, Fe, Mg, Mn and Zn are presented in Fig.1.

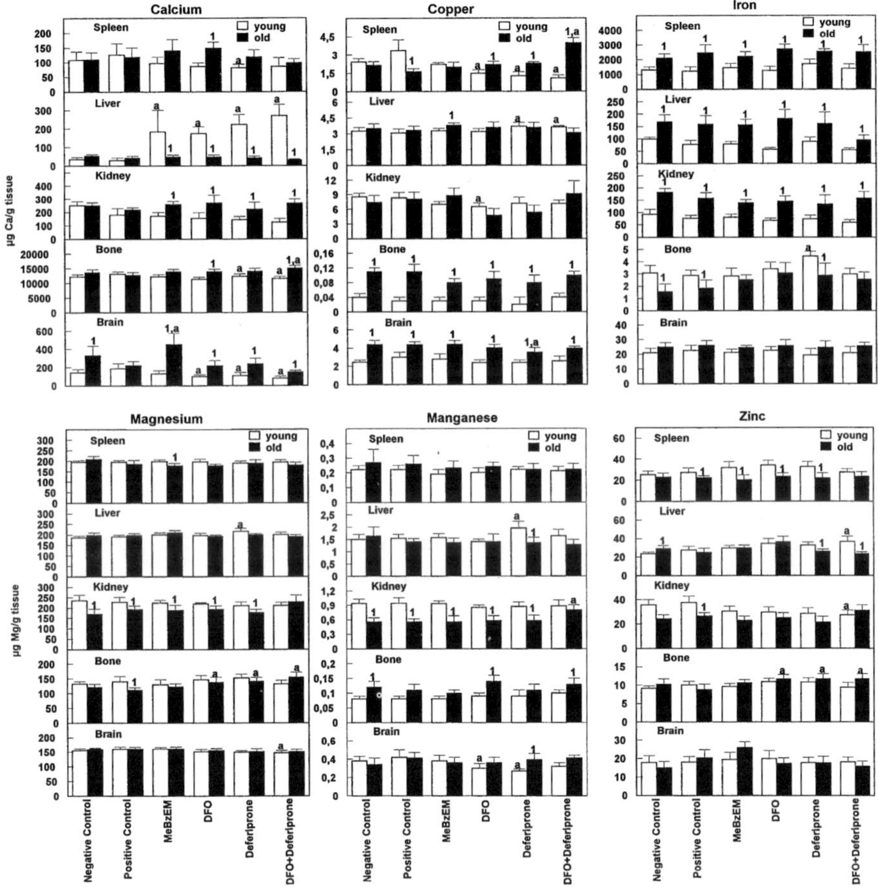

Fig. 1. Element concentrations in spleen, liver, kidney, bone and brain from young and old Al-loaded rats following administration of DFO, deferiprone, or DFO plus deferiprone for 5 days. [1] For each element, indicates significant differences ($p < 0.05$) in relation to the age (young vs. old rats receiving the same chelation therapy). [a] Indicates significant differences compared with the respective positive control group, $p < 0.05$.

The results show that the influence of age on tissue levels of various essential elements in Al-loaded rats not subjected to chelation therapy was quite different depending on the respective element.

In the positive control groups, no age-related differences were noted in tissue Ca concentrations, while Fe was the most affected element. Iron levels in spleen, liver and kidney were significantly higher in old than in young rats. On the other hand, the effects of chelation therapy on Ca, Cu, Fe, Mg, Mn and Zn tissue concentrations of Al-loaded rats were rather limited in both age groups.

According to the present results, no remarkable negative effects on the tissue distribution of a number of essential elements would be expected if the above chelating agents were used for Al mobilization and removal.

Acknowledgement
This study was supported by the DGICYT, Ministry of Education, Spain, through grant PM95-0062. The authors thank Anabel Diez for valuable technical assistance.

References

1.-Yokel RA, Burgess E, Day JP, Domingo JL, Flaten TP, Savory J. Prevention and treatment of aluminium toxicity including chelation therapy: status and research needs. *J Toxicol Environ Health* 1996; 48: 667-83.
2.- Domingo JL . Adverse effects of aluminium-chelating compounds for clinical use. *Adverse Drug React Toxicol Rev* 1996; 15: 145-65.
3.-Gomez M, Esparza JL, Domingo JL, Corbella J, Singh PK, Jones MM. Aluminium distribution and excretion: a comparative study of a number of chelating agents in rats. *Pharmacol Toxicol* 1998; 82: 295-300.
4.-Gomez M, Esparza JL, Domingo JL, Corbella J, Singh PK, Jones MM. Comparative aluminium mobilizing actions of deferoxamine and four 3-hydroxypyrid-4-ones in aluminium-loaded rats. *Toxicology* 1998; 130: 175-81.
5.-Gomez M, Esparza JL, Domingo JL, Corbella J, Singh PK, Jones MM. Chelation therapy in aluminium-loaded rats: influence of age. *Toxicology* 1999; 137: 161-68.
6.-Sanchez DJ, Gomez M, Llobet JM, Corbella J, Domingo JL . Effects of aluminium on the mineral metabolism of rats in relation to age. *Pharmacol Toxicol* 1997; 80: 11-7.

Metal Ions in Biology and Medicine; vol 6. Eds. J.A. Centeno, Ph. Collery, G. Vernet, R.B. Finkelman, H. Gibb, J.C. Etienne. John Libbey Eurotext, Paris © 2000, pp. 597-600.

Zn action on cysticercosis caused by *Taenia crassiceps* in mice

Maria Dolores Lastra, Edda Sciutto, Rodolfo Pastelin, Ana Esther Aguilar and Gladis Fragoso

Laboratorio de investigación en Inmunología, Departamento de Biología, Facultad de Química, UNAM, Circuito Escolar, Ciudad Universitaria, Mexico, D.F. cp 04510; fax: 56 22 37 40; Email: lastraa@servidor.unam.mx

Introduction. Zinc is a trace element with a pivotal role in the immune system, influencing T cells maturation and functions, elevating the antibody response and increasing the phagocytic capacity in mice perinatal stages. Infection status often agrees with zinc concentrations. Zn supplementation may improve immune responses to parasite infections (1, 5). *Taenia solium* cysticercosis is a parasitic disease that still seriously affects human health and causes important economic losses in non-developing countries in Latin America, Asia and Africa, where conditions of poverty, poor hygiene and feeding habits that favor parasite transmission, persist. In this context, host nutrition could be an important factor influencing the host-parasite relationship, as has been observed in other gastrointestinal helminth infections (1). In the nutritional status, the micronutrients are known to be required for a fully functional immune system (2), in particular zinc dietary is an essential trace element required for a range of immune functions, including T-cell, macrophage and natural killer cell activity, and its deficiency is related with high frequency of several infections (3).
To further improve knowledge about parasite infections and its relation with zinc, this study assesses the zinc (500 mg/L) supplementation impact, in an experimental Taenia crassiceps model of cysticerci, evaluating the metal effects over antibody responses, parasite load, and presence .CD3 ,CD4 and CD8

Methods. Mice A syngenic BALB/cAnN strain of mice, previously characterized as susceptible to cysticercosis was used (1, 4). Pregnant mice received 500 mg/l of zinc in drinking water and water without and excess of zinc (control group). zinc concentration used was previously determined (4). zinc treatment were maintained during the gestation, lactation and during the time of the experiments.

Female BALB/cAnN mice were distributed in four groups:

- Group I: Zn supplemented (Zn^+) mice, non infected
- Group II:Zn supplemented (Zn^+) mice, infected with 10 *T. crassiceps* cysticerci
- Group III: non-supplemented (Zn-) control mice, non-infected
- Group IV : non-supplemented control mice (Zn-), infected

Infection. Parasite for infections were harvested from the peritoneal cavity of mice 1-3 mo after inoculation of 10 small non-budding cysticerci (2-3 mm in diameter), per mice. (Fig 1)

Antibody response. Specific antibody levels were determined by ELISA following the previously described procedure (1). Optical density readings at 405 nm were carried out in a Humareader ELISA processor (Human Gessellchaft Fur Biochemica und Diagnostica, Taunusstein, Germany). (Fig 2)

Proliferation assay. Spleen cells from 3 control and zinc treated mice, non infected and 5 days after infection with *T. crassiceps* cysticerci, were cultured in enriched RPMI 1640 medium with mitogen or Ag. After 72 h, the cultured cells were pulsed (1 μCi per well) for a further 18 hr (Methyl ^3H thymidine) (Amersham, Life, Science, U. K.). Then, all cells were harvested and the amount of incorporated label was measured by counting in a 1205 β-plate spectrometer (Wallac). (Fig 3)

Flow cytometry. After 72 h of *in vitro* culture with mitogen or antigen, splenocytes were harvested and CD8, CD4 and CD3 expression was determined by three-color fluorescence-activated cells sorting following the procedure previously described (1). Cells were stained with the following monoclonal antibodies: fluorescein isothiocyanate-conjugated anti- CD8, phycoerythrin-conjugated anti-CD4 and Cychrome anti- CD3 (all from Pharmingen, Cal). Ten thousand cells were analyzed with a lymphocyte gate as defined by light scatter in a FACScan (Becton Dickinson, Cal). Results were expressed as percent of positive cells.

Statistical analysis. The statistical analysis of the difference between mean values of binding activity in ELISA, and proliferation assays was carried out by the unpaired T test Welch's (Alternative T Test). All statistical analyses were performed by the Instat Software Program (GraphPad, Cal). Data were considered as statistically significant at $p<0.05$.

Results. The increased resistance showed by the diminution of parasite load in Zn+(II) treated animals is not due is not due to the IgG antibody response (Fig. 1, 2). After 6 days of infection T-cell proliferation response to concanavaline A was lightly depressed both in Zn- and Zn+ supplemented mice (II, IV), while specific T cell proliferation induced by cysticercal antigens was only depressed in Zn- mice(IV). Infected Zn+ mice (II) exhibited a lower decrease in T cell response ($p<0.05$) in early infections, than Zn- infected mice(IV) (Fig 3).

In addition, spleen cells from group IV showed a significant decrease of CD3+, CD4+CD8-, and CD4-CD8+ cells, both *in vivo* and when kept in culture with RPMI or with specific cysticercal antigens added *in vitro*. However, this effect was not observed in infected mice Zn+(II) (data not shown).

These results suggest the need to study the role of zinc supplementation in increasing the mice resistance to murine cysticercosis.

References

1. Fragoso G, Lamoyi E, Mellor A, Lomeli C, Govezensky G, Sciutto E: Genetic control of susceptibility to Taenia crassiceps cysticercosis. Parasitology 112:119-124,1996.
2. Chandra RK: Nutrition and the immune system: an introduction. Am J Clin Nutr 66:460S-463S, 1997
3. Wellinghausen N, Kircher H and Rink L: The immunobiology of zinc. Immunol Today 11:80-82, 1997
4. Lastra MD, Pastelin R, Herrera M, Orihuela VD, Aguilar AE: Increment of immune responses in mice perinatal stages after zinc supplementation. Arch Med Res 28: 67-72, 1997
5. Shankar AH, Prasad AS: Zinc and immune function: the biological basis of altered resistance to infection. In: Black RE (Ed) Zinc for Child Health, Am J Clin Nutr 68 (suppl):447S-463S, 1998

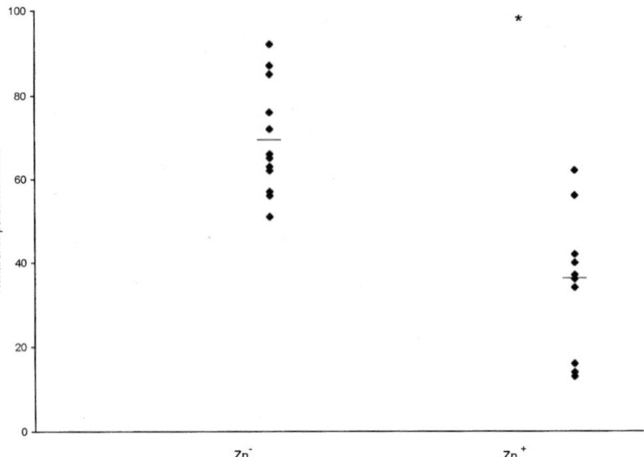

Figure 1. Individual number of parasites recovered from each BALB/c mouse infected with *Taenia crassiceps* cysticerci and supplemented with Zn

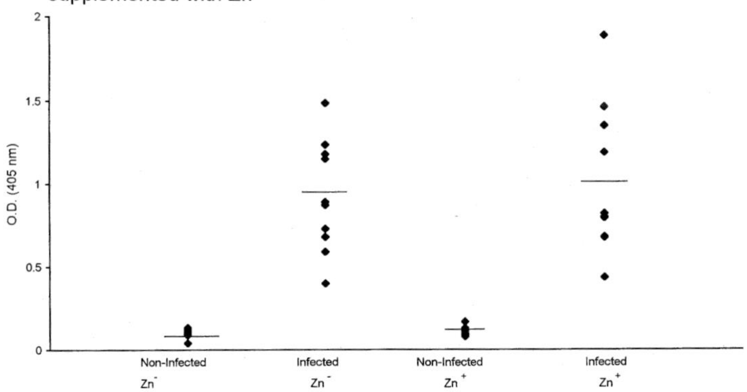

Figure 2. Individual antibody response against *Taenia crassiceps* antigens

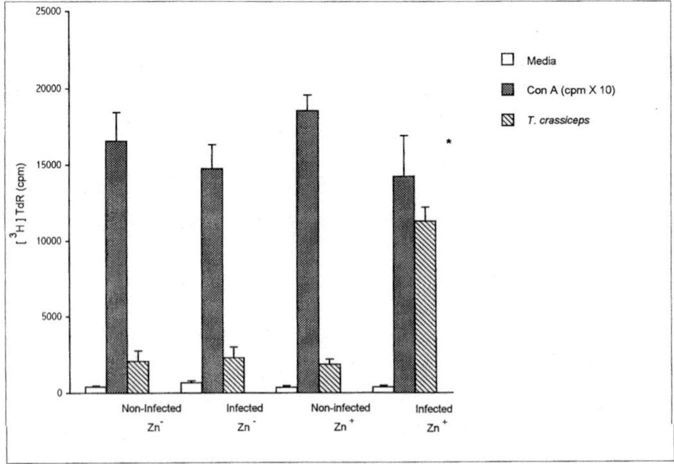

Figure 3. Proliferation response of spleen cells from non infected and infected mice coming from non Zn treated mothers (Zn-) and Zn treated mothers (Zn+)

Metal Ions in Biology and Medicine; vol 6. Eds. J.A. Centeno, Ph. Collery, G. Vernet, R.B. Finkelman, H. Gibb, J.C. Etienne. John Libbey Eurotext, Paris © 2000, pp. 601-603.

Chelating therapy. Evaluation of new copper chelators using hepatocyte suspension

Raya A.[1], Llobet J.M.[1,2], Gómez J.[1], Domingo J.L.[2], Corbella J.[1]

[1] Toxicology Unit, School of Pharmacy, University of Barcelona, Avda. Joan XXIII s/n, 08028, Barcelona, Spain; [2] Laboratory of Toxicology and Environmental Health, School of Medicine, Rovira i Virgili University, Sant Llorenç 21, 43201, Reus, Spain

Introduction

Wilson´s disease (WD) is a genetic disorder that is a fatal unless detected and treated before serious illness develops from copper poisoning. WD affects one in thirty thousand people world wide. The genetic defect causes excessive copper accumulation, mainly in liver and brain.
Now, D-Penicillamine (DPA) and Triethylentetraamine (TRIEN) are used in clinical therapy with good results, however most of patients suffer some adverse effects. Walshe introduced these chelating agents in 1956 and 1969 respectively. Ever since, a lot of chelating agents has been evaluated to looking for a necessary improvement of the treatment. Other therapeutic options are Zn and tetrathiomolybdate (TTM). In our knowledge, TTM is still under clinical evaluation.

The present work is aimed to test the usefulness of the rat hepatocyte suspension as a screening method for a list of potential copper chelating agents. Selected compounds may be used in *in vivo* experiments.

The use of hepatocyte suspension as a model is really advantageous because we are working with a live system, and also the hepatocyte is the main copper target cell. So, it seems one of the *in vitro* methods with possibilities to give us useful information for further extrapolation to human.

Materials and methods

Animals: Cu unloaded male Sprague-Dawley rats, 200-250g weigh.
Chemicals: DPA, N-Ac DPA, L-cysteine (L-Cys), N-Ac L-Cys), TTM, 1,4,7,11-tetraaza undecane. 4 HCl (TAUD), tetraethylenepentamine. 5HCl (TETREN), TRIEN, 1,5,8,12-tetraazadodecane (TADD), 1,4,7,10-tetraazaciclododecane (CYCLEN), 1,4,8,11-tetraazaciclododecan-5,7-dione (TACDD), isopentyl dimercaptosuccinate (Mi-DMSA) and 3-dimercapto-1-propane-sulfonic acid (DMPS).
Cell suspension procedure: isolation from the rat liver was carried out following the Seglen method described in 1973,
Analytical Procedures: Cu levels were determined by inductively coupled plasma spectrometry with mass detection (ICP-M), (Perkin Elmer ELAN 6000).

Experimental assays: In order to establish the definitive assay structure, we determine the Cu background in the liver cell of unloaded rats. The founded value was 3.15µM, (the analytical value in attack solution was 8ng/ml, 40 times the detection limit).Then, we use unloaded liver rats in all assays.

Assay 1. Checking the procedure:
This assay was aimed to determine the optimal chelating agent concentration and the best incubation time. We try with DPA, because is the clinical first choice treatment. The test concentrations for the chelating agent were approximately 10 and 25 times the copper concentration: 30 and 80 µM, respectively.
Incubation conditions: 1 and 2h of incubation time, 37°C, slow and continuous waving. Continuous carbogen gas (O_2/CO_2, 19:1) flow was supplied to incubation flasks. The viability of cells was tested using the Trypan Blue (TB) exclusion method and the LDH leakage method. The Cu content into the cells was measured after the incubation time.

Assay 2. Screening test:
Taking the assay 1 results, we design the screening experiment using the chelating agent list. Assay conditions: 1h of incubation time, and 80 µM of each tested compound. All the other conditions remain unchanged.

Results and discussion

Assay 1. Checking the procedure
Due to few of place in the paper, in Table 1 we present the viability results of higher chelating agent concentration test.

Table 1. Viability data *vs* incubation time. Chelating agents 80 µM.

	Trypan blue		LDH (U/L) in cells		LDH (U/L) extracell.	
	t =1h	t =2h	t =1h	t =2h	t =1h	t =2h
Control	91%	88%	19,670.0	24,108.7	965.09	1,124.33
DPA	89%	82%	18,046.3	23,238.8	631.54	1,184.57

As can observe the % of viability and the LDH leakage data was coincident, and indicates good preservation of cell integrity. However, we can found the best results in 1h incubation tubes, in comparison all 2h data suggest a light integrity loss. There are no differences related to chelating agent concentration (30 and 80 µM).

In Table 2 we show the different Cu content in the cells after incubation period.

Table 2. Copper level variations (% from control)

D-PA concentration	Incubation time	
	t =1h	t =2h
30µM	24.49%	22.51%
80µM	38.10%	31.68%

The greatest variation in Cu level is found in samples corresponding to 80 μM of DPA and 1h of incubation time. These good results of the method using DPA are very hopeful due its correlation with their in vitro usefulness. After that, we assume the method as able to be used as screening test.

ASSAY 2. Screening test.

The variation of Cu levels (% of control) corresponding to the tested chelating agents are showed in Table 3.

Table 3. Variation of the Cu concentration level in cells after incubation time

	% of variation
DPA	38.1
N-Ac DPA	0.27
L-Cys	39.1
N-Ac L-Cys	5.8
TTM	27.1
TAUD	21.7
TETREN	7.6
TRIEN	8.4
TADD	0.90
CYCLEN	31.5
TACDD	2.5
Mi-DMSA	1.2
DMPS	2.8

The viability tests carried out at the end of incubation period don't show any signs of cell disruption.

DPA, L-Cys, TTM, TAUD and CYCLEN treatment provokes a significant decrement in Cu cellular levels (20-40%). TETREN and TRIEN only reach low levels of response (7-8%). Other compounds testes don't archive significant response.

Compounds as TETREN, TRIEN, TAUD and DPA have also got good results in some in vivo studies (Jones et al. 1995). DPA and TRIEN are used in human therapy.

Then, L-Cys and CYCLEN may be used in further *in vivo* experiments to check their capabilities.

All this data confirm the usefulness of this method to be used as a screening test.

Using this method we hope to be able to check a huge list of potential useful compounds avoiding a lot of animal lives. After the first screen using rat hepatocytes, we can assay *in vivo* only the compounds with good perspectives.

References

- Jones M., Singh P., Zimmerman L., Gomez M., Albina ML., Domingo JL. (1995). *Effects of some chelating agents on urinary copper excretion by the rat.* Cem. Research in Toxicol. 942-948.
- Seglen PO. (1973). *Preparation of rat liver cells.III Enzymatic requeriments for tissue dispersion.* Exp. Cell. Res. 82, 391-398.
- Walshe JM. (1996). *Treatment of Wilson´s Disease: the historical background.* Q J Med. 89, 553-555.

Metal Ions in Biology and Medicine; vol 6. Eds. J.A. Centeno, Ph. Collery, G. Vernet, R.B. Finkelman, H. Gibb, J.C. Etienne. John Libbey Eurotext, Paris © 2000, pp. 604-606.

Superoxide radical, α-tocopherol and cadmium toxicity

Ana Maria Lopes[1], Maria Anastácia Manzano[1], Raul Alves Júnior[1], Jeane Alves Almeida[1], José Luiz Villas Boas Novelli Filho[2], Ethel Lourenzi Barbosa Novelli[1]*

[1] *Departamento de Química e Bioquímica, Instituto de Biociências, Universidade Estadual Paulista, UNESP, Botucatu, São Paulo, Brasil. * Corresponding author – E-mail: drno@uol.com.br. [2] Faculdade de Medicina, Universidade Estadual Paulista, UNESP, Botucatu, São Paulo, Brasil*

Abstract: A rat bioassay validated for the identification of the effects of α-tocopherol on cadmium toxicity revealed increased creatinine, lipoperoxide and lactate dehydrogenase activities while superoxide dismutase were decreased in rats treated with cadmium. Tocopherol induced increased serum high-density-lipoprotein and depressed the toxic effects of cadmium on creatinine and lactate dehydrogenase activity. Tocopherol protected tissues from toxic effects of cadmium by an action on superoxide dismutase activity and by a direct-antioxidant action decreasing lipoperoxide formation.
Keywords: cadmium, α-tocopherol, superoxide radical, antioxidant, rats.

Introduction

Contamination with cadmium compounds have high potential risk for the health of populations (1,2,3) and for this reason, treatment of their toxic effects urgently should be established. Oxygen is an essential element for aerobes as it is the terminal acceptor of electrons during oxidative phosphorylation. However, in certain conditions such as in engage of cadmium exposure (3), the electron flow may become uncoupled, leading to production of reactive oxygen species (ROS).

Vitamin E, d-α-tocopherol is an essential fat-soluble vitamin that has the highest biological antioxidant activity. So, a beneficial effect of therapeutic supplementation with tocopherol may be considered, since populations are exposed to many forms of cadmium compounds.

This study was carried out to determine whether α-tocopherol intake can protect tissues against damage induced by cadmium, and to clarify the contribution of superoxide radical (O_2^-) in this process.

Material and Methods

Cadmium chloride was tested for tissue damage by a single intraperitoneal injection Cd^{++} (2mg/Kg). To determine the potential therapeutic effect of vitamin E, a group of the Cd^{++} ($CdCl_2$) treated rats received drinking solution of *D,L* α-tocopherol (40mg/L) for 15 days.

Serum was used for total protein (4), lipoperoxide (5), creatinine (6), HDL-cholesterol (7), vitamin E (6), lactate dehydrogenase (6) and superoxide dismutase (7) determinations.

Results and Discussion

Cadmium induced increased serum creatinine and total lactate dehydrogenase (Table 1), reflecting renal and cardiac damage. Serum creatinine indicates the degree of impairment of the glomerular function, and the rate of deterioration or improvement (8). LDH is used for myocardial ischemia diagnosis (9).

Vitamin E deficiency is uncommon but several studies suggest an inverse association between α-tocopherol plasma concentration and cardiovascular diseases (10). Table 1 shows that the average daily oral tocopherol intake (group C) was 7 mg (calculated as α-tocopherol concentration in drinking solutions' s consumption). Rats given tocopherol showed increased vitamin E serum concentration, indicating that it is absorbed by the intestinal mucosa and reached blood stream

The increased lipoperoxide and decreased SOD levels indicated the generation of superoxide radical in cadmium treated rats. Tocopherol induced increased serum high-density-lipoprotein and depressed the toxic effects of cadmium alone, since creatinine and lactate dehydrogenase determinations were recovered to the control values.

The most obvious effect noted in rats following $CdCl_2$ injection was the increased ratio Lipoperoxide/α-tocopherol. This relation is an approach to evaluate the balance between lipid oxidative damage (lipoperoxide) and antioxidants (quantitatively α-tocopherol accounts for most of the antioxidant protection) (11). The ratio lipoperoxide/α-tocopherol was 29% higher in the cadmium alone (B) than in control rats, and 67% lower in rats with α-tocopherol intake (C) than in controls (A). The obtained results (Table 1) supports an imbalance of the oxidant/antioxidant system in $CdCl_2$ which indicates a situation of oxidative stress in Cd^{++} treated rats.

Tocopherol decreased lipoperoxide and led the SOD activities to approach those of the control values.

We concluded that superoxide radical is produced as a mediator of cadmium toxicity. Tocopherol possesses a significant anti-radical activity and inhibits the cadmium effect on superoxide dismutase activity. Tocopherol also protected tissues from toxic effects of cadmium by a direct-antioxidant action decreasing lipoperoxide formation.

References

1- Novelli ELB, Lopes AM, Rodrigues AS, Novelli Filho JLVB, Ribas BO. Superoxide radical and nephrotoxic effect of cadmium exposure. *Int J Environ Health Res* 1999; 9: 109-16.

2- Novelli ELB, Rodrigues NL, Ribas BO. Superoxide radical and toxicity of environmental nickel exposure. *Human & Experimental Toxicol* 1995; 14: 248-51.

3- Novelli ELB, Vieira EP, Rodrigues NL, Ribas BO. Risk assessment of cadmium toxicity on hepatic and renal tissues of rats. *Environ Res* 1998; 79: 102-5.

4- Lowry DH, Rosembrough NJ, Farr AL. Protein measurement with folin phenol reagent. *Journal Biological Chemistry* 1951; 193: 265-75.

5- Barber AA. Lipid peroxidation in rat tissue homogenates: interaction of iron and ascorbic acid as the normal catalytic mechanism. *Lipids* 1966; 1: 146-51.

6- Moura RA. Técnicas de Laboratório. São paulo: Atheneu,1992.

7- Otero J, Toni P, Garcia Morato YV. Superoxo dismutasa: metodo para su determinacion. Revis Iberoamen Invest Clin 1983; 2: 121-27.

8- Gaw A, Cowan RA, Oreilly DST. Clinical Biochemistry. New York: Churchil Livingstone, 1995.

9- Miller O. O laboratório para o Clínico. São Paulo: Atheneu, 1993.

10-Witting PK, Bowry VW, Stocker R. Inverse deuterium kinetic isotope effectfor peroxidation in human low-density lipoproptein (LDL): a simple test for tocopherol mediated peroxidation of LDL lipids. *FEBS Letters* 1995; 375: 45-9.

11-Oteiza PI, Uchitel OD, Carrasquedo F, Dubrovski AL, Roma JC, Fraga CG. Evaluation of antioxidants, protein, and lipid oxidation products in blood from sporadic amiotrophic lateral sclerosis patients. *Environ Res* 1997; 22: 535-39.

Table 1 Drinking solution ingestion, lipoperoxide/tocopherol relation, total protein, creatinine, HDL-cholesterol, Vitamin E, superoxide dismutase (SOD) and lactate dehydrogenase (LDH) determinations in control (A), rats treated with cadmium in absence (B) and presence of α-tocopherol intake (C).

Determinations	Groups			Statistical conclusions
	A	B	C	
Drinking solution Ingestion(mL/24h)	42.9±3.2	32.1± 2.3	36.7± 2.2	A > (B = C)
Lipoperoxide/ tocopherol	0.017	0.022	0.0056	B > A > C
Total protein (g/dL)	8.7± 1.2	8.5± 0.9	8.3± 1.1	A = B = C
Creatinine (mg/dL)	0.58± 0.01	1.1± 0.01	0.67± 0.03	B > (A = C)
HDL-cholesterol (mg/dL)	41.3± 3.2	43.4± 2.9	58.3± 4.3	C > (A = B)
Vitamin E (mg/dL)	2.5± 0.1	2.3± 0.2	3.9± 0.2	C > (A = B)
Lipoperoxide (ng/mL)	426.6± 24.6	508.6± 11.2	218.7± 9.9	B > A > C
SOD (U/mg protein)	61.4± 1.7	45.8± 2.2	64.1± 2.3	B < (A = C)
LDH (UI)	109.5 ± 9.1	205.5± 6.4	121.1± 6.8	B > (A =C)

Supported: FAPESP (Fundação de Amparo a Pesquisa do Estado de São Paulo), CAPES (Coordenadoria de Aperfeiçoamento de Pessoal de Ensino Superior) and CNPq (Conselho Nacional de Desenvolvimento Científico e Tecnológico).

Metal Ions in Biology and Medicine; vol 6. Eds. J.A. Centeno, Ph. Collery, G. Vernet, R.B. Finkelman, H. Gibb, J.C. Etienne. John Libbey Eurotext, Paris © 2000, pp. 607-609.

Ligands with carboxylic or phosphonic groups as secuestering agents for beryllium(II)

Alfredo Mederos, Sixto Domínguez, Erasmo Chinea and Ana Valle

Departamento de Química Inorgánica, Universidad de La Laguna, Tenerife, Canary Islands, Spain; amederos@ull.es

Abstract

Beryllium(II) inhibits numerous enzymes that compete with magnesium(II). In the presence of magnesium(II), at pH 4-6, nitrilotripropionic acid (NTP) practically only sequester beryllium(II). Methylenediphosphonic acid (MDP) sequester beryllium(II) at physiological pH. NTP and MDP now are the best sequestering agents.

Introduction

Beryllium is the most toxic non radiactive element in the Periodic Table. Due to its low density, high strength and high thermal conductivity, beryllium is a component of materials indispensable in today's nuclear, aeroespace and nuclear industries. The most notable biochemical effects resulting from beryllium contamination in mammalians include permanent cell modification, alteration of DNA replication, interference in enzimatic reactions and impairment of cell division. Efforts to discover a therapeutic agent that may neutralise the biological activity of beryllium compounds have so far been unsuccessful, so there is renewed interest in the element´s coordination chemistry, notwithstanding the risks associated with handling its compounds[1,2].
The great toxicity of the beryllium is perhaps one of the most important reasons why the experimental studies of its interaction with ligands present in biological systems or in the environment are very limited indeed[1,2]. Therefore, in the last years there is renewing interest in the search for suitable ligands as antidotes for beryllium poisoning. Two types of the ligands have concentrate the attention as sequestering agents: 1) ligands with carboxylic groups. 2) ligands with phosphonic groups.

Hydrolysis

Good sequestering agents for beryllium(II) are the ligands that hinder the formation of the hydrolytic species in aqueous solution. The $[Be(H_2O)_4]^{2+}$ cation exists only in very acidic solutions. In less acidic media, several polynuclear hydrolytic species are formed, being the trimer $[Be_3(OH)_3]^{3+}$, the specie predominant over almost all of the pH range up to precipitation of $Be(OH)_2$, which takes place at pH > 5[3]. The trimeric cation $[Be_3(OH)_3(H_2O)_6]^{3+}$ has been characterized with picrate salt in solid state . Beryllium hydroxide have anphoteric character. New polinuclear anions $[Be_4(OH)_{10}]^{2-}$ and $[Be_2(OH)_7]^{3-}$ have recently been characterized by X-ray diffraction analysis.

Polyaminocarboxylic acids

EDTA and others tetramethylcarboxylic acids (H_4L) derived from aliphatic diamines such as 1,2-PDTA (1,2-propylene-diamine-tetraacetic) and CDTA (trans-1,2-cyclohexanediamine-tetraacetic), are not good sequestering agents for Beryllium(II), since at pH >5 the specie H_2L^{2-} competes favorably with the complex BeL^{2-} and it does not hinder the

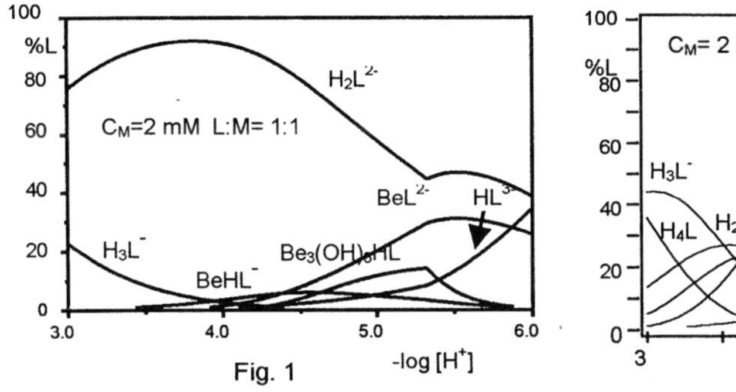

Fig. 1

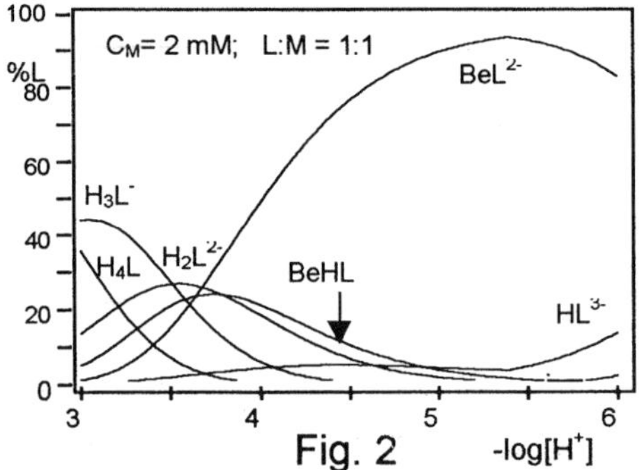

Fig. 2

formation of the hydrolytic species of Be(II) (Fig. 1). Contrarily, tetramethylcarboxylic acids derived from aromatic diamines, such as 3,4-TDTA (3,4-toluenediamine-tetraacetic) and *o*-PhDTA (*o*-phenylene-diaminetetraacetic) are good sequestering agents for beryllium(II) at pH 4.5-6 (or above 6 with excess of ligand) (Fig. 2), since these ligands sequester beryllium(II) at a sufficiently low pH to impede the hydrolysis of this small cation. The potentially tetradentate ligands nitriloaceticdipropionic (NADP) and nitrilotripropionic (NTP) acids have similar behaviour.

It has already been pointed out that one of the causes of the toxicity of beryllium(II) is to inhibit numerous enzymes competitive to magnesium. We therefore considered it worthwhile to analyze the selective uptake of beryllium(II) in the presence of magnesium(II). The chemical speciation diagrams as a function of pH (ligand: Be(II): Mg(II), 1:1:1) show that *o*-PhDTA and 3,4-TDTA (Fig. 3a) between pH 4-6 simultaneously sequester Be(II) and Mg(II), whereas NTA and NADP (Fig. 3b) practically only sequester Be(II)![1,2]. The advantages of NTP and NADP acids to sequester specifically Be(II) are evident. The beryllium(II) in the $[Be(NTP)]^-$ complex lies at the center of a slightly distorted tetrahedron toward C_{3v}[1,2].

Ligands with phosphonic groups

Recently, the interaction of Beryllium in aqueous solution (25°C; I=0.5M made up with $NaClO_4$ and $(CH_3)_4HCl$) with the ligands phosphonoacetic acid (PA), methylenediphosphonic acid (MDP) and phosphonopropionic acid (PP)[4] have been investigated using both potentiometric and multinuclear magnetic resonance measurements (^{31}P, ^{13}C, ^{1}H and ^{9}Be). Comparing ligands with phosphonate groups with ligands with carboxylate groups (for ex., MDP and malonic acid) the stability constants of the complexes formed indicate that the ligand with phosphonate groups are more stable than the corresponding ligands with carboxylate groups. The species distribution diagram (Fig. 4) indicates that MDP (H_4L), sequester beryllium(II) at low pH, hindering the formation of the hydrolytic species of the beryllium(II). MDP sequester beryllium(II) at physiological pH (Fig. 4).

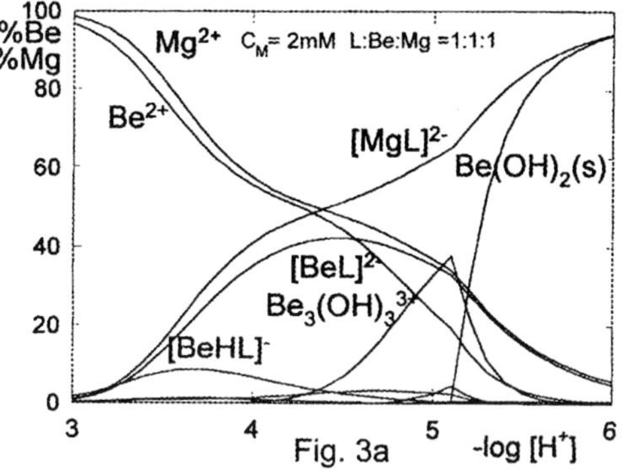

Fig. 3a

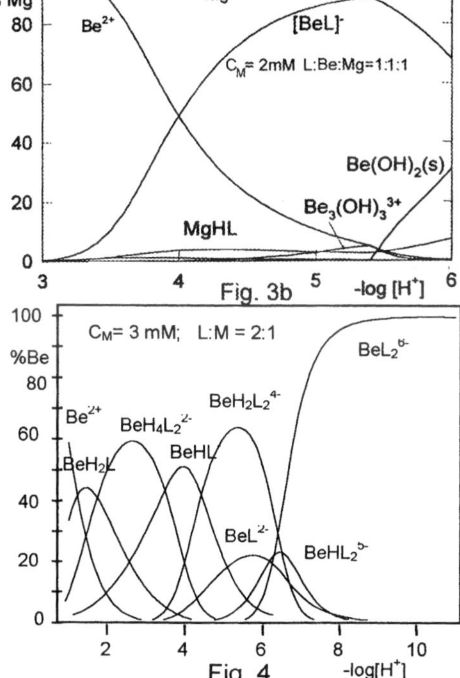

Fig. 3b

Fig. 4

Acknowledgements

We wish to thank the Ministerio de Educación y Cultura, Spain (grant PM98-0148) for the finantial support.

[1] Chinea, E., Domínguez, S., Mederos, A., Brito, F., Arrieta, J.M., Sanchez, A., and Germain, G, Inorg. Chem., 1995, **34**, 1579.

[2] Mederos, A., Domínguez, S., Chinea, E., Brito, F., Midollini, S, and Vacca, A., Bol. Soc. Chil. Quim., 1997,**42**, 281.

[3] Alderighi, L., Bianchi, A., Mederos, A., Midollini, S., Rodríguez, A., and Vacca, A., Eur. J. Inorg. Chem., 1998, 1209.

[4] Valle, A., Chinea, E., Domínguez, S., Mederos, A., Midollini, S., and Vacca, A., 1999, Polyhedron, 1999,**18**, 3253.

Metal Ions in Biology and Medicine; vol 6. Eds. J.A. Centeno, Ph. Collery, G. Vernet, R.B. Finkelman, H. Gibb, J.C. Etienne. John Libbey Eurotext, Paris © 2000, pp. 610-612.

Omeprazol changes the absorption and disposition of orally administered cadmium and zinc in mice

J.A. Sørensen[1], O. Andersen[2], J.B. Nielsen[1]

[1] *Department of Environmental Medicine, University of Southern Denmark, Odense University, Winsløwparken 17, DK-5000, Odense C, Denmark;* [2] *Institute of Life Sciences and Chemistry, Roskilde University Centre, Box 260, DK-4000, Roskilde, Denmark*

Abstract

The proximal part of duodenum is important for cadmium and zinc absorption (3,4). The absorption of both metals are expected to depend on solubility characteristics, which are pH dependent. It was therefore of interest to investigate the effect of gastrointestinal pH on intestinal absorption of zinc and cadmium. Omeprazol, an antacid drug for patients with peptic ulcer disease apparently not affecting other physiological parameters in the gastrointestinal tract, was used as a relevant modifier of intestinal acidity. Effects of repeated daily administrations of Omeprazol on the gastrointestinal absorption site and the time course for whole-body and organ deposition of orally administered zinc chloride or cadmium chloride in mice was investigated. Omeprazol significantly changed the intestinal deposition profiles for cadmium and zinc and reduced the absorption of both metals. Already 24 hours after administration of the metals, a pronounced effect on the intestinal absorption of both metals was observed. Hepatic and renal depositions of cadmium were reduced in accordance with the reduced whole-body deposition of cadmium. However, the ratio between liver and kidney deposition of zinc was significantly decreased by Omeprazol treatment indicating that Omeprazol may have systemic effects on zinc kinetics.

Introduction

The chemical environment created by the food components and the intestinal secretions at the site of absorption affects the absorption of trace elements (2). Omeprazol is a potent acid pump inhibitor (H+, K+, ATPaseinhibitor) and has been demonstrated to affect gastrointestinal acidity in several different experimental models (1). The extent to which Omeprazol changes absorption of essential and toxic metals has not previously been studied.

Materials and methods

Female NMRI mice were orally exposed to $ZnCl_2$ or $CdCl_2$ (stomach tube or drinking water), which was labelled with ^{65}Zn or ^{109}Cd. One group served as control group and the other groups received 0.01mg Omeprazol/mouse (0.8 µmol/kg) through stomach tube twice a day. In order to determine the intestinal labelling profile of Cd and Zn, mice were killed after specific time periods and the intestines were cut into segments of 2 cm lengths and counted in the Searle 1195R gamma counter.

Experiment 1: For three days groups of mice (n=10) received drinking water containing either 2 µmol $ZnCl_2$/l labelled with ^{65}Zn or 0.04 µmol $CdCl_2$/l labelled with ^{109}Cd. The animals were killed at day three and the intestinal labelling profile determined.

Experiment 2: Groups of mice (n=10) received a single oral dose of 30 µmol/kg $ZnCl_2$ labelled with ^{65}Zn or a single oral dose of 2 µmol $CdCl_2$/kg labelled with ^{109}Cd. At day eightteen, the animals were killed. Whole-body retention was calculated for each animal and expressed as medians in percent of the original dose.

Results

A marked decrease in intestinal zinc deposition was seen in jejunum (segment 4-10) from mice given Omeprazol as compared to controls (Figure 1). Throughout the remaining part of the small intestine Omeprazol did not affect the intestinal labelling profile (data not shown). In the single dose experiment, Omeprazol significantly reduced WBR of zinc from day 1 and throughout the experimental period (Table 1). Omeprazol significantly reduced the duodenal deposition of cadmium at day 3 as compared to controls (Figure 2). The single dose experiment demonstrated a significantly lower WBR of Cd in mice given Omeprazol as compared to controls (Table 1). This is also reflected in a statistically significant 3 times lower deposition of cadmium in the gastrointestinal tract, the liver and the kidneys (data not shown).

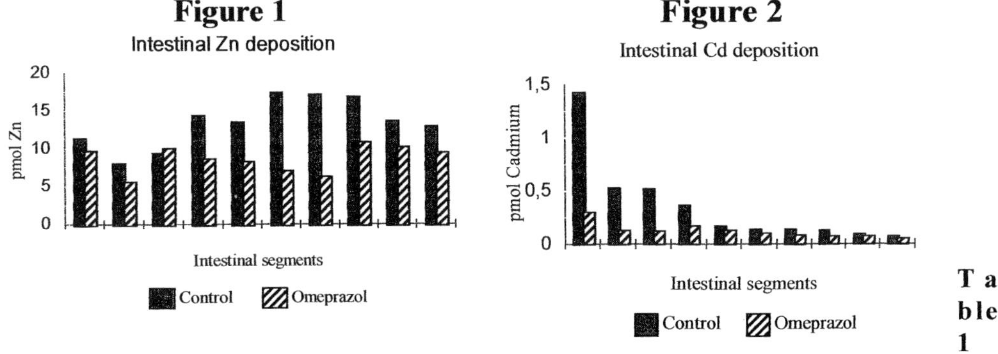

Figure 1

Figure 2

Table 1

% GI deposition	Zinc		Cadmium	
days	Control	Omeprazol	Control	Omeprazol
0	100	100	100	100
1	16	8,6	14,6	7,6
2	13,6	7,6	4	1,8
3	12	7	1,3	0,5
5	10,6	6,2	0,9	0,3
7	9,5	5,6	0,9	0,3
10	8,4	5	0,8	0,3
14	7,6	4,6	0,8	0,2

Discussion

The intestinal zinc deposition was most prominently altered in jejunum (Figure 1) where a slower, more prolonged absorption have been suggested to occur (4). This is reflected in the reduced WBR in the omeprazol treated group.Zinc is probably absorbed throughout the small intestine both passively and actively. The alteration of pH by Omeprazol treatment apparently reduces the zinc absorption by reducing the absorption i jejunum. Patient who are already marginally deficient in zinc, may have this condition aggravated by treatment of omeprazol.

Omeprazol treatment reduced the WBR of cadmium and significantly reduced the duodenal preference of cadmium deposition. Cadmium is probably absorbed passively. The change in pH probably reduces the solubility of Cd and thereby the absorption. For patients who are at risk of having consumed Cd contaminated food, treatment with omeprazol would be an option to lower the gastrointestinal absorption of cadmium.

References

1. Larsson, H., Mattson, H., Sundell, G., Carlsson, E. Animal Pharmacodynamics of Omeprazol. A survey of it pharmacological properties in vivo. Scand. J. Gastroenterol. 1985, 20 (suppl 108), 23-35.

2. Sandström,B. Factors influencing the uptake of trace elements from the digestive tract. Proceedings of Nutrition Society 1988, 47, 161-167.

3. Sørensen, J.A., Nielsen, J.B., Andersen, O. Identification of the gastrointestinal absorption site for cadmium chloride in vivo. Pharmacology and Toxicology 1993, 73, 169-173.

4. Sørensen, J.A., Nielsen, J.B., Andersen, O. An in vivo study of the gastrointestinal absorption site for zinc chloride in mice. J Trace Elem Med Biol 1998, 12, 16-22.

Metal Ions in Biology and Medicine; vol 6. Eds. J.A. Centeno, Ph. Collery, G. Vernet, R.B. Finkelman, H. Gibb, J.C. Etienne. John Libbey Eurotext, Paris © 2000, pp. 613-615.

Chelating properties towards Fe(III), Al(III), Ga(III) and biological evaluation of two *N*-substituted 3-hydroxy-4-pyridinones

M. Amélia Santos*[a], Raquel Grazina[a], Ana Q. Neto[a], Guilhermina Cantinho[b], Lurdes Gano[c] and Luciana Patrício[c]

[a] Centro de Química Estrutural, Complexo I, Instituto Superior Técnico, Av. Rovisco Pais, 1049-001 Lisboa, Portugal; [b] Instituto de Medicina Nuclear, Faculdade de Medicina de Lisboa, R. Egas Monis, 1600 Lisboa, Portugal; [c] Instituto Tecnológico e Nuclear, Estrada Nacional n° 10, 2686-953 Sacavém, Portugal

Abstract.- The interaction of two 3-hydroxy-4-pyridinones *N*-substituted with an alkylamino (HL^1) and an alkylcarboxyl group (H_2L^2) witth Fe(III), Ga(III), Al(III) have been studied in aqueous solution. There is a clear effect of the *N*-substituents on the vitro and in vivo interactions: H_2L^2 is more hydrophilic and better chelating agent then HL^1, but they have the same relative order of magnitude of metal ion stability (Fe(III)>Ga(III)>Al(III)). Both the chelators show interferences in the typical biological behavior of the ^{67}Ga-citrate in mice: HL^1 enhanced the urinary while H_2L^2 induced a lower blood clearance but a higher bone uptake, namely when the radionuclide is previously loaded.

The development of chelating agents for selective sequestering metal ions of the group 13 has been the object of current interest due to the role these species in the genesis of diseases [*e.g.* Fe(III), Al(III)] or the diagnostic of diseases [*e.g.* ^{67}Ga(III)]. Thus, a large number of hydroxypyridinone derivatives have been developed and studied in their interaction with those M^{3+} metal ions [1-3]; the 1,2-dimethyl-3-hydroxy-4-pyridinone, HL^3, is currently used in the treatment of iron-overload [4].

As part of an ongoing project aimed at developing sequestering agents for the group IIIA metal ions, we have recently synthetized two ring-*N* functionalised 3-hydroxy-4-pyridinone: the 1-(3′-aminopropyl)-3-hydroxy-2-methyl-4-pyridinone (**HL^1**) and the 1-(2′-carboxyethyl)-3-hydroxy-2-methyl-4-pyridinone (**H_2L^2**) and studied their interaction with Ga(III) and the lipo-hydrophilic balance of the ligands [5]. We describe herein an overall study of their chelating properties towards this set of

R, N, CH_3, OH, O

HL^1 R= ⁄⁄⁄ NH_2

H_2L^2 R= ⁄⁄ COOH

HL^3 R= $-CH_3$

trivalent metal ions in aqueous solution. Some *in vivo* studies were also undertaken to complement the preliminar biodistribution evaluation of ^{67}Ga-citrate in mice.

The ability of ligands for complexation with the three metal ions is summarised in Table I which presents the global formation constants and the percentage of the major species (with reference to the total metal concentration), at physiological pH [6]. The protonation constants and the formation constants for thc complexes were determined by potentiometry (SUPERQUAD program), but the ferric complexes, because the ligand-to-metal ratio 1:1 species were fully formed at the initiation of the potentiometric titration. The ferric complexes of H_2L^2 were studied by spectrophotometry (PSEQUAD program), while a mixed method was used for HL^1 (the formation constants of 1:1 species were determined by spectrophotometry and then used, at fixed values, for the subsequent potentiometric calculation of the 2:1 and 3:1 species. The hydroxo complexes were included in the calculations, with fixed values.

Table I – Stepwise protonation constants (log*ic*) of the ligands, HL^1, H_2L^2, HL^3 as well as global formation constants (log β) of the Fe(III), Ga(III) and Al(III) complex species with major contributions (%) at the physiological pH.[a] and pM values. $C_{Ligand} = 2 \times 10^{-3}$ M and the L:M = 3:1; $I = 0.1$ M KNO_3.

Ligand *R*	log K_i	Complex $M_pH_qL_r$ (p,q,r)	log β $Fe_pH_qL_r$ (%)	log β $Ga_pH_qL_r$ (%)	log β $Al_pH_qL_r$ (%)	pM[b] *(Fe)*
HL^1	10.07	(1,2,2)	--	--	39.12	
	9.09				*(~50)*	17.4
-(CH2)3NH2	3.20	(1,3,3)	61.75 *(>90)*	60.15 *(~90)*	54.26 *(~50)*	
H_2L^2	9.83					
	4.13	(1,0,3)	37.97	36.84	35.82	21.5
-(CH2)2CO2H	3.34		*(~75)*	*(~70)*	(~75)	
HL^3 *-CH3*	9.86[c] 3.70	(1,0,3)	37.2[c], 35.88[d]	38.42[c], 35.76[d]	32.62[c], 32.62[d]	18.3[c]

[a] ref. 6; [b] pM = -log [M] at physiological pH (7.4), 1 μM M, 10 μM C_L; [c] ref. 2; [d] ref. 3.

A compative analysis of the results indicate that both the ligands present good ability for complexation with these M^{3+} ions. In a wide range of pH centered around the physiological region, the major complex species are $M(HL^1)_3^{3+}$ and ML^2_3. For comparison of the different compound ability, pM values were used instead of the stability constants due to differences between the protonation constants. Thus, at physiological pH, the acid derivative H_2L^2 presents the highest affinity for these metals ions.(pFe is about 4 orders of magnitude higher then the amino derivative). This behavior is explained by the presence of the protonated amine group, which induces a electron-withdrawing effect on the ligand *O*-negative charge and also a coulombic repulsion over the coordinating M^{3+} ion. Conversely, at physiological pH, the acid derivative has a negatively charged group (COO^-) which, by opposite reasons, increases the metal binding interaction. The order of stability for both of these ligands with the three group 13 metals is Fe(III) > Ga(III)> Al(III), according to expectations based on reports of similar complexes.

Biodistribution studies were carried out in female Charles River mice at 30 and 60 min and 48 h after i.v. administration of ^{67}Ga-citrate, according the protocol previously described [5]. For comparative purposes with the normal biodistribution profile of ^{67}Ga-citrate in mice, separated groups of animals were intraperitoneally co-injected or injected 30 min. after or 30 min. before ^{67}Ga-citrate administration with 100 μg of each one of the ligands under study.

The present study made evident that the administration of both chelating agents interfere in the typical ^{67}Ga-citrate biological distribution. The amount of ^{67}Ga removed from the soft tissues and its favourite tissue uptake was dependent both on the chelator and on the moment of administration relatively to the ^{67}Ga injection (see Table II).

Table II – Radioactivity ratio between the uptake in bone and muscle at 48 h after ^{67}Ga citrate administration (n=6) according to different moments of ligand administration

Injected ligand	Moment of ligand administration	Radioactivity ratio bone/ muscle
^{67}Ga citrate	--	2.27
^{67}Ga + HL^1	co-injection	6.62
	30 min. after	1.85
	30 min. before	4.38
^{67}Ga + H$_2$L^2	co-injection	6.62
	30 min. after	6.16
	30 min. before	7.12

While ligand HL^1 enhanced the urinary excretion and induced an increase on ^{67}Ga removal from muscle, H$_2$L^2 administration led to a lower blood clearance and a significant increase on bone uptake when co-injected or injected after ^{67}Ga administration. Nevertheless, when administered before ^{67}Ga, both ligands led to a pronounced bone uptake and a higher bone/muscle radioactive ratio, namely at 48 h (see Table II. This could be related to high affinity of the chelators for sequestering the nuclide, namely H$_2$L^2, which pGa (20.1) [5] is even higher than that of the ferritin (19.2) [7]. Thus, they seem to assume behaviour similar to that of a bone-scanning agent and ^{67}Ga-L^2 complex can be thought as a potential drug for the diagnosis of bone diseases.

References

[1] Rai BL, Rekhordi LS, Khodr H, Jin Y, Lin Z, Hider R. Synthesis, Physicochemical Properties and Biological Eval. N-substituted-2-alkyl-3-hydroxy-4-pyridinones. *J. Med.Chem.* 1998; 41: 3347-59.

[2] Clevette D, Lyster D, Nelson W, Rihela T, Webb G , Orvig C. Solution Chemistry of Gallium and Indium 3-hydroxy-4-pyridinone complexes in Vitro and in Vivo". *Inorg. Chem* 1990; 29: 667-72.

[3] Clarke ET, Martell AE. 1-Methyl-3-hidroxy-2-pyridinone complexes of the trivalent metal ions of Fe(III), Al(II), Ga(III), Al(III), In(III). *Inorg. Chim. Acta* 1992; 196: 185-194.

[4] Kontoghiorges G J. New Orally Active Iron Chelators. *Lancet* 1985; 817.

[5] Santos MA, Grazina R, Neto AQ, Cantino G, Gano L, Patrício L. Synthesis, Chelating Properties Towards Gallium and Biological Evaluation of two N-substituted 3-Hydroxy-4-pyridinones. *J. Bioinorg. Chem.* (in press).

[6] For the sake of simplicity, this table does not include the values obtained for the species MH_iL_j, (i, j = 1, 2) with minor contributions, at pH=7.4; the all set of values and the speciation curves are in a full paper (in prep).

[7] Harris WR, Pecoraro VL. Thermodynamic Binding Constants for Gallium Transferrin. *Biochemistry* 1983; 22: 292-99.

Acknowledgments: The authors are grateful to *Fundação Calouste Gulbenkian* and *FCT* for financial support (project PRAXIS/PCEX/QUI/85/96).

Metal Ions in Biology and Medicine; vol 6. Eds. J.A. Centeno, Ph. Collery, G. Vernet, R.B. Finkelman, H. Gibb, J.C. Etienne. John Libbey Eurotext, Paris © 2000, pp. 616-618.

Screening and testing strategy for biological activity of rhenium cluster compounds

N.I. Shtemenko, I.V. Pyroshkova-Patalakh, A.V. Shtemenko, O.V. Kozhura

Board of Biophysics and Biochemistry of Dniepropetrovsk State University, 320625 Dniepropetrovsk, 13 Naukoviy by-street, Ukraine

Search biologically active compounds among rhenium clusters with carboxylic and amino acid ligands is very perspective as these substances have some common structural and chemical properties with antitumour compounds of inorganic nature [1,2] but have much more lower toxicity [3]. Recently it was shown that binuclear oxo-complex of rhenium with nicotinamide (ANA) with composition $Re_2(Ph_3P)_2(ANA)_2O_3Cl_4$ may be biologically active as it selectively induced K^+ and Li^+ ions transport through artificial bilayer lipid membrane [4]. Investigation of the influence of a range of chemical compounds on velocity of acidic haemolysis of red blood cells (RBS) is a known convenient model to elucidate whether structural differences in these substances would be screened through mode of action with native membrane of RBS. The aim of recent investigation was to try to compare some new rhenium cluster compounds with organic ligands in this model and to try to choose among them the most promised ones.

Rhenium cluster compounds of four types: $(AH)_m[Re_2Cl_8]_nH_20$ (I), cis-$[Re_2(HA)_2Cl_4]Cl_2$ (II), trans-$[Re_2(HA)_2Cl_4]Cl_2$ (III) shown on the figure 1 and $Re_2A_2Cl_4Cl_2$ (IV), where AH – carboxylic or amino acid, m – 1,2; n – 0;1 were synthesized according to procedures, elaborated by us . Method of preincubation of erythrocytes by I-IV with following measurements of velocity of haemolysis was performed. Average resistance (AR) of RBS was calculated in percents to control experiments, where all procedures without I-IV were repeated. As substances I-III are hydrolyzed in water solutions with different velocity, experiments with freshly prepared (i) solutions, with solutions 48h after (ii) and 72h after (iii) preparation were made. Model of haemolytic anemia in vivo and experiments with Guerink carcinoma were accomplished according to described procedures.

Due to high lability of chlorine–ions in I formation of II occurred during dissolving of I in nitromethane solutions (fig.1). Products of thermal treatment (195 – 225 C) of I in inert atmosphere were clusters of III type. All types of the complexes had different velocity of hydrolysis and cis – trans isomerization.

Substances of type I are very unstable in water. All of them revealed a week stabilizing effect of RBS in high concentrations and I c, d in the most of experiments with different concentrations. As there exists a range of stability in water – Id>Ic>Ib>Ia – it is possible to suggest that the size of amino acid radical plays important role in interactions between cluster and cell.

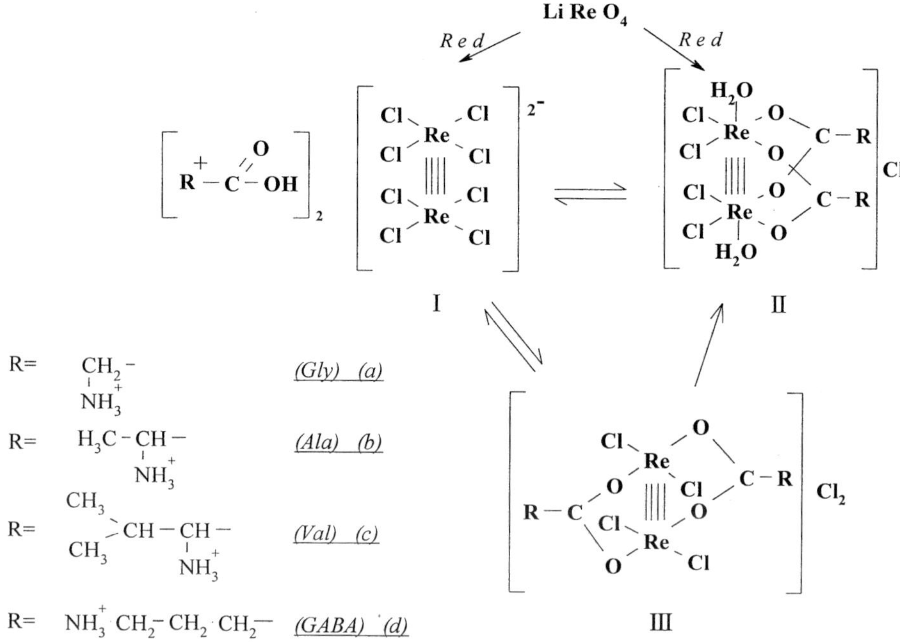

$LiReO_4$

R= $CH_2(NH_3^+)-$ *(Gly) (a)*

R= $H_3C-CH(NH_3^+)-$ *(Ala) (b)*

R= $(CH_3)_2CH-CH(NH_3^+)-$ *(Val) (c)*

R= $\overset{+}{N}H_3\,CH_2-CH_2\,CH_2-$ *(GABA) (d)*

I II III

Figure 1. Structure and interconversion of three types of rhenium cluster compounds with amino acids

Substances of type II were investigated especially thoroughly as among them the strongest stabilizers were found. Preincubation of RBS with i-solutions of II b and II c led to significant increasing of haemolysis that may be compared with effect of steroids on RBS (fig.2, i). It is necessary to note, that the form of stabilizing curve (dependence of AR from concentration of solutions) is common for all investigated clusters of rhenium that confirms the role of cluster fragment in biochemical processes involved in the process of haemolysis prevention. To our surprise ii-solutions of all II acted as haemolytics (fig.2, ii) and iii-solutions of the same substances was very mild reagents in the model (fig.2, iii). We guess that 48h is enough for formation of clusters with hydroxyl groups that revealed destructive properties and after 72h they convert to products of following hydrolysis. Process of isomerization of II to III may be possible too as all compounds of type III was practically inactive in the model (is not shown).

Among cluster compounds of type IV which are stable in water there were no destructors of RBS and stabilizing effect correlated with hydrophobicity of radical of the acid. The most essential activity showed IY with isobutyric acid as a ligand IV e (is not shown).

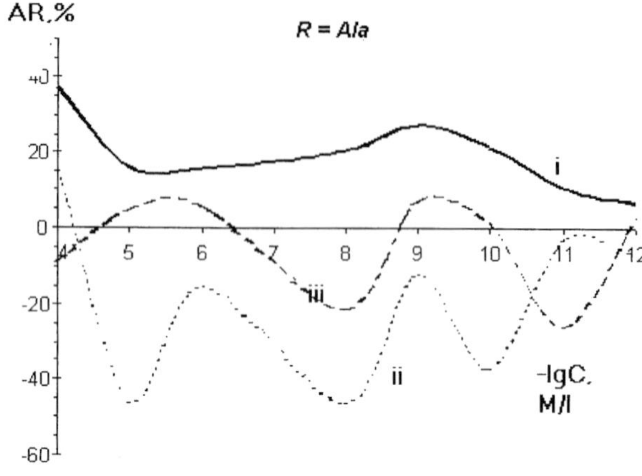

Figure 2. Average resistance (AR) of RBS under influence of preincubation in solutions with II b of different concentrations and different time after preparation

Behavior of cluster compound in the RBS-model does not predict the destiny of a substance in medicine but is a rather thin instrument for demonstration of sensitivity of biological objects to peculiarities of structure and properties of chemical compounds with close structure.

IV was absolutely untoxic in experiments in vivo on mice and its limited solubility in water made us to use liposomic forms of injection; II d with good solubility showed low toxicity. Both complexes were active in the in vivo model of haemolytic anemia; they increased stability of erythrocytes and quantity of haemoglobine. II d showed to be active in growth preventing of Guerink carcinoma.

REFERENCES:

1. Шалимов С.А., Кейсевич Л.В., Литвиненко Л.А., Волченскова И.И., Никишин П.Ф., Потебня П.Ф., Потебня Г.П. Лечение неоперабельных опухолей органов брюшной полости . Киев: Преса Украины. – 1998.
2. Keppler B. K., Berger M.R., Klenner T., Heim M.E. Metal Complexes as Antiturmour Agents *Advances in Drug Reserch* 1990; 19: 243 –310.
3. Eastland G.W.Jr., Yang G., Thompson T. Studies of rhenium carboxylates as antiturmour agents. Part II. Antiturmour studies of bis(mu-ropionato)diaquatetrabromodirhenium (III) in tumor-bearing mice *Methods Find Exp. Clin. Pharmacol* 1983; 7 : 435-438.
4. Бовыкин Б.А., Штеменко А.В., Сытник Т.В., Часова Э.В. О необычном поведении комплексного соединения рения с бислойными липидными мембранами *Украинский биохимический журнал* 1996; 3 : 107 –111.

Metal Ions in Biology and Medicine; vol 6. Eds. J.A. Centeno, Ph. Collery, G. Vernet, R.B. Finkelman, H. Gibb, J.C. Etienne. John Libbey Eurotext, Paris © 2000, pp. 619-621.

Zinc and copper in cardiovascular diseases

S. Rovesti, M. Bergomi, G. Vivoli

Department of Hygiene, Microbiology and Biostatistics, University of Modena and Reggio Emilia, Via Campi 287, 41100 Modena, Italy

Abstract. Animal and human studies suggest that trace elements such as Zn and Cu may be implicated in the pathogenesis of cardiovascular diseases, but the physiopathological role of these elements is still controversial. Aim of the review is to provide an update on this topic. High serum Cu and ceruloplasmin levels and low serum Zn levels were found significantly associated with an increased risk of mortality from cardiovascular diseases, especially coronary heart disease. Most recent epidemiological studies have shown that serum or plasma levels of Cu and ceruloplasmin were significantly higher in patients with cardiovascular disorders than in healthy subjects, even though the biological significance of circulating levels of Cu is still debated due to the complexity of homeostatic mechanisms. An imbalance of Zn and Cu status has also been associated with human hypertension as well as other important risk factors for coronary heart disease such as an unfavorable serum lipid profile. Among the possible mechanisms by which Zn and Cu are implicated in the pathogenesis of cardiovascular diseases, increasing attention has focused on their hypothesized role in preventing oxidative stress. The antioxidant properties of Zn and its involvement in preserving vascular endothelium integrity may have important implications for acute and chronic vascular processes. Although controversy still surrounds oxidant-antioxidant role of copper, there is evidence that an adequate copper status is required to maintain the antioxidant defenses.

The traditional risk factors for cardiovascular diseases do not fully explain the varied incidence of diseases, suggesting the involvement of other factors. Among the potential risk factors related to diet and life-style, some minerals and trace elements seem to be involved in the pathogenesis of these pathological conditions [1-3]. Of the trace elements of nutritional interest, particular attention was recently devoted to copper (Cu) and zinc (Zn). As suggested by *in vivo* and *in vitro* experimental studies, both Cu and Zn play a role in the structural and functional integrity of cardiovascular system [4,5].
Cross-sectional studies disclosed raised serum Cu levels in patients with acute myocardial infarction and chronic manifestations of atherosclerosis. Serum Zn concentration is decreased in many acute and chronic medical conditions, especially in acute myocardial infarction. It has been hypothesized that the high serum Cu levels and low serum zinc levels

may be secondary to compartmentalization caused by inflammation or injurious processes [2]. In large prospective population studies high serum copper or ceruloplasmin and low serum Zn appeared to predict incidence and death caused by vascular disease, with particular reference to coronary artery disease [2]. However, the biological significance of circulating Cu levels is still controversial due to the complexity of homeostatic mechanisms, and it has been suggested that high serum levels may mask soft tissue depletion. In agreement with this hypothesis, epidemiological studies measuring Cu and Zn concentrations in human organs, mostly implied a direct relation between Cu deficiency in specific organs and the development of cardiovascular disease [1].
Epidemiological surveys on subjects of different ages, showed that serum Cu levels were positively related to some risk factors of cardiovascular disease, such as systolic blood pressure, LDL cholesterol, smoking and body mass index [6-9]. Conflicting results emerged from epidemiologic studies on the potential involvement of Zn and Cu in blood pressure regulation. Some authors found different seric or urinary levels of Zn and Cu in hypertensive and normotensive subjects, while others failed to detect any significant difference.
The main findings of our studies on this topic are summarized in the following table.

Hypertensive (H) subjects	Key findings	Ref. no.
50 treated H	↑Zn-S; BP directly related to Cu-S	10
63 untreated borderline H	↑Cu-U; ↓AP-S and LDH-S	11
31 untreated borderline H	↓AP-S and LDH-S; DBP inversely related to Cu-Zn SOD; SBP inversely related to lysyl oxidase	12
60 untreated borderline H	↑Risk of hypertension with increasing of Cu-S; BP inversely related to lysyl oxidase	13

S: serum; U: urine; AP: alkaline phosphatase; LDH: lactic dehydrogenase; SOD; superoxide dismutase; DBP: diastolic blood pressure; SBP: systolic blood pressure.

Our epidemiological studies carried out, with the case-control design, on patients with different ages, stages of hypertension and drug intake, suggest that in hypertension might occur a modification in the homeostasis of zinc and copper. The impaired activity of Cu-dependent enzymes such as Cu-Zn SOD and lysyl oxidase in hypertensive subjects is of particular interest. Experiments in Cu deficient-animals showed a reduced activity of Cu-Zn SOD and lysyl oxidase, with impairment of elastin and collagen, as well as reduced endothelium control of vascular tone through both the protection of nitric oxide against inactivation and the prevention of lipid peroxidation damage to endothelial cells. Cu deficiency was also associated with increased circulating cholesterol levels, higher susceptibility of LDL to oxidation, impaired activity of some coagulation factors, electrocardiographic and blood pressure changes [2,5].
Although much controversy surrounds the oxidant-antioxidant role of copper, as recently reviewed, many data support the hypothesis that Cu is an antioxidant element and that oxidative damage is crucial in atherogenesis [2] .
Recent studies have shown that Zn is essential for maintaining vascular endothelium integrity. There is also increasing evidence in animal models that, in addition to its function as a membrane stabilizer, Zn may have a physiological role as an antioxidant [4], although the role of low Zn status in human cardiovascular disease is not clearly defined. A high

intake of Zn can lower HDL cholesteerol and compromise antioxidant defences probably due to the antagonistic effect of Zn and Cu status [2].

In conclusion the results of experimental and epidemiological studies available to date, give further support to the hypothesis that an imbalance of Zn and Cu homeostasis is probably involved in the pathogenesis of cardiovascular diseases.

References

1. Houtman JPW. Trace elements and cardiovascular diseases. *J Cardiovasc Risk* 1996; 3: 18-25.
2. Strain JJ. Trace elements and cardiovascular disease. In: Sandström B, Walter P, eds. *Role of Trace Elements for Health Promotion and Disease Prevention.* Bibl Nutr Dieta. Basel: Karger, 1998 (No 54): 127-40.
3. Fields M. Role of trace elements in coronary heart disease. *Br J Nutr* 1999; 81: 85-6.
4. Hennig B, Toborek M, McClain CJ. Antiatherogenic properties of zinc: implications in endothelial cell metabolism. *Nutrition* 1996; 12: 711-7.
5. Klevay LM, Medeiros DM. Deliberations and evaluations of the approaches, endpoints and paradigms for dietary recommendations about copper. *J Nutr* 1996; 126: 2419S-26S.
6. Kromhout D, Wibowo AAE, Herber RFM, Dalderup LM, Heerdink H, de Lezenne Coulander C, Zielhuis RL. Trace metals and coronary heart disease risk indicators in 152 elderly men (the Zutphen Study). *Am J Epidemiol* 1985; 122: 378-85.
7. Salonen JT, Salonen R, Korpela H, Suntioinen S, Tuomilehto J. Serum copper and the risk of acute myocardial infarction: a prospective population study in men in eastern Finland. *Am J Epidemiol* 1991; 134: 268-76.
8. Elcarte López T, Villa Elízaga I, Gost Garde JI, Elcarte López R, Martín Pérez A, Navascués Pujada J, Navarro Blasco I, Aparicio Madre MI. Cardiovascular risk factors in relation to the serum concentrations of copper and zinc: epidemiological study on children and adolescents in the Spanish province of Navarra. *Acta Paediatr* 1997; 86: 248-53.
9. Klipstein-Grobusch K, Grobbee DE, Koster JF, Lindemans J, Boeing H, Hofman A, Witteman JCM. Serum caeruloplasmin as a coronary risk factor in the elderly: the Rotterdam Study. *Br J Nutr* 1999; 81: 139-44.
10. Bergomi M, Rovesti S, Vivoli G. Zinc and copper in hypertension. In: Vernet J-P, ed. *Heavy Metals in the Environment,* vol 1. Edinburgh (UK): CEP Consultants, 1989: 114-7.
11. Vivoli G, Borella P, Bergomi M, Fantuzzi G. Zinc and copper levels in serum, urine, and hair of humans in relation to blood pressure. *Sci Total Environ* 1987; 66: 55-64.
12. Vivoli G, Bergomi M, Rovesti S, Pinotti M, Caselgrandi E. Zinc, copper, and zinc- or copper-dependent enzymes in human hypertension. *Biol Trace Elem Res* 1995; 49: 97-106.
13. Bergomi M, Rovesti S, Vinceti M, Vivoli R, Caselgrandi E, Vivoli G. Zinc and copper status and blood pressure. *J Trace Elem Med Biol* 1997; 11: 166-9.

Metal Ions in Biology and Medicine; vol 6. Eds. J.A. Centeno, Ph. Collery, G. Vernet, R.B. Finkelman, H. Gibb, J.C. Etienne. John Libbey Eurotext, Paris © 2000, pp. 622-624.

Copper and atherogenesis

G.A.A. Ferns[1, 2], D.J. Lamb[3], T.Y. Avades[1] and A. Taylor[1, 2]

[1] School of Biological Sciences, University of Surrey, Guildford, Surrey GU2 5XH, UK; [2] Department of Clinical Biochemistry, Royal Surrey County Hospital, Egerton Rd, Guildford, Surrey GU2 5XX, UK; and [3] Department of Chemical Pathology, Glenfield General Hospital, University of Leicester, Groby Rd, Leicester LE3 9QP, UK

Introduction The positive association between serum copper (Cu) levels and coronary heart disease (CHD) has been known for several years [1]. It has been proposed that this relationship is due to the elevated levels of low density lipoproteins (LDLs) associated with low plasma Cu levels [2]. However the epidemiological evidence is conflicting [3]. Oxidative modification of LDL is thought to play a key role in atherogenesis. Copper ions can catalyse this process in vitro, and there is evidence that transitional elements within the artery wall can also do so [4,5]. We have found that caeruloplasmin, the major copper-containing plasma protein can stimulate smooth muscle cell proliferation [6], a process considered to be important in atherogenesis. However Cu is also an important constituent of superoxide dismutase (SOD), an enzyme involved in free radical scavenging, a role that may be protective in preventing CHD. We have reported that Cu supplements reduce atherosclerosis in the cholesterol-fed rabbit [7], being associated with reduced monocyte binding to arterial endothelium and reduced lesion size. In the present study we have examined the effects of Cu depletion on atherosclerosis in these animals.

Methods NZW rabbits were placed on a Cu-deficient diet çontaining 0.25-1.0% cholesterol. Dietary cholesterol content was adjusted to achieve a plasma cholesterol of approximately 25-30 mmol/L. Cu was administered in the drinking water. Animals received Cu at: 0, 2.5, 10 and 70 mg/ day. Some animals received pencillamine plus the Cu-free diet. Animals remained on the diets for 3 month, and were then killed. The thoracic aortae were halved longitudinally; one half was stained and atherosclerosis quantified using oil red-O staining and image analysis. The other half was divided for the measurement of Cu, cholesterol and SOD activity.

Results The results of quantitation of lesion area were as follows: Group (a) Cu-free 63±4%, (b) Cu-free plus Penicillamine 57±9%, (c) 2.5 mg Cu/ d, 65±6%; (d) 10 mg Cu/ d, 43±7%, and (e) 70 mg Cu/ d, 53±6% (mean±sem) (Figure 1). The levels of tissue SOD in iu/mg wet tissue were respectively: (a) 182±17, (b) 198±46, (c) 262±47, (d) 260±18, and (e) 298±37 (mean±sem) with a significant difference between groups (a) and (d) ($P<0.05$) (Figure 2), and a positive correlation between tissue copper and tissue SOD activity for the groups combined ($r=0.655$, $p<0.05$).

Figure 1. The effects of copper intake on atherosclerotic lesion development in the cholestrol-fed rabbit

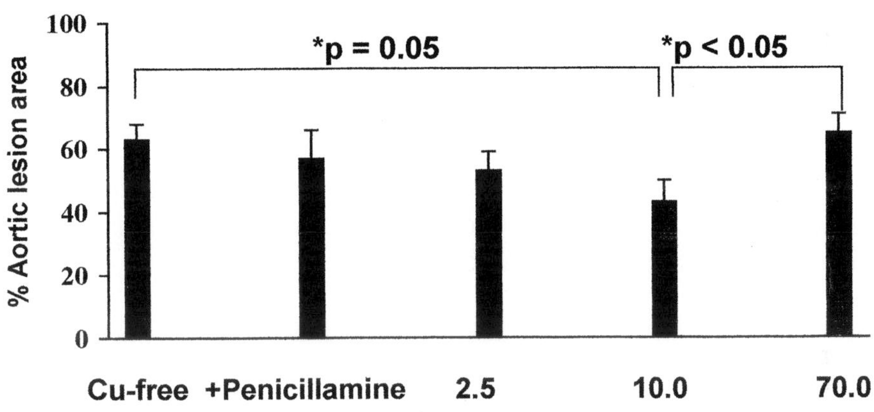

Figure 2. The effects of copper intake on aortic superoxide dismutase activity in the cholesterol-fed rabbit

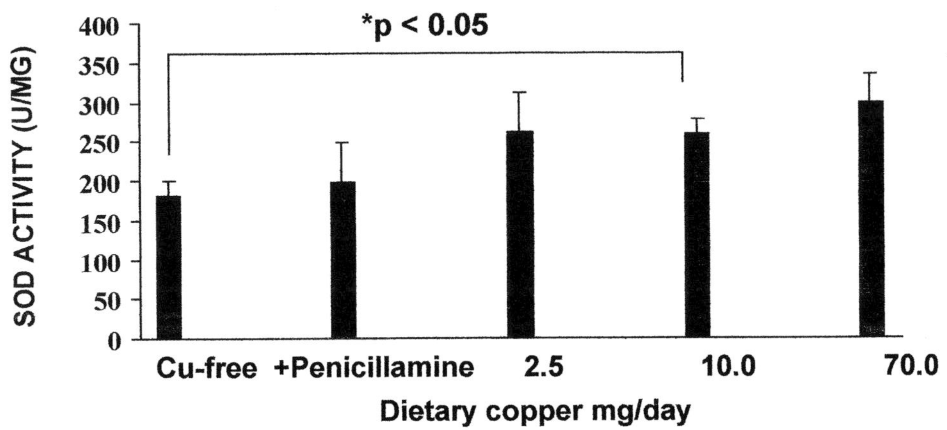

Conclusion Cu has the potential to play an important role in CHD through its effects on the cellular elements of the arterial wall, leucocyte and platelet function and lipoprotein metabolism. Copper deficiency is associated with elevated serum cholesterol concentrations and impaired endothelium-dependent arterial relaxation, and has been shown to cause an increased accumulation of arterial lipid peroxides, possibly due to decreased CuZnSOD activity. However, there is persuasive evidence that LDL modification is important in the early phases of atherogenesis. Copper is very effective in catalysing this modification in vitro, although the mechanisms by which this occurs are still obscure. Whether copper is involved in lipoprotein modification in vivo is still unproven, however copper ions are present within the artery wall, and may be released following arterial injury or from caeruloplasmin in areas of low pH (for example beside an activated macrophage). The epidemiological evidence supports the notion that copper may promote atherosclerosis, although some of these data are difficult to interpret and are not entirely consistent. The association between copper status and risk of coronary heart disease may ultimately be biphasic where both copper deficiency and overabundance may contribute to separate risk factors resulting in increased atherosclerotic lesion development

References

[1] Klevay LM. Coronary heart disease. The zinc/ copper hypothesis. Am J Clin Nutr 1975; 28, 764-774.

[2] Klevay LM. Ischaemic heart disease: Updating the zinc/ copper hypothesis. In: ed. Naito HK. Nutrition and Heart Disease (Monographs of the American College of Nutrition. vol 5). New York: S.P. Medical and Scientific Books, 1983, 61-67.

[3] Ferns GAA, Lamb DJ, Taylor A . The role of copper ions in atherogenesis: the blue Janus. Atherosclerosis 1997; 133, 139-152.

[4] Lamb DJ, Mitchison MJ, Leake DS. Transitional metal ions within human atherosclerotic lesions can catalyse the oxidation of low density lipoprotein by macrophages. FEBS Lett 1995; 374, 12-16.

[5] Evans PJ, Smith C, Mitchison MJ, Halliwell B. Metal ion release from mechanically-disrupted human arterial wall. Implications for the development of atherosclerosis. Free Rad Res 1995; 23, 465-469.

[6] Lamb DJ, Ferns GAA. Caeruloplasmin increases rabbit aortic smooth muscle cell proliferation. Clin Sci 1998; 94, 13p (abstract)

[7] Lamb DJ, Reeves GL, Taylor A, Ferns GAA. Dietary copper supplementation reduces atherosclerosis in the cholesterol-fed rabbit. Atherosclerosis 1999; 146, 33-43.

Metal Ions in Biology and Medicine; vol 6. Eds. J.A. Centeno, Ph. Collery, G. Vernet, R.B. Finkelman, H. Gibb, J.C. Etienne. John Libbey Eurotext, Paris © 2000, pp. 625-628.

Are iron, ferritin and hemoglobin involved in atherogenesis?

Wei Li[1], John M. Carstensen[2], Xi Ming Yuan[1]

[1] *Pathology II and* [2] *Oncology, Linköping University Hospital, Linköping, S-581 85, Sweden*

Introduction: Although body-iron and iron containing proteins have been implicated in atherogenesis earlier,[1] mainly based on the epidemiological studies, the exact role of them in the initiation and progression of atherogenesis is still unclear.[2]

Oxidized low-density lipoprotein (oxLDL) is believed to play an important role in atherogenesis. It is generally accepted that transition metals, particularly iron, in combination with a reducing agent are required for cellular LDL oxidation. Although iron, even in a catalytic form, has been demonstrated in atheroma gruels, its origin, precise localization, and implications within human atheroma are unknown.

It has been suggested that the serum iron level could be a critical factor for determining oxidative stress in atherogenesis, however, the results from epidemiological studies remain controversial. It is known that serum iron accounts only for a very limited portion of the body iron (0.004%) and is readily bound by serum macromolecules, such as transferrin, ferritin, haptoglobin, hemopexin and albumin. The majority of body iron is located intracellularly, e.g., in the form of hemoglobin and intracellular ferritin (68% and 27% of body iron, respectively).

We have hypothesized that lysosomal iron, as an important form of tissue iron, may be exocytosed from macrophages that have been iron-loaded by phagocytosis and degradation of iron-rich structures, e.g., senescent erythrocytes, or apoptotic cells. Such cells may acquire and store certain quantities of the redox-active iron that, if released, may promote LDL oxidation, uptake by macrophages, and oxidative stress related cellular damage.

We aimed to (i) characterize the regulation of ferritin expression in the iron-laden macrophages, (ii) study the interaction between such cells and lipoproteins and effect of vitamin E and desferroxamine, (iii) search for the evidence of erythrophagocytosis in human atheroma, (iv) examine the possible relationship between hemoglobin and cardiovascular death in a Swedish cohort.

Methods: Human monocyte-derived macrophages (HMDMs) were obtained from human buffy coat. HMDMs were first exposed to iron salts ($FeCl_3$, or hemoglobin, or heme), or UV-irradiated erythrocytes (UVRBC) for 12 hours, in some groups α-tocopherol (a-T) were also added (**Fig. 1 A and B**). Following carefully rinsing, LDL (50 - 100 µg/ml) was added in fresh culture medium without or with α-tocopherol (a-T) and incubated for another 24 - 48 h (**Fig. 1 A and B**). The conditioned medium and cell pellets were collected for iron measurement by atomic absorption spectroscopy, LDL oxidation was measured using assays of lipid peroxides (LPO) and thiobarbituric acid-reacting substances (TBARS). At indicated time points, lipid accumulation in the cell was evaluated using Nile red staining.[3] Ferritin mRNA in HMDMs was evaluated by Northern and dot blot analysis. Electrophoresis Mobility Shift Assay (EMSA) was used for determination of the binding of iron regulatory proteins (IRP-1 and IRP-2) to the iron responsive elements (IREs) within the ferritin mRNAs. Cellular ferritin examined using both ELISA and immunoprecipitation.

Arterial wall segments with fatty streaks or advanced lesions were collected from coronary arteries and thoracic aortas of 12 clinical autopsy cases. Normal appearing regions from the same cases together with normal coronary arteries from seven young forensic autopsy cases, without any sign of atherosclerosis, were used for comparison. Immunohistochemistry of CD 68 (macrophage marker), hemoglobin and ferritin were applied to serial sections of these arterial wall segments using an avidin-biotin complex (ABC) technique. Apoptotic cells were in situ assayed by the TUNEL-technique and Apostain (detection of apoptotic single strand DNA, ssDNA). We also applied the Pearl's method, energy dispersive X-ray microanalysis, and a modified Timm sulphide silver method (SSM) to demonstrate the occurrence of iron in human atherosclerotic lesions.

Results: We found that iron-uptake into macrophages, via transferrin-receptors (iron-loading) or phagocytosis of red blood cells via scavenger receptors (erythrophagocytosis), leads to accelerated synthesis of ferritin at both the mRNA and protein levels. The binding activity of iron regulatory proteins (IRP-1 and IRP-2) was increased by desferrioxamine and decreased by hemin and iron salts.

The binding and uptake of UV-irradiated erythrocytes by human macrophages and J-774 cells were greatly stimulated compared to that of native erythrocytes. The uptake resulted in lysosomal accumulation of iron in a low-molecular weight form, as shown by autometallography. Ensuing exocytosis of iron to the culture medium was demonstrated by atomic absorption spectroscopy.[4]

After 24 h LDL-exposure iron-laden cells ($FeCl_3$ or UVRBC, 12 h) showed increases in TBARS and LPO in culture medium, while α-tocopherol together with LDL exposure declined the lipid peroxidation (**Fig.1, A**). Neutral lipids and phospholipids accumulated in a granular, lysosome-like pattern in the iron-laden cells with a foam cell-like morphology. The enhanced ceroid-formation in iron-laden cells indicates the occurrence of poor degradation of LDL in such macrophage-foam cells.[3] The LDL together with α-tocopherol-treatment also results in a decrease in lipid accumulation in iron-laden HMDMs after another 48 h incubation (**Fig. 1, B**). The capacity of macrophages to oxidize LDL was much enhanced following erythrophagocytosis, and the process was shown to involve secretion of iron. Consequently, LDL oxidation was greatly inhibited by desferrioxamine.[3,5] The exposures of iron-laden macrophages to oxLDL also resulted in enhanced exocytosis of iron and ferritin, while high-density lipoprotein (HDL) inhibited such exocytosis.

OxLDL is taken up by macrophages through scavenger receptor-mediated endocytosis, which then leads to cellular damage, including apoptosis. We found that oxLDL-induced cellular damage in macrophages is associated with iron-mediated intralysosomal oxidative reactions, which cause partial lysosomal rupture and ensuing apoptosis. These series of events can be prevented by pre-exposing cells to the iron-chelator, desferroxamine (DFO), whereas it is augmented by pretreating the cells with a low molecular weight iron complex. Since both DFO and the iron complex would be taken up by endocytosis, and thus directed to the lysosomal compartment, the results suggest that the oxidized lipid-induced damage of macrophages is associated with iron-mediated intra-lysosomal oxidative reactions.[6,7]

We next investigated the presence of low molecular weight iron and ferritin in human atheroma, and their possible relation to the apoptotic process. With the very sensitive Timm sulphide-silver method, we found foam cells to contain heavy metals with a mainly lysosomal localization in human atheroma. Pronounced ferritin and hemoglobin accumulation, lysosomal low-molecular-weight iron, and apoptosis mainly concerned CD 68-positive cells (macrophages) in the atherosclerotic lesions (**Fig. 2**). No ferritin- or CD 68-positivity was found in normal coronary arteries from the young forensic-autopsy cases, while a moderate number of such cells were observed in the intima of very early atherosclerotic lesions (Type I) (**Fig. 2**). In the intima, cytosolic ferritin and iron with a lysosomal type distribution were found in many CD 68-positive macrophages, which were frequently surrounded by erythrocytes. A substantial number of apoptotic cells within the intima, media, and adventitia were registered in atherosclerotic lesions examined, although mainly in the vulnerable macrophage-enriched areas of the atheroma shoulder **(Fig. 2)**.[8]

In a 90000 Swedish cohort, serum iron and hemoglobin concentrations distinctly differ between men and women by age levels. In both men and women, hemoglobin positively but serum iron negatively are correlated with relative death rate of ischemic heart disease and acute myocardial infarctions, which show a concentration-dependent patterns. Furthermore, serum iron strongly enhanced the effect of hemoglobin on cardiovascular death.

Coclusions: 1. Following the degradation of iron-containing structures, erythrophagocytosis or phagocytosis of apoptotic cells, iron, mainly bound in ferritin, but also in low-molecular weight form, may store within the lysosomal apparatus of macrophages. The process accompanied with enhanced ferritin synthesis and mRNA expression. 2. Iron, even in a form of ferritin, may be exocytosed by the iron-laden macrophages. This may result in ensuing LDL oxidation and foam cell-formation, which can be prevented by α-tocopherol and desferroxamine. Moreover, such lysosomal iron may also sensitise lysosomes to oxidative stress and induce apoptosis of macrophage/foam-cells that may result in instability and rupture of atherosclerotic plaques. 3. Iron, hemoglobin and ferritin accumulated in atherosclerotic lesions, mostly in macrophage-rich areas of the atheroma shoulder. Erythrophagocytosis and hemoglobin degradation may serve as one of principle sources for iron and ferritin accumulation in atherosclerotic lesions. 4. Hemoglobin may be an additional risk factor for explaining 'iron hypothesis' in atherogenesis.

References

1. Sullivan JL. Iron and the Genetics of Cardiovascular Disease Circulation 1999 100: 1260-1263.

2. Yuan XM, and Brunk UT: Iron and LDL oxidation in atherogenesis. *APMIS* 1998, 106:825-842.

3. Yuan XM, Brunk UT, and Olsson AG: Effects of iron- and heamoglobin-loaded human monocyte-derived macrophages on oxidation and uptake of low density lipoprotein. *Arterioscler Thromb Vasc Biol* 1995; 15:1345-1351.

4. Yuan XM, Olsson AG, and Brunk UT: Macrophage erythrophagocytosis and iron exocytosis. *Redox Report* 1996; 2:9-17.

5.Yuan XM, Li W, Olsson AG, and Brunk UT: Iron in human atheroma and LDL oxidation by macrophages following erythrophagocytosis. *Atherosclerosis* 1996; 124:61-73.

6. Li W, Yuan XM, Olsson AG, and Brunk UT: Uptake of oxidized LDL by macrophages results in partial lysosomal enzyme inactivation and relocalization. *Arterioscler Tromb Vasc Biol* 1998, 18:177-184.

7. Li W, Yuan XM, and Brunk UT: OxLDL-mediated cytotoxicity to macrophages is mediated by lysosomal leak and is modified by intralysosomal iron. *Free Radic Res* 1998, 29:389-398.

8. Yuan XM: Apoptotic macrophage-derived foam cells of human atheromas are rich in iron and ferritin, suggesting iron-catalysed reactions to be involved in apoptosis. *Free Radic Res* 1999;30:221-232.

TBARS (505/549)
LPO
80,0
60,0
40,0
20,0
0,0
nmol /mg protein
1 2 3 4 5 6 7
FeCl3 (50µM)
UV-RBC (20%.50µl)
a-T (40µM)
12 hours
LDL (100µg/ml)
a-T (40µM)
24 hours
Fig. 1 A
Netrual lipid
Phospholipid
1250
1000
750
500
250
0
Fluorescence per HMDM (A.U.)
1 2 3 4 5 6 7 8
FeCl3 (50µM)
UV-RBC (20%.50µl)
a-T (40µM)
12 hours
LDL (100µg/ml)
a-T (40µM)
48 hours
Fig. 1 B
CD68
Ferritin
Hb
ssDNA

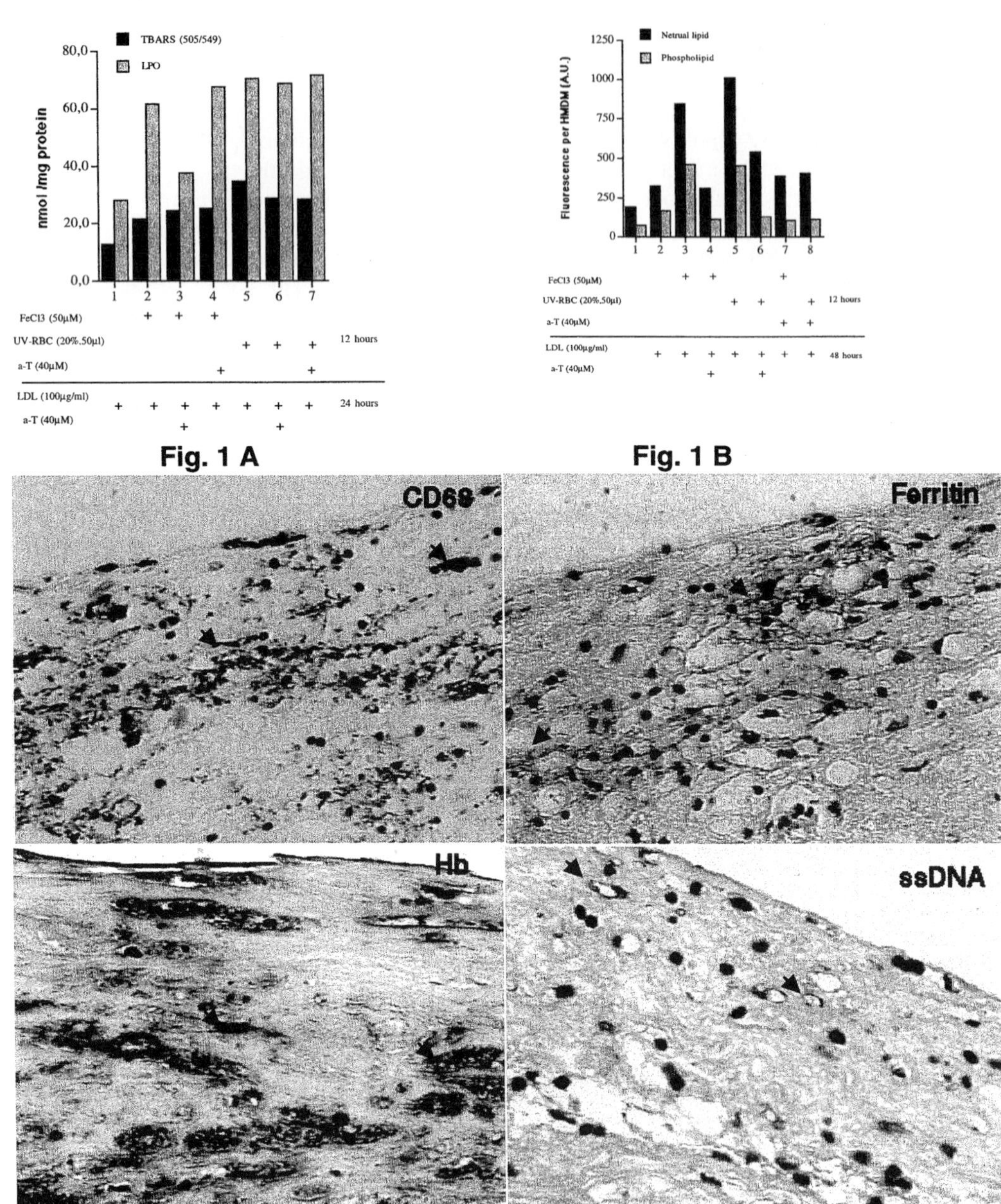

Fig. 2

Metal Ions in Biology and Medicine; vol 6. Eds. J.A. Centeno, Ph. Collery, G. Vernet, R.B. Finkelman, H. Gibb, J.C. Etienne. John Libbey Eurotext, Paris © 2000, pp. 629-631.

Serum selenium and acute myocardial infarction (AMI)

Pérez Beriain R.M., García de Jalón A., Pérez Beriain T., Calvo Ruata M.L., Escanero Marcén J.F., Cabeza Sánchez A.

Servicio de Bioquímica Clínica, Sección de Nutrición y Metales, Hospital Universitario Miguel Servet, Calle Calamita n° 3, 50009 Zaragoza, Spain

INTRODUCTION

Acute myocardial infarction (AMI) is defined as the necrosis of the cardiac muscle owing to an interruption in the bloodflow in the coronary arteries.

There seems to exist a relationship between selenium deficiency and a greater risk of diseases of the myocardium [1,2,3].

Selenium deficiency has been implicated in the aetiopathogeny of Keshan disease, an endemic cardiomyopathy observed in China, and in other cases of congestive cardiomyopathy in subjects on artificial nutrition [4].

In the bibliography a positive correlation is expresed between the selenium concentration in serum and the right ventricular ejection fraction, as well as very low values for blood selenium for patients suffering from AMI [5]. But others authors think selenium status does not appear to be an important determinant of risk of myocardial infarction [6].

Other studies show that persons with selenium <45 μg/l have 2.9 times greater risk of suffering from a coronary disease [7].

AIMS

To study the relationship between the acute myocardial infarction and serum concentrations of selenium in our country.

MATERIALS AND METHODS

Samples were analysed from 73 patients, aged between 45 and 87,at the moment of arrival at the Accident and Emergency Unit under suspicion of AMI and whose diagnosis was confirmed by clinic tests, cardiac enzymes and electrocardiogram findings, and the serum concentration of selenium was determined.

As a control group, we selected the serums of 182 apparently healthy people who were aged between 45 and 80.

The determination was carried out using atomic absorption spectrophotometry (AAS) with a graphite camera and a Zeeman background corrector (*Perkin Elmer 4110 ZL*), using Pd $(NO_3)_2$ solution as matrix modifier.

The statistical calculations were carried out using SPSS statistics program. The statistical test used, was the Student T-test for equality of means.

RESULTS

The distribution of the selenium levels (probability interval or mean +/- 2 times Standard Deviation (S.D.)) in the differents groups (95% from the patients in the AMI group, and 95% from the subjects in the control group), are defined to the following illustration (fig. 1).

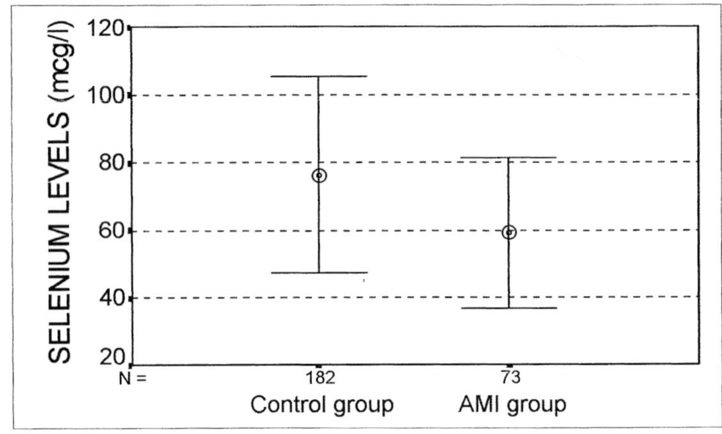

Figure 1.

The results of the serum concentrations of selenium in the groups (table II) were as follows:

	N	Mean (μg/l)	S.D.	I.C. (95%)
Control group	182	76.4	14.5	74.3 - 78.6
AMI group	73	59.2	11.1	56.6 - 61.8

Table 1.

The means comparison using the Student T test shows a statistically significant difference with a $p<0.001$.

The error bars represent confidence interval for the mean, with a confidence level of 95% (fig. 2).

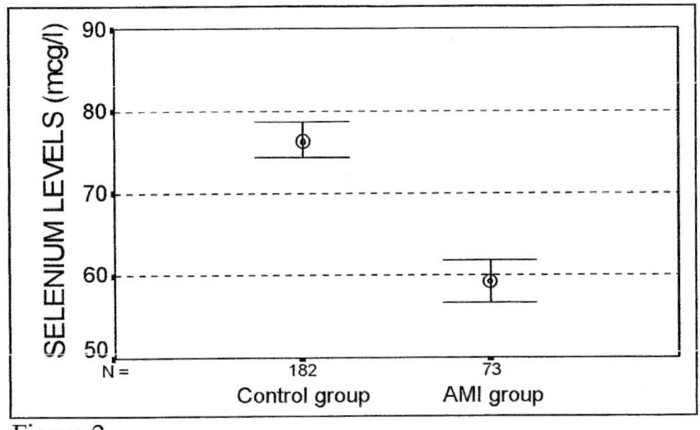

Figure 2.

CONCLUSIONS

We can conclude that in our country the individuals with acute myocardial infarction showed lower serum concentrations of selenium than those serum concentrations of selenium in the normal population, although greater than values considered to be pathological (< 30 μg/l).

REFERENCES

1. Sartiano GP, Lynch WE, Hopkins CB, Darby TD. *Erythrocyte and plasma selenium measurements in cosgestive cardiomyoopathy*. N Engl J Med 1982 Aug 26; 307(9) : 558. (Letter).
2. Goldman IS, Kantrowitz EN. *Cardiomyopathy associated with selenium deficiency*. N Engl J Med 1981 Sep 17; 305(12) : 701. (Letter).
3. Johnson RA, Baker SS, Fallon JT, Maynard EP, Ruskin JN, Wen Z, Ge K, Cohen HJ. *An occidental case of cardiomyopathy and selenium deficiency*. N Engl J Med 1981 May 14; 304(20) : 1210-2. (Letter).
4. Ge K, Yang G. *The epidemiology of selenium deficiency in the etiological study of endemic diseases in China*. Am J Clin Nutr. 1993 Feb. 57(2 Suppl) : 259S-263S.
5. Oster O, Prellwitz W, Kasper W, Meinertz T. *Congestive cardiomyopathy and the selenium content of serum*. Clin Chim Acta 1983 Feb 29; 128(1) : 125-32.
6. Kardinaal AF, Kok FJ, Kohlmeier L, Martin-Moreno JM, Ringstad J, Gomez-Aracena J, Mazaev VP, Thamm M, Martin BC, Aro A, Kark JD, Delgado-Rodriguez M, Riemersma RA, van't Veer O, Huttunen JK. *Association betwwen toenail selenium and risk of acute myocardial infarction in European men. The EURAMIC Study*. Am J Epidemiol. 1997 Feb 15; 145(4) : 373-9.
7. Neve J. *Selenium as a risk factor for cardiovascular diseases*. J Cardiovasc Risk. 1996 Feb. 3(1) : 42-7.

ACKNOWLEDGMENTS

This work has been supported by the Asociación para la Promoción de la Fundación Miguel Servet.

Metal Ions in Biology and Medicine; vol 6. Eds. J.A. Centeno, Ph. Collery, G. Vernet, R.B. Finkelman, H. Gibb, J.C. Etienne. John Libbey Eurotext, Paris © 2000, pp. 632-634.

Manganese intake and hypertension. An experimental approach in DOCA-salt hypertensive rats

P. Laurant[1], E. Gaillard[1], E. Chanut[2], S. Bobillier-Chaumont[1], C. Jacquot[2], J.H. Trouvin[2], A. Berthelot[1]

[1] *Laboratoire Physiologie, Pharmacologie et Nutrition Préventive Expérimentale, Faculté Médecine Pharmacie, Besançon, France;* [2] *Laboratoire Pharmacologie, Faculté de Pharmacie, Chatenay-Malabry, France*

Introduction

Manganese (Mn) is an essential element which is present in trace amounts in all mammalian cells. Several studies have focused upon the role of Mn on the cardiovascular system. Mn decreases cardiac contractility, heart rate and has antiarrhythmic effects (Kliegfield *et al.*, 1981; Horner & Kliegfield, 1982, Brurok *et al.*, 1997). In isolated blood vessels, increasing Mn concentration decreases vascular tone and contractility induced by several agonists (Kasten *et al.*, 1994).The mechanisms by which Mn modifies cardiac and vascular function are not well understood. The calcium antagonistic properties of Mn may play a role since Mn acts as a calcium entry-blocker decreasing intracellular calcium levels (Nasu, 1995). It has been shown that Mn prevents superoxide degradation of nitric oxide (NO) and that Mn induces endothelium- and NO-dependent vascular relaxation, decreasing peripheral resistance and thus, lowering blood pressure (Kasten *et al.*, 1994). They are few reports on the effects of Mn on blood pressure in clinical and experimental hypertension. Some experimental studies reveals that intravenous administration of Mn increases, lowers or does not change blood pressure levels (Jamieson *et al.*, 1983; Dudek & Pytkowski, 1991; Kasten *et al.*, 1994; Jynge *et al.*, 1997). Given the essential role of Ca in the hypertensive state and the *in vitro* effect of Mn on cardiovascular function, we suggest that Mn may have possible beneficial effect on high blood pressure. This paper presents some experimental evidence concerning the effects of dietary Mn intake on blood pressure, vascular reactivity and central catecholamine levels in some brain structures implicated in the control of blood pressure of experimental mineralocorticoid-salt (DOCA-salt) hypertensive rats.

Dietary Mn intake and blood pressure in DOCA-salt hypertensive rats

A Mn-enriched diet (6g/kg), given for 11 weeks, inhibits the rise in blood pressure (fig 1), attenuates the development of DOCA-salt hypertension in rats, has no effect on heart rate and inhibits development of cardiac hypertrophy. These findings suggest, as will be discussed below, that Mn lower peripheral resistance in blood vessels of DOCA-salt rats by decreasing vascular tone and reactivity.

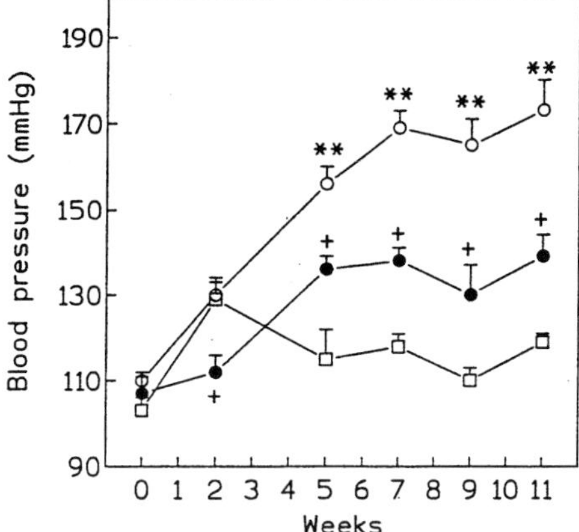

Figure 1 Systolic blood pressure measured in conscious, restrained and prewarmed control normotensive (80 mg/kg Mn) (□), DOCA-salt hypertensive (80 mg/kg Mn) (○), and Mn-enriched DOCA-salt (6 g/kg Mn)(●) rats. Data are means ± SEM. n = 10-15 rats per group. Asterisks indicate a significant difference in blood pressure. **$p < 0.01$ versus normotensive rats; $^{+}p < 0.05$ versus normotensive and DOCA-salt hypertensive rats.

Dietary Mn intake and vascular function

DOCA-salt hypertension is characterised by increased peripheral resistance which results from enhanced vascular responsiveness to endogenous agonists and impaired endothelium-dependent relaxation. Our *ex vivo* experimental studies on isolated aortae and perfused mesenteric vascular beds from DOCA-salt rats showed that a Mn-enriched diet decreases reactivity to endogenous agonists such as norepinephrine, attenuated the vascular responsiveness to $CaCl_2$, and "normalised" the endothelium- and NO-dependent relaxation to acetylcholine in conductance artery (aorta) and resistance arteries (mesenteric vascular bed). Although the precise effect of Mn on blood vessels remains to be defined, Mn may affect Ca influx, intracellular release/reuptake or cellular efflux of Ca (Nazu, 1995). The beneficial effect of Mn on blood vessels in DOCA-salt hypertensive rats may also be explained by stimulating NO synthase and/or guanylate cyclase pathways in vascular cells since Mn is known to be a cofactor of guanylate cyclase (Wedler, 1994), and to help superoxide dismutase activity, resulting in potentiation of NO action in vascular tissus (Kasten et al., 1994).

Dietary Mn intake and central catecholamine production

The central nervous system regulates vasomotor tone, cardiac output, heart rate and hydromineral metabolism. We have shown that DOCA-salt hypertension in rats increases norepinephrine and dopamine levels in the pons-medulla, cortex and hypothalamus indicating alteration in central catecholaminergic activity which could alter cardiovascular function and, consequently elevate blood pressure (Talman 1985). The Mn-enriched diet decreases norepinephrine content in the pons-medulla and hypothalamus of DOCA-salt rats. It is suggested that the hypothalamic noradrenergic pathway may play an important role in the pathophysiology of DOCA-salt hypertension and, that treatment which could inhibit the central noradrenergic activity, such as Mn supplementation, may prevent the rise in blood pressure in this form of hypertension.

Conclusion

A high Mn intake attenuates the development of DOCA-salt hypertension in rat. This beneficial effect on blood pressure may be related to change in vascular function (decrease in adrenoceptor affinity, improvement of endothelium-dependent relaxation, decrease in Ca-induced contractility), and to change in central cerebral norepinephrine content. It is suggested that Mn may exert peripheral and central actions to attenuate DOCA-salt hypertension.

References

Brurok H, Schjott J, Berg K, Karlsson JOG, Jynge P. (1997). Manganese and the heart: acute cardiodepression and myocardial accumulation of manganese. *Acta Physiol. Scand.* 1997; 159 : 33-40.

Dudek H, Pytkowski B. Effect of in vivo manganese administration on calcium exchange and contractile force of rat ventricular myocardium. *Basic Res. Cardiol.* 1991; 86 : 515-522.

Horner WH, Kliegfield P. Antidisrhythmic and dose-related hemodynamic effects of manganese. *J. Cardiovasc. Pharmacol.* 1982; 4 : 1949-1956.

Jamieson DD, Quinn RJ, Le Coutier A. Antagonism by manganese of isoprenaline dilatation of the guinea-pig isolated trachea. *Clin. Exp. Pharmacol. Physiol.* 1983; 10 : 511-519.

Jynge P, Brurok H, Asplund A, Towart R, Refsum H, Karlsson JO. Cardiovascular safety of MnDPDP and $MnCl_2$. *Acta Radiol.* 1997; 38: 740-749.

Kasten TP, Settle SL, Misko TP, Currie MG, Nickols GA. Manganese potentiation of nitric oxide-mediated vascular relaxation. *Eur. J. Pharmacol.* 1994; 253 : 35-43.

Nasu T. Actions of manganese ions in contraction of smooth muscle. *Gen. Pharmac.* 1995; 26 : 945-953.

Talman WT. Cardiovascular regulation and lesions of the central nervous system. *Ann. Neurol.* 1985; 18 : 1-12.

Wedler FC. Biochemical and nutritional role of manganese: an overview. In Klimis-Tavantzis ED, ed. *Manganese in health and diseases*. Boca Raton: CRC Press, 1994 : 1-37.

Metal Ions in Biology and Medicine; vol 6. Eds. J.A. Centeno, Ph. Collery, G. Vernet, R.B. Finkelman, H. Gibb, J.C. Etienne. John Libbey Eurotext, Paris © 2000, pp. 635-637.

Environmental cadmium exposure and hypertension and cardiovascular risk

Muneko Nishijo[1], Hideaki Nakagawa[1], and Teruhiko Kido[2]

[1] *Department of Public Health, Kanazawa Medical University, Daigaku 1-1, Uchinada, Ishikawa 920-0293, Japan;* [2] *School of Health Sciences, Faculty of Medicine, Kanazawa University, Kodatsuno 5-11-80, Kanazawa, Ishikawa 920-0942, Japan*

Introduction

In animal experiments, blood pressure elevations are found with low cadmium(Cd) concentrations but also decreases with high Cd concentrations. Also the possibility of A-V block induced by Cd was reported in an in vitro study. In men, in general populations with low level of Cd exposure, the relationships between body Cd concentrations and hypertension or cardiovascular diseases have been reported in some studies. However, the effects of moderate or heavy Cd exposure on blood pressure in the environmental or industrial fields are controversial.

Therefore, we undertook to clarify the influence of Cd exposure on blood pressure levels and the cardiovascular system in the inhabitants living in a Cd polluted area and itai-itai disease patients who are most heavily exposed to Cd and suffer from renal tubular dysfunction and osteomalacia.

A review of previous epidemiological surveys

Previous large scale epidemiological surveys of blood pressure levels or prevalence of hypertension among inhabitants living in the Jinzu River basin or the Kakehashi River basin were reviewed.

Nogawa and Kawano[1)] found that the systolic blood pressure of 471 women aged >=40 years suspected of having bone damage and renal tubular dysfunction was significantly lower in each 10 year age group as compared to 2308 women in a control area, with diastolic blood pressure also tending to be lower.
The Japanese Environmental Agency [2)] conducted a health impact survey in 7 Cd polluted areas in Japan, and found that the prevalences of hypertension in the inhabitants with proteinuria and glucosuria living in the Kakehashi River basin and Jinzu River basin were lower than those in the control areas.

The relationship between blood pressure and renal dysfunction induced by Cd

Itai-itai disease is prevalent in the Jinzu River basin in Toyama Prefecture which is the area most severely affected by Cd in Japan. The total of 64 itai-itai disease patients, all women, received detailed examination including measurement of blood pressure, renal function tests, blood gas analysis, urinalysis and blood chemical measurements at our University hospital. Also in the Kakehashi River basin in Ishikawa Prefecture which is the second large scale Cd polluted area in Japan, a high prevalence of renal tubular dysfunction has been reported, and the cases of renal tubular dysfunction found in health impact survey have been followed up. At this time, blood pressure, creatinine clearance(CCr), %TRP, fractional excretion of sodium (FENa), Base excess(B.E.), urinary beta2-microglobulin(b2MG) and urinary Cd were measured in itai-itai disease patients, and compared with these parameters of 43 female inhabitants living in the Kakehashi River basin(Kakehashi inhabitants) and 13 female controls.

In the subjects with CCr<35ml/min, systolic and diastolic blood pressure levels of itai-itai disease patients were lower than those of Kakehashi inhabitants. Although their renal tubular dysfunctions were more severe than Kakehashi inhabitants, there was no significant difference of FENa between them(Table 1). In the subjects with CCr>=35, systolic blood pressure of itai-itai disease patients was significantly decreased as compared with Kakehashi inhabitants, and diastolic blood pressure was decreased as compared with controls. At this time also, there was no difference in FENa among these three groups(Table 1).

Mortality analysis for cardiovascular diseases

We followed the 3178 Kakehashi inhabitants(1424 men and 1754 women) for 15 years who participated in the health impact survey in 1981-2, and investigated the standardized mortality ratio(SMR) for cardiovascular diseases when the subjects were divided into 2 groups according to urinary b2MG.

As shown in Table 2, SMR for heart failure of the subjects with urinary b2MG>=1mg/gCr was higher than those of the Japanese general population or the subjects with urinary b2MG<1 mg/gCr in both sexes. In the men, a significant increase of SMR for cerebrovascular diseases due to increased cerebral infarction mortality was observed. However, SMRs for ischemic heart diseases or cerebral hemorrhage were not increased in either sex.

Discussion

On the basis of the epidemiological studies in Japan, moderate or heavy environ -mental Cd exposure was suggested to decrease blood pressure of inhabitants. Moreover, blood pressure levels of itai-itai disease patients who show more progressive renal tubular dysfunction were lower than Kakehashi inhabitants. This suggests that the severe renal tubular dysfunction induced by Cd is related to the decrease of blood pressure. However, the increase of excretion of Na in the renal tubule is considered not to be the main mechanism decreasing blood pressure, because there was no significant difference in FENa between the itai-itai disease patients and Kakehashi inhabitants.

With regard to mortality of Kakehashi inhabitants, the SMR's of the diseases related to hypertension, ischemic heart diseases or cerebral haemorrage, were not increased. However an excess of death due to heart failure was observed, but this does not mean increased mortality from heart diseases. Because, at that time in Japan, it was customary to ascribe the cause of death to heart failure in cases with no clear-cut cause of death or gradual deterioration culminating in death.

In conclusion, renal tubular dysfunction induced by moderate or heavy environmental Cd exposure is suggested to decrease blood pressure.

Table 1 Comparisons of blood pressure level and renal function tests between itai-itai disease patients and inhabitants living in Kakehashi River basin

	Itai-itai disease patients		Kakehashi Inhabitants		Controls	
	mean	S.D.	mean	S.D.	mean	S.D.
CCr<35	(N=44)		(N=13)		-	
Age	72.2	5.3*	76.3	5.6	-	-
BMI	22.1	2.8	20.9	3.6	-	-
Systolic blood pressure	112.3	21.0**	140.3	23.3	-	-
Diastolic blood pressure	60.9	14.5*	70.5	14.1	-	-
Urinary b2-MG(mg/gCr)	195.0	0.25**	20.4	0.93	-	-
Urinary Cd (mg/gCr)	21.4	0.3***	11.0	0.3	-	-
%TRP	48.7	19.4*	70.2	13.4	-	-
Serum creatinine	2.8	1.7*	1.7	0.8	-	-
Serum Cl	113	3.8**	109	4.3	-	-
B.E.	-7.3	4.0**	-2.9	3.5	-	-
FENa	4.8	3.2	3.4	1.6	-	-
CCr>=35	(N=20)		(N=30)		(N=13)	
Age	65.9	8.4*	72.6	7.0	67.7	6.9
BMI	23.2	3.2	22.6	4.3	24.4	2.6
Systolic blood pressure	118.8	14.8**	136.2	18.1	133.8	16.2
Diastolic blood pressure	71.7	11.2&	74.3	10.0	81.7	11.7
Urinary b2-MG(mg/gCr)	118.9	0.24*&	7.4	0.64&	0.24	0.48
Urinary Cd (mg/gCr)	23.3	0.17&	12.3	0.18&	5.3	0.12
%TRP	65.7	13.7**&&	79.2	9.5	86.3	4.9
Serum creatinine	1.4	0.32&	1.1	0.21&	0.8	0.1
Serum Cl	110	2.4*&	107	1.3	107	3.1
B.E.	-3.7	2.6**	-0.89	1.7	-	-
FENa	2.0	0.7	1.8	0.8	2.0	0.5

*:P<0.05, **:P<0.01, ***:P<0.001 : Comparison with Kakehashi inhabitants
&:P<0.05, &&:P<0.01 : Comparison with controls

Table 2 The SMR for cardiovascular diseases among inhabitants living in Kakehashi River basin

	Men				Women			
Urinary b2MG	<1mg/Cr		>=1mg/gCr		<1mg/Cr		>=1mg/gCr	
	Obs.	SMR	Obs.	SMR	Obs.	SMR	Obs.	SMR
All causes	367	83 -*	140	127 ** &&	271	82 -*	199	146***&&&
Ischemic heart diseases	17	54 -*	3	38	14	60	10	99
Heart failure	38	93	22	179***&	40	104	46	248*&
Cerebrovascular diseases	48	73	31	161*&&&	46	74 -*	37	128 &
Cerebral haemorrage	14	99	4	99	14	93	3	51
Crebral infarction	30	63	27	147	23	61 -*	29	147

*:P<0.05, **:P<0.01, ***:P<0.001: Comparison with Japanese general population
&:P<0.05, &&:P<0.01, &&&:P<0.001: Comparisons between b2-MG categories

References

1) Nogawa K and kawano S: A survey of the blood pressure of women suspected of "Itai-itai" disease. Juzen Med J, 1969, 3:357-363. (in Japanese, with English abstract)

2) Japan Public Health Association Cadmium Research Committee: Studies of health effects of cadmium. Kankyo Hoken Report, 1989, 53:69-345. (in Japanese)

Metal Ions in Biology and Medicine; vol 6. Eds. J.A. Centeno, Ph. Collery, G. Vernet, R.B. Finkelman, H. Gibb, J.C. Etienne. John Libbey Eurotext, Paris © 2000, pp. 638-640.

The effect of cadmium and zinc ions on vascular tonus

Gülsen Öner[1], Ibrahim Bilgen[1], Mustafa Edremitlio lu[2], Zeliha Alkan[3]

[1] Akdeniz University, Faculty of Medicine Department of Physiology Antalya; [2] K r kkale University Faculty of Medicine Department of Physiology, K r kkale; [3] Ministry of Health, Ankara, Turkey

Abstract:

Rats receiving 15 ppm $CdCl_2$ in drinking water for 30 days displayed hypertension and nephrotoxicity associated with endothelial dysfunction. ncreased sensitivity to Phenylephrine(PE) and decreased relaxant response to Acethylcholine(Ach) in the aortic ring of Cadmium(Cd) treated rats were partially reversed by preincubation of rings with L-Arginine(Arg) .Cd induced nephrotoxicity and vessel tone changes were completely prevented by zinc enriched diet.

Key words: Cd,zinc,NO,EDHF ,hypertension, L-arginine,nephrotoxicity

Introduction:

Endustrialisation benefits society but also punishes it through environmental pollution.One of the most toxic component of the environmental pollutants is Cd. Its nephrotoxicity has been emphasised as one of the most important deteriorative effects. Because Cd is accumulated in the body, its deposition in the kidney is directly correlated with both the exposure, duration and the amount of ingestion [1,2].

Cd induced impairment in kidney functions are often associated with hypertension which also has a high frequency in industriliazed countries [3]. The etiology of hypertension focused on the impairment of vessel tone which depends on the fine balance between endothelial dilators and constrictors [4].NO receives special attention among the endothelial dilators and is produced from L-Arg by NO synthase enzyme which is influenced by some metal including Cd [1,5]. Cd causes a cencentration dependent constriction in resistance arteriols in skeletal muscles [6] in addition,it impaires the functions of kidney which has a vital role in blood pressure regulation[7,8]. However the presence of controversial reports about the role of Cd in hypertension in humans[9] draws a veil over the clinical importance of Cd toxicity and causes underestimation of this topic.

The hypertensive action of Cd and its prevention must be studied in detail to reap the benefits of industrial development without being subjected to its risks.So,we aimed to study 1- The effect of Cd on vessel tone 2- The mechanism by which Cd induces endothelial dysfunction and its reversibility in rats.

Material and Methods:

60 two month old male Wistar rats were divided into four groups. Animals in the first and second group received normal rat food while other two groups were fed a diet containing 200 ppm zinc. 15 ppm $CdCl_2$ was added into the drinking water of the second and fourth groups for 30 days. On day 30 ,8 animals from each group were anaesthetized with 1 g/kg urethane i.p and used for the measurement of systolic and diatolic blood pressure and kidney functions as described previously [7,8].The remaining rats were killed by blow on the head and the aortic rings were prepared and

studied according to the method of Li et al[10].A force displacement transducer(FDT 1-A MAY) connected to a Labcard computer system were used to record the isometric tension of the rings. A resting tension of 1 g was maintained for the optimum observation of maximal contractile response and expressed as mg.

After 1 h equilibrium period a) 8-10 rings from each group were used to study the cumulative concentration response curve(CRC) for phenylephrine (10^{-8} -10^{-5} M), b)The precontracted rings with 10^{-6} M PE (a submaximal contraction dose) were used to study CRC for Acethylcholine(10^{-8} - 10^{-4} M) in the absence and presence of 10^{-2}M L-Arg. and CRC for sodium nitroprusside(SNP)(10^{-9} -10^{-5} M), c)The effect of L-Arg addition on the component of Ach induced relaxation response in the rings preincubated with10^{-4}M L-NAME, 10^{-5}M indomethacine(IND) and 10^{-2} M of Tetraaethylammonium(TEA) for 10 min.

Mann Whitney U test and paired Samples t were used for the analysis of intergroups and intragroup significance respectively . $p<0.05$ considered as significant.

Results and Discussion:

As seen in table I obvious Cd accumulation in blood and renal cortex was the evidence of Cd toxicity which was also further supported by increased arterial pressures and decreased glomerular filtration rate.

Figure I shows that rings from Cd exposed rats are more sensitive to the cumulative doses of PE than those of controls($p<0.01$).The mean pD_2 value for PE was 7.1±0.06 in controls and 7.4 ±0.1 in Cd treated rings. On the other hand dilation to Ach was significantly lower in Cd treated rings(Fig.2).Unchanged dilation response against SNP doses excluded possibility of Cd induced alteration in smooth muscle cells response.Blokade of basal NO production by 10^{-4} M L-NAME increased response to 10^{-6}M PE from 23,41±4.73 % to 39.23±6.44% and 77.13±19.83% in Cd and zinc exposed rats respectively($p<0.01$).This elevated response to PE which indicates increased basal NO production can be a compansatory result of Cd induced increased sensitivity to constrictors to maintain normal vessel tone. Partial reversal of impaired Ach response with L-Arg addition supported the deficiency of NO precursor due to overuse (Fig.2)in cadmium exposed rings.L-Arg addition into the bath increased the magnitude but also changed the contributors of Ach induced relaxation.Consisting with the previous data Ach elicited mainly L-NAME sensitive relaxation in normal thorasic aorta. However, the share of NO decreased significantly and TEA sensitive component (EDHF) occured after L-arg preincubation in all rings irrespective of treatment.These L-Arg dependent changes in the characterisation of endothelial relaxation are interesting and needed to study in detail. Co-administration of zinc prevented both Cd induced nephrotoxicity and endothelial dysfunction. As a results our findings suggested that Cd induced Prostanoid decrease may cause of less response to Ach which was reversed partially with L-arg, however zinc enriched diet completely prevented the toxicity of Cd .

References:

1-Ramirez DC, Martinez LD, Marchevsky E, Gimenez MS: Biphasic effect of cadmium in non-cytotoxic conditions on the secretion of nitric oxide from peritoneal macrophages. *Toxicol* 1999;139 (1-2):167-77

2-Bomhard EM, Maruhn D, Rinke M :Time course of chronic oral cadmium nephrotoxicity in Wistar rats: excretion of urinary enzymes. *Drug Chem Toxicol* 1999 ;22(4):679-703
3-Zemel MB,Dietary pattern and Hypertension The DASH study Nutr Rev 1998,55(8):303-305
4-Boulanger CM.Secondary Endothelial Dysfunction,Hypertension and Heart failure J Mol Cell Cardiol 1999,31(1)39-49
5-Tian L and Lawrance DA:Metal induced modulation of nitric oxide production in vitro by murine macrophages Lead,Nickel and Cobalt utilize different mechanism.Toxicol Appl Pharmacol 1996 141(2):540-7
6- Zhang C,Thind GS,Joshua IG Fleming JT :Cadmium induced arteriolar constriction in skeletal muscle microsirculation Ame J Hypertens 1993,6(supl 4):325-29
7-ÖnerG,Senturk UK,Izgut-Uysal VN:The role of atrial Natriureti Peptide in cadmium induced hypertension . J Trace Elem.Exp Med 1995,8:147-53
8-ÖnerG, enturk UK,and Izgut -Uysal VN:Role of cadmium inducedlipid peroxidation in the kidney response to atrial natriureti hormone Nephron 1996,72:257-62
9-Spieker C,Zidek W,Zumkley H Cadmium and Hypertension Nephron 1987,47 Suppl1:34-6
10-Li Q,Zhang J,Pfaffendor M,and van Zwieten PA: Comparative effects of Angiotensine II and its degradation products angiotensin III and angiotensin IV in rat aorta. Brit J Pharmacol 1995 ,116:2963-70

Rats treated with	Blood Cd^{++} µg/ml	Sistolic pressure mmHg	Diastolic pressure mmHg	GFR µl/min.	% Component of Relaxant response to Ach(10^{-5}M) Without L-Arginine			With L-Arginine		
					NO	PGs	EDHF	NO	PG	EDHF
Control	1.87± 1.64	87± 4	65 ± 4	520.22 ± 68.8	100.62 ±1.55	35.51 ±0.09	None	33.60** ±3.81	48.18 11.38	33.57 ±4.53
Cd^{++}	6.08±* 2.62	118 ± 3 *	92 ± 1*	225.63 ± 23,8*	99.19 ± 1.11	13.61* ±9.29	None	81.73* ±4.9	46.10** ±4.02	39.46 ±2.27
Zinc	2.14 ± 1.14	95 ± 4	69 ± 3	564.37 ±99.0	101.25 ±1.65	38.79 ±13.37	None	79.80* ±10.53	30.42 ±17.61	27.64 ±4.54
Zn+ Cd	3.73± 1.95	97 ± 3	75± 4	517.3 ±57.9	97.51 ±0.56	47.5± 8.26	None	67.22* ± 7.52	36.47 ±10.39	34.20 ±16.77

Table - I : Mean±SE :Cd and Zinc induced changes on studied parameters($P<0.05$ vs. respective control* and L-Arg**)

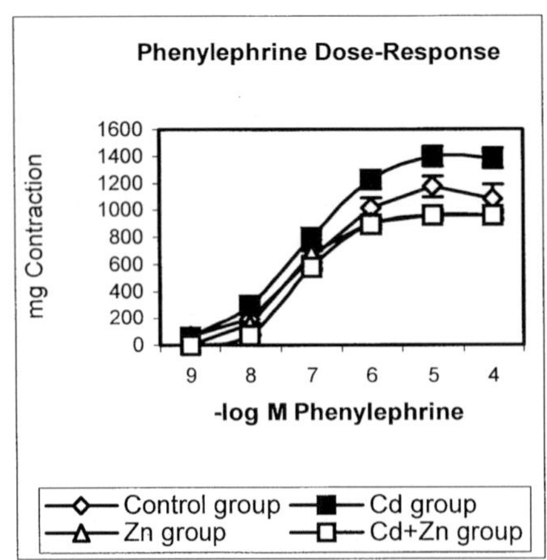

Fig. 1. The CRC for cumulative doses of PE

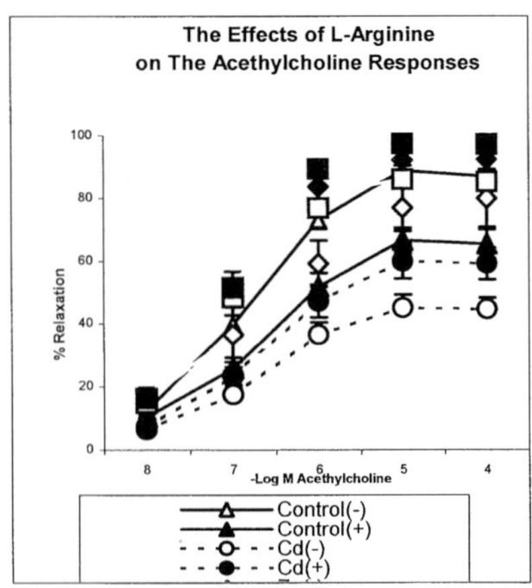

Fig. 2. The CRC for Ach in the presence (+)and absence(-) L-Arg.

Metal Ions in Biology and Medicine; vol 6. Eds. J.A. Centeno, Ph. Collery, G. Vernet, R.B. Finkelman, H. Gibb, J.C. Etienne. John Libbey Eurotext, Paris © 2000, pp. 641-645.

Cardiovascular modulation by cadmium ions

V.N. Puri

Division of Pharmacology, Central Drug Research Institute, Lucknow-226 001, India

Cardiovascular diseases are the major killer worldwide and mortality and morbidity are the major concerns for medical care providers and medical management executives. Rapid industrialization has seen massive consumption and exposure of various metals including Cadmium (20000 tons) in electroplating, galvanization, plastic, paints, pigments, batteries, coal and fossil fuels, cigarette, fertilizer and pesticide etc. industry. Several studies have documented the association of increased blood pressure with increasing consumption of cadmium ions in experimental animals and human beings [1-5]. Pressure effects of cadmium could be due to very complex interactions between autonomic, pressure peptide and newer adhesion molecules interplay at cell membrane surface or various types of voltage sensitive and insensitive channels. We are interested in elucidating the mechanism of action of cadmium induced hypertension. Additionaly hypertensive rat model could be used as screening model for newer hypotensive agents.

Hypertension (50-60 million in USA alone) is painless multifactorial polygenic disorder. Hypertension is also known as "silent killer" without any shape. Persistent hypertensive disease produces target organ damage, heart, kidney and brain. Hypertension is produced in humans and experimental animals due to involvement of both central and peripheral mechanisms. Several lines of experimental evidences [1,2,4] have suggested that cadmium ions injected in the conscious or anaesthetized (acute, chronic) rats of different species Charles Foster, Evans. Sprague Dawley (S-D) both male and female produced increase in blood prssure on oral and systemic administration. It is very interesting to observc that most of the publications from Schroder [1], Perry [3], Puri [4] and Revis [6] and repeat publications have always found hypertensive response. However, Poster et al [7] group failed to observe hypertensive response in rats on chronic oral feeding of cadmium ions. It is, therefore, clear that ultimate resultant effect of cadmium is hypertensive response. Cadmium induced hypertension is due to the involvement of both Central and peripheral inputs. Cadmium (1 mg/kg i.v.) administered to urethane anaesthetized Charles Foster rats produced initial transient lowering of blood pressure followed by persistant hypertensive response. Cadmium (1 ug i.c.v) administration produced hypertensive response in rats. In spinal transected rats cadmium (1 mg/kg i.v.) increased the blood pressure but the magnitude of increase in BP was much less than that observed in whole animal. All these results proved that cadmium ions are active on cardiovascular controlling center of medulla oblongata of rat. Additional experiments were done to study the dose response relationship between cadmium and blood pressure in rats. It was observed that cadmium ions (0.32, 1.0, 3.2 mg/kg i.v.) and (1, 3.2, 10 ug i.c.v) produced dose dependent hypertensive response in Sprague-Dawley rats [8]. It was interesting to note that I performed the study in India as well as in USA J.H.M.H.C. Gainesville, Florida and have observed hypertensive response in S-D rats. It was further observed that cadmium induced hypertensive response is observed for 2 weeks time in rats. Several experiments in rats were done to elucidate the mechanism of cadmium induced hypertension Charles Foster rats were treated with cadmium (1 mg/kg i.p.x4 days) Blood pressure was recorded and serum was used for estimation of catecholamines BP was raised to statistically significant levels (106 ± 4.6 control vs 153 ± 20.8 cad test) ($P < 0.01$). Hypertensive response was associated with increased levels of adrenaline and noradrenaline. Studies done by Fadloun & Leach [2] supports our observation. However, the effect of metal apapears to be presynaptic in nature. Reserpinization could have antagonized the hypertensive effect of cadmium in rats, but cadmium failed to antagonize the pharmacological response. Alpha 1 adrenergic and alpha2 drenergic blocker prazosin, priscolene [9], yohimbine respectively, antagonized noradrenaline response but cadmium induced hypertensive response was not attenuated to statistically significant levels. Cadmium and tyramine interaction in rats did not support that postsynaptic adrenergic receptor involvement in the hypertensive response produced by cadmium ions. Role of Beta receptor modulation by cadmium is underway.

Various components of Renin Angiotensin System (RAS) plays a very important role in the production of hypertension [10]. RAS modulation by cadmium have been desccribed in the literature but the reports are not consistent [11,12,13] therefore effects of actue and chronic cadmium administration on cardiovascular and RAS in rats were studied. Acute administration of cadmium (1 mg/kg i.p.) did not induce sisgnificant changes in plasma renin activity (PRA), while serum angiotensin converting enzyme (ACE) was statistically significantly (P<0.01) reduced, blood pressure was elevated [14]. epeated administration of cadmium (1 mg/kg i.p. x 5) and (captopril 20 mg/kg p.o. plus cadmium 1mg/kg i.p. x 5) did not produce significant changes in the PRA in S-D rats [15]. Cadmium produced inhibition of ACE at different time interval in rats was seen with captopril a known inhibitor of ACE. However, captopril produced lowering of BF while cadmium was hypertensive in nature [16]. These results provide evidence that cadmium induced hypertensive response in rats did not involve RAS. Additional studies are needed to study the effect of cadmium on substrate angiotensinogen, prorenin, ACE polymorphism and angiotensin II release and response. Cadmium an inorganic metal has been reported to be the blocker of voltage sensitive calcium channel [17,18]. However, blockers of calcium channels verapamil nifedapine, amlodapine are established hypotensive agents both in experimental animals and human being [19] by reducing the entry of calcium ions and peripheral vascular resistance. In light of the available information we examined the role of calcium channel blocker in cadmium induced hypertension in rats.

It was observed that Verapamil (2.5 mg/kg i.v.) reduced the hypertensive response induced by cadmium (0.1, 0.3, 1.0 mg/kg i.v.) in urethane anesthetized (S -D) rats [20]. Pharmacodynamic responses of 2 blockers of calcium channel could have resulted in additional hypotensive response in rats. However, such observations were not obtained suggesting a very complex interactions between 2 blockers on cellular enzyme system, lipid membranes, cytosolic and nuclear structures on metal receptors to produce pharmacological responses in the rats. Area need more rapid attention.

Cadmium induced hypertensive rat model was developed (cadmium 1 mg/kg i.p. x 7 days) in this Institute. 4 groups of S- D rats were tested for the effecct of saline, captopril (10 mg/kg i.p.) and saline and Prazosin (10 mg/kg i.p.) on blood pressure and heart rate response on pentobarbitone anesthetized (50 mg/kg i.p.) rats. It was observed that in saline treated rats converting enzyme inhibitor captopril did produce lowering of blood pressure 49 ± 15 mm Hg which lasted about 30 min. However, Captopril in cadmium hypertensive rats produced

56±1 mm Hg blood pressure lowering which lasted uptill 5 hrs 35±7.8 mm Hg or beyond Heart rates were decreased, but the effect was not statistically significant compared to the salien treated rats. Prazosin alpha adrenergic blocker also produced significant lowering of blood pressure which lasted for over 3 hours of observation period. Heart rate was decreased by Prazosin treatment. These results clearly indicate that 2 separate group of hypotensive agents produced qualitatively and quantitatively significant hypotensive effects, thus cadmium induced hypertensive rat model could be used for screening the novel and effective hypotensive agents. It is proposed that cadmium antagonists which are the blocker of calcium channel, angiotensin converting enzyme and other biological systems associated with multifactorial disease of hypertension would be better agents. In addition such agents could reduce the burden of cadmium from the body thus reducing the quantities of cadmium ions which are known to produce cardiovascular abnormalities. In near future cadmium stabilizers might appear as better treatment modalities for the treatment of hypertension and its complications like left ventricular hypertrophy.

It is thus concluded the cadmium induced hypertension in rats has complex mechanism. This model could be used for screening newer hypotensive agents. Cadmium mobilizers design and development are the challenges to combinatorial chemists and biologists.

REFERENCES

1. Schroeder H.A. Cadmium Hypertension in rats. Am. J. Physiol., 1964: 207 62-70.

2. Fadloun Z., Leach G.D.H. Effect of cadmium ions on blood pressure, dopamine b- hydroxylase activity and the responsiveness of in vivo preparation to sympathetic stimulation, noradrenaline and tyramine. J. Pharma. Pharmacol., 1981: 33: 660-64.

3. Kopp S.J., Glonek T., Perry H.M., Erlanger M., Perry E.F. Cardiovascular actions of cadmium at environmental exposure levels. Science, 1982: 217 837-83

4. V NPuri V.N., Sur R.N. Cardiovascular effects of cadmium on intravenous and intracerebroventricular administration in rats. Can. J. Physiol. Pharmacol., 1983: 61: 1430-32

5. Bakshi S.K., Chawla K.P., Khandekar R.N., Raghunath R. Cadmium and Hypertension. JAPC, 1994: 42 449-50.

6. Revis N.W. A possible mechanism for cadmium induced hypertension in rats. Life Sciences, 1978: 22: 479-485.

7. Poster M.C., Miya T.S., Bousquet W.F. Cadmium inability to induce hypertension in rats. Toxicol. & Appl. Pharmacol., 692-697.

8. Puri, V.N, Cadmium induced hypertension. Clin. Exp. Hyper. 1999: 21: 79-84.

9. Puri V.N., Sur R.N. Effect of cadmium clonidine intraction in rats. Pharmacol. Res. Commun., 1986: 18: 1119-1122.

10. Dzau V.J. Evolving concepts of renin angiotensin system. AJH, 1988: 1: 334S-337S.

11. Eakin D.J., Whanger P.D., Weisig P.H. Cadmium and Nickil influence blood pressure, plasma renin and tissue metal concentration. Am. J. Physiol., 1980: 238: E55-E62.

12. Perry A.M.S., Erlanger M. Circulating renin activity in rat following doses known to induce hypertension. J. Lab. Clin. Med., 1973: 82: 399-404.

13. Thind G.S., Kaufman G., Stephan K.F., Blackmore W.S. Vascular reactivity and mechanical properties of normal and cadmium hypertensive rabbits. J. Lab. Clin. Med., 1970: 76 560-581.

14. Puri V.N. Acute effects of cadmium on renin angiotensin system in rats. Bioch. Pharmacol., 1992: 44187-188.

15. Puri V.N., Tandon V., Effect of repeated administration of cadmium, captopril and combination on plasma renin activity in rats. Pharmacol. Res., 1997: 16: 411-414.

16. Puri V.N. Effect of cadmium and captopril on serum angiotensin converting enzyme activity in rats. Ind. H.J., 1997: 49: 297-299.

17. Nowycky M.C., Fox A.P., Tsien K.W. Three types of neuronal calcium channels with different sensitivity. Nature, 1985: 316: 443-444.

18. Kiss T., Osipenko O.N. Toxic effects of heavy metals, on ionic channels. Pharmacol. Review, 1994: 46:245-267.

19. Cohn J.N. Calcium, vascular smooth muscle and calcium entry blocker in hypertension. Ann. Int. Med., 1983: 98:806-809.

20. Puri V.N. Effect of verapamil on cadmium induced hypertension in rats. Ind. J. Exp. Biol., 1996: 34-1268-1270.

Metal Ions in Biology and Medicine; vol 6. Eds. J.A. Centeno, Ph. Collery, G. Vernet, R.B. Finkelman, H. Gibb, J.C. Etienne. John Libbey Eurotext, Paris © 2000, pp. 646-648.

Impaired endothelial-mediated vascular function in vessels of rats poisoned with lead and cadmium

Anna Skoczyńska, Joanna Wróbel, Ryszard Andrzejak

Department of Internal and Occupational Diseases, Wroclaw Medical University, Pasteur 4, PL-50-367, Wroclaw, Poland

Introduction

Our previous studies demonstrated an increase response of the postsynaptic alpha receptors in mesenteric bed of rats poisoned with lead (5) or cadmium (6). Lead and cadmium in low doses caused hypertension and cadmium enhanced the hypertensive action of lead (3). Endothelial dysfunction coupled with hypertension was described. It was known, that lead and cadmium could induced dysfunction of endothelium. Moreover a lead/cadmium interaction on vascular endothelium related to cytotoxic action of these metals was shown (2). An existence of lead/cadmium interaction effect on the basal tone and/or contractility of vessels could be expected, all the more, that the lead/calcium interaction on the neurotransmitters release is known yet. The aim of this study was to evaluate the impact of lead and cadmium treatment on the endothelial modulation of the vascular response to norepinephrine (NE) and angiotensin II (A II) in rat.

Material and methods

Male Buffalo rats aged 8 weeks were administered intragastrically to lead (35 mg/kg) and/or cadmium (5 mg/kg), once a week for a period of 7 weeks. The superior mesenteric artery was cannulated and perfusated as described earlier (6). Changes in mesenteric vascular resistance due to NE (0.4 μg) and next A II (0.4 μg) were measured:

- before and during the infusion of ketoprofen (LEK; 200 μg/ml/min). This infusion was continued up to time the perfusion pressure returned to the basal values. After the infusion of ketoprofen has been ended, 15-minutes Krebs solution, and next 15-minutes losartan (Merc Sharp; 50 μg/ml/min.) infusions were continuing and NE and A II injections were repeated
- before and during the infusion of N-ω-nitro-L-arginine (L-NOARG; 22.0 μg/ml/min)

Statistical analysis: Two-way ANOVA for repeated measures was applied.

Results and discussion

An inhibitory effect of PGs synthesis blocker on the vasoconstriction induced by A II was observed, table 1. Toda described similar changes and explained it with inhibition of cyclo-oxygenase (6). However ketoprofen attenuated this effect A II lower in vessels of rats poisoned simultaneously with lead and cadmium. We suggest, that the release of vasoactive PGs as a consequence of endothelial A II receptor stimulation, changed more under the influence of lead and cadmium administered to rats simultaneously, than under the influence of metals administered singly. Ketoprofen attenuated also the pressor effect of NE, but this inhibition was less potent in arteries of cadmium poisoned rats. This result indicated, that treatment with cadmium modified the influence of PGs on effect of NE.

Table 1. Relative (in % of response obtained before ketoprofen infusion) changes of perfusion pressure induced by NE or A II injected during ketoprofen infusion

	Ketoprofen infusion (200 μg/ml/min)	
	NE (0.4 μg)	A II (0.4 μg)
Control rats (n = 9)	28,1 ± 19,5	37,2 ± 17,9
Cd – rats (n = 8)	58,2 ± 33,0*	30,3 ± 14,6
Pb – rats (n = 8)	33,3 ± 8,9	40,6 ± 14,5
Pb+Cd. rats (n = 7)	39,0 ± 10,2	63,32 ± 15,9*

* Significantly different from the control group, $p < 0.05$

The inhibition of the vasodilatory components of the pressor response to AII and NE, was obtained by using NO synthesis blocker. L-NOARG acting with some delay, enhanced the pressor action of NE. However, in rats poisoned with cadmium, L-NOARG enhanced the vascular response to NE the most efficiacious, table 2.

Table 2. Relative changes of perfusion pressure induced by NE or AII injected during L-NOARG infusion

	L-NOARG infusion (22 μg/ml/min)	
	NE (0.4 μg)	A II (0.4 μg)
Control rats (n = 9)	117.2 ± 23.3	103.5 ± 43.4
Cd – rats (n = 8)	140.9 ± 38.5	128.7 ± 37.7
Pb – rats (n = 8)	129.0 ± 35.3	88.8 ± 39.1
Pb+Cd.rats (n = 7)	128.3 ± 42.6	97.1 ± 47.3

L-NOARG potentiated the A II induced vasoconstriction only in cadmium poisoned rats, indicating a greater influence of nitric oxide in cadmium treated rats vasculature. The decreasing response to A II injected on the L-NOARG infusion in both lead and lead plus cadmium poisoned rats suggest, that lead interacts with the NO-mediated component of A II induced vascular response.

It was observed by others, that losartan was able to reduce the *ex vivo* vasoconstriction induced by NE in aortic rings from hypertensive rats. This effect was not observed in endothelium denuaded rings, suggesting a mediatory role of an endothelium-derived factor in this action of losartan. (1). In our study losartan nearly abolished the response to A II and reduced the NE induced vasoconstriction, table 3.

Table 3. Relative changes of perfusion pressure induced by NE or AII injected during losartan infusion

	Losartan infusion (50 μg/ml/min)	
	NE (0.4 μg)	A II (0.4 μg)
Control rats (n = 9)	48.3 ± 31.1	14.9 ± 21.9
Cd. – rats (n = 8)	58.6 ± 25.5	0.21 ± 0.08
Pb – rats (n = 8)	46.7 ± 17.0	20.6 ± 33.7
Pb+Cd. rats (n = 6)	50.4 ± 13.9	20.0 ± 32.5

In conclusion, this study indicates that the NE or A II induced responses in vessels of metal treated rats were mediated by endothelial prostanoids synthesis (in cadmium group) and/or NO synthesis (in lead group). Because losartan abolished the difference in response of metal treated and control rats to NE we suggest, that the observed earlier, increasing reactivity of lead and cadmium poisoned rats vessels to NE, could be coupled with AT1 receptor.

Literature:

1. Cachofeiro V., Maeso R., Munoz G.R., Lahera V. The potential role of nitric oxide in angiotensin II-receptor blockade. Blood Press. Suppl. 2, 29-35, 1996
2. Kaji T, Suzuki M, Yamamoto C, Mishima A, Sakamoto M, Kozuka H. Severe damage of cultured vascular endothelial cell monolayer after simultaneous exposure to cadmium and lead. Arch Environ Contam Toxicol 28: 168-172, 1995
3. Perry HM, Erlanger MW Perry EF. Effect of second metal on cadmium-induced hypertension. Arch Environ Health 38: 80-85, 1983
4. Skoczyńska A., Juzwa W., Smolik R., Szechiński J., Běhal F. Response of the cardiovascular system to catecholamines in rats given small doses of lead. Toxicology, 39, 275-289, 1986
5. Skoczyńska A. Andrzejak R., Smolik R., Andrzejak D. Effect of oral cadmium administration on the reactivity of isolated mesenteric vessels to norepinephrine (NE) in rats. Metal Ions Biol Med., 686-690, 1998
6. Toda N., Ayaziki K., Okamura T. Modyfication by endogenous prostaglandins of angiotensin II – induced contraction in dog and monkey cerebral and mesenteric arteries. J Pharmacol Exp Ther, 252, 374-379, 1990

Metal Ions in Biology and Medicine; vol 6. Eds. J.A. Centeno, Ph. Collery, G. Vernet, R.B. Finkelman, H. Gibb, J.C. Etienne. John Libbey Eurotext, Paris © 2000, pp. 649-651.

Role of divalent cations in cardioprotection

Dipak K. Das and Nilanjana Maulik

University of Connecticut School of Medicine, Cardiovascular Research Center, Department of Surgery, Farmington, Connecticut, USA

ABSTRACT. We have recently found that Ba^{2+} in the micromolar range inhibits phosphoinositide-specfic phospholipase C (PtdIns-PLC) activity in vascular smooth muscle cells. In this study we show that, in the presence or absence of Ca^{2+}, Ba^{2+} dose-dependently inhibits myocardial PtdIns-PLC activity when measured in vitro in microsomal fractions using phosphatidylinositol 4,5-bisphosphate as substrate. The LD_{50} was approximately 30 µM Ba^{2+} for both basal and Ca^{2+}-stimulated PtdIns-PLC activity, and at concentrations above 100 µM, Ba^{2+} totally blocked the Ca^{2+}-stimulated PtdIns-PLC activity. 100 µM Ba^{2+} reversibly blocked the increase in cytosolic Ca^{2+} during ischemia and reperfusion as shown by measuring fura 2 fluorescence ratios at 340 and 380 nm. Ba^{2+} pre-perfusion also attenuated the amount of lactate dehydrogenase released in the coronary effluent during reperfusion, indicating a reduced cellular injury.

INTRODUCTION. While disturbed Ca^{2+} homeostasis is one of the causes for myocardial ischemia reperfusion injury, the mechanism involved for intracellular Ca^{2+} overloading remains controversial (1). We have shown that inhibition of α_1-receptor-stimulated phosphoinositide-specific phospholipase C (PLC) reduces the early rise in cytosolic Ca^{2+} in concert with the reduction of cellular injury (2). We hypothesized that α_1-stimulated phosphoinositide hydrolysis together with Ca^{2+}-stimulated PLC activity may form a positive feed-back mechanism to sustain high levels of cytosolic Ca^{2+}, leading to sarcolemmal and sarcoplasmic reticulum dysfunction. In this study, we have tested the ability of Ba^{2+}, a divalent cation that antagonizes Ca^{2+} at many Ca^{2+}-binding sites, to disrupt this putative positive feed-back mechanism and prevent ischemia/reperfusion-induced Ca^{2+} overloading.

MATERIALS AND METHODS. Sprague-Dawley rats of 300 gm body weight were anesthetized with 120 mg/kg sodium pentibarbital (i.p.) and the hearts isolated and perfused by Langendorff Technique (3). Hearts were subjected to 30 min ischemia followed by reperfusion. At indicated times, 100 µM Ba^{2+} was added to the perfusion buffer. Hearts were sectioned at the atrio-ventricular junction after 5 min perfusion, and ventricular muscle was frozen in liquid N_2 for subsequent analysis of PLC (4). Cytosolic Ca^{2+} concentrations were determined by perfusing the hearts in presence of 0.5 mM fura 2 acetoxymethylester using a Calcium Analyzer (CAF-100, JASCO, Inc., MD).

RESULTS: We first tested the effect of Ba^{2+} on basal (without Ca^{2+}) and Ca^{2+}-stimulated PLC activity using phosphatidylinositol 4,5-biphosphate as substrate. Figure 1 shows the effect of 300 µM Ba^{2+} on the enzyme activity in purified microsomal fraction isolated from left ventricles of control hearts. The results showed a significant inhibition of basal Ba^{2+} in conjunction with more than 10-fold reduction in the IP_3 generation in buffer containing 10 µM Ca^{2+}. Figure 2A shows the dose-dependency of Ca^{2+} stimulation on myocardial PLC activity over the physiologic range of Ca^{2+} concentrations (0.1-10 µM). At two different stimulatory Ca^{2+} concentrations, we studied the dose-dependent relationship between Ba^{2+} concentration and PLC inhibition (Figure 2B). The LD_{50} for Ba^{2+} inhibition was 30 µM at both 1 and 10µM Ca^{2+}.

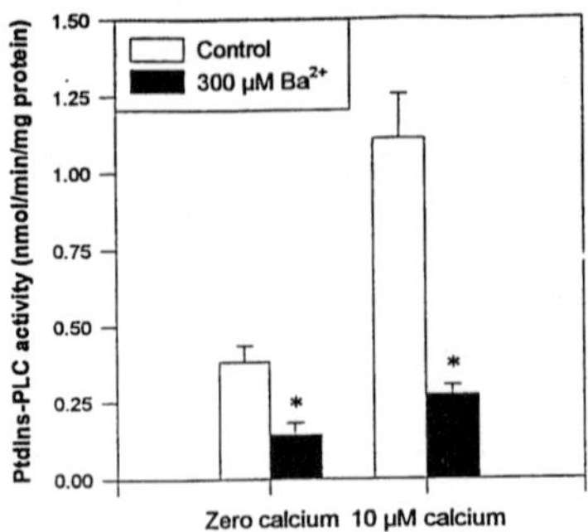

*Figure 1. Effect of 300 μM Ba^{2+} on PLC activity. Myocardial microsomal fraction (200 μg protein) in zero Ca^{2+} buffer or buffer containing 10 μM Ca^{2+} (free ionic concentrations) was used and enzyme activity was calculated as radioactivity incorporated into IP_3 from 20 μM phosphatidyl[^3H]inositol 4,5-bisphosphate Data are Means± SEM of 6 experiments; *p<0.01 vs. control (no Ba^{2+}).*

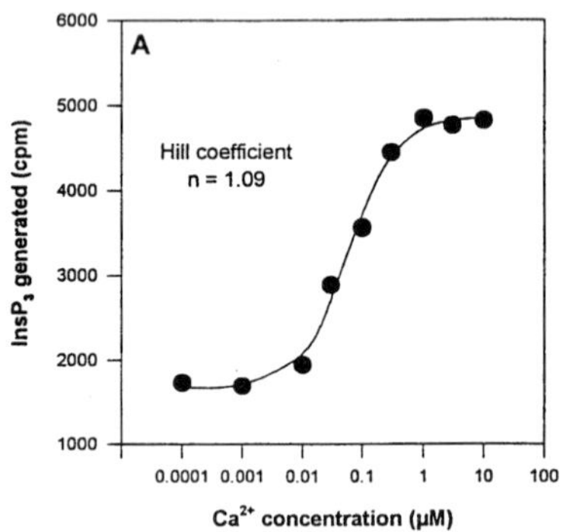

Figure 2. A. Ca^{2+} stimulation of myocardial PLC activity. Enzyme activity was measured in vitro as in Figure 1 and free Ca^{2+} concentration in the assay buffer was varied from 10^{-10}M ("zero" Ca^{2+}) to 10^{-4} M by changing $CaCl_2$ and EDTA concentrations.

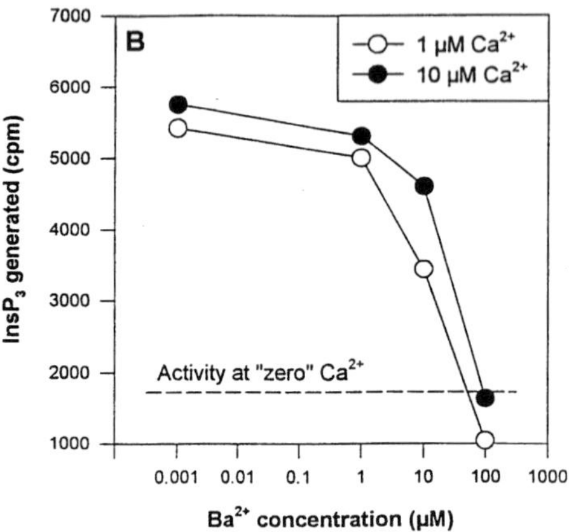

B. Dose-dependency of Ba^{2+} concentrations indicated are free ion concentrations in the assay buffer. Each point represents a separate experiment.

Using Langendorff set-up coupled to JASCO Ca^{2+} analyzer, we have been able to document apparent increase in free cytosolic Ca^{2+} during ischemia and reperfusion as shown in Figure 3 (top tracing). The use of a perfusion buffer containing 100 μM Ba^{2+} for 10 min before the onset of global ischemia and during the first 10 min of reperfusion produced a marked inhibition of the rise in Ca^{2+} fluorescent signal (Figure 3, bottom trace). The effect of Ba^{2+} appeared to be reversible and dependent of the duration of Ba^{2+} perfusion. The middle tracing of Figure 3 shows a partial reduction in Ca^{2+} increase obtained if Ba^{2+} perfusion is followed by a short 5 min washout prior to ischemia. Ba^{2+} perfusion also produced a decrease in heart rate (by approx. 30%) during pre-ischemia and more rapid restart of rhythmic contractions during reperfusion (usually in the first 1 min after start of reperfusion), although the macroscopic appearance of Ba^{2+} perfused hearts at the end of 30 min ischemia was similar to that of control hearts (partial contracture). The apparent reduction of cellular injury and enhanced functional recovery during reperfusion was confirmed by experiments exhibiting reduced lactate dehydrogenase release in the coronary effluent of Ba^{2+}-perfused hearts (Figure 4).

DISCUSSION. A large number of divalent cations have been employed to study the molecular actions of Ca^{2+} by using their ability to specifically interfere with Ca^{2+}-protein binding and channel transport systems. Of these cations, Sr^{2+} appears almost always behave as an agonist, mimicking Ca^{2+} activities, but most other cations such as Ni^{2+}, Co^{2+}, Mn^{2+}, and Ba^{2+} vary widely in their abilities to act as Ca^{2+} agonists or antagonists at different sites. Ba^{2+} is cytotoxic at higher

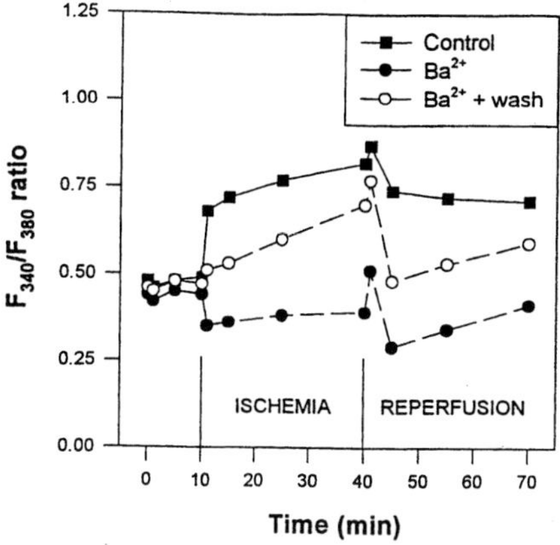

Figure 3. Effect of 100 µM Ba^{2+} on cytosolic Ca^{2+} during ischemia and reperfusion. Fura 2 fluorescence ratios were recorded in isolated rat hearts subjected to 30 min ischemia and 30 min reperfusion. The perfusion buffer contained 100 µM Ba^{2+} for different periods as follows: -o- from 10 min prior to ischemia until 10 min of reperfusion; -o- from 10 min prior to ischemia until 5 min prior to ischemia; -[ ]- no perfusion with Ba^{2+}-containing buffer. Results are Means of 3 separate experiments per group.

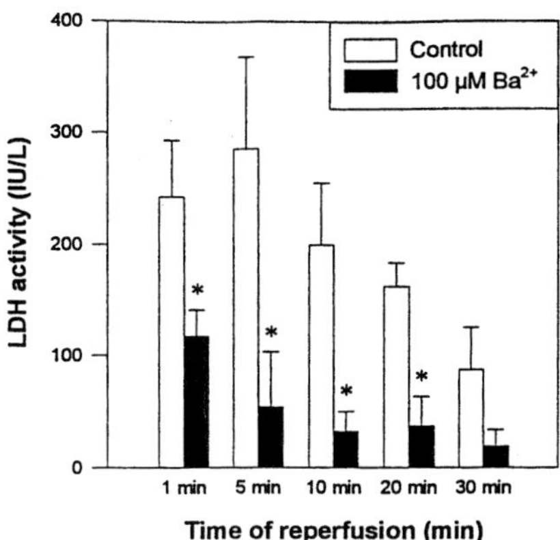

*Figure 4. Effect of Ba^{2+} on lactate dehydrogenase release. Lactate dehydrogenase activity was assayed in the coronary effluent of Ba^{2+} perfused hearts (protocol as in Figure 3, -o-) and control hearts (protocol as in Figure 3, -[ ]-) prior to ischemia and at various times during reperfusion. Results are Means ± SEM (n=6). *$p<0.05$ vs. control*

concentration (LD_{50} is 19.2 mg/kg) and leads to muscle contracture. In the heart, Ba^{2+} produces contracture at 0.5-2 mM apparently through a direct effect on actin-myosin tension development. However, recent studies have shown that at lower concentrations (10^{-4}M or lower) Ba^{2+} has different effect on actin-myosin interaction, being rather inhibitory and decreasing the myofilament's Ca^{2+} sensitivity (5). This would make micromolar Ba^{2+} an ideal candidate to counteract the effects of myocardial Ca^{2+} overloading. Since Ca^{2+} stimulation of PLC may induce a sustained high level of PLC activity during ischemia and reperfusion, the fact that 100 µM Ba^{2+} lowers the PLC activity to values below basal values (at "zero" Ca^{2+}) even when 10 µM Ca^{2+} is used in the assay (Figure 2B) suggests that at this concentration, Ba^{2+} may effectively disrupt any putative positive feed-back involved in maintaining enhanced PLC activity. The observed Ba^{2+} effect of blocking Ca^{2+} overloading resembles the recently described action of Ba^{2+} as well as other divalent cations to block so-called Ca^{2+} paradox (6). We can, therefore, conclude that the evidence presented in this report suggests that Ba^{2+}, at micromolar, non-toxic concentrations (i) dose-dependently inhibits PLC activity and (ii) reversibly blocks ischemia/reperfusion-induced Ca^{2+} overloading. These observed phenomena may be causally related and may underlie a cardioprotective role of Ba^{2+} during ischemia and reperfusion.

REFERENCES.

1. Opie LH, 1989. Reperfusion injury and its pharmacologic midification. Circulation 80: 1049-1076.
2. Prasad MR et al., 1991. Role of phospholipase A2 and C in myocardial ischemic reperfusion injury. Am J Physiol 260: H877-H883.
3. 3. Liu X et al., 1993. Attenuation of myocardial reperfusion injury by reducing intracellular calcium overloading with dihydropyridines. Biochem Pharmacol 45: 1333-1342.
4. Grundeman RLF et al., 1991. Length-dependent activation by Ba2+ and Sr2+ of skinned cardiac and skeletal muscle of the rabbit. Am J Physiol. 260: C609-C617
5. Nayler et al., 1983. Cobalt manganese and calcium paradox. J Mol Cell Cardiol 15: 735-747.

Metal Ions in Biology and Medicine; vol 6. Eds. J.A. Centeno, Ph. Collery, G. Vernet, R.B. Finkelman, H. Gibb, J.C. Etienne. John Libbey Eurotext, Paris © 2000, pp. 652-654.

Zinc and copper imbalance as high risk to myocardial infarction in Indians

Satish K. Taneja[1], Sanjam Girhotra[1] and Kiran Pal Singh[2]

[1] Department of Zoology, Panjab University Chandigarh-160014; [2] Department of Endocrinology, M.D. Oswal Cancer Research Foundation, Ludhiana-141066 India

Abstract : Imbalance of Cu-Zn status has been reported to exert strong influence in the etiology of myocardial infarction (MI).To assess the degree of ionic imbalance, logistic regression (LR-MI) model is suggested for the diagnoses of individuals at high risk to this disease.

Introduction : Zn and Cu are essential trace metals whose patterns in the tissues of subjects died of artherosclerosis, hypertension or myocardial infarction (MI) differ from those of healthy controls. Either high Cu and low Zn (1-3) or high Zn and low copper (4-5) reserves have been reported to exert strong influences on individual risk factors of cardiovascular diseases. We investigated if the ionic imbalance of these two metals in the body can serve as predictive indicator to identify the individuals at high risk to MI.

Materials and Method : For this purpose, Zn and Cu concentrations in hair and urine of patients diagnosed and hospitalized for MI (MI patients) and their descendent (MI descendents) were estimated in atomic absorption spectrophotometer as described previously (6). The Data were compared and analyzed statistically with their BMI and age matched healthy volunteers with no family history of MI or NIDDM (control group and control descendents).

Results and Discussion : Mean BMI, Zn and Cu concentration in hair and urine of BMI patients, MI descendents and their age matched control is given in the table - I.

Table I : Mean BMI, Zn and Cu in hair and urine of control group, control desendents, MI descendents and MI patients.

Group	BMI (Kg/m^2)	Hair Zn (μmol/g)	Urine Zn (μmol/l)	Hair Cu (μmol/g)	Urine Cu (μmol/l)
Control	21.37±0.87	3.79±0.45	5.92±0.36	0.19±0.02	0.33±0.04
Con-Desc	19.79±0.43	3.57±0.15	5.76±0.15	0.23±0.01	0.32±0.02
MI-Desc	22.02±0.88	4.73±0.30[a]	12.00±0.35[a]	0.10±0.1[a]	0.34±0.02
MI-Pat	23.78±0.64	7.44±0.33[b]	22.38±1.03[b]	0.05±0.01[b]	0.15±0.02[b]

Mean ± S.E. of 30 (15 males, 15 females) observations each. Mean values within a column not showing a common superscript letter were significantly different ($p < 0.001$). Con-Desc, Control Descendent; Mi-Desc, MI Descendent; MI-Pat, MI Patients.

The data revealed that Zn and Cu concentrations in hair and urine of control were within the normal range but there was consistent rise in the levels of Zn and fall of Cu in hair and urine from control to MI descendents to MI patients. The graded increase of Zn in hair and urine in MI descendents (potentially susceptible) to MI patients from that of control suggests that humans destined to contract MI have consistently an oprating mechanism of excessive Zn absorption at young age, the part of which is retained and rest is excreted out. The excessive bioavailability of Zn in humans (7-8) and genetically and dietary obese mice (9) has been reported to increase body fat deposition - a high risk factor of MI. The continuous influx of excessive Zn in tissues causes Cu deficiency over a period of time through Zn - Cu antagonistic interaction (10) as observed in hair and urine of MI descendent and MI patients in this study. Cu deficiency is known to cause hypertension, hypercholesterolemia and increase in low density lipoprotein increasing thereby the risk factor of MI (4,5).

Two factors could possibly be responsible for the excessive absorption of Zn in MI susceptible subjects, either the consumption of diet rich in Zn and low in copper or over expression of genes responsible for the synthesis of Zn metallothionein either independently (11) or under the influence of stress hormone - glucocorticoid from adrenal cortex (12). The possibility of excessive dietary Zn intake in MI susceptible subjects is unlikely to exist because the control, MI descendents and MI patients were sharing the same type of food and some being the member of the same family enshowing normal and other altered Zn and Cu concentrations in their hair and urine in the samples investigated in this study. The over expression of genes for Zn metallothionein, therefore, seems responsible for this ionic imbalance. Whether their over expression occurs independently or under the influence of hypersecretion of stress hormone of adrenal cortex is not clear and needs further investigation. However, the stress hormone as a cause of cardiovascular disease including MI is one of the recognized factors where its level in diseased patients has been seen to be significantly higher than those of healthy volunteers.

On subjecting the logistic regression to the data assigning response variable Y as `O' to control group and `I' to MI patients, a model referred here as LR - MI model was obtained having impact values as constant, -3.342; BMI; - 0.776; hair Zn; - 2.441 ; urine Zn , + 3.441; hair Cu, - 15.078 and urine Cu, - 24.153 for the equation $Y = e^x/1+e^x$ where $x = (-3.342) + [-0776 \times BMI (kg/m^2)] + [-2.441 \times hair Zn (\mu mol/g)] + [3.441 \times urine Zn (\mu mol/l)] + [-15.078 \times hair Cu (\mu mol/g)] + [-24.153 \times urine Cu (\mu mol/l)]$.

On substituting the values of Zn and Cu concentration of each volunteer, the response variable "Y" as O for all healthy volunteers and 0.999 or 99.9% susceptibility for all patients were obtained. The model was tested by blind trials and the susceptibility was obtained as expected. The value of Y in MI descendents ranged between 0 to 100%. The highly susceptible individuals of this group (above 85%) displayed hypertriglyceridemia, and high VLDL fraction in the blood plasma approaching conditions close to ischemic heart disease. This suggests that the individuals with higher susceptibility are likely to contract the disease relatively at young age and the onset of the disease would depend upon the degree of ionic imbalance owing to the degree of stress and the type of food the susceptible individual consumes during intervening period. The model when cross checked with a published data, it gave results as expected.

In this model, urine Zn is the only positive impact factor, Cu in hair and Cu in urine have significant and Zn in hair has insignificant opposing effects. Taking this into account we treated one MI volunteer patient with Cu supplementation at the rate of 5 mg Cu as CuCl two times a day for 21 days. His serum cholesterol fell from 246 mg/100ml to 189 mg/100 ml and triglyceride from 324 mg/100 to 210 mg/100 ml of serum. This suggests that the increasing prevalence of coronary heart disease in Indians and increased mortality at young age may be associated with imbalance of Cu and Zn attributed to the intake of Zn in high amount in food raised through extensive use of micronutrients in which Zn stands out prominently and such food items that promote absorption of Zn. The Cu therapy to the Indians at high risk to coronary heart disease is likely to reduce the severity by checking Zn influx and raising Cu bioavailability to their tissues.

References :

1. Wecker W E C, Ulmer D D, Vallee B L. Metalloenzymes and myocardial infarction. 11. Malic and lactic dehydrogenase activities and zinc concentrations in serum. *N Engl J Med* 1956; 255: 449-465.

2. Lopez C, Ocon D C, Mengo M S, Frasquet I, De Armenia U A. Study of Zinc and copper serum levels in dyslipidemias. *Therapie* 1991; 46: 17-20.

3. Reunaneu A, Knekt P, Marniemi J, Maki J, Maatela J. Serum calcium, magnesium, copper and zinc and risk of cardiovascular death. *Eur J Clin Nutr* 1996; 50: 431-437.

4. Klevay L M. Coronary heart disease: The zinc copper hypothesis. *Amer J Clin Nutr* 1975; 8: 764-774.

5. Davydenko N V, Smirnova I P, Kvasha E A, Gorbas I M The relationship between the Cu & Zn intake with food and the prevalence of ischemic heart disease and its risk factors. *Liksprava* 1995; 73-77 (abs.)

6. Taneja S K, Mahajan M, Gupta S, Singh K P. Assessment of copper and zinc status in hair and urine of young women descendants of NIDDM patients. *Biol Trace Elem Res* 1998; 62, 255-264.

7. Prentice A. Does mild zinc deficiency contribute to poor growth performance ? *Nutr Rev* 1993; 51: 268-270.

8. Chen M D, Lin P Y, Cheng V, Lin W H. Zinc supplementation aggravates body fat accumulation in genetically obese mice and dietary obese mice. *Biol Trace Elem Res* 1996; 52: 125-132.

9. Prasad A S, Brewer G J, Schoomaker B E, Rasbani P. Hypocupremia induced by Zinc therapy in adults. *J Amer Med Ass* 1978; 240: 2166-2168.

10. Dalton T, Fu K, Palmiter R D, Andrews GJ. Transgenic mice that over-express metallothionein I resists dietary Zinc deficiency.*J Nutr* 1996; 126 : 825-833.

11. Kelly E J, Quaije C J, Froelick G J, Palmiter R D. Metallothionein I and II protect against Zinc deficiency and Zinc toxicity in mice. *J Nutr* 1996; 126 : 1782-90.

Metal Ions in Biology and Medicine; vol 6. Eds. J.A. Centeno, Ph. Collery, G. Vernet, R.B. Finkelman, H. Gibb, J.C. Etienne. John Libbey Eurotext, Paris © 2000, pp. 655-657.

Reducing bioavailability of lead-contaminated urban soil with mineral or biosolid treatment

Judith Hallfrish, Qi Xue, Claude Veillon, Kristine Patterson, Joan M. Conway, Sally Brown and Rufus Chaney

Beltsville Human Nutrition Research Center, ARS-USDA, Beltsville, MD 20705, University of Maryland, College Park, MD 20742, University of Washington, Seattle, WA 98195
Corresponding author: Judith Hallfrisch, B 308, R 126, Beltsville Human Nutrition Research Center, ARS, USDA, Beltsville, MD 20705; hallfrisch@bhnrc.arsusda.gov

Corresponding author: Judith Hallfrisch, B 308, R 126, Beltsville Human Nutrition Research Center, ARS, USDA, Beltsville, MD 20705; hallfrisch@bhnrc.arsusda.gov

INTRODUCTION

Lead poisoning, or plumbism was described by Nicander over 2000 years ago and may be responsible for the fall of the Roman Empire (1). In the United States, lead-containing paint was not banned until 1978, thus not only are many mining and gardening sites contaminated with lead, but in many cities housing still contains lead-based paint which has contaminated the surrounding soil (2). Lead-based paint and industrial lead contamination present a danger to the health and mental development of many poor urban children (3-4). Because removal is not feasible in many areas, soil remediation using mineral and organic treatments may provide a more effective method to reduce danger. Lead bioavailability was assessed by measuring the incorporation of Pb into bone and other tissues, bone density (BMD), and bone mineral content (BMC).

METHODS

Soils were collected in Baltimore, MD from three gardens identified as high in Pb by the Kennedy Krieger Institute. Concentrations ranged from 616-2085 ppm Pb (5). Soil containing approximately 2000 ppm Pb was incubated for 30 days with the following treatments: New York control compost, raw, pelleted and ashed NY compost, control NY compost with lime, iron-rich Baltimore compost, Baltimore compost with lime, and a commercial compost (NVIRO). Soils were dried and sieved before feeding as 5% of the diet to 84 Sprague-Dawley rats for 30 days. Lead acetate (at 0, 10 and 20 ppm in diets of 95% AIN93G and 5% sand) was used as the standard curve for incorporation of Pb into tissues. Whole body (WB) bone mineral density (BMD) and bone mineral content (BMC) were determined by dual energy x-ray absorptiometry (DXA) the day before termination on 5 rats/group (6). One femur was excised for mineral analysis and the other was scanned by DXA for BMD and BMC. Waller-Duncan test was used for mean separation if analysis of variance F-value was significant ($p < 0.05$).

RESULTS

Table 1. Mineral content as determined by analysis (/g) and DXA

Treatment	Femur		Blood	Liver	Kidney	WB		Femur	
	Pb	Mg	Pb			BMD	BMC	BMD	BMC
Unit	:g	mg	:g	:g	:g	g/cm5	g	g/cm5	g
AIN93G	0.6	3.96	0	.02	0.5	.236	3.28	.088	.020
+10 ppm Pb	34	3.98	115	.89	6.7	.233	3.10	.103	.013
+20 ppm Pb	67	4.19	174	1.11	8.5	.231*	2.94	.118	.045
Baltimore soil	145	4.06	229	3.10	14.6	.242	3.47	.104	.031
+Fe compost	73*	3.88*	193	1.91*	9.8*	.245	3.52	.096	.021
+lime	82*	3.56*	215	2.02*	10.4*	.240	3.18	.109	.044
+NY compost	104*	3.77*	245	2.29*	13.7	.245	3.52	.097	.028
+lime	91*	3.65*	182*	2.03*	9.6*	.242	3.51	.123	.062
+NY raw	87*	3.70	203	1.84*	12.8	.240	3.30	.100	.034
+NY pelleted	87*	3.97	210	1.78*	10.2	.244	3.20	.098	.029
+NY ashed	97*	3.82*	246	1.90*	12.5	.249	3.53	.097	.046
+NY NVIRO	111*	3.17*	341*	2.52	17.4*	. 241	2.92	.099	.014

*different from Baltimore soil ($p < 0.05$).

Bone calcium and zinc did not differ among groups, even though diet levels varied significantly. Lead incorporation into bone was reduced by all treatments. Pb was reduced in kidneys of rats consuming high iron compost and by the addition of lime. Liver Pb was reduced by all treatments except the NY NVIRO which also increased kidney and blood lead. BMD and BMC of femurs did not vary, but whole body BMD was highest in rats consuming ashed compost and significantly lower in control rats than in rats consuming the Baltimore soil. WB-BMD of rats consuming soil tended to be higher than of control rats. Liver and kidney Zn and Mg did not vary according to treatment. Kidney Ca was elevated by NVIRO.

CONCLUSIONS

Results indicate that bioavailability of Pb can be substantially reduced by application of a variety of biosolid treatments. Lime may further reduce lead incorporation. Since all diets contained adequate levels of minerals before the addition of amended soils, the results reflect a conservative estimate of the reduction of bioavailability in children for whom calcium, magnesium, and iron intakes may not be optimal (7). DXA did not provide consistent data. Further analyses of the interactions of various minerals in the bone and other tissues may provide useful information about the optimal combinations of minerals for maximal reduction of lead bioavailability.

BIBLIOGRAPHY

1. Quarterman J. Lead. Chapter 4. In: Mertz W (ed). Trace elements in human and animal nutrition, Volume 2, London: Academic Press, 1986 : 281-317.
2. Chaney RL, Sterrett SB, Mielke HW. The potential for heavy metal exposure from urban gardens and soils. In: Preer JR (ed). Proc Symp Heavy Metals in urban gardens. Washington, DC: Univ Dist Columbia Extension Service, 1984 : 37-84.
3. Kim R, Hu H, Rotnitzky A, Bellinger D, Needleman H. A longitudinal study of chronic lead exposure and physical growth in Boston children. Environ Health Perspect 1995; 103 : 952-957.
4. Todd AC, Wetmur JG, Moline JM, Godbold JH, Levin SM, Landrigan PJ. Unraveling the chronic toxicity of lead: an essential priority for environmental health. Environ Health Perspect 1996; 104 Suppl 1: 141-146.
5. Brown SL, Xue Q, Chaney RL, Hallfrisch JG. Effect of biosolids processing on the bioavailability of Pb in urban soils. In: Biosolids management innovative treatment technologies and processes. Proc. Water Environment Research Foundation Workshop #104, Chicago, 1997 : 43-54.
6. Mitlak BH, Schoenfeld D, Neer RM. Accuracy, precision, and utility of spine and whole-skeleton mineral measurements by DXA in rats. J Bone Miner Res 1994; 9: 119-126.
7. Hamilton JD, O'Flaherty EJ. Influence of lead on mineralization during bone growth. Fundam Appl Toxicol 1995; 26 : 265-271.

Metal Ions in Biology and Medicine; vol 6. Eds. J.A. Centeno, Ph. Collery, G. Vernet, R.B. Finkelman, H. Gibb, J.C. Etienne. John Libbey Eurotext, Paris © 2000, pp. 658-660.

Stabilization of chromate wastes

Gutiérez-Ruiz M.E.[1], Hernández Claudia[1] and Ramirez Peralta Miguel Angel[2]

[1] *LAFQA, Instituto de Geografía, Ciudad Universitaria, Coyoacan, México, D.F. 04510. E-mail: ginny@servidor.unam.mx;* [2] *Perry Ingenieros Proyectos S.A. E-mail: perrying@df1.telmex.net.mx*

ABSTRACT

Solid wastes rich in Cr (VI) were accumulated during several years. The aquifers are polluted with sodium chromate. A technology to stabilized the wastes was developed in order to diminish the environmental impact and the risk to the population- It is a good example of friendly solution to manage hazardous wastes, because: a) two hazardous wastes are treated at the same time, b) the water used in the process comes from polluted aquifers, c) no water discharges are produced, d) only industrial sulfuric acid is used, and e) the process is economically viable for a medium sized industry.

INTRODUCTION

Chromium compounds produced in Mexico, through oxidizing in a furnace, mineral chromites with sodium carbonate. Solid wastes rich in Cr (VI) were accumulated during several years. One plant is located in the State of Mexico (No. 1) and the other is located in the State of Guanajuato (No. 2). In both places, the aquifers are polluted with sodium chromate, and the yellow water from the chromium dissolution is spread in soil and wastes [1,2,3]. In order to control the contamination in the State of Mexico, the Plant No. 1 was closed, building an industrial grave to deposit 400,000 tons. As a consequence of the lack of protection underneath the deposit the chromium dispersion persisted. In the other site, Plant No. 2, the original process was changed to use chromate solution imported from USA. In this place, the wastes were deposited in a free space that belongs to the company, forming a huge mountain. The deposit is protected with a membrane liner and drainage system connected with a water treatment plant, but the chromate salts tint the surface of the deposit with a yellow color, causing apprehension in the population [2].

Salinity and chromium pollution are impacting soils and groundwater. A study was carried out to approach a definitive solution. After study different conditions[4], the best economical and environmental option was the reduction of Cr(VI) with spent sulfuric acid contaminated with SO_2, carbon and long-chain hydrocarbons. The method was studied in the laboratory and experiments were carried out in a pilot plant. At the present, the engineering of the process plant is being developed and the plant will be operating in next year.

EXPERIMENTAL

Composition of wastes:

In both plants the same process was used, but the composition of the wastes is different. This fact is due to differences in furnace temperature, soda concentration, and fate of sodium sulfate and aluminum hydroxide. In Plant 1, Na_2SO_4 was separated and soil was added to wastes, while in Plant 2, the $Al(OH)_3$ was separated (Table I).

Table I. Wastes mineral composition (X-ray Diffraction)

PLANT 1	PLANT 2
Na_2CrO_4	**Na_2CrO_4**
$MgCr_2O_4.7H_2O$	
$FeO(Cr,Al)_2O_3$	**$FeO(Cr,Al)_2O_3$**
Na_2SO_4	
$KAl_2SiO_3AlO_{10}(OH)$	$4CaO.Al_2O_3.Fe_2O_3$
$CaSO_4.2H_2O$	$1.3(K,Na)_2O.\ 0.6(Mg,Fe)O.\ 3.3(Fe,Al)O_2.5H_2O$
$CaCO_3.H_2O$	**$CaCO_3$**
$\alpha Al_2 2^{\circ}{}_4 3$, α $Al(OH)_3$	$MgSO_4$
SiO_2	**SiO_2**
$MgFe_2O_4$	
$MgAl_2Ti_3O$	
$Al_2O_3.4SiO_2.nH_2O$	
$Ca_2Fe(PO_4)_2(OH).1.5H_2O$	
$FeAl_2(PO_4)_2$	
$Fe(OH)SO_4.2H_2O$	
$Na_2Fe(SO_4)_2(OH)$	
$Al_2SiO_5(OH)_4$	

Process description

Step 1. Grinding a portion of solid wastes to 200 mesh and mixing with water (1:1.5, wastes: polluted water)

Step 2. Measurement of the following parameters: carbonates, pH, total Cr(VI) (polarographic method) and oxidation capacity of Fe^{2+} (volumetric titration)

Step 2. Determination of acidic/reduction potential of the acid wastes

Step 3. Carbonates destruction and acidification with spent sulfuric acid and industrial sulfuric acid. Doses determine per oxidation capacity of solid wastes and acidic/reduction potential of spent acid.

Step 4. Liberation of chromate and reduction

Step 5.Transportation of reduced materials to the final deposit

Step 6. Basic mineral dissolution and neutralization (slow reaction)

Step 7. Solar water evaporation

RESULTS

According to the Toxicity Characteristic Leaching Procedure described in NOM-053 (Mexican legislation) and Method 1312 (EPA-USA), the stabilized wastes are no-hazardous. The Cr (VI) concentration extracted with acetic acid buffer is less than 5 mg/L and the pH vary from 6 to 7 with a mean value of 6.35 (Table II). The particle size, the pH and the control of temperature are very important factors to get a complete Cr (VI) liberation and reduction.

The wastes of the plant No.1 after reduction can be used in brick manufacturing, as it was probed during the preliminary experiments[5]. The stabilized wastes of the plant No.2 cannot be reused because they are rich in sodium and iron and they are very poor in aluminum (Table II).

Table II. Wastes composition before and after treatment

	No. 1		No. 2	
	BEFORE	AFTER	BEFORE	AFTER
pH (1:5, solid: $CaCl_2$ 0.1 M)	8.11±0.1	6.14±0.1	11.31±0.1	6.35±0.1
Total Na (%w/w)	0.26±0.02	-	2.38±0.25	-
Total Cr (%w/w)	1.24±0.03	-	1.87±0.02	-
TotalAl (%w/w)	25.90±0.2	-	7.65±0.45	-
Total Fe (%w/w)	2.53± 0.1	-	15.54±0.24	-
Cr (VI) ppm	2,991	4.12	9,980	2.36

This method is a good example of friendly solution to manage hazardous wastes, because: a) two hazardous wastes are treated at the same time, b) the water used in the process comes from polluted aquifers, c) no water discharges are produced, d) only industrial sulfuric acid is used, and e) the process is economically viable for a medium sized industry. Before selecting any method to process hazardous waste, it is very important to characterize the wastes, study changes in the matrix and to calculate the direct and indirect environmental impacts, specially related with energy, water and reagents consumption.

REFERENCES

1. BGS *Effects of wastewater reuse on urban groundwater resources, Leon Mexico. Phase 1 Report. Ed. British Geological Survey Tech. Rep. WD/94/25. Keyworth, Nottinghnshire, England.* 1994

2. Gutiérrez-Ruiz M. *Cromo en Leon.* Memorias 1er. Simposio Nacional sobre Residuos Peligrosos. PUMA-UNAM-Mexico. 1996 : 124-145

3. Gutiérrez-Ruiz M. Bocco G. Castillo-Blum S. *Contaminación por cromo en el norte de la ciudad de México, un enfoque interdisciplinario.* Boletín del Instituto de Geografía-UNAM Mexico 1987 ; 16 : 77-125

4. Gutiérrez-Ruiz M., Castillo-Blum S., Rosales-Aguilera, E. *Chromate contamination north of Mexico City.* UNEP Industry and Environment 1989 ; 12 : 51-56

5. Gonzalez M., Gutiérrez-Ruiz M., Lozano R. Flores L. *Chromium Species Transformation during the Stabilization Process of Industrial Wastes and Brick Manufacturing.* Proceeding 4th International Conference Environmental Contamination Barcelona. 1990 : 132-134

Metal Ions in Biology and Medicine; vol 6. Eds. J.A. Centeno, Ph. Collery, G. Vernet, R.B. Finkelman, H. Gibb, J.C. Etienne. John Libbey Eurotext, Paris © 2000, pp. 661-663.

A new bacteria resistant to several metal ions and able to reduce hexavalent chromium

Rita Branco, Maria Carmen Alpoim, and Paula Vasconcellos Morais

Departamento Bioquímica, Faculdade de Ciências e Tecnologia da Universidade de Coimbra, 3001 Coimbra, Portugal

Strains identified as *Ochrobactrum* spp. were able to grow with as much as 5 mM Cr(VI) under aerobic conditions. All the strains were able to reduce completely 1 mM Cr(VI) without simultaneous chromium uptake. Cr(VI) reducing efficiency was reduced with increasing Cr(VI) concentrations. Strains were also able to resist to 1 mM Ni^{2+}, Co^{2+} and Zn^{2+} and to several antibiotics.

Introduction

Cr(VI) compounds often cause environmental pollution since they are powerful oxidants that are easily reduced inside the cells resulting in irreversible cell damage [1]. Bacterial resistance to chromium and other toxic metals has been widely reported [2, 3]. Active exclusion of chromium from the citosol or external reduction of Cr(VI) to the less toxic Cr(III), or both, achieves this resistance. Genetic studies have found plasmids that determine for chromate resistance [4]. Because biological reduction of Cr(VI) usually generates an insignificant quantity of chemical sludge, biological means to detoxify the Cr(VI) has been receiving considerable attention. In this study we characterised a chromium-resistant-reducing bacterium isolated from a contaminated sludge to be used as a biological tool in bioremediation.

Material and Methods

Bacteria and growth conditions: A chemiotaxonomic group with 5-bvl-1 as the representative strain of the cluster and *Ochrobactrum antropi* type strain LMG 3331 and strain LMG 3301 were cultivated in Nutrient Agar (NA; Difco) at 30°C for maintenance. All strains were maintained at –80°C in Nutrient Broth (NB; Difco) containing 15% glycerol.

Bacteria characterisation: Strains were characterised by their, morphology, Gram staining, API 20 NE (bioMerieux, France) whole–cell protein profile (SDS-PAGE) and by their fatty acid methyl esters profile (FAME) [5]. Resistance to tetracycline, kanamycin, chloramphenicol ampicillin and naladix acid were tested using standard antibiotic discs sensitivity testing method (Difco) in Muller-Hinton medium incubated at 30°C during 24h.

Cr(VI) resistance and reduction: Nutrient Broth or buffered NB (NB with 60 mM HEPES) and Buffered Minimal Medium (MM) with 0.5% glucose (Degreese minimal medium [6] without phosphate buffer and with 60 mM HEPES) were used in resistance and reducing experiments. Strains were tested for their resistance to Cr(VI) by growth with increasing Cr(VI) concentrations, at 30°C with 135rpm for 90h, in aerobic and anaerobic conditions. Cr(VI) reducing ability of the bacteria was tested with Cr(VI) concentrations ranging from 1 to 3 mM, at 30°C with 135 rpm for 140 h.

Cr(VI) reduction was assayed using the diphenylcarbazide method [7] and total chromium was assayed by atomic absorption.
Resistance to other metal ions: Strains were tested for their resistance to 1 mM Ni^{2+}, Co^{2+} and Zn^{2+} by growth in buffered MM at 30°C with 135 rpm for 140 h.

Results

The bacteria isolated from activated sludge were gram-negative motile rods, with 18:1 as major fatty acid. The representative strain (5-bvl-1) belongs to the species *Ochrobactrum antropi* according to the results from API 20 NE and FAME analysis (MIDI identification System). Strain was resistant to tetracycline, kanamycine, chloramphenicol and naladix acid.
Fig. 1 shows the effects of different Cr(VI) concentrations on growth of strain 5-bvl-1. Increasing Cr(VI) concentrations led to a decrease in cell viability. Strain 5-bvl-1 was also able to resist to 1 mM Ni^{2+}, Co^{2+} and Zn^{2+}.

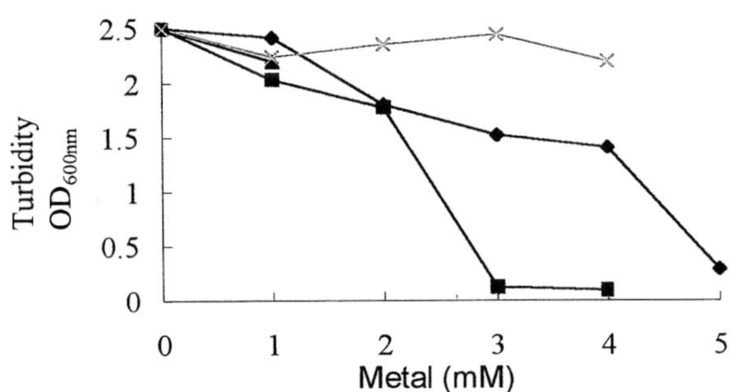

Fig. 1. Metal ion resistance of strain 5-bvl-1 measured by maximal turbidity in medium MM at 600 nm in presence of increasing concentrations of Cr(VI) (♦), Ni^{2+} (■), Co^{2+} (▲), and Zn^{2+}(×).

Strain 5-bvl-1 showed Cr(VI) reduction ability (Fig.2), but the ability of the strain to reduce Cr(VI) depended on the medium composition i.e. the reduction in buffered MM was greater than in the other media. The rate of Cr(VI) reduction was dependent on Cr(VI) concentration i.e. the time required to reduce Cr(VI) increased in proportion to the amount of Cr (VI) added. Cr(VI) reduction led to a decrease in pH and this decrease was also dependent on the amount of Cr(VI) added (results not shown). The total chromium in the medium remained unchanged and as shown in Fig. 2, Cr(VI) reduction is not followed by chromium uptake.

Discussion

This is the first report of an *Ochrobactrum* chromium resistant bacterium. This strain, isolated from activated sludge collected at a waste water treatment plant in a chromium contaminated area, was able to grow with as much as 5 mM Cr(VI) whereas the other strains of this genus such as the strains *O. anthropi* LMG 3331 and

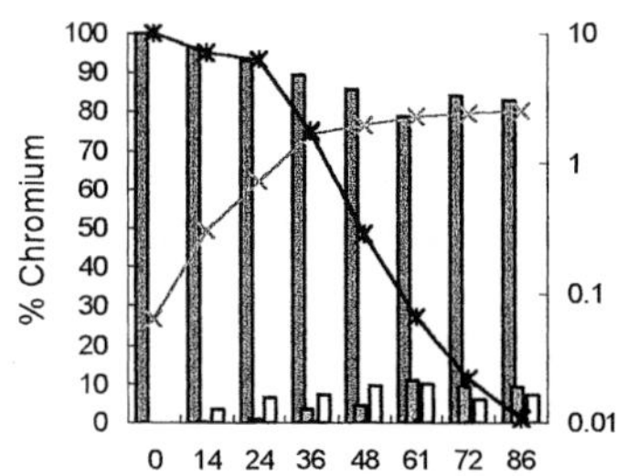

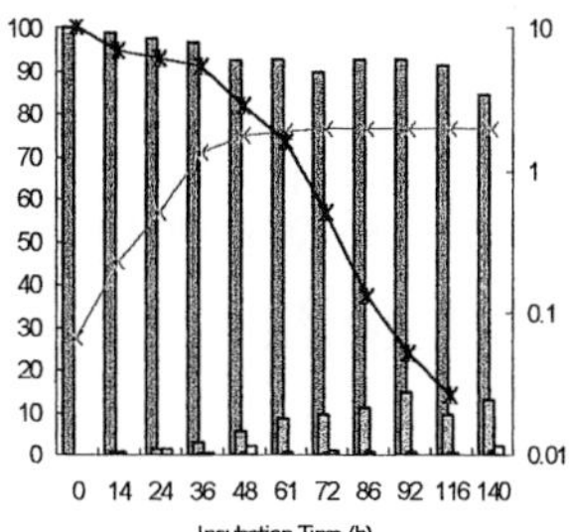

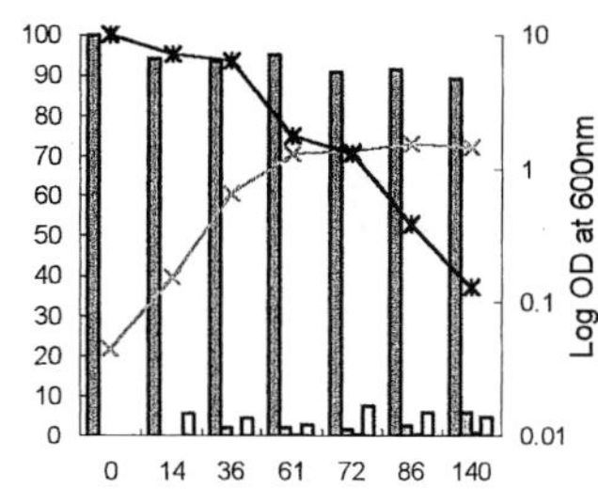

Fig. 2. Resistance, reduction and uptake of chromium by strain 5-bvl-1. Symbols: grey bars, total chromium in supernatant; green bars, uptake of chromium; yellow bars, chromium removed during cell washing; red line, Cr(VI) in the supernatant; blue line, growth measured as increasing turbidity.

LMG 3301 can not tolerate even 1 mM Cr(VI). Although these bacteria have plasmids of different sizes, it is not known if chromate resistance is plasmid determined because all attempts to cure the strain were unsuccessful. This strain reduce Cr(VI), under aerobic conditions, when reached the stationary phase, because Cr(VI) disappearance does not go along with a corresponding decrease in total chromium in the medium. We do not know yet the molecular basis of this reduced uptake of chromium by the strain, but it may be due either to modification of specific carriers, external reduction of Cr(VI) to the octahedral coordinated Cr(III) or to an efficient efflux system. The reduced uptake of chromium may probably explain the resistance of the strain to Cr(VI) as previously suggested for *P. fluorescens* [2]. Furthermore, the Cr(VI) reduction led always to a decrease in pH, being the percentage of reduction much greater in buffered medium than in unbuffered medium. A generalised resistance to several toxics may be committed either to a general physiological mechanism developed in response to a toxic environment or to the presence of resistance genes.

1.Langand, S. The carcinogenicity of chromium compounds in man and animals. In: Metabolism and Toxicity. 1983. D. Burrows (ed.)CRC Press, Inc. Boca Roton, Fla, pp. 13-30.

2.Lovely, D. R. Dissimilatory metal reduction. *Ann. Rev. Microbiol.*, 1993; 47: 263-290.

3.Wang, Y-T, Shen, H. Bacterial reduction of hexavalent chromium. *J. Indust. Microbiol.*, 1995; 14: 159-163.

4.Silver, S. Bacterial heavy metal resistance: new surprises. *Annu. Rev. Microbiol.*, 1996; 50: 753-789.

5.Ferreira A, Morais P, da Costa, M. Computer-aided compairison of protein electrophoretic patterns for grouping and identification of heterotrophic bacteria from mineral water. *J Appl Bacteriology* 1996; 80: 479-486.

6.Degryse, E. Glansdorff, N., and Piérard, A. A comparative analysis of extreme thermophilic bacteria belonging to the genus *Thermus*. *Arch Microbiol* 1978; 189-196.

7.Ishibashi Y, Cervantes C, Silver, S. Chromium reduction in *Pseudomonas putida*. *Appl Environ Microbiol* 1990; 2268-2270.

Metal Ions in Biology and Medicine; vol 6. Eds. J.A. Centeno, Ph. Collery, G. Vernet, R.B. Finkelman, H. Gibb, J.C. Etienne. John Libbey Eurotext, Paris © 2000, pp. 664-668.

Influence of amino acids on the heavy metal toxicity in *Escherichia coli K12* cells

L.A. Khassanova[1], Z.M. Khassanova[2], A. Yu. Ivanov[3], L. Yu. Markelia[2], A.V. Gavrjushkin[4], G.F. Combs Jr.[5]

[1] *Department of Environmental Protection of Bashkir State University, 32, Frunze Street, 450072 Ufa, Russia;* [2] *Department of Botany of Bashkir State Pedagogical University, 3a, October Revolution Street, 450025 Ufa, Russia;* [3] *Institute of Cell Biophysics, Russian Academy of Sciences, 142292 Pushchino, Russia;* [4] *State Research Institute of Applied Microbiology, 142279 Obolensk, Russia;* [5] *Division of Nutritional Sciences, Cornell University, Ithaca, NY, USA*

ABSTRACT

The method of electroorientational (EO) spectroscopy was used to study the influence of amino acids (AAs): cysteine (CYS), methionine (MET), selenomethionine (SeMET), arginine (ARG), glutamine (GLN) on the toxicity of mercury and copper for plasma membrane (PM) of *Escherichia coli* K12 cells. The *Escherichia coli* K12 cells were pre-incubated with AAs during 15 min and then were treated with various heavy metals (HMs) for an additional 15 min. The damaging effect of each HM was assessed at medium pH conditions corresponding to the highest concentration of hydroxylated forms of metal ions and, consequently, the maximal toxic effect of each HM. Among the studied AAs, CYS and SeMET more effectively prevented PM damage of *Escherichia coli* K-12 cells induced by $HgOH^+$ (pH 6.0) and $CuOH^+$ (pH 7.0) ions. The observed strong and pH-independent protection by CYS and SeMET may be explained by the presence of reactive SH- and $SeCH_3$ groups capable of reacting with the potentially damaging HM species.

INTRODUCTION

The early and nonspecific responses of bacterial cells to HM action involve changes in membrane permeability resulting from the modification of membrane-associated proteins with inactivation of their functional groups involved in the maintenance of membrane structure. Among the main physico-chemical determinants of HM injury are pH, water alkalinity/hardness, the presence/absence of hydrated forms of metal ions, and the presence/absence of HM-chelates. Thus the greatest cellular toxicities of mercuric ions are observed in acidic media, while cupric ions are the most toxic effect in neutral media (Khassanova et al., 1996; Khassanova et al., 1998). Increases in pH leads to intensification of the formation of metal-organic complexes (Albert, 1989; Ershov et al., 1989; Gromov, 1989; Ivanov et al., 1997; Khassanova et al., 1998). Such complexes can be formed by AAs, which act by way of their large number of functional groups. Depending on pH and presence of dissociable functional groups, AA can act as anions, cations or electroneutral ions (Eichhorn, 1978), thus influencing on the oxidative capacities of formed HM complexes (Farell et al., 1990; Mohapatra et al., 1997). The role of some AA in the reduction of HM toxicity for growth characteristics of *Anabaena variabilis* and *Chlorella vulgaris* was reported earlier (Mohapatra et al., 1997; Kosakowska et al., 1986). However the influence of AA on the HM injury effects for PM of bacterial cells has not been studied previously.

MATERIALS AND METHODS

Escherichia coli K 12 cells were grown in shaken flasks (150 rpm) at 37^0C in M9 medium with 0.1% yeast extract for 5 h, which corresponded to the exponential growth phase. Cells were twice washed with distilled water, recovered by low speed centrifugation and kept at 4^0C during the experimental period (2-4 h) at the concentration of 10^{10} cells/ml. The required pH were prepared by adding 0.01 N HCl and 0.01 M TRIS (tris-(hydroxymethyl)-aminomethane) («Reachim», Russia), and electric conductivity was standardized by adding 0.01 M NaCl (0.00215 Sm/m). The cells were pre-incubated with various AAs for 15 min and then were treated by a HM (0.01 M) for an additional 15 min. The damaging effect of each HM was assessed at medium pH corresponding to the highest concentration of their respective hydrated form, to yield the maximal toxic effect of each metal ion. The pH of the medium was monitored continuously using with an ionometer «pH-340» (Russia), electric conductivity was measured with a conductometer «OK-102/1» («Radelkis», Hungary), and cell suspension optical density was controlled with a photoelectric colorimeter «FEC-56 M» (Russia) (cuvette - 1 cm, filter - 540 nm). Cell electro-orientational (EO) spectra were registered by determining the relative changes of the cell suspension optical density in a uniform field of alternating electrical current with an intensity of 60 V/cm and a frequency of 5-7-10 MHz (Miroshnikov et al., 1986). The EO-spectra were plotted using a device developed at the State Research Center of Applied Microbiology (Obolensk, Russia) for this purpose. Distilled water with electric conductivity not more than 0.00013 Sm/m and the following AAs were used: L- cysteine (CYS, MW 121.2), L-methionine (MET, MW 149. 2), L-selenomethionine (SeMet, MW 196.1) («Sigma», USA), L-arginine (ARG, MW 174.2) and L-glutamine (GLU, MW 146.2). The HM salts were: $HgCl_2$, $CuCl_2$ («Aldrich», USA). All measurements were made at room temperature.

RESULTS AND DISCUSSION

The EO spectra (Fig.1, a,b) of intact (0), Hg (1 a), Cu (1 b), CYS (2 a,b) treated cells and cells exposed to Hg or Cu after pre-incubation with CYS (3 a,b) showed decreases in absolute EO values upon cell exposure to mercury and copper ions.

The EO values at electric field high frequencies, especially at 7-10 MHz, are determined by their cytoplasm and PM properties (Miroshnikov et al., 1986). Therefore, the EO changes observed in response to HM treatment can be attributed to damage to the PM barrier, involving the leakage of free ions and other low-molecular substances out of the cytoplasm and resulting in decreased cell electric conductivity. Pre-incubation with CYS significantly reduced the damaging effects of mercuric and cupric ions, as evidenced by decreases in EO absolute values.

The EO values presented on the figures 2-3 (a,b) show the protective properties of several AAs on the PMs of cells treated with Hg at pH 6.0 and Cu at pH 7.0. The changes in EO values (fig.2 a,b) of *E. coli* cells treated with Hg show that pre-incubation with only CYS, Se-MET and ARG at a molar ratio (AA:Hg - 2.0:1.0 and AA:Hg - 10:1.0) rendered protection to the cell PM. In contrast, EO values of cells treated with Cu (fig. 3, a) showed that pre-incubation with each AA at a molar ratio (AA:Cu - 2.5:1.0) confered protection on cell PM permeability. This protection was greatest for CYS, followed by SeMET, ARG, and GLN and MET, respectively. Increases in AA:HM molar ratios 10.0:1.0 significantly reduced Cu PM toxicity, although the differences in the protective effects of AAs were reduced.

a.

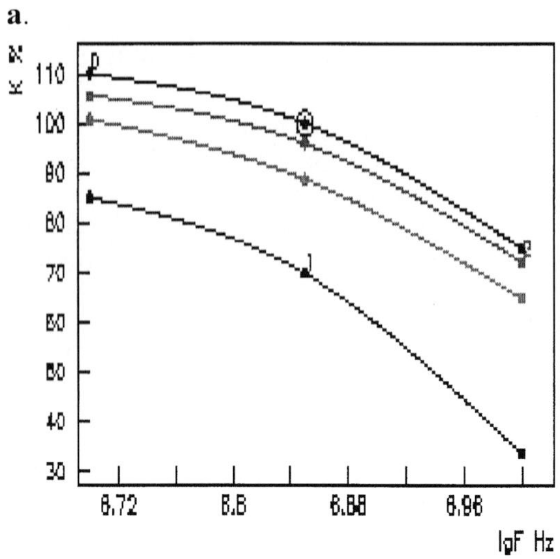

b.

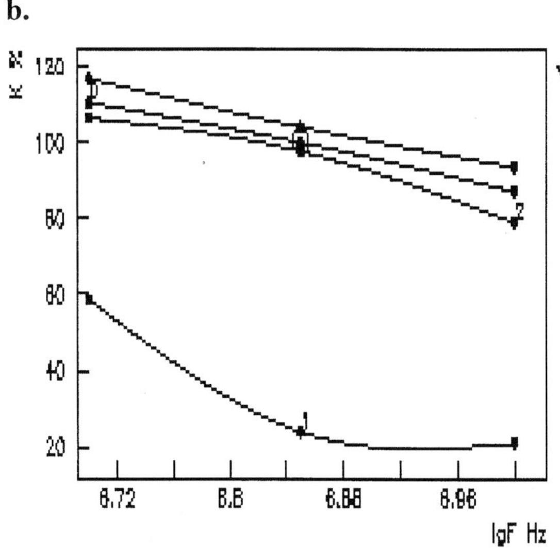

Fig.1 a, b. EO- spectra of *Escherichia coli* K 12 intact (0) and treated cells by: a) 5 μM Hg (1), 50 μM CYS (2) and Hg after pre-incubation with CYS (3), pH 6.0. b) 10 μM Cu (1), treated with 50 μM CYS (2) and Cu after pre-incubation with CYS (3), pH 7.0. $K=(\Delta D_i/\Delta D_o) \times 100\%$, where ΔD_i is the change of the cell suspension optical density at applied electric field; ΔD_o is the same for the intact cell suspension at electric field frequency 7 MHz.

Pre-inculation with CYS or SeMet consistently conferred strong and pH-independent protection of PM against both Hg and Cu. In the case of CYS, this effect would appear to result from the presence in that AA of the highly reactive thiol (SH-) group. Heavy metals are known to have special affinities to such sulfur (S)-containing functional groups (Ershov et al., 1989). Thus, the lack of PM protection from MET can be explained by lack of availability of

a.

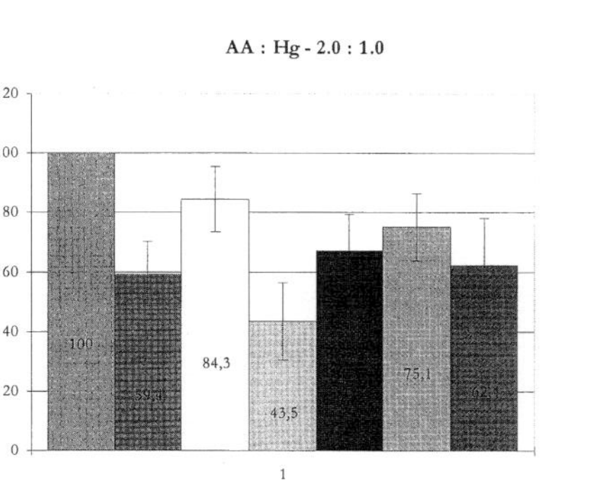

b.

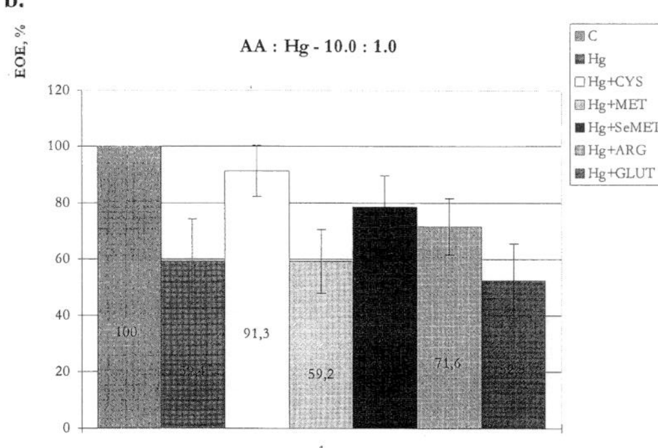

Fig. 2.a-b. EOE values (7.0 MHz) of *Escherichi coli* cells treated by mercury ions (5 μM) and pre-incubated with different AAs at a molar ratio AA:Hg - 2.0:1.0 (a), 10:1.0 (b); pH 6.0.

a.

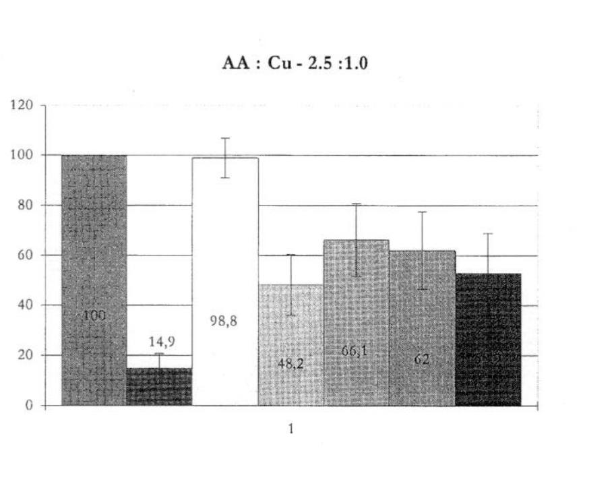

b.

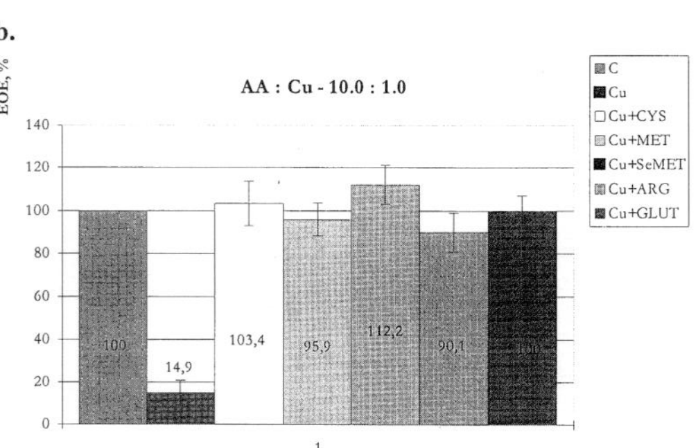

Fig. 3, a-b. EOE values (7.0 MHz) of *Escherichia. coli* cells treated by copper ions (10 μM) and pre-incubated with different AAs at a molar ratio AA: Cu - 2.5: 1.0 (a), 10: 1.0 (b). pH 7.0.

its carbon-bonded S atom (Eichhorn, 1978). That PM protection from Hg and Cu damage was observed for SeMet is less clear, as that AA lacks a functional group comparable to that or CYS. It is possible, therefore, that the protection observed after SeMet-pre-incubation may have been due to its catabolism to the highly reactive selenolate ion (CH_3Se^-), which is known to redox-cycle (Chaudiere et al., 1992; Spallholz, 1997; Spallholz et al., 2000).

The amplification of PM-protection at pH 7.0 is most likely caused by the lowering of proton densities of the functional groups of those AAs. Such effects would be expected to simplify the metal-ligand coordination and, consequently, to increase the metal binding forces (Martin, 1993). The protection by AA effect against Cu-induced membrane damage may be related to the relatively great ability of that metal to form complex (Eikhenberger, 1993). Thus, the protective effects of AA would appear to be mainly due to the nature of their functional groups, and to their abilities to form stable neutral or negatively charged HM-complexes that do not affect the PM-binding of biomolecules.

REFERENCES

GROMOV B.V., PAVLENKO G.V. Bacterial ecology. Edition of the Leningrad State University (Leningrad). 1989, 248 p.

ALBERT A. Selective toxicity. Medicine (Moscow). 1989, 2: 432 p.

EIKHENBERGER E. Correlation between necessity and toxicity of metals in water ecosystems. *Some questions of metal toxicity*. Mir (Moscow). 1993: 62-88.

IVANOV A. Yu. et al. Toxic effect of hydroxylated metal ions on the plasma membrane of bacterial cells. *Microbiologiya* (Moscow). 1997, 66: 588-594.

KHASSANOVA L.A. et al. Electrophysical analysis of metal ions-induced toxic shock in phototrophi microorganisms. *Metal Ions in Biology and Medicine*. John Libbey Eurotext (Paris). 1996, 4: 229-233.

KHASSANOVA Z.M. et al. Significance of environmental conditions in the mercury toxicity for *Escherichia coli* K-12 cells. *Metal Ions in Biology and Medicine*. John Libbey Eurotext (Paris). 1998, 5: 337-343.

EICHHORN G.M. Inorganic biochemistry. Mir (Moscow). 1978, 1: 711 p.

ERSHOV Yu. A., PLETNEVA T.V. Mechanisms of the inorganic compounds toxicity. Medicine (Moscow). 1989, 253 p.

FARELL R.E., GERMIDA J.J., HUANG MING P. Biotoxicity of mercury as influenced by mercury (II) speciation. *Appl. Environ. Microbiology.* 1990, 56: 3006-3016.

MOHAPATRA D.K. et al. Biotoxicity of mercury to *Chlorella vulgaris* as influenced by amino acids. *Acta biologica Hungarica*. 1997, 48: 497-504.

KOSAKOWSKA A. et al. Effect of amino acids on the toxicity of heavy metals to phytoplancton. *Bull. Environ. Contam. Toxicol.* 1988, 40: 532-538.

MIROSHNIKOV A.I., FOMCHENKOV V.M., IVANOV A.Yu. Electrophysical analysis and cell separation. Nauka (Moscow). 1984, 198 p.

MARTIN R. Bioinorganic chemistry of the toxic metal ions. *Some questions of metal toxicity*. Mir (Moscow). 1993: 25-62.

CHAUDIERE J., COURTIN O., LECLAIRE J. Glutathione oxidase activity of selenocystamine: a mechanistic study. *Arch. Biochem. Biophys*. 1992, 296: 328-336.

SPALLHOLZ J.E. Free radical generation by selenium compounds and their prooxidant toxicity. *Biomed. Environ. Sci.* 1997, 10: 260-270.

SPALLHOLZ J.E., SHRIVER B.J., REID T.W. Dimethyldiselenide generates superoxide in an invitro chemiluminescence assay. *Free Rad. Biol. Med.* 2000, 27 (in press).

Metal Ions in Biology and Medicine; vol 6. Eds. J.A. Centeno, Ph. Collery, G. Vernet, R.B. Finkelman, H. Gibb, J.C. Etienne. John Libbey Eurotext, Paris © 2000, pp. 669-671.

Study of transport processes of metal in cucumber plants by TXRF-spectrometry

Gyula Záray[1], Anita Varga[1], Ferenc Fodor[2]

[1] *Department of Chemical Technology and Environmental Chemistry, Eötvös University, P.O. Box 32, Budapest, H-1518, Hungary;* [2] *Department of Plant Physiology, Eötvös University, P.O. Box 330, Budapest, H-1445, Hungary*

Abstract: Transport processes of some essential (K, Ca, Fe, Mn, Zn) and toxical (Cd, Ni, Pb or V) elements were studied in cucumber plants grown in modified Hoagland nutrient solutions containing iron in chemical form of Fe(III)-citrate, Fe(III)-EDTA or $FeCl_3$. The xylem sap samples were directly analyzed by TXRF-spectrometry after addition of internal standard. The transport rate of the four toxical elements within the xylem chanel increase in order of $V \ll Pb < Cd < Ni$. Cd hampers the water uptake and thereby the amount of all transported essential elements. Pb leads to a slight increment in the transport rate of the five essential elements. Ni hinders the transport of K and Zn. Due to the low accumulation and transport of V in the plant its presence results in the smallest influence on the transport processes of the essential elements.

Introduction:

One of the most fruitful ways to obtain valuable information about the interaction of heavy metal pollutants with inorganic and organic molecules of plants is the quantitative determination of all chemical compounds of plants by growing them under controlled environmental conditions in the presence and absence of heavy metals. The changes in the chemical composition of plants caused by heavy metals can be established through the analysis of various plant parts (leaves, stems, roots, etc.) and the xylem or phloem fluids.

To study the element transport in plants in most cases the xylem fluids were investigated [1,2]. Although the sample volume can be increased by simultaneous collection of xylem fluid from more plants cultivated under the same environmental conditions the total volume, especially in heavy metal contaminated plants, does not exceed 1 cm^3. Therefore multielemental trace analysis of low-volume xylem fluids or biological tissues requires powerful microanalytical techniques like

ICP-mass spectrometry combined with the electrothermal vaporization system [3] or the total reflection X-ray fluorescence (TXRF) spectrometry [4].

Since the comparison and the evaluation of the literature data are difficult due to the differences in growing circumstances and ages of the plants, chemical form of contaminants, etc., we have decided to study the influence of Cd, Ni, Pb and V on cucumber plants, which were simultaneously grown at the same experimental conditions (lighting, temperature, growing time, concentration of elements in the nutrient solutions). In this study we present the results of TXRF investigation of the xylem fluids of cucumber plants evaluating the effect of these four heavy metals on the uptake and transport processes of essential elements.

Experimental: Cucumber seedlings (Cucumis sativus L.) were cultivated in modified Hoagland nutrient solutions containing Cd,Ni, Pb or V in concentration of 10^{-5}M. At the second leaf stage, 3-3 plants were cut 5 mm above the root collar and the xylem saps were collected for 60 min from the freshly cut surfaces into polyethylene vials using micropipettes. After determination of their weights the xylem sap samples were stored at -22°C.

For the TXRF investigations of xylem fluids, 190 μl of each sample was spiked with a standard solution of Ga to a final concentration of 1 μg/cm^3. From each of these spiked and mixed solutions 25 μl was dropped onto a quartz glass carrier and dried in a clean box applying a ceramic-coated hot plate at 80°C for 30 min. From each solution three parallel samples were prepared. The analysis were carried out by an EXTRA IIA TXRF-spectrometer (produced by Atomika Instruments GmbH, Oberschleissheim, Germany).

Results and discussion: The transported amounts of the xylem sap increase in the presence of Pb and V contamination related to the control plants independently from the chemical form of iron. In the case of Ni pollution, however, a relatively high decrease (30-50%) can be observed. Addition of Cd resulted in a drastic reduction of the xylem fluid in the case of Fe(III)-EDTA and Fe(III)-citrate, while in the presence of $FeCl_3$ the bleeding was completely blocked and it was not possible to collect xylem sap at all.

The amounts of heavy metals transported in the xylem sap during a 1 hour bleeding period are listed in the following table:

Iron form	ng metal / hour related to 1g of fresh root			
	Cd	**Ni**	**Pb**	**V**
Fe(III)EDTA	254.5 ± 22.5	277.6 ± 6.9	32.42 ± 1.60	n. d.
Fe(III)-citrate	243.9 ± 6.7	346.3 ± 11.2	224.7 ± 10.1	n. d.
$FeCl_3$		509.5 ± 10.3	265.6 ± 4.5	n. d.

Independently on the iron form, Ni shows the highest transport rate. The contamination of V in the xylem samples was below the detection limit. The transport of essential elements investigated (first of all Fe) was strongly reduced by Cd. The transport of K, Zn and Fe was partly blocked by Ni. However, Pb-contamination resulted in a moderate increment in the transport of K, Ca, Zn and Mn. The effect of V added as $VOSO_4$ can be neglected.

Conclusions: The influence of heavy metals on the transport of essential elements depends on all the variable parameters (pollutants, essential elements and the chemical form of iron). The general effect of heavy metals investigated changes in the following sequences: Cd > Pb ~ Ni » V. The explanation of these phenomena requires the determination of the transport partners in the xylem (e.g. metalloproteins, complexes formed with malic, citric or fumaric acids).

Acknowledgements: This research work was supported by the National Scientific Research Foundation (Hungary) through Grants T014861 and T02913.

References:

[1] L.D. Noodén, C.S. Mauk, Physiol. Plant. 70 (1987) 735.
[2] S.Satoh, C.Iizuka, A.Kikuchi, N.Nakamura, T.Fujii, Plant. Cell Physiol. 33 (1992) 841.
[3] C.J.Park, J.C. van Loon, P. Arrowsmith, J.B. French, Anal. Chem. 59 (1987) 2191.
[4] Gy. Záray, A. Varga F. Fodor, E. Cseh, Microchem. J. 55 (1997) 64.

Metal Ions in Biology and Medicine; vol 6. Eds. J.A. Centeno, Ph. Collery, G. Vernet, R.B. Finkelman, H. Gibb, J.C. Etienne. John Libbey Eurotext, Paris © 2000, pp. 672-674.

Phytoremediation of metal-contaminated soils: Jackson state university research initiatives

Gregorio B. Begonia[1], Maria T. Begonia[1], Gloria L. Miller[1], and Murty Kambhampati[2]

[1] *Department of Biology, Jackson State University, Jackson, MS 39217 USA and* [2] *Department of Biology, Southern University, New Orleans, LA 70126 USA*

ABSTRACT

Phytoextraction is becoming popular as a cost-effective and environmentally sound phytoremediation strategy for reducing toxic metal levels from contaminated soils. Cognizant of the potential of this phytoremediation technique as an alternative to expensive remediation technologies, a series of experiments were conducted to evaluate the suitability of some plants as phytoextraction species. Based from a ≥60% translocation index (shoot metal uptake * 100 / total plant metal uptake), four species (*Ipomoea lacunosa*, *Sesbania exaltata*, *Brassica napus*, *Brassica campestris rapifera*) exhibited tolerance and significant accumulation of Pb or Cd into their shoots. In another experiment, the translocation of Pb to the shoots of *I. lacunosa* was enhanced by the addition of 5 mM ethylenediaminetetraacetic acid (EDTA). At each level of applied Pb, the amount of residual soil Pb after harvest decreased with increasing concentration of EDTA. Research initiatives are underway which are geared toward maximization of metal translocation to the shoots of other promising species.

INTRODUCTION

There has been an increasing interest in phytoremediation as a plant-based alternative for cost-effective and environmentally sound clean up of metal-contaminated soils [1]. Phytoextraction is a phytoremediation strategy that utilizes plants to remove toxic metals from contaminated soils [2]. In phytoextraction, an efficient plant species must be able to absorb a substantial amount of the toxic metal into its roots and preferentially translocate the metal into the harvestable above-ground biomass for easier harvesting. Through a multiple cropping scheme, suitable species can be planted in succession ultimately leading to the reduction of soil metal concentrations to environmentally acceptable levels.

In addition to a plant's ability to produce high biomass and tolerate toxic metal levels, the success of phytoextraction is also dependent upon the availability of the metal in the soil for plant uptake. For instance, Pb has limited solubility in soils and availability for plant uptake due to complexation with organic matter, sorption on oxides and clays, and precipitation as carbonates, hydroxides and phosphates [3]. The soluble Pb levels of most soils remain very low and do not allow substantial uptake by the plant.

Another requisite to metal phytoextraction is to increase and maintain metal concentrations in the soil solution. Chelates have been used to increase the solubility of metal cations in soils and nutrient solutions and are reported to have significant effects on metal accumulation in plants [4,5]. Recent studies [6,7] also demonstrated that addition of synthetic chelates to Pb-contaminated soils dramatically increased Pb concentration in soil solution. This increase of Pb concentration in soil solution triggered a surge of Pb accumulation in corn, peas and *B. juncea* grown on Pb-contaminated soils.

Using hydroponics [5] and artificial soil media [8], we identified *I. lacunosa* as one of the promising species for phytoextraction because of its high biomass under elevated Pb levels, and ability to accumulate high amounts of Pb into its shoots. This paper summarizes the current status of our screening efforts to find metal accumulating plant species. The other objective was to determine whether EDTA amendment can enhance the shoot uptake of Pb by *I. lacunosa* when grown on a Pb-contaminated soil.

MATERIALS AND METHODS

Seeds of plant species were planted in pots containing various kinds of growing media. Different aqueous solutions (0-500 ppm) of Pb or Cd were periodically added to the growing medium during the plant's active vegetative growth stage. In other experiments, aqueous solutions of Pb (0-2000 ppm) and EDTA (0-5 mM) were added once before planting to determine whether EDTA can further enhance the uptake of metals by the shoots.

Plants were maintained either in a greenhouse or laboratory supplemented with high intensity lamps (PAR: 800 μmol photons $m^{-2}s^{-1}$). A complete nutrient solution was added periodically based on evaporative demand. In screening experiments, treatments were arranged in a completely randomized design (CRD) with 5 replications. The chelate experiment was arranged in a 4Pb x 5 EDTA factorial in a Randomized Complete Block (RCB) design with 5 replications.

Shoot and root dry biomass were obtained at harvest. Dried plant tissues were ground in a Wiley mill equipped with a 60-mesh screen. Metals from ground plant tissues and soil samples were extracted using HNO_3-H_2O_2 digestion protocols [8, 9] and microwave digestion techniques, respectively. Metal contents of digested samples were quantified using atomic absorption spectrophotometry.

RESULTS AND DISCUSSION

Based from shoot uptake data, our screening efforts yielded four species that have great potential for phytoextraction of Pb or Cd from contaminated soils. Since total metal removal is a function of the metal concentration in the harvestable biomass, a suitable species must produce high biomass at the contaminated site. *I. lacunosa* not only produced high biomass but was able to tolerate elevated levels of Pb/EDTA from the soil. There were no discernible toxic effects of Pb/EDTA on *I. lacunosa* except for a slight reduction in biomass at the highest Pb/EDTA treatment combination.

Another requisite to the success of phytoextraction is the enhancement of metal accumulation in the harvestable biomass. Pb uptake in the shoot increased with increasing level of soil-applied Pb. For each concentration of soil-applied Pb, there was an increasing amount of Pb accumulated in the shoots as the concentration of EDTA was increased. This was especially true with the addition of 5 mM EDTA. For instance, when 5 mM EDTA was added in combination with either 500, 1000, or 2000 ppm Pb, the shoot accumulated an average 60% of the total Pb taken up by the whole plant. There were no significant effects of chelate amendments on the amount of Pb accumulated in the roots. However, there was a decreasing concentration of Pb remaining in the soil after harvest, as the concentration of applied EDTA was increased. We believe that EDTA especially at the highest concentration (e.g., 5 mM) enhanced Pb desorption from soil to soil solution, facilitated transport into the xylem, decreased binding of Pb by the root tissue, and increased Pb translocation from the roots to shoots as previously demonstrated in EDTA-mediated phytoextraction studies using corn, peas and *Brassica juncea* [6,7].

LITERATURE CITED

1.Salt D, Blaylock M, Kumar P, Dushenkov V, Ensley B, Chet I, Raskin I. Phytoremediation: A novel strategy for the removal of toxic metals from the environment using plants. *Biotechno*l 1995;13: 468-474.

2.Kumar P, Dushenkov V, Motto H, Raskin I. Phytoextraction: The use of plants to remove heavy metals from soils. *Environ Sci Technol* 1995; 29: 1232-1238.

3.McBride M. Environmental chemistry of soils. New York: Oxford University Press, 1994.

4.Checkai R, Corey R, Helmke P. Effects of ionic and complexed metal concentrations on plant uptake of cadmium and micronutrient metals from solution. *Plant Soil* 1987; 99: 335-345.

5.Ghosh S, Rhyne C. A search for lead hyperaccumulating plants in the laboratory. *J Mississippi Acad Sci* 1998; 43:11-12.

6.Huang, J, Chen J, Berti W, Cunningham S. Phytoremediation of lead-contaminated soils: Role of synthetic chelates in lead phytoextraction. *Environ Sci Technol* 1997; 31: 800-805.

7.Blaylock, M, Salt D, Dushenkov V, Zacharova O, Gussman C, Kapulnik Y, Ensley B, Raskin I. Enhanced accumulation of Pb in Indian mustard by soil-applied chelating agents. *Environ Sci Technol* 1997; 31: 860-865.

8.Begonia, G. Comparative lead uptake and responses of some plants grown on lead contaminated soils. *J Mississippi Acad Sci* 1997; 42: 101-106.

9.Begonia G, Davis C, Begonia M, Gray C. Growth responses of Indian mustard [*Brassica juncea* (L.) Czern.] and its phytoextraction of lead from a contaminated soil. *Bull Environ Contam Toxicol* 1998; 61: 38-43.

Metal Ions in Biology and Medicine; vol 6. Eds. J.A. Centeno, Ph. Collery, G. Vernet, R.B. Finkelman, H. Gibb, J.C. Etienne. John Libbey Eurotext, Paris © 2000, pp. 675-677.

Microbial characterisation of chromium-contaminated sludge from a wastewater treatment-plant

Romeu Francisco, Maria Carmen Alpoim, and Paula Vasconcellos Morais

Departamento Bioquímica, Faculdade de Ciências e Tecnologia da Universidade de Coimbra, 3001 Coimbra, Portugal

A group of 48 strains resistant to Cr(VI) was isolated. Isolates formed 9 clusters and 10 unclustered strains according to SDS-PAGE, and 8 clusters after FAME analysis. All isolates were able to grow in the presence of 1mM Cr(VI) and all showed ability to reduce the concentration of Cr(VI) present in the growth medium. This study showed diversity within the Cr(VI) resistant bacteria that can be used in environmental cleanup of industrial wastes.

Introduction

Surface waters that receive large quantities of industrial waste waters, contain high concentrations of heavy metals including the highly toxic chromium (VI) (Cr(VI)). The potential for the biological transformation of the very toxic Cr (VI) to the less toxic Cr (III) was recently discovered. In order to know the capacities of the well-adapted chromium resistant bacteria, we characterised the microbial community of a treatment plant from chromium contaminated industrial tanning area.

Material and Methods

Isolation of bacterial strains: samples were collected from activated sludge collected in wastewater treatment plant in a chromium-contaminated area. Samples were enriched in the presence of 2 mM Cr (VI). After 3 days incubation at 25°C, aliquots were plated in Nutrient Agar (NA; Difco) and incubated for 48 h, at 30°C. All colonies differing in morphology were isolated, purified and maintained at –80°C in Nutrient Broth (NB; Difco) containing 15% glycerol.

Bacteria characterisation: all isolates were characterised by their, morphology, Gram staining, whole–cell protein profile (SDS-PAGE) and by their fatty acid methyl esters profile (FAME) [1].

Cr(VI) resistance and reduction: all isolates were tested for their resistance to Cr(VI) by growth in NB with increasing Cr(VI) concentrations, at 30°C with 135rpm for 90h, in aerobic and anaerobic conditions. Cr(VI) reducing ability of the isolates was tested in NB with 1 mM Cr(VI) at 30°C with 135 rpm for 72h. The reduction was assayed using the diphenylcarbazide method [2].

Results

A group of 48 strains resistant to Cr(VI) was isolated. The numerical analysis of the protein electrophoregrams of all the bacteria isolated formed 9 clusters and 10 unclustered strains at 75% or higher similarity level. Two major clusters included 49% of the bacteria. The 8 clusters formed after FAME numerical analysis were in agreement with the SDS-PAGE clusters except for cluster G. Cluster I from SDS-PAGE includes clusters A and B from FAME analysis (Table 1).

Table1: Constitution of the populations formed after numerical analysis of the protein electrophoregrams based on 75% similarity or higher and the FAME cluster correspondence.

Protein cluster	Nº isolates	FAME cluster	MIDI identification	Isolates
I	7	A	*Ochrobactrum anthropi*	5-bvl-2b, 5-pte, 5-bvlme-b1, 5-bvl-2a, 5-bvl-1
		B	*Ochrobactrum anthropi*	6-btpll, 12B-c2
un	1	NT	NT	5-bvlme-a
un	1	un	unknown	3'b-2b
II	3	C	unknown	1'-G, 12B-b, 2
un	1	un	NT	12B-c1
un	1	C	unknown	Cas3-d
III	2	D	unknown	2'-P, 5-bvlme-b2
IV	15	E	*Acinetobacter* sp., *A. radioresistens*, or *A. calcoaceticus*	4'-X, 7, Cas3-a1, Cas3-b, 4'-a2, Cas3-c1, Cas3-c2, 4'-Xb, 12A-b, 6-abat, 12A-a2, 4, 12B-d, 6-bo-1
		D	*Acinetobacter johnsonii*	3b-b2
V	1	un	*Clavibacter michiganense* insidiosum	3'-a
	1	un	*Clavibacter michiganense* nebraskense	Cas3-a2
VI	3	F	*Aureobacterium barkeri*	3b-b1, 3'b-1, 12B-a1
un	1	H	*Flavobacterium aquatile*	3ba
VII	2	H	*Flavobacterium aquatile*	3b-a, 3'b-2a
un	1	un	*Comamonas* sp.	8
un	1	H	*Aureobacterium barkeri*	3a
VIII	2	G	*Clavibacter michiganense* nebraskense	Bran3-a2, Bran3-b
un	1	un	*Clavibacter michiganense* nebraskense	Bran3-a1
IX	2	G	*Clavibacter michiganense* nebraskense	12A-a1
		un	unknown	6-bo-2
un	1	G	*Clavibacter michiganense* nebraskense	9
un	1	un	*Clavibacter michiganense* nebraskense	1

un: unclustered; NT: not tested;

Using the MIDI identification system only clusters C and D and 4 unclustered strains were not identified, based on a similarity index greater than 0.6 (Table 1). All tested bacteria were able to grow under aerobic conditions in 1mM Cr(VI). Furthermore, cluster I and VI and two unclustered bacteria were able to grow in 2 mM Cr(VI). Only the strains from cluster I were able to grow under anaerobic conditions in the presence of 1 mM Cr(VI). All tested bacteria showed ability to reduce the concentration of Cr(VI) present in the growth medium (Table 2).

Discussion

Isolated strains were able to stand the presence of 2 mM Cr(VI) during enrichment. After isolation all the strains but 4 were able to grow in the presence of 1 mM Cr(VI). Furthermore, all the strains from SDS-PAGE cluster I (FAME cluster A), one strain from cluster IV, 2 strains from cluster VI and unclustered 5bvlm-a and 3a were able to grow in the presence of 2 mM Cr(VI). These results show once more that resistance to Cr(VI) can be found in several taxonomic groups [2, 3]. Strains from the major cluster E were identified as *Acinetobacter*. The members of this genus are usually found in sewage [4] and this results suggest that the presence of Cr(VI) does not affect this population, although it is one of the populations with a lower ability to reduce Cr(VI) concentration in the medium. The second large cluster (SDS-PAGE cluster I) was identified as *Ochrobactrum anthropi*, a α *Proteobacteria* phylogenetically related to *Brucella*. The α *Proteobacteria* are not usually the major

Table 2: Growth of bacteria isolates from sludge when incubated in NB at 30°C with Cr(VI) under aerobic and anaerobic conditions, and maximal reduction when incubated aerobically in NB at 30°C.

SDS-PAGE cluster	Maximal reduction (%)	Aerobic growth		Anaerobic growth	
		1mM CrVI	2mM CrVI	0mM CrVI	1mM CrVI
I	17,3	++	++[b]	++	+
5-bvlme-a	NT[a]	++	++	++	+
3'b-2b	NT	++	-	++	+
II	6,6	++	-	++	-
12B-c1	NT	++	-	++	-
cas3-d	NT	++	-	++	-
III	12,1	++	-	++	-
IV	10,9	++	-	++	-
V	29,3	++	-	+	-
VI	NT	++	++	++	-
3ba	23,5	++	+	++	-
VII	24,7	++	-	++	-
8	7,8	++	-	++	-
3a	39,1	++	+	++	-
VIII	10,8	+	-	+	-
bran3-a1	9,5	+	-	++	-
IX	10,6	+	-	++	-
9	15,4	++	-	++	-
1	10,3	+	-	++	-

[a]NT: not tested; [b]except strains from FAME cluster B; ++: growth with OD going above 0,5; +: growth was noticed but OD did not go above 0,4; -: no growth was observed during the incubation period.

group of the microbial population of sludge, but their ability to multiply within cultured epithelial cells (Velasco, 1998) and to grow in the presence of Cr(VI), could justify their presence in this tanning sewage. This population includes two clusters, defined by FAME analysis, with different abilities to grow in the presence of Cr(VI) probably as result of a different membrane fatty acid composition. This study isolated Cr(VI) resistant bacteria that can be used in environmental cleanup of industrial wastes.

1.Ferreira A, Morais P, da Costa, M. Computer-aided compairison of protein electrophoretic patterns for grouping and identification of heterotrophic bacteria from mineral water. *J Appli Bacteriology* 1996; 80: 479-486.

2. Ishibashi Y, Cervantes C, Silver, S. Chromium reduction in *Pseudomonas putida*. *Appl Environ Microbiol* 1990; 2268-2270.

3. Peitzch N, Eberz G, Nies D H. Accaligens eutrophus as a bacterial chromate sensor. *Appl Environ Microbiol* 1998; 64: 453-458.

4.Snair J, Amann R, Huber I, Ludwig W, Schleifer K-H. Phylogenetic analysis and in situ identification of bacteria in activated sludge. *Appl Environ Microbiol* 1997; 63: 2884-2896.

5. Velasco J, Romero C, Goni-López I, leiva J, Diaz R, Moriyón I. Evaluation of the relatedness of *Brucella* spp. and *Ochrobactrum anthropi* and description of *Ochrobactrum intermedium* sp. nov., a new species with a closer relantionship to *Brucella* spp. *Int J Syst Bacteriol* 1998; 48: 759-768.

Metal Ions in Biology and Medicine; vol 6. Eds. J.A. Centeno, Ph. Collery, G. Vernet, R.B. Finkelman, H. Gibb, J.C. Etienne. John Libbey Eurotext, Paris © 2000, pp. 678-681.

Comparative study of *Escherichia coli* K-12 and *Lactobacillus plantarum* 195 cells exposed to $HgOH^+$ ions

A. Yu. Ivanov[1, 5], L.A. Khassanova[2, 5], A.V. Gavrjushkin[3], Ph. Collery[5], J.C. Etienne[5], Z.M. Khassanova[4, 5], C. Choisy[2]

[1] Institute of Cell Biophysics, Russian Academy of Sciences, 142292 Pushchino, Russia; [2] Department of Environmental Protection of Bashkir State University, 32, Frunze Street, 450072 Ufa, Russia; [3] State Research Institute of Applied Microbiology, 142279 Obolensk, Russia; [4] Department of Botany of Bashkir State Pedagogical University, 3a, October Revolution Street, 450025 Ufa, Russia; [5] Institut International de Recherche sur les Ions Métalliques, 45, rue Cognacq Jay, Centre Hospitalier Régional Universitaire, 51092 Reims cedex, France

ABSTRACT

The influences of $HgOH^+$ (1-100 μM) on the plasma membranes (PMs) of *Escherichia coli K-12* and *Lactobacillus plantarum* 195 cells were studied by the method of electroorientational spectroscopy (0.5–10 MHz). It was shown that PM damage increased with increasing concentrations of $HgOH^+$. However *L. plantarum* 195 was more resistant than *E. coli* K-12 to the toxic effect of $HgOH^+$. Inhibition of cell wall synthesis of *L. plantarum* 195 achieved by cell washing at 0°C decreased the resistance of their PM to $HgOH^+$. We propose that the observed differences in the sensitivity of *E. coli* K-12 and *L. plantarum* 195 cells may be due to differences in the composition and sizes of their respective cell walls which may affect the accessibility of $HgOH^+$ ions to their PMs.

INTRODUCTION

The toxic effects of heavy metals on bacterial cells and microalgae have been shown to increase considerably when those metals are present in hydrated, univalent form (e.g., $MeOH^+$) (Ivanov et al., 1996 a,b, 1997; Khassanova et al., 1996 a, b). For example, electrophysical analyses of the effects of mercuric ions on *Escherichia coli* K-12 cells have demonstrated dramatic toxic effects of hydrated, univalent forms of that metal on the PM (Khassanova et al., 1998). The susceptibilty of microorganisms to such metal ion damage is known to be determined by the structure and composition of the cell wall, which is thought to affect the accessibility of metal ions to the PM. *Lactobacillus* spp. have highly developed cell walls, the synthesis of which can be controlled *in vitro*. However the resistance of these cells to mercuric ions has not been studied. The aim of the present investigation was to compare the barrier properties of PMs of *Lactobacillus plantarum* 195 cells to those of *Escherichia coli* K-12 cells, which different in size, as they affect resistance to hydrated mercuric ions ($HgOH^+$).

MATERIALS AND METHODS

Escherichia coli K-12 cells were cultured for 8 h in M9 medium in the presence of peptone (10g/l), and *Lactobacillus plantarum* 195 cells were cultured in Rogosa medium (De Man et al., 1960) for 3 h. Both bacterial cultures were grown in shaken flasks (150 rpm) at 37°C. Cells were separated from the growth media by low speed centrifugation, and they were washed in distilled water and incubated in $HgCl_2$ solutions at pH 4.9-5.1, under which conditions the metal is exists in hydrated form ($HgOH^+$). *Lactobacillus plantarum* 195 cells treated to produce cells with incomplete cell walls (1) by performing the washing step described above at 0°C, which arrested further cell wall construction. *Lactobacillus plantarum* 195 cells with complete cell walls (2) were obtained by performing the washing step room temperature.

Solutions with Hg concentrations from 1 to 100 μM were compared with a control solution of NaCl (electroconductivity 0.0035 Sm/m). The electroconductivity of the various $HgCl_2$ solutions were adjusted by adding 10 mM NaCl, adjusting to pH 4.9-5.1 using 0.10 N HCl. Prior to any measurements the cell suspensions (10^7 cells/ml) were exposed to $HgCl_2$ for 15 min at 20°C. The distilled water used in these experiments had electroconductivity less than 0.00013 Sm/m.

The responses of *E. coli* K-12 and *L. plantarum* cells to $HgOH^+$ were determined by electroorientation (EO) spectroscopy. The EO spectra were obtained by measuring the relative changes in the optical density of cell suspension which took place as the cells oriented in a uniform field of alternating current (frequency 0,5-10 MHz; intensity 60 V/cm). Cell PM damages were judged by the EO spectra shifts from the high frequency area to the low frequency area, calculated as the cell EO-effect value: $\Delta\beta/\beta o = (\beta c\text{-}\beta o)/\beta o$ (Khassanova et al., 1998).

RESULTS AND DISCUSSION

The EO spectra of *E. coli* K-12 and *L. plantarum* 195 cells, both intact and treated with different concentrations of $HgOH^+$ ions, are shown on the figure 1 (a,b,c). Spectra changes were observed for all Hg-treated cells. However for *E. coli* K-12 cells and *L. plantarum* 195 cells with incomplete cell walls, these changes took place at lower Hg concentrations than for intact *L. plantarum* 195 cells with complete cell walls.

The concentration-dependencies of cell PM damage (parameter $\Delta\beta/\beta o$) for all $HgOH^+$-treated cells are shown in figure 2. Increases in $HgOH^+$ concentration led to PM damage. *Escherichia coli* K-12 cells were more sensitive to the $HgOH^+$ action. The order of sensitivity was: *E. coli* K-12 > *L. plantarum* 195 with incomplete cell wall > *L. plantarum* 195 with complete cell wall. These differences in the cell sensitivity may be due to the compositional differences in their respective cell walls.

The cell walls of the microorganisms used in this study differ in several important ways. For example, the *E. coli* K-12 cell wall is known to contain one layer of murein, which makes up 10% of the cell wall mass, while the *L. plantarum* 195 cell wall has a thicker murein layer accounting for 30-40% of its cell wall mass. Moreover, inter-peptide connections, which are characteristic of the *L. plantarum* 195 cell wall, are absent in *E. coli* K-12. The special feature of *L. plantarum* 195 cells is the existence of theichoic acids, which are bound to murein through the phosphate. Theichoic acids are not observed in Gram-negative bacteria. However on the surface of *E. coli* murein layer are large amounts of lipids, which comprise some 80% of cell wall mass (the so-called external membrane). The special feature of the external membrane of Gram-negative bacteria is the presence of a great quantity of transmembrane proteins, i.e. porines, which allow low molecular weight, hydrophilic substances to pass through freely (Kvasnikov et al., 1975; Schlegel, 1985). These compositional differences in cell surface layers may confer differential accessibility of metal ions to the respective PMs, which would explain the differential sensitivity to Hg-toxicity demonstrated for *E. coli* K-12 and *L. plantarum* 195 cells in the present study.

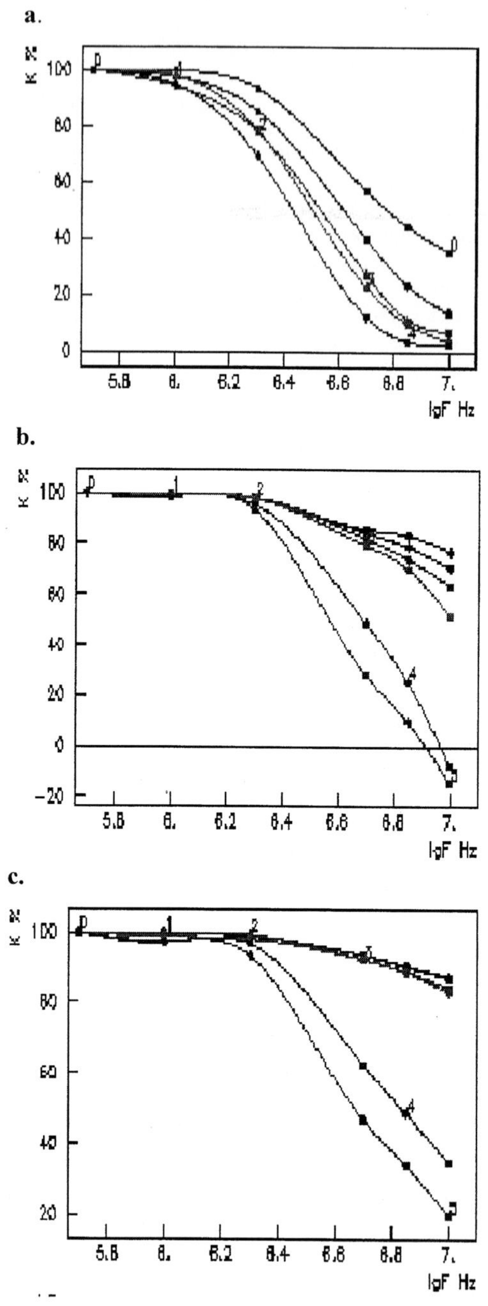

Fig.1. EO spectra of *E. coli* K-12 (a), *L. plantarum* 195 with incomplete cell wall (b), *L. plantarum* 195 with complete cell wall (c), treated with various concentrations of Hg ions: a-b 1.0, 5.0, 10, 50, 100 (1-5), c- 1.0, 5.0, 10, 100 (1-4) μM and control (0). K = $(\Delta D_i / \Delta D_o) \times 100\%$, where ΔD_i is the change in the optical density of cell suspension in the electric field; ΔD_o is the same for the cell suspension incubated under standard conditions at an electric field frequency 0.5 MHz.

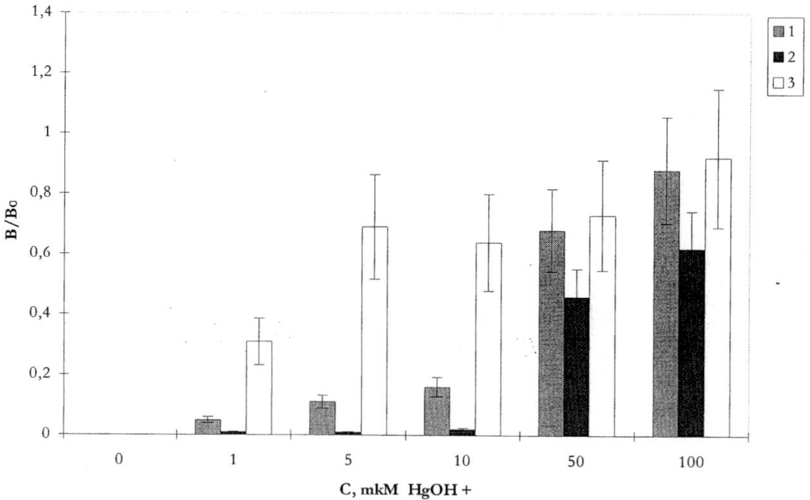

Fig.2. Δβ/βo of *L. plantarum* 195 with incomplete cell walls (1), *L. plantarum* 195 with complete cell wall (2) and *E. coli* K-12 (3), treated by different concentrations of $HgOH^+$.

ACKNOWLEDGEMENTS

The authors would like to acknowledge Dr. Sh. Validov from the Institute of Biochemistry and Physiology of Microorganisms of Russian Academy of Sciences and the Foundation of Pr. Z. Khassanova for their supports in realization of this work.

REFERENCES

DE MAN J.C., ROGOSA M., SHARPE M.E. A medium for the cultivation of *Lactobacillus. J. Appliyed Biol.* 1960, 23: 293-300.

IVANOV A. Yu. et al. Microorganisms as tool of studying copper metal ions-induced in electrophysical cell properties. *Cell. Mol.Biol.* 1996, 42: 825-831.

IVANOV A. Yu. et al. Control by electrical parameters of *Escherichia coli* K-12 membrane damages resulting from metal ions. *Metal Ions in Biology and Medicine*. John Libbey Eurotext (Paris). 1996, 4: 234-237.

IVANOV A. Yu. et al. Toxic effect of hydroxylated metal ions on the plasma membrane of bacterial cells. *Microbiologiya* (Moscow). 1997, 66: 588-594.

KHASSANOVA L.A. et al. Electrophysical analysis of metal ions-induced toxic shock in phototrophic microorganisms. *Metal Ions in Biology and Medicine.* John Libbey Eurotext (Paris). 1996, 4: 229-233.

KHASSANOVA L.A. Electrophysical analysis and physiological-biochemical particularities of cell damages by heavy metal ions. Thesis (St. Petersburg). 1996.

KHASSANOVA Z.M. et al. Significance of environmental conditions in the mercury toxicity for *Escherichia coli* K-12 cells. *Metal Ions in Biology and Medicine*. John Libbey Eurotext (Paris). 1998, 5: 337-343.

KVASNIKOV E.I., NESTERENKO O.A. *Lactobacteria* and paths of their utilization. Nauka (Moscow). 1975, 389 p.

SCHLEGEL H.G. Allgemeine Mikrobiologie. Georg Thieme Verlag (Stuttgart, New York). 1985, 567 p.

Metal Ions in Biology and Medicine; vol 6. Eds. J.A. Centeno, Ph. Collery, G. Vernet, R.B. Finkelman, H. Gibb, J.C. Etienne. John Libbey Eurotext, Paris © 2000, pp. 682-684.

Effects of cadmium and lead on the bioluminescence of *Vibrio fischeri*, and the growth and O_2, uptake of microorganisms

Paul B. Tchounwou, and Lamar Reed

Environmental Toxicology Research Laboratory, NIH-Center for Environmental Health, School of Science and Technology, Jackson State University, Jackson, MS 39217, USA

Abstract: Several studies on heavy metal pollution have indicated that cadmium (Cd) and lead (Pb) rank among the most toxic elements of great environmental and human health concerns. Microorganisms are known to be excellent test organisms because of the relative ease for handling and suitability for analysis. In this research, we tested the toxic effects of Cd and Pb against a marine bacterium (*V. fischeri*), and a heterogenous population of bacteria derived from the Pearl River in Jackson, Mississippi. Using the level of bioluminescence, and the kinetics of dissolved oxygen (DO) uptake and growth as measures of toxicity, Cd and Pb concentrations effecting 50% reduction in these parameters (EC_{50}) were determined as toxic end-points. Bacterial bioluminescence was assessed using the Microtox Assay. Optical density (measure of growth) and oxygen uptake were measured over a 20hrs time period. Pb-EC_{50}s of 0.34 $\pm$ 0.03, 3.10 $\pm$ 0.01and 3.80 $\pm$ 0.02 mg/L were recorded for bioluminescence, growth and dissolved oxygen uptake, respectively. Cd-EC_{50}s were significantly higher ($p<0.05$) than those reported for Pb, indicating that lead was more toxic than cadmium. As expected, study results also indicated that *V. fischeri* was more sensitive (about 5X with Cd, and 10X with Pb) to metal toxicity than the mixed population of Pearl River bacteria. Reductions in bioluminescence, growth, and oxygen uptake were directly correlated to metal concentrations, with toxic levels ranging from slightly toxic in lower concentrations, to extremely toxic in higher ones. Upon 20 hrs of exposure, a strong correlation ($r^2=0.98$) was found between the times required to produce 50% reduction in DO concentrations (T_{50}s), and the concentration levels of heavy metals, indicating a time-response relationship with respect to metal toxicity.

Introduction: Assessing the potential effects of toxic pollutants on the environment is becoming extremely important. Results of laboratory assessments of such contaminants have helped in regulating their use and disposal, and in protecting the quality of the environment. Bioassays used in aquatic toxicology have taken a prominent position among analytical tests for identifying and measuring environmental hazards [1]. Such bioassays have been developed for testing a variety of organic and inorganic chemicals, as well as effluents, surface waters and sediment samples for acute and chronic toxicity. Many bioassays using higher organisms such as fish, protozoa, and algae have been executed, but are labor intensive, time consuming, costly, complex, and often requiring a great deal of equipment [2]. More importantly, these aquatic bioassays do not provide quantitative information on the impact of pollutants on biological treatment systems. In the view of national and international regulations, regulatory agencies are also supporting the development of new toxicity screening procedures which are sensitive, inexpensive, and easier to perform. The use of bacterial *in vitro* assays such as the Microtox Assay have become an attractive alternative to traditional and costly fish and invertebrate methods for toxicological screening. These new assays have been developed to assess the toxicity of various environmental agents, validated and recognized by several standards organizations [3].The purpose of this study was to apply selected microbial test protocols (bioluminescence, growth, and oxygen uptake measurements) to assessing the toxicity of hazardous metals including cadmium and lead.

Experimental Design and Research Methods: The Microtox assay was carried out with a Microtox Model 500 Toxicity Analyzer System (Azur Environmental, Carlsbad, CA). Tests were carried out as described by Azur Environmental [4]. The procedure measured the relative acute toxicity of metal (cadmium or lead) producing data for the calculation of metal concentration effecting 50% reduction in light output (EC_{50}). For each test run, 2 controls without lead, 8 sample/lead dilutions and 2 replicates were done. Tests were carried out on 45.00, 22.50, 11.25, 5.63, 2.81, 1.41, 0.70, and 0.35% of the original metal concentration (4ppm). The sensitivity of the strain of bioluminescent bacteria (*Vibrio fischeri*) was tested for quality control purposes. For growth and oxygen uptake experiments, one liter water sample was collected aseptically from the Pearl River in Jackson, Mississippi. Upon return to the laboratory, bacterial cultures were done by transferring 10 mL of water sample to 990 mL of sterile quarter strength nutrient broth, and incubating the mixture at room temperature (25°C$\pm$0.5°C). A series of 12 autoclaved 1L-capacity reaction beakers containing 500 mL of sterile 1/4 nutrient broth were used. An initial stock of 1000 ppm of Pb or Cd was used to make a serial dilution of 1, 2, 3, 4, 5, and 6 ppm of Pb or Cd. A control growth medium without metal was also made, and the experiment was run in duplicate and repeated two times. Inoculation was made by adding 5 mL of bacterial culture to each of the 12 test containers, followed by a gentle shaking to insure a complete mixing. Growth and oxygen uptake measurements were done continuously every 2 hours for a 20 hrs time period, following previously described protocols [5]. All experiments were done in duplicate and repeated at least once. Descriptive statistics were applied to calculate the means$\pm$SD of all data sets associated with specific metal concentrations. Specific growth and oxygen depletion rates were computed as slopes of graphical representations of raw data versus times. The toxic end-points expressed as 50% growth inhibition concentration or as 50% oxygen depletion concentration (EC_{50}s) were next derived from graphical presentations of these specific rates versus metal concentrations. Furthermore, activity quotients were calculated to determine the degree of toxicity associated with lead exposure. Linear regression analysis was performed to determine the relationship between lead concentrations and the times required for 50% reduction in oxygen uptake (TD_{50}s).

Results and Discussion: Bioluminescence was used as endpoint for measuring the effect of Cd and Pb to *Vibrio fischeri*. For both Cd and Pb, a strong dose-response relationship was determined. The concentration of Cd and Pb effecting 50% reduction in bioluminescence (EC_{50}) were computed to be 0.79$\pm$0.12 mg/L and 0.34$\pm$0.03 mg/L, respectively; indicating that Pb was more toxic than Cd. A strong dose-response relationship was also found in the tests with the mixed population of microorganisms, using growth and oxygen uptake rate as toxicity end-points. Data obtained from growth experiments showed an overall increase in bacterial growth with the increase in holding/incubation time. These data also showed significant reductions in maximum growth rates with increasing concentrations of cadmium or lead. EC_{50} values were computed to be 4.50$\pm$0.04 mg/L, and 3.50$\pm$0.02 mg/L for Cd and Pb, respectively. Experiments assessing the effects of cadmium and lead on the rates of dissolved oxygen uptake by the mixed population of microorganisms indicated significant decreases in individual rates of oxygen uptake with increasing concentrations of cadmium or lead. The mean values of EC_{50} were 5.00$\pm$0.42 mg/L for Cd, and 3.80$\pm$0.04 mg/L for Pb. These data indicated that the mixed population of microorganisms was about 5 times (Cd), and about 10 times (Pb) less sensitive to metal toxicity than the marine bacterium, *Vibrio fischeri* [5]. A strong correlation (r^2=0.98) was found between TD_{50}s (times required to produce 50% reduction in oxygen uptake) and metal concentrations, indicating a time-response relationship with regard to cadmium or lead toxicity [5]. These data support conclusions from previous studies acknowledging bacterial bioassays as viable alternatives to the traditional and costly fish and invertebrate-based assays [6-9]. Among the microbial tests, the Microtox assay has been widely applied to assess the toxicity of a wide range of natural and anthropogenic pollutants [10,11].

Conlusions: Results of this study indicated that Cd and Pb exerted significant toxicity to both *Vibrio fischeri*, and the heterogenous population of microorganisms derived from the Pearl River in Jackson, MS. This toxicity was evidenced by significant reductions in bioluminescence (*V. fischeri*), growth and oxygen uptake rates (mixed population). Also, the data obtained from this research clearly point out the significance of using microbiological systems for acute toxicity testing in aquatic toxicology. Bioassays employed in the present investigation fulfilled the requirement criteria of fast toxicity screening based on their simplicity, speed, cost effectiveness and the fact that bacteria grow rapidly, represent a low trophic level, and thus provide sensitive early warning data of environmental impacts at higher trophic levels. Of the three biosystems evaluated, the Microtox was the most sensitive; yielding EC_{50s} that were only about one tenth of values recorded in batch cultures (growth inhibition and oxygen depletion tests). In batch systems, no significant difference ($p > 0.05$) in EC_{50}s was recorded, indicating that the growth inhibition end-point could be used to predict metal toxicity on the respiration of microorganisms, and vice versa. Although batch systems were time consuming (20 hrs exposure time), and relatively less sensitive than the Microtox, they provided valuable information on the toxic effects of Cd and Pb on microbial growth and respiration. Also, they appeared to be easier to perform, and requiring less expensive equipment (turdibimeter, and dissolved oxygen meter), compared to the high cost of the Microtox analyzer. In this investigation, cadmium and lead were selected as reference toxicants because of their wide distribution in the environment, and their high degree of toxicity to biological systems [12].

Acknowledgments: This research was supported in part by a grant from the U.S. Department of Army (Grant No. DE-W-7505-ENG48) to Lawrence Berkeley National Laboratory, and Subcontract No. 6482515 to Jackson State University, and in part by a grant from the U.S. Department of Energy through the Environmental Technology Consortium, under Cooperative Agreement No. DE-FC04-90AL66158.

References

[1] Bulich AA, Huynh H, Ulitzur S. The use of luminescemt bacteria for measuring chronic toxicity. In: Ostrander GK, ed. *Techniques in Aquatic Toxicology*. Boca Raton: CRC Press - Lewis Publishers. 1996.

[2] Marking LL, Kimerele RA. Aquatic Toxicology Symposium Summary. ASTM 667, American Society for Testing and Materials, Philadelphia, PA. 1979.

[3] ASTM.Test Method for Assessing the Microbial Detoxification of Chemically Contaminated Water and Soil Using a Toxicity Test with a Luminescent Marine Bacterium. ASTM D-5660. American Society for Testing and Materials, Philadelphia, PA. 1995.

[4] Azur Environmental. Microtox - Acute Toxicity Basic Test Procedures. Carlsbad, CA. 1995.

[5] Tchounwou PB, Reed L. Assessment of lead toxicity to the marine bacterium, *Vibrio fischeri*, and to a heterogeneous population of microorganisms derived from the Pearl River in Jackson, Mississippi, USA. *Rev Environ Hlth* 1999; 14(2) : 51-61.

[6] Dombroski EC, Gaudet ID, Florence LZ. A comparison of techniques used to extract solid samples prior to acute toxicity analysis using the Microtox test. *Environ Toxicol Water Qual* 1996; 11 : 121-128.

[7] Ribo JM. Interlaboratory comparison studies of the luminescent bacteria toxicity bioassay. *Environ Toxicol Water Qual* 1997; 12 : 283-294.

[8] VanDam RA, Camilleri C, Finlayson CM. The potential of rapid assessment techniques as early warning indicators of wetland degradation: A review. *Environ Toxicol Water Qual* 1998; 13 : 297-312.

[9] Ghosh SK, Doctor PB, Kulkarni PK. Toxicity of zinc in three microbial test systems. *Environ Toxicol Water Qual* 1996; 9 : 13-19.

[10] Kaiser KLE, Lum KR, Palabrica VS. Review of field applications of the Microtox test in Great Lakes and St. Lawrence river water. *Water Pollut Res J Can* 1988; 23 : 270-278.

[11] Qureshi AD, Flood KW, Thompson SR, Jinhurst SM, Inniss GS, Rokosh DA. Comparison of a luminescent bacterial test with other bioassay for determining toxicity of pure compounds and complex effluents. In: Pearson JG ed. *Proceedings of Fifth Conference on Aquatic Toxicology and Hazard Assessment*. American Society for Testing and Materials, Philadelphia, PA. 1982; 179-195.

[12] Tchounwou PB, Siddig AA, Marian ML. Post-remediation monitoring for soil, sediment and water contamination by lead from a controlled Superfund site in Mississippi. *Environ Toxicol Risk Assess* 2000; (In Press).

Metal Ions in Biology and Medicine; vol 6. Eds. J.A. Centeno, Ph. Collery, G. Vernet, R.B. Finkelman, H. Gibb, J.C. Etienne. John Libbey Eurotext, Paris © 2000, pp. 685-687.

Cytoplasmic protein binds *in vitro* to a sequence in the 3'untranslated region of a novel form of human ferritin heavy chain mRNA

Maire Percy[1, 2, 3], Elisa Chan[3], Hien Chau[3], Simon Wong[3], and Theo Kruck[1, 3]

[1] *Departments of Physiology and* [2] *Obstetrics and Gynaecology, University of Toronto;* [3] *Surrey Place Centre, 2 Surrey Place, Toronto, Ontario, Canada, M5S 2C2*

ABSTRACT

Background: Human brain ferritin heavy (Ft H) chain mRNA differs from liver Ft H mRNA by virtue of an extension of 279 nucleotides (nt) at the end of the 3'untrans-lated region (3'UTR) in which there are 3 putative hairpin loops (L1, L2 and L3). L1 and L2 are conserved in the 3'UTR of human cyclooxygenase-2.

Aim: To determine if cytoplasmic protein in immortalized human B lymphoblasts (LB cells) binds *in vitro* to the L1+L2 sequence of brain Ft H mRNA.

Methods: A native RNA oligonucleotide probe corresponding to L1+L2 was 5'-end-labelled with [γ^{32}P]ATP. Binding between labelled RNA and protein in cytoplasmic lysate of LB cells was studied using band-shift assays with UV cross-linking. Effects of treating lysate with heparin and iron salts were examined.

Results: Addition of RNA probe to LB cell extracts results in the formation of 4 protein-RNA complexes (120, 90, 68 and 56 kDa). Pre-treatment of lysate with heparin alters the electrophoretic mobility of protein-RNA complexes and enhances protein-RNA binding. Pre-treatment with iron salts (0.062 to 3mM) abolishes protein-RNA binding. Heparin and iron effects are independent of new protein synthesis.

Conclusions: LB cell cytoplasm contains a set of proteins that bind to a putative regulatory sequence in the 3'UTR of Ft H mRNA. Such protein-mRNA binding is modulated by heparin and iron, and appears to be distinct from that which occurs between iron regulatory proteins (IRPs) and iron responsive elements (IREs).

Introduction:

A novel human Ft H mRNA species, abundant in adult human brain, lung and white blood cells, was recently discovered. It differs from well-characterized mRNA encoding Ft H chain in liver by virtue of an extension of 279 nt in the 3'UTR that contains 3 putative hairpin loops (L1, L2 and L3). L1 and L2 are conserved in the 3'UTR of the inducible, inflammatory enzyme cyclooxygenase-2 and are distinct in sequence from the IRE motif [1]. Immortalized human LB cells express brain Ft H mRNA and Ft H protein. We asked if cytoplasmic protein in LB cells would bind to the L1+L2 sequence of Ft H mRNA under *in vitro* conditions that permit binding between IRPs and IREs in the 3' or 5'UTRs of various proteins involved in iron metabolism [2,3].

Materials and Methods:

Cytoplasmic extract was prepared from cultured LB cells established from a healthy female. A native RNA oligonucleotide corresponding to nts 1013 to 1095 of brain Ft H mRNA [1] was custom synthesized and 5'end-labelled with [γ^{32}]ATP using T4 polynucleotide kinase. A band-shift assay, in which RNA-protein complexes are cross-linked by UV light, was used to characterize protein-mRNA binding. Complexes were resolved by denaturing polyacrylamide gel electrophoresis. Effects of pre-treating lysate with heparin (often used to reduce "non-specific RNA-binding"), iron salts, actinomycin D (an inhibitor of RNA synthesis), or cycloheximide (an inhibitor of new protein synthesis) on protein-RNA binding were examined. Radioactive bands were visualized by autoradiography.

Results and Discussion:

Fig. 1 demonstrates typical results. Addition of RNA probe to LB cell extract results in the formation of 4 different protein-RNA complexes (120, 90, 68 and 56 kDa) (panels A and B). Specificity of RNA binding is evident from non-competitive inhibition (panel B). Pre-treatment of lysate with heparin (5 mg/ml) alters the mobility of all 4 protein-RNA complexes and enhances the autoradiographic density of the two slowest migrating bands (panel C). Pre-treatment of lysate with iron salts (0.062–3 mM) abolishes protein-RNA binding (panel C). Heparin and iron effects are independent of new protein synthesis. The demonstrated protein-mRNA binding may reflect a new regulatory mechanism that enables Ft H expression and/or localization to be rapidly regulated in response to iron and other signals that mimic *in vitro* heparin effects.

Figure 1: Representative examples of UV cross-linking analysis of binding between cytoplasmic protein in LB cells and labelled RNA probe.

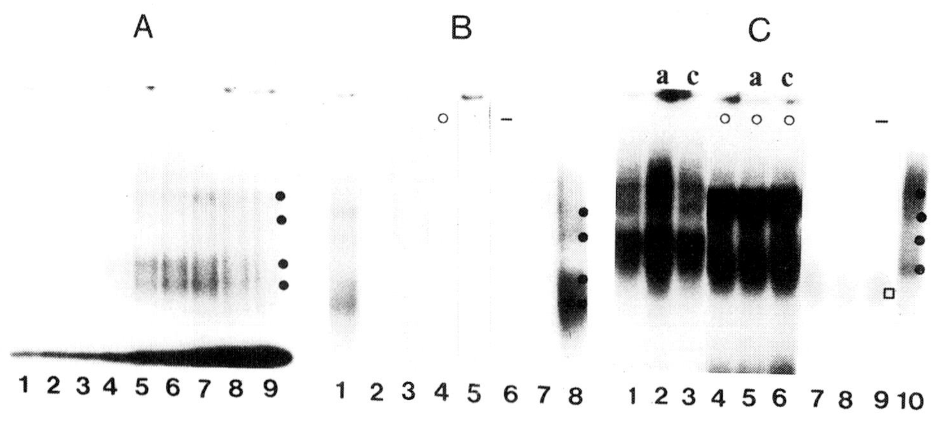

Legend:

In standard experiments, heparin is added after the RNA. In panel A, the dark band at the bottom is unbound RNA probe. In panels B and C, unbound probe was run off the gel to prevent interference with detection of protein-RNA complexes.

Symbols: –, no lysate; o, heparin added before the RNA; c, cycloheximide added before the RNA; a, actinomycin D added before the RNA; ●●●●, positions of the 4 protein-RNA complexes; □, position of RNA probe when lysate is treated with iron salts.

A): Representative band-shift experiments showing that protein-RNA complexes (●●●●) form over a wide range of lysate concentrations. Molecular sizes of complexes are: 120, 90, 68 and 54 kDa. Two-fold serial dilutions of lysate ranged from 1:1 (slot1) to 1:256 (slot 9).

B): Representative composite of control experiments showing that the autoradiogram bands (●●●●) are protein-RNA complexes. Slots 1 and 8: standard experiments. Slot 2: lysate pre-treated with proteinase K. Slot 3: no UV cross-linking. Slots 4 and 5: RNA probe replaced with radioactive ATP; slot 4, heparin added before the radioactive ATP; slot 5, heparin added after UV cross-linking. Slot 6: RNA probe, no lysate. Slot 7: lysate pre-treated with a 100-fold excess of unlabelled RNA probe (non-competitive inhibition experiment).

C): Representative composite of effects of various agents on protein-RNA complex formation. Slots 1-3, heparin added after UV cross-linking. Slots 4-6, heparin added before the RNA (o). Slots 2 and 5: lysate pre-treated with actinomycin D (a). Slots 3 and 6: lysate pre-treated with cycloheximide (c). Slot 7, lysate treated with 3 mM ferrous ammonium sulphate. Slot 8, lysate treated with 3 mM ferric chloride. Slot 9: ferric chloride and RNA probe, but no lysate. Slot 10, lysate pre-treated with 3 mM HCl. Heparin pre-treatment of lysate alters the electrophoretic mobility of the two lower molecular weight complexes and increases the signal intensity of the top two complexes; these effects are independent of new protein and RNA synthesis. Iron compounds abolish protein-RNA binding and result in apparent dimerization of the RNA probe.

Supported by the Rehabilitation Institute (Toronto) and SURF (Caltech).

References:

1. Percy ME, Wong S, Bauer S, Liaghati-Nasseri N, Perry MD, Chauthaiwale VM, Dhar M, Joshi JG. Iron metabolism and human ferritin heavy chain cDNA from adult brain with an elongated untranslated region: new findings and insights. *Analyst* 1998, 123:41-50.
2. Leibold EA, Munro HN. Cytoplasmic protein binds *in vitro* to a highly conserved sequence in the 5'untranslated region of ferritin heavy- and light-subunit mRNAs. *Proc Natl Acad Sci U S A*, 1988, 85, 2171-5.
3. Mullner EW, Neupert B and Kuhn LC. A specific mRNA binding factor regulates the iron-dependent stability of cytoplasmic transferrin receptor mRNA. *Cell* 1989, 58, 373-82.

Metal Ions in Biology and Medicine; vol 6. Eds. J.A. Centeno, Ph. Collery, G. Vernet, R.B. Finkelman, H. Gibb, J.C. Etienne. John Libbey Eurotext, Paris © 2000, pp. 688-690.

Hemochromatosis (HFE) gene analysis of formalin-fixed samples suspect for elevated iron content and hemochromatosis

R.M. Przygodzki[1], Z.D. Goodman[2], L. Rabin[2], J.A. Centeno[3], Y. Liu[1], A.E. Hubbs[1], T.J. O'Leary[1]

[1] *Department of Cellular Pathology, Molecular Division,* [2] *Department of Hepatic and Gastrointestinal Pathology,* [3] *Department of Environmental and Toxicologic Pathology, Armed Forces Institute of Pathology, 6825 16th St., N.W. Washington, D.C., 20306 USA*

Background: Classic hereditary hemochromatosis (HH) is the most prevalent monoallelic genetic disease in Caucasians. The genetic predisposition to HH is linked to the human major-histocompatibility-class I-like protein designated HFE, located on chromosome 6p21.3 [1, 2]. The majority of patients with HH are of Celtic ancestry [2]. It is estimated that 1 in 10 white Americans carries at least one allele with this polymorphism [3]. Several polymorphisms in the hemochromatosis (*HFE*) gene have been identified, of which two are more commonly recognized, i.e. codons 282 and 63 [1]. The most common polymorphic alterations occur at codon 282 (basepair G745A), producing an amino acid change from cysteine to tyrosine. The less prevalent codon 63 (basepair C187G) alteration produces an amino acid change from histidine to aspartic acid. Histologically, there is increased stainable iron on liver biopsy, initially periportally, and later in all parts of the tissue. Scarring and cirrhosis occurs in the advanced stages of this disease when hepatic iron concentrations exceed 20000µg/g dry weight. Clinical evidence of increased transferrin saturation or serum ferritin levels may suggest HH.

Aims: Restriction enzyme digestion of the *HFE* PCR product derived from a peripheral blood sample is the usual diagnostic approach. We, however, sought to investigate whether archival formalin-fixed, paraffin-emdedded biopsy samples sent for consultation to the AFIP with a suspicion for hemochromatosis may indeed display *HFE* alterations. Further, the establishment of the genetic status in a given consult case may be peformed using this methodology on samples that are too small for hepatic iron concentration analysis.

Design: Sixty-one archival hepatic needle biopsy cases from patients suspect for HH on the basis of elevated serum ferritin or transferrin saturation levels, or Prussian blue hepatic iron staining, comprised the study. In addition, twenty-one samples underwent quantitative hepatic iron measurement by flame atomic absorption spectrophotometry [4, 5]. DNA extraction was performed as previously described [6]. PCR amplification for the codon 63 and 282 polymorphisms of the *HFE* gene was performed using flanking intron primers. For the codon 282 polymorphism detection, primers were designed that would avoid the 5569 basepair polymorphism [7, 8]. The PCR products were then cycle-sequenced using the large dye terminator kit (Perkin-Elmer, Foster City, CA) and run on a PE Biosystems 377 automated sequencer (Perkin-Elmer) to determine the genotype(s) present.

Results: Sixteen (26%) cases showed genotypic HH (11 codon 282; 2 codon 63, 3 compound heterozygotes). Seventeen (28%) cases had a single heterozygous alteration (6 codon 282; 11 codon 63), whereas 28 (46%) cases were wildtype. Genotypic HH patients had both markedly higher serum ferritin (wildtype and heterozygous mean of 1090 μg/L versus mutant 1265 μg/L) and hepatic iron index (wildtype and heterozygous mean of 2.07 versus 3.29 for mutant). In addition, they were significantly more likely to have hepatic iron concentrations > 4000 μg/g liver (dry weight) ($p=0.009$ by 2-tailed Fisher's exact test). The observation of a hepatic iron concentration > 2500 μg/g dry weight had a sensitivity and specificity of 1.00 and 0.64 for identification of genotypic HH, though the patient number was small. The low patient number was due to inadequate biopsy tissue amounts for the hepatic iron quantitation assay. If a threshold of 4000 μg/g dry weight was used, the sensitivity and specificity were 0.89 and 0.73, respectively. Prussian blue staining of 4+ had a sensitivity and specificity of 0.83 and 0.74 for identification of genotypic HH; if staining of 3+ or 4+ was used, then the sensitivity and specificity were 0.77 and 0.58, respectively.

Conclusions: Patients whose biopsies were either clinically and/or histologically suspect for HH had a 54% chance of demonstrating *HFE* alterations, and a nearly 1/4 risk of genotypic HH. Neither mild to moderate iron stain positivity nor iron quantity in liver biopsy materials precluded *HFE* alteration, although high hepatic iron was strongly associated with genetic HH. *HFE* genotyping of minute archival liver samples is a feasible alternative to blood sampling in patients with liver disease requiring biopsy, and when liver biopsy samples are too small for hepatic iron concentration assessment.

References:

1. Feder JN, Gnirke A, Thomas W, Tsuchihashi Z, Ruddy DA, Basava A, Dormishian F, Domingo R, Jr., Ellis MC, Fullan A, Hinton LM, Jones NL, Kimmel BE, Kronmal GS, Lauer P, Lee VK, Loeb DB, Mapa FA, McClelland E, Meyer NC, Mintier GA, Moeller N, Moore T, Morikang E, Wolff RK, et al. A novel MHC class I-like gene is mutated in patients with hereditary haemochromatosis [see comments]. *Nat Genet* 1996; 13(4):399-408.
2. Ajioka RS, Jorde LB, Gruen JR, Yu P, Dimitrova D, Barrow J, Radisky E, Edwards CQ, Griffen LM, Kushner JP. Haplotype analysis of hemochromatosis: evaluation of different linkage- disequilibrium approaches and evolution of disease chromosomes. *Am J Hum Genet* 1997; 60(6):1439-47.
3. Edwards CQ, Griffen LM, Goldgar D, Drummond C, Skolnick MH, Kushner JP. Prevalence of hemochromatosis among 11,065 presumably healthy blood donors. *N Engl J Med* 1988; 318(21):1355-62.
4. Pestaner JP, Ishak KG, Mullick FG, Centeno JA. Ferrous sulfate toxicity: a review of autopsy findings. *Biol Trace Elem Res* 1999; 69(3):191-8.
5. Centeno JA, Pestaner JP, Mullick FG, Virmani R. An analytical comparison of cobalt cardiomyopathy and idiopathic dilated cardiomyopathy. *Biol Trace Elem Res* 1996; 55(1-2):21-30.
6. Przygodzki RM, Finkelstein SD, Langer JC, Swalsky PA, Fishback N, Bakker A, Guinee DG, Koss MN, Travis WD. Analysis of p53, K-ras-2, and C-raf-1 in pulmonary neuroendocrine tumors: Correlation with histologic subtype and clinical outcome. *Am J Pathol* 1996; 148(5):1531-41.
7. de Villiers JN Kotze MJ. Significance of linkage disequilibrium between mutation C282Y and a MseI polymorphism in population screening and DNA diagnosis of hemochromatosis. *Blood Cells Mol Dis* 1999; 25(3-4):250-2; discussion 253-4.
8. Jeffrey GP, Chakrabarti S, Hegele RA, Adams PC. Polymorphism in intron 4 of HFE may cause overestimation of C282Y homozygote prevalence in haemochromatosis [letter] [see comments]. *Nat Genet* 1999; 22(4):325-6.

Metal Ions in Biology and Medicine; vol 6. Eds. J.A. Centeno, Ph. Collery, G. Vernet, R.B. Finkelman, H. Gibb, J.C. Etienne. John Libbey Eurotext, Paris © 2000, pp. 691-693.

Direct protein to protein copper(I) transfer

Paul Cobine, Christopher E. Jones, Lisa N. Deecke, Wasantha A. Wickramasinghe and Charles T. Dameron

The National Research Centre for Environmental Toxicology, The University of Queensland, 39 Kessels Road, Coopers Plains, Brisbane, Australia, 4108

Introduction

The Gram positive bacterium *Enterococcus hirae* has a simple copper metabolic pathway that is analogous to the pathway in mammalian cells and utilizes copper chaperones, homologous to those in mammals, to transfer and insert copper into apo-enzymes. A number of critical enzymes and proteins utilize copper ions in either a catalytic or structural capacity. Copper chaperones are part of the mechanism by which copper is delivered to and inserted into these proteins [1, 2]. The copper homeostasis gene products of *E. hirae* are translated from the *cop* operon which encodes *copZ-copY-copA-copB* [3]. The respective gene products are a copper chaperone, CopZ; a copper regulated repressor, CopY; and two ATPase pumps CopA and CopB. The current understanding of the *cop* system is that cellular copper levels are regulated by the import and export pumps (CopA and CopB) whose expression is control by CopY [4, 5]. Copper regulates the expression of the operon. CopZ delivers copper(I) to the repressor CopY causing it to lose its DNA binding activity and, thereby, promotes the transcription of the operon. In the delivery process copper(I) is transferred from an exposed site in CopZ to a solvent shielded site in CopY that is luminescent. Using the movement of copper(I) to a larger protein and the increase in copper(I)-thiolate specific luminescence during the metal transfer has enabled us to develop two independent *in vitro* copper transfer assays [5] that are being used to develop an understanding of metal transfer processes.

The copper chaperones are a homologous group of proteins having a $\beta\alpha\beta\beta\alpha\beta$ global fold and an exposed -CxxC- metal binding loop [6]. Despite this conservation of exposed binding site and tertiary fold, metallochaperones function specifically. The second metal binding module Menkes protein (MNKr2), a homologue of CopZ, is unable to act as a chaperone for CopY. The existence of charged faces in the metallochaperones and their importance in the interaction with target proteins had been proposed [6, 7]. We demonstrate that the addition of 2 pairs of lysines to a face of MNKr2 enables it to dock and transfer copper(I) to CopY, a gain of function mutation.

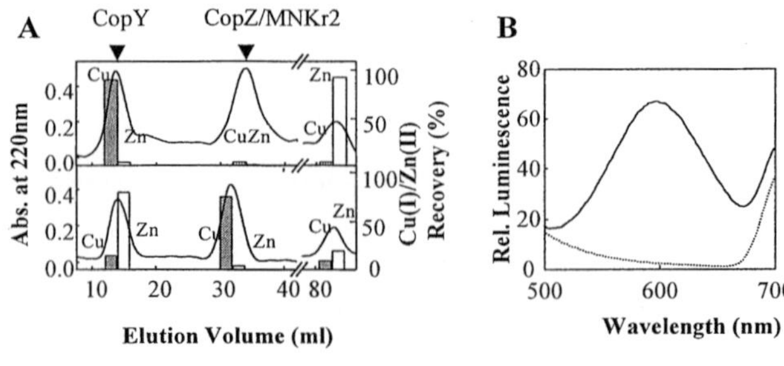

Figure 1: A) Gel filtration of Cu(I):chaperone with larger target. CopZ transfer Cu(I) (top) while MNKr2 (bottom) retains Cu(I).
B) The transfer from Cu(I)CopZ monitoring the formation of a luminescent Cu(I)CopY (solid line). While MNKr2 retains the copper in a poorly shielded metallochaperone binding site(dashed).

Results and Discussion

The CopZ-CopY-interaction results in transient docking and copper transfer from a small protein to a larger one and is monitored by gel filtration, Figure 1A [5]. The transfer of Cu(I) to CopY displaces a Zn(II) molecule, required for DNA binding activity. Copper moves from an exposed binding site in CopZ to a copper-thiolate binding site in CopY that is shielded from solvent interactions. Secluded Cu(I)-S sites are luminescent and have been studied in proteins such as metallothionein and ACE1 [8]. The transfer of copper from the chaperone to its target is easily monitored by emission at 600 nm Figure 1B. In contrast the homologue MNKr2 retains copper in its exposed metal binding site Figure 1A &B. These *in vitro* results define a specificity for chaperone-target interaction.

The NMR structure of CopZ shows that it has a distinct charge distribution. It is the charge distribution that is widely regarded as the key to the specificity of the chaperone-target interaction [2, 6, 7, 9]. Further emphasis is placed on the distribution of charge by the site-directed mutations of Atx1p [9]. The mutations made at specific lysine residues of Atx1p led to a loss of chaperone function in Atx1p-Ccc2p assay. Primary sequence alignment show that these residues are absent in CopZ, Figure 2. A CopZ lysine rich face lies along the β-sheet of the chaperone [6]. Replacement of residues 31,32(Q,R) and

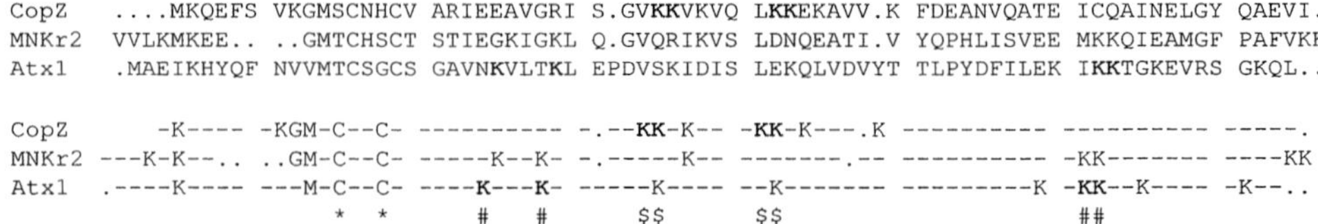

Figure 2: Sequence alignment of metallochaperones from *E. hirae*, *H. sapiens* and *S. cerevisiae*.
* conserved -CxxC- motif, $ position of the lysine residues engineered into MNKr2, # residues mutated by Portnoy *et al* [9].

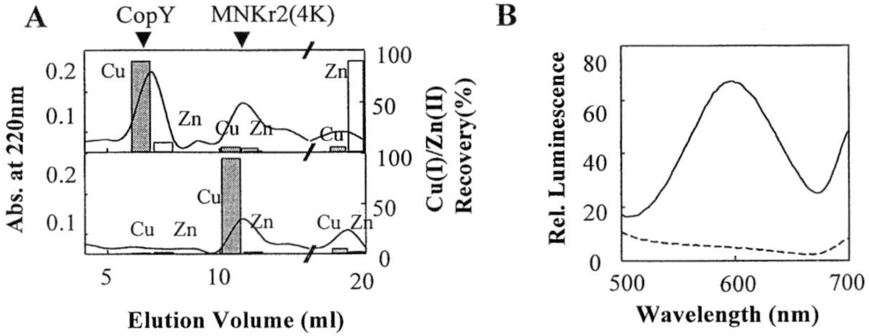

Figure 3: A) Gel filtration of MNKr2(4K) incubated with CopY (top) and alone (bottom)
B) Relative luminescence of CopY/MNKr2(4K) (solid) vs Cu(I):MNKr2(4K)(dashed)

37,38 (D,N) in MNKr2 with lysine yielded a mutant protein carrying the lysine arrangement of CopZ. The mutant, MNKr2(4K) expressed to the same level as the wild type and was purified in the same manner [10]. The addition of the lysine residues had no apparent effect on the native metal binding properties of the protein. MNKr2(4K) was assessed on its ability to transfer Cu(I) to CopY. In contrast to MNKr2 the addition of a lysine face in MNKr2(4K) resulted in transfer of Cu(I) to CopY. Transfer was demonstrated by both gel filtration and luminescence assays, Figure 3. It was apparent that the inclusion of the lysine face provides a significant increase in recognition of the target protein. The development of a more sensitive assay is required to further understand the mechanics of this transient interaction. These results however do provide us with a starting point for the elucidation of the mechanism of recognition.

References

[1] Valentine, J.S. and Gralla, E.B. (1997) Science 278, 817-818.
[2] Harrison, M.D., Jones, C.E., Solioz, M. and Dameron, C.T. (2000) TIBS 25, 29-32.
[3] Strausak, D. and Solioz, M. (1997) J. Biol. Chem. 272, 8932-8936.
[4] Solioz, M., Odermatt, A. and Krapf, R. (1994) FEBS Lett. 346, 44-47.
[5] Cobine, P., Wickramasinghe, W.A., Harrison, M.D., Weber, T., Solioz, M. and Dameron, C.T. (1999) FEBS Lett. 445, 27-30.
[6] Wimmer, R., Herrmann, T., Solioz, M. and Wuthrich, K. (1999) J. Biol. Chem. 99, 22597-22603.
[7] Rosenzweig, A.C., Huffman, D.L., Hou, M.Y., Wernimont, A.K., Pufahl, R.A. and O'Halloran, T.V. (1999) Structure 7, 605-617.
[8] Dameron, C.T., Winge, D.R., George, G.N., Sansone, M., Hu, S. and Hamer, D. (1991) Proc. Natl. Acad. Sci. USA 88, 6127-6131.
[9] Portnoy, M.E., Rosenzweig, A.C., Rae, R., Huffman, D.L., O'Halloran, T.V. and Culotta, V.C. (1999) J. Biol. Chem. 274, 15041-15045.
[10] Harrison, M.D., Meier, S. and Dameron, C.T. (1999) Biochim. Biophys. Acta 1453, 254-260.

Metal Ions in Biology and Medicine; vol 6. Eds. J.A. Centeno, Ph. Collery, G. Vernet, R.B. Finkelman, H. Gibb, J.C. Etienne. John Libbey Eurotext, Paris © 2000, pp. 694-697.

Phosphorylation of the metal-activated transcription factor in response to metals

Timothy K. Adams and Jonathan H. Freedman

Nicholas School of the Environment, Duke University, Durham, NC 27708, USA

INTRODUCTION

The primary mechanism for metal detoxification is chelation by metallothionein (MT). Metallothioneins are small (~60 amino acid residues) cysteine-rich proteins that are ubiquitous among eukaryotes [1]. Vertebrate MTs complex seven atoms of zinc and/or cadmium per polypeptide [2]. In a broad spectrum of animal tissues and cultured cells, elevated concentrations of many transition metals elicit rapid induction of MT mRNAs and proteins [1,2]. The induction of MTs by physiological concentrations of zinc and copper, and the high affinities of MT for these metals suggest that it plays a key role in metal homeostasis [1,2]. The observations that cadmium and other non-essential metals (mercury, lead] are strong inducers of MT transcription and have high affinities for the protein [1,2], suggests that MT also functions in metal detoxification.

Regulation of MT transcription by metals is mediated by the binding of specific transcription factors to one or more promoter elements, designated metal responsive elements (MREs). Gel mobility shift, DNase I footprinting and *in vitro* transcription assays have been used to identify several potential MRE-binding transcription factors in mice, rats and humans [3]. A protein in mice, designated MTF-1 (MRE-binding transcription factor), that is responsible for zinc-inducible MT-I transcription has been isolated [4]. MTF-1 binding to MREs is also induced by oxidative stress [5]. MTF-1 contains six zinc finger domains and several *trans*-activation domains: acidic-rich, proline-rich and serine/threonine-rich. The serine/threonine domain contains several potential protein kinase C and casein kinase II phosphorylation sites. Deletion analysis of MTF-1 suggests that interactions among all of the functional domains are required for metal-inducible transcription [6].

Schaffner *et al* [4] proposed that MTF-1 regulates transcription by acting as a zinc sensor, which in the absence of metal cannot bind to MREs. As cells accumulate zinc, the metal binds in the finger domains causing a conformational change in the protein and subsequent binding to DNA. When MT levels are sufficient, it removes the zinc from MTF-1, thereby inactivating the transcription factor.

An alternative model posed by Palmiter [7], hypothesizes a zinc sensitive inhibitor which complexes with MTF-1 rendering it inactive. As cellular zinc levels increase, the metal binds with the inhibitor releasing it from MTF-1, allowing the transcription factor to active MT expression.

Typically, zinc is used as an inducer to investigate the interactions among MREs, MTF-1 and MT transcription. There is a paucity of information regarding the molecular mechanism of MT transcriptional activation by cadmium or other transition metals. Electrophoretic mobility shift and transcriptional analyses with MT promoter fragments demonstrate that cadmium-activation of MT expression is mediated by MREs [8]. Furthermore, cadmium exposure does not induce MT-I or MT-II transcription in mouse embryonic stem cells in which both alleles of the MTF-1 gene are disrupted [9]. This suggests that cadmium-induced MT transcription is controlled through the interaction between MTF-1 and MREs. Current models describing the regulation of MT transcription however, do not adequately explain MTF-1 activation by metals other than zinc.

Here we investigate a third model in which transition metals activate signal transduction cascades that ultimately cause a change in MTF-1 phosphorylation. It is the change in MTF-1 phosphorylation that affects its ability to activate MT transcription.

EXPERIMENTAL PROCEDURES

Expression Plasmid

An ~2Kb cDNA fragment that includes the coding region for the mouse MTF-1 (gift of Dr. William Schaffner) was directionally cloned into the pCDNA3.1-myc-his expression vector (Invitrogen). Transfection of cultured cells with this construct results in the constitutive expression of an MTF-1-myc-his fusion protein. The fusion peptide contains a His_6-tag, which can be used for protein purification, and a myc epitope, to identify the expressed protein by Western immunoblot analysis.

Cell Culture and Transfection

COS-7 cells were maintained in complete Dulbecco's Modified Eagle's medium containing 10% fetal bovine serum, 5% non-essential amino acids, 5% L-glutamine and 5% penicillin/streptomycin at 37°C in 5% CO_2. For transfection studies, cells were grown to 50% confluency in 150-mm plates. The medium was removed, and the cells were then washed with Opti-MEM reduced serum medium. Transient transfection with the MTF-1-myc-his expression plasmid was accomplished by lipofection. After six hours, the transfection medium was replaced with complete medium, and the cells were then incubated for an additional 72 h. Following this incubation, the cells were washed with phosphate free medium, and then phosphate free medium containing ^{32}P-orthophosphate (0.25 mCi/ml) was added. Transfected and non-transfected cells were then incubated for 5 h in the presence of either 10μm $CdCl_2$, 100μm $ZnCl_2$ or no added metal.

Extracts/Purification/Analysis

Cells were lysed in a 1% Triton-X/8M urea buffer. The MTF-1-myc-his protein was then purified using Ni-NTA affinity chromatography (Qiagen). Eluted proteins were resolved by SDS-PAGE and subsequently transferred to PVDF membranes. The identification and quantification of ^{32}P-labeled proteins were accomplished by autoradiography and PhosphorImager analysis. The location of the fusion protein was determined by Western immunoblot analysis, using either anti-myc or anti-poly-His_4 antibodies, and enhanced chemiluminescence (ECL). To assess phosphorylation status of the MTF-1 fusion protein, autoradiographs and Western blots were aligned.

	^{32}P-Labeled Proteins				**Western Immunoblot**			
MTF-1	-	+	-	+	-	+	-	+
Zinc	-	-	+	+	-	-	+	+

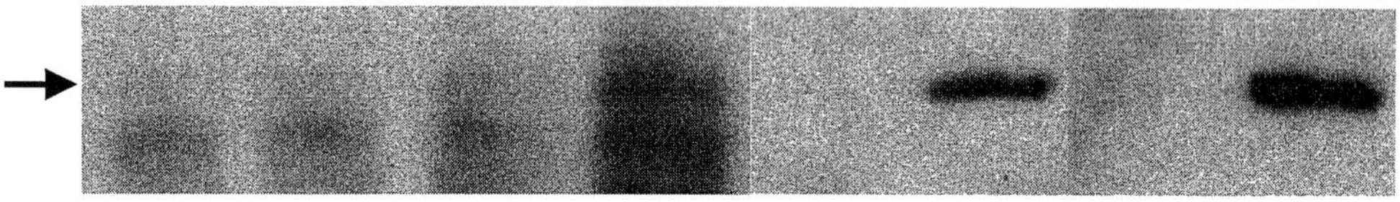

Figure 1. Ni-NTA purified, ^{32}P-labled proteins were separated by SDS-PAGE and immobilized on PVDF membranes. *left panel*; autoradiogram following a 60 min exposure. *right panel*; MTF-1-myc-his visualized by ECL using a mixture of anti-myc or anti-poly-His_4 antibodies. The *arrow* indicates the position of the MTF-1-myc-his fusion protein.

RESULTS/DISCUSSION

Western blot analysis confirms that there is a high level of MTF-1 fusion protein expression in both metal-treated and non-exposed cells (Fig. 1). In the absence of added metal, MTF-1 is phosphorylated. Cadmium exposure did not appear to affect the level phosphorylation, compared to non-exposed cells (results not shown). In contrast, the level of phosphorylation/per unit protein increased when cells are exposed to zinc (Fig. 1). These results support a model in which the phosphorylation of MTF-1 may affect its ability to act as a transcriptional activator.

Palmiter proposed the MTF-1-inhibtor model based on the ability of a soluble factor to restore zinc-inducible MT transcription in a variant cell line that constitutively expressed MT [7]. Based on the observation that MTF-1 is phosphorylated *in vivo*, we suggest that this factor may be a protein kinase or phosphatase. This kinase or phosphatase may be near the end of potentially many different signal transduction pathways. Independent pathways may respond to different metals and other MT inducers. Once the kinase or -phosphatase is activated, it induces MT transcription by modifying MTF-1. The modification may be an increase in level of MTF-1 phosphorylation, or a change in the specific amino acid residue that is phosphorylated. Further, the specific modification may depend on the individual inducer.

REFERENCES

1. Hamer, DH. Metallothionein. *Annu Rev Biochem* 1986; 55: 913-951.
2. Kagi, JHR Schaffer, A. Biochemistry of metallothionein. *Biochemistry* 1988; 27: 8509-8515.
3. Searle, PF. Zinc dependent binding of a liver nuclear factor to metal response element MRE-a of the mouse metallothionein-I gene and variant sequences. *Nucleic Acids Res* 1990; 18: 4683-4690.
4. Radtke, F, Heuchel, R, Georgiev, O, Hergersberg, M, Gariglio, M, Dembic, Z Schaffner, W. Cloned transcription factor MTF-1 activates the mouse metallothionein I promoter. *EMBO J* 1993; 12: 1355-1362.
5. Dalton, TP, Li, Q, Bittel, D, Liang, L Andrews, GK. Oxidative stress activates metal-responsive transcription factor-1 binding activity. Occupancy *in vivo* of metal response elements in the metallothionein-I gene promoter. *J Biol Chem* 1996; 271: 26233-26241.
6. Radtke, F, Georgiev, O, Muller, HP, Brugnera, E Schaffner, W. Functional domains of the heavy metal-responsive transcription regulator MTF-1. *Nucleic Acids Res* 1995; 23: 2277-2286
7. Palmiter, RD. Regulation of metallothionein genes by heavy metals appears to be mediated by a zinc-sensitive inhibitor that interacts with a constitutively active transcription factor, MTF-1. *Proc Natl Acad Sci USA* 1994; 91: 1219-1223.
8. Datta, PK Jacob, ST. Activation of the metallothionein-I gene promoter in response to cadmium and USF *in vitro. Biochem Biophys Res Commun* 1997; 230: 159-163.
9. Heuchel, R, Radtke, F, Georgiev, O, Stark, G, Aguet, M Schaffner, W. The transcription factor MTF-1 is essential for basal and heavy metal-induced metallothionein gene expression. *EMBO J* 1994; 13: 2870-2875.

Metal Ions in Biology and Medicine; vol 6. Eds. J.A. Centeno, Ph. Collery, G. Vernet, R.B. Finkelman, H. Gibb, J.C. Etienne. John Libbey Eurotext, Paris © 2000, pp. 698-700.

Activation of estrogen receptor-alpha by the heavy metal cadmium

Adriana Stoica[1], Benita S. Katzenellenbogen[2], Mary Beth Martin[1]

[1] Department of Biochemistry and Molecular Biology, Vincent T. Lombardi Cancer Center, Georgetown University, Washington, DC, 20007, USA; [2] Department of Molecular and Integrative Physiology, University of Illinois, Urbana, IL 61801, USA

Estrogens are a family of steroidal hormones that are synthesized in a variety of tissues but are produced primarily in the ovaries. The principal function of estrogens is to promote the growth and differentiation of the sexual organs and other tissues related to reproduction. The disruption of the reproductive system of male and female animals in the wild has been attributed to environment contaminants which mimic the effects of estradiol. It has been suggested that the high incidence of hormone related cancers and diseases is also due to the presence of environmental estrogens. In fact, a number of chemicals in the environment demonstrate estrogen-like activity when tested in biological systems (1).

The biological effects of estrogens are mediated by estrogen receptors (ER) alpha and beta. The estrogen receptor isoforms belongs to a family of closely related genes that include the glucocorticoid, progesterone, mineralocorticoid, thyroid, retinoic acid, and vitamin D receptors (2). All receptors in this gene family appear to have similar structural and functional domains. The estrogen receptor is divided into domains, termed A through F, based on regions of sequence homology between the human estrogen receptor and the chicken estrogen receptor (3). Region A/B is the variable N-terminal region of the receptor which is important in transactivation of transcription (3). The central region, domain C, is a short well conserved cysteine rich region which corresponds to the DNA binding domain. The cysteine residues are capable of forming 2 zinc fingers. The DNA binding fingers are formed when the cysteines tetrahedrically coordinate with a zinc ion allowing the intervening amino acids to form fingers which interact specifically with DNA (4;5). The most structurally and functionally complex region of the receptor is the C-terminal domain which corresponds to regions D, E, and F. Region E is the hormone binding domain which is composed of alpha helices that form a hydrophobic ligand binding pocket. Similar to other receptors (6-12), the hormone binding domain of the estrogen receptor contains twelve alpha-helices (H1-H12) folded into a three-layered antiparallel alpha-helical sandwich. The central core layer contains three alpha-helices (H5/6, H9, and H10) sandwiched between two additional layers of helices composed of H1-4, H7, H8, and H11. The central core of the hormone binding domain is flanked by helix H12. It has been proposed that the hormone binding domain functions in a manner similar to a "mouse trap" (6). Upon binding, the ligand induces a conformational change resulting in the formation of a salt bridge between H4 and H12 repositioning helix H12 over the central core and consequently entrapping the hormone. Ultimately, the repositioning of helix H12 results in the formation of a transcriptionally active receptor. In addition to transcriptional activation, the C-terminal region is also responsible for hormone induced dimerization of the receptor (13).

Although steroid receptors are zinc binding proteins, several other metals interact with steroid receptors and influence their structure and function. Nickel, copper, cadmium, and cobalt have been shown to substitute for zinc in the zinc finger of ERα and to influence the binding of the DNA binding domain to an estrogen response element (14). The replacement of zinc with either nickel or copper inhibits the binding of the DNA binding domain to an estrogen response element, whereas, replacement of zinc with either cadmium or cobalt has no effect on specific DNA binding.

In addition to the DNA binding domain, metals have been shown to bind to the hormone binding domain of receptors and to block binding of the ligand. In the case of ERα, calcium has been shown to reversibly block the binding of estradiol (15). Interaction of arsenite, cadmium, and selenite with cysteines in the hormone binding domain of the glucocorticoid receptor has also been shown to inhibit the binding of dexamethasone to the receptor while zinc had no effect on ligand binding (16).

Studies from this laboratory have shown that the cadmium mimics the effects of estradiol in the estrogen responsive breast cancer cell line, MCF-7 (17). Similar to treatment with estradiol, treatment of cells with cadmium decreased the amount of estrogen receptor protein and mRNA. The effects of cadmium on ER expression occurred at the level of transcription as evidenced by an inhibition of ER gene transcription. Treatment of cells with cadmium also increased the expression of several estradiol inducible genes. The amount of progesterone receptor protein and mRNA increased significantly following exposure to the metal. The amount of cathepsin D also increased after treatment with the metal. Although cadmium had an inhibitory effect on the transcription of the ER gene, it stimulated the transcription of the genes for progesterone receptor and pS2. The effects of cadmium were blocked by an antiestrogen demonstrating that the effects of the metal are mediated by the estrogen receptor. More important than its effects on gene expression, cadmium also stimulated the proliferation of MCF-7 cells. To understand the mechanism by which cadmium activates ERα, the ability of cadmium to bind to and activate wild type and various mutants of ERα was examined. When tested in transient co-transfection assays in COS-1 cells, cadmium concentrations as low as 10^{-10} M activated ERα. Scatchard analysis employing either purified human recombinant ERα or extracts from ER-containing MCF-7 cells demonstrated that ^{109}Cd binds to the estrogen receptor with an equilibrium dissociation constant of approximately 4 to 5×10^{-10} M. Cadmium also blocked the binding of estradiol to ERα ($K_i = 0.48 \times 10^{-9}$ M), suggesting that the heavy metal interacts with the hormone binding domain of the receptor. To study the role of the hormone binding domain in cadmium activation, COS-1 cells were transiently co-transfected with GAL-ER, a chimeric receptor containing the DNA binding domain of the transcription factor GAL4 and the hormone binding domain of ERα, and a GAL4-responsive reporter gene. Treatment of the transfected cells with either 10^{-6} M cadmium or 10^{-9} M estradiol resulted in a four-fold increase in reporter gene activity. The effect of cadmium on the chimeric receptor was blocked by the antiestrogen, ICI-164,384, suggesting that cadmium activates ERα through an interaction with the hormone binding domain of the receptor. Transfection and binding assays with ERα mutants identified C381, C447, E523, H524, and D538 as possible interaction sites of cadmium with the hormone binding domain of the receptor. When C381 and C447 were mutated to alanines, the ability of cadmium to bind to the receptor was not altered, but the ability of cadmium to transactivate the receptor was lost. Mutation of either E523, H524, or D538 resulted in the complete loss of binding and activation. The precise role of these amino acids in the interaction and activation of the estrogen receptor by cadmium remains unknown. It is not known whether these amino acids participate directly in the formation of the metal binding site or indirectly in the recruitment of cadmium to the binding site within the receptor. Although the mechanism by which the metal activates the estrogen receptor remains to be established, the studies described above provide evidence that cadmium is a potent nonsteroidal estrogen. The metal binds with high affinity to the hormone binding domain of the estrogen receptor and consequently activates the receptor.

Reference List

1. **Colborn T, von Saal FS, Soto AM** 1993 Developmental effects of endocrine-disrupting chemicals in wildlife and humans. Environ Health Persp 101:378-384

2. **Beato M** 1989 Gene regulation by steroid hormones. Cell 56:335-344

3. **Kumar V, Green S, Stack G, Berry M, Jin J.R., Chambon P** 1987 Functional domains of the human estrogen receptor. Cell 51:941-951

4. **Miller J, McLachlan AD, Klug A** 1985 Repetitive zinc-binding domains in the protein transcription factor IIIA from Xenopus oocytes. EMBO J 4:1609-1614

5. **Krust A, Green S, Argos P, Kumar V, Walter P, Bornert JM, Chambon P** 1986 The chicken oestrogen receptor sequence: Homology with v-erbA and the human oestrogen and glucocorticoid receptors. EMBO J 5:891-897

6. **Wurta JM, Bourguet W, Renaud JP, Vivat V, Chambon P, Moras D, Gronemeyer H** 1996 A canonical structure for the ligand-binding domain of nuclear receptors. Nature Structural Biology 3:87-94

7. **Renaud JP, Rochel N, Ruff M, Vivat V, Chambon P, Gronemeyer H, Moras D** 1996 Crystal structure of the RAR-gamma ligand-binding domain bound to all-trans retinoic acid. Nature 378:681-689

8. **Bourguet W, Ruff M, Chambon P, Gronemeyer H, Moras D** 1995 Crystal structure of the ligand-binding domain of the human nuclear receptor RXR-alpha. Nature 375:377-382

9. **Brzozowski AM, Pike ACW, Dauter Z, Hubbard RE, Bonn T, Engstrom O, Ohman L, Greene GL, Gustafsson J, Carlquist M** 1997 Molecular basis of agonism and antagonism in the estrogen receptor. Nature 389:753-758

10. **Wagner RL, Apriletti JW, McGrath ME, West BL, Baxter JD, Fletterick RJ** 1995 A structural role for hormone in the thyroid hormone receptor. Nature 378:690-697

11. **Tanenbaum DM, Wang Y, Williams SP, Sigler PB** 1998 Crystallographic comparison of the estrogen and progesterone receptor's ligand binding domain. Proc Natl Acad Sci USA 95:5998-6003

12. **Shiau AK, Barstad D, Loria PM, Cheng L, Kushner PJ, Agard DA, Greene GL** 1998 The structural basis of estrogen receptor/coactivator recognition and the antagonism of this interaction by tamoxifen. Cell 95:927-937

13. **Kumar V, Chambon P** 1988 The estrogen receptor binds tightly to its responsive element as a ligand-induced homodimer. Cell 55:145-156

14. **Predki PF, Sarkar B** 1992 Effect of replacement of "Zinc fingers" Zinc on estrogen receptor DNA interactions. J Biol Chem 267:5842-5846

15. **Maaroufi Y, Hardouze AB, LeClercq G** 1997 Decrease of hormone binding capacity of estrogen receptor by calcium. J Receptor Signal Transduction Research 17:833-853

16. **Simons SSJr, Chakraborti PK, Cavanaugh AH** 1990 Arsenite and cadmium(II) as probes of glucocorticoid receptor structure and function. J Biol Chem 265:1938-1945

17. **Garcia-Morales P, Saceda M, Kenney N, Kim N, Salomon DS, Gottardis MM, Solomon HB, Sholler PF, Jordan VC, Martin MB** 1994 Effect of cadmium on estrogen receptor levels and estrogen-induced responses in human breast cancer cells. J Biol Chem 269:16896-16901

Metal Ions in Biology and Medicine; vol 6. Eds. J.A. Centeno, Ph. Collery, G. Vernet, R.B. Finkelman, H. Gibb, J.C. Etienne. John Libbey Eurotext, Paris © 2000, pp. 701-703.

Molybdenum-induced endocrinopathy in thiomolybdate-treated sheep: a histological and immunocytochemical study

Susan Haywood[1], Zuhal Dincer[1], and Bharat Jasani[2]

[1] *Department of Veterinary Pathology, University of Liverpool, L69 3BX UK;* [2] *Department of Pathology, University of Wales College of Medicine, CF4 4XN, UK.*

Molybdenum (Mo) is a trace element essential for the activity of xanthine oxidase, sulphite oxidase and aldehyde oxidase. Genetically conditioned and nutritional deficiencies are extremely rare and there is little substantiated information on Mo toxicity in man, until recently, when a case of acute toxicity with neurological and reproductive endocrine complications was reported from consumption of a Mo supplement[1]. Mo toxicity has been recognised in animals, although information is still scarce. Mo supplementation has been reported to reduce fertility in cows and heifers apparently by interfering with release of pituitary luteinizing hormone[2]. More recently, copper poisoned sheep treated with ammonium tetrathiomolybdate TTM became infertile with elevated concentrations of Mo in the brain[3] and experimental studies confirmed that Mo is retained for long periods in brain, pituitary and other endocrine glands[4].

It is hypothesised that Mo (as molybdate) may severely affect the brain and/or neuroendocrine axis and the present study aimed to explore any histological and immunocytochemically detectable changes in the damaged pituitaries, ovaries and testes and adrenal glands of thiomolybdate treated sheep.

Materials and Methods

Tissues were utilised from five cases of TTM dosed sheep with six undosed control sheep.

Histopathology

Pituitary, adrenal, ovarian and testicular tissue sections were stained with H&E for morphological examination and in addition the pituitaries were stained with Periodic Acid Schiff-Orange G (Pearse, 1953) to differentiate acidophils from basophils.

Immunocytochemistry

Anterior pituitary hormones were identified using antihuman antibody to ACTH, LH, FSH and GH to examine any qualitative or quantitative changes in the immunoreactive cell population. The sheep sections were assayed against human anterior pituitary hormone for cross immunoreactivity.

Results

Histology

There was marked diminution of the distal lobe of the adenohypophysis with histologically a reduced number of chromophobe cells compared to chromophils. By contrast surviving chromophils particularly the acidophils were disproportionately enlarged with cytoplasmic granular swelling and polar displacement of the nucleus. Chromatin condensation and nuclear compaction, cellular shrinkage and loss also observed.

The testes contained a high proportion of degenerate seminiferous tubules with marked attenuation of lining epithelium and diminished spermatogenesis. The ovaries contained multiple large cystic degenerate follicles and marked numbers of atretic follicles. The adrenal glands showed some cortical loss and irregularity with lipid depletion.

Immunocytochemistry

Cross reactivity was present against human antibody with ACTH, LH, FSH, GH in the undosed sheep in descending order of strength. The immunoreactive cell distribution, indicative of overall population, was generally much more sparse and irregular in the TTM-treated sheep than in the untreated controls (Figures 1 and 2). However, paradoxically, all TTM sheep showed some apparent enhancement of immunoreactivity on an individual cell basis, indeed background degranulation was occasionally seen in the vicinity of the stained cells. (Table 1)

Table 1. Anterior pituitary hormone reactivity (individual cells) in TTM-treated sheep compared with undosed sheep.

Hormone	Undosed sheep	TTM-dosed sheep
ACTH	+++	+++ [+]
LH	++	++ [+]
FSH	+	+ [+]
GH	+/-	[+]

+++ Strong ++ Moderate + Weak [+] enhanced

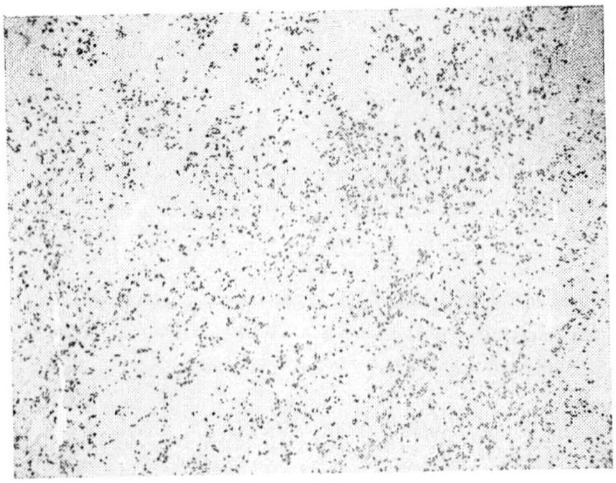

Figure 1. Pituitary sheep: ACTH immunoreactivity

Figure 2. Pituitary TTM sheep; Sparse ACTH immunoreactivity

Discussion

The results support the concept of a pituitary endocrinopathy with secondary target organ failure. However the immunocytochemical findings indicate that the pituitary hormone-producing cells are not primarily affected with respect to their synthetic activity but seemingly as a consequence of their failure to release their constituents with resulting involution and consequent hormone depletion. From this it can be inferred that the adenotrophic-releasing hormones secreted by the neuroendocrine cells of the hypothalamus are non operative either due to an absolute deficiency or dysfunction at the receptor site. Since Mo has been shown to traverse the blood-brain barrier and be retained in brain it could be that the primary lesion may reside in the hypothalamus. Search is being made for a lesion in the central nervous system.

Finally this study confirms and expands earlier findings that Mo reduces fertility in cows and heifers[2] and sheep[3,4] apparently by direct effect on the neuroendocrine axis. By extension molybdate species may likewise be toxigenic to man and its usefulness as a therapeutic agent in Wilson disease[5] needs to be reassessed.

References

1. Momcilovic B. A Case report of acute human molybdenum toxicity from a dietary molybdenum supplement (1999), Arch Indust Hyg Toxicol. **50** (3): 289-297.
2. Phillippo M, Humphries W R, Atkinson T, Henderson G D & Garthwaite P H. The effect of dietary molybdenum and iron on copper status, puberty, fertility and oestrus cycles in cattle. *Journal of Agricultural Science* (1987) **109**: 321-336.
3. Haywood S, Dincer Z, Humphries W R. Endocrinopathy and brain copper elevation in tetrathiomolybdate-treated sheep. In *Trace Elements in Man and Animals.Proceedings of the Eighth International Symposium on Man and Animals.* TEMA-8 (1993). Eds. M Anke, D Meissner and C F Mills. Verlag Media Touristik, 601-602.
4. Haywood Susan, Dincer Zuhal, Holding J & Parry Nicola M. Metal (molybdenum, copper) accumulation and retention in brain, pituitary and other organs of ammonium tetrathiomolybdate-treated sheep. *Brit J. Nutr.* (1998) **79**: 329-331.
5. Walshe J M. Tetrathiomolybdate ($M.S_4$) as an anti-copper agent in man. Scheinberg I H, Walshe J M, eds. *Orphan Diseases and Orphan Drugs* (1986) 68-75.

Summary

Molybdenum is an essential trace element but little is known of its toxic effects in man. Ammonium tetrathiomolybdate (TTM) induced a late onset pituitary endocrinopathy in sheep and Mo retention was confirmed in pituitary and brain. This study examines the morphological changes in TTM-affected pituitaries, and target organs, related to qualitative and quantitative changes in adenotrophic immunoreactive cells. Marked atrophic changes were identified in the adenohypophysis and target organs. There was overall depletion of ACTH, LH, FSH (GH), although individual surviving cells showed apparent enhanced immunoreactivity. Concluded that changes were the outcome of failure hormone-releasing factors and that a Mo-induced lesion may be in the hypothalamus.

Metal Ions in Biology and Medicine; vol 6. Eds. J.A. Centeno, Ph. Collery, G. Vernet, R.B. Finkelman, H. Gibb, J.C. Etienne. John Libbey Eurotext, Paris © 2000, pp. 704-706.

Role of HEXXH motif of zinc metalloproteases in activity of *Escherichia coli* E14 encoded lit protein

Stephen I.N. Ekunwe

Jackson State University, Department of Biology, Jackson, MS. 39217; e-mail: ekunwest@stallion.jsums.edu

Abstract

e14 encoded Lit (late inhibitior of T4 development) protein of *Escherichia coli* (*E. coli*) K-12 strain, upon activation by a phage polypeptide determinant, Gol (grow-on-lit) peptide, internal to the major head protein of phage T4, has been shown to cleave elongation factor Tu (EF-Tu). Lit protein possesses the signature zinc binding sequence HEXXH of zinc metallopeptidase super-family. From studies of the role zinc plays in catalysis of zinc metallopeptidases, it is thought that the histidine (Hs) residues in the HEXXH sequence are the primary ligands to the metal ion while the glutamic acid (E) residue plays a catalytic role, serving as a general base. The aim of this study was to determine if the HEXXH sequence plays any role in the activity of Lit protein, and then to carry out studies to determine if Lit protein may be classified as a zinc metallopeptidase. This aim was accomplished by replacing the first H and the E in the HEXXH sequence with alanine (A) by site-directed mutagenesis. Inhibitor experiments were also done with the protein. While the role H plays is not very clear at this time, replacement of E causes Lit protein to lose activity. Lit protein was also found to be sensitive to inhibitors of zinc metallopeptidases, suggesting that Lit protein may be a member of that family.

Introduction

The role of metal ions in biology and medicine has been known for a long time. Zinc has been reported to be an essential and integral component of over 300 enzymes called zinc metallopeptides. Zinc plays a role in both enzyme catalysis and structure. Zinc metallopeptides constitute a large family of enzymes whose members are involved in numerous diverse processes such as: extracellular matrix maintenance, reproduction and embryonic development. Members have also been reported to play roles in hypertension, arthritis, cancer, lethality of snake venom, tetanus and botulism toxins[1]. Zinc metallopeptides possess the HEXXH sequence. Thermolysin, Astacin, Serratia, Matrixin and Reprolysin sub-families have been reported[1]. The best known bacterial enzyme of this super-family is thermolysin. Other bacterial enzymes exist that possess the HEXXH sequence characteristic of members of this family. *e14* encoded Lit protein of *E. coli* K-12 strain is one such enzyme. It participates in one of the best understood phage exclusion systems, the *e14* exclusion of bacteriophage T4. This exclusion is due to the cleavage of EF-Tu by activated Lit protein. Lit protein is activated when it interacts with Gol peptide[2]. The role the HEXXH sequence plays in the activity of Lit protein is the focus of this study. Finally, studies were done to determine whether Lit protein belongs to the zinc metallopeptidase super-family.

Materials and Methods

In this project, a 998 base pair *lit* gene fragment was PCR engineered and cloned into pUC8 vector and then sub-cloned into pET-30b vector (Novagen) containing the cleavable N-terminus His-tag/S-protein tag which facilitate affinity purification, and detection of the fusion protein respectively. The resulting plasmid construct, pEKS, was used to transform competent *E. coli* strain, JM109DE3*lit*^{0}pLysS. Clones that over-produced Lit protein were selected, and used to produce Lit protein which was then purified on a nickel affinity column. *In-vitro* cleavage assay of EF-Tu was used to monitor activity of Lit protein. The assay involved reacting Lit protein with Gol peptide (Multiple Peptides, California, USA) and previously purified EF-Tu. EF-Tu cleavage product, EF-Tu*, was identified by sodium dodecyl sulfate (SDS) gel electrophoresis.

The HEXXH sequence in Lit protein should make Lit protein sensitive to inhibitors of metallopeptidases such as ethylenediaminetetraacetic acid (EDTA) and 1,10-phenanthroline. The effect of these inhibitors on the activity of Lit protein was studied by first incubating Lit protein with each inhibitor separately: EDTA (5 mM), 1,10-phenanthroline (0.1mM) at room temperature for 10 minutes prior to assaying for activity as described above.

The hypothesis that changing residues in the HEXXH sequence of Lit protein would affect its activity was tested by making the following mutations: H160A (cat160gct), E161A (gaa161gca) using the PCR-based QuikChange site-directed mutagenesis method (Stratagene). The DNA of pEKS was the template DNA. The PCR product was used to transform competent *E. coli* strain JM109DE3*lit*^{0}pLysS and *lit*^{0} transformants were selected. From these clones, "mutant" Lit protein was produced, purified and tested for activity as usual.

Results and Discussion

Activity of Lit protein was inhibited by EDTA and 1,10-phenanthroline (Figure 1a). Both EDTA and 1,10-phenanthroline are metal chelators. 1,10-phenanthroline has a strong affinity for zinc[3,4]. The activity of Lit protein was not inhibited by inhibitors of both acid and thiol proteases. Lit protein from the mutant strains were tested for activity. Most of the protein resulting from mutation H160A was is in inclusion bodies where it is not readily available for reaction. This makes it difficult to determine whether this residue plays a similar role in HEXXH of Lit protein as it does in the canonical HEXXH sequence of zinc enzymes where it is required to ligand zinc[5]. Mutation E161A on the other hand, produced Lit protein, most of which was recovered from the soluble fraction of disrupted cells. This protein did not cleave EF-Tu (Figure 1b). Alanine in place of glutamic acid residue in this sequence could not serve as a catalytic base[5,6]. This result suggests that the glutamic acid residue in the HEXXH sequence of Lit protein plays a role in its activity. More work is being done with residues ^{164}H within the HEXXH sequence, ^{159}H and ^{169}H outside the sequence. Ultimately, detailed structural studies will be needed to fully understand the role this sequence plays in the activity of Lit protein and to determine whether Lit protein is a zinc metalloprotease.

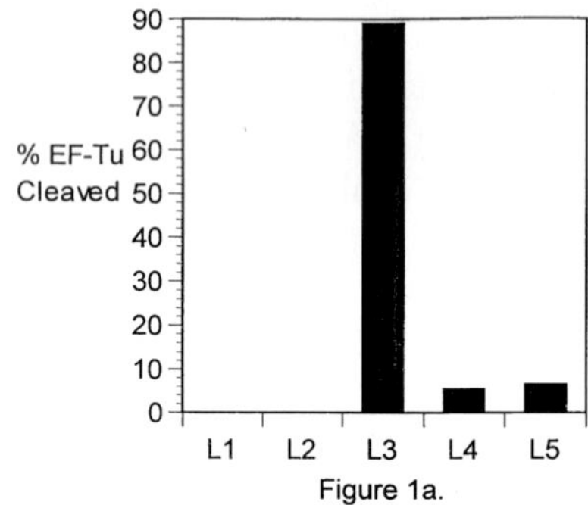

Figure 1a: Effect of inhibitors. L1: Lit only; L2: Lit + EF-Tu; L3: Lit + EF-Tu + Gol; L4: L3 + EDTA; L5: L3 + 1,10-phenanthroline.

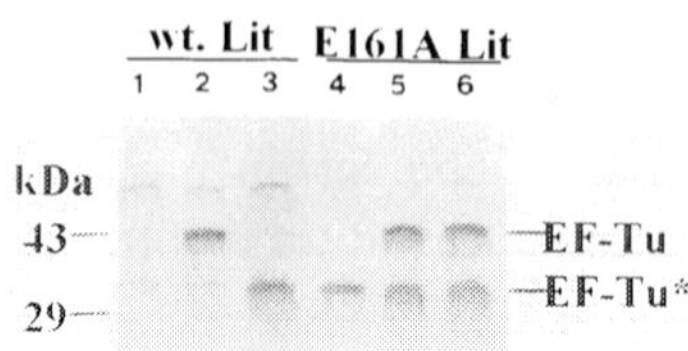

Figure 1b.

Figure 1b shows gel of activity assay. Lane 1, Lit only. Lane 2, Lit + EF-Tu. Lane 3, Lit + EF-Tu + Gol. EF-Tu has been cleaved in Lane 3. Lanes 4,5,6 show a similar experiment using Lit protein with E161A mutation. EF-Tu is not cleaved.

Acknowledgement

I thank my colleague Ernest B. Izevbigie for valuable suggestions in the preparation of this manuscript. I also thank Larry Snyder, my Ph. D. dissertation mentor for providing the funding and guidance that made this work possible.

References

1. Hooper NM. Families of zinc metalloproteases. *FEBS Lett* 1994; 354: 1-6.
2. Georgiou T, Yu Y-T, Ekunwe S, Buttner MJ, Zuurmond A-M, Kraal B, Kleanthous C, Snyder L. Specific peptide-activated proteolytic cleavage of *Escherichia coli* elongation factor, Tu. *Proc. Natl. Acad. Sci.* USA 1998; 95: 2891-2895.
3. Drum DE, Vallee BL. Differential chemical reactivities of zinc in horse liver alcohol dehydrogenase. *Biochemistry* 1970; 9: 4078-4086.
4. Giedroc DP, Keating KM, Williams KR, Konigsberg WH, Coleman JE. Gene 32 protein, a single-stranded DNA binding protein from bacteriophage T4, is a zinc metalloprotein. *Proc. Natl. Acad. Sci.* USA 1986; 83: 8452-8456.
5. Jiang W, Bond JS. Families of metalloendopeptidases and their relationships. *FEBS Lett* 1992; 312: 110-114.
6. Cha J, Auld DS. Site-directed mutagenesis of active site glutamate in human matrilysin: investigation of its role in catalysis. *Biochemistry* 1997; 36: 16019-16024.

Metal Ions in Biology and Medicine; vol 6. Eds. J.A. Centeno, Ph. Collery, G. Vernet, R.B. Finkelman, H. Gibb, J.C. Etienne. John Libbey Eurotext, Paris © 2000, pp. 707-709.

Effects of Zn administration on interleukin-1 gene expression of murine macrophages

Ana Esther Aguilar, Rodolfo Pastelin, Silvia Pérez and Maria Dolores Lastra

Laboratorio de Investigación en Inmunología, Departamento de Biología, Facultad de Química, UNAM. Circuito Escolar, Ciudad Universitaria, México, D.F. CP 04510, fax 56 22 37 40. email: lastraa@servidor.unam.mx

Introduction. Trace elements particularly Zn, have a great influence in the development and maintenance of the immune system(1).The role of Zn in the improvement of impaired immunity is well documented.(2) The macrophage a pivotal cells in many immunologic functions is adversely affected by zinc deficiency, which can dysregulate intracellular killing, cytokine production and phagocytosis. The zinc supplementation improves lymphocytes, particularly T cells activities, and macrophages functions such as phagocytosis and the cells metabolic activity(3). The macrophage appears to be a cell susceptible, to Zn intervention(4). Interleukin-1 (IL-1) secretion is characteristic of macrophage activation(5), thus its modulation by Zn could result in the immune response elevation. We addressed this question by designing a model of BALB/c mice supplemented with Zn (500 mg/L) during the gestation, lactation and postweaning stages (6 wk and 9 wk treatment)(6). We investigated the possibility of IL-1 modulation, by zinc.

Methods. IL-1 was determined in serum by an ELISA immunoenzymatic assay (Genzyme mouse interleukin-1α ELISA kit) and in the macrophages supernatant by the procedure described in Pastelin R. *et al* (Zinc role on macrophages interleukin12 and tumor necrosis factor alpha secretion during mice perinatal stages).

Reverse transcription polymerase chain reactions assays (RT-PCR), were performed to asses the effects of oral Zn supplementation over IL-α mRNA expression, in peritoneal macrophages from mice supplemented with Zn since the gestation to the lactation periods, and from gestation to postweaning, controls were stablished. Total RNA was extracted from the macrophages suspension by the thiocyanate method. RNA purity and concentration were confirmed, 1UA at 260 nm equates 40 μg/mL and the relation 260/280 proved the product was a mRNA free of proteins.

The amplification by PCR was performed (Gene Amp PCR Reagent kit, Perkin-Elmer). Reverse transcription from RNA to cDNA was conducted in a thermalcycler (PCR System 2400 Perkin Elmer). PCR products were separated by electrophoresis in 1.5 % agarose gels and 40 mV, with MW indicators, stained with ethidium bromide, and finally, photographed.

Results. IL-1 serum concentrations demonstrated an increase of about 20% after 6 weeks of zinc supplementation and with a significant ($p<0.05$) decrease of 30% , after 9 weeks. (Fig 1)

In mice (6 weeks Zn treatment) IL-1 concentration evaluated by an ELISA, showed a significative increase (100 %) in the supernatant from LPS stimulated macrophages, with a pronounced drop after the postweaning period (9 weeks Zn treatment). (Fig 2)

In summary, we report that Zn can enhance the IL-1 gene expression on macrophages activated by LPS. Kinetic studies of IL-1 gene expression evaluated by RT-PCR, showed a maximum level of induction 4h after treatment with LPS, followed by a decrease to basal levels within 10h. (Fig 3)

Results suggest an important role of zinc in macrophages stimulation, which carefully monitored could result in modulation of IL-1 secretion, and even modification of its serum concentrations.

References

1.Prasad AS: Marginal deficiency of zinc and immunological effects. In Prasad AS (Ed), Essential and Toxic Trace Elements in Human Health and Disease: An Update 380: 1-22 Wiley-Liss Inc, 1993
2.Wellinghausen N, Kircher H and Rink L: The immunobiology of zinc. Immunol Today 11:80-82, 1997
3.Shankar AH, Prasad AS: Zinc and immune function: the biological basis of altered resistance to infection. In: Black RE (Ed) Zinc for Child Health, Am J Clin Nutr 68 (suppl):447S-463S, 1998
4.Peters AMJ, Bertram P, Gahr M, Speer CP: Reduced secretion of interleukin-1 and tumor necrosis factor-α by neonatal monocytes. Biol Neonate 63: 157-162, 1993
5.Dinarello CA: Biology of interleukin 1. Faseb J 2:108-115, 1988
6.Lastra MD, Pastelin R, Herrera M, Orihuela VD, Aguilar AE: Increment of immune responses in mice perinatal stages after zinc supplementation. Arch Med Res 28: 67-72, 1997

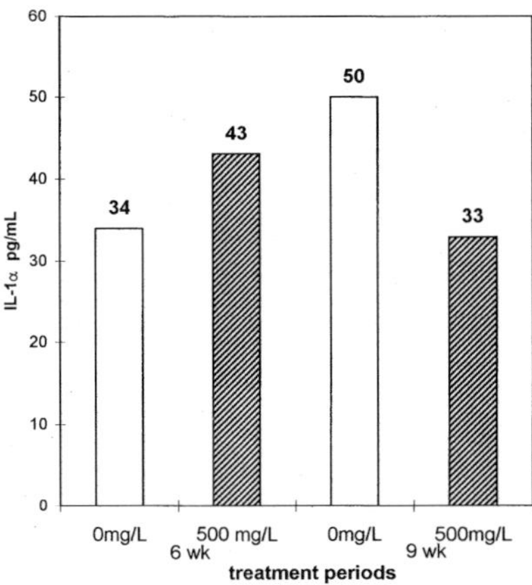

Figure 1. IL-1 levels in serum. Mice were supplemented with Zn (500 mg/L) during the gestation, lactation and post weaning stages, (6 and 9 wk).

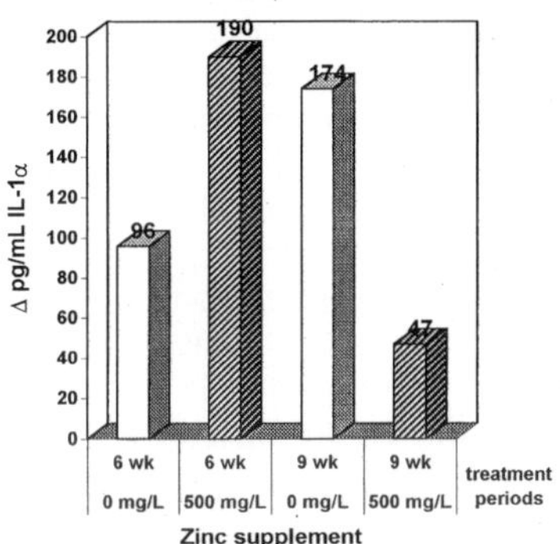

Figure 2. Zn supplementation effect over IL-1 production in LPS stimulated peritoneal macrophages. Results from the IL-1 assay are expressed as the media of the cytokine concentration in pg/mL in Zn exposed macrophage cultures – pg/mL of the cytokine concentration in basal cultures

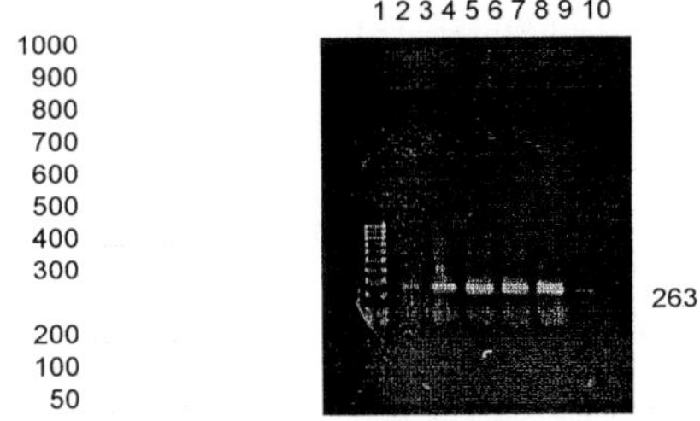

Figur 3. Kinetics of IL-1 mRNA expression. mRNA is expressed from 0 hours (lanes 3 and 8) , 2h(lanes 4), 4h (lane 5), 6h(lane 6), 8h(lane 7) the product has about 260 pb, and persists for 12 hours, its intensity being stronger at 4 hours (lane 5).Lane 2, MW markers.

Metal Ions in Biology and Medicine; vol 6. Eds. J.A. Centeno, Ph. Collery, G. Vernet, R.B. Finkelman, H. Gibb, J.C. Etienne. John Libbey Eurotext, Paris © 2000, pp. 710-713.

Nitric oxide modulation of interleukin-1β-evoked intracellular Ca^{2+} release in brain striatal slices

A. Meini, A. Benicci, G.P. Sgaragli, M. Palmi

Istituto di Scienze Farmacologiche, Università di Siena, via E.S. Piccolomini, 170 53100 Siena, Italy

Our previous work on the sequencing of the fever process showed that administration of interleukin-1β (IL-1β) and other pyrogens into the lateral ventricle of rabbits was accompanied by an increase in Ca^{2+} concentration [Ca^{2+}] in cerebrospinal fluid (CSF). The changes in brain [Ca^{2+}] were shown to be strictly correlated with the temperature gain and the increase in prostaglandin E_2 in CSF of these animals [1]. Acetylsalicylic acid, dexamethasone, lipocortin 5-(204-212), a gluco-corticoid-derived peptide, the ventricular-cisternal perfusion with EGTA and the specific IL-1 receptor antagonist, IRAP all counteracted the increase in [Ca^{2+}] as well as hyperthermia evoked by IL-1β [1] [2]. These data corroborate the involvement of Ca^{2+} in thermoregulation and establish the role of this ion in the intracellular signalling pathways that control the pyrogenic response to IL-1β.

The aim of the present study was to provide evidence of the involvement of nitric oxide (NO) in IL-1β-induced Ca^{2+}release and to investigate the source of the increased Ca^{2+} release. Ca^{2+} efflux was measured in 350 μm slices of rat striatum pre-loaded with $^{45}Ca^{2+}$ (6.02 x 10^{-6} M) for 30 min and superfused with oxygenated (95% O_2 + 5% CO_2) Ca-EGTA (mM concentration: 135 NaCl, 10 D-Glucose, 5 HEPES, 4.6 KCl, 1 $MgCl_2$, pH=7.2) buffered physiological salt solution at a constant rate of 0.5 ml/min. Following the method previously described [2], Ca^{2+} release was determined and expressed as the percentage of residual radioactivity present in the tissue at each sampling interval (Fractional Release, FR). Baseline spontaneous FR, corresponded to FR values of 10 fractions collected during the 30-min preceding the drug perfusion period.

Diethylamine/NO complex sodium (Dea/NO), dibutyryl cyclic GMP (di-cGMP) and IL-1β alone or in combination with N-ω-Nitro-L-Arginine Methyl Ester (L-NAME) were perfused over 30 min. To investigate on intracellular stores involved in IL-1β-induced Ca^{2+} release, we checked the effect of depletion of intracellular Ca^{2+} pools by bradykinin, an inositol-(1,4,5)-trisphosphate receptor ($InsP_3R$) activator and by caffeine a ryanodine receptor (RYR) agonist. Striatal slices were pre-incubated with caffeine or bradykinin in the 30 min interval of the $^{45}Ca^{2+}$ loading period and then perfused in the presence of thapsigargin with a Ca^{2+}-free medium.

As shown in Fig. 1, baseline spontaneous FR of $^{45}Ca^{2+}$ from slices of rat striatum in the absence of stimulation was constant. Addition of

IL-1β to the perfusion liquid induced a slow and delayed increase in the rate of spontaneous Ca^{2+} efflux that started about 30 min after cytokine addition and increased in strength after wash-out. When the effect of exogenous NO, supplied by Dea/NO was checked, we found that, similarly to IL-1β, this compound induced a sustained raise of Ca^{2+} release. The presence of L-NAME, a well-known inhibitor of nitric oxide synthase (NOS), completely reversed Ca^{2+} release induced by IL-1β. On the contrary, the enantiomer D-NAME, which is not a substrate of NOS, did not antagonize this effect (data not shown). Di-cGMP, similarly to IL-1β induced a progressive and sustained increase of Ca^{2+} release which was delayed and dose-dependent (Fig. 2). As reported in Fig. 3, tissues pre-treated with caffeine but not those pre-treated with bradykinin showed a marked reduction, compared to not pre-treated tissues, of IL-1β-induced Ca^{2+} release.

These results sustain the hypothesis that NO was the intracellular mediator of IL-1β effect on Ca^{2+} response. Thus in rat striatum, where a population of NOS–containing neurons has been evidenced [3], a downregulation of NOS activity by the competitive inhibitor L-NAME was seen to antagonise the effect of IL-1β on Ca^{2+} release while a nucleophile(amine)/NO complex, Dea/NO, which is known to decompose with generation of NO at physiological pH [4], mimicked the effect of IL-1β on Ca^{2+} efflux.

Although the signalling pathways involved in NO-mediated intracellular Ca^{2+} release from both the $InsP_3$ and the RY-Ca^{2+} pools are still largely unknown, NO-mediated generation of cGMP and activation of a G kinase are generally accepted as part of the overall mechanism [5]. Indeed in striatum we found that the membrane-permeant analogue of cGMP, di-cGMP, induced an increase of Ca^{2+} release. Finally the finding that pre-treatament with caffeine but not that with bradykinin greatly decreased Ca^{2+} release suggests that the RY Ca^{2+} stores are mainly involved in the IL-1β effect on Ca^{2+} response. IL-1β, beside being an endogenous pyrogen contributes to many neurological diseases such as multiple sclerosis, AIDS, dementia complex, stroke and Alzheimer's disease [6], thus our results may support the hypothesis that the NO/cGMP/Ca^{2+} pathway is part of the signalling cascade subserving multiple functions of IL-1β.

REFERENCES

1) **Palmi M**, Frosini M, Becherucci C, Sgaragli GP, Parente L. Increase of extracellular brain calcium involved in interleukin-1β-induced pyresis in the rabbit: antagonism by dexamethasone. *Br J Pharmacol* (1994); 112:449-452.
2) **Palmi M**, Frosini M, Sgaragli GP. Interleukin -1β stimulation of $^{45}Ca^{2+}$ release from rat striatal slices. *Br J Pharmacol* (1996); 118:1705-1710.
3) **Strijbos PJLM**, Leach MJ, Garthwaite J. Vicious cycle involving Na^{+} channels, glutamate release, and NMDA receptors mediates delayed neurodegenaration through nitric oxide formation. *J Neurosci* (1996); 16:5004-50013.
4) **Maragos CM**, Morley D, Wink DA, Dunams TM, Saavedra JE, Hoffman A, Bove AA, Isaac L, Hrabie JA, Keefer LK. Complexes of $^{\bullet}NO$ with nucleophiles as agents for the controlled biological release of nitric oxide. Vasorelaxant effects. *J Med. Chem.* (1991); 34:3242-3247.
5) **Clementi E**. Role of nitric oxide and its inrtacellular signalling pathways in the control of Ca^{2+} homeostasis. *Biochem Pharmacol* (1998); 55:713-718.
6) **Rotwell NJ**. Functions and mechanism of interleukin-1 in the brain. *Trends Pharmacol Sci* (1991); 12:430-436.

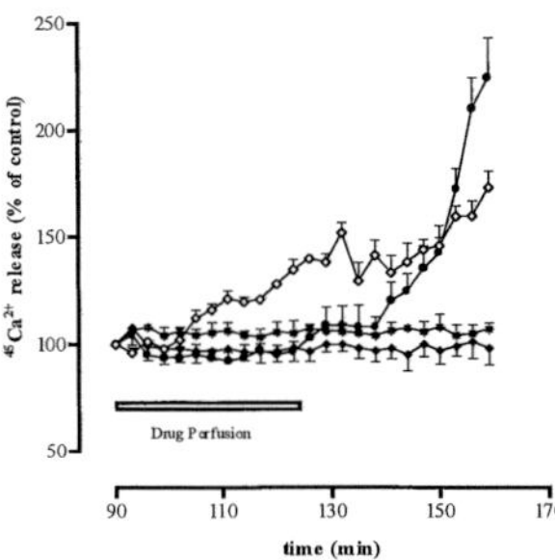

Fig. 1. Effect of 10 ng/ml IL-1β (•), 1 mM Dea/NO (◊) and 10 ng/ml IL-1β plus 3 mM L-NAME (♦) on release of $^{45}Ca^{2+}$ from rat striatal brain slices. Control (*) represents release in the absence of stimulation. Release is expressed as a percentage of the residual radioactivity present in the tissue at each sampling interval (fractional release, FR,). Values (mean of triplicate determinations from 3-5 separate experiments) with S.E. mean (S.E.M.) show percentage deviations in $^{45}Ca^{2+}$ efflux above baseline release. Baseline release (100%) is the mean release in 10 fractions collected in the 30 min interval preceding drug perfusion. Groups data of $^{45}Ca^{2+}$ release were compared statistically by ANOVA for the treatments: IL-1β vs Control, FR $= p < 0.01$, Dea/NO vs Control, FR $= p < 0.01$, IL-1β vs IL-1β + L-NAME, FR $= p < 0.01$.

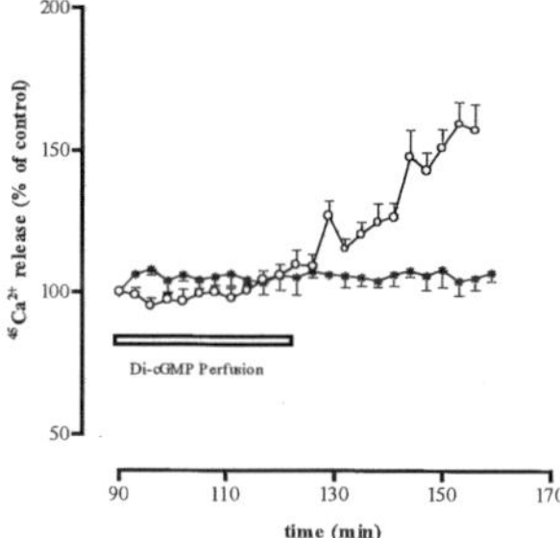

Fig. 2. Effect of 100μM di-cGMP (O) on release of $^{45}Ca^{2+}$ from rat striatal brain. For details see legend to Fig. 1. Group data of $^{45}Ca^{2+}$ release were compared statistically by ANOVA for the treatments: di-cGMP vs control (*), FR=$p<0.001$

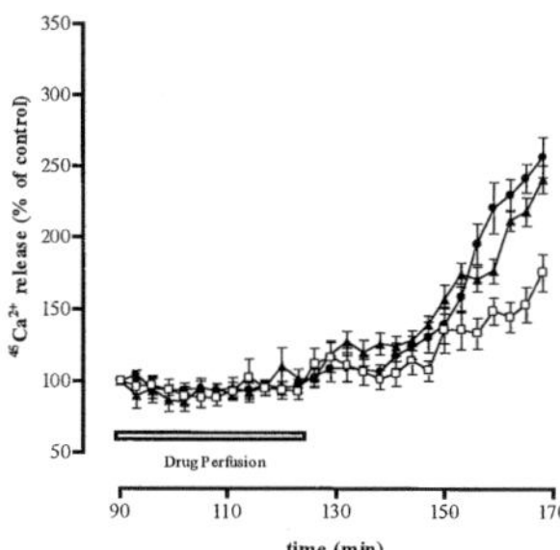

Fig. 3. Effect of tissue pre-incubation with 20 mM caffeine (□) or 5μM bradykinin (▲) on $^{45}Ca^{2+}$ release induced by 10 ng/ml IL-1β (•). Striatal slices were pre-incubated with caffeine or bradykinin in the 30 min interval of the $^{45}Ca^{2+}$ loading period and then perfused in the presence of 0.1μM thapsigargin with a Ca^{2+}-free medium. For details see legend to Fig. 1. Group data of $^{45}Ca^{2+}$ FR were compared statistically by ANOVA for the following treatments: caffeine pretreated vs bradykinin pretreated tissues, FR $= p < 0.001$.

Metal Ions in Biology and Medicine; vol 6. Eds. J.A. Centeno, Ph. Collery, G. Vernet, R.B. Finkelman, H. Gibb, J.C. Etienne. John Libbey Eurotext, Paris © 2000, pp. 714-716.

Vanadium-induced alterations in cytoskeleton and protein tyrosine-phosphorylation in osteoblast cell lines

A.M. Cortizo[1], S.M. Kreda[2]

[1] *Bioquímica Patológica, Facultad de Ciencias Exactas, Universidad Nacional de La Plata, Argentina;*
[2] *CF/Pulmonary Research and Treatment Center, University of North Carolina at Chapel Hill, NC, USA*

Abstract

This study investigates the effect of vanadate and vanadyl on protein-tyrosine phosphorylation(PTP) and cytoskeleton reorganization in two osteoblastic cell lines. Vanadium induced changes in cell morphology and formation of focal adhesion and stress fibres organization. These alterations correlated with an increase in the PTP levels of several proteins in osteoblasts in culture.

Introduction

Vanadium compounds elicited insulin-mimetic and growth factor-like properties in different biological systems [1]. These compounds are specially stored into the bone [2], where they can regulate glucose metabolism, cell progression and differentiation, morphological transformation and caused cytotoxic effects [3]. Bone remodelling is a dynamic process resulting from the balance between bone formation by the osteoblasts and bone resorption by osteoclasts. The coupling between these processes is believed to be regulated by growth factors synthesised and stored in the bone and/or external stimulus acting by different mechanisms [4]. Vanadium, by inhibiting protein tyrosine phosphatases inhibits the dephosphorylation and consequently increases the levels of phosphorylated tyrosine residues of different proteins [5]. However, how vanadium can induce both, growth promotion and cytotoxicity in bone is still unknown.

In this study we investigate the protein tyrosine phosphorylation and cytoskeleton reorganization, evaluated through the actin, tubulin and focal adhesion kinase, in two osteoblast-like cells incubated with vanadate and vanadyl.

Materials and Methods

Serum starved UMR106 osteosarcoma and MC3T3E1 osteoblast-like cells were incubated with different doses (0-5 mM) of sodium vanadate (Vi) or vanadyl sulphate (VO) for 6 hours and the cytoskeleton alterations were analysed by immunofluorescence. Cells growth on glass coverslips were fixed, permeabilised and stained for F-actin, α-tubulin, and focal adhesion kinase (FAK) [6]. Confluent cells were treated with 1-5 mM vanadium for 10 min and analysed by SDS-PAGE and Western blot using and antiphosphotyrosine antibody, revealed by a biotin-enhanced system with alkaline phosphatase reactive [7]. The blots were semiquantitated by scanning and analysed using the Scion-beta 2 program.

Results and Discussion

Serum-starved cultures for 24 hours showed fewer stress fibres compared to controls (10% FBS). Vi and VO induced changes in the cell morphology and cytoskeleton reorganization in a dose-dependent manner. The cells appeared less flat with a decrease in the number and length of intercellular processes. The nuclei and cytoplasms became smaller and condensed. The intensity of tubulin and actin staining associated with stress fibres greatly increased. In addition, few number of cells were surviving after 5 mM vanadium treatment.

Serum-starved control cultures displayed FAK mainly localized in the nuclei in both osteoblastic lines (Figure 1). Cells treated with increasing concentrations of vanadate for 6 hours show that FAK was mainly associated to the stress fibres and accumulated into the tips of the actin filaments. The amount of stress fibres formed in response to vanadate treatment was greater than the induced by vanadyl. These results seems to indicate that in osteoblast-like cells, the vanadium-caused changes in cell morphology are associated with reorganization of specific cytoskeleton proteins and the assembly of focal adhesion.

Figure 1: Immunofluorescence for FAK.

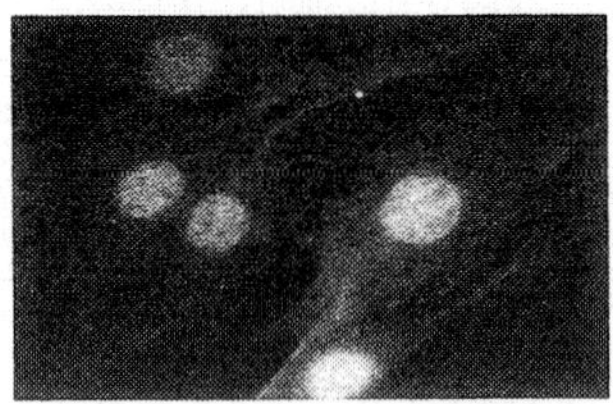

Control MC3T3E1 **100μM Vi-treated cells**

Both vanadate and vanadyl induced a rapid and marked increase in PTP on proteins of 85-150 kDa (Figure 2). In comparison, 10^{-6}M insulin and 0.5% FBS increased the phosphorylation of two additional bands with apparent mass of 145 and 170 kDa. Further experiments are in progress in order to characterise those proteins that become tyrosine phosphorylated by vanadium-induced formation of focal adhesion.

Figure 2. Western blot of phosphotyrosine proteins.

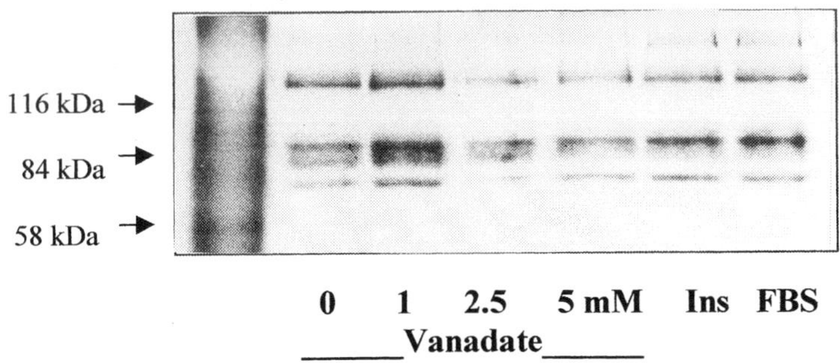

These mechanisms may explain at least in part, the cell toxicity caused by vanadium in bone producing cells.

Acknowledgements

This work was partially supported by grants from Facultad de Ciencias Exactas, UNLP; CICPBA, CONICET and Agencia Nacional de Promoción Científica y Técnica. AMC is a member of the Carrera del Investigador, CICPBA, Argentina.

References

1. Stern A, Yin X, Tsang S-S, Davison A, Moon T. Vanadium as a modulator of cellular regulatory cascades and oncogene expression. *Biochem Cell Biol* 1993; 71: 103-112.
2. Nielsen FH. In: Sielgel H and Siegel A (eds). *Vanadium and its role in life*. New York: Marcell Dekker. 1995: 543-573.
3. Etcheverry SB, Cortizo AM. Bioactivity of vanadium compounds on cells in culture.In: Nriagu JO (ed). *Vanadium in the Enviroment*. New York: John Wiley & Sons, Inc. 1998: 359-394.
4. Ng KW, Romas E, Donnan L, Findlay DM. Bone biology. *Bailliere Clin Endocrinol Metab* 1997; 11: 1-22.
5. Gresser MJ, Tracey AS. Vanadate as phosphate analogs in biochemistry. In Chasteen ND (ed.). *Vanadium in Biological Systems*. The Netherlands: Kluver Academic Prublishers. 1990: 63-79.
6. Aplin AE, Juliano RL. Integrin and cytoskeleton regulation of growth factor signaling to the MAP kinase pathway. *J Cell Science* 1999; 112: 695-706.
7. Sálice VC, Cortizo AM, Gómez Dumm CL, Etcheverry SB. Tyrosine phsophorylation and morphological transformation induced by four vanadium compounds on MC3T3E1 cells. Mol Cell Biochem 1999; 198: 119-128.

Metal Ions in Biology and Medicine; vol 6. Eds. J.A. Centeno, Ph. Collery, G. Vernet, R.B. Finkelman, H. Gibb, J.C. Etienne. John Libbey Eurotext, Paris © 2000, pp. 717-719.

Hemochromatosis mutations and familial Alzheimer disease

Sharon Moalem[1], Maire Percy[1], David Andrews[2], Simon Wong[1], Theo Kruck[1], Arthur Dalton[3], Pankaj Mehta[3], Bettye Fedor[3], and Andrew Warren[4]

[1] Department of Physiology, University of Toronto, Toronto, Canada; [2] Department of Statistics, University of Toronto, Toronto, Canada; [3] New York State Institute for Basic Research in Developmental Disabilities, Staten Island, NY USA; [4] Johns Hopkins Medical School, Baltimore MD, USA, Surrey Place Centre, 2 Surrey Place, Toronto, Ontario, Canada, M5S 2C2

ABSTRACT

Background: Mutations in the class I-like major histocompatibility complex gene called HFE are associated with hereditary hemochromatosis (HHC), a disorder of excessive iron uptake. Aberrations of iron metabolism have been described in Alzheimer disease (AD). The present study is of interest because of the documented evidence of oxidative damage and vascular disturbances in AD and the possibility of metal ion involvement in disease pathogenesis.

Aim: To compare the prevalence of two common HFE mutations - C282Y and H63D- in patients with familial AD (FAD) and healthy normal individuals of similar age and gender distribution.

Methods: DNA samples from patients with FAD ($n = 26$) and healthy normal volunteers ($n = 41$) were screened for C282Y and H63D mutations using PCR analysis. As the apolipoprotein E E4 allele (ApoE E4) is a known risk factor for AD, DNA samples were ApoE genotyped for comparison. Data were analyzed by Chi squared analysis and interpreted at the 0.05 level of significance without Bonferroni corrections.

Results: Relative to the healthy normals, ApoE E4 was over-represented in both males and females with FAD. HFE mutations, however, were over-represented in males and under-represented in females with FAD. When subjects were stratified according to gender, and the presence or absence of HFE mutations or the ApoE E4 allele, only two comparisons were significant. Among males, the percentage with FAD who lacked HFE mutations and the ApoE E4 allele was significantly less than in the normals in this category ($p = 0.0001$). Among females, the percentage with FAD who lacked HFE mutations but were ApoE E4 positive was significantly greater than in the normals in this category ($p = 0.036$). Results were similar for C282Y and H63D in combination or for H63D alone.

Conclusions: Among ApoE E4 negative males, the absence of HFE mutations may be protective against FAD. Furthermore, the ApoE E4 allele may be most predisposing to FAD among HFE mutation negative females. The possibility that HFE mutations may provide an important new genetic linkage in AD should be followed up.

Introduction:

The question of metal ion involvement in the pathogenesis of Alzheimer disease has yet to be sufficiently explored. There have been many studies that have found evidence of oxidative damage and increased amounts of metals such as iron, and aluminum in the brains of patients suffering from Alzheimer disease [1]. There have also been reports of vascular disturbances that are thought to contribute and/or exacerbate the degree to which this form of dementia progresses [2]. Hereditary hemochromatosis (HHC) is a disorder of excessive iron uptake and deposition. Point mutations in a class I-like major histocompatibility gene called HFE are associated with HHC [3]. In this report, we compare the frequencies of two common HFE point mutations associated with HHC (C282Y and H63D), and ApoE, a known risk factor for Alzheimer disease [4], in a well-characterized group of Caucasian individuals with familial Alzheimer disease (FAD). HFE wild-type protein reduces the affinity of transferrin receptor for transferrin. C282Y and H63D mutant proteins do not have this negative modulatory effect [5].

Materials and Methods:

DNA samples from patients with FAD ($n = 26$) and healthy normal volunteers from the same geographical region ($n = 41$) were screened for C282Y and H63D mutations using PCR analysis. As the apolipoprotein E E4 allele (ApoE E4) is a known risk factor for AD, DNA samples were ApoE genotyped for comparison. Data were analyzed by Chi squared analysis and interpreted at the 0.05 level of significance without Bonferroni corrections.

Results and Discussion:

Relative to the healthy normals, ApoE E4 was over-represented in both males and females with FAD. HFE mutations were over-represented in males and under-represented in females with FAD. When subjects were stratified according to gender, and the presence or absence of HFE mutations or the ApoE E 4 allele, only two comparisons were significant. Among males, the percentage with FAD who were HFE mutation and E4 negative was significantly less than in the normals ($p = 0.0001$). Among females, the percentage with FAD who were HFE mutation negative and ApoE E4 positive was significantly greater than in the normals ($p = 0.036$). Results were similar for C282Y and H63D in combination or for H63D alone. These observations support the proposition that there is a complex association between HFE mutations and the ApoE E4 allele in FAD that is different in males and females. Among ApoE E4 negative males, the absence of HFE mutations may be protective against FAD and, conversely, the presence of HFE mutations may be predisposing to FAD. Furthermore, the ApoE E4 allele may be most predisposing to FAD among HFE mutation negative females. Because transferrin is the major iron binding protein for aluminum as well as iron, C282Y and H63D also would be expected to enhance aluminum uptake and deposition [6]. Given our findings, this could possibly help explain some of the observations of increased metal ions, such as iron and aluminum, found in the brains of patients with AD [7]. Furthermore, it is relevant to note that injections with the trivalent metal chelator, desferrioxamine, which binds to and removes iron, aluminum, and other transition metals, has been found to retard the development and progression of AD, as well as reducing overall mortality in AD [8]. From a therapeutic development standpoint, research into new strategies to reduce oxidative damage in AD is highly warranted. As well, the possibility that HFE mutations may provide an important new genetic linkage in AD should be followed up.

Excerpted from: Moalem S, Percy ME, Andrews DF, Wong S, Kruck TPA, Dalton AJ, Mehta P, Fedor B, Warren AC. Are hemochromatosis mutations involved in Alzheimer disease? Am J Med Genet, in press.

Supported by the Alzheimer Society of Canada, the Rehabilitation Institute (Toronto), a Margaret and Howard Gamble Research Grant, National Institute on Aging: grant numbers R31-AGO8849, R01-AG11290 and PO1-AG11531, and a grant from the Alzheimer's Association.

References:

1. Perl DP, Good PF. Aluminium and the neurofibrillary tangle: results of tissue microprobe studies. *Ciba Found Symp* 1992;169:217-36.
2. Crawford F, Abdullah L, Schinka J, Suo Z, Gold M, Duara R, Mullan M. Gender-specific association of the angiotensin converting enzyme gene with Alzheimer's disease. *Neurosci Lett* 2000; 280:215-219.
3. Feder JN, Gnirke A, Thomas W, Tsuchihashi Z, Ruddy DA, Basava A, Dormishian F, Domingo R Jr, Ellis MC, Fullan A, Hinton LM, Jones NL, Kimmel BE, Kronmal GS, Lauer P, Lee VK, Loeb DB, Mapa FA, McClelland E, Meyer NC, Mintier GA, Moeller N, Moore T, Moriang E, Prass CE, Quintana L, Starnes SM, Shatzman RC, Brunke KJ, Drayama DT, Risch NJ, Bacon BR, Wolff RD. A novel MHC class I-like gene is mutated in patients with hereditary hemochromatosis. *Nat Genet* 1996; 13:399-408.
4. Roses AD. Apolipoprotein E and Alzheimer's disease. The tip of the susceptibility iceberg. *Ann N Y Acad Sci* 1998; 855:738-43.
5. Feder JN, Penny DM, Irrinki A, lee VK, Lebron JA, Watson N, Tsuchihashi Z, Sigal E, Bjorkman PJ, Schatzman RC. The hemochromatosis gene product complexes with the transferrin receptor and lowers its affinity for ligand binding. *Proc Natl Acad Sci USA* 1998; 95:1472-7.
6. Golub MS, Han B, Keen CL. 1999. Aluminum uptake and effects on transferrin mediated iron uptake in primary cultures of rat neurons, astrocytes and oligodendrocytes. *Neurotoxicology* 1999; 20:961-70.
7. Bouras C, Giannakopoulos P, Good PF, Hsu A, Hof PR, Perl DP. A laser microprobe mass analysis of brain aluminum and iron in dementia pugilistica: comparison with Alzheimer's disease. *Eur Neurol* 1997; 38:53-8.
8. Crapper-McLachlan DR, Dalton AJ, Kruck TP, Bell MY, Smith WL, Kalow W, Andrews DF. Intramuscular desferrioxamine in patients with Alzheimer's disease. *Lancet* 1991; 337:1304-8.

Metal Ions in Biology and Medicine; vol 6. Eds. J.A. Centeno, Ph. Collery, G. Vernet, R.B. Finkelman, H. Gibb, J.C. Etienne. John Libbey Eurotext, Paris © 2000, pp. 720-722.

Genotoxic effect of dichromate and permanganate

Wen-Hsun Yang*, Di Chang, Kimberly Johnson, and Jen-Rong Yang

Biology Department, Jackson State University, Jackson, Mississippi, USA

Abstract: Potassium dichromate and permanganate are the most common oxidizing chemicals used in research laboratories and industry. Consequently their biosafety profile is of great concern to many users. In order to estimate the damaging effect of those chemicals on genetic material, the strand-breaking assay on Simian Virus *(SV40)* DNA as well as the mutagenic and lethal assays on *Salmonella Test Strain TA102 (TA102)* were performed. The results of this study show there is a proportional increase in the occurrence of single- and double-strand breaks in the *SV40* viral DNA as the concentration of either dichromate or permanganate is increased from 1 mM to 64 mM. This is indicated by a proportional increase in the percentages of Form II (circular) and Form III (linear) DNA found at the expense of Form 1 (superhelix) viral DNA. The genotoxic assay using dichromate and permanganate in the *TA102* bacteria showed a differential response of the bacteria to those chemicals. As the concentration of permanganate was increased from 1 mM to 64 mM, a proportional increase in the lethal effect (without mutagenic effect) was seen. In contrast, the mutagenic effect of dichromate, indicated by the increase in the number of revertants, was seen at concentrations ranging from 1 mM to 8 mM, while the lethal effect was seen at higher concentrations ranging from 34 mM to 64 mM. These results suggest that dichromate and permanganate have similar damaging effects on DNA molecules. The damage to DNA in the presence of permanganate was repaired by normal cellular mechanisms. However, the damage to DNA in the presence of dichromate was incorrectly repaired with mutation.

Introduction: Chromium is listed as one of the most abundant metals in the Earth's crust (number ten in order), whereas manganese occurs in lesser quantity (Bartlett and James 1987). Chromium is usually not detectable in the Mississippi River or the Pearl River. However, manganese is measurable at a level of 0.010 and 0.076 ppm, respectively in those two rivers (Yang *et al.* 1994). The importance of these two elements in the metal industry for enhancing the quality of iron or aluminum alloys is well known. Manganese is also an important cofactor in many enzymes. For example, as a cofactor in the water-splitting enzyme, manganese contributes significantly in the production of energy-phosphates along with the production of protons and oxygen molecules in the Photosystem II. Manganese also serves as an important cofactor for phosphate-transferring enzymes such as creatine kinase and pyruvate kinase, and for the urea-splitting enzyme, arginase. In contrast, the biochemical effects of chromium are not as brilliantly displayed as manganese. Chromium is known as a cofactor for stimulating glucose uptake into cells and as a trace element necessary for the growth of bone and connective tissue. However, in general, chromium is recognized in biology and medicine for its carcinogenic effect (Benicelli *et al.*, 1983; Daniel *et al.*, 1985) rather than for its beneficial effects.

Materials and Methods: In order to assay DNA strand breaks induced by test chemicals, 1.7204 µg/10 µl of *SV40* DNA was prepared in TBNE buffer [1.24% Trishydroxide-methyl-aminomethane (Tris base), 0.2922% sodium chloride, and 0.38% Ethylenediamine tetraacetic acid (EDTA), pH 7.5]. After the addition of equal amounts of the test chemicals, at the different experimental concentrations, to the *SV40* DNA preparation, the mixtures were then placed in microtubes and incubated for 1 hour in a refrigerator at 4°C. 10 ul of this mixture was then mixed with an equal volume of loading medium (0.025% Bromophenol blue, 0.025% Xylene cyanol, and 2.5% Ficol "Type 400"). 15 µl of the final mixtures were then loaded into wells formed in a 0.8% agarose gel chamber containing TBE buffer (1.08% Tris base, 0.55% Boric acid, and 0.0761% EDTA with pH 7.6). Submersive gel-electrophoresis was performed for 4 hours at a constant voltage of 80 DCV (40 mA) in the TBE buffer. After staining for 2 to 4 hours with ethidium bromide (0.5 µg/ml water) the gel was destained for 20 to 30 minutes in a 1 mM magnesium sulfate solution. Then the gel was placed on an ultraviolet transilluminator for fluorescent photography at a wavelength of 300 nm. A Polaroid camera with Kodak #22 Wratten filter was used for photography. A sensitive Polaroid film, type 55 P/N black and white film, was used for documenting the Form I (superhelix), Form II (circular form) and Form III (linear form) DNA bands formed on the gel. A LKB Gelscan XL laser beam densitometer was used to scan and convert DNA bands on film into corresponding peaks in graphical form. After integration and data-management in a computer, the peak areas in the densitograph were calculated as percentage proportions of the 3 different DNA forms. For assays of the genotoxic effects of these chemicals *in vivo*, *TA102* was obtained courtesy of Dr. Ames (University of California, Berkeley) and used in a genotoxic assay modified from the original method of Ames *et al* (1975). *TA102* was streak cultured in MG agar plate (1.5% agar, 2% dextrose, 0.00978% $MgSO_4$, 0.183% citric acid, 1% K_2PO_4, and 0.229% $NaHNH_4PO_4$). Histidine (260 µM), biotin (3 µM) and tetracycline (10 µg

/ml) were added to maintain the growth of the test strain. For preparation of frozen stocks, a single colony of the test bacteria strains was cultured in 40 ml of Oxoid Nutrient broth #2 until early stationary phase was reached. The culture was performed in a shaker incubator at 300°C and 200 rpm. The 40ml culture was then mixed with 7 ml glycerol and dispensed 1 ml per microtube for storage at -80°C in a deep freezer. For the mutagenecity assay, one volume of the frozen stock was diluted into 80 volumes of fresh Nutrient broth #2 for culture in a shaker incubator. After 5 to 6 hours of incubation at 30°C and 200 rpm in a shaker incubator, the mid-logarithmic phase of growth was reached. 0.1 ml of cultures were incubateded for 30 minutes with equal volume of various concentrations of potassium dichromate or permanganate in test tubes at 25°C. Thereafter, 0.5 ml of a salt solution containing 0.1 mM phosphate buffer (pH 7.4), 33 mM potassium chloride and 8 mM magnesium chloride was added . Finally 2 ml of top agar (50°C containing 0.5% saline solution, 0.6% agar, 0.5 mM histidine and 0.5 mM biotin), was added to the mixtures in tubes for vigorous mixing for 30 seconds before making a coat on top of an MG plates. Numbers of colonies formed by reverse mutation on the MG plates were recorded after 48 hours of incubation at 37°C.

Results and Discussion: The *SV40* viral DNA incubation assay (Table 1) clearly shows a proportional increase in Form II DNA, probably caused by single-strand breaks in the DNA, as the concentration of dichromate or permanganate is increased from 1 mM to 32 mM. In addition there is a proportional increase in Form III DNA, probably caused by double-strand breaks, as the concentrations of these two chemicals are increased from 4 to 32 mM (Table 1). Previous studies on restriction endonuclease (Adler *et al*., 1973) and on radiation (Dizdaroglu *et al*., 1977) suggested that either enzymatic hydrolysis or free radical attack may lead to strand breaks in Form I (Superhelix) of *SV40* DNA. These strand breaks can then result in the formation of either Form II (circular) or Form III (linear) DNA. The present study suggests that superoxide, hydrogen peroxide, or hydroxyl radicals formed as a result of interaction with highly oxidized, unstable chemicals (dichromate or permanganate) within an aqueous system can also induce the formation of strand breaks in SV40 viral DNA. In addition, superoxide radicals and hydrogen peroxide molecules formed in the mitochondria during aerobic metabolism was previously shown to cause various nonenzymatic reactions in biological system (Forman and Boveries 1982). In our genotoxic studies using the *TA102* bacteria, severe DNA damage was found when the concentration of dichromate or permanganate was increased. At a concentration of 64 mM or higher, the lethal effect was nearly 100%. However, at a lower concentration of permanganate (1mM to 8 mM), the lethal effect was less. In contrast, dichromate was mutagenic at the lower concentrations (1 mM to 8 mM) with a high number of revertants formed (Table 2). These results suggest that the DNA repair mechanism may function differently in the presence of dichromate and permanganate. Faulty repair of DNA strand breaks in the presence of dichromate may result in mutations. By contrast, accurate repair of DNA strand breaks in the presence of permanganate may diminish the likelihood of mutagenic effects. Bianchi *et al*. (1983) showed that chromium [Cr(VI)] was directly mutagenic in a number of strains of *Salmonella typhimurium*; they detected base pair substitutions in *TA1535* and *TA100* bacteria as well as frameshift mutations in *TA1538* and *TA98* bacteria. The results obtained using the *TA102* bacteria by Benicelli *et al*. (1983), Daniel *et al*. (1983) and in the current experiment also confirm that Cr(VI) is able to produce base pair substitutions (AT→ GC). By contrast, neither permanganate nor other manganese ions have previously been observed to have a mutagenic effect; the present study corroborates the results of those previous studies.

Acknowledgements: This work was supported by the Defense Department of Energy under contract #DE-ACO#76SF0098 (to the University of California at Berkeley); subcontract #46170 to Jackson State University.

Literature Cited:

Ames, B.N., McCann, J. and F. Yamasaki,, Mutation Res. 31: 347-364 (1975)

Adler, S.P., and D.Nathans, B. Biochim. Biophys. Acta. 299: 177—188(1973)

Bartlett, R. J. and B. R. James, In "Chromium in the Natural and Human Environments. Volume 20" (Nriagu, J. O. and E. Nieboer) 267-303 (1987).

Benicelli.C., A. Camoirano, S. Petruzzeli, P. Zanacchi, and S. De Flora. Mutation Res. 122: 1-5 (1983)

Bianchi, V., L. Celotti, G. Lanfranchi, F. Majone, G. Martin, A. Montaldi, G., Sponza, G. Tamino, P. Vernier, A. Zantedeschi, and A. G. Levis. Mutation Res. 117: 279-300 (1983)

Daniel, R. M., and H.V. Phi. Mutation Res. 155: 49-51 (1985)

Dizdaroglu, M., Schulte-Frohnlinde, D., and von Sonntag, C, Int. J. Biol., 32: 481-490, (1977).

Forman H. J., and A. Boveris, In "Free Radicals in Biology. Vol. V." (Pryor, W.A. ed.) pp 65-90 (1982).

Yang, W.H. A. Baaree, J. and A. Yee, High selenium concentration and selenite hyperresistant bacteria in the lower stream of Mississippi River. In "Mississippi Water Resource Conference (Daniel, B. J. ed.) 24: 37-47 (1994).

Table 1. Strand-breaking effects of Potassium Dichromate and Potassium Permanganate on *SV40* DNA*.

Chemicals Group No.	Chemical conc mM (%)	Percentages of *SV40* DNA forms produced Form I (Superhelix)	Form II (Circular)	Form III (Linear)	Strad-break effect
Negative control	0.00 (0.00)	97.3	2.7	0	
Dichromate-1	1.00 (0.0294)	94.6	5.8	0	Single**
D-2	2.00 (0.0626)	89.1	6.8	4.1	S & D***
D-3	4.00 (0.1177)	86.5	8.5	5.0	"
D-4	8.00 (0.2354)	84.6	9.5	5.9	"
D-5	16.0 (0.4707)	83.2	10.1	6.7	"
D-6	32.0 (0.9414)	79.7	11.8	8.5	
Negative Control	0.00 (0.00)	92.9	7.1	0	
Permanganate-1	1.00 (0.0158)	88.2	11.8	0	Single
P-2	2.00 (0.0316)	67.7	21.9	10.7	S & D
P-3	4.00 (0.0632)	44.3	29.7	10.1	"
P-4	8.00 (0.1264)	35.0	24.4	17.6	"
P-5	16.0 (0.2528)	49.2	33.3	18.1	"
P-6	32.0 (0.5056)	36.6	35.1	28.3	"

* After 1 hours incubation of test chemicals with *SV40* DNA at 4°C, gel-electrophoresis of the incubated materials were performed for 2 hours at 80 DCV(40 mA). DNA bands formed by electrophoresis were stained with ethidium bromide for fluorescent photography. Densitometer was used for quantitation of DNA bands into peak areas.

** Single strand-break effect.

*** Single and double-strand break effect.

Table 2. Genotoxic effects of Potassium Dichromate and Potassium Permanganate on TA102 bacteria.

Chemical and Group No.	Chemical conc. MM (%)	No. of revertants Ân±Sn*	Statistics t-value**	Genotoxic effect
Dichromate-1	1.000 (0.0294)	162.3 ± 37.8	(5.57)	Mutagenic
D-2	2.00 (0.0588)	365.7 ± 210.5	(2.69)	Mutagenic
D-3	4.00 (0.1177)	686.0 ± 92.4	(12.10)	Mutagenic
D-4	8.00 (0.2354)	381.0 ± 6.2	(59.68)	Mutagenic
D-5	16.0 (0.4707)	56.7 ± 21.9	(1.38)	
D-6	32.0 (0.9414)	2.7 ± 2.5	(-7.42)	Lethal
D-7	64.0 (1.8828)	0.0 ± 0.0	(-8.38)	Lethal
Permanganate-1	1.000 (0.0158)	32.4 ± 14.6	(-0.61)	
P-2	2.00 (0.0316)	28.7 ± 12.8	(-1.09)	
P-3	4.00 (0.0632)	24.5 ± 12.0	(-1.65)	
P-4	8.00 (0.1264)	14.2 ± 9.5	(-3.36)	Lethal
P-5	16.0 (0.2528)	11.3 ± 11.4	(-3.36)	Lethal
P-6	32.0 (0.5056)	3.2 ± 5.3	(-7.69)	Lethal
P-7	64.0 (1.0112)	0.0 ± 0.0	(-8.38)	Lethal
Negative Control (Dist. Water)		38.2 ± 7.9		
Positive Control (Daunomycin 0.5 μg/100 ml)		741.0 ± 161.5	(4.35)	Mutagenic

* Mean ± standard deviation (Ân ± Sn) of 3 experimental culture plates.

** Estimated t-values were statistically calculated from the difference of test samples from the the negative standard acccording to the formula of $t=[(\hat{A}n - \hat{A}_1) - 0] / [(Sn^2)/3 + (S_1^2)/3]^{1/2}$, and compared with the critical value ($t_{df=3, \alpha=0.05} = \pm 2.132$) for test of their significance in a statistical test.

Metal Ions in Biology and Medicine; vol 6. Eds. J.A. Centeno, Ph. Collery, G. Vernet, R.B. Finkelman, H. Gibb, J.C. Etienne. John Libbey Eurotext, Paris © 2000, pp. 723-725.

Zinc, copper, calcium and phosphorus levels and growth of preterm neonates fed on preterm milk and preterm formula

B. Sharda

Dept of Pediatrics and Neonatology, RNT Medical College, Udaipur, India

Clinical researchers have been surprisingly slow to move into the area of pre-term nutrition, for premature babies – born into the world months ahead of time, ill, with poor reserves and with a need for rapid growth – it might be suspected that nutritional care would be of immense importance for the quality of their survival. Pre-term neonates are at increased risk of copper and zinc depletion if sufficient quantities of these nutrients are not provided in a bio-available form in postnatal life. An abnormally low concentration of zinc in mother's milk has been associated with clinical nutritional zinc deficiency in pre-term and term newborns. The potential for copper depletion may be greater in rapidly growing neonates. The purpose of this study was to observe the growth and estimate zinc, copper, calcium, and phosphorus levels of pre-term neonates of different gestational age and birth weight while feeding on pre-term mother's milk and pre-term formula from birth to 90 days of age.

Forty eight pre-term neonates were divided into two groups. Group I–28 neonates – 15 pre-term appropriate for gestational age (PreAGA) and 13 pre-term small for gestational age (PreSGA) and fed on pre-term mother's milk. Group II – 20 neonates–10 PreAGA and 10 PreSGA and fed on pre-term formula (DEXOLAC Special Care). Ten term appropriate for gestational age (TAGA) neonates, their mothers and 10 non-pregnant women served as control. Gestational age estimated either singly or in combination of date of last menstrual period, fetal ultrasonography, and postnatal clinical examination. Neonates classified into pre-term (<37 weeks or 259 days) and term (37-41 weeks or 259-293 days). Neonates with the birth weight of <10th percentile for their gestational age were labeled as SGA and with birth weight 10-90th percentile as AGA. Weight was recorded by electronic machine with minimum capacity of 5g. Length was recorded by infantometer (cm) and cranial circumference by steel tap (cm). Neonates' serum, mothers' serum, and breast milk zinc, copper, and calcium was analyzed by atomic absorption spectrophotometer and phosphorus by spectrophotometer. Preparation of glassware, precautions, storage, and analysis of samples were as described earlier[1]. Neonates' weight, length, and cranial circumference were serially recorded along with neonates' serum, mothers' serum, and breast milk zinc, copper, calcium, and phosphorus at birth, 30th, 60th, and 90th day of age in each group and p value calculated.

Table I. Zinc, copper, calcium, & phosphorus in serum and milk

Category	Material	Zinc(ug/dL)	Copper(ug/dL)	Cal (mg/dL)	Phos(mg/dL)
PreAGA	serum	106.26±4.53b	67.4±7.40d	9.17±0.36f	7.16±0.26
PreSGA	neonate	81.07±3.59	48.1±4.99	9.29±0.31	7.10±0.25
TAGA		123.4±5.32a	79.8±5.45c	9.92±0.24e	7.22±0.26
p= a v/s b <0.001; c v/s d <0.001; e v/s f <0.001; others are non-significant.					
PreAGA	serum	77.47±4.88b	181.5±7.16d	8.53±0.20f	6.69±0.19
PreSGA	mother	63.50±4.97	183.8±7.67	8.59±0.18	6.48±0.20
TAGA		59.00±3.53a	201.6±7.89c	9.00±0.18e	6.82±0.15
p= a v/s b <0.001; c v/s d <0.001; e v/s f <0.001; others are non-significant.					
PreAGA	milk	469.5±12.26b	48.6+2.37d	35.3±0.9	13.24±1.10
PreSGA	mother	476.0±8.70	49.4±2.17	35.7±1.06	13.78±1.08
TAGA		499.2±9.60a	56.0±4.47c	35.7±0.68	14.84±0.54
p= a v/s b <0.001; c v/s d <0.05; others are non-significant.					

Table II. Serial changes in wt, length, & cranial circumference in group I & II

	Weight (g)			Length (cm)			Cranial circum (cm)		
Gr	30th day	60th day	90th day	30th day	60th day	90th day	30th day	60th day	90th day
I	690±64	1530±109	2200±172	3.5±0.28	7.6±0.48	11.1±0.53	1.9±0.13	3.9±0.14	.8±0.16
II	800±77	1735±99	2621±53	3.3±0.45	7.0±0.54	10.3±0.60	1.8±0.22	4.0±0.26	6.0±0.17
p=	<0/001	<0.001	<0.001	<0.05	>0.05	<0.05	>0.05	>0.05	>0.05

Results of these observations are presented in Table I and II. Quantitative variables were expressed as mean ±SD and were compared using student's 't' test. Serum copper was significantly high and zinc was low in pregnant women compared with non-pregnant women ($p < 0.001$). Mother's of TAGA neonates had significantly high copper and low zinc levels than mothers of TSGA, PreAGA, and PreSGA neonates (p <0.05, <0.02, and <0.01). Maternal serum copper was significantly low and zinc high in mothers delivering pre-term neonates of various gestational ages. Breast milk copper level was significantly high in TAGA mothers compared with PreSGA mothers ($p < 0.05$) and in mothers delivering neonates <1.5 kg compared with mothers delivering neonates >2.5 kg ($p < 0.01$).

Breast milk zinc content was low in PreAGA and PreSGA mothers and in mothers delivering neonates <2.5 kg compared with term delivery mothers ($p < 0.001$). Low serum calcium and phosphorus has been observed in pregnant mothers (PreAGA and PreSGA) compared with non-pregnant women. Low serum calcium has been observed in PreAGA mothers compared with TAGA mothers. Pre-term neonates of group II showed higher wt gain at 30th, 60th, and 90th day (p <0.001) compared with group I.

Discussion: The important finding of this study is that serum zinc and copper levels of PreAGA, PreSGA, and neonates weighing <2.5 kg were significantly low compared with TAGA and neonates weighing >2.5 kg. Breast milk zinc in PreAGA and PreSGA was significantly low and so was serum zinc in PreAGA and PreSGA mothers. Pre-term neonates who are exclusively breast fed develop zinc deficiency due to low breast milk zinc[2] SGA infants are reported to have better weight and linear growth during first 6 months of life if they receive zinc supplementation[3]. Similarly increase zinc intake during early infancy was reported to be beneficial to very low birth weight infants. Calculated daily intake of copper and zinc for infants from breast milk were markedly lower than those of recommended dietary allowances [4]. Pre-term infants fed on the non-supplemented formula had a marginal copper supply and their first balances were negative. Pre-term neonates on pre-term formula (group II) showed higher wt gain at 30th, 60th, and 90th day of age compared with mothers' milk (group I). There was no change in cranial circumference and length in both groups.

Conclusion: Serum zinc, copper, & calcium level is low in pre-term. Serum zinc & copper is low in SGA. Low serum zinc, calcium, & phosphorus and high serum copper is observed in pregnant mothers compared with non-pregnant women. Low serum copper & calcium & high serum zinc is observed in mothers of pre-term neonates. Zinc & copper level is high in term mother's milk and in colostrum. Pre-term neonates on special formula (group II) showed higher wt gain compared with mother's milk (group I) while increase in length & cranial circumference is same. Serum zinc, copper, & calcium levels are low in pre-term neonates. Pre-term neonates on special formula showed higher wt gain as compared to pre-term milk.

References:

1. Sharda B,Adhikari R,Ajmera M,Gambhir R,Singh PP. Zinc&copper in preterm neonates: Relationship with breast milk. Indian J Pediatr 1999;66:685-695.
2. Heinen F, Matern D, Pringsheim W, Leititis JU, Brandis M. Zinc deficicnecy in an exclusively breast-fed pre-term infant. Eur J Pediatr 1995;154:71-75.
3. Castillo-Duran C, Rodrigues A, Venegas G, Alvarez P, Icaza G. Zinc supplementation and growth of infants born small for gestational age. J Pediatr 1995;17:206-211.
4. Ohtake M, Tamura T. Changes in zinc and copper concentration in breast milk and blood of Japanese women during lactation. J Nutr Sci Vitaminol 1993;39:189-200.

Metal Ions in Biology and Medicine; vol 6. Eds. J.A. Centeno, Ph. Collery, G. Vernet, R.B. Finkelman, H. Gibb, J.C. Etienne. John Libbey Eurotext, Paris © 2000, pp. 725-729.

Selenium-rubidium interaction in breast milk at high dietary selenium intake

V.E. Negretti de Brätter, P. Brätter, E. Pinto de López, L. García de Torres

Hahn-Meitner-Institut Berlin, Dept. Trace Elements in Health and Nutrition, Glienicker Str. 100, D-14109 Berlin, Germany; Hospital General de San Felipe, Departamento de Neonatología, Edo. Yaracuy, Venezuela

Summary

Breast milk samples, serum and erythrocytes were collected from mothers living in seleniferous areas of Venezuela and analyzed by means of instrumental neutron activation analysis to determine the elements Se, Rb and Zn. Three regions were defined according to the mean daily Se-intake level (205, 274 and 552 μg per day). Maternal dietary Se-intake is positively correlated with the Se-concentration in Serum, erythrocytes and breast milk. The significant decrease of Rb found in breast milk , erythrocytes and serum was significantly correlated with the increase of Se in this body fluids. Because the maternal dietary Rb-intake was nearly constant (about 1,6 mg per day) in all regions we suggest that the Se-Rb-interaction takes place at the gastrointestinal side. In contrast to Rb the Zn-concentration of serum and erythrocytes was not influenced by the selenium intake. The significant decrease of the Zn-binding ligand citrate in breast milk at high maternal Se-levels was shown to be linked with metabolic changes in the mammary gland (4). The mechanisms of the interaction Selenium with Rb and Zn are obviously different. ***Keywords:*** Selenium, rubidium, zinc, breast milk, high dietary Se-intake, erythrocytes, serum, lactating women, mammary gland, humans .

Introduction

Breast milk is the most complete feed during early infancy. The success of lactation with respect to trace elements should be stated using the maternal nutritional adequacy of the milk. The essential major and trace elements in human milk are not greatly affected by maternal diet, with the exception of selenium and iodine. Factors influencing the concentration of zinc in breast milk have been studied but very little is known about rubidium. The essentiallity of Rb in humans has been mentioned (1, 2) but there is a lack of knowledge about the biological role of rubidium. A positive correlation between selenium and rubidium levels in the pineal body has been reported (3). The present work was aimed to study the effects of a high dietary selenium intake on the content of Rb in breast milk.

Material and Methods

A total of 143 women (mean age 21.3± 4.6 a, range 18-23 a) living in the Venezuelan states of Yaracuy and Portuguesa were examined. Their consent was obtained according to the ethical guidelines of the Helsinki Declaration. The subjects were on the same socio-economic level and have lived a minimum of 3 years in the region. To exclude seasonal variations the sample collection was carried out within a period of 3 weeks. The sample period each day was from 8 to 12 o'clock in the morning. In order to obtain more accurate information milk samples were collected within the lactation period 20-24 days post-partum. Details of individuals, sample collection and pre-analytical steps can be seen elsewhere (4). Determination of Se, Rb and Zn in serum, erythrocytes and breast milk including Rb and Se in total diets was performed by instrumental neutron activation analysis (INAA). The method of analysis and the check of the accuracy of the element determination are well described elsewhere (4,5,6).

Results

From our former studies in Venezuela and based on the analysis of total diet (5) and on the measured selenium content in breast milk, toe-nails and red blood cells three regions of different Se-intake level were well defined (4, 6): the state Yaracuy defined as region 1 and in the state Portuguesa the two regions 1 and 2. Dietary Se-intake, Rb-intake and contents (mean ± SD) of selenium, rubidium and zinc in erythrocytes and breast milk of lactating mothers of these regions are given in Tab.1. With exception of Zn significant regional differences were obtained for Se and Rb in erythrocytes and serum (Tab.1).

Table 1. Regional dietary Se-intake and contents (mean ± SD) of selenium, rubidium and zinc in serum, erythrocytes and breast milk of lactating mothers

	Yaracuy Region 1	Portuguesa Region 2	Region 3	Significance* Reg. 3 *vs.* Reg. 1
Se -serum (µg/L)**	0.233 ± 0.050 (n=41)	0.325 ± 0.095 (n=8)	0.556 ± 0.220 (n=14)	< 0.0001
Zn -serum (µg/L)**	0.728 ± 0.110 (n=41)	0.747± 0.150 (n=8)	0.732 ± 0.120 (n=14)	n.s.
Rb -serum (mg(kg)	1.81 ± 0.45 (n=29)	1.59 ± 0.39 (n=20)	1.38 ± 0.34 (n=13)	< 0.01
Se- erythrocytes (mg/kg)	1.59 ± 0.76 (n=29)	2.28 ± 0.53 (n=8)	5.15 ± 1.24 (n=14)	< 0.001
Rb- erythrocytes (mg/kg)	11.1 ± 2.7 (n=28)	10.8 ± 3.4 (n=8)	6.9 ± 1.7 (n=12)	< 0.001
Zn- erythrocytes (mg/kg)	42.49 ± 5.21 (n=29)	38.69 ± 4.96 (n=8)	42.81 ± 4.91 (n=14)	n.s.
Se-breast milk (µg/kg)	503.0 ± 283.0 (n=55)	626. 0 ± 232.0 (n=37)	1113 ± 365 (n=34)	< 0.001
Rb-breast milk (mg/kg)	6.85 ± 1.77 (n=55)	5.34 ± 1.23 (n=39)	4.25 ± 1.11 (n=34)	< 0.0001
Zn -breast milk (mg/kg)	30.7 ± 11.2 (n=55)	25.0 ± 11.2 (n=37)	22.9 ± 9.7 (n=34)	< 0.01
Mean dietary intake				
Se (µg per day)	205	274	552	< 0.0001
Rb (mg per day)	1.6	1.6	1.6	n.s.

*Mann-Whithney U-test; n.s.= non significant: **wet weight; the large SD is due to the wide range of the inter-individual variation

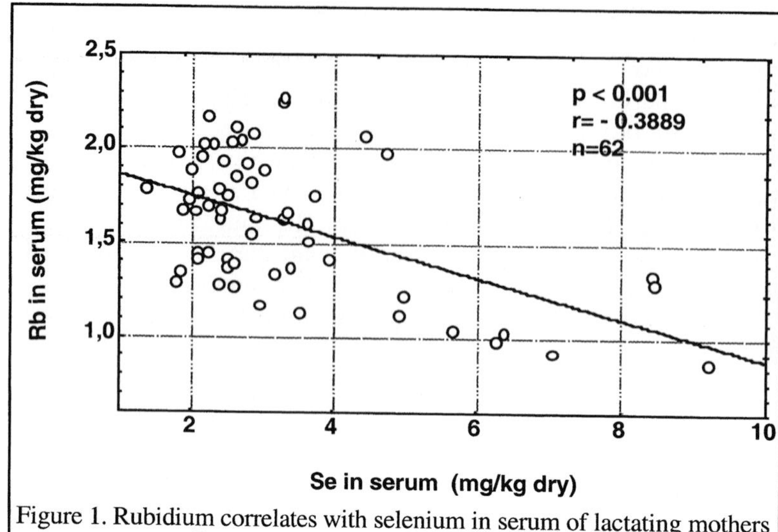

Figure 1. Rubidium correlates with selenium in serum of lactating mothers (Spearman's rank correlation coefficient)

In contrast to Zn (Tab.1),Rb shows a significant negative correlation with selenium in serum (Fig. 1). Rb is significantly negative correlated with selenium not only in erythrocytes (Fig.2) but also in breast milk (Fig.3).

Discussion

The maternal dietary Se-intake and the Se-content in serum, erythrocytes and in breast milk are significantly positive correlated (4,6). The significant decrease of Rb found in breast milk (Fig.3), erythrocytes (Fig.2) and serum (Fig.1) was significantly correlated with the increase of Se in these body fluids. An influence of dietary Rb-intake can be excluded because of the comparable Rb-intake levels (1.6 mg per day) in all regions. Nearly all the ingested Rb is absorbed in the small intestine and transferred into the plasma. Rb resides in the body predominantly inside the cells. The red blood cell compartment is assumed to exchange only with the plasma based on kinetics similar to that of potassium (7).

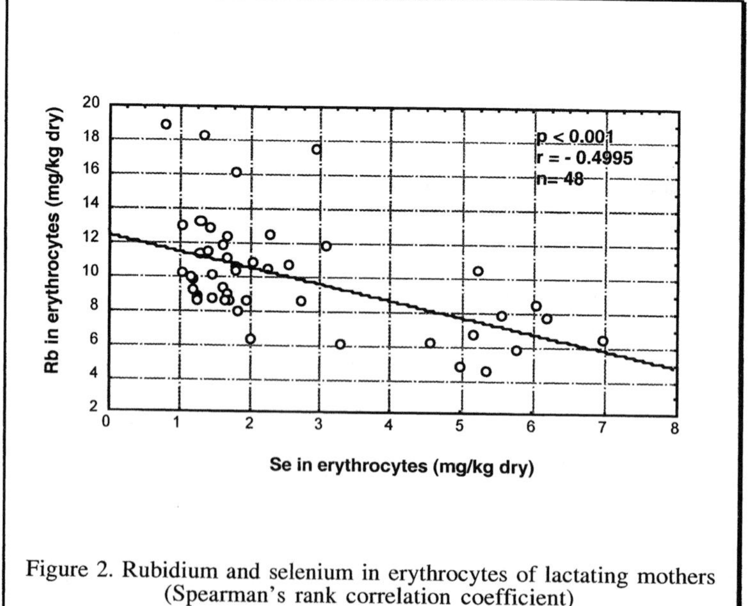

Figure 2. Rubidium and selenium in erythrocytes of lactating mothers (Spearman's rank correlation coefficient)

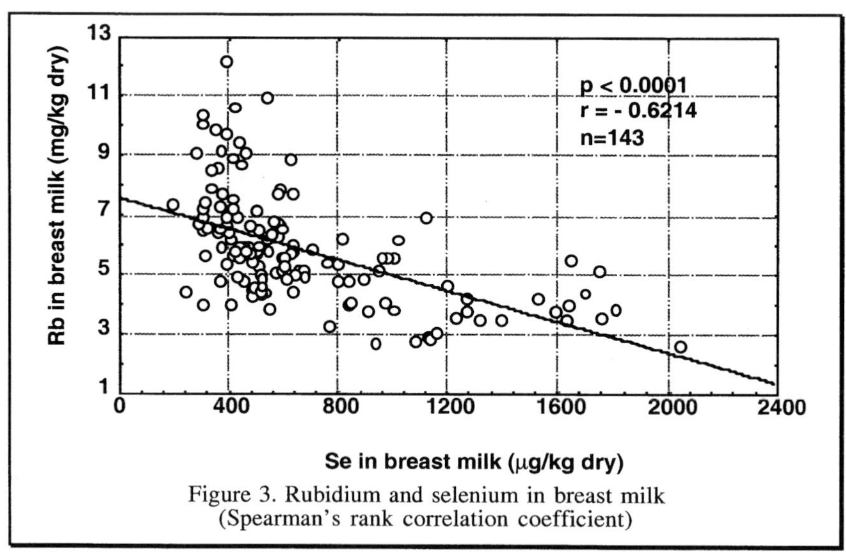

Figure 3. Rubidium and selenium in breast milk
(Spearman's rank correlation coefficient)

The breast milk reflects the Rb-level of the mammary gland and therefore changes in the plasma Rb-concentration as well.
We suggest that the Rb-Se-interaction takes place in the small intestine and not in the mammary gland as it was found for Zn (4). In contrast to Rb, Zn-concentration of serum and erythrocytes (Table 1) was not influenced by the maternal Se-intake. On the other hand, a decrease of Zn in breast milk was observed. At high maternal Se-status the significant decrease of citrate, as the main Zn-binding ligand in breast milk, was shown to be linked with metabolic changes in the mammary gland (4).

References

1- I. Lombeck, K. Kasperek, L. E. Feinendegen, H. J. Bremer. Rubidium-A possible essential trace element (1980) Biol Trace Elem. Res.; 2:193-198

2- E. Selin, V. Teeyasoontranont. Rubidium: a comparison of potassium or an essential trace element of ist own? (1991) Beitr. Infusionsther. Basel. Karger; 27: 86-103

3- U. Demel, A. Höck, K. Kasparek, L.E. Feinendegen. Trace element concentration in the human pineal body. Activation analysis od cobalt, iron, rubidium, selenium, zinc, antimony and cesium (1982) Sci. Tot. Envir. 24:135

4- P. Brätter, V. E. Negretti de Brätter, S. Recknagel and R. Brunetto. Maternal selenium status influences the concentration and binding pattern of zinc in human milk (1997) J, Trace Elements Med. Biol. 11:203-209

5- V. E. Negretti de Brätter, P. Brätter, W. Oliver, N. Alvarez. Study of the trace element status and the dietary intake of mineral and trace elements in relation to the gastric cancer incidence in Táchira, Venezuela (1998) In. Metal Ions in Biology and Medicine (Eds. P. Collery, P. Brätter, V. Negretti de Brätter, L. Khassanova, J. C. Etienne) John Libbey Eurotext, Paris:557-565

6- P. Brätter, V. E. Negretti de Brätter, U. Rösick, H. B. von Stockhausen. Selenium in the nutrition of infants: influence of the maternal selenium status (1991) In: Trace Element in Nutrition of Children-II (Ed. R. K. Chandra) Nestlé Nutrition Workshop Series, Vol. 23: 79-90

7- R. W. Legget, L. R. Williams. A biokinetik model for Rb in humans (1988) Health Physics;55;4:685-702

Metal Ions in Biology and Medicine; vol 6. Eds. J.A. Centeno, Ph. Collery, G. Vernet, R.B. Finkelman, H. Gibb, J.C. Etienne. John Libbey Eurotext, Paris © 2000, pp. 730-732.

Physiologically based pharmacokinetic modeling of the lactational transfer of methylmercury

John C. Lipscomb[1], Janusz Z. Byczkowski[2] and Terry Harvey[1]

[1] *US EPA, National Center for Environmental Assessment, Cincinnati, Ohio, 45268, USA; and [2] TN and Associates, Cincinnati, Ohio, 45246, USA*

ABSTRACT

The developmental neurotoxicity of methylmercury (MeHg) in the human has been well-characterized following catastrophic events in Minimata Bay, Japan and in Iraq. The most common route of MeHg exposure in humans is through the intake of contaminated foodstuffs, especially fish. While the precautions against the ingestion of potentially-contaminated foods during pregnancy are well-recognized, precautions against the ingestion of MeHg during lactation are not so uniformly recognized. However, the continued development of the central nervous system during the early postnatal period serves to elongate the period during which this critical system is susceptible to toxic insult. AIM: This model was developed for quantitative assessment of the lactational transfer of MeHg to the human. METHOD: An available physiologically based pharmacokinetic model was refined to include parameters specific for the elimination of MeHg in breastmilk. The completed model was calibrated with experimental data allometrically scaled from rodents to humans verified by comparing its predictions against data for MeHg distribution and elimination in mothers and their nursing infants. RESULTS: Model predictions closely paralleled actual data. The model incorporates current and previous maternal exposures to MeHg to predict the kinetics of MeHg excretion in breastmilk and the daily intake by the nursing infant. CONCLUSIONS: The model may be used to quantify MeHg intake by the nursing infant under different rates of maternal MeHg ingestion.

EXPOSURE, TOXICITY AND LACTATION

Mercury (Hg) from both natural and anthropogenic sources is ubiquitous in environment. The elemental form, Hg^0, becomes dispersed in the earth's atmosphere and slowly oxidizes to divalent Hg^{2+}. Methylation, mostly by anaerobic bacteria in marine and fresh water sediments, produces organic forms, of which methylmercury (MeHg) is the most common. As a result of bioaccumulation, MeHg accounts for most of the mercury content found in animals (primarily fish) - that serve as food sources for humans. Generally, elemental and inorganic forms of mercury are not readily absorbed from the gastrointestinal tract (bioavailability of less that 5%), and thus are not as highly bioconcentrated in animals as is MeHg (nearly complete) [1].

MeHg is well-known as a developmental neurotoxicant. Its effects can be profound, and increase in severity with increasing exposure. The continued development of the central nervous system beyond parturition prolongs the period of susceptibility. Thus, MeHg consumed by the mother may be transferred from the bloodstream to the milk via one or more of several mechanisms [2,3] and the suckling infant may thus be exposed to maternally-derived MeHg [1,4]. This phenomenon has been previously investigated by applying physiologically based pharmacokinetic (PBPK) modeling techniques to data describing the pharmacokinetics of halogenated industrial solvents [5,6].

PHARMACOKINETIC DATA AND EXISTING MODELS

Tragically, there are multiple data sets of mercury concentrations in blood, hair and milk of mothers and in fetal blood of newborns exposed in utero. Due to the recognized susceptibility of the developing human, a large amount of data was collected when pregnant women were inadvertently exposed to MeHg. Some data demonstrated the temporal distribution in blood and deposition in hair, as well as the concentration of MeHg in milk and in umbilical (neonatal) blood. The richness of these data sets has allowed the construction and testing of PBPK models which estimate the distribution of MeHg in the human, such as that of Clewell et al. [7]. This model served as the template to which an additional submodel addressing lactational transfer was added.

MODEL CONSTRUCTION AND OPERATION

The model consisted of three interlinked submodels. The Mother Submodel was comprised of 12 compartments, in which the distribution of mercury over time was evaluated. Eight compartments (plasma, kidney, rapidly perfused, slowly perfused, fat brain-blood, placenta, liver and gut) were described as flow-limited and four (hair, red blood cells, brain tissue, and feto-placental unit) were described as diffusion-limited. Breast milk was separately described as a fraction of the rapidly-perfused compartment, with 10% of the blood flow being equilibrated with milk. Milk:plasma partition coefficients were derived from published data [2] describing blood and milk mercury concentrations. For this paper, the fetus submodel will not be described. The conversion of MeHg to inorganic mercury was described as a first-order process taking place in hair, brain, liver and intestine with fecal constituents. The Infant Submodel was comprised of six compartments and included an infant body weight growth algorithm. When exercised to simulate a dietary exposure to MeHg, the model accurately predicted the concentrations of MeHg in maternal blood, hair and milk, and infant blood as compared to reported levels [8]. Several maternal model parameters including volume of the fat compartment, plasma and red blood cell volumes, and MeHg blood:milk partition coefficient highly impacted the distribution of MeHg to milk and the subsequent exposure to the nursing infant. One of the critical assumptions made in the model was the relationship between the concentration of mercury forms (organic and inorganic) distributed between plasma and red blood cells. Assumptions made about this relationship may impact the model's ability to predict the concentration of mercury in breastmilk. However, predicted MeHg concentrations in infant blood (derived from lactational transfer) made under the assumptions and in a simulated exposure similar to the Iraqi exposure were quite similar (within approximately 17%) to those concentrations reported in the literature. This model may prove useful in estimating the lactational exposure of the infant to MeHg consumed by the nursing mother.

REFERENCES

1. Agency for Toxic Substances and Disease Registry (ATSDR), *Toxicological Profile for Mercury (Update)*, U.S. Department of Health and Human Services, Public Health Service, Atlanta, GA, 1999.

2. Fujita M, and Takabatake E. Mercury levels in human maternal and neonatal blood, hair and milk. *Bull Environ Contam Toxicol* 1977; 18 : 205-209.

3. Grandjean P, Weihe P, White RF, Milestone development in infants exposed to methylmercury from human milk. *NeuroToxicol* 1995; 16 : 27-34.

4. Abadin HG, Hibbs BF and Pohl HR. Breast-feeding exposure of infants to cadmium, lead, and mercury: a public health viewpoint. *Toxicol Ind Health* 1997; 13 : 495-517.

5. Byczkowski JZ. Linked physiologically based pharmacokinetic model and cancer risk assessment for breast-fed infants. *Drug Inf J* 1996; 30 : 401-412.

6. Byczkowski JZ, Kinkead ER, Leahy HF, Randall GM, Fisher JW. Computer simulation of lactational transfer of tetrachloroethylene in rats using a physiologically based model. *Toxicol Appl Pharmacol* 1994; 125 : 228-236.

7. Clewell HJ, Gearhart JM, Gentry PR, Covington TR, VanLandingham CB, Crump KS, Shipp AM. Evaluation of the uncertainty in an oral reference dose for methylmercury due to interindividual variability in pharmacokinetics. *Risk Analysis* 1999; 19 : 547-558.

8. Amin-Zaki L, Elhassani S, Majeed MA, Clarkson TW, Doherty RA, Greenwood MR, Giovanoli-Jakubczak T. Perinatal methylmercury poisoning in Iraq. *Am J Dis Child* 1976; 130: 1070-1076.

Metal Ions in Biology and Medicine; vol 6. Eds. J.A. Centeno, Ph. Collery, G. Vernet, R.B. Finkelman, H. Gibb, J.C. Etienne. John Libbey Eurotext, Paris © 2000, pp. 733-735.

Serum concentrations of trace elements in aging, health and disease

Michael Krachler[1], Gerhard H. Wirnsberger[2], Erich Rossipal[3], Wolfgang Domej[4]

[1] Institute for Analytical Chemistry, [2] Department of Internal Medicine, Division of Nephrology, [3] Department of Pediatrics, [4] Department of Medicine, Karl-Franzens University Graz, Austria

Mostly reference ranges for concentrations of trace elements in sera are reported exclusively for healthy adults. However, the metabolism of particular trace elements is known to be quite different in newborns, infants, and adults resulting in divergent serum concentrations of trace elements in these subjects. Pregnancy also changes the maternal serum trace element pattern.
Data for this paper were compiled from several studies performed previously [1-8] by our group to provide concentration ranges of selected trace elements in sera of different population groups and patients at various disease states.

Methods

Blood was drawn into polyethylene tubes or with a Vacutainer® system and was centrifuged 10 min at 1800 g at 4°C. Trace elements were determined in digests of sera/plasma by inductively coupled plasma mass spectrometry (ICP-MS) after microwave assisted acid digestion with high purity reagents. Several whole blood and serum reference materials were analyzed with every batch of samples to guarantee the accuracy and precision of the applied analytical procedures.

Results and Discussion

Concentration differences of selected trace elements, focussing on the four trace elements Cu, Rb, Sr and Zn, will be discussed in detail. For example, Cu is mobilized during pregnancy in mothers resulting in serum Cu levels that are twice as high as found in non pregnant healthy women. Umbilical cord serum Cu concentrations are, however, distinctly lower than in all other subjects. It is well known that the huge amount of Cu provided by the mother during pregnancy is stored in the fetal liver. This vital Cu depot is depleted by the young infant during its first year of life. Figure 1 indicates that feeding of young infants with formulae causes a distinct alteration of the serum trace element status in comparison to breast-fed infants. Generally, this difference will be more pronounced the more prominent the gap of concentrations in formulae and milk will be. Probably, young infants do not have adequate mechanisms of homeostasis developed yet to prevent surplus intake of trace elements from formulae nor to prevent elevated serum levels.

Table 1. Serum concentrations (µg/L, mean ± standard deviation) of the two trace essential elements copper and zinc in various subjects.

	number of subjects	Cu	Zn
newborns			
mixed umbilical cord sera	20	400 ± 130	930 ± 220
venous umbilical cord sera	9	470 ± 150	910 ± 260
arterial umbilical cord sera	9	410 ± 110	840 ± 230
infants, 3 months			
formula-fed	6	780 ± 180	460 ± 30
breast-fed	5	730 ± 90	420 ± 50
pregnant women	29	2030 ± 520	650 ± 180
hemodialysis patients[a]	68	1050, 580 - 1700	890, 650 - 1200
patients suffering from internal diseases	66	1480 ± 670	710 ± 170
reference range for healthy adults		600 - 1400	600 - 1200

[a] median, observed range

Table 2. Serum concentrations (µg/L, mean ± standard deviation) of the two trace elements rubidium and strontium in various subjects.

	number of subjects	Rb	Sr
newborns			
mixed umbilical cord sera	20	320 ± 120	20 ± 7
venous umbilical cord sera	9	310 ± 40	20 ± 5
arterial umbilical cord sera	9	270 ± 50	19 ± 6
infants, 3 months			
formula-fed	6	260 ± 80	40 ± 25
breast-fed	5	390 ± 90	12 ± 3
pregnant women	29	200 ± 60	22 ± 9
hemodialysis patients[a]	68	190, 150 – 220	44, 38 - 50
patients suffering from internal diseases[b]	66	160	28
reference range for healthy adults		150 – 560	28 - 44

[a] median, observed range [b] median

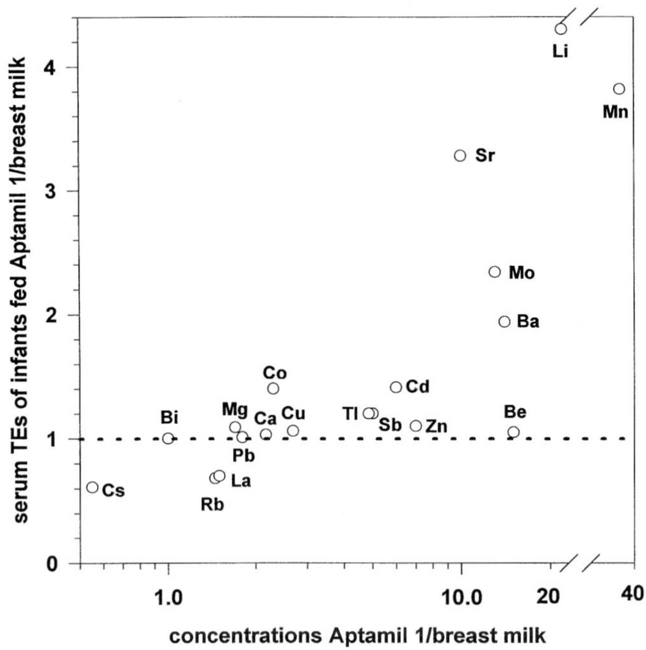

Fig. 1 Correlation between concentrations of selected trace elements in the formula Aptamil 1 and human milk and serum trace element concentrations of the infants.

Conclusions: Serum concentrations of trace elements in newborns, infants, adults, healthy and diseased subjects are significantly different from each other. Thus reference ranges for serum trace elements should be set up more carefully considering age and the clinical status of a person.

References:

1. M. Krachler, G. Wirnsberger and K.J. Irgolic, *Biol Trace Element Res* 58: 209-221, 1997.
2. M. Krachler, H. Scharfetter and G.H. Wirnsberger, *Nephron*, 83: 777-782, 1999.
3. M. Krachler, E. Rossipal, D. Micetic-Turk, *Biol Trace Element Res* 68: 121-135, 1999.
4. W. Domej, M. Krachler, C. Schlagenhaufen, M. Trinker, G.J. Krejs, K.J. Irgolic, *J Trace Elements Med Biol* 11: 232-238, 1997.
5. M. Krachler, E. Rossipal, D. Micetic-Turk, *Eur J Clin Nutr* 53: 486-494, 1999.
6. M. Krachler and K.J. Irgolic, *J Trace Elements Med Biol* 13: 157-169, 1999.
7. M. Krachler, M. Lindschinger, B. Eber, N. Watzinger and S. Wallner, *Biol Trace Element Res* 60: 175-185, 1997.
8. M. Krachler, E. Rossipal, D. Micetic-Turk, *Trace Elem Electrolytes* 16: 46-52, 1999.

Metal Ions in Biology and Medicine; vol 6. Eds. J.A. Centeno, Ph. Collery, G. Vernet, R.B. Finkelman, H. Gibb, J.C. Etienne. John Libbey Eurotext, Paris © 2000, pp. 736-737.

Aging of human bones. An infrared study

Mariana Petra, Jane Anastassopoulou, Athanassios Dovas,
Dimitrios Yfantis and Theophilos Theophanides

National Technical university of Athens, Chemical Engineering Department, Radiation Chemistry and Biospectroscopy, Zografou Campus, 15 780 Zografou, Athens, Greece

Introduction

Fourier transform infrared spectroscopy is increasingly recognized as a method for the investigation of mineralized human bones. Human bones from the ancient region of Avdira, Greece, of 2500 years old have been studied together with recent ones using Fourier Transform Infrared (FT-IR) spectroscopy. Avdira is an ancient Greek city, where Demokritos, discovered the atom (άτομο, α-τέμνω, cannot cut more) and he coined the word atom as the smallest particle of a chemical element that can take part in a chemical reaction without being permanently changed and which has the characteristics of the bulk material. The ancient bones were given to us from the Archeological Museum of Kavala, a nearby city, for this study. Bone decomposition is a slow chemical process and it takes centuries to end up in phosphates (PO_4^{3-}) and carbonates (CO_3^{2-}), which have characteristic vibrational spectra[1,2]. Comparison of these spectra of recent and old human bones might help us understand the aging process of the bones in humans and also identify the structures of these phosphates and carbonates[3]. Phosphates are very important in the diets of plants and animals. Nature converts with time old bones into an assimilative form of phosphorous that can be used to maintain ATP in living plant cells. ATP is the major energy storage in chemical form in cells.

Experimentals

The FT-IR spectra were recorded with a BOMEM Michelson 100 spectrophotometer with a resolution of 2 cm^{-1} and 25 scans were recorded. The new human bones were obtained from the feet of patients who were operated due to an accident. The samples were washed with hydrogen peroxide 30% and acetone, alternatively to eliminate the organic part, i.e. blood chromophores and fat tissue contents. Finally the samples were dried under vacuum and KBr pellets were prepared.

Results and Discussion

The data of the FT-IR spectra are in Table. The old human bones contained water molecules and their hydroxyl hydrogen bonded vibrations were observed at 3618 cm^{-1} and 3385 cm^{-1}, whereas the new bones do not show the free hydroxyl vibration of OH. On the other hand, the spectra of the old bones do not show the organic part at all. This is because the organic part is characterized from the methyl and methylene vibrations ($-CH_3$, $-CH_2$) at 2928 and 2856 cm^{-1}, the protein vibrations near 1700 cm^{-1} and the sugar vibrations near 1160 cm^{-1}, which are not present in the spectra of the old bones, due to assimilation process. Only the bands of the phosphate and carbonate[4] groups are present in the spectra of these bones. It is shown in Table that the carbonates are in form of calcite and aragonite, that both are crystalline forms of carbonates. This finding is very interesting, since these forms are found in nature. The samples are being examined farther with other techniques.

Table. Comparison of some characteristic infrared bands of old and new human bones together with their assignment (cm^{-1})[5]

Old human bones	New human bones	Assignments
3618		νH_2O free
3385	3350	νNH_2 &νOH, H-bond
	3005	$\nu_{sym}{=}CH_2$
	2928	$\nu_{sym}CH_3$
	2856	$\nu_{sym}CH_2$
	1743	NH-protein, esters
1649	1650	δH_2O
	1466	δCH_3 aragonite
1451	1457	δCH_2, scissor
1419		$\nu_3CO_3^{2-}$ calcite
	1376	δCH_3 asym
	1238	$\nu_3PO_4^{3-}$
	1160	CO sugar
	1098	$\nu_1$calcite
1032	1026	$\nu_3PO_4^{3-}$
964		$\nu_1PO_4^{3-}$
913		$\nu_1PO_4^{3-}$
871	872	$\nu_2CO_3^{2-}$ calcite
795		
695	666	δO-P-O, $\nu_4PO_4^{3-}$

References

1. Walters M A, Leung Y C, Blumenthal NC, Le Geros R Z, Konsker K A, A Raman and infrared Spectroscopic investigation of biological hydroxyapatite, *J. Inorg. Biochem.*, 1990: **39**, 193-200.
2. Penel G, LeRoy G, Bres E, New preparation method of bone samples for Raman microspectroscopy. *Appl. Spectrosc.*, 1998: **52/2,** 312-313.
3. Edwards H G M, Williams A C, Farwell D W, Palaiodental using Ft-Raman spectroscopy *Biospectroscopy*, 1995: **1**, 29-36.
4. Wenthrup-Byrne E, Armstrong C A, Armstrong R, Collins B M, *J Raman Spectrosc.* 1997: **28**,151-158.
5. Theophanides T, Vibrational Spectroscopy of Metal Nucleic Acids Systems, in *Infrared and Raman Spectra of Biological Molecules*, 1979 (ed. T. Theophanides), D. Reidel Publishing Co, Dodrecht, Holland, pp. 205-223.

Metal Ions in Biology and Medicine; vol 6. Eds. J.A. Centeno, Ph. Collery, G. Vernet, R.B. Finkelman, H. Gibb, J.C. Etienne. John Libbey Eurotext, Paris © 2000, pp. 738-740.

Interaction of aluminum and some essential elements following aluminum exposure in pregnant and nonpregnant rats

M. Bellés, D.J. Sánchez, M.L. Albina, J.L. Domingo and J. Corbella

Laboratory of Toxicology and Environmental Health, School of Medicine, "Rovira i Virgili" University, San Lorenzo 21, 43201 Reus, Spain

It is now well established that oral aluminum (Al) administration during pregnancy can produce a syndrome that includes growth retardation, delayed ossification, and perhaps malformations at high doses that also lead to reduced maternal weight gain [1,2]. Competition with essential trace elements is one of the possible mechanisms that have been proposed to explain Al-induced developmental toxicity [3]. It seems particularly relevant during periods of rapid growth in late gestation and early infancy when heavy demands are made on trace element metabolism. However, an important issue that has not been addressed yet, is the possible mobilization of maternal Al body stores in bone and transfer to the fetus along with calcium and other essential elements, phenomenon that was already demonstrated for lead [4].

In recent years, a number of studies on the interaction of Al with essential trace elements have been carried out [3,5,6]. However, information about the effects of oral Al on the mineral status of pregnant animals is rather scarce [7,8]. Although in a recent review Borak and Wise [9] suggested that environmental and dietary Al exposure would be unlikely to pose risks of Al accumulation to pregnant animals or their fetuses, the abundant data on Al-induced developmental toxicity in mammals cannot be undervalued [1,2]. The aim of the present study was to determine the interactions of Al with six essential trace elements: calcium (Ca), magnesium (Mg), manganese (Mn), copper (Cu), zinc (Zn) and iron (Fe) in various tissues of pregnant and nonpregnant rats orally exposed to Al for 20 consecutive days.

Materials and Methods

Animals and Chemicals. Aluminum hydroxide was purchased from E. Merck (Darmstadt, Germany). Adult male and female Sprague-Dawley rats (220-250 g) were obtained from Criffa (Barcelona, Spain). Following an acclimation period of two weeks. One-half of the female rats were mated with males (2:1) overnight and examined the following morning for copulatory plug. The day on which a vaginal plug was found was designated as day 0 of gestation.

Experimental. Thirty plug-positive females were randomly divided into three groups which consisted of 10 animals each. The other half of female rats was also randomly divided into three groups (n = 10). All groups of pregnant and nonpregnant rats received $Al(OH)_3$ by gavage for 20 consecutive days at 0, 200 and 400 mg/kg/day. Aluminum hydroxide solutions were prepared in tap water and administered at a volume of 1 ml/350 g body weight.

At the end of the exposure period, all animals were placed in metabolism cages and urines were collected during 24 h for Al and essential element analyses. Subsequently, pregnant and nonpregnant rats were sacrificed by overexposure to diethyl ether. Samples of liver, bone (femur), spleen, kidneys and brain were removed and analyzed for Al concentrations, as well as for the levels of Ca, Mg, Mn, Zn, Cu and Fe. The urinary and tissue concentrations of Al, Ca, Mg, Mn, Zn, Cu and Fe were analyzed as described previously [6].

Results and Discussion

In the present study no maternal toxicity was evidenced following exposure of pregnant rats to 200 and 400 mg/kg/day of $Al(OH)_3$ on gestation days 1-20. However, the investigation of potential changes on essential trace element metabolism could be valuable to get an overall information on Al-induced disturbances during pregnancy.

The Al concentrations and the levels of Ca, Mg, Mn, Zn, Cu and Fe in liver, bone, spleen, kidneys and brain of pregnant and nonpregnant rats exposed to 0, 200 and 400 mg/kg/day of $Al(OH)_3$ during 20 days are depicted in Figures 1 - 7. In turn, Figure 8 shows the urinary concentrations of Al, Ca, Mg, Mn, Cu, Zn and Fe.

The results of the current investigation show remarkable differences between pregnant and nonpregnant rats in tissue Al concentrations after oral Al exposure for 20 days. While in pregnant rats given 400 mg $Al(OH)_3$/kg/day the highest and the lowest Al levels were found in kidneys and brain, respectively, in nonpregnant animals exposed to the same doses of $Al(OH)_3$ brain and liver were the tissues showing the highest and the lowest Al accumulation. Notwithstanding, no significant differences between pregnant and nonpregnant rats were found in the urinary levels of Al. With regard to the essential trace elements, tissue accumulation was most affected in pregnant than in nonpregnant animals. In pregnant rats, the hepatic and renal concentrations of Ca, Mg, Mn, Cu, Zn and Fe, as well as the levels of Ca and Mg in bone, and the concentrations of Cu in brain were significantly higher in the Al-exposed groups than in the control group. However, in nonpregnant rats only Ca concentrations in spleen and kidneys, Cu levels in kidneys, and Fe concentrations in bone and spleen were significantly higher at 200 and 400 mg/kg/day of $Al(OH)_3$ than in the control group.

In summary, the current results in pregnant rats together with those of previous studies indicate that although high oral doses of $Al(OH)_3$ do not show any evidence of maternal (and developmental) toxicity, oral Al exposure during pregnancy can produce changes in the tissue distribution of various essential elements.

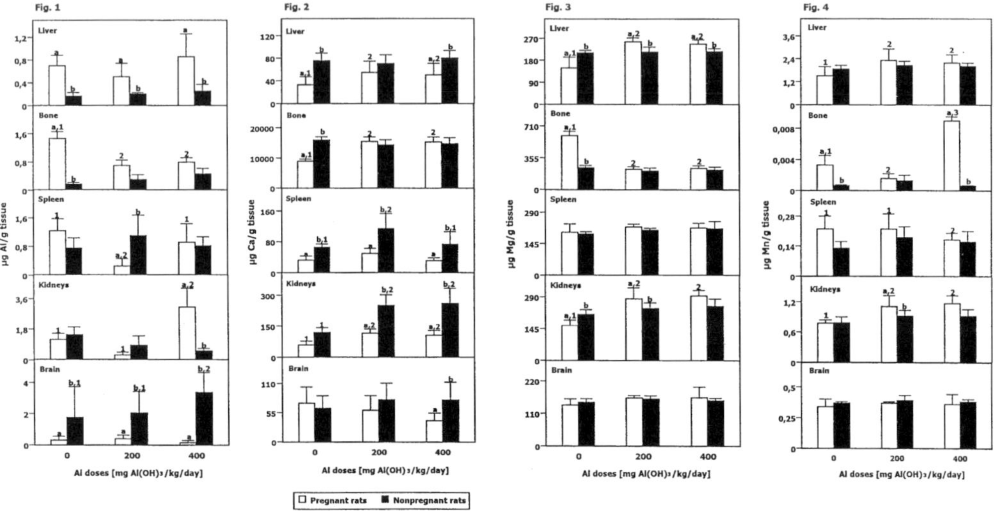

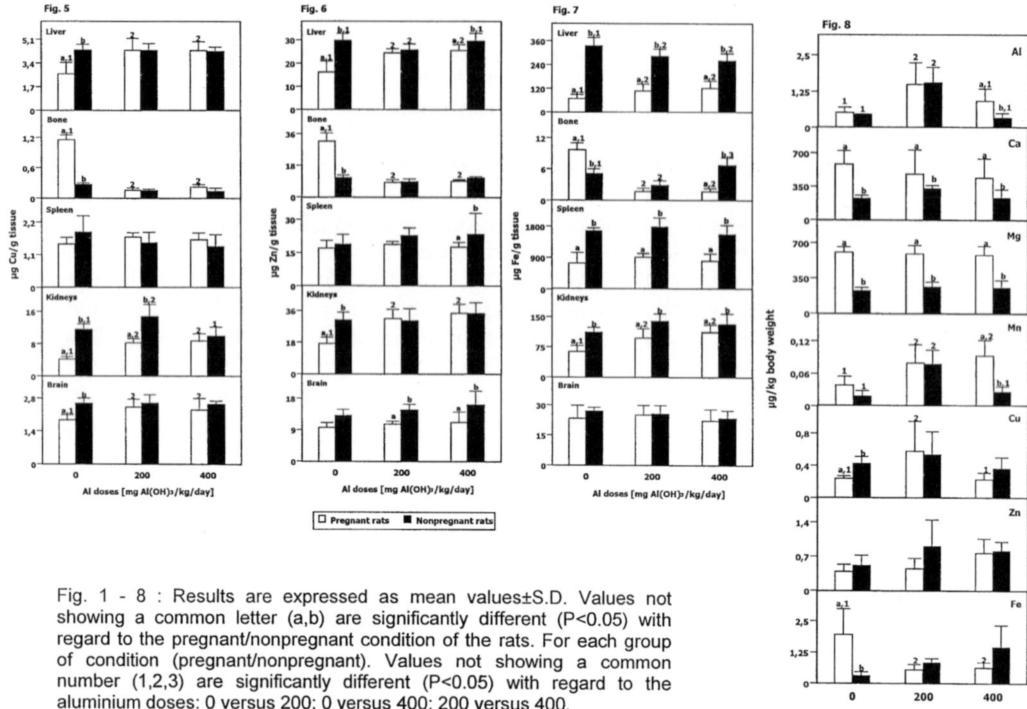

Fig. 1 - 8 : Results are expressed as mean values±S.D. Values not showing a common letter (a,b) are significantly different (P<0.05) with regard to the pregnant/nonpregnant condition of the rats. For each group of condition (pregnant/nonpregnant). Values not showing a common number (1,2,3) are significantly different (P<0.05) with regard to the aluminium doses: 0 versus 200; 0 versus 400; 200 versus 400.

Acknowledgements

This work was supported the DGICYT, Ministry of Education, Spain, grant PM96-0030.

References

1. Domingo JL. Reproductive and developmental toxicity of aluminum: A review. *Neurotoxicol Teratol* 1995; 17:515-21.

2. Golub MS, Domingo JL. What we know and what we need to know about developmental aluminum toxicity. *J Toxicol Environ Health* 1996; 48:585-97.

3. Chmielnicka J, Nasiadek M. Tissue distribution and urinary excretion of essential elements in rats orally exposed to aluminium chloride. *Biol Trace Elem Res* 1991;31:131-38.

4. Silbergeld EK. Lead in bone: implications for toxicology during pregnancy and lactation. *Environ Health Perspect* 1991;91:63-70.

5. Greger JL, Bula EN, Gum ET. Mineral metabolism of rats fed moderate levels of various aluminum compounds for short periods of time. *J Nutr* 1985; 115:1708-16.

6. Sanchez DJ, Gomez M, Llobet JM, Corbella J, Domingo JL. Effects of aluminum on the mineral metabolism of rats in relation to age. *Pharmacol Toxicol* 1997; 80:11-17.

7. Golub MS, Han B, Keen CL. Developmental patterns of aluminum and five essential mineral elements in the central nervous system of the fetal and infant guinea pig. *Biol Trace Elem Res* 1996; 55:241-51.

8. Muller G, Burnel D, Gery A, Lehr P. Element variations in pregnant and nonpregnant female rats orally intoxicated by aluminum lactate. *Biol Trace Elem Res* 1993; 39:211-19.

9. Borak J, Wise Sr JP. Does aluminum exposure of pregnant animals lead to accumulation in mothers or their offspring?. *Teratology* 1998; 57:127-39.

Metal Ions in Biology and Medicine; vol 6. Eds. J.A. Centeno, Ph. Collery, G. Vernet, R.B. Finkelman, H. Gibb, J.C. Etienne. John Libbey Eurotext, Paris © 2000, pp. 741-743.

Deferiprone (L1) does not protect against aluminum-induced maternal and embryo/fetal toxicity in mice

J. Corbella[1], D.J. Sánchez[2], M.L. Albina[2], M. Bellés[2] and J.L. Domingo[2]

[1] *Toxicology Unit, Hospital Clínic Provincial, c/Casanova, Barcelona, Spain and* [2] *Laboratory of Toxicology and Environmental Health, School of Medicine, "Rovira i Virgili" University, San Lorenzo 21, 43201 Reus, Spain*

In humans, aluminum (Al) absorption and accumulation can occur via the diet, including water and therapeutic preparations administered in large quantities such as antacids and buffered aspirins, the inhalation of particulate Al and, controversially, through the skin. Aluminum toxicity occurs in individuals with renal insufficiency who are treated by dialysis with Al-contaminated solutions or oral phosphate binding agents that contain Al [1,2].

There are clear evidences that dietary silicon can reduce the gastrointestinal absorption of Al and increase its elimination [3,4]. However, in a recent study silicon was not effective in protecting against the Al-induced developmental toxicity in mice [5]. On the other hand, it has been demonstrated that a number of chelating agents may act as antagonists of the embryo/fetal toxicity of certain metals [6]. Recently, the protective activity of desferrioxamine (DFO), an efficient chelator available for the treatment of iron and Al overload, on Al-induced developmental toxicity was evaluated in mice. Notwithstanding, s.c. administration of DFO (40 mg/kg/day) on gestation days 6-18 offered only a very modest encouragement as a protective agent for pregnant mice i.p. exposed to Al chloride on gestation days 6-15 [7].

Since deferiprone is also an effective chelating agent in mobilizing iron and Al following exposure to these elements [8], in the present study we investigated whether oral administration of deferiprone could ameliorate the developmental toxic effects of Al in mice.

Materials and Methods

Animals and chemicals. Virgin male and female Charles River CD1 mice, average weight of 26-31 g were purchased from Criffa (Barcelona, Spain). Following an acclimation period of one week, female mice were mated with males (2:1) overnight and examined the following morning for copulatory plugs. The day on which a vaginal plug was found was designated day 0 of gestation. Animals were assigned to experimental groups by stratified randomization so that body weights were equivalent across all groups on gestation day 0.

Aluminum was administered as Al nitrate nonahydrate (E. Merck, Darmstadt, Germany), while 1,2-dimethyl-3-hydroxypyrid-4-one (deferiprone, L1) was a gift from Professor Mark M. Jones (Vanderbilt University, Nashville, TN). Solutions of Al nitrate and deferiprone were prepared in deionized water and the concentrations adjusted so that a 30-g mouse would receive a volume of 0.20 ml.

Experimental. Plug-positive female mice were randomly divided into five groups which consisted of one control group, one group given 1327 mg/kg of Al nitrate nonahydrate (one-third of the oral LD_{50}) on gestation day 12, one group given 902 mg/kg of sodium nitrate on gestation day 12, one group given deferiprone (24 mg/kg/day) on days 12-15 of gestation, and one group given 1327 mg/kg of Al nitrate nonahydrate on gestation day 12 followed by deferiprone (24 mg/kg per administration) at 2, 24, 48, and 72 hr after Al exposure (days 12-15 of gestation). Aluminum nitrate, sodium nitrate and deferiprone were given orally (gavage). The dose of sodium nitrate was equimolar (in nitrate) to that of Al nitrate nonahydrate. On gestation day 18, animals were sacrificed with diethyl ether and uterine contents and external, internal, and skeletal anomalies were evaluated.

Results and Discussion

There were no deaths or early deliveries in any group. In the group given Al nitrate only, maternal toxicity was evidenced by one abortion, significant reductions in food consumption (gestation days 12-15 and 0-18) and body weight gain (gestation days 12-15). Body weight at termination and corrected body weight change were even more affected (reduced) in the group given Al plus deferiprone than in that exposed to Al only (Figure I).

FIG. I Maternal effects

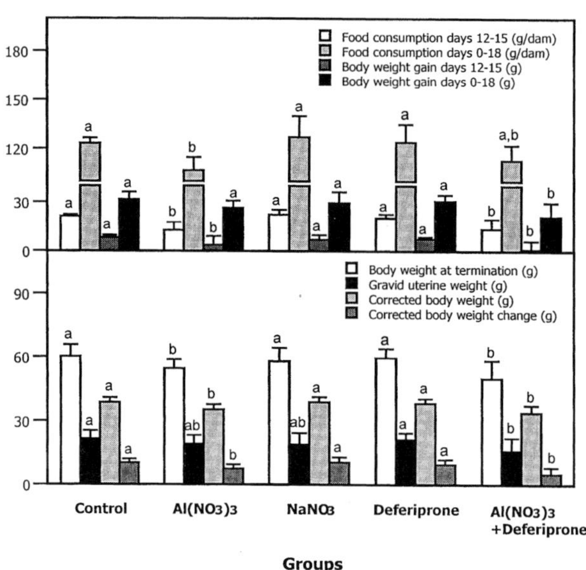

Results are expressed as mean values±SD. Values not showing a common letter (a,b) are significantly different at $P<0.05$. Corrected body weight: (Body weight at sacrifice)-(Gravid uterine weight). Corrected body weight change: (Corrected body weight)-(Body weight on gestational day 0) calculated as percentage of corrected body weight.

There were not significant differences between Al, deferiprone, and the concurrent administration of both chemicals on the number of viable and non-viable implants per litter, or the sex ratio. However, fetal body weight was significantly lower in the group given Al nitrate only (Figure II). No protective activity of deferiprone on the Al-induced reductions in fetal weight was noted.

Administration of Al nitrate, deferiprone, and Al nitrate plus deferiprone did not cause external or internal malformations and variations. The most common morphological defects were reduced ossification of a number of bones found in the skeletal examination (Figure III). Again, no protective effects of deferiprone on the Al-induced skeletal defects could be observed.

FIG. II. Fetal body weight (g)

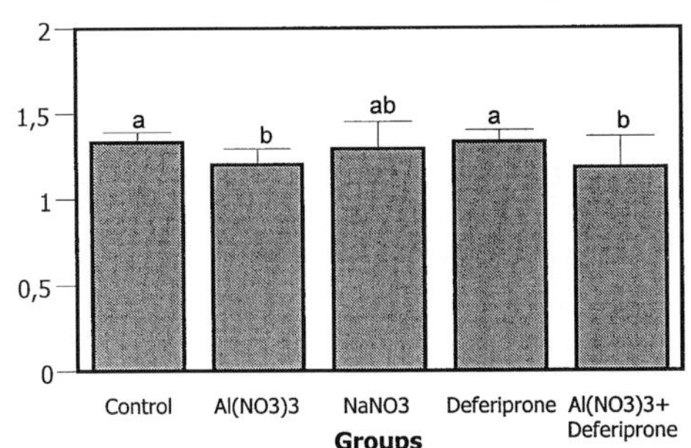

FIG.III. Skeletal alterations

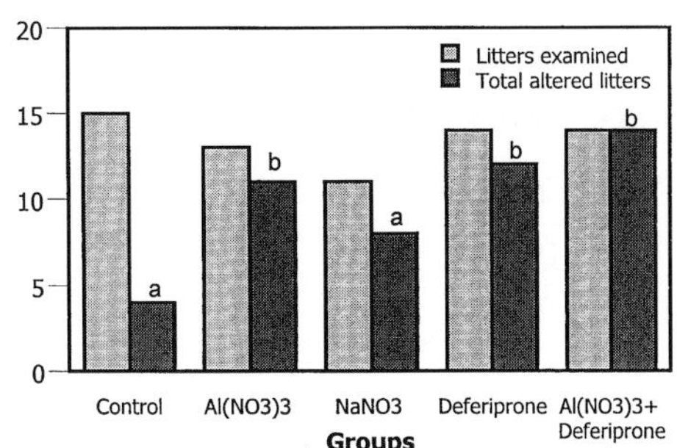

Results are expressed as mean values±SD. Results are expressed as mean values.
Values not showing a common letter (a,b) are significantly different at $P<0.05$.

According to the present results, administration of deferiprone at 24 mg/kg was not a developmental toxicant by itself. However, no protective activity of the chelator on Al-induced maternal and developmental effects could be noted. By contrast, a more pronounced decrease in maternal weight gain and corrected body weight change, as well as an increase in the number of litters with fetuses showing skeletal variations were observed in the group given Al and deferiprone. These results indicate that this chelating agent should not be used to protect against Al-induced developmental toxicity from potential maternal Al intoxication.

The current results together with recent data showing the lack of protective effects of dietary silicon [5] and DFO [7] on Al-induced developmental toxicity in pregnant mice seem to suggest that women should avoid the consumption of high doses of Al-containing compounds during gestation. However, taking into account the known variation interspecies, the extrapolation of the present results in mice to pregnant women would require further investigations in more than one species.

Acknowledgements

This work was supported the DGICYT, Ministry of Education, Spain, grant PM96-0030.

References

1. Alfrey AC. Aluminum and renal disease. In: Bourke E, Mallick NP, Pollak VE, editors. *Moving points in nephrology*. Basel: Karger, 1993: p 110-24.
2. Andreoli SP, Bergstein JM, Sherrard DJ. Aluminum intoxication from aluminum-containing phosphate binders in children with azotemia not undergoing dialysis. *N Engl J Med* 1984; 310:1079-84.
3. Yokel RA, Ackrill P, Burgess E, Day JP, Domingo JL, Flaten TP, Savory J. Prevention and treatment of aluminum toxicity including chelation therapy: status and research needs. *J Toxicol Environ Health* 1996; 48:667-83.
4. Bellés M, Sanchez DJ, Gomez M, Corbella J, Domingo JL. Silicon reduces aluminum accumulation in rats: relevance to the aluminum hypothesis of Alzheimer disease. *Alzheimer Dis Assoc Disord* 1998; 12:83-87.
5. Bellés M, Albina ML, Sanchez DJ, Domingo JL. Lack of protective effects of dietary silicon on aluminum-induced maternal and developmental toxicity in mice. *Pharmacol Toxicol* 1999; 85:1-6.
6. Domingo JL. Developmental toxicity of metal chelating agents. *Reprod Toxicol* 1998; 12:499-10.
7. Albina ML, Bellés M, Sanchez DJ, Domingo JL. Prevention by desferrioxamine of aluminum-induced maternal and developmental toxic effects in mice. *Trace Elem Electrolytes* 1999; 16:192-98.
8. Kontoghiorghes GJ. Comparative efficacy and toxicity of desferrioxamine, deferiprone, and other iron and aluminum chelating drugs. *Toxicol Lett* 1995; 80:1-18.

Metal Ions in Biology and Medicine; vol 6. Eds. J.A. Centeno, Ph. Collery, G. Vernet, R.B. Finkelman, H. Gibb, J.C. Etienne. John Libbey Eurotext, Paris © 2000, pp. 744-746.

Age-related differences in the treatment by chelating agents of aluminum-loaded uremic rats

M. Gómez[1], J.L. Esparza[1], J.M. Llobet[2], J. Corbella[2] and J.L. Domingo[1]

[1] *Laboratory of Toxicology and Environmental Health, School of Medicine, "Rovira i Virgili" University, 43201 Reus; and* [2] *University of Barcelona, Barcelona, Spain*

Aluminum (Al) toxicity has been a common problem in patients with chronic renal failure undergoing hemodialysis. At present, the most effective method to remove Al from the body is by chelation with desferrioxamine (deferoxamine, DFO) [1]. In spite of the beneficial effects of DFO for the treatment Al overloading, the high cost of the drug, the need for parenteral administration, as well as a number of serious side effects of DFO [2], are important reasons to search for orally effective, cheaper and less toxic Al chelators than DFO.

In recent years, a great deal of interest has been shown in 3-hydroxypyrid-4-ones (HPs), new iron and Al chelators. Among these compounds, only 1,2-dimethyl-3-hydroxypyrid-4-one (deferiprone, L1) has been administered to humans, whereas clinical studies with others were stopped [3]. Recent studies in our laboratory compared in healthy rats the relative efficay of nine HPs with different lipophilicities on the urinary excretion and tissue distribution of Al, showing that oral administration of L1 could be a potential alternative treatment to parenteral DFO in Al removal [4,5]. On the other hand, it has been demonstrated that age is one of the factors influencing the efficiency of chelation therapy in metal accumulation and toxicity [6]. The purpose of the present study was to compare in two age groups of uremic rats the efficacy of parenteral DFO, oral L1, and a combined administration of DFO (parenteral) and L1 (oral) on the urinary excretion and tissue accumulation of Al.

Materials and Methods

Animals and chemicals Male Sprague-Dawley rats were obtained from Criffa (Barcelona, Spain). Young rats were 21 days of age upon arrival (70-80 g), while adult rats were 6 months of age (360-510 g). To induce uremia, animals were subjected to a two stage 5/6 nephrectomy (5/6 N_x). Aluminum nitrate nonahydrate was obtained from E. Merck (Darmstadt, Germany) and deferoxamine (DFO) was from Ciba (Barcelona). 1,2-Dimethyl-3-hydroxypyrid-4-one (deferiprone, L1) was a generous gift from Prof. Mark M. Jones, Vanderbilt University (Nashville, TN, USA).

Experimental Fifty animals in each age group received i.p. injections of Al nitrate nonahydrate at doses of 45 mg/kg/day for five consecutive weeks (5 days per week). An additional group of uremic rats received i.p. injections of 0.9% saline (negative control group). Animals in the positive control groups received deionized water by gavage and s.c. injections of 0.9% saline for 5 days. Rats in the experimental groups were given s.c. solutions of DFO in 0.9% saline at 0.89 mmol/kg, oral solutions of L1 in deionized water at 0.89 mmol/kg, or combined administrations of DFO (s.c.) and L1 (gavage) at doses of 0.45 mmol/kg for 5 days. During chelation therapy, rats were placed in individual plastic metabolism cages and urines were collected daily for 5 consecutive days. Twenty-four hours after the last administration of the chelators, rats were anesthetized with diethyl ether and killed. Samples of the following tissues were collected: spleen, brain, liver, kidney and bone (femur). Aluminum concentrations in tissues and urine were analyzed as described previously [4].

Results

Significant age differences in the cumulative (5 days) Al urinary excretion were only noted in the control group and the group given DFO plus L1, in which adult rats excreted more Al than young animals. Moreover, while in young rats the efficacy of combined DFO/L1 treatment was lower than that of DFO or L1, in the adult group administration of DFO plus L1 had a similar efficacy than that of DFO and higher to that of L1 (Fig. 1). With regard to Al tissue accumulation, the most notable reduction was found in the liver of young rats. No significant age differences between groups were noted in the remaining tissues (Fig. 2).

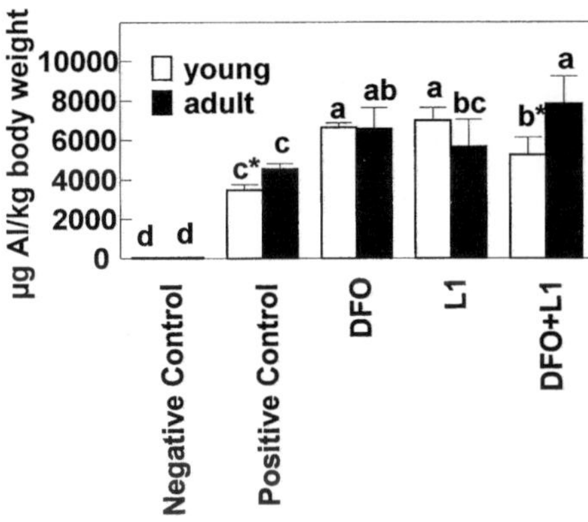

Fig. 1. The effect of the indicated treatments on the cumulative amount of Al (mg/kg body weight) excreted into urine during the total period (5 days) of collection. Bars indicate S.D. Values not showing a common superscript (a,b,c) are significantly different from the respective positive control groups (young and adult) at P < 0.05. An asterisk (*) indicates significant age-related (young vs. adult) differences at P < 0.05.

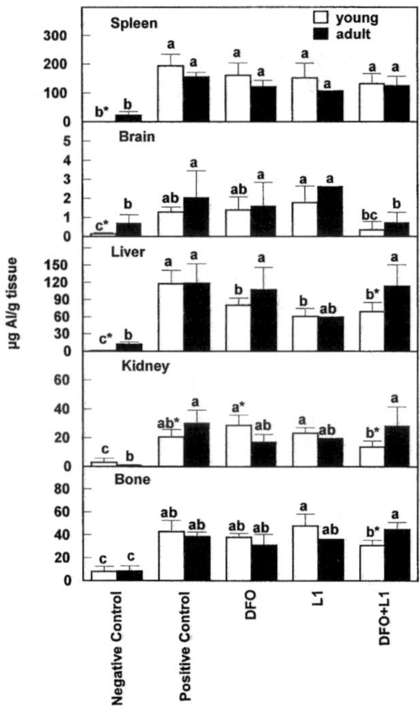

Fig. 2. The effect of the indicated treatments on Al concentrations (mg/g tissue) into spleen, brain, liver, kidney and bone of rats killed at the end of the chelation therapy. Bars indicate S.D. For each tissue, values not showing a common superscript (a,b,c) are significantly different from the respective positive control groups (young and adult) at P < 0.05. An asterisk (*) indicates significant age-related (young vs. adult) differences at P < 0.05.

Discussion

In recent years, it has been shown that DFO and L1 have a comparable effect on Al removal when used in equimolar doses [4,5,7]. Although information concerning the effects of L1 on Al mobilization in Al-loaded uremic rats is very scarce [7,8], in a previous study a remarkable death rate was observed in uremic rats given L1 (s.c. or p.o.) at 1.35 mmol/kg/day for 5 days [7]. On the other hand, in a recent study, we found that L1 was most effective than DFO in enhancing urinary Al excretion, but not in reducing tissue Al levels in two age groups of Al-loaded healthy rats [9]. These effects were similar for young and adult animals. In the current study, in general terms, the effects of DFO and L1 in increasing the urinary Al excretion and in reducing Al concentrations in various tissues were quite comparable.

In summary, the results of the current study show that a combined therapy with DFO and L1 of each drug is also effective in mobilizing Al from the body of Al-loaded uraemic rats. However, further studies are needed to establish the safety and efficacy of the administration of a longer combined therapy. On the other hand, although also effective in adult animals, the efficacy of DFO plus L1 was lower in adult than in young rats.

Acknowledgements
This study was supported by the DGICYT, Ministry of Education, Spain through grant PM95-0062.

References

1. Jablonski G, Klem KH, Danielsen C Ch, Moselkide L, Gordelazde JO: Aluminium-induced bone disease in uremic rats: effect of deferoxamine. *Biosci Reports* 1996, 16, 49-63.
2. Domingo JL: Adverse effects of aluminium-chelating compounds for clinical use. *Adverse Drug React Toxicol Rev* 1996, 15, 145-65.
3. Kontoghiorghes GJ: New concepts of iron and aluminium chelation therapy with oral L1 (deferiprone) and other chelators. *Analyst* 1995, 120, 845-85.
4. Gómez M, Esparza JL, Domingo JL, Corbella J, Singh PK, Jones MM: Aluminium distribution and excretion: a comparative study of a number of chelating agents in rats. *Pharmacol Toxicol* 1998, 82, 295-300.
5. Gómez M, Esparza JL, Domingo JL, Singh PK , Jones MM: Comparative aluminium mobilizing actions of deferoxamine and four 3-hydroxypyrid-4-ones in aluminium-loaded rats. *Toxicology* 1998, 130, 175-81.
6. Kargacin B, Kostial K, Arezina K, Singh PK, Jones MM, Cikrt M: Influence of age and time of administration of dithiocarbamate analogues on cadmium retention in rats. *J Appl Toxicol* 1991, 11, 273-77
7. Gómez M, Domingo JL, del Castillo D, Llobet JM, Corbella J: Comparative aluminium mobilizing actions of several chelators in aluminium-loaded uraemic rats. *Hum Exp Toxicol* 1994, 13, 135-39.
8. Elorriaga R, Fernandez-Martín JL, Menendez-Fraga P, Naves ML, Braga S Cannata JB: Aluminium removal: short-and long-term preliminary results with L1 in rats. *Drugs Today* 1992, 28(A), 177-82.
9. Gómez M, Esparza JL, Domingo JL, Singh PK, Jones MM: Chelation therapy in aluminium-loaded rats: influence of age. *Toxicology* 1999, 137, 161-68.

Metal Ions in Biology and Medicine; vol 6. Eds. J.A. Centeno, Ph. Collery, G. Vernet, R.B. Finkelman, H. Gibb, J.C. Etienne. John Libbey Eurotext, Paris © 2000, pp. 747-750.

Zinc role on macrophages interleukin 12 and tumor necrosis factor alpha secretion during mice perinatal stages

Rodolfo Pastelin, Ana Esther Aguilar, Maria Cabañas and Maria Dolores Lastra

Laboratorio de Investigación en Inmunología, Departamento de Biología, Facultad de Química, UNAM. Circuito Escolar, Ciudad Universitaria, México, D.F., CP 04510, fax 56223740. Email: lastraa@servidor.unam.mx

Introduction. Zinc is a crucial nutritional component required for the normal function of the immune system. Lack of the metal is associated with various immunodeficiency conditions, particularly in perinatal stages (1,2).The cell that appears to be directly susceptible to zinc modulation is the macrophage, that produces interleukin 12 (IL-12) and tumor necrosis alpha (TNFα), among other monokines. IL-12, has been shown to regulate the proliferation and function of T and NK cells: the activities of IL-12 suggest that it may play a role in the host resistance against predominantly intracellular microbial infections, and cancer(3,4,5). Because IL-12 appears to play a central role in a variety of immunological processes, it is critically important to understand the regulation of its synthesis and its modulators. IL-12, TNF alpha, IL-1 and IL-6 are produced within the first few hours of endotoxemia (6).

With this in mind, we studied zinc supplementation effects (500 mg/L) from gestation to lactation on BALB/c mice, over IL-12 serum concentration , and TNFα production in peritoneal macrophages, stimulated with LPS. (Table I)

Methods. An ELISA immunoenzymatic assay (Biosource Int Cytoscreen mouse IL-12 kit) was employed to assess IL-12 in serum after mice LPS inoculation. Briefly, 96 well flat-bottomed microtritation plates coated with anti-IL-12 monoclonal antibody (anti IL-12) were used. IL-12 from the samples was captured in the wells, by the monoclonal antibody. A policlonal biotinilated antibody anti IL-12, was added and linked to the IL-12 present in the solid phase, after incubation and washings. The reaction was made visible by adding avidine-peroxidase that bonded to the biotine; this in turn reacted with its substrate producing a cromogen, whose absorbance was read at 450 nm in a Biomek spectrophotometer.

The TNFα concentration, was determined in the LPS stimulated macrophages supernatants. Cells were obtained from the peritoneum. Polystyrene microplates (Genzyme mouse TNFα ELISA kit) , were used; 5 X 10^5 cells were deposited in each well. Lypopolyssacharide (LPS) and supplemented RPMI were added, controls were stablished. Microplates were incubated at 37 C in a 5% CO_2 atmosphere; supernatants were harvested and centrifuged. Macrophages supernatants and standards were added to wells , and the same procedure described for IL-12 was followed for the determination of TNFα, in the LPS activated macrophages, supernatant.

Results. Results are expressed as pg/mL IL-12 , and as delta for TNF alpha (pg/mL TNFα, from LPS stimulated cells – pg/mL TNFα, from non LPS stimulated cells). Results demonstrate that IL-12 concentration was significantly increased (two fold) in mice 3 weeks old (group I) receiving zinc in vivo, over a period of 6 weeks, (since gestation).(Fig 1)

Since IL-12 is a monokine capable of steering T helper cells function towards Th1, interleukin 12 elevation due to Zn supplementation is an event of paramount importance that could lead, within limits, to a positive modulation of the immune response.

Results for TNFα production showed a 30% increase in Zn treated mice , group I , 3 weeks old (6 wk treatment), and a 20% elevation, in group II mice, 6 weeks old (9 wk treatment). (Fig 2)

The beneficial effects of TNF in resistance to infections are thought to be the result of modest amounts of TNF production at local sites of infection. In contrast, the production of larger amounts of TNF which leads to a systemic distribution could be dangerous. Thus the repercussions of a prolonged TNF increase, related to Zn administration, should be closely supervised. (Fig 2)

Results suggest that zinc administration should be carefully monitored, since the host ability to self regulate the monokines bioactivity may be positively modulated.

References

1.Wellinghausen N, Kircher H and Rink L: The immunobiology of zinc. Immunol Today 11:80-82, 1997
2.Lastra MD, Pastelin R, Herrera M, Orihuela VD, Aguilar AE: Increment of immune responses in mice perinatal stages after zinc supplementation. Arch Med Res 28: 67-72, 1997
3.Gately MK, Renzetti LM, Magram J, Stern AS, Adorini L, Gubler U, Presky DH: The interleukin-12/Interleukin-12-Receptor System: Role in Normal and Pathologic Immune Responses. Annu Rev Immunol 16:495-521, 1998
4.Skeen MJ, Miller MA, Shinnick TM, Ziegler HK. Regulation of murine macrophage IL-12 production. J Immunol 156: 1196-1205, 1996
5.Heinzel FP, Hujer AM, Ahmed FN, Rerko RM: In vivo production and function of IL-12 p40 homodimers. J Immunol 158:4381-4388,1997
6.Bazzoni F and Beutler B: The tumor necrosis factor ligand and receptor families. New Engl J Med 334:1717-1725, 1996

GROUP	ZINC TREATMENT PERIODS mg/L		
	GESTATION progenitors → F_1	LACTANCY progenitors→ F_1	POSTWEANING F_1
	3 weeks	3 weeks	3 weeks
CONTROL	0	0	
I	500	500	
CONTROL	0	0	0
II	500	500	500

Table I. Experimental design. Group I: mice supplemented with Zn (500 mg/L) during the lactation and gestation periods (6 wk treatment, 3 weeks old). Group II: mice Zn supplemented, during the gestation, lactation, and postweaning periods (9 wk treatment, 6 weeks old). Controls did not receive Zn.

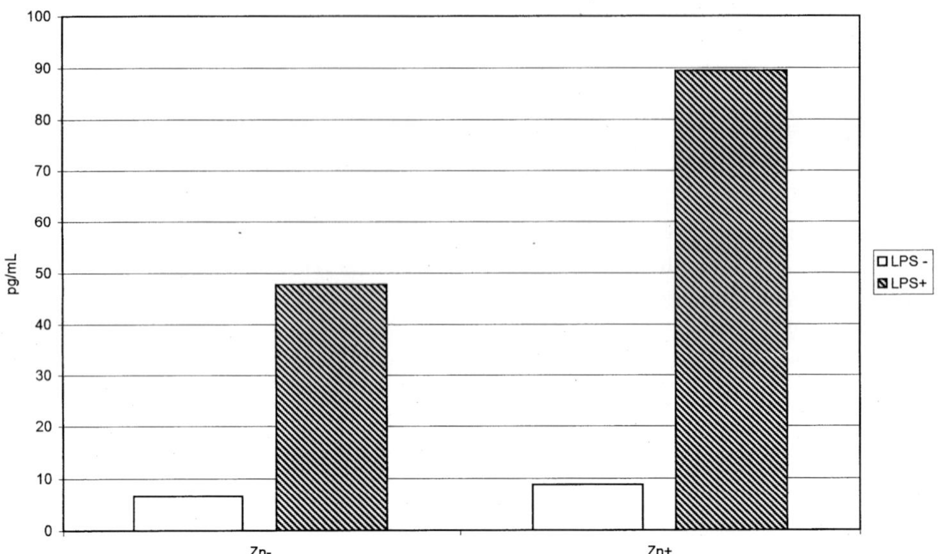

Figure 1. Zn supplementation effect over IL-12 serum levels.

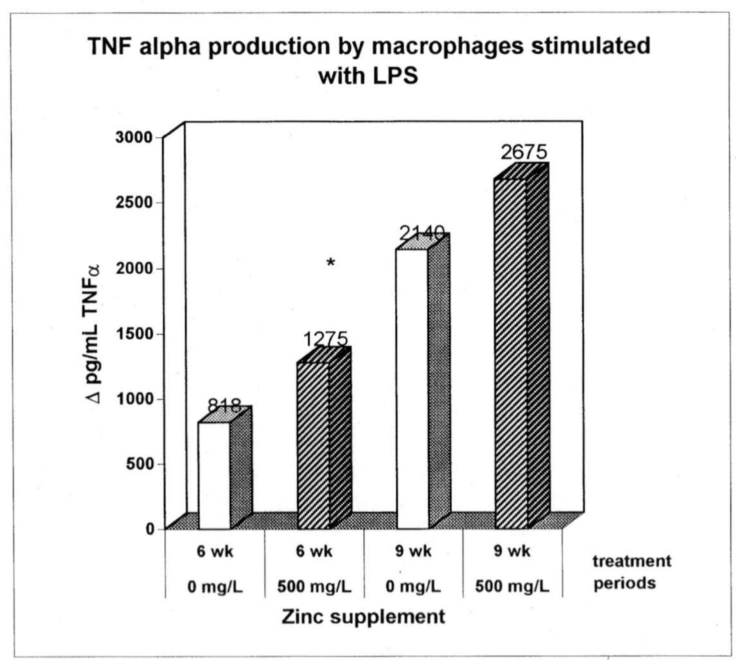

Figure 2. Zn supplementation effect over TNFα production, in LPS stimulated peritoneal macrophages. TNFα concentrations in mice 3 & 6 weeks old.* Statistical differences ($p < 0.05$)

Metal Ions in Biology and Medicine; vol 6. Eds. J.A. Centeno, Ph. Collery, G. Vernet, R.B. Finkelman, H. Gibb, J.C. Etienne. John Libbey Eurotext, Paris © 2000, pp. 751-754.

Iodine, molybdenum and selenium balance study in extremely low birth weight infants

A. Raab[1,2], A. Loui[2], P. Brätter[1], M. Obladen[2]

[1] Hahn-Meitner-Institut Berlin, Department of Trace Element Research for Health and Nutrition, Glienicker Str. 100, D-14109 Berlin, Germany; [2] Charité Virchow-Klinikum, Department of Neonatology, Augustenburger Platz 1, D-13353 Berlin, Germany

Abstract

Extremely low birthweight (ELBW) infants are in danger of trace element deficiency in their early postnatal life because of low stores at birth, immature digestive system and high growth rate. The demand of rapidly growing infants for essential trace elements including selenium, iodine and molybdenum may easily exceed their nutritive supply. Among other functions, selenium is necessary for the cell defense against free radicals that are produced in the enhanced cell synthesis of ELBW infants. Iodine is essential for thyroid function and postnatal brain development. Molybdenum plays a vital role in the metabolism of purines and sulfur amino acids.

To assess the Se, I and Mo supply and requirements of ELBW infants two balance studies were performed in ten premature infants (birthweight less than 1000 g) at 7 and 12 weeks after birth. All infants were fed fortified human milk but without addition of trace elements. Urine and feces were collected during a period of 72 h and aliquots of them were analyzed together with food samples. The trace elements iodine and molybdenum were measured by inductively coupled plasma mass spectrometry, selenium was determined by means of instrumental neutron activation analysis. From the analytical results and the clinical protocol the daily intake and the excreted amounts of the trace elements were calculated.

In each of the two periods two infants were found in negative balance of iodine because of high renal iodine losses. Their intestinal iodine absorption was significantly lower than the mean net absorption. Two of the infants (one in both studies, another one in the first period only) showed negative balance for molybdenum because of low breast milk content. Four other babies were found in negative balance of molybdenum because of high renal losses. In contrast to I and Mo the selenium balance was positive in all infants of this study and its retention was about 70 % in both periods.

We conclude, that due to negative balance, ELBW infants are at risk for iodine and molybdenum deficiency.

Introduction

Extremely low birth weight infants (ELBW) are born with low stores of iodine, selenium and molybdenum. Because of their immature digestive system and high growth rate they are in danger of postnatal trace element deficiency. The consequences of I deficiency are widely known. So far no case of Se or Mo deficiency has been described in preterm infants, however less is known about these essential trace in ELBW infants. We hypothesized that German ELBW infants fed with breast milk do not reach a positive metabolic balance of I, Se and Mo.

Patients

The study was carried out in the Department of Neonatology, Charité Virchow-Hospital Berlin from January to September 1998. The protocol was approved by the local ethic committee, written informed consent was obtained from the parents. During the duration of the study 19 infants less than 1000 g birthweight were born, 10 of them met the study criteria and parental approval was given. 72 h balance studies (complete collection of urine and feces and a portion of the feeding) were performed at two time points in these infants. Their mean birthweight was 845 ± 76 g and mean gestational age 25.9 ± 0.6 wk. the infants received parenteral trace element supply (containing iodine: 7.88 nmol/ml and selenium: 25.3 nmol/ml) during 16 ± 10 d and reached full enteral feeding at a mean of 27 ± 9 d. At a mean age of 52 ± 7 d (balance period I) they had reached a mean weight of 1397 ± 138 g and were fed 155 ± 14 ml/kg/d breast milk with fortifier. During balance period II (age 80 ± 10 d) their mean weight was 1997 ± 253 g and they had a mean intake of 145 ± 12 ml/kg/d. Their average weight gain during the whole study was 11.0 ± 1.0 g/kg/d.

Methods

Selenium, iodine and molybdenum concentrations were measured at the Department of Molecular Trace Element Research for Health and Nutrition, Hahn-Meitner-Institut Berlin.

I and Mo were measured in alkaline solution (1 % (v/v) ammonia) by inductively coupled plasma mass spectrometry (ICP-MS). Selenium was measured by instrumental neutron activation analysis (INAA) via Se-75. Certified reference material was used for quality control (e.g. for iodine BCR 63 (n=10) 0.79 ± 0.03 µg/g (0.81 ± 0.05), molybdenum Ghent Serum (n=10) 7.10 ± 0.016 ng/g (6.7 - 8.3), selenium (Seronorm Serum) (n=10) 64.6 ± 8.02 µg/g (70 - 92)).

Absorption was calculated as total intake minus fecal excretion and retention as total intake minus fecal excretion minus urinary excretion, respectively. The results (Tab. 1) are given as mean ± SD. Statistical calculations were done using Spearman rank calculation.

Results and Discussion

Selenium

The Se concentration in breast milk during balance period I was 0.14 ± 0.02 µmol/l and 0.20 ± 0.12 µmol/l during balance period II. The Se intake was positively correlated with absorption (r_s=0.860, $p<0.0001$) and retention (r_s=0.884, $p<0.0001$). Serum Se was negatively correlated with age (r_s=-0.449, $p<0.05$) and weight (r_s=-0.560, p=0.01) despite nearly constant absorption and retention during both balance periods. For erythrocytes (RBC) no correlation was existent , because of a large portion of trans-

fused adult erythrocytes (average cumulated volume 65.7 ± 31.6 ml/kg). Se concentration in RBC's was 742 ± 323 nmol/l (balance period I) and 882 ± 216 nmol/l (balance period II). None of the 10 infants was in negative Se balance during both observation periods.
Balance data about Se in preterm infants are scare. The results for absorption and retention of our study are in agreement with the findings of Ehrenkranz et al. (1), who used Se-74 as an extrinsic tracer. Serum Se is declining during the first weeks of life in the ELBW infants. A similar relationship was reported for term infants born in selenium rich regions of Venezuela [2]. This decline is probably a physiological process independent of the Se intake and therefore the Se serum concentration can not be used as a marker for the Se status during this period of life.

Iodine

The breast milk concentration of iodine was 1.13 ± 0.63 μmol/l during balance period I and 0.91 ± 0.47 μmol/l during balance period II. During balance period II three infants consumed breast milk with an iodine concentration of 26.7 μmol/l. Because the reason of this high iodine intake remained unclear, these infants were excluded from the calculation of the iodine balance period II. Iodine intake correlated with absorption (r_s= 0.983, $p<0.0001$) and retention (r_s= 0.637, $p<0.01$).
Our balance data for iodine in ELBW infants are similar to results published by Delange et al. (3). Delange found that about 40 % of the preterm infants were in negative iodine balance. In both observation periods of our study two different infants were found in negative iodine balance, because of high renal losses.

Tab. 1: Selenium, iodine and molybdenum balance data

	Selenium	Iodine	Molybdenum
balance period I			
Intake (nmol/kg/d)	24.2 ± 2.9[a]	170.3 ± 92.9[a,b]	12.58 ± 7.99[a]
Absorption (nmol/kg/d)	18.6 ± 3.4[a]	157.9 ± 93.5[a]	10.43 ± 8.22[a]
Retention (nmol/kg/d)	13.7 ± 3.3[a]	52.3 ± 75.9[b]	7.37 ± 9.01[a]
Serum (nmol/l)	250 ± 27	632 ± 152	7.81 ± 2.87
balance period II			
Intake (nmol/kg/d)	31.6 ± 16.0[a]	137.7 ± 69.7*[a,b]	4.74 ± 2.39[a]
Absorption (nmol/kg/d)	25.6 ± 16.2[a]	122.6 ± 65.2*[a]	2.78 ± 2.38[a]
Retention (nmol/kg/d)	21.3 ± 16.1[a]	44.0 ± 69.5*[b]	-0.32 ± 2.26[a]
Serum (nmol/l)	207 ± 58	681 ± 305*	6.06 ± 2.37

* n=7, intake (n=3): 3510, absorption (n=3): 3485, retention (n=3): 3265
a: r>0.8, p<0.0001, b: r>0.6, p<0.01

Molybdenum

Mo concentration in milk was 77.7 ± 52.2 nmol/l (balance period I) and 29.3 ± 18.4 nmol/l (balance period II). Absorption (r_s=0.983, p<0.0001) and retention (r_s=0.853, p<0.0001) correlated with intake. The excretion via feces and urine was nearly constant during both balance periods. During each study period 3 infants were in negative Mo balance. Two others showed negative balance during period I or II.

Friel et al. (4) carried out Mo balance studies in LBW infants. Their gestational age (29.8 ± 2.5 wk) was higher than in our study. In addition the Mo intake (35.4 ± 13.5 nmol/kg/d) of the breastfed group was much higher than that of our infants. Friel found a retention of 11.6 ± 16.8 nmol/kg/d (~ 32 %). The retention in our study was very variable ranging from -250 to 87 %. We found no correlation between the inorganic Mo -present as contamination of iron supplements - and the absorption or the retention of Mo. The finding of Werner et al. (5) concerning a higher bioavailability of inorganic Mo could not be confirmed. The same applies for the high plasma Mo levels published by Bougle et. al. (6). They reported a Mo concentration of 194 ± 30 nmol/l (no information about quality control). Our values in the range of 2.8 to 13.1 nmol/l are more than one order of magnitude lower and comparable to findings of Versieck in adults (3.12 - 8.94 nmol/l) (7).

Literature

1. Ehrenkranz RA, Gettner PA, Nelli CM, Sherwonit EA, Williams JE, Ting BT, Janghorbani M. Selenium absorption and retention by very-low-birth-weight infants: studies with the extrinsic stable isotope tag 74Se. J Pediatr Gastroenterol Nutr 1991; 13:125-133.
2. Brätter P, Negretti de Brätter V, Rittner M, Pinto de López E, Garcia de Torres L. Zeitlicher Verlauf von Spurenelementkonzentrationen in Serum und roten Blutzellen gesunder Neugeborener und Säuglinge. in Anke M et al. Mengen- und Spuren-Elemente, Verlag H Schubert, Leipzig 1996: 180-190.
3. Delange F, Bourdoux P, Chanoine P, Ermanns AM. Physiopathology of iodine nutrition during pregnancy, lactation, and early postnatal life. in Berger H. Vitamins and Minerals in Pregnancy and Lactation Nestle Nutrition Workshop Series 16 (Joint Symposium, Nestle Hoffmann-La Roche) Raven Press, New York 1988: 205-214.
4. Friel JK, MacDonald AC, Mercer CN, Belkhode SL, Downton G, Kwa PG, Aziz K, Andrews WL. Molybdenum requirements in low-birth-weight infants receiving parenteral and enteral nutrition. JPEN J Parenter Enteral Nutr 1999; 23: 155-9.
5. Werner E, Giussani A, Heinrichs U, Roth P, Greim H. Biokinetic studies in humans with stable isotopes as tracers. Part 2: Uptake of molybdenum from aqueous solutions and labelled foodstuffs. Isotopes Environ Health Stud 1998; 34: 297-301.
6. Bougle D, Foucault D, Voirin J, Bureau F, Duhamel JF. Molybdenum in the premature infant. Biol Neonate 1991; 59: 201-3.
7. Vanhoe H, Versieck J, Moens L, Dams R. Role of inductively coupled plasma mass spectrometry in the assessment of reference values for ultra-trace elements in human serum. Trace Elements and Electrolytes 1995; 12: 81 - 88.

Metal Ions in Biology and Medicine; vol 6. Eds. J.A. Centeno, Ph. Collery, G. Vernet, R.B. Finkelman, H. Gibb, J.C. Etienne. John Libbey Eurotext, Paris © 2000, pp. 755-757.

Effects of the concurrent exposure to manganese and hydrocortisone in pregnant mice

M. Torrente[1, 2], M.L. Albina[1], M.T. Colomina[1, 2], J.L. Domingo[1] and J. Corbella[1]

[1] *Laboratory of Toxicology and Environmental Health Faculty of Medicine; and* [2] *Psychobiology Unit, Dept. of Psychology, "Rovira i Virgili" University, San Lorenzo 21, 43201 Reus, Spain*

Manganese (Mn), a widely distributed metal in soils, sediments, rocks, water and biological materials, is an essential trace element required by mammals for certain physiological functions. Both, deficiency and excess, have been reported to cause central nervous system (CNS) disturbances [1]. It has been shown that Mn can cross the placental and the hematoencephalic barriers and to accumulate in the fetus. Although no behavioral or neurochemical effects were found in rats prenatally exposed to Mn, a diminished depth in cortical layers was recently reported [2].
On the other hand, maternal stress has been shown to enhance the developmental toxicity of some elements such as arsenic, aluminum or mercury [3,4]. The effects of stress are mainly mediated by glucocorticoids, which have been reported to increase the vulnerability of neurons to metabolic insults, potentially by altering the neuronal defense capacity against oxidative damage [5]. In the present study, the effects of concurrent Mn and hydrocortisone treatment were evaluated in pregnant mice. In order to reduce other maternal effects derived from stress (such as food consumption), hydrocortisone was used to assess glucocorticoid mediated effects by stress. The doses of Mn were dictated by previous data, which showed a gradient of toxic effects ranging from no observed to moderate or severe [6]. Hydrocortisone (HC) was administered at doses resembling to those found in a situation of mild to moderate stress [7].

MATERIAL AND METHODS

Animals: Sexually mature male and female Swiss mice (28-30 g) were obtained from Criffa (Barcelona, Spain). Animals were quarantined for 7 days after shipping. One male and two females were mated overnight and examined the following morning for copulatory plug. The day on which a vaginal plug was found was designated as day 0 of gestation.

Treatment: Eighty pregnant mice received $MnCl_2$ (sc) at doses of 0, 1, 2, and 4 mg/kg from days 6 to 18 of gestation. Each group was divided in two subgroups and animals in the subgroups received 0 and 5 mg of HC during the same period. On gestation day 18, animals were sacrificed and the uterus were removed. Live fetuses from each dam were processed for external, skeletal and visceral anomalies.

Parameters evaluated: Maternal body weight and food consumption were monitored daily during the treatment period. After cesareans, gravid uterine weight, total number of implantations, resorptions, live and dead fetuses, sex ratio and fetal body weight were recorded. External, visceral and skeletal abnormalities were evaluated.

Statistical procedure: A two-way (Mn x HC) analysis of variance (ANOVA) for repeated measures using the day as repeated measure was used to evaluate body weight change and food consumption during the treatment period. A two-way (Mn x HC) analysis of variance (ANOVA) was also used to evaluate the remaining data. A LSD (Least Significant Differences) test was used to assess differences between groups when necessary. The litter was the unit of comparison for developmental data. Differences were considered to be significant at $p<0.05$.

RESULTS

Maternal body weight gain during the treatment period and body weight at termination were reduced in animals receiving Mn at the highest dose (4 mg/kg), as well as in animals treated with HC, alone or combined with Mn (Fig. 1). Significant interactions between Mn and HC on maternal body weight were found for all gestation periods evaluated. Gravid uterine weight and relative liver and kidney weight were significantly reduced for animals receiving Mn at the highest dose.

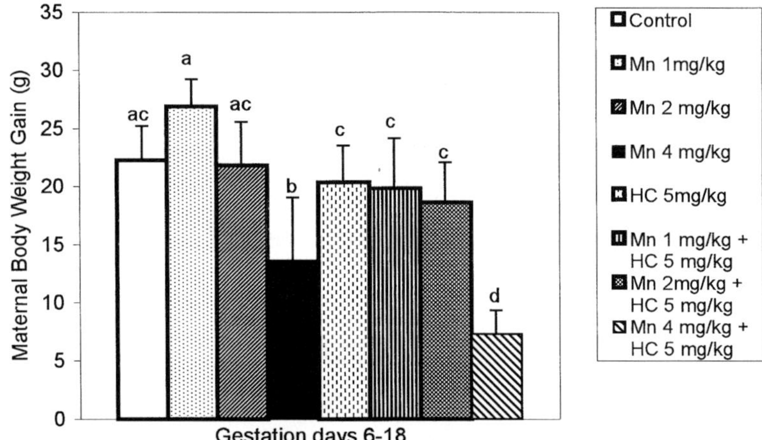

Fig. 1: Maternal body weight gain on gestation days 6-18. Different letters indicate significant differences between groups at $p < 0.05$.

In turn, an increased number of resorptions and a decreased number of live fetuses were observed in animals treated with Mn at 4 mg/kg. These effects were increased by the concurrent administration of HC (Fig. 2). No external, internal or skeletal malformations were observed. Only some skeletal variations (delayed ossification and wavy ribs) were observed in animals treated with Mn at 2 and 4 mg/kg (data not shown).

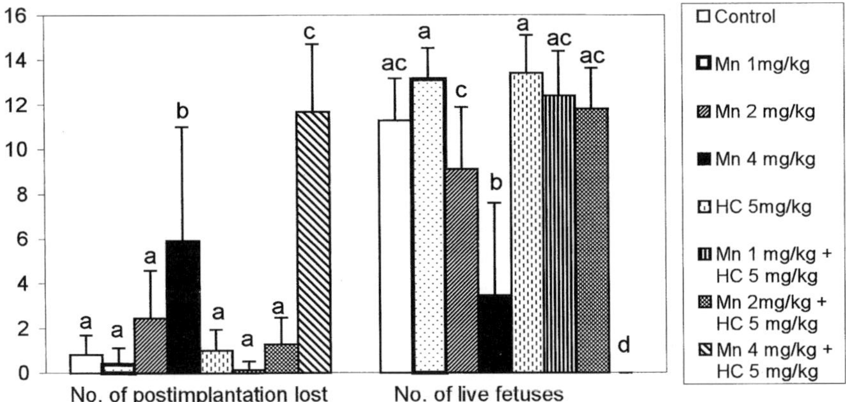

Fig.2: Number of postimplantation loss and live fetuses. Different letters (a,b,c,d) indicate significant differences between groups at $p < 0.05$.

DISCUSSION

In the current study, $MnCl_2$ administration during organogenesis (days 6-15) and during the late gestation period (days 16-18) caused maternal and developmental toxicity at 4 mg/kg/day. Previous investigations in our laboratory showed maternal toxic effects of $MnCl_2$ at 8 and 16 mg/kg/day, but not at 4 mg/kg/day, when administered during the organogenesis period (days 6-15). These differences might indicate a maternal toxic effect produced during late gestation. Embryo/fetal toxicity was also observed at the highest dose of Mn. However, no external, internal, or skeletal malformations were found, which is in accordance with previous reports [6].

Although significant interactions between Mn and HC were found on maternal body weight gain (gestation days 6-18), gravid uterine weight, as well as in postimplantation loss, it was only evidenced in the groups receiving the highest dose of Mn (4 mg/kg). It agrees with recent studies in which stress interacted with other metals (Hg, As, Al). Interactions were only observed in the groups receiving metal doses that were toxic by themselves [3,4].

REFERENCES

1. Prahlad K, Seth PK, Chandra SV. Neurotoxic effects of manganese. In: Bondy SC, Prasad KN, eds. Metal neurotoxicity. Florida: CRC Press, 1988:19-33.
2. Pappas BA, Zhang D, Davidson CM, Crowder T, Park GAS, Fortin T. Perinatal manganese exposure: Behavioral, neurochemical, and histopathological effects in the rat. *Neurotoxicol Teratol* 1997; 19:17-25.
3. Colomina MT, Albina ML, Domingo JL, Corbella J. Effects of maternal stress on methylmercury-induced developmental toxicity in mice. *Physiol Behav* 1995; 58:974-984.
4. Colomina MT, Esparza JL, Corbella J, Domingo JL. The effect of maternal restraint on developmental toxicity of aluminum in mice. *Neurotoxicol Teratol* 1998; 6:651-656.
5. McIntosh LJ, Hong KE, Sapolsky RM. Glucocorticoids may alter antioxidant enzyme capacity in the brain: baseline studies. *Brain Res* 1998; 791:209-214.
6. Sanchez DJ, Domingo JL, Llobet JM, Keen CL. Maternal and developmental toxicity of manganese in the mouse. *Toxicol Lett* 1993; 69:45-52.
7. Magariños AM, McEwen BS. Stress induced atrophy of apical dendrites of hippocampal CA3c neurons: Comparison of stressors. *Neuroscience* 1995; 69:83-88.

Metal Ions in Biology and Medicine; vol 6. Eds. J.A. Centeno, Ph. Collery, G. Vernet, R.B. Finkelman, H. Gibb, J.C. Etienne. John Libbey Eurotext, Paris © 2000, pp. 759-761.

The international tissue and tumor repository for chronic arsenosis in humans (ITTRCA)

Norbert P. Page[1], Jose A. Centeno[1], Florabel G. Mullick[1], Leonor E. Martinez[2], Elena Ladich[1], Herman Gibb[3], Claudia Thompson[4], David Longfellow[5], and Robert Finkelman[6]

[1] The Armed Forces Institute of Pathology (AFIP), Washington, D.C.; [2] Mexican Institute Social Security Cd Juárez Chih. México; [3] U.S. Environmental Protection Agency, Washington D.C.; [4] The National Institute for Environmental Health Sciences, Research Triangle Park, North Carolina; [5] U.S. National Cancer Institute, Bethesda, Maryland; and [6] U.S. Geological survey, Washington, D.C.

The AFIP has recently established the *International Tissue and Tumor Repository for Chronic Arsenosis (ITTRCA).* The goals of ITTRCA are to: 1) provide a central repository to store tissues for current and future research needs, 2) develop a standardized classification for arsenic-induced lesions, 3) provide consultation on diagnostic (morphologic) criteria, education, and research on the chronic effects of arsenic, and 4) to foster research among national and international scientists working on arsenic health effects by facilitating the use of tissues and other pathological materials. The need for such as repository and standardization of diagnostic criteria was identified by the September 1997 workshop on Arsenic: Health Effects, Mechanisms of Action, and Research Issues (Abernathy, et al., 1999).

The environmental exposure to arsenic is now a well-recognized international health concern and considerable research is underway to elucidate the magnitude of the problem (Guha Mazumder et al., 1999). However, the mechanisms by which arsenic induces cancer and other health effects remain unclear. In addition, there are numerous uncertainties as to the metabolism and retention of arsenic in the body and the cellular and biochemical interactions. The lack of a central repository and diagnostic center for such materials and data has hampered the conduct of meaningful pathogenesis and epidemiologic studies on chronic arsenosis. Accordingly, the development of a tissue repository would be of great value to national and international researchers and organizations involved in the study of arsenosis.

Tissues and other materials provided for arsenic-exposed cases will be obtained from national and international contributors, identified, and archived in an environmentally-controlled repository already developed by the AFIP. The materials collected and stored include preserved tissues, paraffin blocks, microscope slides, fluids (whole blood, serum, urine), hair, finger and toe nails, medical and pathological records, photographs and clinical/chemical laboratory analyses. Methods, protocols, and guidance will be provided for identification, collection, handling, shipment, and storage of tissue specimens.

Materials collected and archived must be obtained and processed using methods that will assure adequate preservation for long-term storage as well as usability for sophisticated special stains and laboratory analysis. It is essential that the methods used to preserve and ship tissues and other materials do not result in future interference with analytical chemical techniques or special pathology stains or diagnostic procedures. Cases received and accessioned by the ITTRCA will be validated by providing pathological diagnoses, chemical/toxicologic analysis, molecular biology test for DNA changes, and any other diagnostic technique required for consultation purposes.

The ITTRCA could serve as a resource for studies of analytical toxicology, molecular biology, and P53 mutation analysis, among other possible research endeavors. The AFIP, like many research establishments, has available advanced and sophisticated techniques for fundamental research including electron microscopy, magnetic resonance imaging, morphometrics, digital imaging processing, molecular microspectroscopic techniques, immunoperoxidase, polymerase chain reaction, and DNA/RNA probes. Many of these specialized laboratory tests and techniques are especially applicable to arsenic toxicology, e.g., immuno-histologic evaluation of skin lesions, speciation measurements of metabolic profile, ultrastructural and chemical-spectra imaging.

Access to the materials will be well controlled to insure the integrity of the specimens and adherence with confidentiality requirements. A Steering Committee, consisting primarily of scientists from the sponsoring agencies, assists AFIP by providing guidance on management and direction, evaluation of requests for access and availability to the materials, and promoting the project on an international basis.

A major objective is to make the archived materials available to national and international researchers through consultation, contributions, and requests for the development of research projects. Requests for the use of these materials will be accompanied by a research protocol and evaluated by the Registry's Advisory Committee and by the AFIP Research and Tissue Utilization Committees.

The data obtained from the study of submitted specimens will be summarized and collected in a computerized database, tentatively named the ***Chronic Arsenic Effects Registry (CAER)***. The CAER will be developed as a component of the ITTRCA. To improve the use and accessibility to the information gathered through this Registry, efforts will be initiated to develop a WEB Site to share basic and fundamental information on the capabilities and use of materials available at the Registry.

ITTRCA will be maintained and administered by the Armed Forces Institute of Pathology (AFIP) using techniques and procedures already developed for the *National Pathology Repository (NPR)* at AFIP. The AFIP currently has over 175 cases pertaining to arsenic exposure, most involving acute effects toxicity. While these will serve as the nucleus for the ITTRCA, new cases will be sought especially those involving chronic exposures to arsenic.

Support for the ITTRCA is provided by the U.S. Environmental Protection Agency, U.S. National Cancer Institute, and the National Institute for Environmental Health Sciences. The U.S. Geological Survey has established a companion repository for environmental samples, such as soil and plants, from areas with high arsenic concentrations.

References:

1. Abernathy CO, Liu YP, Aposhian HV, Beck B, Fowler B, Goyer R, Menzer R, Rossman T, Thompson C, Waalkes M. Arsenic: health effects, mechanism of actions, and research issues. Environ Health Perspect 1999 Jul; 107(7):593-7.
2. Guha Mazumder DN, De BK, Santra A, Dasgusta J, Ghosh N, Roy BK, Ghoshal UC, Saha J, Chatterjee A, Dutta S, Haque R, Smith AH, Chakraborty D, Angle CR, Centeno JA. Chronic Arsenic Toxicty: Epidemilogy, Natural History and Treatment. In Arsenic Exposure and Health Effects (Chappell WR, Abernathy CO, Calderon RL, editors), 1999 Elsevier Science B.V. UK; 335-347.

Metal Ions in Biology and Medicine; vol 6. Eds. J.A. Centeno, Ph. Collery, G. Vernet, R.B. Finkelman, H. Gibb, J.C. Etienne. John Libbey Eurotext, Paris © 2000, pp. 762-764.

Influence of disturbances in the hypognaesemia on the disturbances in the cardiac rhythm of operated patients

W. Piekoszewski[1], Z. Kopański[2], K. Sadlik[1], T. Lewandowski[2], M. Schlegel-Zawadzka[3]

[1] *Institute of Forensic Research,* [2] *Clinical Military Hospital,* [3] *Jagiellonian University; Kraków, Poland*

INTRODUCTION

Correct concentrations and proportions of the respective bioelements are one of the real elements of efficient homeostasia in man. The violation of these proportions develops a cascade of disturbances which are the cause of different ailments. Magnesium is one of the basic intracellular elements. Its concentration in the blood amounts to 100 mg on average. It may then be deduced that the determination of the content of magnesium in the blood has no great significance in the evaluation of the magnesium metabolism in the organism. However, according to Durlach, it is not because the magnesium content in the blood is stable, that allows us to define even its small variations [1]. The studies of magnesium in this compartment above all allow us to reveal the disturbances of the metabolism of that element when they affect a pathological population, i.e. a defined group of patients. Until most recently however, the influence has rarely been considered in the changes in the concentration of that bioelement in the formation of a risk in common surgery patients with post-operative cardiological complications. That inclined the authors to present their own studies, the aim of which was to establish the degree of dependence between the magnesium concentration in the serum and the risk of generation of heart rhythm disturbances in the post-operative period in patients subjected to operations of the organs of the abdomen.

MATERIAL AND METHOD

The analysis included 98 patients (58 men and 40 women) aged 45 to 76 years, operated on for different abdominal diseases. The group was comprised of 36 persons operated for cholecystolithiasis, 29 for cancer of the large intestine, 20 for acute apendicitis, 7 for ovarian tumours, 6 for cancer of the stomach.

In all the patients studied the level of magnesium in the serum was estimated before the procedure as well as in the following days up to their discharge from the clinic. Conditions were standardised.

In the analysis of the heart rhythm disturbances (HRD) occurring after the procedure, the following divisions were considered: rhythm different from sinusoidal; additional atrial and additional ventricular contractions.

The magnesium concentration in the serum was determined using the flame atomic absorption spectrometric method.

RESULTS

In patients having undergone procedures on abdominal organs the magnesium concentration in the serum varied from 4.03 to 23.11 ug/ml (average 16.86±6.26 ug/ml). It was confirmed that the surgical procedure was predisposed to the generation of magnesium deficiencies in the serum yet idiopathically compensated within 7 days.

Heart rhythm disturbances (HRD) in the post-operative period occurred in 31 patients (31.6%). The differences in the average magnesemia between the group of patients with cardiological complications and the group of persons without these complications are presented in Table I.

Table I. Changes of the megnesium concentration in the serum of patients with post-operative heart rhythm disturbances.

Group of patients	Number of patients	Magnesium concentration in the serum [ug/ml] Average±SD
Patients with HRD	31	14.78±6.21
Patients without HRD	67	18.94±4.51

• to ** - statistically significant differences

In our own studies we also estimated the critical value below which appears a statistically significantly high risk of development of post-operative heart rhythm disturbances in patients subjected to common surgical procedures. That value amounted to 13.72 ug/ml with an average error of 8.48 %.

DISCUSSION

According to our studies the level of magnesemia in the first days after the operation decreases, after which it gradually increases - reaching average values close to the pre-operative values on the 7th post-operative day. It was shown that at the moment the HRD were generated, the average magnesium concentration in the serum of patients with this complication statistically significantly decreased in comparison with the persons in whom those disturbances did not occur. The characteristically low magnesium level in the post-operative period, predicting a statistically very high risk of developing HRD, amounted to 13.72 ug/ml. It was not clear, however, whether the hypomagnesemia favoured the development of a defined form of heart rhythm disturbances.

The significance of magnesium in the generation of heart diseases has already been evaluated in many works. In studies using animals it was indicated that magnesium acted extensively on the peripheral and coronary vessels, had antiarrhythmic properties, as well as diminished the injury of the myocardian caused by reperfusion. Yet the clinical significance of those observations is still unclear. Some of the clinical tests in the fresh myocardiac infarct point to the existence of a toward the diminution of mortality with the administration of magnesium intravenously. In the studies of a group from Leicester, a 24 % diminution of that risk was observed. A favourable affect of magnesium on the decrease in the number of HRD also appeared. However, not all clinical studies underline such positive action of intravenous infusions of magnesium during the course of heart diseases [1].

The studies we conducted indicate that the post-operative monitoring of the magnesium concentration in the serum is a procedure worth being recommended for patients subjected to common surgical procedures, since the decrease of the magnesemia level may be a risk factor for the development of HRD.

REFERENCES

1. Durlach J. Magnesium in clinical practice. John Libbey, London Paris 1988.
2. Mertz W. The essential trace elements. *Science* 1981; 213:1332-1338.
3. Woods KL. Possible pharmacological actions of magnesium in acute myocardial infarction. *Br J Clin Pharmacol*, 1991; 32:3-10.
4. Rasmussen HS, McNair P, Norregard P, Backer V, Lindeneg O, Balslev S. Intravenous magnesium in acute myocardial infarction. *Lancet*, 1986; I:234-6.
5. Teo KK, Yusuf S, Collins R, Held PH, Peto R. Effects of intravenous magnesium in suspected acute myocardial infarction: overview of randomised trials. *BMJ*, 1991; 303:1499-1503.

Metal Ions in Biology and Medicine; vol 6. Eds. J.A. Centeno, Ph. Collery, G. Vernet, R.B. Finkelman, H. Gibb, J.C. Etienne. John Libbey Eurotext, Paris © 2000, pp. 765-767.

Fungal cytotoxicity and toxigenicity induced by metal ions: effect on human and animals

R. Cuero[1], H. Ibarguen[2] and G. Mmbjjwe[1]

[1] *Prairie View A&M University, CARC, Prairie View, Texas 77446, USA;* [2] *University of Texas, M.D. Anderson Cancer Center, Department of Clinical Investigation, Houston, Texas 77030, USA*

ABSTRACT

Metal ions (Zn^{+2}, Cu^{+2}, and Fe^{+2}) stimulated growth and induced cytotoxicity and toxigencity in fungi, **Fusarium graminearum**, **F. Moniliforme**, and **Aspergillus flavus,** grown in soil or liquid cultures. Cytotoxiciy was detected in human lung cells after 96 h; most of the cells died (98%). The effect of zinc concentration was further determined on fungal DNA profile. Zinc and copper also showed differential effects on growth of toxigenic fungi and on the production of their concomitant mycotoxin. These effects were related to changes in the fungal DNA and RNA characterization.

INTRODUCTION

Fungal spores are almost always present in the air, in field crops during growth and harvesting, and in internal surfaces of damp dwelling, as sources of spores. Inhalation of these fungal spores can lead to adverse health conditions such as respiratory allergy, particularly in atopic individuals (1), fungal infection particularly in immunosuppressed individuals such as cancer patients, or direct toxicity to the lung due to mycotoxins. Mycotoxicoses have been demonstrated in animals, **Fusaria** species have been reported causing mycotis keratitis in human (2), and as producer of mycotoxins (3). Microorganisms such as fungi, become in direct contact with toxic metal ions from excessive pesticide, organic fertilizers from sewage sludge and animal manure, and from industrial chemical contamination in the soil. Therefore, the purpose of this study was to determine the effects of metal ions on fungal growth, DNA/RNA characterization, cytotoxicity and toxigenicity in relation to human and animal health.

MATERIALS AND METHODS

Human Lung Cell Culture. The human lung squamous carcinoma cell line, A549 (ATCC No. CCL 185) grown as monolayer with a doubling time between 24-30h was used, and grown according to standard procedures by American Type Culture Collection (ATCC). The cells growth was monitored with an inverted microscope, and counted in an automated coulter counter.

Fungal Spore Extract and the Bioassay. F. graminearum spores previously collected from indoor air of university residences, and subsequently cultured in agar (1 week), then inoculated in sterile zinc-amended soil (2 months), and finally transferred into czapeck liquid culture amended with the respective metal ion. A 0.5 mM of Zn^{+2} sulfate was used to treat the **F. graminearum** liquid culture for the lung cells bioassay. While 5 ppm concentration of metal ions was used for other experiments with toxigenic fungi. Four total treatments including their respective controls at pH 7, were used. All treatments were done in triplicates.

Fungal Growth and Toxin Analysis. Three strains of **A. flavus** (one toxigenic and two atoxigenic), a toxigenic **F. graminearum**, and **F. moniliforme** were used to determine the effects of metal ions on fungal toxigenicity. Fungal growth and concomitant mycotoxins were analyzed in liquid cultures by biomass dry weight, and their mycotoxins by ELISA method; liquid cultures were analyzed after a week incubation.

Fungal DNA/RNA Determination. Standard extraction for fungal liquid cultures was done, and the DNeasy and RNeasy QIAGEN kits, and standard electrophoretic procedures, were used.

RESULTS AND DISCUSSION.

Figures 1A & 1B, clearly show the high degree of toxicity against human lung cells (98% mortality after 96 h.), exhibited by extract of **F. graminearum** grown in soil containing 5 ppm zinc, as compared to control without zinc.

Each metal ion showed differential stimulating fungal growth in liquid culture, depending on the fungal strains. Copper and iron exhibited higher stimulating growth effect (15-40%) than zinc. Previous reports have also shown the effects of metal ions on fungal toxic metabolites, under different conditions (3, 4). Fungal DNA and RNA increase corresponded with increase in fungal growth and toxin producion mediated by the metal ions (Fig 2). Thus indicating the phenotypic effects of these metal ions on microbial nucleic acid and metalloenzymes such as polymerase (3, 5).

REFERENCES

1. Smith J, Anderson G, Lewis C, Murad. Cytotoxic fungal spores in the indoor atmosphere of the damp domestic environment. FEMS Microbiol Let 1992; 100:337-344

2. Cuero R. Ecological distribution of Fusarium solani: mycotic keratitis. J. Cl. Microbiol 1980; 12(3):455-461
3. Cuero R, Duffus E, Williams M. Effects of zinc and associated mycoflora on fungal growth and toxins production. Mycotoxins and Phycotoxins 1998. Developments in Chemistry, Toxicology and Food Safety; 33:311-319
4. Jackson M, Slinger P, Bothast R. Erects of zinc, iron, cobalt, and manganese on **Fusarium moniliforme** NRRL 1361 growth and fusarin C biosynthesis in submerged cultures. App Environ Microbiol; 55:649-655
5. Failla M. Zinc: functions and transport in microorganisms. In: E. Weinberg (ed.). Microorganisms and Minerals; Chapter 4: 151-214. Marcel Dekker, N.Y.

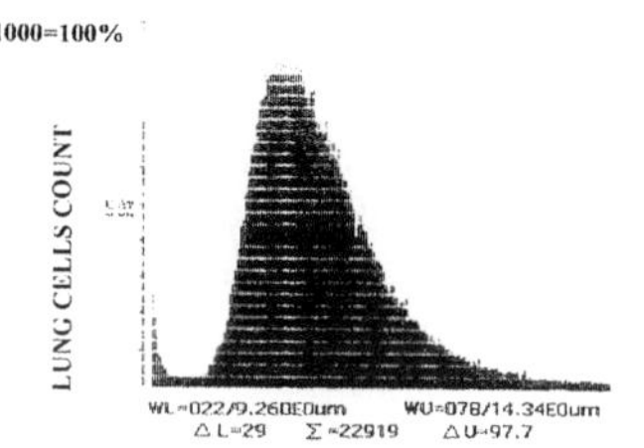

FIG. 1-A. LUNG CELLS GROWN WITH EXTRACT OF F. GRAMINEARUM WITHOUT ZINC (CONTROL), AFTER 96 HOURS.

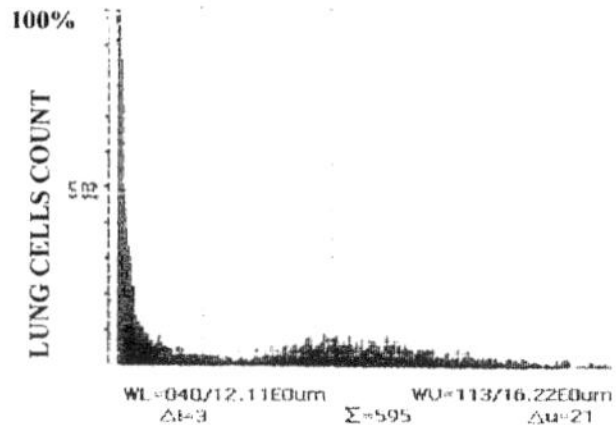

FIG.1-B. LUNG CELLS AFTER TREAT MENT WITH EXTRACT OF F. GRAMINEARUM GROWN WITH ZINC, AFTER 96 HOURS. TOTAL DEAD OF LUNG CELLS (98%).

RNA of F. GRAMINEARUM

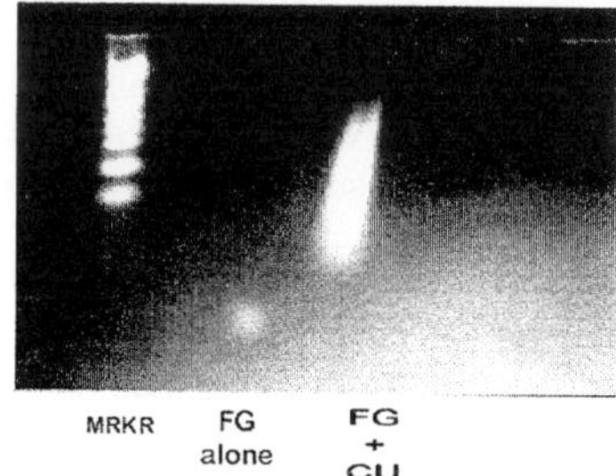

Fig.2. Increased RNA concentration of toxigenic F. GRAMINEARUM grown in copper (5 ppm) amended substrates, as compared to F. GRAMINEARUM alone grown without copper.

Metal Ions in Biology and Medicine; vol 6. Eds. J.A. Centeno, Ph. Collery, G. Vernet, R.B. Finkelman, H. Gibb, J.C. Etienne. John Libbey Eurotext, Paris © 2000, pp. 768-770.

Toxicity of mercury, lead and silver in intestinal cancer patients

C. Díez[1], I. Manso[1], J. Rabadán[2] and M.C. Martín Mateo[1]

[1] Department of Biochemistry, [2] Thoracic Surgery Division, University of Valladolid, Spain

Abstract

It is known that trace metals have a catalytic function on the generation of oxygen free radicals (OFRs) which have been associated with carcinogenic diseases. OFRs′ effect is based on their role as molecular marks, which are responsible for the typical mutations in cancer cells and for oxidation damage that causes lipid peroxidation, membrane weakening and finally cellular lysis, hemolysis in red blood cells (RBCs).

This study has been conducted using RBCs of two groups: cancer patients and healthy blood donors (control group). RBCs were incubated "in vitro" for 6 hours with mercury (10^{-5}M), lead (10^{-4}M) and silver (10^{-5}M) with two different buffers: barbital (BS) and phosphate (PBS). The possible inhibitory effect on hemolysis was also studied adding the aminoacid cysteine to the metal solution.

High metal toxicity is shown by an increased percentage of hemolysis and metahemoglobin and a decreased percentage of oxihemoglobin.

Mercury and silver were the most hemolizant metals (97.67±2.11% by Hg^{+2} and 97.31±1.41% by Ag^{+} after 6 hr. of incubation) followed by lead (87.78±4.44% after 6 hr.). Hemolysis induced in PBS resulted in a reduction from the same study in BS: 97.67±2.11% to 83.89±8.49% for mercury, 97.31±1.41% to 92.77% for silver and the difference was particularly significant in lead, 87.78±4.44% to 7.41±0.59%.

The addition of cysteine into RBCs had a remarkable inhibitory effect on the three metal-induced hemolysis: 97.67±2.11% to 2.23±0.70% for mercury, 97.31±1.41% to 4.04±1.05% for silver and 87.78±4.44% to 6.38% for lead.

The comparative study among cancer patients and control group, focused on how these metals inducing hemolysis, presented no difference for mercury and lead, although there was a significant increase in silver in cancer patients and its inhibition by cysteine was less than in the healthy blood donors.

Introduction

Trace elements are toxic mainly because of their ability to induce OFRs [1]. These act as molecular marks that activate protooncogenes, who are responsible for the typical, uncontrollable growth of cancer cells, and inactivate suppressor genes of tumours [2].

Lipid peroxidation is also the consequence of the attack of free radicals to membrane lipids, thus destroyed by their rigidity [3].

Lead and mercury induce hemolysis in RBCs because they react rapidly with sulfhydryl groups in the RBC membrane. They also lead to the decrease of activity by enzymes in the pentose phosphate shunt which maintains the antioxidant defence of the membrane.

The test oxidation damage by OFRs is shown by: increased percentage of hemolysis, decreased percentage of oxihemoglobin, that transports oxygen in RBCs and increased percentage of metahemoglobin, non functional to transport oxygen.

Materials and methods

Two groups were studied in these experiments: one of 18 patients with intestinal cancer and the other of 20 healthy blood donors (control group).

The method followed was according Caffrey [4]. Blood samples were treated with equal volumes of citrate buffer (40mM), sodium chloride (155mM) and sodium phosphate (20mM). The samples were centrifuged to separate the RBCs and were then washed with BS or PBS (pH 7.4). The 6 ml. erythrocyte solution was adjusted to a 1.5% hematocrite and was then incubated for 6 hr. at 37°C with of Hg^{+2}, Ag^{+}, Pb^{+2} and Cys.

The percentage of hemolysis was determined from spectrophotometric readings at 410 nm., of centrifuged samples supernatant taken every hour. The remaining cells, washed with BS or PBS, were used to determine the percentage of oxihemoglobin and metahemoglobin from spectrophotometric readings at 560, 576 and 630 nm. inserted in the equations proposed by Benesch and coll. [5].

The optimal concentrations of metals and of cysteine were determined previously (unpublished results).

Results

The hemolysis induced by mercury, silver and lead, after 6hr. of incubation with different conditions of study, is shown in Fig. 1, 2 and 3 respectively.

The percentages of oxihemoglobin and metahemoglobin, studied in the donors with and without cysteine, are shown in Fig.4 for mercury, Fig.5 for silver and Fig.6 for lead.

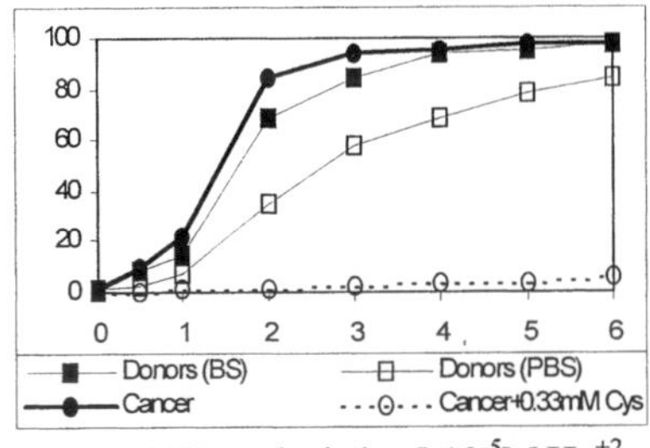

Fig.1.%Hemolysis by 5 10^{-5}M Hg^{+2}

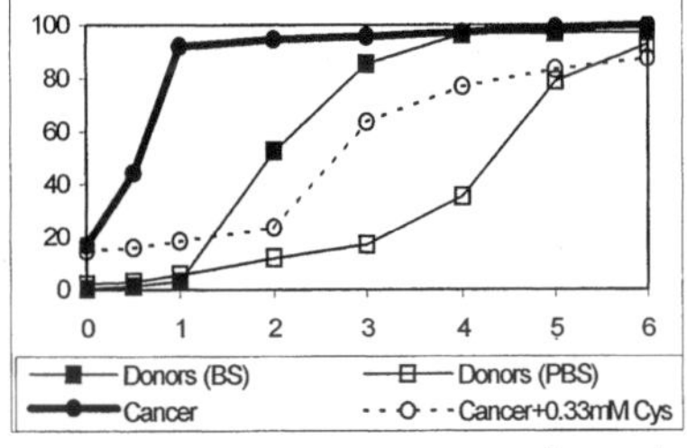

Fig.2.%Hemolysis by 13 10^{-5}M Ag^{+}

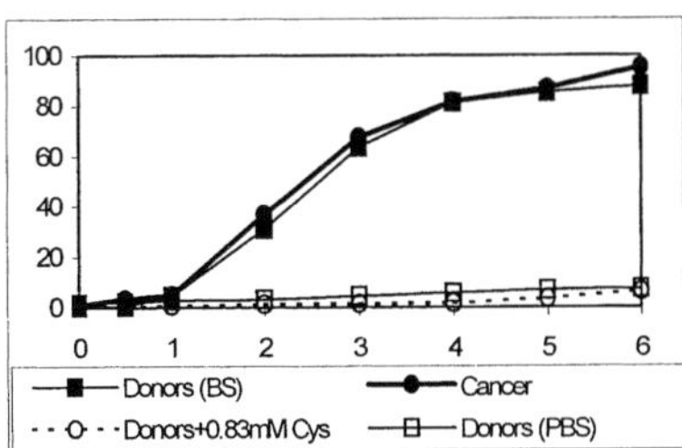

Fig.3.%Hemolysis by 5 10^{-4}M Pb^{+2}

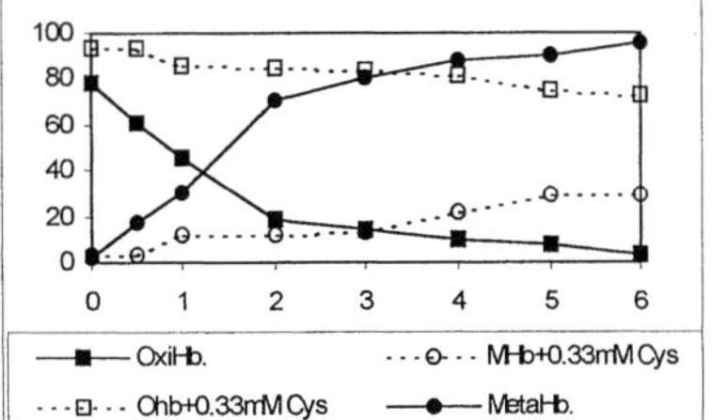

Fig.4.%OxiHb,MetaHb by 5 10^{-5}M Hg^{+2}

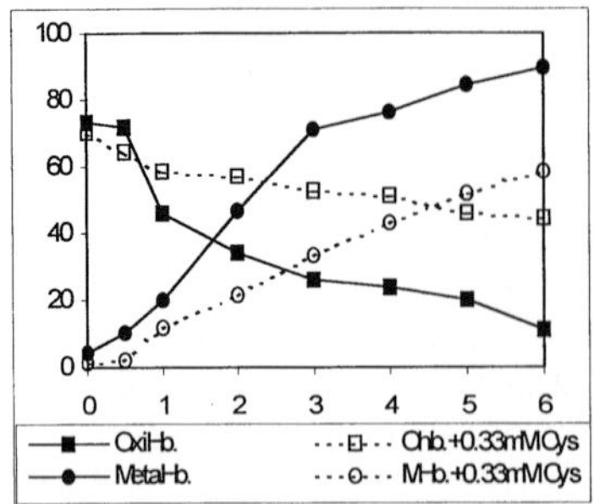

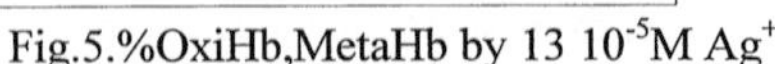

Fig.5.%OxiHb,MetaHb by 13 10^{-5}M Ag^{+}

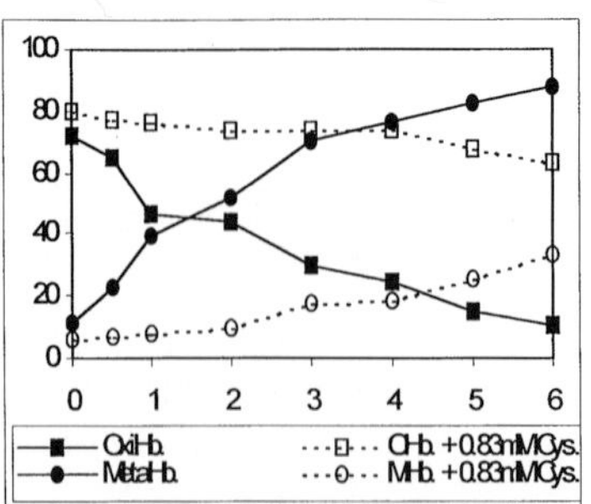

Fig.6.%OxiHb,MetaHb by 5 10^{-4}M Pb^{+2}

Discussion

The three metals, that we have studied, have a very hemolizant effect; however, mercury (Fig.1) and silver (Fig.2) are the most powerful in RBCs in both groups.

The level of hemolysis induced by each metal in PBS is lower than that in BS [4], because the metals first precipitate in the PBS solution and are unable to act. Lead (Fig.3) was almost entirely inhibited whereas the others demonstrated only a partial decrease.

Cysteine almost entirely inhibits the hemolysis induced by mercury, silver and lead (Fig.1,2,3) because it forms mercaptides among metals and its sulfhydryl groups, competing with the membrane groups that join metals, and preventing their attack.

The results of the experiments conducted with mercury and lead demonstrated only a minor difference in hemolysis level between the two groups. Silver (Fig.2), however, affected the hemolysis level in cancer patients to a much higher degree from the beginning of the tests. This could be explained by the lack of defences of the RBCs of cancer patients which could enhance the ability of OFRs to attack cell membranes. Similarly, the inhibition level in the presence of cysteine is much lower in cancer patients than in control subjects. Healthy blood donors have more cysteine in their plasma and present a higher inhibition rate whereas cancer patients have lost its cysteine and they are more exposed to the attack of OFRs and to the consequent hemolysis.

High metal toxicity is shown by a decreased percentage of oxihemoglobin and an increased percentage of metahemoglobin that are studied here in the RBCs of blood donors with each metal (Fig.4 for mercury, Fig.5 for silver and Fig.6 for lead). The changes in both percentages are softer when cysteine (inhibitor) is added. There are not significant differences in the RBCs of cancer patients (unpublished results).

References

1. Barnes G, Frieden E. Trace metals ion induced hemolysis. *Biochemica et biophysica acta* 1973; 302: 457-458.
2. Galeotti T, Borrello S, De Leo M. E, Rhia F. On the role of free radicals in the development of Cancer. In: Richelieu Press, ed. *Free radicals in the Environment, Medicine and Toxicology* 1994: 509-512.
3. Chiu D, Kuipers F, Lubin B. Seminars in Hematology 1989; 26: 257-276.
4. Caffrey J. M. and coll. Biological Trace Elements Research 1986; 11: 19-27.
5. Benesch R. E, Benesch R, Young S. Equations for the Spectrophotometric Analysis of Hemoglobin Mixtures. *Analitycal Biochemistry* 1973; 55: 245-248.

Metal Ions in Biology and Medicine; vol 6. Eds. J.A. Centeno, Ph. Collery, G. Vernet, R.B. Finkelman, H. Gibb, J.C. Etienne. John Libbey Eurotext, Paris © 2000, pp. 771-773.

Effect of Na^+ ion concentration in solutions on Cu^{2+}-induced DNA structural transitions

Elene Hackl, Yurij Blagoi

Institute for Low Temperature Physics and Engineering, National Academy of Sciences of Ukraine, 47 Lenin Ave., 310164 Kharkov, Ukraine; E-mail: e_hackl@usa.net

In our previous works [1.2] we have shown that on the DNA interaction with Cu^{2+} ions in aqueous solution at 29^{0}C DNA may transit into the compact state remaining in the B-form. This transition is of high positive cooperativity. In the number of works devoted to DNA condensation it is noted that the degree of charge neutralization on DNA phosphates necessary to induce DNA condensation may be achieved only in the case of action of condensing agents with valence 3 and more (see review [3] and references therein). But condensing agents may provoke DNA condensation not only through an electrostatic mechanism; they may also act by perturbing hydration structure [4], crossbridging neighboring helices, or perturbing DNA helix structure [5]. In particular, in [6], where the DNA condensation under divalent metal ions action was also studied, it was shown, that Mn^{2+} ions can produce toroidal condensates of supercoiled plasmid DNA but not of lineared one. Condensation mechanism with Mn^{2+} ions is not primarily electrostatic, but instead depends on supercoiling and destabilizing the DNA secondary structure due to Mn^{2+} binding to the DNA bases [6].

The importance of the electrostatic interaction in the condensation process is usually confirmed by existence of the strong dependence of the condensing agents binding to DNA (or of the condensation degree) on monovalent salt concentration in solution (irrespective of the kind of condensing agent - multivalent cations, polyamines, cationic lipids, etc. [3, 6-9]). To test whether the Cu^{2+}-induced DNA condensation in aqueous solution shown by us in [1,2] has primarily electrostatic mechanism, in the present work we studied Cu^{2+} ions interaction with DNA and DNA structural transitions taking place as a result of such interaction in solutions with different concentrations of monovalent sodium ions (i.e. on the presence of competition between mono- and divalent counterions).

Materials and methods

In the work the native calf thymus DNA with molecular weight of 1.9×10^7 Da, the protein content being lower than 0.1%, RNA being lower than 0.2 %, hypochromic effect being 36 %, was used. DNA samples were dissolved in cacodylate buffer, Na^+ concentration being 5×10^{-3} M, pH 7 ± 0.1. The biopolymer concentration in solution determined by UV spectroscopy was in the range of $(4.5 \div 4.8) \times 10^{-2}$ M of phosphorus.

Infrared spectra of DNA complexes with Cu^{2+} ions in solutions in the region of phosphate groups absorption (1000-1400 cm^{-1}) were recorded by the infrared spectrophotometer UR-20 (Karl Zeiss, Jena). To take spectra the special CaF_2 cuvettes with path lengths of 62 and 50 μm were used. The cuvettes were thermostated at 29±0.1^{0}C.

Results and discussion

IR spectra of DNA and DNA complexes with Cu^{2+} ions in aqueous solutions with different Na^{+} ion concentrations (0.05 ÷ 1 M) were taken. In the absence of Cu^{2+} ions IR spectra of DNA in the region of phosphate groups absorption have 3 main absorption bands at 1053 cm^{-1} (vibrations of the C-O-P sugar-phosphate backbone), 1090 cm^{-1} (ν_S - symmetrical vibrations of phosphate groups) and 1223 cm^{-1} (ν_{aS} - antisymmetrical vibrations of phosphate groups). The positions of these bands correspond to the IR spectrum of the native DNA in B-form in aqueous solution [1, 2]. Comparison of the IR spectra of DNA in solutions with different Na^{+} ion concentrations shows that the increase of the monovalent ion concentration in solution (in the absence of Cu^{2+} ions) does not lead to the spectrum modifications. This evidences that even at the significant increase of the monovalent ion concentration in solution DNA does not transit into the compact form without Cu^{2+} ions. On the DNA interaction with Cu^{2+} ions shifts of the absorption bands to higher frequencies and the sharp increase of intensities of bands ν_S and ν_{aS} occur, at that DNA remains in B-form. The character of changes in the spectra was similar in all solutions of different Na^{+} contents. In [1, 2] we attributed these spectral changes (first of all, the sharp increase of absorption band intensities) to the DNA transition into the compact form under the action of Cu^{2+} ions. Thus, the results obtained permit to say that Cu^{2+}-induced DNA condensation occurs in solutions of high monovalent ions (Na^{+}) concentrations too.

Fig. 1 shows the dependencies of the relative change of the intensity (R) of the absorption band ν_S on the total Cu^{2+} ions concentration ($[Cu^{2+}]$) in solutions with different Na^{+} contents. As is seen from Fig., a general view of all dependencies R ($[Cu^{2+}]$) is similar.

With the increase of Na^{+} ion concentration in solution the interval of Cu^{2+} ion concentrations, in which the rise of R value occurs, increases (Fig.1, *insert*). This means that the increase of Na^{+} ion concentration in solution results in decreasing the cooperativity of the Cu^{2+}-induced DNA condensation. For comparison, in Fig.1 (*insert*, curves 2-4) the concentration intervals ΔC for the number of condensing agents are shown (ΔC is the interval of condensing agent concentrations, in which the DNA condensation (intra- or intermolecular) occurs). As is seen from Fig., the more the condensing agent valence (Cu^{2+}<$CoHex^{3+}$<$spermine^{4+}$) the narrower the interval of condensing agent concentrations in which DNA condensation occurs, i.e. the higher cooperativity of the condensation process. Besides, regardless of the condensing agent valence, cooperativity of the DNA condensation process decreases with the increase of the Na^{+} ion concentration in solution. The decrease of cooperativity of the DNA condensation process with the rise of the Na^{+} ion concentration in solution may be explained by competition between Cu^{2+} and Na^{+} ions for binding sites on DNA phosphate groups. Such competition must result in the decrease of binding constants of Cu^{2+} ions interacting with DNA in solutions of high Na^{+} concentrations. Indeed, estimation of binding constants (K_{bind}) of Cu^{2+} ions interacting with DNA on condensation process performed using the model proposed in [2] shows that, when increasing Na^{+} ion concentration in solution, K_{bind} decrease significantly (not illustrated).

It also follows from Fig. 1, that the maximum increase of absorption band ν_S intensity (R_{max} value) is practically equal for DNA - Cu^{2+} complexes in solutions with different Na^{+} ion concentrations. Thus, the degree of the Cu^{2+}-induced condensation (which is proportional to the R_{max} value) depends on the Na^{+} concentration in solution very weakly in the interval of the monovalent ion concentrations studied. Similar results were obtained by Ma and Bloomfield: for Mn^{2+}-induced DNA condensation they have shown that the scattering intensity of DNA solution with Mn^{2+} ions decreases only slightly with increasing NaCl or $MgCl_2$ concentrations

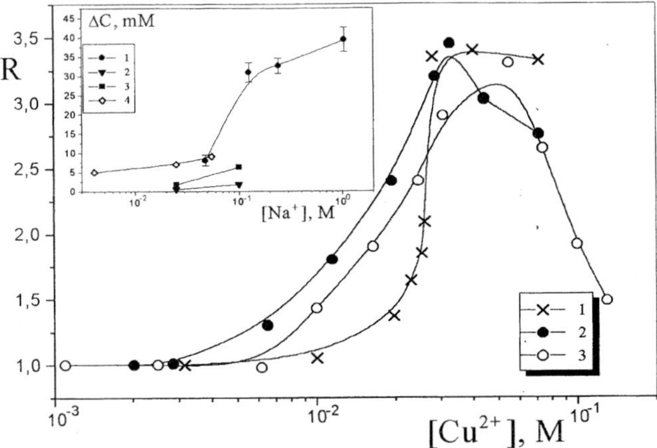

Fig. 1. Dependencies of relative change of intensity (R) of absorption band ν_S on total Cu^{2+} ions concentration for DNA complexes with Cu^{2+} ions in aqueous solutions containing different Na^+ ion concentrations, M: 5×10^{-2} (1), 0.242 (2), 1.045 (3). $R=D_i/D_0$, where D_0 is optical density at maximum of absorption band at given frequency for DNA without Cu^{2+} ions, D_i is the same value for DNA complex with Cu^{2+}.

Insert: Dependencies of interval of condensing agent concentrations, in which DNA condensation (intra- or intermolecular) occurs, (ΔC) on total concentration of Na^+ ions in solution for DNA condensation under the action of: 1 – Cu^{2+}, 2 – spermine^{4+}, 3 – CoHex^{3+}, 4 – spermidine^{3+} (dependencies 2-4 were calculated from data cited in [8-9]).

[6]. This is in marked contrast to DNA condensation induced by +3 or +4 agents, the degree of which decreases sharply at addition of mono- or divalent cations [3,7,8]. This implies that both Mn^{2+}-induced DNA condensation shown in [6] and Cu^{2+}-induced one shown by us in [1,2] are not dominated by electrostatics.

Thus we have obtained, that the degree of the Cu^{2+}-induced DNA condensation depends on the Na^+ concentration in solution very weakly. At the same time, with the increase of Na^+ content in solution cooperativity of the DNA condensation decreases as well as K_{bind} of Cu^{2+} ions interacting with DNA on the condensation process. The results obtained permit to suppose that the mechanism of DNA condensation under Cu^{2+} ion action is not completely electrostatic.

References

1. Hackl E, Kornilova S, Kapinos L, et.al. Study of Ca^{2+}, Mn^{2+}, Cu^{2+} ion binding to DNA in solutions by means of IR-spectroscopy. *J Mol Struct* 1997; 408 / 409: 229-32.
2. Kornilova S, Hackl E, Kapinos L, et.al. DNA interaction with metal ions. Cooperativity of metal ion binding at DNA compactization. *Acta Biochim Polon* 1998; 45: 107-17.
3. Bloomfield V. DNA condensation by multivalent cations. *Biopolymers* 1998; 44: 269-82.
4. Rau D, Parsegian V. Direct measurement of the intermolecular forces between counterion-condensed DNA double helices. Evidence for long range attractive hydration forces. *Biophys J* 1992; 61: 246-59.
5. Bloomfield V. Condensation of DNA by multivalent cations: considerations on mechanism. *Biopolymers* 1991; 31: 1471-81.
6. Ma Ch, Bloomfield V. Condensation of supercoiled DNA induced by $MnCl_2$. *Biophys J* 1994; 67: 1678-81.
7. Braunlin W, Anderson C, Record M.T.Jr. Competitive interactions of $Co(NH_3)_6^{3+}$ and Na^+ with helical B-DNA probed by ^{59}Co and ^{23}Na NMR. *Biochemistry* 1987; 26: 7724-31.
8. Pelta J, Livolant F, Sikorav J. DNA aggregation induced by polyamines and cobalthexamine. *J Biol Chem* 1996; 271: 5656-62.
9. Pelta J, Durand D, Doucet J, Livolant F. DNA mesophases induced by spermidine: structural properties and biological implications. *Biophys J* 1996; 71: 48-63.

Metal Ions in Biology and Medicine; vol 6. Eds. J.A. Centeno, Ph. Collery, G. Vernet, R.B. Finkelman, H. Gibb, J.C. Etienne. John Libbey Eurotext, Paris © 2000, pp. 774-776.

Sm(III) hydrolysis and complexation with α-aminoacids

Julia Torres[1], Carlos Kremer[1], Eduardo Kremer[1], Sixto Domínguez[2], Alfredo Mederos[2], Erich Königsberger[3]

[1] *Cátedra de Química Inorgánica, Facultad de Química, CC1157, Montevideo, Uruguay;* [2] *Departamento de Química Inorgánica, Universidad de La Laguna, 38200 La Laguna, Tenerife, Canary Islands, Spain;* [3] *Department of Physical Chemistry, University of Leoben, Franz-Josef-Strasse 18, A-8700 Leoben, Austria*

Abstract

Sm (III)-glycine and Sm(III)-alanine systems were studied by potentiometry and ^{1}H-NMR spectroscopy. Mono and binuclear complexes were observed in solution for both systems, even though hydrolysis competes with the formation of these coordination compounds.

Introduction

Some radionuclides have already been used to treat skeletal metastases; among them, ^{153}Sm (β emitter, $t_{1/2}$ = 46.27h) has shown excellent nuclear and chemical properties. In fact, coordination compounds of ^{153}Sm, such as ^{153}Sm-EDTMP, have just been successfully used as radiotherapeutic agents [1]. On the other hand, the intake of α-aminoacids (Haa) by abnormal cells is enhanced due to the special metabolism of tumour cells. So, it is possible to hypothesise that the captation of Sm(III) complexes of these Haa by cancer cells should be preferential. It is important that such complexes are stable in the medium in which they will be used. In this sense, the thermodynamic stability of the coordination compounds in physiological conditions (37°C, 0.15M ionic strength), should be evaluated. In addition, it must be taken into account that Sm(III) can undergo hydrolysis reactions which will interfere with the formation of the desired complexes. Data dealing with these hydrolysis reactions and also with solubility of $Sm(OH)_3$ are available in various media, but in conditions of temperature and ionic strength different from the physiological ones [2]. This communication deals with hydrolysis of Sm(III) and complexation of Sm(III) with Haa (glycine=Hgly and alanine=Hala) in different media, some of which simulate the physiological environment. So, potentiometric studies in aqueous solution at 25.0 or 37.0°C and 0.15 or 0.5M NaCl or $NaClO_4$ ionic strength were carried out. Besides, as precipitation of $Sm(OH)_3$ was observed beyond pH 6, the determination of its $^{*}K_{s0}$ was achieved.

Results and discussion

The monohydroxo complex was the only species detected before precipitation in the Sm(III) concentration interval under investigation (4-40 mM). Results (only for some selected experimental conditions) are depicted in Table I; $*K_1$ corresponds to the equilibrium quotient of the process:

$$Sm^{3+} + H_2O \rightleftharpoons [Sm(OH)]^{2+} + H^+ \quad , *K_1$$

This complex is the predominant species only in a very short pH interval (see Fig. 1). These results were consistent with previously reported data [2]. Hydrolysis studies were also carried out employing NaCl as supporting electrolyte. These experiments resulted in higher values of log $*K_1$ probably due to the presence of chloride ions as ligands which could be responsible of an electron-withdrawing effect.

T (°C)	Medium	^{a}log $*K_1$	Average log $*K_{s0}$
37	$NaClO_4$ 0.15M	-6.83±0.02	16.32 ± 0.06
	NaCl 0.15M		16.66 ± 0.05
25	$NaClO_4$ 0.15M	-8.43±0.02	
	NaCl 0.15M		16.42 ± 0.02

Table I. Sm(III) hydrolysis and solubility studies of $Sm(OH)_3$ (s). [a]Around 40 experimental points in the 3.5-6.5 pH interval were used for each log $*K_1$ calculation.

The pale yellow solid formed in conditions that simulate physiological ones was fully characterised as $Sm(OH)_3$ by IR spectra, elemental and thermal analyses and X-Ray powder diffraction. Solubility measurements of this solid (results also depicted in Table I) agreed within the experimental error. We found acceptable agreement at 25°C with reported data for different media [2]. $*K_{s0}$ corresponds to:

$$Sm(OH)_3\,(s) + 3\,H^+ \rightleftharpoons Sm^{3+} + 3\,H_2O \quad , *K_{s0}$$

The obtained potentiometric results of Sm(III)-Haa systems, are depicted in Table II and Figure 1. $\beta_{mn\text{-}p}$ correspond to the equilibrium quotients of the process:

$$m\,Sm^{3+} + n\,Haa \xrightleftharpoons{\beta_{mn\text{-}p}} [Sm_m(H_{(n-p)/n}aa)_n]^{(3-p)+} + p\,H^+$$

It is worth noting that in both systems mono and dinuclear species are formed at pH lower to around 6.5, where $Sm(OH)_3$ (s) is precipitated. Almost all complexes of Sm(III) with these Haa are formed with the zwitterionic form of the ligands. For the $[Sm(Haa)]^{3+}$ coordination compounds, not very high formation constants were found, which means that these complexes are not very stable. Besides, $[Sm(Haa)_3]^{3+}$ complexes were also detected (for Hgly, this complex is partially deprotonated). The latter are in equilibrium with their dimeric form $[Sm_2(Haa)_6]^{6+}$. In Sm(III)-Hala system, the dimeric form only appears at higher concentrations of ligand and metal, whereas at lower concentrations, only $[Sm(Hala)]^{3+}$ is formed.

$[Sm^{3+}]$ (mM)	Sm(III)-Hgly system	Sm(III)-Hala system
5-7	log β_{110}=1.60±0.09	logβ_{110}= 1.14±0.06
	log $\beta_{13\text{-}1}$=1.36±0.05	logβ_{130}=2.3±0.2
	log β_{260}=13.3±0.1	logβ_{260}= 6.9±0.1

Table II- Potentiometric results on Sm-Haa systems in $NaClO_4$ 0.15M, 37°C.

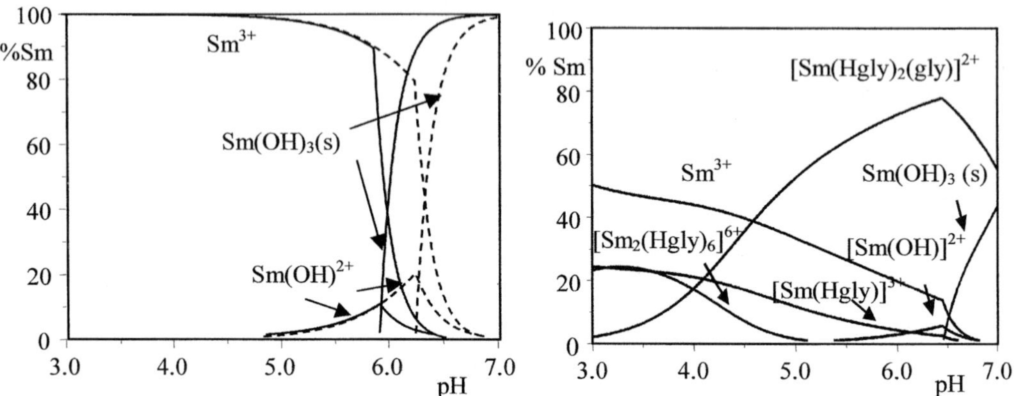

Figure 1. Species distribution diagrams, 37°C, 0.15M $NaClO_4$. On the left, Sm(III) hydrolysis (total $[Sm^{3+}]$=5mM (dashed line) and 50mM (continuous line)). On the right, Sm(III)-Hgly system (total $[Sm^{3+}]$= 7mM, total [Hgly]=21mM).

The presence of different complex species of samarium(III) was also confirmed by ^{1}H-NMR studies in D_2O. For example, varying the Sm:Hgly molar ratio, it was possible to see how CH_2 singlet of Hgly was shifted showing equilibrium between the different species. In spite of the fact that different concentrations of Sm were used for potentiometric measurements and ^{1}H-NMR studies, comparable results were obtained.

Acknowledgements

We would like to thank Álvaro Mombrú and Elena Pardo from Crystallography Lab, Physics Department, Facultad de Química, for the X-Ray powder diffraction diagrams. Part of this work was supported by C.S.I.C. (Comisión Sectorial de Investigación Científica). We also thank Ministerio de Educación y Cultura, Dirección General de Enseñanza Superior e Investigación Científica, Spain, through grant PM98-0148.

References

[1]Volkert WA, Hoffman TJ. Therapeutic radiopharmaceuticals. *Chem. Rev.* 1999; **99**: 2269-92.

[2] Kragten J, Decnop-Weever LG. Hydroxide complexes of lanthanides-II. *Talanta* 1979: **26**: 1105-9.

Metal Ions in Biology and Medicine; vol 6. Eds. J.A. Centeno, Ph. Collery, G. Vernet, R.B. Finkelman, H. Gibb, J.C. Etienne. John Libbey Eurotext, Paris © 2000, pp. 777-779.

The interaction mechanism of heavy metals with bilayer lipid membranes and their toxicity

Kylyvnyk K.E., Sushenko C.A., Bovykin B.A.

The Ukrainian State Chemical Technology University Dnepropetrovsk, Ukraine

Among environmental pollutants it is necessary to single out the heavy metals. They have high stability and toxicity and, forming complexes, are transmitted between components of the ecosystem, and penetrate through the food chain into human nutrition.

The mechanisms of the toxic activity of metals are manifold. But almost always the penetration of ions through plasmatic membrane and their interaction with components of a cell (core, Golgi complex, endoplasmic reticulum etc.) is necessary.The first barrier to an ion's penetration of an organism is the plasmatic membrane of a cell. The biochemical activity of heavy metals largely depends on their state (ionic shape or complex, saturated or unsaturated), on the pH of medium, and the presence of other substances.

In our work we attempted to connect the interaction mechanism of ions with a cell membrane with the metal toxicity.

As the model of plasmatic membranes we have used the bilayer lipid membranes (BLM) which are formed from phospholipids of ox brain by the well-known Mueller's method. The membranes were formed on the small aperture (Ø 1,1 mm) in a Teflon septum separating two aqueous solutions. By the change in the electrical characteristics of a membrane (resistance, capacity and membrane potential) we determined the interaction mechanism of ions with the BLM (adsorption; adsorption with a partial permeability, permeability).

For measurement of membrane resistance we used the method of cyclic volt-ampere characteristics (VAC) [2].

The membrane potential was measured by the usual method, i.e. by connecting the high-resistance voltmeter in a mode of voltage measurement. Also the potential was determined by the method of the current minimum of the second harmonic [3].

The influence of heavy metal ions on the elastic properties of BLM was investigated by the method of third harmonic current [4], which measures the Young elasticity module in a direction perpendicular to the membrane.

Nitrates of the investigated metals were added to the solution washing one side of the membrane and the change in membrane potential and electroconductivity were registered. We used solutions with __ 2÷4 for prevent hydrolysis of the salts.

In our opinion, there is a direct link between the mechanism of the ions' interaction with the BLM and their toxicity. Namely: the ions possessing a small toxicity (for example, Zn, for which the maximum concentration limit for drinking water is 5mg/l) in physiological conditions are only adsorbed on a membrane surface. In nitrate solutions the hydrated cations of such metals, even in high concentration, do not change the membrane's electroconductivity but are only adsorbed on its surface. With an increase of the charge of the metal ions the adsorption ability grows. The univalent cations (except _g$^+$ and _l$^+$) are adsorbed very poorly on the membrane surface.

With the increase of cation's charge the adsorption ability grows sharply which results in loss of membrane stability. To obtain a membrane potential of 60-70 mV the concentration of divalent ions should be $C_{(Zn - Cd)} = 1...5*10^{-2}$ _. Trivalent cations in the same conditions already at concentration 10^{-5}(Ga) and 10^{-4} (Al) generated potential 100-120 mV. The higher an ion's toxicity, the lower its concentration necessary to produce that potential at which the membrane becomes unstable (100 mV and more). With increased toxicity and membrane potential a change in elastic properties of a membrane is observed (decrease of elasticity). The maintenance of elasticity in a certain range is extremely important for normal functioning of living cell. This description shows the first mechanism of interaction of a metal's ions with a membrane.

The second mechanism of the metal ion interaction with the membrane is observed when the ion exist as hydrophilic-hydrophobic complexes or form such complexes with components of the solution or membrane. By virtue of hydrophilic-hydrophobic properties such complexes will penetrate through the membrane and if a charge is present, this results in the change of the membrane electroconductivity.

So, for example, the ions of copper and gallium are only adsorbed on the membrane surface, but with the formation of complexes, the slope of the volt-ampere characteristics is increased, which testifies to the change of the membrane electroconductivity. The addition of $[Ga(HINA)_3]Cl_3$ complex of concentration of $5*10^{-4}$ M (here HINA is hydrazide isonicotinic acid) increased the conductivity by more than two orders. The same effect was achieved also by addition of 10^{-5} _ $[Zn(BMC)_2]Cl_2$ (BMC is N-methyl-2- benzimidazolyl carbamate).

The third mechanism was the sum of the two previous and was observed when the adsorption and penetration of an ion through the membrane was simultaneous.

In all cases a change in elastic properties of the membrane is observed. The adsorption of solvated cations results in the ordering of the membrane structure around the adsorbed ion. As the result, the temperature of phase transitions changed and the elasticity of the membrane decreased (for divalent ions up to 5 %, for trivalent - up to 10 %). If the metal ion existed in the form of a hydrophilic-hydrophobic complex the change of elasticity is more significant, at the expense of the interaction of hydrophobic ligands with the membrane.

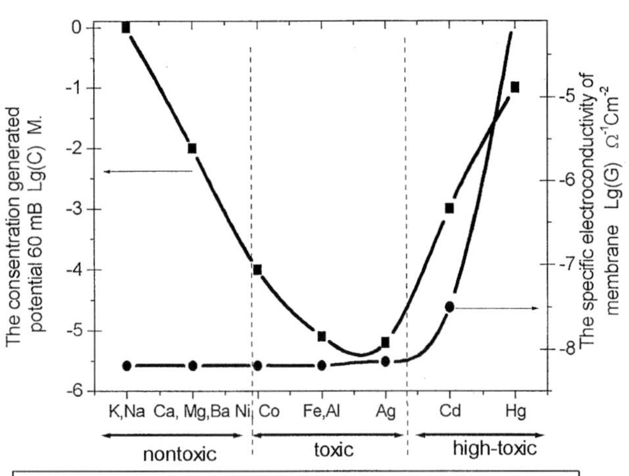

The change of interaction between ions and BLM while metal toxity increasing

Also the pH of the solution and the presence of extraneous ions is very important. The true concentration of an ion decreased with the increasing of the solution pH at the expense of the formation of hydrates and the influence on the membrane was weakened.

The presence of halogenide ions in the solution has a dual influence. So, in the case with Ag^+ the addition of Hal^- ions resulted in formation of the nonsoluble precipitates and the influence on the membrane weakened. If instead of Ag^+ we take Hg^{2+} ions, which in nitrate solutions only adsorbed on a membrane the opposite effect was observed. The addition of Hal^- ions resulted in formation of covalent ions ($HgHal^+$), which penetrated through the membrane, changing electroconductivity.

With a transition from models to biological membranes, the interaction of ions with protein components is added, basically at the expense of their sulphide and hydrosulfide groups.

1.Mueller P. Methods for the formation of single biomolecular lipid membranes in auqueous solution.//J.Chem-1963-67,N2.-P.534-535.

2.Tien H.T. Cyclic voltammetry of bilayer lipid membranes// J. Phis. Chem. 1984. Vol.88, N15, P.3172-3174.

3.Соколов В.С., Кузьмин В.Г. Измерение разности поверхностных потенциалов бислойных мембран по второй гармонике емкостного тока //Биофизика,1980,25,168.

4.Пасечник В.А., Гианик Т. Упругие свойства бислойных мембран в направлении, перпендикулярном плоскости мембраны.//Коллоидный журнал,1977,39,с.1182-1185.

Metal Ions in Biology and Medicine; vol 6. Eds. J.A. Centeno, Ph. Collery, G. Vernet, R.B. Finkelman, H. Gibb, J.C. Etienne. John Libbey Eurotext, Paris © 2000, pp. 780-782.

Lead tissue accumulation effects on rats administered treated sewage water

Ioannis Papagiannis, Fotini Mane and Vicky Kalfakakou

Experimental Physiology Lab. Environmental Physiology Unit, Faculty of Medicine, University of Ioannina, Ioannina 45 110, Greece

Background: Chronic exposure to lead (Pb) is related to neuromuscular syndromes, anaemia, mitochondrial, impairment, kidney dysfunction, infertility, growth retardation, cardiovascular injuries and bone fragility. Domestic treated sewage is considered a water resource in times where clear water is lacking despite the fact that sometimes sewage contains toxic metals such as Pb. **Aim**: The investigation of accumulation rate of Pb in tissues and organs of rats administered sewage as drinking water in relation to functional parameters of these organs. **Methods**: Rats divided in 5 groups were administered sewage effluent undiluted, pH: 8.0 and pH≤7.0 and diluted 1:5 and 1:10 with tap water.The control group received just tap water. The experiment lasted 24 months during which every 6 months creatinine, hepatic enzymes, blood indices analyses and electrocardiogram recordings were performed to animals. Body weight and survival time, were registered every 2 weeks. Also every 6 months 3 animals from each group were sacrificed and tissue Pb determination was performed by means of atomic absorption spectrophotometry. **Results**: Lead concentration in effluents was at 0,01± 0,003 mg/l. The highest Pb concentration appeared in bones (31.91 μg/g), heart 5.06 μg/g), spleen (3.82 μg/g) and kidney (3.8 μg/g). Accumulation rate of Pb was increased during the last 6 months of exposure. White blood cell counts were significantly decreased while serum glucose was increased in the undiluted pH: 8 sewage received group. In the above group as well as in groups received acidified sewage (pH≤7.0) and diluted 1:5, body weight and survival time were significantly decreased.

Conclusions: Chronic exposure to low Pb concentrations results in Pb tissue accumulation and is related to systemic dysfunction's and decreased survival time in rats.

Introduction

Lead (Pb) is considered one of the 10 most dangerous pollutants (1): Lead inhibits important biochemical procedures by replacing essential metals and by producing toxic free radicals (2,3). Chronic exposure to Pb through drinking water causes mitochondrial impairment, encephalopathy and peripheral paralysis, anemia, hypertension and myocardiopathy, osteomalakia, renal failure and infertility (4,5).

Domestic sewage are enriched by 1.9- 6.1 Pb mg / habitant / day (6).

In the present study treated domestic effluents were administered to rats as drinking water, for 24 months, in order to study Pb effects on the animals' physiology.

Materials and Methods

Wistar rats (N=100, male, 2 months old) divided in groups were administered water as follows: P_1: treated effluent, pH: 8.0, P_2: treated effluent diluted 1:5 with tap water, P_3: treated effluent diluted 1:10 with tap water. P_4: treated effluent, pH≤7.0, P_5: control group, received tap water. Every 6 months, 3 animals from each group, after anesthetization, ECG-recordings, blood urine and tissue samples were taken. General blood tests as well as plasma creatinine, sugar and hepatic aminotransferases (ALT, AST) determinations were performed. Lung, heart, spleen, liver, kidney, testis, urinary bladder, tibial bone and muscle and brain tissue samples as well as plasma, total and filtered effluent and tap water samples were analysed for Pb by means of a Perkin-Elmer 560 Atomic Absorption Spectrophotometer. Body weight and survival time were registered every 2 weeks. Tissue pathology was inspected after hematoxyline- eosine and rhodamine staining.

Results and Discussion

Lead levels in treated effluent were: **a.** Filtered sample: 0.004±0.001 mg/l. **b.** Total sample: 0.01±0.003 mg/l. The metal after 24months of rats exposure was selectively accumulated in bones (31.91 µg/g), heart (5.06 µg/g), spleen (3.82 µg/g) and kidney (3.8 µg/g). Lead Accumulation Indices (Pb-AI) are shown in the table.

$$\text{Pb-AI} = \frac{\text{Pb tissue conc. at 24 months}}{\text{Pb tissue conc. at 0 months}}$$

In brackets are the percentages of Pb- AI change in reference to control group.

LEAD ACCUMULATION INDICES (Pb – AI)

	P1 (pH:8.0)	P4 (pH<7)	P2 (1:5)	P3 (1:10)	P5 (control)
Spleen	3,60 (68,4)	2,68 (25,3)	2,54 (19,0)	2,80 (31,0)	2,14
Kidney	3,30 (131,6)	1,97 (38,5)	1,67 (17,1)	1,38 (-3,0)	1,42
Urinary bladder	2,70 (25,9)	2,34 (8,8)	2,02 (-6,0)	2,14 (-0,4)	2,15
Testis	4,33 (73,2)	3,81 (52,5)	2,61 (4,7)	2,93 (17,3)	2,50
Liver	5,37 (95,8)	3,77 (37,4)	3,40 (23,9)	3,63 (32,4)	2,74
Heart	8,28 (133,8)	5,07 (43,3)	4,66 (31,8)	3,99 (12,7)	3,54
Lungs	2,81 (66,5)	3,25 (92,9)	2,07 (22,8)	2,01 (19,1)	1,69
Brain	3,05 (62,8)	2,49 (32,6)	2,30 (22,5)	1,82 (-3,2)	1,88
Tibial bone	3,50 (70,5)	2,62 (27,8)	2,33 (13,4)	2,42 (17,8)	2,05
Tibial muscle	3,31 (59,3)	2,48 (19,3)	2,18 (4,9)	2,28 (9,6)	2,08

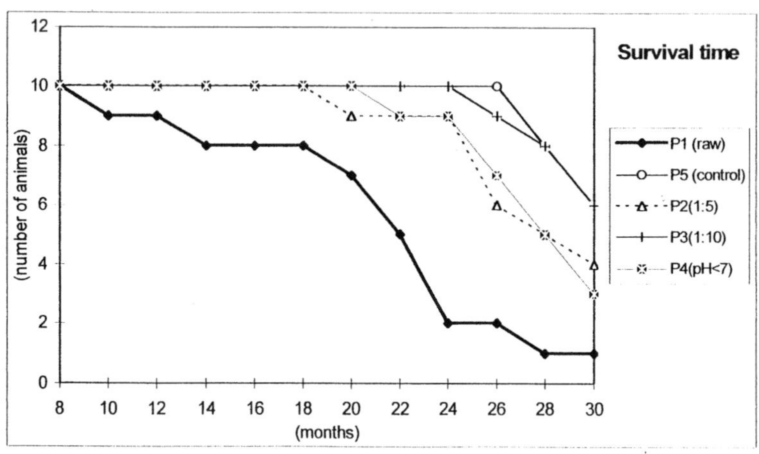

Heart, kidney, liver and bone of P_1 group presented the higher Pb-AI percentile changes.
ECG recordings revealed ventral extrasystoles, S-T falls and A-V blocks, maybe due to calcium increased influx to the sarcoplasmic reticulum (7).
Serum creatinine and ALT levels were increased also in P_1 group, indicating renal and hepatic dysfunction probably due to glutathione –S-transferase inhibition (8).
Tissue pathology showed metal deposits mainly across lamina propria of renal tubules and liver sinuses, followed by cellular degeneration and necrotic changes (9).
Lead in lungs was significantly accumulated in P4 group rats. Survival time is shown in the figure and it seems that is significantly and positively related to lower Pb concentrations and pH≤7.0 of the drinking water.

Conclusions

Chronic exposure of rats to low Pb levels of treated effluents as drinking water causes a rather selective Pb accumulation in heart, kidney liver and bone. Accumulation indices are proportionally related to functional disturbances such as cardiac rate and conductivity, creatinine and hepatic enzymes and inversely related to survival time.

References

1. EPA, 1986b. Quality criteria for water. US environmental Protection Agency, Office of Water Regulations and Standards. Publication 440/5-86-001.
2. Fujiwara Y., Watanabe S., Sakamoto M., Kaji T.: Repair of wounded monolayers of cultured vascular endothelial cells after simultaneous exposure to lead and zinc. *Toxicol. Lett.*, 1998, 94(3):181-188.
3. Vij AG., Satija NK. and Flora SJ.: Lead induced disorders in hematopoietic and drug metabolizing enzyme system and their protection by ascorbic acid supplementation. *Biomed. Environ. Sci.*, 1998, 11(1): 7 - 14.
4. Moore MR., Meredith PA., Goldberg A., Carr KE., Toner PG., Lawrie TD.: Cardiac effects of lead in drinking water of rats. *Clin. Sci. Mol. Med.*, 1975, 49(4): 337-341.
5. Hu H.: Bone lead as a new biologic marker of lead dose: recent findings and implications for public health. *Environ. Health Perspect.* 1998, 106(4): 961-967.
6. Jenkins D., Russell L.L.: Heavy metals contribution of household washing products to municipal wastewater. *Wat. Envir. Res.*, 1994, 66(6):805 – 813.
7. Lal B., Murthy RC., Anand M., Chandra SV., Kumar R., Tripathi O., Srimal RC.: Cardiotoxicity and hypertention in rats after oral lead exposure. *Drug. Chem. Toxicol.*, 1991, 14(3): 305-318.
8. Daggett DA., Nuwaysir EF., Nelson SA., Wright LS., Kornguth SE. and Siegel FL.: Effects of triethyl lead administration on the expression of glutathione S-transferase isoenzymes and quinone reductase in rat kidney and liver. *Toxicology*, 1997, 117(1): 61 - 71.
9. Papagiannis IL.: Biophysiological effects of secondary biological treatment plant effluent administration, as drinking water, to rats in relation to heavy metals accumulation. Doctorate thesis, 2000, Greece.

Metal Ions in Biology and Medicine; vol 6. Eds. J.A. Centeno, Ph. Collery, G. Vernet, R.B. Finkelman, H. Gibb, J.C. Etienne. John Libbey Eurotext, Paris © 2000, pp. 783-785.

Cadmium toxicity in *P. argyrostoma*

Bartolomé Ribhas-Ozonas, Olga García-Arribas, Mar Pérez-Calvo

Department of Toxicology, Institut of Health Carlos III, Ministry of Health, 28220-Majadahonda, Madrid, Spain

Abstract

To realize the biotest on diptera larvae of *Parasarcophaga argyrostoma*, the larvae are exposed to $CdCl_2$ at different concentrations: 1, 25, 50, 75, 100 µg Cd/g diet, are weighed at the beginning and 24, 48 and 72 hours, after the toxic exposure. The weight of the larvae at different times and concentrations exposed to the toxic, give us the % of growth inhibition, and after several experiments, the repetitivity, linearity and sensitivity. The results suggest that the cadmium exposure of *P. argyrostoma* larvae shows the alteration of weight and % weight increase at the concentration between 10-75 µg Cd/g diet. The 50% weight inhibition during development is attained with the dose of 25 µg Cd^{2+}/g diet at 72 hours. The non observed effect level (NOEL) per os is fixed to 10 µg Cd^{2+}/g diet. The non observed adverse effects level (NOAEL) should be fixed also at 10 µg Cd^{2+}/g diet. The acute lethal dose is established at 400 µg Cd^{2+}/g diet. The bioassay is an interesting alternative method for the substitution of laboratory mammals and this work should encourage and conduct to apport new data for the next homologation of this technique, because of its rapidity, reliability and utility to detect the hazard of poisoning for any compound in environmental pollution.
Keywords: Cadmium toxicity, cadmium exposure, bioassay, biotest, alternative method.

Introduction

Cadmium is a heavy metal of increasing prevalence in our environment, due to the production of metallic pieces, paints, batteries and industrial development (Shaikh and Smith, 1980). The anthropogenic activity which induced mobilization of cadmium (Cd) into the biosphere is approximately 30 times the global emission rate from natural sources (Nriagu and Pacyna, 1988).
Cadmium accumulates in plants, soils and food. The general population is mainly exposed by the oral route, and through tobacco smoke inhalation, by water ingestion and animal consumption. (Lauwerys et al, 1990). Cadmium has been reported to produce several toxic effects in animals and men. Several studies made in rats confirm that the cadmium toxicity produces nephropaty, hypertension, proteinuria and decreases the body weight. (Lall et al, 1997).

To investigate the cadmium toxicity there is applied the biotest on diptera larvae *P. argyrostoma*. (Labrousse and Matile, (1996). Insect larvae have already been used to detect the presence of toxins in human cadavers, being very important in forensic investigations (Kintz et al., 1990). The presence of different toxic heavy metals in nutrition has been studied using diptera larvae through the evaluation of the mercury in fish using sarcophagous dipter larvae. There has been studied the biological effects of heavy metals on the development of *Aedes aegypty* (Díptera: Culicidae) larvae (Rayars Keller A. et al, 1998).

Material and Methods

The larvae of *Parasarcophaga argyrostoma* obtained from the incubation of pupae in a breeding cage at 30°C with high degree of humidity, and a 12/24 h light cycle.
To realize the biotest there are used different cadmium concentrations (100, 75, 50, 25, 1 µg/g diet) homogenized with beef meat in plastic boxes and each one with ten larvae like the controls submitted to the same process. The larvae are weighed at the beginning of the experiment and at 24, 48 and 72 hours after the exposure.

The growth test is realized by weighing the animals one by one at time zero, 12 hours after lying on the fresh beef meat; this initial weight represents 100% of growth. The beef meat was first homogenized with a Waring Blendor and afterwards distributed in fractions of 9g, into little plastic boxes and each one newly homogenized with the concentration of the toxic compound, $CdCl_2$ at 100, 75, 50, 25, 10 µg Cd/g diet. The plastic boxes are perforated allowing an aerobic environment for the larvae growth. Then ten larvae were laid on each plastic box containing homogenized diet, and submitted to the before mentioned conditions.

Results

Kinetics of larval growth.
This graphic is obtained by weighing the larvae one by one at differents times: at the beginning of the experiment and at 24, 48 and 72 hours.

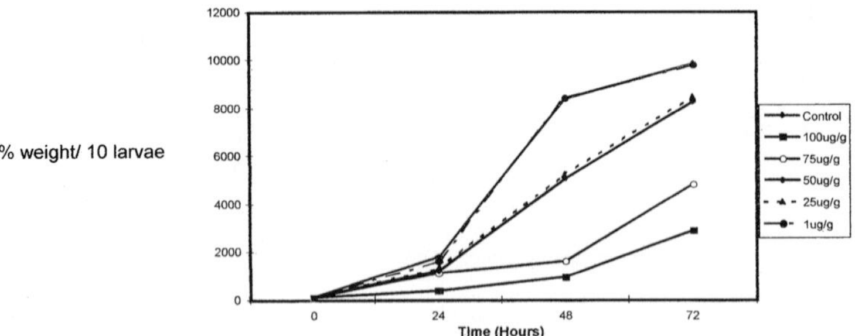

Fig.1. Kinetics of larval growth expressed as the percent of weight increase. The % weight is refered to 10 larvae. The inicial weight of the 10 larvae represents 100%, the rest of weights are percentages of this initial value.

The kinetics of poisoning shows linear growth, but it must be noted that the percentage of weight increase differed from one concentration of Cd^{2+} to another. When the Cd concentration is higher the % weight increase becomes lower. Between 10-75 $\mu gCd^{2+}/g$ diet the larvae show growth inhibition. The 50% inhibition during development is attained with the dose of 25 $\mu gCd^{2+}/g$ diet at 72 H.

Sensitivity

This is the dose-response curve for cadmium chloride. Diptera larvae are exposed to different concentrations of metal ion (100, 75, 50, 25, 1) $\mu gCd^{2+}/g$ diet. It represents % larval weight at different concentrations of cadmium.

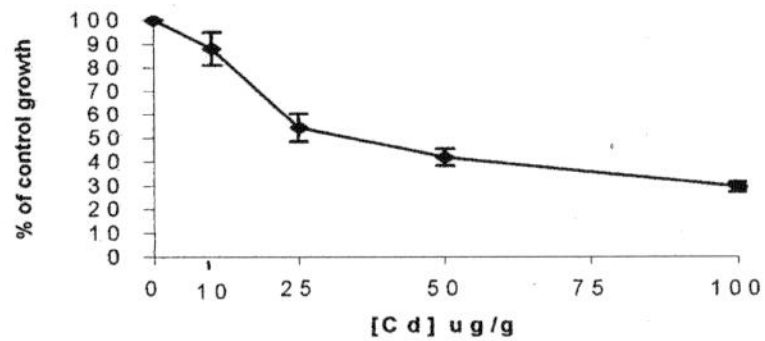

Fig. 2. Dose-response curve for 10 larvae submitted to different cadmium concentrations. The control represents the 100 % weight increase at different times. The weight increase values for cadmium exposure are expressed as percentages of the control ones.

When cadmium concentration of the diet increases, the % weight of the larvae became lower. At cadmium concentration of 1 $\mu g/g$ diet the larval growth is not affected, its behaviour is similar to the control. The larvae do not detect Cd^{2+} below this concentration. Figure1 shows the kinetics of poisoning and figure 2 expresses the dose-response curve, both are complementary.

Reproducibility

There is shown the reproducibility assay. It is evaluated based on five experiments running on differents days.

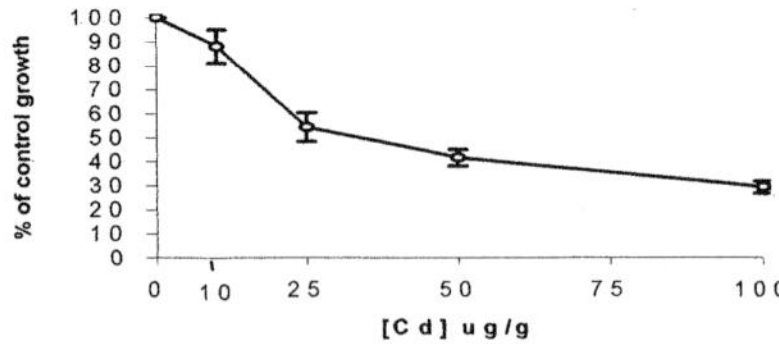

Fig .3. The curve of reproducibility shows the mean of the standard deviation of five experiments running with ten larvae per dose of toxic concentration (10, 25, 50, 100) μg Cd^{2+}/g. The percentage of growth of the control (beef meat alone) represents 100% growth. The rest of values are calculated as percentages of this standard value.

Discussion

The proposed bioassay is extremely simple in its theory and practice. An important asset is the technical simplicity, which eliminates extraction and purification steps. The development of this technique doesn't require high level training. It is very easy to perform. The biotest is inexpensive because it doesn't need complex materials or equipment, moreover it's easy to breed the insects at low cost.
The larvae used in this assay can be fed easily with a wide variety of protein samples. It doesn't require a special breeding, being very useful for toxicological experimentation. We intend to use it to detect poisons of mineral and organic compounds in different animal species (fish, birds, mammals etc.). It would be specially interesting to detect hazard of poisoning in wildlife animals, protected animals, because of the increasing use of (pesticides, heavy metals, new synthetic compounds, etc). There can be used a high number of animals (140 or more) per experiment and each one with two assays, which render the results statistically more reliable than other techniques.

The biotest is also an interesting alternative method for the substitution of laboratory mammals (mices, rats, rabbits, etc), that are used generally for animal experimentation to make toxicity assays. It's a versatile technique, because it can be applied to detect different types of toxics (metals, pesticides, sea toxins, etc). In this work we have used the heavy metal cadmium as toxic because of its frecuency in water pollution, wastes, air and nutrition. This element is widely distributed in the environment arising from industrial emissions and wastes. Actually we go on with the experiments testing different kinds of toxins. The *P. argyrostoma* bioassay is a rapid technique. The experiment lasts 72 hours. At this time we have obtained the larval weight at time 0, 24, 48, 72.

We study with this data the % growth increase, linearity, sensitivity and repetitivity. It's a sensitive test because of its capacity to detect different concentrations of cadmium per 25 μg/g units. When the toxic concentracion is lower, the % growth increase is higher, and at 1μg/g , the cadmium does not affect the larval growth, and its behabiour is similar to the control. Concentrations greater than 100 μg/g are lethal for the larvae. The non observed adverse effects level (NOEL) is fixed at 10 μg Cd^{2+}/g diet. The non observed adverse effects level (NOAEL) should be fixed also at 10 μg Cd^{2+}/g diet. The acute lethal dose is established at 400 μg Cd^{2+}/g diet.
Finally the *P. argyrostoma* life cycle is 40 days which allows to study several generations in a few months and to establish the toxicity, determining the % growth increase, linearity, sensitivity and repetitivity. There can also be observed the physiological alterations after the toxic effect during different generations. Its short life cycle is very useful to make " in vivo" experiments under the effects of different toxics and to evaluate genotoxic effects.

References

Kintz, P., Godelar, B., Tracqui, A., Mangin, P., Lugnier, A.A., and Chamount, A. J. (1990). Fly larvae: a new toxicological method of investigation in forensic medicine. J. Forensic Sci. 35, 204-207.

Labrousse, H., and Matile, L. (1996). Toxicological biotest on diptera larvae to detect ciguatoxins and various other substances. Toxicon 34, 881-891.

Lall, S.B., Das, N., Rama, R., Peshin, S.S., Khattar, S., Gulati, K. and Seth S.D. (1997). Cadmium induced nephrotoxicity in rats. Indian. J. Exp. Biol. 35, 151-154.

Lauwerys, R., Amery, A., Bernard, A., Bruaux, P., Buchet, J-P., Claeys, F. et al. (1990). Health effects of Environmental Exposure to Cadmium. Environ. Health. Persp. 87, 283-289.

Nriagu, J.O., and Pacyna, J.M. (1988). Quantitative assessment of worldwide contamination of air, water and soils by trace metals. Nature 333, 134-139.

Rayms-Keller, A., Olson, K.E., McGaw, M., Oray, C., Carlson, J.O., and Beaty, B.J. (1998). Effects of heavy metals on Aedes aegypty (Diptera: Culicidae) larvae. Ecotoxicol. Environ. Saf. 39, 41-47.

Shaikh, Z.A., and Smith, J.C. (1980). Metabolism of orally ingested cadmium in humans. In *Mechanism of Toxicity and Hazard Evaluation* (B. Holmstedt, R. Lauwerys, M. Roberfroied, Eds.), pp. 569-574. Elsevier/ North Holland Biomedical Press.

Metal Ions in Biology and Medicine; vol 6. Eds. J.A. Centeno, Ph. Collery, G. Vernet, R.B. Finkelman, H. Gibb, J.C. Etienne. John Libbey Eurotext, Paris © 2000, pp. 786-788.

The effect of heavy metal-binding metallothionein on Zn, Cu and Cd accumulation in rat kidney

Shigeru Saito[1], Masaaki Kurasaki[3], Masashi Okabe[2], and Katsumi Yoshida[1]

[1] *Dept. of Preventive Medicine, St. Marianna University School of Medicine, Kanagawa 216-8511, Japan;* [2] *Dept. of Public Health and Environmental Medicine, The Jikei University School of Medicine, Tokyo 10-8461, Japan;* [3] *Dept. of Environmental Medicine and Informatics, Graduate School of Environmental Earth Science, Hokkaido University, Sapporo 060-0810, Japan*

Introduction

Metallothionein (MT) is characterized by a low molecular weight (6500-7000 Da), a high affinity for heavy metals such as Zn, Cd and Cu, a high cysteine content and a lack of aromatic amino acids [1]. A remarkable feature of all MT is its inducibility by several heavy metals such as Zn, Cd and Cu, hormones, cytotoxic agents, various physiological conditions associated with physical or chemical stresses and X-ray irradiation [1]. They are believed to be involved in the homeostasis of the cellular concentrations of essential heavy metals such as Zn and Cu, and in the detoxification of heavy metals such as Cd [2]. However the renal or hepatic heavy metal metabolism has not been investigated in detail. In order to understand the roles of MT on heavy metal accumulation in renal cytosol of rats, the relative Zn, Cd and Cu-binding capacities of heavy metal-induced MT (the ratio of heavy metal content in MT to heavy metal increment in renal cytosol) after Zn, Cd and Cu injection were determined by a dose-response and time-course studies.

Materials and Methods

Animal. Fifty-four male Sprague-Dawley rats, weighing 125-150 g were divided into 18 groups of 3 rats were housed at a constant temperature of 21.5 ± 1.5°C on a 12-hr light/12-hr dark cycle for two weeks prior to starting the experiments. In a dose-response study, $ZnSO_4$, $CuSO_4$ and $CdCl_2$ were dissolved in saline solution to obtain 1, 5, 10 or 20 mg Zn/kg, 2, 4 or 6 mg Cu/kg and 1 , 2 or 3 mg Cd/kg, respectively. Zn (20 mg/kg), Cu (6 mg/kg) and Cd (3 mg/kg) were maximum tolerated doses. Each rat was injected with a single intraperitoneal injection of saline or heavy metal doses and killed 14 hr after injection by anesthesia with diethyl ether. In a time-course study, $ZnSO_4$, $CuSO_4$ and $CdCl_2$ were dissolved in saline solution to obtain 10 mg Zn/kg, 4 mg Cu/kg and 2 mg Cd/kg, respectively. Each rat was injected with a single intraperitoneal dose of heavy metals and killed 7, 14 and 21 hr after injection. The control rat group was untreated.

Heavy metal contents in kidney. To analyse the heavy metal contents in kidney, 0.5 g of both right and left kidneys (1.8-2.3 g) were minced before sampling to assure the homogeneity.

The tissue was digested with mixed acids (1 ml conc. H_2SO_4, 5 ml conc. $HClO_4$ and 10 ml conc. HNO_3) as reported previously [3]. The contents of Zn and Cu were measured with a Hitachi Flame Atomic Absorption Spectrophotometer, and the Cd content was assayed using a computer-controlled sequential Inductively Coupled Plasma Mass Spectrometer.

Heavy metal contents in MT. One gram of both right and left kidneys was minced before sampling to assure the homogeneity, cut into pieces and homogenized (5:1=v:w) in ice-cold 50 mM Tris/HCl, pH 8.1, with a polytron three times for 30 seconds intervals. The homogenate was centrifuged at 10,000 x g for 30 min at 4°C with a Kubota centrifuge, model KR/200B. The supernatant was centrifuged at 110,000 x g for 60 min at 4°C using a Hitachi ultracentrifuge. An aliquot (3 ml) of the cytosol was applied to a Sephadex G-75 column (1.0 x 100 cm) equilibrated with 10 mM Tris/HCl, pH 8.1, and eluted with the same buffer at 4°C. The eluent was collected in 1.5 ml fractions and assayed for Zn, Cu and Cd concentrations with a Hitachi Flame Atomic Absorption Spectrophotometer, model 180-30. Heavy metal contents in MT were calculated from an elution volume of 51-69 ml (Kd = 0.55) corresponding to metallothionein fraction [3, 4].

Statistics. The data with 95% confidence interval from the comparison of two regression slopes were statistically analysed using the Statview II program on a Macintosh computer. If 95% confidence intervals did not overlap, the difference between the values was considered significant at $P<0.05$. The data were also compared by an unpaired student's t-test. A probability value of $P<0.05$ was accepted as significant.

Results and Discussion

This investigation studied the roles of MT on Zn, Cu and Cd accumulation in rat kidney after injection of the heavy metals. The Zn, Cu and Cd contents of the cytosol and kidney increased following increasing doses of Zn, Cu and Cd, respectively. In kidneys, approx. 65% of the Zn content, 60% of the Cu content and 65% of the Cd content in kidneys were detected in the cytosol after Zn, Cu and Cd injection, respectively [5]. Zn, Cu and Cd contents in the kidney increased during the period after Zn, Cu and Cd injection. In the kidneys approx. 65% of the Zn content, 65% of the Cu content and 65% of the Cd content were detected in the cytosol after Zn, Cu and Cd injection, respectively. From the elution profiles of sephadex G-75 column, the amounts of the Zn and Cu increments were attributable to the MT and high molecular weight protein fraction, while most of the Cd increment was attributable to the MT fraction [5]. The results in the dose-response study were similar to those in the time-course study.

In the dose-response study, the relationships between the Zn, Cu or Cd contents in the cytosol and the MT were examined in the kidneys (table 1). There were close relationships between heavy metal contents in the cytosol and metallothionein of all heavy metal-injected rats. Each significant correlation was observed between the Zn, Cu or Cd contents in the cytosol and MT. The slopes of regression lines of Zn, Cu and Cd (Zn; $Y= 0.45X-8.08$, Cu; $Y=0.43X-0.24$ and Cd; $Y=0.84X+0.05$) were determined to be Zn; 0.45, Cu; 0.43 and Cd; 0.84. These data demonstrated that 45 and 43% of the Zn and Cu increments in the renal cytosol after Zn and Cu injection were bound to MT, respectively. These values were lower than those reported for the hepatic cytosol in the dose-response study by Zn and Cu injection [6]. On the other hand, 84% of the Cd increment in renal cytosol after Cd injection was bound to MT. This value was similar to that reported for the hepatic cytosol in the dose-response study by Cd injection [6]. In the dose-

Table 1.

Comparison of regression line parameters (intercept, slope with 95 % of confidences intervals; 95 % C.I., correlation coefficient; r and P value for r) between Zn, Cu and Cd-injected groups.

Group	intercept	slope (95% C.I.)	correlation coefficient (r)	P value for r
(I) Dose-response study				
Zn	-8.08	0.45 (0.39-0.50)*	r = 0.980	P<0.001
Cu	-0.24	0.43 (0.39-0.48)*	r = 0.988	P<0.001
Cd	0.05	0.84 (0.82-0.86)	r = 0.999	P<0.001
(II) Time-course study				
Zn	-7.33	0.46 (0.40-0.51)*	r = 0.980	P<0.001
Cu	0.06	0.39 (0.37-0.40)*	r = 0.988	P<0.001
Cd	0.05	0.86 (0.80-0.93)	r = 0.999	P<0.001

Significantly different from Cd-injected group; *P<0.05.

response and time-course studies there was no significant difference
between the slopes of Zn and Cu, while a significant difference was observed between the slopes of Zn and Cd (P<0.05). We observed that these results in the time-course study were a good agreement with those in the dose-response study. Our results suggest that the role of MT in Zn or Cu accumulation in the kidney of Zn or Cu-injected rat is different from that of MT in Cd accumulation in the kidney of Cd-injected rat. In conclusion, the present results suggest that approx. 45, 40 and 85% of the Zn, Cu and Cd increments in the renal cytosol after Zn, Cu and Cd injection are bound to Zn, Cu and Cd-induced MT, respectively. An order of the relative heavy metal-binding capacities of Zn, Cu and Cd-induced MT in vivo was determined to be Cd > Zn ≅ Cu in kidney [5].

References

[1] Kägi JHR Evolution, structure and chemical activity of class I metallothioneins. An overview. In : Eds. Suzuki KT, Imura N, & Kimura M. *Metallothionein III*, Birkhäuser Verlag Basel/Switzerland, 1993 : 29-55.

[2] Kojima Y, Kägi JHR. Metallothionein. *Trends Biochem Sci* 1978 ; 3 : 90-93.

[3] Saito S, Okabe M, Kurasaki M. Localization of renal Cu-binding metallothionein induced by Au injection into rats. *Biochim Biophys Acta* 1997 ; 1335 : 353-58.

[4] Saito S, Hunziker PE; Differential sensitivity of metallothionein-1 and –2 in liver of zinc-injected rat toward proteolysis. *Biochim Biophys Acta* 1996 ; 1289 : 65-70.

[5] Saito S, Okabe M, Yoshida K, Kurasaki M. The effect of heavy metal-induced metallothionein on Zn, Cu and Cd accumulation in rat kidney. *Pharmacol Toxicol* 1999 ; 84 : 255-60.

[6] Saito S, Kojima Y. Differential role of metallothionein on Zn, Cd and Cu accumulation in hepatic cytosol of rats. *Cell Mol Life Sci* 1997; 53 : 267-70.

Metal Ions in Biology and Medicine; vol 6. Eds. J.A. Centeno, Ph. Collery, G. Vernet, R.B. Finkelman, H. Gibb, J.C. Etienne. John Libbey Eurotext, Paris © 2000, pp. 789-790.

The DNA catalysis of a carnosine-based reaction and the inhibitory effect of Ni(II)

Bijan Farzami[1], Ali Shamsaie[1], Hasan Farsam[2] and Zahra Bathaee[3]

[1] Department of Biochemistry, Tehran Medical Sciences University, P.O. Box 14155-5399, Tehran, Iran; [2] Department of Pharmaceutical Chemistry, Faculty of Pharmacy, Tehran Medical Sciences University, Tehran, Iran; [3] The Institute of Biochemistry and Biophysics, Tehran University, Tehran, Iran.

Abstract:
A highly sensitive fluorometric method using the fluorescence indicator dichlorofluorescein(DCF) was employed to study the interaction between DNA, Carnosine and Nickel(II).In our experiments, DNA posed a unique enzyme-like catalytic function in the oxidative conversion of nonfluorescent dichlorofluoroscin(LDCF) to the fluorescent DCF. Nickel induced an strong inhibition in the reaction which could be ascribed to the formation of a triad complex between DNA, Carnosine and Ni(II).

Introduction:
The activation and oxidation of diacetyldichlorofluorescin(LDADCF) to nonfluorescent dichlorofluorescin(LDCF) and to fluorescent dichlorofluorescein has been used to detect ultramicro quantities of hydroperoxides[1-3]. We employed this method to study the interaction between DNA, nickel and Carnosine, an endogenous dipeptide (β-alanyl-L-histidine) with antioxidant and free-radical scavenging roles[4].

Material and Methods:
2′,7′- dichlorofluorescin diacetate(LDADCF) and Carnosine were from Sigma Chemical Company. Hydrogen peroxide, Hematin and nickel chloride were from Merck (Germany) .
DNA was solvent-extracted and purified from calf thymus.

Preparation of dichlorofluorescin:
Stock solution of LDADCF (1mM) was made in ethanol and stored in the dark. LDADCF is stable for month under this condition. Activation of LDADCF to LDCF for assay required dilution : 1 vol of the ethanol Solution with 4 volume of 0.01 N Sodium hydroxide. The mixture was allowed to stand at room temperature for 30 minute. LDCF has a high rate of autoxidation , so it is required to be freshly prepared and discarded after use each day.

Preparation of hematin solution:
The hematin solution (0.01 mg/ml) was prepared by dissolving 1mg of hematin in 0.5 ml of 0.2 N NaOH and then diluted to 100 ml with 50 mM Tris-HCl buffer, pH=7.5 . This solution was made fresh each day. Hematin was used to accelerate the reaction.

Assay condition:
100 ml of Tris-HCl buffer (pH=7.5) was mixed with 14 ml of hematin solution and boiled or 15 minute. While Purging with nitrogen, this solution was cooled on ice. To prepare the Medium for our reactions, a 2.7 ml volume of this solution was mixed with 200 μL of activated dichlorofluorescin (4×10^{-5} M) and 100 μL Hydrogen peroxide (9×10^{-6} M). Ultimately, the needed amounts of reactants (DNA, carnosine and Ni) was added. Then the mixture was incubated under a nitrogen atomosphere in a sealed vial at 50°C for 45 minute. The reaction was cooled to the room temperature and the relative fluorescence determined using a spectrofluorophotometer (Shimadzu) with a 4 ml fluorescence cell. The excitation and emission wave lengths were 500 and 520 nm, respectively, both with 2-nm band width. [1-3]

Results and Discussion:
In our experiments, the simultaneous use of DNA and carnosine in the above mentioned reaction condition produced enhancement in the rate of oxidation of LDCF to DCF (depicted in fig.1 by an increase in the relative fluorescence). It could indicate the catalytic role of DNA in some energy-transfer reaction between carnosine and other components of the cell in a similar fashion as DCF in

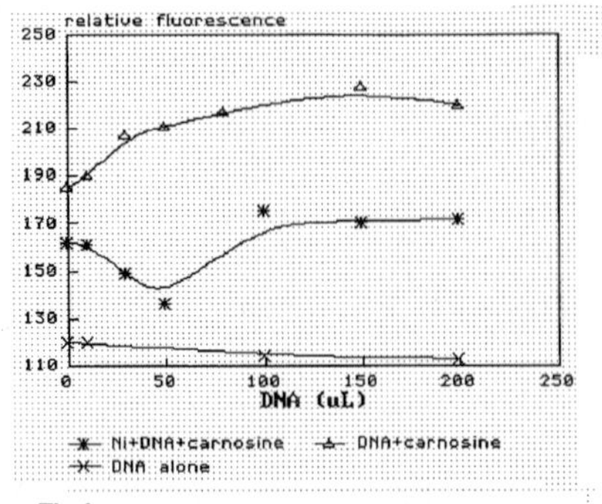

Fig.1- The trend of inhibition by Ni(II) in DNA activated carnosine reaction

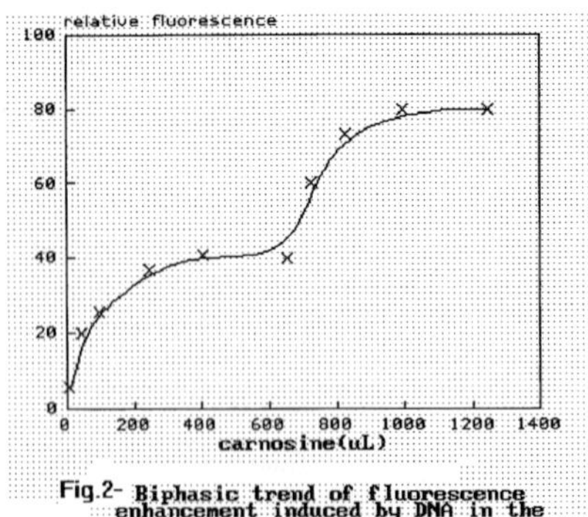

Fig.2- Biphasic trend of fluorescence enhancement induced by DNA in the carnosine-DCF reaction

our reaction. The combined effect of DNA-carnosine complex produced a biphasic saturation trend (fig.2) which was similar to Michaelis-Menton's saturation curve and could be treated likewise.Two V_m's were obtained : V_m1= 45 pico mole/min. and V_m2= 75 pico mole/min., with K_m1 value of 9 μM and K_m2 value of 79 μM. The use of $NiCl_2$ induced strong inhibition in the rate of DNA-carnosine catalysis which was specific in that, it was not effective in systems where DNA or carnosine alone were under study (fig.1) . This effect could be assigned to the formation of a trimolecular complex between carnosine, Ni and DNA that could inhibit the energy transfer action of DNA-carnosine complex.

Further study should be undertaken to elucidate the exact molecular mechanism of DNA catalysis and the inhibiting role of Ni.

References:

1-Sanches Ferrer A et al, Fluorescence detection of enzymatically formed hydrogen peroxide in aqueous solution and in reversed micelles, Analytical Biochemistry, 1990, 187, 129-132

2- Cathcart R, Schwiers E, Ames B N, Detection of picomole levels of hydroperoxides using a fluorescent dichlorofluorescein assay, Analytical Biochemistry, 1983, 134, 111-116

3- Keston A S, Brandt R, The fluorometric analysis of ultramicroquantities of hydrogen peroxide, Analytical Biochemisty, 1965, 11, 1-5

4- Hipkiss A R, Carnosine, a protective, anti-aging peptide?, The International Journal of Biochemistry & Cell Biology, 1998, 30, 863-868

Acknowledgement:

2′,7′- dichlorofluorescin diacetate(LDADCF) was kindly donated by Prof. Philippe Collery. Thanks to Prof. Moosavi's Lab collaborations during our studies.

Metal Ions in Biology and Medicine; vol 6. Eds. J.A. Centeno, Ph. Collery, G. Vernet, R.B. Finkelman, H. Gibb, J.C. Etienne. John Libbey Eurotext, Paris © 2000, pp. 791-793.

Selenium intake in the traditional Cretan Mediterranean diet

M. Simonoff, C. Sergeant, R. Ortega, Ch. Hamon, G. Simonoff

Laboratoire de Chimie Nucléaire Analytique et Bioenvironnementale, CNRS UMS 5084, Le Haut Vigneau, B.P. 120, 33175 Gradignan cedex, France

Abstract

Diets consumed by Mediterranean populations and especially the Cretans are a subject of particular interest since the rate of chronic diseases is low and life expectancies are among the highest. Numerous recent studies have indicated possible roles for free radical mediated processes in human pathology with respect to the suppressive action of antioxidants such as Selenium, vitamins E, C, and carotenoids. Dietary habits of rural traditional Cretan families have been investigated in order to evaluate the food consumption of each kind of products and permit comparison with previous studies. Selenium has been measured by Neutron Activation Analysis and PIXE (Proton-Induced X-Ray Emission) in more than 200 samples corresponding to an intake of 75 µg per day.

Introduction

Dietary factors have been implicated in the cause and prevention of important diseases including cancer, coronary heart disease and cataracts, as shown in many recent studies. Diets consumed by Mediterranean populations have been a subject of special interest, since in certain regions bordering the Mediterranean Sea the rates of chronic diseases are among the lowest in the world and life expectancies are among the highest [1-2-3-4].This situation is particularly apparent in the Greek Island of Crete. The diet of Cretans for centuries is characterised by high intakes of olive oil, vegetables and fruits, limited quantities of meat and eggs.

Possible roles for free radical - mediated processes in human pathology are suspected. This has led to a considerable interest in the substances thought to prevent the deleterious effects of these substances in vivo, namely the antioxidants. Moreover, the extent of fat intake is important for the consequences on membrane composition and peroxidation processes. The biochemistry of free radical reactions, the manner in which they damage cells and the nature of the antioxidant inhibiting effect on these reactions with cellular constituents have been the subject of a number of recent reviews [5]. Some of the antioxidants are micronutriments derived directly from the diet (vitamins E, C, and carotenoids); others, such as trace elements, are essential components of antioxidant enzymes. These include Selenium for glutathione peroxidase, Cu, Zn, Mn for superoxide dismutase, and Fe for the activity of catalase.

To obtain more information about the traditional Cretan diet and especially Selenium intake, we measured the selenium content of more than two hundred food samples collected in several markets and rural areas of Crete and calculations were carried out on the average Selenium intake in the traditional Cretan diet on the basis of the household food consumption of families living in small rural villages.

Materials and Methods

Selenium was measured by nuclear activation analysis (NAA) in Berlin (Hahn-Meitner Institute) and Proton-Induced X-Ray Emission, (Van de Graaff Accelerator,

Centre d'Etudes Nucléaires in Bordeaux) after digestion and preliminary chemical concentration using ^{75}Se for yield determination [6-7-8].

Dietary habits of families living in different rural areas of the Island and claiming to have persisted in their ancestral nutritional traditions have been investigated in two ways:

- the help of a semi-quantitative food-frequency questionnaire
- the total consumption of the families for one year based on private production.

Results and Discussion

An average consumption per year was determined for 28 vegetables, 16 fruits, 5 pulses, 7 dried fruits, and 12 varieties of meat and fish. The following table summarizes the daily food intake of the most frequently consumed foods, expressed in grams per day.

Food	Our results Crete	Greece (*) Crete	Greece (*) Corfu	Yugoslavia (*) Dalmatia	Greece (**) Elderly people
Bread	370	380	450	435	260
Rice	27	30	15	64	
Vegetables	463	191	191	200	267
Potatoes	142	190	150	214	64
Pulse	43	30	30	7	56
Fruits	304	464	462	6	238
Meat, Chicken	22	35	35	117	100
Mutton, Goat	38				
Fish	25	18	60	96	38
Eggs	22	25	5	31	12
Feta	112	248	84	438	222
Cretan yogurt	79				
Dried fruits	49				
Honey	21				
Olive oil	99	95	75	88	46
Wine	104				106
Total	1920	1706	1557	1696	1408

(*) Ref. 2 and 9 - (**) Ref. 10

Table : Food intake in grams per day

The traditional Mediterranean diet is rich in vegetables and fresh fruits, bread, potatoes, olive oil, feta, Cretan yogurt, pulses and dried fruits. Our results for food consumption are in good agreement with previous studies such as the Seven Countries Study [2-9] or, more recently, with reports concerning elderly Greeks [10]. During the last 30 years the traditional diet of Crete has undergone modification from the influence of new commercial trends, tourism and other nutritional habits, resulting in an increase in the consumption of meat, sweets, and ice cream, and a decrease in the use of olive oil, frequently replaced by satured fats.

Our estimate indicated a daily Selenium intake of 75 µg. The 1989 Recommended Dietary Allowances for Selenium is 70 and 55 µg for adult men and women respectively [11].

Our results indicate that the daily intake of Selenium from the traditional Cretan diet is one of the highest in Europe. In comparison, values for other European countries are the following : Germany, 59 µg; England, 60 µg; Belgium, 47 µg [12]; northern Italy, 43 µg; France 47 µg [7-13]; Finland, 31 µg in 1980, followed by 55 µg subsequent to importation of wheat [14]. It appears probable that Selenium effectively provides specific antioxidant protection even though the high proportion of fresh plants, fruits, cereals and olive oil guarantees a high intake of caroten, vitamin C, tocopherols and other substances such as polyphenols and anthocyanins that may be beneficial. All these antioxidant factors, as well as the content of the different fatty acids (saturated and unsaturated) have been calculated or measured in the present work.

Acknowledgments

We are grateful to the Greek Embassy, Monasteries, Pépinières Christian Deschamps, Drs Matthaiadis and Tsaoussidos for providing support, cooperation and local technical assistance. We thank particularly Dr. Gawlik, Pr. Brätter and EU Program HMC and PECO for access facilities to NAA in HMI in Berlin.

References

[1] - World Health Organization. World health statistics annual, 1993, Geneva WHO

[2] - Keys A, ed. Coronary heart disease in seven countries. *Circulation* 1970 ;41 (suppl 1) : 1-211

[3] - World Bank. World development report : investment in health. Washington, DC : World Bank, 1993

[4] - WHO, FAO. Food and health indicators in Europe : nutrition and health, 1961-1990 (computer program). Copenhagen : World Health Organization Regional Office for Europe, 1993

[5] - B. Halliwell and J.M.C. Gutteridge 1989 : *Free radicals in Biology and Medicine 2nd ed. Oxford : Clarendon.*

[6] - Simonoff M, Hamon C, Moretto P, Llabador Y, Simonoff G (1988). High sensitivity PIXE determination of selenium in food and biological samples using a preconcentration technique. *Nucl. Instr. and Meth.* B31 : 442-448

[7] - Simonoff M, Moretto P, Llabador Y, Simonoff G. (1988) : Selenium in food and nutrition in France. Trace Element - *Analytical Chemistry in Medicine and Biology, Vol 4., Editors : P. Brätter, P. Schramel,* 1988. *Walter de Gruyter & Co., Berlin-New York - Printed in Germany*

[8] - Simonoff M, Sergeant C, Garnier N, Moretto P, Llabador Y, Simonoff G, Conri C. (1992) : Antioxidant status (Selenium, vitamins A and E) and aging. *Free Radical and Aging I. Emerit and B. Chance editors, Birkhauser Expererentia* Supp. 62 (1992) p. 368-397

[9] - Kromhout D, Keys A, Aravanis C, et al. Food consumption patterns in the 1960's in seven countries. *Am. J. Clin. Nutr.,* 1989; 49 : 889-894

[10] - Trichopoulou A, Kouris-Blazos A, Vassilakou T, et al. Diet and Survival of elderly Greeks : o link to the past. *Am. J. Clin. Nutr.* 1995 (suppl); 1346S-1350S

[11] - RDA Recommended Dietary Allowances 10th, ed. National Research Council Washington DC, 1989

[12] - Robberecht H, and Deelstra H.A. Dietary selenium intake in Belgium. *Z. Lebensm. Unters Forsch.,* 1984; 178 : 266-271

[13] - Simonoff M, Simonoff G. Le Sélénium et la vie. Masson, 1991 (245 pages)

[14] - Mutanen M. Dietary intake and sources of selenium in young Finnish women. *Human Nutrition : Applied Nutrition,* 1984; 38A : 265-269

Metal Ions in Biology and Medicine; vol 6. Eds. J.A. Centeno, Ph. Collery, G. Vernet, R.B. Finkelman, H. Gibb, J.C. Etienne. John Libbey Eurotext, Paris © 2000, pp. 794-796.

Reference ranges for trace elements in urine, erythrocytes, and hair by high-resolution inductively coupled plasma-mass spectrometry

F. Leung, P. Edmond, C. Bradley

Trace Elements Laboratory, London Health Sciences Centre, London, Ontario, Canada

INTRODUCTION

Inductively coupled plasma-mass spectrometry (ICP-MS) is becoming more often used for total elemental analysis for biological samples due to its high sensitivity, multielement measurements, isotope ratio capabilities, and as a detector for speciation of elements when coupled to a liquid chromatographic system [1]. These tests are becoming commercially available from several laboratories which apply quadrupole mass filter instruments (QICP-MS) due to its relatively lower cost and ease of operation. The main problem with QICP-MS is its limited mass resolution (power of m/Δm 300) which cannot resolve spectral interferences caused by atomic or molecular ions from biological samples of the same nominal mass as the analytes. With the development of high-resolution ICP-MS (HR-ICP-MS), mass resolution powers up to 10,000 are achieved using a double focusing, magnetic and electric sector field analyzer which can resolve most of the polyatomic interferences [2]. We compared panels of trace elements from human erythrocytes, urine and hair specimens using HR-ICP-MS with reference data provided by four clinical laboratories which used QICP-MS.

SUBJECTS AND METHODS

Healthy adults (n=104, age 25 to 54 yrs) with no known diseases from an urban college and hospital laboratory volunteered to provide samples of blood (n=48), hair (n=56) and urine (n=45) for mineral and trace element analysis. We applied a HR-ICP-MS instrument, the ELEMENT (Finnigan MAT, Bremen, Germany) at three resolution modes of low (m/Δm 300), medium (m/Δm 3,000) and high (m/Δm 10,000). Urine samples were diluted 10 fold with 1% nitric acid in type 1 (Milli-Q) water before analysis. Erythrocytes were separated from whole blood collected in Vacutainer tubes (heparin, navy-top, Becton Dickinson). Prior to analysis, an aliquot of erythrocyte (0.4 mL) was digested with equal amounts of concentrated nitric acid: hydrogen peroxide, and then diluted 20-fold with Milli-Q water. Hair was washed with 0.1% triton X, rinsed x3 with Milli-Q water, dried in an oven at 70°C for 30 min., and digested with concentrated nitric acid for 1 h. It is diluted 10-fold with Milli-Q water before analysis by HR-ICP-MS.

RESULTS AND DISCUSSION

Many factors such as the lifestyles of the population studied, dietary intake, environmental exposure, geographical region of a country, methodology, and instrumentation used for the testing can contribute to the reference values established for an analyte from any laboratory. Table 1 lists the results for 15 trace elements measured for erythrocytes. These were compared to other reference values from clinical laboratories which measured erythrocyte and whole blood. Erythrocyte antimony is 3 to 65-fold lower, arsenic is approximately 10-fold lower, chromium is 20 to 900-fold lower, thallium is 12-fold lower, and vanadium is significantly lower when compared by HR-ICP-MS to other reference laboratories using QICP-MS for erythrocytes. Nickel values in serum and whole blood are reported to range from <0.05-1.08 [3], and are similar to the present erythrocyte values. They are significantly lower than two other reported clinical whole blood values.

Urine samples, 24 h were analyzed for 26 elements, and those with marked lower values are listed in Table 2. The use of HR-ICP-MS for the analysis of urine elements showed results for chromium of up to 187-fold, iron of up to 100-fold, manganese of up to 75-fold, uranium of up to 200-fold, and vanadium of up to 1750-fold lower when compared to four other clinical laboratory reference values. The higher values used by these laboratories may reflect the lack of resolution for these elements when determined by QICP-MS.

With hair analysis, the matrix effect is smaller which results in a better correlation between many of the 38 elements analyzed, but there are still several elements listed in Table 3 which are markedly higher, probably due to spectral interferences which cannot be corrected at low resolution.

CONCLUSIONS

A number of mineral and trace element reference values determined by HR-ICP-MS on human erythrocytes, urine and hair samples were markedly lower when compared to QICP-MS results. This indicates that for these elements, the high resolution system is capable of resolving many of the interferences encountered at low resolution. There was also a wide variability of reference ranges for these elements among the assessed clinical laboratories. One must be alert to such differences in values, and need to interpret the findings with caution as they may have limited clinical relevance.

REFERENCES

1. Bayon MM, Cabezuelo ABS, Gonzalez EB, Alonso JIG, Sanz-Medel A. Capabilities of fast protein liquid chromatography coupled to a double focusing inductively coupled plasma mass spectrometer for trace metal speciation in human serum. *J Anal At Spectrom* 1999;14:947-951
2. Marchante-Gayon JM, Muniz CS, Alonso JIG, Sanz-Medel A. Multielemental trace analysis of biological materials using double focusing inductively coupled plasma mass spectrometry detection. *Anal Chim Acta* 1999;400:307-20
3. Sunderman, Jr. FW. Nickel In: Werner M. ed. *CRC Handbook of Clinical Chemistry*, IV, CRC Press, Inc., Boca Raton, Florida, 1989, 261-4

Table 1. Erythrocyte and Whole Blood* Elements in μg/L (unless specified)

ELEMENT	HR-ICP-MS	LAB. A	LAB. B	LAB. C	LAB. D
Antimony	0-0.2	0-13	0-1000*	0-0.6	0-3*
Arsenic	0-1.46	0-14	0-2000*	na	0-52*
Cadmium	0-3.3	0-9	0-10*	0-1.9	0-12*
Chromium	0.08-3.0	30-60	700-2700	na	12-213*
Copper	550-930	635-890	500-2000	590-960	552-1410*
Manganese	15-40	15-39	100-400	15-48	11-53*
Mercury	0-5	0-10	0-50*	0-4	0-5*
Molybdenum	0.43-1.3	na	30-300	0.6-1.8	1-52*
Nickel	0.1-1.8	na	0-100*	na	0-22*
Selenium	200-400	225-375	400-2000	230-420	42-514*
Thallium	0-0.08	na	0-15*	0-1.0	0-3.0*
Vanadium	0.05-0.21	35-80	2000-7000	19-39	0-154*
Zinc (mg/L)	11.5-16.4	9.5-14.5	10-40	8.5-11.9	3.5-7.5*

*In whole blood, na = not available, Identities of Clinical Labs A-D are available from authors.
Laboratory A-D results are determined with a QICP-MS
Other elements [Lead 0-100, and Magnesium 38-66 mg/L] are comparable by HR-ICP-MS and by QICP-MS

Table 2. Urine Elements in μg/day (unless specified)

ELEMENT	HR-ICP-MS	LAB. A	LAB. B	LAB. C	LAB. D
Aluminum	0-25	0-60	0-50	0-52	0-96
Arsenic	0-60	216-456	0-1000	0-31	<75
Chromium	0.2-0.8	73.6-150	30-120	5-42	20-135
Cobalt	0.1-1.25	0-8	0-80	0.1-17	na
Copper	3.5-18	16-33.6	10-70	1-54	29-136
Iron	3-20	20.8-64	300-2000	na	na
Manganese	0.1-0.8	4-11.2	5-60	2.6-7	1-6.7
Selenium	30-130	na	350-1000	21-213	56-280
Silver	0-0.07	0-4	na	na	na
Tin	1-7	0-102	na	0-11	0-5.6
Uranium	0-0.015	na	na	0-3	0-1.6
Vanadium	0.02-0.20	8-27.2	50-350	1-17	na

na=not available

Other elements determined by HR-ICP-MS are similar to QICP-MS values as follows:
Boron 0.8-10 mg/d, Barium 0-5, Beryllium 0-2.9, Cadmium 0-2, Calcium 50-250 mg/d, Lead 0-4, Mercury 0-4, Magnesium 25-170 mg/d, Molybdenum 20-180, Nickel 0-5, Strontium 40-230, Sulphur 50-800 mg/d, Thallium 0-0.6 and Zinc 100-600.

Table 3. Hair Elements in μg/g (unless specified)

ELEMENT	HR-ICP-MS	LAB. A	LAB. B	LAB. C	LAB. D
Arsenic	0-0.15	0-0.15	0-5.0	0-1.1	0-0.05
Boron	0.4-3.4	0.80-2.8	0-100	0.01-4.0	0.55-1.6
Chromium	0.05-0.35	0.80-1.25	0.2-3.0	0.01-0.6	0.8-1.6
Iron	4.5-15	5-14	20-200	5.5-13.7	8-15
Lead	0-1.5	0-4.5	0-4	0-5	0-0.5
Manganese	0.08-0.5	0.3-0.75	0.2-4	0.07-1	0.12-0.2
Molybdenum	0.025-0.1	0.03-0.08	0-1.5	0.02-1	0.025-0.08
Nickel	0-0.35	0-0.7	0-5	0-1.1	0-0.35
Selenium	0.5-1.8	0.95-1.7	0-25	0.2-5.5	1.05-1.35
Vanadium	0.002-0.03	0.009-0.08	0.3-3	0.01-0.55	0.015-0.026

Elements which show similar results using either system include: Aluminum 0-8, Antimony 0-0.04, Barium 0-1.5, Beryllium 0-0.004, Bismuth 0-0.095, Cadmium 0-0.15, Calcium 400-1500, Cobalt 0.002-0.05, Copper 15-100, Iodine 0.1-1.2, Lithium 0.006-0.1, Magnesium 40-120, Mercury 0-1, Palladium 0-0.2, Phosphorus 125-200, Platinum 0-0.004, Potassium 5-60, Silicon 5-35, Silver 0-0.25, Sodium 5-65, Strontium 0.3-5.38, Sulphur 45-55 mg/g, Thallium 0–0.002, Thorium 0-0.004, Tin 0.05-0.4, Titanium 0-0.4, Uranium 0-0.08, Zinc 140-200

Metal Ions in Biology and Medicine; vol 6. Eds. J.A. Centeno, Ph. Collery, G. Vernet, R.B. Finkelman, H. Gibb, J.C. Etienne. John Libbey Eurotext, Paris © 2000, pp. 797-808.

The role of copper 3,5 diisopropyl salicylate on the growth of Ehrlich ascitis carcinoma

Nadia I. Zakhary[1]; Nagia Moharam[2]; Mostafa El-Kabany[3]; Camilia Adly[4]; Saad El-Guindy[1]; Mohamed S. Ahmed[1]; Mahmoud El-Merzabani[1]; Abdel Fatah Badawi[5] and Sarah Abdel Raouf.

[1] *Cancer Biology Department, NCI, Cairo University;* [2] *Zoology Department, Faculty of Science, Cairo University;* [3] *Pathology Department, NCI, Cairo University;* [4] *Chemistry Department, Faculty of Science, Damieta University;* [5] *Applied Organic Chemistry, Egyptian Petrolium Research Institute.*

ABSTRACT :

The present study was designed, aiming at highlighting the effect of copper II (3,5 diisopropyl salicylate)$_2$ (CuDIPS) on the growth of Ehrlich ascitis carcinoma cell line (EAC) in vitro, as well as its protective effect against the in-vivo damage caused by the later. The in vitro study was performed by inoculating different concentrations of (CuDIPS) with 2 x10^6 EAC. The (CuDIPS) affected, significantly the viability of EAC cells. The percentages of nonviable cells has been correlated with increasing concentrations of (CuDIPS) The in vivo studies revealed that, this compound could be safely used upto 250 mg/kg.b.w.. (CuDIPS) delayed the growth of solid tumour induced by subcutaneous inoculation of 2.5x10^6 EAC cells. For biochemical, histopathological and histochemical studies, 80 female Swiss albino mice, weighing 18-20 gm. each, were divided into the following four groups; 1) control group of untreated mice, 2) EAC group of mice that were intraperitoneally (i.p.) injected with 2.5x10^6 EAC cells, 3) (CuDIPS) group of mice that were i.p. injected with 25 mg/kg b.w. of (CuDIPS) day after day, for a period of one week and 4) EAC +(CuDIPS) group of mice that were i.p. inoculated with EAC and injected with (CuDIPS) using doses mentioned before. Biochemical analysis comprised the determination of glucose-6-phosphatase (G-6-Pase), adinosine triphosphatase (ATPase) and nucleic acids (DNA and RNA)), total protein as well as the levels of iron, calcium and magnesium. Histopathological changes were examined microscopically and correlated with histochemical features of the proliferative activity using argyrophilic stains for nucleolar organising regions (Ag NORs).

IN CONCLUSION: the present study revealed that CuDIPS had a negative influence on the growth of EAC cells, beside counteracting its biochemical damaging effects and proliferative activity.

INTRODUCTION :

Many drugs have been introduced in the field of anticancer agents. Although they were successfully used to control tumour growth, yet their side effects limited their use at their optimal doses. Previous studies were carried out to study the effect of organic and inorganic complexes in controling tumour growth (1,2,3,4,5). It was reported that copper complexes of nonsteroidal anti-inflammatory drugs had anticancer effects (6). Copper (II) (3,5-diisopropylsalicylate)$_2$ (Cu DIPS), is a low molecular weight lipophilic copper coordinator complex, that counteracts the superoxide action (7). It was experimentally found that CuDIPS possessed antitumour activities when subsequently adminstred into the site of Ehrlich solid tumour (8). It was observed that, there is a significant reduction of the tumour growth with an increase in survival rates as compared with the saline treated controls.

In addition to the conventional pathological parameters, several experimental techniques have been shown to provide biological information in several malignancies. Nuclear DNA contents have been considered as a useful index of estimating biological malignancy, because the proliferating potential of cancer cells is strongly associated with nuclear DNA (9). Moreover, nucleolar organizer regions (NORs) are DNA loops that code ribosomal RNA (rRNA). These NORs are closely related to production of ribosome and protein through transcription of rRNA and reflect the activity of the nucleolus and the whole cell. Argyrophilic NORs (AgNORs) stain is the way to depict, specifically, proteins binding to NORs and is associated with fission and proliferating activity of the cells (10).

The present study was designed aiming to inviestigate for the effect of CuDIPS on the growth of EAC, as well as its role in counteracting the damaging effects due to the later. This was carried out by a series of in vitro and in vivo studies.

MATERIAL AND METHODS:

I-In vitro study:

The effect of CuDIPS on the viability of EAC cells was studied according to the method of El-Merzabani et al .,(11)

II-In vivo studies:

A-Solid tumour: 30 female albino mice, wighing 18-20 g each, were used for this study. Ten were left untreated as controls. Twenty mice were s.c. injected in their right thigh with $2.5\text{x}\ 10^6$ EAC. The next day they were divided into two groups, each containing 10 mice. One group was s.c injected with 25 mg CuDIPS/kg at the same site of EAC inoculation for three times, day after day, and the other group was left without further treatment. The size of solid tumour was measured using Vermir caliper, starting from the ninth day-post EAC. And the tumour volume was calculated, according to the following equation(12);

Tumour volume (mm3)= $4/3\ \pi\ (A/2)^2\ (B/2)\ =0.52\ A^2B$; where A and B are the minor and major axis respectively.

Animals were sacrificed after 24 days and the solid tumours, whether treated or not with CuDIPS was homogenised in slaine (1:10 w/v) for biochemical investigations that included determination of DNA, RNA and total protein contents. Tissues from thighs of normal untreated mice, were subjected to the same biochemical analysis.

B-Ascitic tumour:

The LD 50 of CuDIPS was calculated. Eighty mice were divided into the following the groups:-

1-Control group, 2- EAC-bearing mice were in i.p. injected with $2.5\text{x}10^6$ EAC.
3- CuDIPS group: mice were i.p. with 25 mg CuDIPS/kg b.w.for three times day after day. and 4- EAC+ CuDIPS : mice were i.p injected with EAC and CuDIPS with the same doses mentioned before, the following parameters were investigated:-

1) Survival time. 2) Changes in body weight. 3) Biochemical studies. Liver was homogenized in saline (1:10w/v) and used for determination of: a) glucose-6-phosphatase activity (G-6-Pase), according to Swanson (13). b) adenosine triphosphatase (ATPase) activity, according to EL-Aaser and EL-Merzabani (14) . c) extraction of nucleic acids according to Melmed et al. (15) and determination of DNA and RNA content according to Dische and Schwartz (16) and Mejboum

(17), respectively. d) total protein content according to Lowry et al. (18). And, e) iron, calcium and magnesium levels using atomic absorption technique. 4) Histopathological examination for hepatic tissue sections stained with haematoxylin and eosin stains (19). 5) Histochemical profile for cell proliferation using sections stained with silver nitrate for AgNORs using the technique of Crocker and Nar (19).

RESULTS:

I. In vitro experiments: The effect of CuDIPS on the viability of EAC cells was studied and the results were expressed as percentages of non-viable cells (NVC). Increasing the concentration of CuDIPS in the EAC media was accompanied by an increase in the percent of NVC, (table 1and figure 1).

II. In vivo studies : A) Solid tumours:

1- Tumour volume (TV): Tumour volume of the group untreated with CuDIPS, progressively increase in size. However, treatment with 3 successive doses of CuDIPS resulted in a significant decrease in tumour volume, regardless the observation period (figure 2).

Table (2) represents a significant increase in the DNA and RNA, contents of the solid tomour. On the other hand, total protein was not significantly changed as compared to control tissue. Nevertheless, treatment of tumour bearing mice with CuDIPS resulted in significant decreases in DNA, RNA and total protein content as compared with untreated tumour, while non significant changes in DNA, RNA but a significant decrease in total protein content was observed when compared to control tissue.

B) Ascitic tumour

Figure (3), represents the effect of different treatments on the percent of changes in body weight of mice. The untreated EAC bearing mice showed progressive increase in the body weight reaching 100% on the 24th day. Treating EAC bearing mice with CuDIPS led to retardation in their growth. The percent of change in healthy control and CuDIPS were only 32.4% and 25.9%, respectively; at the 24th day.

Figure (4) represented the survival of mice under different treatments. All mice injected with CuDIPS alone, as well as healthy control mice lived for more than 60 days. None of the untreated EAC bearing mice survived more than 26 days post inoculation. However 50% of EAC + CuDIPS group survived for more than 26 days. 20% of them showed complete cure and survived for more than 60 days.

Table (3) reprents the G-6-phase activity in liver homogenates of mice under different treatments. Regarding the day 14 post inoculation, the G-6-phase activity was elevated in the EAC group but not in the CuDIPS and EAC + CuDIPS gourps as compared with the control group.

Table (4) represents the activity of Atpase groups under different treatment modalties showed significant decrease in ATPase activities as compared with the control group

Table (5) showed significant changes in DNA and significant changes were observed concerning the RNA and protein conternts in the CuDIPS and EAC+ CuDIPS groups as compared with control group.

Concentrations of Fe ,Ca and Mg are shown in table (6). No significant changes were observed concerning the Fe level between the control, CuDIPS and EAC + CuDIPS gruops. Nevertheless, it was significantly elevated in the EAC group. Calcium was also significantly elevated in EAC group as compared with other three groups. Magnesium was elevated in CuDIPS and EAC + CuDIPS groups.

Histopathological findings were parallel to biochemical results. It was found that livers of control untreated group showed normal hepatic architecture with cords of normal hepatocytes. The hepatocytesarranged around central venule and entangled thin walled sinusoids with occasional seen Kupfer cells. This picture was consistent with all control groups among different time schedules. Silver stain for AgNORs revealed an average scores of 1.78 ± 0.23, 2.22 ± 0.17, 2.17 ± 0.22 and 1.92 ± 0.29 among the different control groups of 3,7,10 and 14 days respectively (Fig. 5 a1&a2). On the other hand, mice inoculated with EAC cells showed hepatocytes with moderate cytoplasmic fatty changes and the nuclei exhibited mild pleomorphism with occasional binicleation and prominent nucleoli. Kupfer cells were prominet and hyperplastic. AgNORs scores displayed a significant increase that showed 3.83 ± 0.38, 6.77 ± 1.08, 5.44 ± 0.34 and 6.22 ± 0.92 on different groups among different time intervals (Fig.5 b1&b2). Mice treated with 25 mg/kg b.w. Cu DIPs only displayed rather normal archeticture without evidence of cytoplasmic degeneration or nuclear hyperactivity. Unremarkable, slight kupfer cell hyperplasia was noticed in groups received prolonged treatment. Moreover, Ag NORs scors were near to the control untreated group and recorded 2.6 ± 0.24, 2.77 ± 0.18, 2.22 ± 0.12 and 2.30 ± 0.40 on different time intervals (Fig 5 c1&c2). It was found that when EAC-bearing mice treated with Cu Ips, liver tissue exhibited more or less normal architecture without cytoplasmic degeneration or nuclear activity. Having said that, Kupfer cells were slightly prominent along the hepatic sinusoids. AgNORs scors retained to levels nearer to that of CuDIPs group than to that of EAC group. It was senn that the scores were; 3.26 ± 0.331, 4.81 ± 0.43, 3.65 ± 0.34 and 3.59 ± 0.56 on the different time intervals (Fig. 5 c1&c2). Table (7) represents the results of AgNORs obtained in different groups under the study. It is werth while to mention that all AgNORs scores were closely related and showed a direct correlation with RNA nuclear content determined biochemically, table (5).

Table (1) Effect of CuDIPS on the viability of EAC.

Concentration	CuDIPS $\bar{X}$±SD
0	0
0.8	7.3± 1.4 (6-9)
1.6	13.8± 1.9 (12-17)
3.2	23.2 ±2.2 (20-26)
6.3	31.5± 1.6 (29-33)
12.5	37.0± 1.8 (34-39)
25.0	45.4± 2.1 (43 - 48)
50.0	56.3± 2.2 (53-59)
100.0	61.8± 1.5 (60-64)

Groups sharing same letter are not significantly different.
Results are expressed as percent of non-viable cells.
Results are a mean ± SD of 6 experiments
( ) results are expressed as range.

Figure (5): a-1) section from liver tissue of control healthy untreated group showing normal hepatic architicture with cords of normal hepatocytes around central venule. A-2) Argyrophilic stain for NORs of central group displaying hepatocytes with average scores of 1.83 (⇑) per nucleus. B-1 liver from mice inoculated with EAC cells showing hepatocytes with moderate degree of degeneration and active nuclei. B-2) Silver stain for NORs of same group exihipting AgNORs scores about 3.83 (⇑) per nucleus. C-1) liver from mice only received CuDIPS showing rather normal architcture. C-2) silver stain displayed AgNORs scores of 2.6 (⇑) per nucleus. D-1) liver from EAC bearing mice that treated with CuDIPS showing a considerable recovery without cytoplasmic degeneration a nuclear activity. D-2) silver stain for AgNORs displaying decreasing AgNORs scores of 3.26 (⇑) per nucleus. a,b,c,d = hematoxylin and eosin of original magnification x 200.a2,b2,c2,d2= silver stain for AgNORs of original magnification x 1000.

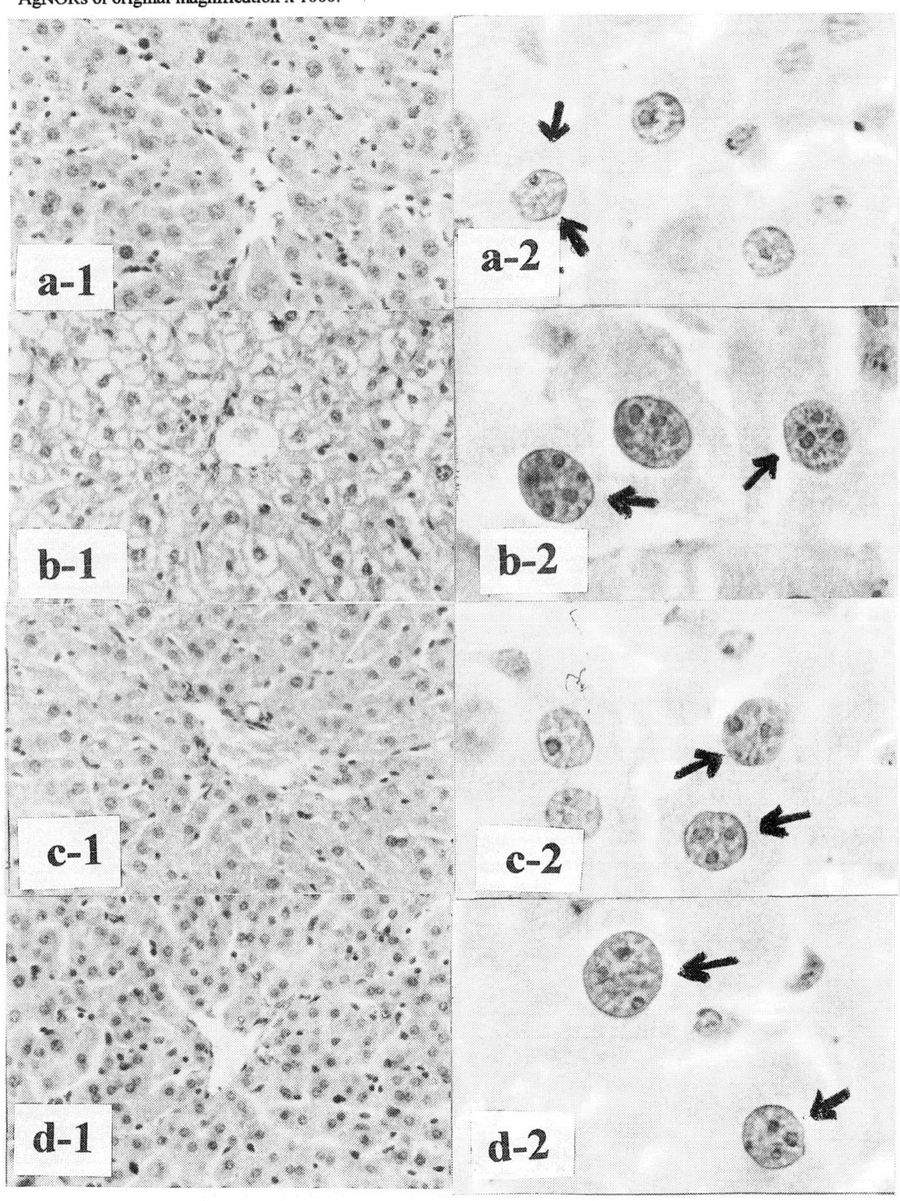

Fig. (1) Effect of CuDIPS on the viability of EAC.

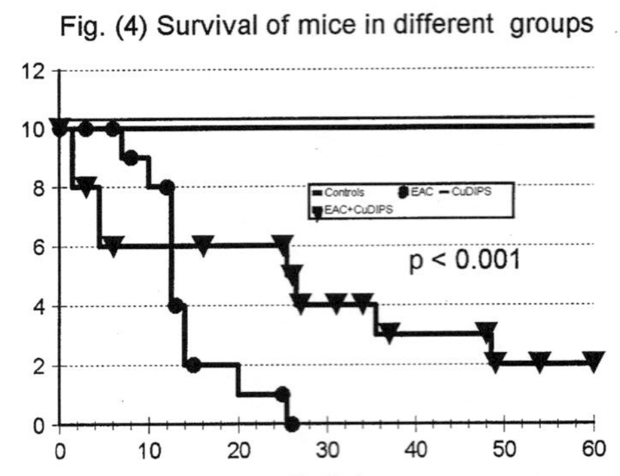

Fig. (2) Volume of solid tumor of Ehrlich treated or not with CuDIPS

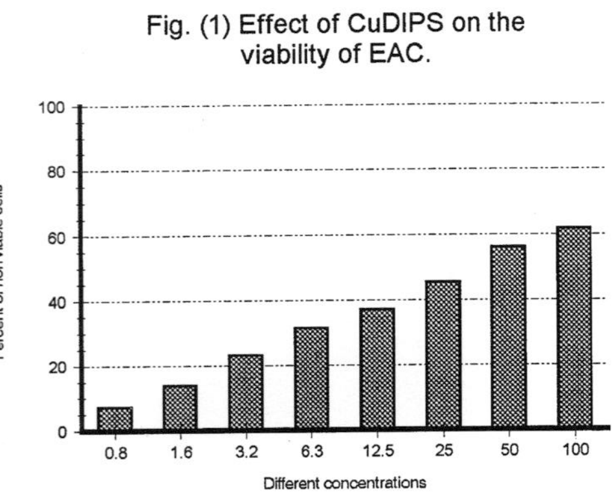

Fig. (3) Percent of change in body weight of mice under different treatments.

Results are represented as percent of change in body weight taking the starting day as zero percent.

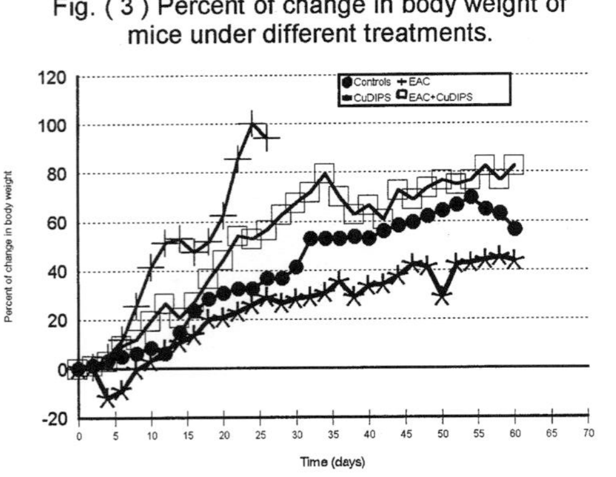

Fig. (4) Survival of mice in different groups

Table (2) DNA, RNA and total protein contents in solid tumour of different groups of mice under investigations.

	Control $\bar{X}$±SD	EST $\bar{X}$±SD	EST+CuDIPS $\bar{X}$±SD	*P - value
DNA	3.44±0.24	3.78±0.25	3.29±0.24	0.002
	(100)	(109.9)	(95.6)	
	(b)	(a)	(b)	
RNA	4.64±0.29	5.39±0.24	4.86±0.27	< 0.001
	(100)	(116.2)	(104.7)	
	(b)	(a)	(b)	
Total protein	83.25±2.87	79.13±3.48	71.13±3.14	< 0.001
	(100)	(95.1)	(85.4)	
	(a)	(a)	(b)	

* p value is significant ≤ 0.05
Groups sharing same letter are not significantly different
Results are expressed as mg / gm wet tissue.
Ten mice are used in each group.
( ) : Results are expressed as percent taking control as 100 percent.

Table (3) Glucose -6 - phosphatase activity level in liver of different groups of mice under investigations measured at different time intervals.

Time (days)	Controls $\bar{X}$±SD	EAC $\bar{X}$±SD	CuDIPS $\bar{X}$±SD	EAC+CuDIPS $\bar{X}$±SD	*P - value
3	3.45±0.31	4.34±0.44	3.78±0.30	4.10±0.42	< 0.001
	(100)	(125.8)	(109.6)	(118.8)	
	(c)	(a)	(bc)	(ab)	
7	3.45±0.37	4.43±0.19	3.67±0.24	4.10±0.15	< 0.001
	(100)	(128.4)	(106.4)	(118.1)	
	(b)	(a)	(b)	(a)	
10	3.36±0.26	4.50±1.07	3.72±0.14	4.13±0.03	< 0.001
	(100)	(133.9)	(110.7)	(122.9)	
	(d)	(a)	(c)	(b)	
14	3.23±0.15	4.48±0.41	3.40±0.19	3.86±0.50	< 0.001
	(100)	(138.7)	(105.3)	(119.5)	
	(c)	(a)	(c)	(b)	

Results are expressed (IU).
Legend as table (2)

Table (4) ATPase activity level in liver of different groups of mice under investigations measured at different time intervals.

Time (days)	Controls $\bar{X}$±SD	EAC $\bar{X}$±SD	CuDIPS $\bar{X}$±SD	EAC+CuDIPS $\bar{X}$±SD	*P - value
3	12.21±0.76	9.42±0.74	11.20±0.90	10.30±0.86	< 0.001
	(100)	(77.1)	(91.7)	(84.4)	
	(a)	(c)	(ab)	(bc)	
7	10.86±0.35	9.09±0.26	10.17±0.26	9.54±0.20	< 0.001
	(100)	(83.7)	(93.6)	(87.8)	
	(a)	(d)	(b)	(c)	
10	11.46±0.29	8.93±0.55	10.59±0.40	9.73±0.41	< 0.001
	(100)	(77.9)	(92.4)	(84.9)	
	(a)	(d)	(b)	(c)	
14	12.00±0.31	9.07±0.68	10.88±0.72	9.61±0.62	< 0.001
	(100)	(75.6)	(90.7)	(80.1)	
	(a)	(c)	(b)	(c)	

Legend as table (3)

Table (5) DNA, RNA and total protien contents in liver of different groups of mice under investigations.

	Controls $\bar{X}$±SD	EAC $\bar{X}$±SD	CuDIPS $\bar{X}$±SD	EAC+CuDIPS $\bar{X}$±SD	*P - value
DNA	2.78±0.17	2.48±0.17	2.46±0.09	2.20±0.17	< 0.001
	(100)	(89.2)	(88.5)	(79.1)	
	(a)	(b)	(c)	(b)	
RNA	10.71±0.39	12.35±0.33	10.83±0.36	11.14±0.24	< 0.001
	(100)	(115.3)	(101.1)	(104.0)	
	(b)	(a)	(b)	(b)	
Total protein	85.75±1.67	75.50±4.01	83.87±2.75	82.13±3.09	< 0.001
	(100)	(88.0)	(97.8)	(95.8)	
	(a)	(b)	(a)	(a)	

Results are expressed as mg / gm wet tissue.
Legend as table (2)

Table (6) Iron, calcium and magnesium concentrations in liver of different groups of mice under investigations.

	Controls $\bar{X}$±SD	EAC $\bar{X}$±SD	CuDIPS $\bar{X}$±SD	EAC+CuDIPS $\bar{X}$±SD	*P - Value
	3.63±0.36	10.57±1.10	3.32±0.34	3.94±0.85	< 0.001
Iron	(100)	(291.2)	(91.5)	(108.5)	
	(b)	(a)	(b)	(b)	
Calcium	1.62±0.57	4.92±0.57	1.65±0.36	0.72±0.12	< 0.001
	(100)	(303.7)	(101.9)	(44.4)	
	(b)	(a)	(b)	(c)	
Magnesium	5.92±0.87	6.90±1.10	12.00±2.94	12.78±0.45	< 0.001
	(100)	(116.5)	(202.7)	(215.9)	
	(b)	(b)	(a)	(a)	

Results are expressed as part permillion (ppm)
Legend as table (2)

Table (7) Ag-NOR score per cell of different groups of mice under investigations.
measured at different time intervals

Time (days)	Controls $\bar{X}$±SD	EAC $\bar{X}$±SD	CUDIPS $\bar{X}$±SD	EAC+CU $\bar{X}$±SD	*P - value
3	1.78±0.23	3.83±0.38	2.56±0.24	3.26±0.31	< 0.001
	(100)	(215.2)	(143.8)	(183.1)	
	(d)	(a)	(c)	(b)	
7	2.22±0.17	6.77±1.08	2.77±0.18	4.81±0.43	< 0.001
	(100)	(305.0)	(124.8)	(216.7)	
10	(c)	(a)	(c)	(b)	
	2.17±0.22	5.44±0.34	2.22±0.12	3.65±0.34	< 0.001
	(100)	(250.7)	(102.3)	(168.2)	
14	(c)	(a)	(c)	(b)	
	1.92±0.29	6.22±0.92	2.30±0.40	3.59±0.56	< 0.001
	(100)	(324.0)	(119.8)	(187.0)	
	(c)	(a)	(c)	(b)	

Legands same as table (2)

DISCUSSION:

In the present study increasing the concentration of CuDIPS in the EAC media was accompanied by a progresive increase in the percent of NVC. This indicates a tumoricidal effect of CuDIPS on EAC cells. These results coincides with those of McAusean (21) who established in vitro, that copper complexes triggered migration of endothelial cells.

Our results showed a progressively increased tumor volume in mice s.c inoculated with EAC. While treatment with CuDIPS decreased the tumour volume.

Treating the EAC group of mice with CuDIPS improved the levels of DNA and RNA in solid tumour, and RNA and protein content in liver homogenates of mice. Our results disagreed with those of El-Kabani et al. (22) who observed no significant changes between EAC group and control group. Nevertheless, they found a significant change in RNA content which correlated with our finding. These results are in agreement with those of Leuthouser and his collegus (8) and Torregrosa et al (23) who showed that subsequent adminstration of CuDIPS directly in the tumour site yeilded both retardation and reduction of tumour growth induced by EAC inoculation. Torregrosa et al. (23) and Shuff et al. (24) illustrated the protective effect of CuDIPS on Ehlich solid tumour and other tumours. Yang et al. (25) reported the ability of copper complexes to inhibit DNA synthesis of tumour cells, which is closely related to the antitumour mechanism of the complex Our results were similar to those of El- Kabani et al. (22) who observed significant decrease in protein content of EAC bearing mice as compared to controls. This could be due to imbalanced growth as previously reported by Ismail (26).The untreated EAC bearing mice showed progressive increase in the body weight reaching 100% on the 24th day, which is due to tumour proliferation and growth. Treating EAC bearing mice with CuDIPS led to retardation in body weights of mice, reaching 52.9% on the same day. Leuthauser et al (8), reported that the growth of EAC inbred mice were retarded by adminstration of CuDIPS, which exhibits superoxide dismutase-like activity. It has been used as anti-inflamatory agent and it is lipid soluble. This property enables the compound to penetrate membranes and become intercellular. The author reported that CuDIPS adminstration lead to reduction in tumour size, delay of metastasis and significant increase in survival of mice.

Mice treated with EAC died after 26 days only but when treated with CuDIPS in addition, the survival was increased more than 60 days.

The present results revealed elevated G-6-Pase activity in liver homogenate of mice bearing EAC. These results coincides with those of El-Kabani et al. (22) who observed an increase in liver G-6 phase activity in EAC inoculated mice. They atributed this increase to increase in glucose utilization due to tumour growth or due to an imbalance of the endocrine system (26,27). The G-6-Pase increased level in EAC groups was slightly decreased when mice were treated with CuDIPS in addition.

The ATPase activity was significantly decreased in livers of EAC bearing mice when compared to controls. Meanwhile, the treatment of EAC bearing mice with CuDIPS in addition, showed slight increase in ATPase activity levels as compared to EAC alone, but it was still decreased than the controls. Our results coincides with those of Zakhary et al. (28) who observed defeciency in ATPase activity in induced tumours. They reported that this is a characteristic feature of liver toxicity or malignant transformation. Mg ,Fe and Ca are known to act on the cell cycle, protein and DNA synthesis (29,30). Some endonucleases are Ca and Mg dependant (31).

Our results showed that mice inoculated with EAC revealed a highly significant increase in iron and calcium contents of their livers. Treatment of EAC bearing mice with CuDIPS showed significant decreases in both iron and calcium as compared to EAC alone In this respect, it is worth mentioning that Winkler et al (32) detected 4- hydroxynonenal in livers of EAC bearing mice. This compound is a major product of lipid peroxidation in rat liver microcosome, and its formation was stimulated by ferrous ions or ferrous histidine.

In our investignation, using material obtained from liver tissue of mice of different groups at different time intervals, histopathological features were of good significance. Control untreated groups and groups received CuDIPS only, were almost similar, concerning normal lobular pattern as well as cytological features. The proliferative activity as reflected by Ag NORs scores, was almost higher in the groups received CuDIPS only than that of untreated groups, but significantly less than that of EAC-inoculated group. Crocker and Nar, (20) reported that Ag NORs scores appeared to reflect cell and nuclear activity, providing a good indication of cell proliferation. Ag NORs scores of tumour inoculated groups retained to the lower level when treated with CuDIPS indicating that the Ag NORs count is a quantitative predictor of the biological behaviours (9).

Our results are in accordance with those obtained by Duran et al. (33) who observed that CuDIPS induced a significant inhibition of malignant conversion during promotion and progression. They reported that this might be due to its biometric superoxide dismutase property (33). It should be noted that the present results revealed that treating mice with CuDIPS was safe enough, as the results of the group treated with CuDIPS alone was around that of the untreated controls. In this respect, it worth mentioning that Crispens and Sorenson (34) evaluated the anticancer activity of CuDIPS. They reported that, toxic effect of the compound could be eliminated by its use as subcutaneous injections rather than intraperitoneal route of administration.

From the previous results, it could be concluded that CuDIPS has tumoricidal effect on malignant cell, examplified by EAC. On the other hand, the study revealed that the complex might be developed for protection of normal tissues in association with malignant tissues.

REFERENCES

1-Osman AM. Mohammed TA and Assem MM.Effect of ascorbic acid and melphalan on the growth of human melanoma cells in vitro. J Egypt. Natl. Cancer. Inst., 2: 421-425,1986.

2-El-Merzabani MM, El-Aaser AA, Osman AM, Ismael N, and Abuel Ela .F Potentiation of therapeutic effect of methane-sulphonate and protection againts its organ cytotoxicity by vitamin c in Ehrlich Ascites carcinoma bearing mice. J. Pharm. Belg., 44:877-884, 1989.

3-Good RA, Lorenz E, Engelman R. and Day NK. Experimental approaches to nutrition and cancer, fats, calories, vitamins and minerals. Med. Oncol. Tumour Pharmacother., 7:183-192, 1990.

4-Leis H.P Jr: The relationship of diet to cancer cardiovascular disease and longevity. Int. Sutg., 76:1-5,1991.

5-Mei W., Dong ZM, Liao BL and Xu HB: Study of immunofuntion cancer patients influenced by supplemental zinc or selenium-zinc combination. Biol. Trace Elem. Res. 28:11-19, 1991.
6-Kasemeier SL, Salari H and Soraenson JR. Anticancer effects of Cu II (3,5-Diisopropyl Salicylate)2 in mice inoculated intramuscularly with Ehlich Ascitis Carcinoma Cells. Biology Of Copper complexes, 361-370,1987.
7-Egner PA, Taffe BG and Kensler TW. Effects of copper complexes on multistage carcinogenessis Biology of copper complexes. P 413:424, 1987.
8-Leuthauser S.W, Oberley L.W, Oberley T.D, Sorenson J.R, and Rama Krishna K. Antitumour effect of a copper coordination compound with superoxide dismutase-like activity. J. Natl Cancer Inst. 66(6): 1077-1081, 1981.
9-Kato M, Saji S, Tsuya H, Miya K, Fukada D, Umemoto T, Kunieda K, Takao H, Sugiyama Y, Tsuji K and Sato M. Clinical study of the relationship between cytological behaviour and postoperative prognosis in colorectal cancer cases with special references to nucelar DNA content and Nucleolar organizer regions.
J. of Surg. Oncol. 64: 36-41, 1997.
10-Underwood JCE, Giri DD. Nucleolar organizer regions as diagnostic discriminants for malignancy.
J.Pathol 155: 95-96, 1988.
11-El–Merzabani MM, El-Aaser,AA, and Attia MA . Screening system for Egyptian plants with potential antitumour activity. J. Planta. Medica,, 36:150-155,1979.
12-Papadopoulos D, Kimler BF, Estes NC, and Durham FJ: Growth delay effect of combined interstitial hyper thermia and brachy therapy in a rat solid tumour model. Anticancer Res., 9: 45-48,1989.
13-Swanson M.A. .Glucouse-6-phosphatase form liver. Method, Enzymol., 2: 541-543,1955.
14-El- Aaser AA and El-Merzabani MM. Simultaneous determination of 5-nucleotidase and Al kaline phosphatase activities in serum.Z. Klin. Chem Klin Biochem., 13:423 -459, 1975.
15-Melmed RM, EL-Aaser AA and Hold SJ. Hypertrophy and hyperplasia of neonatal rat excrine pancreas induced by orally adminstrated soybean trypsin inhibitor. Biochem. Biophy. Acta 321:280-288,1976.
16-Dische A, and Schwarz K. Microchem Acta Z: (1937) 13, Cited in : Radwan A.F. Studies on the effect of soybean feeding on the biochemistry of liver during carcinogenesis.Ph.D Thesis. Faculty of Medicine, Cairo University, (1980).
17-Mejbaum W. Uber diebestimmung kleiner pentosemengen insbesonder in derivatan deradenyl-saure. Z. Physiol.Chem.,285: 117-121,1939.
18-Lowry OH, Rosebrough NJ, Farr AL, and Randall RJ. Protein measurement with the folin phenol reagent. J. Biol. Chem.. 193:265-275, 1951.
19-Conn HL and Darrow MAA. Staining procedures used by the biological stain commissioned 2. Geneva N.Y., Biotech. Publication. 1960.
20-Crocker J and Nar P. Nuclear organizer regions in lymphomas.
J.PAthol. 151:111-118, 1987.
21-Mc Auslan BR, and Reilly W. Exp. Cell. Res. 1980,130,147 sited in biology of copper complexes, 1987.
22-EL-Kabani M, Zakhary NI, Abdel Galil F, EL-Merzabani M and EL-Aaser AA. In-vivo and In-vitro studies on the effect of Zinc sulphate, ascobic acid and Sodium butarate on Ascites Carcinoma cells. J. Egyptian National Cancer Inst., 7: 67-77,1995.

23-Torregrosa D, Kasemeier S.L. Sorenson JR and Chang L.W Effects of Cu(II)(3,5-DIPS) $_2$ on solid ehrlich cell tumour in mice: A pathological study. Biology of coppor complexes,371-103:86,1987.
24-Shuff ST, Chowd H P, Khan MF, and Sorenson JR. Stable superoxide dismutase(SOD)-mimetic ternary human serum albumin–Cu (II) (3,5-diisopropylsalicylate)$_2$ /Cu (II)$_2$ (3,5-diisopropyl–salicylate)$_4$ complexes in tissue distribution of the binary complex..Biochem Pharmacol, 43(7):1601-1612, 1992
25-Yang P, Wang H, Gao F and Yang B. Antitumour activity of the Cu (II) mitoxantrone complex and its interaction with deoxyribonucleic acid . J In Org. Biochem 62 (2): 137–145, 1996.
26-Ismail N. Biochemical studies on the protective effect of vitamin A and C and thiol compounds against the side effects on anticancer drug. Ph. thesis, Faculty of Science, Cairo University, 1987.
27-Osman A. Biopharmacological studies on certain new anti cancer drugs.M.SC. thesis, Cairo University, (1978).
28-Zakhary NI, Badr EL-Din N,EL- Aaser AA, Ibrahim HA abd moharram NZ. Effect of soybean feeding and vitamin C on experimental carcinogensis. 5. Bio chamical changes in the liver of albino mice induced by feeding nitrite and didutylamine. J. Egypt. Natl. Cancer Inst. 4(2):173-186,1989.
29-Collery Ph., Coudoux P and Geoffroy H. Role of magnesium in the development of cancer. Trace substances in enviromental Health. Eds. Hemphil D.D, Missouri, Columbia, XII, 140-147,1978.
30-Bassel P, Zwiller J, Revel MO and Vincendon G. Growth promotion of transformed cells by iron in serum-free culture. Carcinogenesis 6: 355-359,1985.
31-Belokhvostov-AS, and Tomilin-NV. The origin of 5S DNA from tumour Ascitic fluid. EKSP- On Kol., 6(4): 30-33,1984.
32-Winkler-P, Lindner-W Esterbauer-H, Schauenstein-E, Schaur-RJ, and Khoschsorur-GA. Detection of 4-hydroxynonenal as a product of lipid peroxidation in native Ehrlich Ascitis tumour cells. Biochem-Biophys.-acta., 796(3): 232-237,1984.
33-Duran HA, lanfranchi H, Palmieri MA, de Ray BM. Inhibition of benzoyl peroxide- induced tumour promotion and progression by copper (II) (3,5-diisopropylsalicylate)$_2$. Cancer lett, 69(3) :167-172,1993.
34-Crispens CGJR and Sorenson JR. Evaluation of the anticancer activity of CuDIPS inSJL/J mice. Anticancer Res.,8(1):77-79,1988.

Author Index